D1358272

Unit 8   Infection Control 426

**Chapter 21 Infection Control/
Asepsis** 427

**Chapter 22 Standard Precautions
and Isolation** 447

Unit 9   Homeostasis 455

**Chapter 23 Fluid, Electrolyte, and
Acid-Base Balance** 457

**Chapter 24 Medication
Administration** 483

SECTION 3 CONCEPTS
FOR CARE

Unit 10 Fundamental Nursing
Care 526

Chapter 25 Assessment 527

Chapter 26 Pain Management 547

Chapter 27 Diagnostic Tests 573

Unit 11 Special Areas of
Nursing Care 622

**Chapter 28 Nursing Care of the
Older Client** 623

**Chapter 29 Rehabilitation,
Home Health, Long-Term Care,
and Hospice** 653

Unit 12 Leadership/Work
Transition 667

**Chapter 30 Leadership/Work
Transition** 669

Atlas of Nursing Procedures: Basic,
Intermediate, Advanced .687

References/Suggested Readings and
Resources 847

Appendix A: NANDA Nursing Diagnoses 875

Appendix B: Recommended Childhood
Immunization Schedule .877

Appendix C: Abbreviations, Acronyms,
and Symbols 879

Appendix D: English/Spanish Words
and Phrases 884

Glossary 890

Index 903

BASIC NURSING: FOUNDATIONS OF SKILLS & CONCEPTS

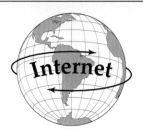

BASIC NURSING: FOUNDATIONS OF SKILLS & CONCEPTS

Lois White, RN, PhD

Former Chairperson and Professor
Department of Vocational Nurse Education
Del Mar College
Corpus Christi, Texas

DELMAR

THOMSON LEARNING™

Australia Canada Mexico Singapore Spain United Kingdom United States

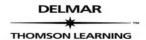

DELMAR

THOMSON LEARNING™

Basic Nursing: Foundations of Skills & Concepts
by Lois White

Business Unit Director:
William Brottmiller

Executive Editor:
Cathy L. Esperti

Acquisitions Editor:
Matthew Filimonov

Senior Developmental Editor:
Elisabeth F. Williams

Editorial Assistant:
Melissa Longo

Executive Marketing Manager:
Dawn F. Gerrain

Channel Manager:
Tara Carter

Project Editor:
David Buddle

Production Coordinator:
Nina Lontrato

Senior Art/Design Coordinator:
Timothy J. Conners

RT42 W435 2002 (handwritten)

Copyright © 2002 by Delmar, a division of Thomson Learning, Inc. Thomson Learning™ is a registered trademark used herein under license.

Printed in the United States
1 2 3 4 5 XXX 06 05 04 02 01

For more information contact Delmar,
3 Columbia Circle, PO Box 15015,
Albany, NY 12212-5015.

Or find us on the World Wide Web at http://www.delmar.com

For permission to use material from this text or product, contact us by
Tel   800-730-2214
Fax 800-730-2215
www.thomsonrights.com

Library of Congress Cataloging-in-Publication Data
White, Lois E. W.
  Basic nursing: foundations of skills & concepts
Lois E. W. White—1st Edition
  p. cm.
ISBN 0-7668-3201-5

NOTICE TO THE READER

Publisher does not warrant or guarantee any of the products described herein or perform any independent analysis in connection with any of the product information contained herein. Publisher does not assume, and expressly disclaims, any obligation to obtain and include information other than that provided to it by the manufacturer.

The reader is expressly warned to consider and adopt all safety precautions that might be indicated by the activities herein and to avoid all potential hazards. By following the instructions contained herein, the reader willingly assumes all risks in connection with such instructions.

The Publisher makes no representation or warranties of any kind, including but not limited to, the warranties of fitness for particular purpose or merchantability, nor are any such representations implied with respect to the material set forth herein, and the publisher takes no responsibility with respect to such material. The publisher shall not be liable for any special, consequential, or exemplary damages resulting, in whole or part, from the readers' use of, or reliance upon, this material.

Contents

Contributors xiv
Procedure Contributors xvi
Reviewers xvii
Preface xviii
How to Use this Text xx

SECTION 1 PERSPECTIVES IN NURSING

UNIT 1 Nurse Skills for Success . .2

Chapter 1 Holistic Care 3

Interrelated Concepts of Health 4
  Holistic Health 4
  Nursing the Whole Person 5
  Wellness 5
  Maslow's Hierarchy of Needs 5
Providing Quality Care 6
  Self-Awareness 6
  Development of Self-Concept 6
Self-Care as a Prerequisite to Client Care 7
  Physical Wellness .7
  Intellectual Wellness 10
  Sociocultural Wellness 10
  Psychological Wellness 10
  Spiritual Wellness 11
Nurture Yourself 11

Chapter 2 Critical Thinking 13

Critical Thinking 13
  New Information .15
  Activity 15
  Student Responsibility 15
Skills of Critical Thinking 15
  Critical Reading 15
  Critical Listening .16
  Critical Writing 17
  Critical Speaking .17
Standards for Critical Thinking 17
  Clarity vs. Lack of Clarity 17
  Precision vs. Imprecision 18
  Specificity vs. Vagueness 18
  Accuracy vs. Inaccuracy 18
  Relevance vs. Irrelevance 18
  Consistency vs. Inconsistency 18
  Logical vs. Illogical 19
  Depth vs. Superficiality 19
  Completeness vs. Incompleteness 19
  Significance vs. Triviality 19
  Adequacy vs. Inadequacy 19
  Fairness vs. Bias .19
Reasoning and Problem-Solving 19
  Purpose 20

The Question at Issue 20
Assumptions 20
Point of View 21
Data and Information 21
Concepts 21
Inferences and Conclusions 21
Implications and Consequences 22
Traits of a Disciplined Thinker 22
  Reason 22
  Humility 22
  Courage 22
  Integrity 22
  Perseverance 22
  Fairmindedness 22
Critical Thinking and the Nursing Process 23

Chapter 3 Student Nurse Skills for Success 25

Develop a Positive Attitude 26
  Create Positive Self-Images 26
  Recognize Your Abilities 27
  Identify Realistic Expectations 27
Develop Your Basic Skills 28
  Reading 29
  Arithmetic and Mathematics 29
  Writing 30
  Listening 30
  Speaking 31
Develop Your Learning Style 32
  Classification of Learning Styles 33
  Strategies for Learning 34
Develop a Time-Management Plan 34
  Analyze Time Commitments 35
  Know Yourself 37
  Clarify the Goal 37
  Set Priorities 37
  Discipline Yourself 37
Develop a Study Strategy 38
  Set Up the Environment 38
  Gather Your Resources 38
  Minimize Interruptions 39
  Get to Know the Textbook 39
  Set Up the Study Plan 39
  Note Taking 41
  Prepare for Exams 42
Practice Thinking Critically 43
Develop Test-Taking Skills 44
  Attitude and Expectations 44
  Preparation 44
  Minimize Anxiety .44
  Improve Test-Taking Skills 45
  Behaviors in the Testing Room 47

UNIT 2 History and Nursing Organizations 49

Chapter 4 Nursing History, Education, and Organizations 51
Historical Overview 51
  Evolution of Nursing 52
  Religious Influences 54
  Florence Nightingale 54
  Nursing and the Civil War 55
  The Women's Movement 56
  Nursing Pioneers and Leaders 56
Practical Nursing Pioneer Schools 57
  Ballard School 57
  Thompson Practical Nursing School 58
  Household Nursing School 58
Nursing in the 20th Century 58
  Flexner Report 58
  Early Insurance Plans 58
  Landmark Reports in Nursing Education 59
  Other Health Care Initiatives 59
  Cost and Quality Controls 60
  Health Care Reform 60
Nursing Education .60
  Types of Programs 60
  Trends in Nursing Education 63
Nursing Organizations 63
  American Nurses Association 63
  National Association of Practical Nurse
    Education and Service, Inc. 63
  National Foundation of Licensed Practical
    Nurses, Inc. .63
  National League for Nursing 66
  National Council of State Boards of Nursing . . .66
The Future of Nursing 67

Chapter 5 The Health Care Delivery System 69
Types of Health Care Services 69
  Primary Care 70
  Secondary Care .70
  Tertiary Care 70
Health Care Delivery System 70
  Providers/Consumers 70
  Settings 72
  Personnel and Services 73
Health Care Team .74
Economics of Health Care 76
  Private Insurance 76
  Managed Care 77
  Federal Government Insurance Plans 78
Factors Influencing Health Care 79
  Cost 79
  Access 79
  Quality 80

Challenges within the Health Care System 80
  Disillusionment with Providers 80
  Loss of Control 81
  Decreased Hospital Use 81
  Changing Practice Settings 81
  Ethical Issues 82
  Vulnerable Populations 82
Nursing's Response to Health Care Challenges . .83
  Nursing's Agenda for Health Care Reform 83
  Standards of Care 83
  Advanced Practice 84
  Public vs. Private Programs 84
  Public Health 84
  Community Health 84
Trends and Issues .85

UNIT 3 Legal and Ethical Issues . .87

Chapter 6 Legal Responsibilities 89
Basic Legal Concepts 90
  Definition of Law 90
  Sources of Law .90
Nursing Practice and the Law 92
  Standards of Practice 92
  Liability 93
  Legal Issues in Practice 93
Nurse-Client Relationship 93
  Torts 93
  Legal Risk 96
  Professional Discipline 97
  Documentation .98
Informed Consent .98
Advanced Directives 100
  Durable Power of Attorney 102
  Living Will 102
Incident Reports .102
Professional Liability 105
Impaired Nurse 105

Chapter 7 Ethical Responsibilities 109
Concepts of Ethics 110
  Ethics in Health Care 110
Ethical Principles .110
  Autonomy 110
  Nonmaleficence 111
  Beneficence 112
  Justice 112
  Veracity 112
  Fidelity 112
Ethical Theories 113
  Teleology 113
  Deontology 113
  Situational Theory 113
  Caring-Based Theory 113
Ethics and Values .114
  Values Clarification 114

Ethical Codes 115
The Client's Rights 115
Ethical Dilemmas 116
   Euthanasia 118
   Refusal of Treatment 119
   Scarcity of Resources 119
Ethical Decision Making 119
   Framework for Ethical Decision Making 119
Ethics and Nursing 120
   Ethics Committees .120
   Nurse as Client Advocate 120
   Nurse as Whistleblower 120

UNIT 4 Communication 123

Chapter 8 Communication 125
Process of Communication 125
   Sender 126
   Message 126
   Channel 126
   Receiver 126
   Feedback 126
   Influences 126
Methods of Communicating 127
   Verbal Communication 127
   Nonverbal Communication 127
Influences on Communication 128
   Age 128
   Education 129
   Emotions 129
   Culture 129
   Language 129
   Attention 129
   Surroundings 129
Congruency of Messages 129
Listening/Observing 130
Therapeutic Communication 130
   Goals of Therapeutic Communication 130
   Behaviors/Attitudes to Enhance
     Communication 131
   Techniques of Therapeutic Communication . .132
   Barriers to Communication 133
Psychosocial Aspects of Communication 134
   Style 135
   Gestures 135
   Meaning of Time 135
   Meaning of Space .136
   Cultural Values 136
   Political Correctness 136
   Importance to Health Care System 136
Professional Boundaries 137
Nurse-Client Communication 137
   Formal/Informal Communication 137
   Social Communication 137

   Interactions 137
   Factors Affecting Nurse-Client
     Communication 138
Communicating with the Health Care Team 140
   Oral Communication 140
   Written Communication 141
   Electronic Communication 141
Communicating with Yourself 142
   Positive Self-Talk 142
   Negative Self-Talk .143

Chapter 9 Nursing Process 145
Historical Perspective .146
Overview of the Nursing Process 146
   Assessment 146
   Diagnosis 149
   Planning and Outcome Identification 152
   Implementation 154
   Evaluation 157
The Nursing Process and Critical Thinking 158
The Nursing Process and Problem Solving 158
The Nursing Process and Decision Making 159
The Nursing Process and Holistic Care 159

Chapter 10 Documentation 163
Documentation as Communication 163
   Documentation Defined 164
   Purposes of Health Care Documentation 164
Principles of Effective Documentation 167
   Elements of Effective Documentation 168
Methods of Documentation 170
   Narrative Charting .171
   Source-Oriented Charting 171
   Problem-Oriented Charting 171
   PIE Charting 171
   Focus Charting 171
   Charting by Exception 171
   Computerized Documentation 173
   Critical Pathway 175
Forms for Recording Data 175
   Kardex 175
   Flow Sheets 175
   Nurses' Progress Notes 178
   Discharge Summary 178
Trends in Documentation 179
   Nursing Minimum Data Set 179
   Nursing Diagnoses .179
   Nursing Intervention Classification 179
   Nursing Outcomes Classification 180
Reporting 180
   Summary Reports 180
   Walking Rounds 181
   Telephone Reports and Orders 181
   Incident Reports 182

Chapter 11 Client Teaching 185
The Teaching–Learning Process 185
  Formal Teaching 186
  Informal Teaching 186
  Learning Domains 187
  Learning Principles 187
  Learning Styles 189
  Barriers to the Teaching–Learning Process . . .189
  Teaching Methods 190
Learning Throughout the Life Cycle 191
  Children 192
  Adolescents 192
  Older Adults 193
Professional Responsibilities Related to
  Teaching 193
  Self-Awareness 194
  Documentation .195
Teaching–Learning and the Nursing Process . . .195
  Assessment 195
  Nursing Diagnosis 200
  Planning 200
  Implementation .201
  Evaluation 202

**UNIT 5 Cultural Aspects of
Nursing** 204

**Chapter 12 Cultural Diversity and
Nursing** 205
Culture 205
  Ethnicity and Race 206
  Cultural Diversity 206
  Components of Culture 207
  Characteristics of Culture 208
Cultural Influences on Health Care Beliefs
  and Practices 208
  Definition of Health 208
  Etiology 208
  Health Promotion and Protection 209
  Practitioners and Remedies 209
  Beliefs of Select Cultural Groups 209
Cultural and Racial Influences on Client Care . .212
  Communication .212
  Orientation to Space and Time 212
  Social Organization 213
  Biological Variation 217
Cultural Aspects and the Nursing Process 218
  Assessment 218
  Nursing Diagnosis 218
  Planning/Outcome Identification 219
  Implementation .220
  Evaluation 220
Sample Nursing Care Plan: The Family with
  Ineffective Coping 221

**Chapter 13 Complementary/
Alternative Therapies** 227
Historical Influences on Contemporary Practices 228
  Ancient Greece .228
  The Far East 228
  China 228
  India 228
  Shamanistic Tradition 229
Modern Trends 229
  Mind/Body Medicine and Research 229
  Holism and Nursing Practice 230
Complementary/Alternative Interventions 230
  Mind/Body (Self-Regulatory) Techniques . . .231
  Body-Movement (Manipulation) Strategies . . .233
  Energetic-Touch Therapies 234
  Spiritual Therapies 237
  Nutritional/Medicinal Therapies 238
  Other Methodologies 239
Nursing and Complementary/Alternative
  Approaches 242

SECTION 2 PHYSICAL AND MENTAL INTEGRITY

**UNIT 6 Human Development
Over the Life Span** 248

Chapter 14 The Life Cycle 249
Basic Concepts of Growth and Development . . .250
  Principles of Growth and Development 250
  Factors Influencing Growth and
    Development 251
Theoretical Perspectives of Human
  Development 251
  Physiological Dimension 251
  Psychosocial Dimension 251
  Cognitive Dimension 252
  Moral Dimension 254
  Spiritual Dimension 255
Holistic Framework for Nursing 256
Stages of the Life Cycle 256
  Prenatal Period .256
  Neonatal Period .257
  Infancy 259
  Toddler Period 262
  Preschool Period 264
  School-Age Period 266
  Preadolescence .268
  Adolescence 270
  Young Adulthood 273
  Middle Adulthood 275
  Older Adulthood 277

UNIT 7 Health Promotion 281

Chapter 15 Wellness Concepts 283
Health 283
Wellness 284
  Emotional Wellness 284
  Mental Wellness 284
  Intellectual Wellness 284
  Vocational Wellness 284
  Social Wellness 285
  Spiritual Wellness 285
  Physical Wellness 285
Health Promotion 285
  Healthy People 2000 285
  Healthy People 2010 286
Illness Prevention 286
  Types of Prevention 288
  Prevention Health Care Team 289
Factors Affecting Health 289
  Genetics and Human Biology 289
  Personal Behavior 289
  Environment Influences 292
  Health Care 292
Making a Genogram 294
Guidelines for Health Living 294

Chapter 16 Stress, Adaptation, and Anxiety 299
Stress 299
  Response to Stress 300
  Manifestations of Stress 301
  Outcomes of Stress 301
Adaptation 302
  Coping Measures 302
  Crisis 303
Anxiety 303
Effects of Illness 305
Effects of Change 306
  Types of Change 307
  Resistance to Change 307
  The Nurse as Change Agent 308
Nursing Process 308
  Assessment 308
  Nursing Diagnosis 309
  Planning/Outcome Identification 309
  Nursing Interventions 309
  Evaluation 311
Personal Stress-Management Approaches for the Nurse 312
Sample Nursing Care Plan: The Client Experiencing Anxiety 314

Chapter 17 Loss, Grief, and Death 317
Loss 318
  Types of Loss 318
Grief 318
  Theories of the Grieving Process 319
  Types of Grief 319
  Factors Affecting Loss and Grief 321
  Nursing Care of the Grieving Client 324
Death 326
  Legal Considerations 327
  Ethical Considerations 327
  Stages of Dying and Death 327
  Nursing Care of the Dying Client 329
  Impending Death 334
  Care After Death 335
  Legal Aspects 336
  Care of the Family 336
  Nurse's Self-Care 336
Sample Nursing Care Plan: The Client with a Terminal Illness/Cancer of the Lung 337

Chapter 18 Basic Nutrition 343
Physiology of Nutrition 344
  Ingestion 344
  Digestion 344
  Absorption 344
  Metabolism 344
  Excretion 345
Nutrients 345
  Water 346
  Carbohydrates 347
  Fats 349
  Protein 350
  Vitamins 352
  Minerals 355
Promoting Proper Nutrition 358
  Four Food Groups (Historical) 358
  Food Guide Pyramid 358
  Dietary Guidelines 360
  Recommended Dietary Allowances 360
  Dietary Reference Intakes 360
Factors Influencing Nutrition 361
  Culture 361
  Religion 363
  Socioeconomics 363
  Fads 363
  Superstitions 364
Nutritional Needs During the Life Cycle 364
  Infancy 364
  Childhood 366
  Adolescence 368
  Young and Middle Adulthood 368
  Older Adulthood 369
  Pregnancy and Lactation 370
Nutrition and Health 371
  Primary Nutritional Disease 371
  Secondary Nutritional Disease 371

Weight Management 371
   Determining Caloric Needs 371
   Overweight 372
   Underweight 372
Food Labeling 373
Food Quality and Safety 373
   Quality of Food 373
   Safety of Food 374
   Food-Borne Illnesses 374
Food Allergies 375
   Allergic Reactions .375
   Treatment of Allergies 375
Nursing Process 376
   Assessment 376
   Nursing Diagnosis .378
   Planning/Outcome Identification 378
   Implementation 378
   Evaluation 381
Sample Nursing Care Plan: The Client
   with Altered Nutrition 382

Chapter 19 Rest and Sleep 385
Rest and Sleep 385
   Physiology of Rest and Sleep 386
   Biological Clock 387
   Factors Affecting Rest and Sleep 388
   Alterations in Sleep Patterns 390
Nursing Process 392
   Assessment 392
   Nursing Diagnosis .393
   Planning/Outcome Identification 393
   Nursing Interventions 393
   Evaluation 395
Sample Nursing Care Plan: The Client
   with Trouble Sleeping 395

Chapter 20 Safety/Hygiene 399
Safety 400
Factors Affecting Safety 401
   Age 401
   Lifestyle/Occupation 402
   Sensory and Perceptual Alterations 402
   Mobility 402
   Emotional State 402
Hygiene 402
   Factors Influencing Hygiene Practice 402
Nursing Process 403
   Assessment 403
   Nursing Diagnosis .405
   Planning/Outcome Identification 408
   Implementation 408
   Evaluation 423
Sample Nursing Care Plan: The Client
   at Risk for Injury .423

UNIT 8 Infection Control 426

Chapter 21 Infection Control/Asepsis . .427
Flora 428
Pathogenicity and Virulence 428
   Bacteria 428
   Viruses 428
   Fungi 429
   Protozoa 429
   Rickettsia 429
Infection and Colonization 429
Chain of Infection 429
   Agent 430
   Reservoir 430
   Portal of Exit 431
   Modes of Transmission 431
   Portal of Entry 432
   Host 432
Breaking the Chain of Infection 433
   Between Agent and Reservoir 433
   Between Reservoir and Portal of Exit 434
   Between Portal of Exit and Mode of
     Transmission 435
   Between Mode of Transmission and
     Portal of Entry 435
   Between Portal of Entry and Host 435
   Between Host and Agent 435
Normal Defense Mechanisms 435
   Nonspecific Immune Defense 436
   Specific Immune Defense 437
Stages of the Infectious Process 438
   Incubation Stage .438
   Prodromal Stage .438
   Illness Stage 438
   Convalescent Stage 438
Nosociomial Infections 438
Nursing Process 439
   Assessment 439
   Nursing Diagnosis .440
   Planning/Outcome Identification 440
   Implementation 440
   Evaluation 442
Sample Nursing Care Plan: The Client
   at Risk for Infection 443

Chapter 22 Standard Precautions
and Isolation 447
Historical Perspective 447
Standard Precautions 449
   Handwashing 449
   Gloves 450
   Mask, Eye Protection, Face Shield 450
   Gown 450
   Client-Care Equipment 450
   Environment Control 450

Linen 450
Occupational Health and Blood-Borne
  Pathogens 450
Client Placement 451
Isolation 451
Client Responses to Isolation 453

UNIT 9 Homeostasis 455

Chapter 23 Fluid, Electrolyte, and Acid-Base Balance 457

Homeostasis 458
Chemical Organization 458
  Elements 458
  Atoms 458
  Molecules and Compounds 460
  Ions 460
Water 461
Gases 461
Acids, Bases, Salts, and pH 462
  Acid 462
  Bases 462
  Salts 462
  pH 462
Buffers 462
  Bicarbonate Buffer System 463
  Phosphate Buffer System 463
  Protein Buffers .463
Substance Movement 463
  Passive Transport 463
  Active Transport .465
Fluid and Electrolyte Balance 465
  Body Fluids 466
  Exchange between the Extracellular and
    Intracellular Fluids 466
  Regulators of Fluid and Electrolyte
    Balance 467
Disturbances in Electrolyte Balance 468
  Sodium 468
  Potassium 468
  Calcium 469
  Magnesium 469
  Phosphate 470
  Chloride 470
Acid-Base Balance 470
  Regulators of Acid-Base Balance 470
  Diagnostic and Laboratory Data 471
Disturbances in Acid-Base Balance 471
  Respiratory Acidosis 472
  Respiratory Alkalosis 472
  Metabolic Acidosis 472
  Metabolic Alkalosis 472
Nursing Process 473
  Assessment 473
  Nursing Diagnosis 475

Planning/Outcome Identification 476
Implementation 477
Evaluation 479
Sample Nursing Care Plan: The Client
  with Excess Fluid Volume 479

Chapter 24 Medication Administration . .483

Drug Standards and Legislation 484
  Standards 484
  Legislation 484
Drug Nomenclature 485
Drug Action 485
  Pharmacology 485
  Pharmacokinetics 487
  Drug Interaction .488
  Side Effects and Adverse Reactions 488
  Food and Drug Administration 488
Factors Influencing Drug Action 488
Medication Orders .489
  Types of Orders .489
Systems of Weight and Measures 490
  Metric Systems .490
  Apothecary System 490
  Household System 491
Approximate Dose Equivalents 491
  Converting Units of Weight and Volume 492
  Drug Dose Calculations 493
Safe Drug Administration 494
  Guidelines for Medication Administration 494
  Documentation of Drug Administration 496
  Drug Supply and Storage 497
Medication Compliance 497
Legal Aspects of Administering Medications . . .498
Nursing Process 498
  Assessment 498
  Nursing Diagnosis 499
  Planning/Outcome Identification 499
  Nursing Interventions 499
Evaluation 519
Sample Nursing Care Plan: The Client
  with Deep Vein Thrombosis 520

SECTION 3 CONCEPTS FOR CARE

UNIT 10 Fundamental Nursing Care 526

Chapter 25 Assessment 527

Health History 528
  Demographic Information 528
  Reason for Seeking Health Care 529
  Perception for Health Status 529
  Previous Illnesses, Hospitalizations, and
    Surgeries 529

Client/Family Medical History 529
Immunizations/Exposure to Communicable
   Diseases 529
Allergies 530
Current Medications 530
Developmental Level 530
Psychosocial History 530
Sociocultural History 530
Complementary/Alternative Therapy Use 530
Activities of Daily Living 530
Review of Systems 530
Physical Examination .531
Inspection 531
Palpation 531
Percussion 532
Auscultation 532
Head-to-Toe Assessment 532
General Survey 534
Vital Signs 534
Pain 538
Height and Weight Measurement 539
Head and Neck Assessment 539
Mental and Neurological Status and Affect . .540
Skin Assessment .540
Thoracic Assessment 541
Abdominal Assessment 542
Musculoskeletal and Extremity Assessment . . .544

Chapter 26 Pain Management 547
Definitions of Pain 548
Nature of Pain 548
Common Myths about Pain 549
Types of Pain 549
Pain Categorized by Origin 549
Pain Characterized by Nature 549
Purpose of Pain 551
Physiology of Pain 551
Stimulation of Pain 552
The Gate Control Theory 553
Conduction of Pain Impulses 553
Factors Affecting the Pain Experience 554
Age 554
Previous Experience with Pain 554
Drug Abuse 554
Cultural Norms 554
JCAHO Standards 554
Nursing Process 554
Assessment 555
Nursing Diagnoses 559
Planning/Outcome Identification 560
Nursing Interventions 560
Evaluation 568
Sample Nursing Care Plan: The Client with
Chronic Pain 569

Chapter 27 Diagnostic Tests 573
Diagnostic Testing 574
Nursing Care of the Client 574
Laboratory Tests 577
Specimen Collection 577
Specific Tests 581
Urine Tests 595
Stool Tests 599
Culture and Sensitivity Tests 599
Papanicolaou Test 600
Radiological Studies 600
Chest X-Ray 604
Computed Tomography 604
Barium Studies 605
Angiography 605
Arteriography 605
Dye Injection Studies 605
Ultrasonography 606
Magnetic Resonance Imaging 607
Radioactive Studies 607
Electrodiagnostic Studies 608
Electrocardiography 608
Electroencephalography 610
Endoscopy 610
Aspiration/Biopsy 610
Bone Marrow Aspiration/Biopsy 614
Paracentesis 614
Thoracentesis 614
Cerebrospinal Fluid Aspiration 614
Other Tests 615

**UNIT 11 Special Areas of
Nursing Care 622**

**Chapter 28 Nursing Care of the
Older Client 623**
Gerontological Nursing 624
Theories of Aging 625
Myths and Realities of Aging 625
Health and Aging 628
Activities of Daily Living 628
Exercise 629
Nutrition 630
Psychosocial Considerations 630
Strengths 630
Health Promotion and Disease Prevention . . .631
Physiologic Changes Associated with Aging . . .632
Respiratory System 632
Cardiovascular System 633
Gastrointestinal System 634
Reproductive System: Female 636
Reproductive System: Male 636
Endocrine System .637
Musculoskeletal System 637

Integumentary System 638
Neurological System .641
Urinary System 642
Sensory Changes 644
Elder Abuse 645
Forms of Abuse 645
Legal Requirements of Reporting 645
Sample Nursing Care Plan: The Client with
Alzheimer's Disease (AD) 646
Financing Elder Care in the 21st Century 649
Medicare 649
Medicaid 650
Omnibus Budget Reconciliation Act 650
Balanced Budget Act of 1997 650

**Chapter 29 Rehabilitation, Home
Health, Long-Term Care, and Hospice . .653**
Legal and Ethical Responsibilities 654
Sources of Reimbursement 655
Medicare 656
Medicaid 656
Private Insurance 656
Licensure, Certification, and Accreditation 656
Licensure 656
Certification 656
Accreditation 656
Rehabilitation 657
The Interdisciplinary Health Care Team 657
Role of the LP/VN 658
Functional Assessment and Evaluation for
Rehabilitation 658
Rehabilitation Settings 659
Home Health Care 659
Role of the LP/VN 659
Long-Term Care 660
Long-Term Care Facilities 660
Subacute Care 660
Continuing Care Retirement Communities . . .661
Assisted Living 661
Adult Day Care 661
Respite Care 661
Foster Care 661
Role of the LP/VN 661
Hospice 662
Sample Nursing Care Plan: The Client
Requiring Rehabilitative Care 662

**UNIT 12 Leadership/Work
Transition 667**

**Chapter 30 Leadership/Work
Transition 669**
Leadership 669
Leadership Styles 669
Leadership Skills 670

Management 670
Task Assignment 671
Tasks of LP/VN 671
Tasks of the UAP 671
Duty Delegation 672
Care Prioritization 673
Workplace Transition 673
The Nursing Team 673
Job Expectations and Responsibilities 674
Organizational Chart .675
From Student to Employee 675
State Board Examination and Licensure 676
The NCLEX-PN 676
Your License 676
Employment Opportunities 676
Hospitals 677
Long-Term Care Facilities/Rehabilitation
Centers 677
Community Health Agencies 677
Private Duty 677
Home Care Agencies 677
Hospice 677
Occupational Health .677
Correctional Facilities 677
School 678
Parish 678
Insurance Companies 678
Preparing for the Job Hunt 678
Identify Your Objective 678
Preparing a Résumé .679
Prepare a Cover Letter 680
Prepare a List of References 680
Prepare a Telephone Call Script 681
Complete a Job Application 681
Prepare for the Interview 681
Prepare a Thank You Note 683
A Final Word about Employment 683

Atlas of Nursing Procedures: Basic,
Intermediate, Advanced 687
References/Suggested Readings and
Resources 847
Appendix A: NANDA Nursing Diagnoses 875
Appendix B: Recommended Childhood
Immunization Schedule 877
Appendix C: Abbreviations, Acronyms,
and Symbols 879
Appendix D: English/Spanish Words and
Phrases 884
Glossary 890
Index 903

Contributors

Joy E. Ache-Reed, RN, MS
Assistant Professor of Nursing
Indiana Wesleyan University
Marion, Indiana
Chapter 12, Cultural Diversity and Nursing

Carol A. Fetters Andersen, RN, MSN
Director of Mental Health Services
St. Anthony Regional Hospital and Nursing Home
Carroll, Iowa
Chapter 28, Nursing Care of the Older Client

Lenore Boris, RN, BSN, MS, JD
New York State Public Employees Federation Organizer (nurse)
Albany, New York
Chapter 30, Leadership/Work Transition

Susan L. Bredemeyer, RN, MS
Assistant Professor
Lutheran College of Health Professions
Fort Wayne, Indiana
Chapter 25, Assessment

Ali Brown, RN, MSN
Assistant Professor
College of Nursing
University of Tennessee
Knoxville, Tennessee
Chapter 9, Nursing Process

Donna J. Burleson, RN, MS
Chair of Health Occupations
Cisco Junior College
Abilene, Texas
Chapter 2, Critical Thinking

Ann H. Cary, RN, PhD, MPH, A-CCC
Professor and Coordinator, PhD in Nursing Program
College of Nursing and Health Sciences
George Mason University
Fairfax, Virginia
Chapter 4, Nursing History, Education, and Organizations

Judy Conlin
Chapter 20, Safety/Hygiene

Jan Corder, RN, DNS
School of Nursing
Northeast Louisiana University
Monroe, Louisana
Chapter 9, Nursing Process

Julie Coy, RNC, MS
Pain Consultation Service
The Children's Hospital
Denver, Colorado
Chapter 19, Rest and Sleep
Chapter 26, Pain Management
Chapter 16, Stress, Adaptation, and Anxiety
Chapter 17, Loss, Grief, and Death

Cheryl Erickson, RN, BSN, MA
Associate Professor
Lutheran College of Health Professions
Fort Wayne, Indiana
Chapter 25, Assessment

Mary Ellen Zator Estes, RN, MSN, CCRN
Former Assistant Professor
School of Nursing
Marymount University
Arlington, VA *and*
Former Critical Care Nursing Education Coordinator
The George Washington University Medical Center
Washington, D.C.
Chapter 25, Assessment

Mary Frost, RN, BSN
Covington, Louisiana
Chapter 13, Complementary/Alternative Therapies

Susan Halley, RN, MS, FNP
Instructor of Nursing
Ball State University
Muncie, Indiana
Chapter 7, Ethical Responsibilities

Lucille Joel, RN, EdD, FAAN
Professor
College of Nursing
Rutgers, The State University of New Jersey
Newark, New Jersey
Chapter 5, The Health Care Delivery System

Denise M. Jordan, RN, BSN, MA
Instructor
Practical Nursing Program
Ivy Tech State College
Fort Wayne, Indiana
Chapter 6, Legal Responsibilities

Mary E. A. Laskin, RN, CS, MN
Clinical Nurse Specialist
Surgical/Orhopedic Services
Kaiser Permanente
San Diego, California
Chapter 26, Pain Management

Judy Martin, RN, MS, JD
Nurse Attorney
Louisiana Department of Health and Hospitals
Health Standards Section
Baton Rouge, Louisiana
Chapter 6, Legal Responsibilities

Linda McCuistion, RN, PhD
Assistant Professor
School of Nursing
Our Lady of Holy Cross College
New Orleans, Louisiana
Chapter 9, Nursing Process

Betty Miller
Staff Development Coordinator
Meadowcrest Hospital
Gretna, Louisiana
Chapter 17, Loss, Grief, and Death

Barbara S. Moffett, RN, PhD
Associate Professor of Nursing
School of Nursing
Southeastern Louisiana University
Hammond, Louisiana
Chapter 9, Nursing Process

Mary Anne Mordcin-McCarthy, RN, PhD
Associate Professor and Director of the Undergraduate Program
College of Nursing
University of Tennessee–Knoxville
Knoxville, Tennessee
Chapter 9, Nursing Process

Barbara Morvant, RN, MN
Louisiana State Board of Nursing
Metairie, Louisiana
Chapter 4, Nursing History, Education, and Organizations

Joan Fritsch Needham, RNC, MS
Director of Education
DeKalb County Nursing Home
DeKalb, Illinois
Chapter 17, Loss, Grief, and Death
Chapter 28, Nursing Care of the Older Client
Chapter 29, Rehabilitation, Home Health, Long-Term Care, and Hospice

Rebecca Osterhaut
Chapter 1, Holistic Care

Brenda Owens, RN, PhD
Associate Professor
School of Nursing
Louisiana State University Medical Center
New Orleans, Louisiana
Chapter 24, Medication Administration

Demetrius Porche, RN, CCRN, DNS
Associate Professor and Director
Bachelor of Science in Nursing Program
Nicholas State University *and*
Adjunct Assistant Professor
Tulane University
School of Public Health and Topical Medicine
New Orleans, Louisiana
Chapter 20, Safety/Hygiene
Chapter 21, Infection Control/ Asepsis
Chapter 22, Standard Precautions and Isolation

Suzanne Riche, RN
Charity School of Nursing
Delgado Community College
New Orleans, Louisiana
Chapter 9, Nursing Process

Maureen Straight, RN, BSN, MSEd
Excelsior College
Albany, New York
Chapter 3, Student Nurse Skills for Success

Susan Stranahan, RN, PhD
Chair, Nursing Department
Indiana Wesleyan University
Marion, Indiana
Chapter 12, Cultural Diversity and Nursing

John M. White, PhD
Former Chairperson, Professor
Biology Department
Del Mar College
Corpus Christi, Texas
Chapter 23, Fluid, Electrolyte, and Acid–Base Balance

Rothlyn Zahourek, RN, CS, MS
Certified Clinical Nurse Specialist
Amherst, Massachusetts
Chapter 13, Complementary/ Alternative Therapies

Procedure Contributors

Gaylene Bouska Altman, RN, PhD
Director of the Learning Lab *and*
Faculty
School of Nursing
University of Washington
Seattle, Washington
Procedures B24, B25, I8

Barbara Brillhart, RN, PhD, CRRN, FNP-C
College of Nursing
Arizona State University
Tempe, Arizona
Procedures B8, B9, B10, B11, B12, B13, B14, B15, I27

Bethany Campbell, RN, MN, OCN
University of Washington Medical Center
Seattle, Washington
Procedure B7

Pat Carroll, RN, C, CEN, RRT, MS
Owner and Consultant
Educational Medical Consultants
Meriden, Connecticut *and*
Per Diem Staff Nurse, Emergency Department
Manchester Memorial Hospital
Manchester, Connecticut
Procedures B2, B33, B38, B39, B40, I8

Beth Christensen, RN, MN, CCRN
Touro Infirmary
New Orleans, Louisiana
Procedures B36, B37, I21, I22, I23, I24

Cheryl L. Cooke, RN, MN
Student Services Coordinator
University of Washington
School of Nursing
Seattle, Washington
Procedure B34

Valerie Coxon, RN, PhD
Affiliate Assistant Professor
University of Washington
Seattle, Washington *and*
CEO
NRSPACE Software, Inc
Bellevue, Washington
Procedure B34

Mary Ellen Zator Estes, RN, MSN, CCRN
Assistant Professor
School of Nursing
Marymount University
Arlington, Virginia *and*
Former Critical Care Nursing Education Coordinator
The George Washington University Medical Center
Washington, D.C.
Procedures B3, B4, B5, B6

Tom Ewing, RN, BSN
Hematology-Oncology
University of Washington Medical Center
Seattle, Washington
Procedure B23

Norma Fujise, RN-C, MS
School of Nursing
University of Hawaii
Honolulu, Hawaii
Procedures I17, I18, I19, I20

Mikel Gray, PhD, CURN, CCCN
Nurse Practitioner/Clinical Investigator
Associate Professor
Department of Urology
University of Virginia Health Sciences Center
Charlottesville, Virginia *and*
Adjunct Professor
Lancing School of Nursing
Bellarmine College
Louisville, Kentucky
Procedures B26, B27, B28, I3, I4, I5, I6, I7

Kathryn Lilleby, RN
Clinical Research Nurse
Fred Hutchinson Cancer Research Center
Seattle, Washington
Procedures B32, B33

Joan M. Mack, RN, MSN, CS
Nebraska Medical Center
Omaha, Nebraska
Procedure B20

Brenda Owens, RN, PhD
Associate Professor
School of Nursing
Louisiana State University Medical Center
New Orleans, Louisiana
Procedures I9, I10, I11, I12, I13, I14, I15, I16, A6

Demetrius Porche, RN, DNS, CCRN
Associate Professor and Director
Bachelor of Science in Nursing Program
Nicholas State University *and*
Adjunct Assistant Professor
Tulane University
School of Public Health and Topical Medicine
New Orleans, Louisiana
Procedures B1, B16, B17, B18, B19, B21, B22, B35, I1, I2, A1

Lorrie Wong, RN, MS
School of Nursing
University of Hawaii
Honolulu, Hawaii
Procedures I17, I18, I19, I20

Martha Yager, RN
Assistant Director of Nurses
Bennington Health and Rehabilitation Center
Bennington, Vermont
Procedures B26, B27, B28, I3, I4, I5, I6, I7

Reviewers

Terri Ardoin, RN, CCM
Louisiana Technical College
Charles B. Coreil Campus
Ville Platte, Louisiana

Kay Baker, RN, MS
Instructional Faculty (Nursing)
Pima Community College
Tuscon, Arizona

Lou Ann Boose, RN, BSN, MSN
Harrisburg Area Community College
Harrisburg, Pennsylvania

Susan Brooks, RN, BSN, MS, MN
Community College of Southern
   Nevada
Las Vegas, Nevada

Gyl A. Burkhard, RN, BSN, MS
Instructor
OCM BOCES
Syracuse, New York

Kay Rice Francis, RN, BSN, MSN
Woman's Health Nurse Practitioner
Nursing Instructor
Lake Michigan College
Benton Harbor, Michigan

Judith L. Gisondi, RN, BSN, MPS
Career Education Center
Hamilton Fulton Montgomery
   BOCES
Johnstown, New York

Ester Gonzales, RN, MSN, MSEd
Del Mar College
Corpus Christi, Texas

Lisa Greenwall
PN Coordinator
Frackville, Pennsylvania

**Sheila Guidry, RN, LPN, BSN,
DSN, PhD**
Wallace Community College
Selma, Alabama

Ruth Hall, BA, MA
Augusta Technical Institute
Augusta, Georgia

Renee Harrison, RN, BSN, MS
Tulsa Community College
Tulsa, Oklahoma

Suellen Klein, RN, BSN, MSN
Nursing Instructor
Lake Michigan College
Benton Harbor, Michigan

**Hope Laughlin, RN, BSN, MS,
MSN, EdD**
Pensacola Junior College
Pensacola, Florida

**Netta Moncur-Bowen, RN, BSN,
MS**
ADN Program
Seminole Community College
Sanford, Florida

Carol J. Nelson, RN, BSN, MSN
Spokane Community College
Spokane, Washington

Dr. Carol Rafferty
Northeast Wisconsin Technical
   College
Green Bay, Wisconsin

Sue Roe, DPA, MS, BNS
Chair, Health Care Management
   and Research Departments and
   Curriculum Committee
Associate Professor
Western International University
Phoenix, Arizona

Gail J. Smith, RN, BSN, MSN
Miami-Dade Community College
School of Nursing
Miami, Florida

Special thanks to the following instructors for participating in the spring 2000 focus group:

Shirley Anderson, MSN
Professor, Nursing Education
Kirkwood Community College
Cedar Rapids, Iowa

Denise Brehmer, RN, MSN
Assistant Professor of Nursing
Ivy Tech State College
Kokomo, Indiana

**Vicki Khouli, RN, BSN, MA,
IBCLC**
Instructor
Ivy Tech State College
Fort Wayne, Indiana

Linda Lauderbaugh
Ivy Tech State College
Kokomo, Indiana

Mary Strong
Kirkwood Community College
Cedar Rapids, Iowa

Mary Tobin
Kirkwood Community College
Cedar Rapids, Iowa

Ann M. L. Woodward
Kirkwood Community College
Cedar Rapids, Iowa

Preface

Basic Nursing: Foundations of Skills & Concepts was developed specifically for practical/vocational students to cover fundamental nursing concepts (nursing process, health care delivery system, documentation, client teaching, and wellness) as well as issues of basic client care (skills such as assessing blood pressure, moving a client, and performing a skin puncture). Practical/vocational nursing students can confront and adapt to certain changes in technology, information, and resources by building a solid foundation of accurate, essential information. A firm knowledge base allows nurses to meet the changing needs of clients.

Underlying Themes

Basic Nursing was organized with two fundamental themes in mind: critical thinking and holistic care.

The ability to think on one's feet is crucial for today's nurses. Roles and responsibilities are continually shifting as the health care environment evolves. Client needs change as well. Unfortunately, given the tremendous amount of information that instructors are expected to teach students, often there is little time left to develop or test a student's ability to think critically. Critical thinking is therefore a central theme in *Basic Nursing: Foundations of Skills & Concepts.*

The concept of holistic care is the second, unifying thread that underlies the entire text. It is important for nurses to learn to respect and treat the client and not just the illness. This is addressed throughout the book in several ways, including stand-alone chapters on wellness and complementary/alternative therapies.

Organization

Basic Nursing's thirty chapters are organized into twelve units and an atlas of procedures grouped at the end of the text for ease of reference.

- **Unit 1, Nurse Skills for Success,** prepares students for success. Nursing is a challenging subject. There is a large body of information that students must master. The pressures of family and academic life often place a daunting challenge in front of students—even at a time when nurses are needed more than ever! Accordingly, concepts of holistic care, critical thinking, and study skills are introduced here.
- **Unit 2, History and Nursing Organizations,** presents a brief overview of the history of nursing and the development of educational programs and nursing organizations.
- **Unit 3, Legal and Ethical Issues,** addresses the unique legal aspects of nursing and the responsibilities of the LP/VN. Ethical issues are also addressed.
- **Unit 4, Communication,** focuses on the process of communication, how communication is vital to the nurse-client relationship, and the technical and legal aspects of documentation. Each component of the nursing process is explained in a clear, concise manner. Client teaching is also presented as a major nursing intervention for clients throughout the life span.
- **Unit 5, Cultural Aspects of Nursing,** discusses issues of diversity and culture within the workplace. Complementary and alternative therapies in addition to the mainstream are also presented.
- **Unit 6, Human Development Over the Life Span,** describes growth and developmental changes over the life cycle.
- **Unit 7, Health Promotion,** addresses wellness concepts and coping behaviors as well as grief, loss, and death. Basic nutrition, rest and sleep, and safety and hygiene are presented as methods of promoting health.
- **Unit 8, Infection Control,** presents the chain of infection, describes various types of pathogenic microorganisms, explains the concepts of asepsis and aseptic technique, and outlines Standard Precautions and isolation measures.
- **Unit 9, Homeostasis,** thoroughly discusses fluid, electrolyte, and acid-base balance. Medication administration is presented in a nursing process format. Also included are legal considerations of medication administration, dose equivalents, and dosage calculations.
- **Unit 10, Fundamental Nursing Care,** includes chapters on assessment, pain management, and diagnositc tests.
- **Unit 11, Special Areas of Nursing Care,** specifically addresses nursing care of the older client. This is vital, given the large numbers of nurses working with older clients in a variety of settings. It assesses the myths and realities of aging, physiologic changes, common health problems, and the changing needs of the older client. Also covered are rehabilitation, home health, long-term care, and hospice.
- **Unit 12, Leadership/Work Transition,** focuses on the skills related to actual working situations and the changes encountered when shifting from the role of student to that of employee. Job skills such as preparing a résumé and applying for a job are detailed.

The **Atlas of Nursing Procedures** addresses nursing skills in three levels: basic, intermediate, and advanced. Procedures are presented in a step-by-step format, with a rationale clearly stated for each step. Numerous figures and illustrations add to the clarity of the presentation.

Back matter in the text includes References/Suggested Readings organized by chapter, which allows the student to find the source of the material presented in each chapter and also to find additional information concerning the topics covered. Resources are also listed by chapter and provide names, addresses, and telephone numbers of organizations specializing in a specific area of health care. Internet addresses are included as available. NANDA diagnoses are included in Appendix A, and the current immunizations schedule in Appendix B. A master listing of all Abbreviations, Acronyms, and Symbols used in the text is provided, as well as an English/Spanish translation list. A glossary of the key terms from all of the chapters is also provided.

Ancillaries

A full supplemental package was created for adopters of *Basic Nursing: Foundations of Skills & Concepts*. It includes:

For the Instructor

An **Instructor's Manual** (ISBN 0-7668-3205-8) provides many resources for the LP/VN instructor. It includes lecture notes, additional student learning activities, additional web and text resources, solutions to case studies, and solutions to review questions.

An **Electronic Instructor's Manual** (ISBN 0-7668-3204-X) also enhances the text. This CD-ROM contains many tools useful for the LP/VN instructor. It includes an image library of over 600 of the illustrations and photographs used in the textbook. These may be easily printed to create unique classroom handouts or placed in Microsoft PowerPoint presentations. Additionally, there is a computerized test bank of over 800 questions on text material.

For the Student

- The **Study Guide** (ISBN 0-7668-3202-3) provides opportunities for additional review on all 30 chapters of the *Basic Nursing* text. The student manual includes key term matching exercises, abbreviation review, exercises and activities, and self-assessment questions.
- The **Procedures Checklists** (ISBN 0-7668-3203-1) may be used to help students evaluate their comprehension and execution of the procedures contained within the core textbook.
- A **Tutorial CD-ROM** (ISBN 0-7668-3823-4) is also available. This CD-ROM contains flashcard activities to review key concepts on a chapter-by-chapter basis.

Finally, an innovative **website** was developed to accompany *Medical-Surgical Nursing: An Integrated Approach* and *Basic Nursing: Foundations of Skills & Concepts* at no additional charge. Accessed at www.DelmarNursing.com, students may—on a chapter-by-chapter basis—view a multimedia presentation that supports and reinforces the concepts in the book. This is perfect for students whose personal lives (sick children, commuting schedules, etc.) occasionally interfere with classroom attendance. A student who misses a lecture or classroom discussion may access the website for timely review.

Acknowledgments

A sincere thank you to the team at Delmar that has worked to make this textbook a reality. Beth Williams, senior developmental editor, a jewel whose humor, knowledge, guidance, and attention to detail produced a first-class textbook, receives a standing ovation. Other members of the team—Matt Filimonov, acquisitions editor; Tim Conners, art coordinator; Nina Lontrato, production coordinator; Dave Buddle, project editor; and Melissa Longo, editorial assistant—have all worked diligently for the completion of this textbook. Thank you.

A special thank you to consultants Captain Alston Kirk, CHC, USN (retired) and John White, PhD for sharing their expertise in religions and anatomy and physiology respectively. Thank you to the contributors and reviewers for your time and expertise in making this book possible.

About the Author

Lois Elain Wacker White earned a diploma in nursing from Memorial Hospital School of Nursing, Springfield, Illinois; an associate degree in science from Del Mar College, Corpus Christi, Texas; a bachelor of science in nursing from Texas A & I University-Corpus Christi, Corpus Christi, Texas; a master of science in education from Corpus Christi State University, Corpus Christi, Texas; and a doctor of philosophy degree in educational administration-community college from the University of Texas, Austin, Texas.

She has taught at Del Mar College, Corpus Christi, Texas, in both the Associate Degree Nursing program and the Vocational Nursing program. For 14 years she was also chairperson of the Department of Vocational Nurse Education. Dr. White has taught fundamentals of nursing, nutrition, mental health/mental illness, medical–surgical nursing, and maternal/newborn nursing. Her professional career has also included 15 years of clinical practice.

Dr. White has served on the Nursing Education Advisory Committee (NEAC) of the Board of Nurse Examiners for the State of Texas and the Board of Vocational Nurse Examiners, which developed competencies expected of graduates from each level of nursing. Serving as an NLN site visitor has given her insight into student and program needs which must be met to provide the best in nursing education. She maintains membership in the Texas Association of Vocational Nurse Educators, Sigma Theta Tau, American Nurses Association, and the National League for Nursing.

Dr. White has been listed in *Who's Who in American Nursing*. She currently serves on the Vocational Nursing Financial Aid Advisory Committee for the Texas Higher Education Coordinating Board.

How to Use This Text

This text is designed with you, the reader, in mind. Special elements and feature boxes appear throughout the text to guide you in reading and to assist you in learning the material. Following are suggestions for how you can use these features to increase your understanding and mastery of the content.

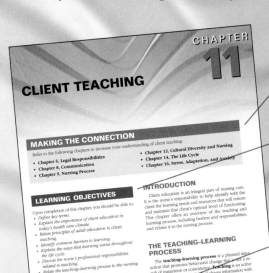

Making the Connection

Read these boxes before beginning a chapter to link material across the holistic care continuum and to tie new content to material you have already encountered.

Objectives

Read the chapter objectives before reading the chapter content to set the stage for learning. Revisit the objectives when preparing for an exam to see which entries you can respond to with "yes, I can do that."

Key Terms

Review this list before reading the chapter to familiarize yourself with new terms and to revisit those terms you already know to link them to the content of the new chapter.

Community/Home Health Care

Read these boxes before making a home visit to a client with a given disorder. You can also use these boxes to prepare for client discharge to ensure that all necessary self-care topics have been covered with a client.

Professional Tip

Use these boxes to increase your professional competence and confidence, and also to expand your knowledge base.

Client Teaching

Read these boxes to gain insight into client learning needs related to the specific disorder or condition. You may want to make your own index cards listing these teaching guidelines to use when you are working with clients.

Infection Control

When reading a chapter, stop and pay attention to these features and ask yourself, "Had I thought of that? Do I practice these precautions?"

Cultural Considerations

Test your sensitivity to cultural and ethnic variations by scanning these boxes and incorporating their guidelines and suggestions into your practice. You may also want to ask yourself what biases or preconceptions you have about different cultural practices before reading a chapter and then read these boxes for information that may help you be more sensitive in your nursing care and approach to clients.

Life Cycle Considerations

Use these boxes to increase your awareness of variations in care based on client age; this will help you deliver more effective and appropriate care.

Safety

Pause while reading to consider these elements and quiz yourself: "Do I take steps such as these to ensure my own and the client's safety? Do I follow these guidelines in every practice encounter?"

Nursing Care Plan

Use these features to test your understanding of application of the content presented. Ask yourself, "Would I have come up with the same nursing diagnoses? Are these the interventions that I would have proposed? What other interventions would be appropriate?"

Case Study

Read over these boxes within text. Draw on the knowledge you have gained and synthesize information to develop your own educated responses to the case study challenges.

Review Questions

When you finish reading a chapter, use these questions to critically test your understanding of concepts covered. You might also read these questions before beginning a new chapter to gauge how much you already know or need to learn about the topic.

Critical Thinking

Visit these boxes after reading the entire chapter to check your acquisition and understanding of the concepts presented.

Web Flash!

Use these boxes to tap into the power of the Internet and enhance your research and technology skills.

Procedures

Reference the procedures as you read the chapters. Study the techniques, review the figures, and be prepared for your clinical days with questions of clarification for your instructor.

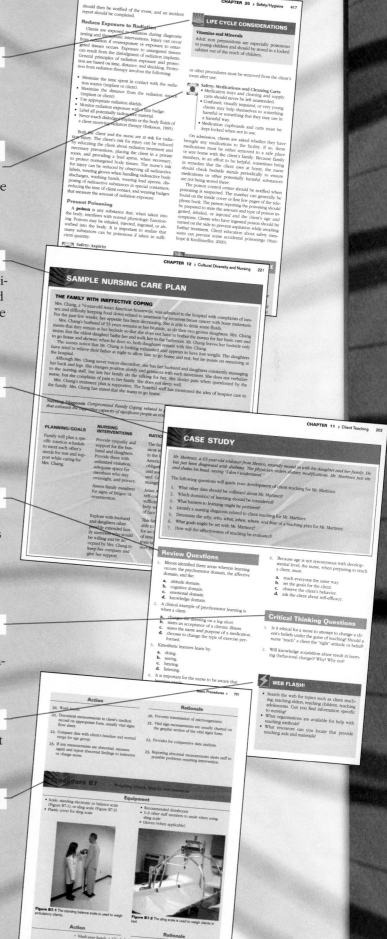

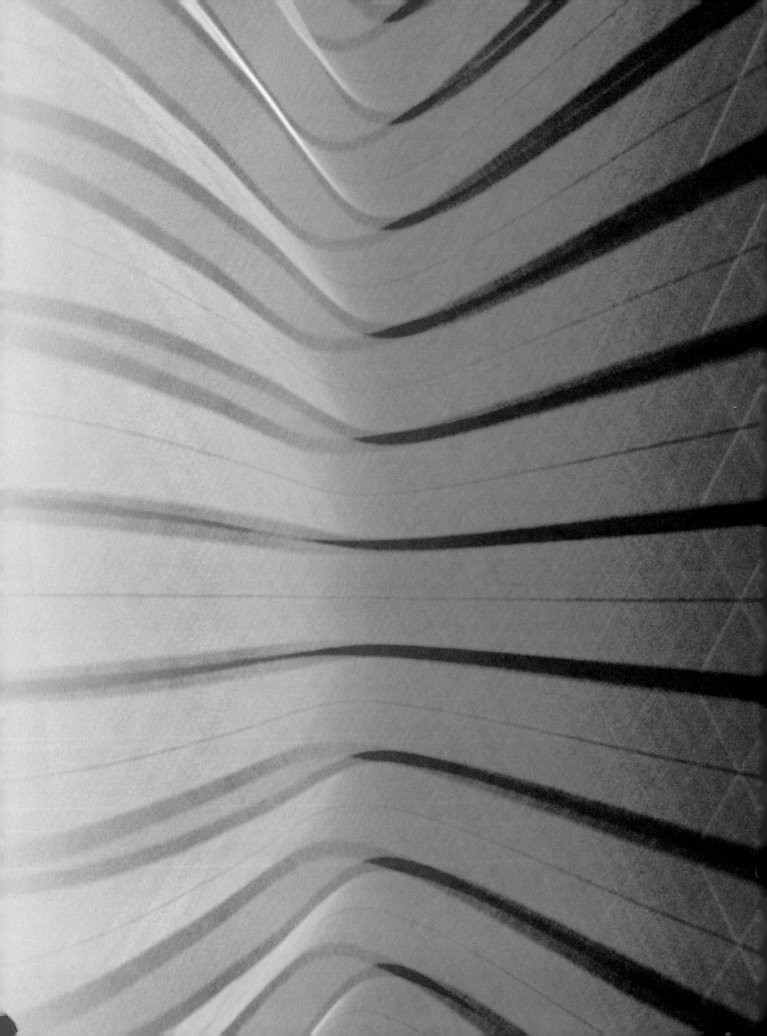

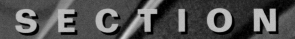

Perspectives in Nursing

Unit 1
Nurse Skills for Success

Unit 2
History and Nursing
Organizations

Unit 3
Legal and Ethical Issues

Unit 4
Communication

Unit 5
Cultural Aspects
of Nursing

UNIT

1
Nurse Skills
for Success

Chapter 1
Holistic Care

Chapter 2
Critical Thinking

Chapter 3
Student Nurse Skills for Success

HOLISTIC CARE

MAKING THE CONNECTION

Refer to the following chapters to increase your understanding of holistic care:

- **Chapter 6, Legal Responsibilities**
- **Chapter 12, Cultural Diversity and Nursing**
- **Chapter 13, Complementary/Alternative Therapies**
- **Chapter 16, Stress, Adaptation, and Anxiety**
- **Chapter 18, Basic Nutrition**
- **Chapter 20, Safety/Hygiene**

- **Chapter 22, Standard Precautions and Isolation**
- **Chapter 23, Fluid, Electrolyte, and Acid-Base Balance**
- **Procedures:** B1, Handwashing; B8, Practicing Proper Body Mechanics

LEARNING OBJECTIVES

Upon completion of this chapter, you should be able to:
- *Define key terms.*
- *Define health as it relates to the whole person.*
- *List and discuss the five aspects of total wellness.*
- *List and discuss Maslow's Hierarchy of Needs.*
- *Describe self-awareness and why it is important to nurses.*
- *Describe self-concept.*
- *Discuss the concept of personal responsibility for one's own illness.*
- *Discover personal attitudes about health and illness and take responsibility for personal well-being.*
- *Identify the components of a healthy lifestyle.*

KEY TERMS

attitude
body mechanics
culture
health
health continuum
holistic
homeostasis
intellectual wellness
Maslow's Hierarchy of Needs
physical wellness
psychological wellness
self-awareness
self-concept
sociocultural wellness
spiritual wellness
wellness

INTRODUCTION

Welcome to practical/vocational nursing. You have chosen one of life's rewarding careers. The next few months of your life will be challenging, exhilarating, frustrating, and full of new experiences. When you consider the difficulty of the nursing program's admission process, being a member of this nursing class is no small achievement. The fact that you have survived admissions demonstrates that you are capable of overcoming the challenges that lie ahead. Balancing family, community, and school responsibilities may prove the most difficult task you have yet to face.

As a nurse, you are a professional caregiver. Your intimate contact with clients allows you the opportunity not only to provide physical and emotional support, but also to teach ways to take an active role in maintaining health.

You may have contact with hundreds of clients, each needing specialized treatment and care. The care you provide will vary from routine, to critical, to emergency. You will be part of a multidisciplinary team of caregivers that includes registered nurses, physicians, nursing assistants, physical therapists, respiratory therapists, laboratory technicians, dietitians, and social workers. All caregivers work together to promote and maintain client health.

Because the caregiver's goal is promoting and maintaining health, understanding the concept of health is paramount. Most simply, health means that an organism is performing its vital functions normally and properly (*Webster's*, 1997).

INTERRELATED CONCEPTS OF HEALTH

In 1948 the World Health Organization (WHO) was founded. The WHO, which functions as an arm of the United Nations, places particular emphasis on combating communicable diseases, educating health care workers, and improving the health of all people of the world. The WHO defines **health** as follows: "Health is a state of complete physical, mental, and social well-being and not merely the absence of disease or infirmity" (WHO, 1974).

Many people believe that health or wellness is only the absence of disease. In its truest form, however, health refers to the total well-being of the whole person.

Holistic Health

Holistic is a term derived from the Greek word *holos,* meaning "whole." Holistic health views the physical, intellectual, sociocultural, psychological, and spiritual aspects of a person's life as an integrated whole. These five aspects cannot be separated or isolated; anything that affects one aspect of a person's life also affects the other aspects. The environment within which a person lives and the manner whereby the person interacts with that environment are also considerations.

The American Holistic Nurses' Association (AHNA) (1994) describes health as the maintenance of harmony and balance among body, mind, and spirit. **Homeostasis** is the balance or stability that the body strives to achieve among these aspects of a person's life by continuous adaptation. Internal physiological homeostasis is a balance of the body's fluids.

Nurses must understand the integration of these aspects of a person's life in order to help clients through healing processes. Figure 1-1 illustrates the holistic perspective.

Holistic Care

Dossey (1998) reports that the use of holistic modalities is gradually becoming integrated into mainstream client care. The National Institutes of Health (NIH) established the National Center for Complementary and Alternative Medicine (NCCAM) to investigate holistic modalities. The NIH defines holistic care as care that "considers the whole person, including physical, mental, emotional, and spiritual aspects." The final goal of investigating holistic modalities is to allow the validated therapies to be further integrated into general client care.

Success in using holistic modalities in client care requires an awareness of a fundamental principle of holism: The nurse *facilitates* the client in attaining the best state for healing to occur. Among the holistic modalities most frequently used in nursing are the following:

- Biofeedback
- Exercise and movement
- Goal-setting
- Humor and laughter
- Imagery
- Journaling
- Massage
- Play therapy
- Prayer

Nurses must be open to new ideas and must not allow holistic modalities to become just another technology. They must work on developing personal healing qualities and become more aware of healing in their own lives. Among other qualities, a healer:

- Demonstrates awareness that self-healing is a continual process.
- Is familiar with self-development.
- Recognizes personal strengths and weaknesses.
- Models self-care.
- Demonstrates awareness that personal presence is as important as technical skills.
- Respects and loves clients.

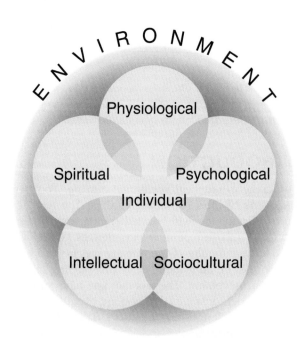

Figure 1-1 Holistic Perspective of Individuals

- Presumes that clients know the best life choices.
- Guides clients in discovering creative options.
- Listens actively.
- Shares insights without imposing personal values and beliefs.
- Accepts client input without judgment.
- Views time spent with clients as an opportunity to serve and share (adapted from Dossey, 1998).

Nursing the Whole Person

Nursing the whole person, or holistic health care, is a comprehensive approach to health care. It considers physical, intellectual, sociocultural, psychological, and spiritual aspects, the response to illness, and the effect of illness on a person's ability to meet self-care needs. Also taken into account is the individual's responsibility for personal well-being. Teaching preventive care is always a focus.

Nurses work with people throughout life to promote wellness and prevent illness (Figure 1-2). The highest level of wellness should be the goal of each nurse and every client.

Wellness

Wellness is a responsibility, a choice, a lifestyle design that helps maintain the highest potential for personal health (Hill & Howlett, 1997). The **health continuum** is a way to visualize the range of an individual's health, from highest health potential to death (Figure 1-3).

An individual's place on the continuum may change daily or even hourly depending on what is happening to that individual. Constant effort is required to balance all aspects of life and to maintain the highest level of health. A person at the highest level of wellness is one who demonstrates good physical self-care, emotional well-being, creative expression, and positive relationships with others.

Wellness incorporates physical, intellectual, sociocultural, psychological, and spiritual wellness. To provide holistic care, all aspects of the individual's wellness must be addressed.

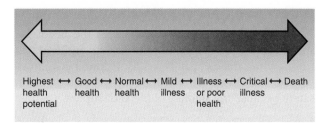

Highest ↔ Good ↔ Normal ↔ Mild ↔ Illness ↔ Critical ↔ Death
health   health   health   illness or poor illness
potential   health

Figure 1-3 Health Continuum

Maslow's Hierarchy of Needs

Abraham Maslow developed a theory of behavioral motivation based on needs. This theory is often referred to as **Maslow's Hierarchy of Needs**. There are five levels in this hierarchy. The basic physiological needs must be met to maintain life. The rest of the needs are related to quality of life. They are safety and security, love and belonging, self-esteem, and self-actualization. The needs of the lower levels must be met before a person is motivated to meet the needs of the next higher level (Figure 1-4).

Many nursing programs use Maslow's Hierarchy of Needs as a basis for planning the care of clients. This ensures that basic physiological needs as well as the other needs are assessed and addressed in individualized care plans.

Physiological Needs

Although Maslow (1954) did not specifically identify the physiological needs, they are generally accepted to be the needs of oxygen, food, water, elimination, rest (sleep)/activity (exercise), and sex. With the exception of sex, all of these needs must be met for the life of the individual to be maintained. Satisfying the sexual need, while not necessary for individual survival, is necessary for survival of the human race. The basic physiological needs must be met before higher-level needs become motivators of behavior. For example, a person who is truly hungry is motivated by that need, and behavior is focused on getting food.

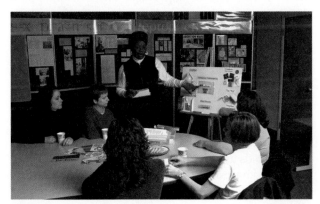

Figure 1-2 Nurses work with clients of all age groups to encourage health and wellness.

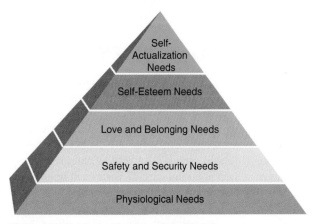

Figure 1-4 Maslow's Hierarchy of Needs

Safety and Security Needs

The next level, safety, encompasses the needs for shelter, stability, security, physical safety, and freedom from undue anxiety. Safety needs include both physical and emotional aspects. Illness is often a threat to safety because the stability of life is disrupted.

Love and Belonging Needs

The third level of the hierarchy, love and belonging, incorporates not only the giving of affection but also the receiving of affection. Having friends and participating with others in groups and organizations are two ways to meet these needs. Meeting these needs is extremely important for mental health.

Self-Esteem Needs

The needs of the self-esteem level are met by achieving success in work and other activities. Recognition from others increases self-esteem and feelings of pride in one's accomplishments.

Self-Actualization Needs

Self-actualization is the highest level of the Maslow hierarchy. A person who has met these needs is confident, self-fulfilled, and creative; looks for challenges; and sees beauty and order in the world.

Maslow contends that because most people are so busy meeting the physiological and the safety and security needs, little time or energy is left to meet the love and belonging, self-esteem, and self-actualization needs; thus, most people are less than satisfied at higher levels of the hierarchy. Even when the lower two levels are met without much trouble, many people have personalities and attitudes that make meeting the needs of the three higher levels difficult if not impossible.

An individual does not move steadily up the hierarchy. As life situations change, a person's unmet needs change, and behavior is motivated by different levels of the hierarchy. For example, if a person who is working to meet the self-esteem need is suddenly laid off at work, the safety and security need of providing financially for self and family suddenly becomes the unmet need that motivates that person's behavior.

PROVIDING QUALITY CARE

The first step in providing quality client care is to be aware of yourself. What kind of personality do you have? Is your self-concept positive, or do you have self-doubts and lack self-confidence? What are your beliefs and attitudes? Knowing the answers to such questions will help you in your role as caregiver.

The next step is taking care of your own needs (see the preceding section on Maslow's Hierarchy of Needs). When you attend to the needs in your own life, you are then free to concentrate on caring for others. Your example of self-care inspires clients to have confidence that you will provide quality care. Thus, self-care is a factor in your effectiveness as a caregiver.

Self-Awareness

Self-awareness is consciously knowing how the self thinks, feels, believes, and behaves at any specific time. Being self-aware is a constant process that is focused on the present. A person's thoughts, feelings, and beliefs are interrelated and greatly influence behavior. Being self-aware influences a person in several ways.

Self-awareness may make a person uncomfortable. Awareness allows the person to either accept or alter feelings, beliefs, and behavior. One can learn to be self-aware. Begin now to concentrate on becoming aware of your thoughts and actions. Take note of your reactions to any given situation. What makes you anxious? What makes you happy? Listen to yourself when you respond to questions and when you visit with friends. Realize that everyone has strengths and weaknesses. Focus on your strengths. Spend your energies on today. Do not dwell on past mistakes; rather try to learn from them, and then forget them. Stop periodically and pay attention to what you feel and believe. Listening not only to the words one speaks but also to the way the words are spoken assists in self-awareness. Use the word *I,* and take ownership of feelings and beliefs. Say, "I am so happy," instead of "That makes me happy."

Self-awareness is extremely important for nurses. Nurses must understand themselves so that their personal feelings, attitudes, and needs do not interfere with providing quality client care. The nurse who is self-aware is more likely to make decisions in response to the client's needs rather than the nurse's own needs. For example, student nurses—and even experienced nurses—are often anxious about caring for a client. By taking some time to practice self-awareness, the nurse might discover that the anxiety stems from never having performed the procedure in question. The nurse can then deal directly with the situation by reviewing the procedure and requesting assistance from an instructor or supervisor. All decisions about client care must be made in response to the client's needs, not the nurse's needs.

Development of Self-Concept

Self-concept is how a person thinks or feels about himself. These thoughts and feelings come from the experiences the person has with others and reflect how the person thinks others view him.

Self-concept begins forming in infancy. An infant whose needs are met feels satisfied and "good." Experiences, both positive and negative, influence a person's self-concept (Figure 1-5). Interactions with significant others, such as parents, extended family, and friends, have a great impact on self-concept. This is true not only during the developing years, but also throughout

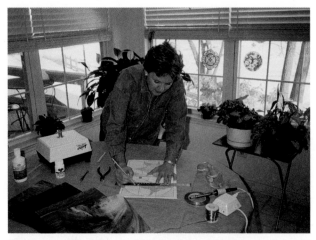

Figure 1-5 Self-concept and self-esteem can be enhanced by learning new skills.

life. Because of its influence on client care, it is important for the nurse to be aware of how her own self-concept has developed. Self-concept develops through feedback from others. The nurse is responsible for providing feedback that will not negatively affect the client's self-concept. A client who is constantly ignored or who receives messages such as "Don't bother me," "Can't you do anything right?", or "You don't have any sense" may very well begin to view himself in these terms, with the likely result being a negative self-concept. On the other hand, a person who is shown caring and who hears messages such as "Let me help you in a minute," "Let's try it this way," or "Have you thought about . . . ?" will move toward a positive self-concept.

SELF-CARE AS A PREREQUISITE TO CLIENT CARE

The most effective means to teach wellness is by positive example. By first practicing good health habits as a nursing student, you will become, by example, an important factor in your clients' overall well-being and good health. Remind yourself and your clients that health is a personal choice and that each person has control over his or her own wellness.

You will be helping clients recognize how their own actions can prevent many of the conditions that cause illness. Choosing to exercise regularly, to eat a balanced diet, to eat breakfast each day, to control fat content, and to select from the basic food groups are good rules for wellness (Figure 1-6). Choosing to not smoke, to practice moderation in the use of alcohol, to avoid all nontherapeutic drugs, and to practice safe sex can help prevent many of the conditions that cause disease and death.

While emphasizing health promotion and client education, the nurse must also encourage and respect the client's responsibility for wellness. This respect allows

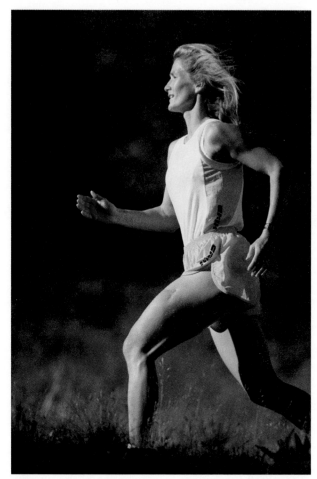

Figure 1-6 Through exercise, this woman is demonstrating a lifestyle choice that will enhance her health status.

the client to become an active partner in, rather than a passive recipient of, health care. It is not enough to tell a client *what* can be done to improve health; the nurse must also be prepared to explain *why*. If a client understands the reason behind an action, the likelihood of compliance increases.

Just as you are aware of yourself as a whole person with many components, help your clients see themselves and their health care as more than physical health. Help clients understand how physical, intellectual, sociocultural, psychological, and spiritual health are all related and can lead to an overall sense of well-being. This is the full meaning of holistic care.

Physical Wellness

Physical wellness refers to a healthy body that functions at an optimal level. To achieve physical wellness a person must practice good grooming; use proper body mechanics; have good posture; refrain from smoking and the use of drugs and alcohol; and have adequate nutrition, sleep, rest, relaxation, and exercise.

Grooming

The nurse communicates a message of health and well-being by being clean and neatly dressed (Figure

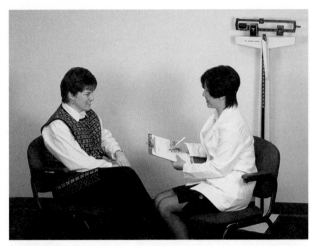

Figure 1-7 The well-groomed nurse sends a message of health and well-being.

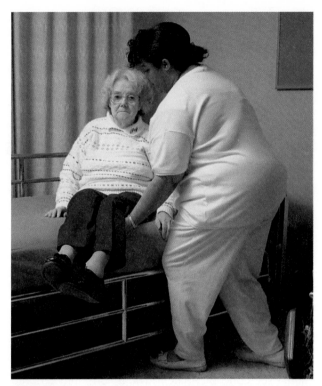

Figure 1-8 Use of Proper Body Mechanics

1-7). A daily bath or shower and the use of a deodorant form the basis of good grooming. Hair should be clean, combed, and neatly styled. Perfume should not be worn, as it may be offensive to clients. Frequent brushing, regular dental checkups, and avoiding refined sugars helps control dental caries.

While important for client safety, good handwashing is also crucial to the nurse's wellness. Antiseptic hand lotion can be used to prevent cracked, dry skin. Fingernails should be kept short, as long nails not only harbor dirt and microorganisms, but also can scratch clients.

Standard Precautions have been established by the Centers for Disease Control and Prevention (CDC) in Atlanta, Georgia. These precautions are designed to protect all health care workers and their clients from the transmission of communicable disease. Good handwashing is an integral part of Standard Precautions. As soon as you have been taught the skill of handwashing, practice it. Make it a part of your daily life. Encourage your clients to establish good handwashing habits.

Jewelry, which can harbor bacteria, and excessive makeup are both inappropriate for the nurse in uniform. Clothing should be clean and free of stains and wrinkles. Clients will have confidence in the nurse who maintains a professional appearance and who practices good hygiene.

Body Mechanics

Wellness involves more than just good grooming practices. It also requires proper **body mechanics**, that is, using the body in the safest and most efficient way to move or lift objects. The use of proper body mechanics is very important because many of the skills and tasks you will perform as a nurse involve lifting or moving clients or objects (Figure 1-8). Bending, lifting, or stooping can cause injury if done incorrectly. One of the first skills you will study involves the practice of proper body mechanics to prevent physical disability, including safe methods for bending, lifting, and moving.

Posture

Good posture is the basis for proper body mechanics. Good posture means the ability to carry oneself well and in correct body alignment. Posture also can send messages about a person. A person who stands with feet spread apart and with hands on hips, for example, may be perceived as aggressive or authoritative, whereas one who holds the arms tightly folded over the chest may be viewed as closed minded.

Observe those around you as they communicate with others. Notice the differences in posture. Does the person who stands in good alignment, with shoulders back and head up, convey self-confidence and capability? Does the individual whose shoulders are drooped and head bowed convey depression, sadness, or lack of self-confidence?

As you continue your studies and begin client care, you will realize that clients appreciate having nurses who appear confident in their own abilities and decision making. When you are with clients, you must be particularly careful of the way you stand. Remember that your posture sends messages about your attitude and feelings. The client should feel that you are confident, caring, relaxed, and willing to listen.

Smoking

Smoking contributes to many health hazards and illnesses. It may also be personally offensive to clients. The odor of cigarette, pipe, or cigar smoke on clothing or the breath (halitosis) may precipitate allergic reactions or lead to a feeling of nausea in some clients.

Most health care facilities have strict rules about smoking. Many facilities are "smoke free." The nurse should never smoke in a client's room. Further, great care should be taken to ensure that no offensive tobacco odors remain should the nurse use or be in close proximity to tobacco products. In each situation, every effort should be made to enforce all safety rules for clients and visitors. "No smoking" signs should be posted and strictly enforced when oxygen is in use.

Drugs and Alcohol

A frightening trend in the United States is the increasing rate of alcohol and drug abuse. Drug abuse has become so widespread within the health professions themselves that impaired caregiver programs have been implemented. Many states now provide access to treatment for the impaired nurse through the state board of nursing. A nurse should never give or make available to another person any drug without the written order of a physician or other person who can legally prescribe medications, such as a nurse practitioner. If you believe that a colleague is abusing drugs, you have an obligation to let your supervisor know so that the colleague can receive help through the impaired nurse program in your state. Should you yourself become addicted, you have a duty to your clients, your peers, and yourself to accept help through a recovery program.

Nutrition

Nursing is emotionally, mentally, and physically demanding. Nurses must be able to think clearly and work efficiently. A balanced diet including fruits and vegetables, whole grains and cereals, milk and milk products, and meats or other protein foods is required for optimal body function.

Nursing students may be tempted to skip meals, omit breakfast, eat snacks, and follow fad diets. This is never a wise practice. While you are in school, your success depends upon you functioning at your best. Skipping meals, especially breakfast, leaves a person tired, weak, and hungry. It is impossible to think effi-

ciently when hungry. Remember Maslow's Hierarchy of Needs: The need for food must be satisfied before you will be motivated to meet the need to learn or to study.

Always eat a balanced breakfast. Pastries and coffee, although satisfying in the moment, elevate the blood sugar level only for a short while before the level plummets. This reaction leaves a person drained, irritable, and hungrier than before. Try to avoid snacking on "junk foods," which contain "empty" calories, or those having very little nutritional value. Instead, plan to eat fruit or high-protein snacks.

Plan a routine for mealtimes, and stick to it. Doing so helps prevent the urge to binge on unhealthy snacks. Also, drink plenty of water. Water is the body's most important nutrient (Figure 1-9). A human being can survive for weeks without food, but only for a few days without water. By weight, approximately 60% of the adult body is water. In order to maintain proper fluid balance and to facilitate the elimination of body wastes, it is necessary to drink plenty of fluids. Most authorities agree that the average adult needs six to eight (8-ounce) glasses of water each day. It is important to maintain a balance in the diet for optimal wellness.

Sleep, Rest, Relaxation, and Exercise

Wellness implies more than eating balanced meals, avoiding harmful substances, and practicing good grooming. Wellness also means taking time to enjoy yourself. It means making time for sleep, rest, relaxation, and exercise.

Sleep is time for the body to replenish its energy reserves and to heal itself. The amount of time needed

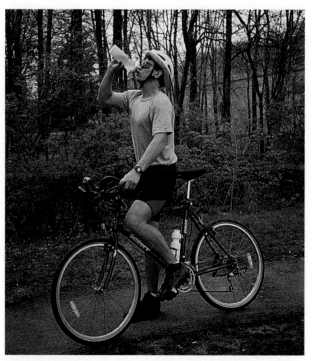

Figure 1-9 Drinking plenty of water is an important element of proper nutrition.

LIFE CYCLE CONSIDERATIONS

Nutrition
- Children's appetites vary with their growth spurts and growth plateaus.
- Healthy eating habits should be established during childhood.
- The amount of food eaten generally declines in the elderly person.
- Proper food choices are more important than quantity for the elderly person.

CLIENT TEACHING

Tips on Maintaining Proper Nutrition
- Read product labels.
- Avoid foods high in fat, sugar, and salt.
- Work to maintain or attain your ideal weight.
- If you drink alcohol, do so in moderation.
- Always eat breakfast.
- Make between-meal snacks healthy, such as raw fruits and vegetables.

may vary with the individual or even with the day. One person may need 8 hours of sleep after a heavy work day but need only 6 after a less strenuous day. An infant, of course, needs more sleep than does a young adult. Sleep is necessary to allow the body's organs to function at their most minimal levels. This period of rejuvenation for the body is necessary for total wellness.

Rest, meaning conscious freedom from activity and worry, is just as important as sleep. Rest is a time of inner quiet and physical inactivity. Only when a person is relaxed and at inner peace can that person rest.

Relaxation means doing something for the fun of it. That which is relaxing to one person may not be relaxing to another. Examples of relaxation activities include reading a novel, reading to children, playing cards or other games, fishing, painting, or sewing or other handwork.

Many experts agree that the best rest follows planned exercise. During exercise, heart rate and breathing increase, circulation improves, and muscles stretch. Exercise is also a time to free the mind of anxiety-producing thoughts. Sometimes after a day's work, a brisk walk frees the mind and allows the body to relax in preparation for rest.

Whichever form of exercise, rest, and relaxation is best for you, make time for it in each day. Rest and relaxation as well as regular sleep and exercise are essential ingredients for wellness and result in reduced fatigue and irritability and possibly increased resistance to colds, flu, and serious infections. Furthermore, the capacity to concentrate increases, which should make a significant difference in your studies.

Intellectual Wellness

Intellectual wellness is the ability to function as an independent person capable of making sound decisions. Such decisions are based on the individual's needs but at the same time take into account the needs of others. Clear thinking, problem-solving skills, good judgment, and the desire to continually learn are all qualities found in the person who is intellectually well.

Nursing requires making many decisions, some of which may mean life or death to the client. The nurse

must have intellectual wellness to be able to make the best decisions possible with regard to client care.

Sociocultural Wellness

Sociocultural wellness is the ability to appreciate the needs of others and to care about one's environment and the inhabitants of it. As a nurse, you will care for clients of all ages and races who speak different languages and come from various cultural groups. Each client's **culture** (behavior, customs, and beliefs of the family, extended family, tribe, nation, and society) influences the way that person views wellness and responds to illness.

It is important that the nurse understand that while everyone's basic needs are the same, the ways that those needs are met may vary based on the client's culture. Today's population is working, playing, and contributing to society for more years than ever before. People are more health conscious, better educated, and more involved in making health choices than perhaps any previous generation. Nurses should encourage such involvement and work to dispel discrimination by accepting each person as an individual.

CULTURAL CONSIDERATIONS

Sociocultural Wellness
Nurses and nursing students come from various cultural backgrounds and are thus excellent resources for you to learn about cultural variations.

Psychological Wellness

Psychological wellness encompasses the enjoyment of creativity, the satisfaction of the basic need to love and be loved, the understanding of emotions, and the ability to maintain control over emotions. Emotions are an integral part of the balance sought in life and are important factors in the way a person relates to others. They are measures of inner thoughts and feelings and are apparent in actions or behaviors.

Wellness requires that individuals recognize emotions and control their reactions in various situations. By controlling their emotions, nurses help create a therapeutic environment within which to help clients.

Another aspect of emotional wellness is a positive attitude. An **attitude** is a feeling about people, places, or things that is evident in the way one behaves. It can be positive or negative. Many books have been written and hundreds of studies have described the role that a positive attitude plays in helping to conquer illness. Many authorities believe having a positive attitude is at least as important as having the best treatment for an illness.

Nursing requires that you see the best in people

during the worst of times. In order to survive and function well, the nurse needs to see life as a challenge and as a gift to cherish and enjoy.

Because a positive attitude is so important when caring for your clients, it is vital that you share yours with them. An attitude can become a habit. If you repeatedly think positively, soon you will unconsciously find yourself seeing the positive aspects in any given situation. For example, you may find yourself at work when the usual number of staff does not show up. You can say to yourself at the beginning of your shift; "There is no way I will ever finish my work on time," or you can tell yourself, "This is the perfect opportunity to get organized early and work together as a team." Either way you will have the same number of staff members. But whereas having a negative attitude will increase your chances of being miserable and unsuccessful, having a positive attitude will help the day go smoother and increase the likelihood of your coworkers being cheerful and willing to help.

Having a positive attitude will also help you in your studies. It will help to open your mind and will spill into your daily life, making that life more enjoyable.

Spiritual Wellness

Spiritual wellness manifests as inner strength and peace. Spirituality is a broader concept than religion and involves one's relationship with self, others, the natural order, and a higher power. It manifests as meaningful work, creative expression, familiar rituals, and religious practices (Wright, 1998). Spirituality involves finding meaning in everything including life, illness, and death. Spiritual needs include love, meaning in life, forgiveness, and hope. The human spiritual dimension is a major healing force. It can mean the difference between life and death, wellness and illness (Dossey, Keegan, & Guzzetta, 1999).

Florence Nightingale spoke boldly about the importance of the spiritual aspect of client care. Dossey and Dossey (1998) state that the richness of a person's interactions with others correlates with positive health outcomes, and that practice of any religion correlates with greater health and increased longevity.

Nurses are not asked to take over the role of spiritual

CLIENT TEACHING

Tips for Wellness

Encourage clients to adopt the following tips for wellness:

- Eat healthy meals and healthy snacks.
- Eat breakfast.
- Do not use tobacco products.
- Exercise regularly.
- Do not use drugs.
- Do not drink alcoholic beverages or drink only in moderation.
- Focus on one problem at a time.
- Get enough sleep every night.
- Practice having a positive attitude.
- Think before speaking.
- Make a list of goals for each day.

counselors. Rather, nurses are encouraged to integrate a holistic approach by extending love, compassion, and empathy; motivating clients to address the spiritual issues; and suggesting how they might do so (Dossey & Dossey, 1998).

Cerrato (1998b) has two suggestions regarding nursing and spiritual wellness: (1) Nurses who have strong religious convictions should not impose those convictions on their clients and (2) nurses should never assume that clients who have no religious interests have no interest in spiritual values. Clients not interested in religion can be encouraged to become involved in some humanitarian endeavor or to look at life's everyday wonders in a different way.

Because they play a key role in helping clients find hope and meaning in life, it is important that nurses understand spirituality. For many, religious practices are an expression of their spirituality. An important function for the nurse is to respect the religious beliefs of clients, provide clients with privacy to practice those beliefs, and make spiritual guidance available through the client's minister, priest, rabbi, or other representative, when requested.

NURTURE YOURSELF

The worthy and demanding profession of nursing requires unselfish caring for others. Those who select nursing as a career generally want to make a difference in people's lives. The demands of clients, employers, and coworkers can cause stress for the nurse. The nurse's personal life may also be a source of stress. Many caregivers do not know how to care for themselves. Those who do not nurture themselves will suffer stress symptoms and illnesses.

PROFESSIONAL TIP

Self-Nurturing
- Develop activities that recharge the body, mind, and spirit.
- Make time for fun. Any activity that brings happiness or joy is beneficial.
- Schedule a few minutes each day to do at least one fun thing.

Persons who are well physically, intellectually, socioculturally, psychologically, and spiritually lead productive, creative lives. They are better able to meet life's challenges and to control their stressors. For nurses, wellness means practicing wellness habits daily. As role models for clients, nurses should be examples of the holistically healthy individual.

SUMMARY

- Wellness includes physical, intellectual, sociocultural, psychological, and spiritual health.
- The keys to wellness are prevention and education.
- Each individual must learn to accept responsibility for his own wellness.
- Nurses are teachers. The most effective means to teach wellness is by positive example.
- There are five levels in Maslow's Hierarchy of Needs: physiological, safety and security, love and belonging, self-esteem, and self-actualization.
- Self-awareness is important for nurses so that their own needs do not interfere with providing quality client care.
- Nurses should get to know themselves by becoming aware of their thoughts, actions, and reactions to situations.
- Good posture is necessary for personal and client safety.
- Dental health is necessary for overall wellness and professionalism.
- Wellness tips include exercising regularly, getting enough sleep, and finding a quiet time each day for relaxing.
- A positive attitude is helpful in looking for the best in everyone.
- All nurses should learn to laugh at themselves and enjoy life's little pleasures.

Review Questions

1. Rest is defined as:

    a. sleeping.
    b. physical inactivity.
    c. playing games with family or friends.
    d. conscious freedom from activity and worry.

2. According to many experts, the best rest follows:

    a. eating.
    b. reading.
    c. exercise.
    d. studying.

3. Regular mouth care and avoiding refined sugars will help control:

    a. acne.
    b. malocclusion.
    c. dental caries.
    d. mononucleosis.

4. What responsibility does the nurse have who believes a colleague is abusing drugs?

    a. Report it to the supervisor.
    b. Ignore it; it is not the nurse's concern.
    c. Tell the colleague to stop or the nurse will call the police.
    d. Assist the nurse to receive help through the local drug treatment program.

5. What can be the result when breakfast is omitted?

    a. The person loses weight faster.
    b. The person is left tired, weak, and hungry.
    c. The person eats more at the noon and evening meals.
    d. The person's mind is sharper, and study time is more productive.

6. Positive or negative feelings about people, places, or things are called:

    a. culture.
    b. empathy.
    c. symptoms.
    d. attitudes.

7. The nurse who smokes may have:

    a. mitosis.
    b. meiosis.
    c. halitosis.
    d. arthrosis.

8. The aspects of total wellness are:

    a. rest, exercise, and good grooming.
    b. physical, psychological, spiritual, intellectual, and sociocultural.
    c. self-awareness; rest; balanced, nutritious diet; good grooming; dental care.
    d. physiological; safety and security; love and belonging; self-esteem; self-actualization.

Critical Thinking Questions

1. What are your own attitudes about health and wellness?

2. What are you doing or what can you do to take responsibility for your own well-being?

 WEB FLASH!

- How many references do you find on the web for "holistic care"?
- Visit the American Holistic Nurses' Association on the Internet.
- Visit the web site of the National Center for Complementary and Alternative Medicine. What is the latest information on holistic modalities?

CRITICAL THINKING

MAKING THE CONNECTION

Refer to the following chapter to increase your understanding of critical thinking:

- **Chapter 8, Communication**

LEARNING OBJECTIVES

Upon completion of this chapter, you should be able to:
- *Define key terms.*
- *State five characteristics of the person who uses critical thinking.*
- *Identify behaviors that illustrate the traits of a nurse who is a critical thinker.*
- *Assess personal strengths and weaknesses in relation to critical thinking skills.*
- *Develop a personal plan for the enhancement of personal critical thinking and reasoning skills.*

KEY TERMS

concept	logic
critical thinking	opinion
discipline	reasoning
disciplined	reflective
judgment	standard
justify	

INTRODUCTION

Thinking as a nurse involves much more than gathering an assortment of facts and skills. Critical thinking in nursing education is not a separate component of the curriculum. It is "an approach to inquiry where both students and faculty examine clinical and professional issues and search for more effective answers" (Miller & Malcolm, 1990).

Nursing is part of a rapidly changing and increasingly complex society. Anyone who expects to have a successful career in nursing, at any level, must be able to compete effectively. This means that practical/vocational nurses must have good problem-solving skills and make quality decisions related to the client care they deliver. Over the past 15 years, increasing attention has been paid to the need for graduates of educational programs at every level and in every **discipline** (branch of learning, field of study, or occupation requiring specialized knowledge) to develop better thinking skills. Nurse educators have been among the leaders in the current movement to find ways to improve the thinking ability of their students. Nurses in clinical practice have also been challenged to improve their ability to reason clearly and logically. Because of these movements, you, as a beginning nursing student, will need to develop your critical thinking skills.

CRITICAL THINKING

The first step in improving the ability to think well is to develop an understanding of **critical thinking**. This involves much more than memorizing a simple definition of this process. The ability to think critically requires a great deal of effort and time. Many questions must be asked as you begin the process of learning to assess your own thinking and the quality of the thinking of others (Figure 2-1). In fact, memorizing an exact definition of critical thinking would be detrimental to the full development of an understanding of this **disciplined** (trained by instruction and exercise) type of thinking. The **concept** of critical thinking includes the basic idea that one becomes a better thinker by developing specific attitudes, traits, and skills. A concept is a mental picture of abstract phenomena that serves to organize observations related to that phenomena. Each person must learn to be **reflective**, or introspective,

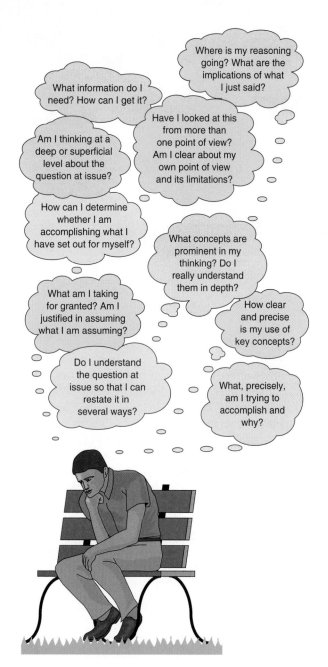

Figure 2-1 Assessing Our Own Thinking (*Courtesy of the Foundation for Critical Thinking, Dillon Beach, CA*)

about his or her own thinking. Critical thinking was briefly described in this way in a workshop presented by Richard Paul (Paul & Willsen, 1993): "Critical thinking is that mode of thinking—about any subject, content, or problem—in which the thinker improves the quality of his or her thinking by skillfully taking charge of the structures inherent in thinking and imposing intellectual **standards** (or a level or degree of quality) upon them." To ensure integrity and consistency of the presentation in this chapter, the criteria, standards, and materials developed by the Center for Crit-

ical Thinking have been used as the organizing framework.

In a newsletter designed for nurse educators interested in the use of critical thinking within the nursing curriculum, Penny Heaslip (1994) presents a definition of critical thinking. This definition serves as a basis for you to develop strategies and tactics as you begin the exciting experience of learning to think more clearly, and in a disciplined manner, about nursing. A comprehensive definition of critical thinking is the disciplined, intellectual process of applying skillful clinical **reasoning** (use of the elements of thought to solve a problem or settle a question) and self-reflective thinking as a guide to belief or action in nursing practice (Heaslip, 1994; Norris & Ennis, 1989; Paul, 1990).

Table 2–1 presents some definitions of critical thinking. Review them and compare the elements that are common to all of them and the elements that are different.

Most of the authors who have written about critical thinking have addressed instructors. This chapter is written for you, the student. It is designed to guide your process of reflecting on and evaluating your own thinking. While your instructors want to help you with the process, you are ultimately responsible for your own thinking.

Many students enter nursing programs unprepared to think critically. Many educators believe this inability may be the result of a lack of instruction in thinking. The result is similar to what would happen to you if you tried to play soccer without knowing the rules or having had a chance to learn the basic skills of the game. Quality thinking is like any skill; it takes practice and discipline to learn. This is a good time to do a self-evaluation related to your current ability to perform the four basic critical thinking processes: reading for meaning, listening critically, writing clearly, and speaking in a logical, coherent manner. These four skills are discussed in the next section. If your basic education program did not emphasize all of these skills, decide now to develop these abilities.

Table 2–1 DEFINITIONS OF CRITICAL THINKING

- "Reflective and reasonable thinking that is focused on deciding what to believe or do" (Ennis, 1985).

- "An investigation whose purpose is to explore a situation, phenomenon, question, or problem to arrive at a hypothesis or conclusion about it that integrates all available information and that can therefore be convincingly justified" (Kurfiss, 1988).

- "The attentive commitment to a self-reflective process of examining one's thoughts, ensuring that the thinking occurring meets intellectual standards" (Heaslip, 1993).

New Information

The quantity of new information that you must be prepared to master may be a barrier to the development of critical thinking skills. Many students (and instructors) focus so intently on the content of a course that they allow little time to think about the material. The ability to think critically about the knowledge base of nursing is essential for learning the content of your nursing courses. The discipline of nursing has an organizing **logic**, or formal principles of a branch of knowledge, that serves to define the appropriate facts and methods required to produce effective nursing practice. This logic serves as a framework within which the student can construct a unique, meaningful system for the practice of nursing. Your nursing program probably has a philosophy and a statement of the main concepts that the nursing faculty use to present the course material in a logical framework.

Activity

If you have not yet reviewed your program's philosophy and main concepts for the purpose of helping you understand your program of study, this would be a good time to do so. Most programs of nursing include a philosophy statement, organizing concepts, and program outcomes in the student handbook or other document provided to students. These resources can help you use your own logic to discover the logic of nursing as presented in your program. Try the following activities:

1. Identify the major concepts (such as nursing, learning, caring) that provide structure for your program's philosophy and organization.
2. Discuss the components, or parts, of each major theme with your classmates and instructors.
3. Use your own words to see how your mental pictures of these ideas may be the same or different from those in your program materials.
4. Review the material you have already covered in your nursing program to identify how the major parts of each course relate to these concepts.
5. Look at the objectives for this course and the topics in this textbook to see how they will relate to the main ideas you have discovered in this activity.

Student Responsibility

Finally, many students find the process of becoming responsible for their own thinking painful. For many students the education processes that were part of their basic school preparation were based on a very structured approach to acquiring selected facts and skills; the students' recall was then tested by "objective" tests. If this was your experience, you may view learning as being the result of the teacher's presenting what must be learned and devising "fair" tests. You may thus believe that your own input to the learning process is of less importance than that of the teacher. You, along with many other students, may find that you are uncomfortable when asked to decide what is important or to be able to defend your **opinions** (subjective beliefs) and **judgments** (conclusions based on sound reasoning and supported by evidence). You may prefer to be told, with no ambiguity, what you need to know.

Nursing, however, does not take place in predictable, highly structured situations. Practical/vocational nurses are required to make decisions at many levels. Knowing how to make good decisions begins with developing the essential skills, traits, and attitudes associated with critical thinking.

SKILLS OF CRITICAL THINKING

Four basic skills are necessary for the development of higher-level thinking skills. These skills are part of the process of developing and using thinking for problem-solving and reasoning. Your abilities in these four areas can be measured by the extent to which you are achieving the universal intellectual standards (UIS). These standards are discussed in the following section and are illustrated in Table 2–2. The four basic skills are critical reading, critical listening, critical writing, and critical speaking.

Critical Reading

Reading for meaning is basic to the acquisition of knowledge from textbooks and journals. The student who can read critically will also do better on tests. Study time will be reduced and retention of material

---

Table 2–2 THE SPECTRUM OF UNIVERSAL INTELLECTUAL STANDARDS

Clear	Unclear
Precise	Imprecise
Specific	Vague
Accurate	Inaccurate
Relevant	Irrelevant
Consistent	Inconsistent
Logical	Illogical
Deep	Superficial
Complete	Incomplete
Significant	Insignificant
Adequate	Inadequate
Fair	Unfair

Adapted from the Foundation for Critical Thinking, Dillon Beach, CA.

will be enhanced. An exercise that can help build reading skills is to use a highlighter pen to mark the main idea of a sentence. Students who have not learned to read critically will find that they have marked most of the text. Joining a study group may help you identify main ideas by comparing with others the various main ideas each of you have derived from the same material. During test reviews, you can make sure to note when misreading or misinterpretation caused you to make an error on the test. By making a conscious effort to identify your individual weaknesses, you will improve your critical reading skills.

Another tactic you can try is to practice restating the main idea to yourself or to another student. As you read the text, have a dialogue with yourself, which could go something like this: "What is the reason for studying this material? How does this relate to what I already know? This does not seem to fit. Did I misunderstand? Can I say this in my own words?" Worrell (1990) has developed a useful tool for guiding your dialogue. It is illustrated in Table 2–3.

Critical Listening

Communication skills, especially listening skills, receive a great deal of emphasis in the nursing curriculum. Even so, many persons do not have effective listening skills. One reason is that many persons have developed the habit of tuning in only occasionally to orally presented material. The result is that the meaning of the oral communication is lost. A way to improve your listening skills is to try to restate the points made in a discussion with another student and have that student give feedback about how accurately you have restated her position. Critical listening also requires that you carry on a mental dialogue with the speaker. For instance, as you listen, focus on what the speaker is saying, listen for key points, notice anything that seems confusing to you as well as those points you already understand (Figure 2-2).

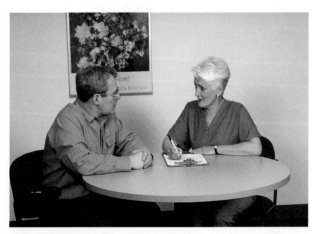

Figure 2-2 Effective listening skills are essential to all client interactions.

Table 2–3 STRATEGIC READING LIST

The following questions serve as a guide for self-talk when reading texts or journal articles. An effective reader is an active, strategic reader! Soon you will find yourself automatically using these and other questions that you have developed, no longer needing the checklist.

PREREADING QUESTIONS

___ 1. Have I previewed (skimmed) the title, headings, subheadings, objectives, and overview?

___ 2. Do the headings/subheadings identify main ideas?

___ 3. What is the chapter about?

___ 4. How is the content related to what I already know?

___ 5. How has the author organized the material? How will this organization help me?

___ 6. Will I need other resources as I read?

___ 7. Based on previewing, what questions should I formulate to guide my reading?

QUESTIONS DURING READING

___ 1. Does this make sense to me?

___ 2. Do I need to look up any unfamiliar words?

___ 3. Do I need to reread difficult material? Or will this be explained further if I read on?

___ 4. Is the author using signal words (*first, next, therefore, as a result*, etc.)?

___ 5. How is this information related to what I know?

___ 6. How is this section linked to the previous section?

___ 7. Can I summarize this section before going any further?

___ 8. Can I answer my prereading questions? Can I formulate new questions?

QUESTIONS AFTER READING

___ 1. Do I understand the main points?

___ 2. Can I outline the content?

___ 3. How is this related to previous learning?

___ 4. How would I use or apply this information?

___ 5. Are there points that I need to clarify? How will I do this?

___ 6. What questions would likely be on an exam from this material?

___ 7. Can I answer my questions, paraphrase the content, and link main points without looking at my notes or text?

From Metacognition: Implications for Instruction in Nursing Education, by P. J. Worrell, 1990, Journal of Nursing Education, *29(4). Reprinted with permission of* Journal of Nursing Education, *SLACK Incorporated, Thorofare, NJ.*

Critical listening requires that you make a conscious commitment to focus on the topic of discussion. This means that you should actively attend to the words and meanings of the speaker. Your ability to recognize things that distract your attention is valuable in increasing your listening skills. Some typical distractions for students include attempting to take word-for-word notes, focusing on the mannerisms or appearance of the speaker, and daydreaming. As in all areas, a good thinker is not afraid to identify weaknesses and strengths in order to improve.

Critical Writing

The ability to state one's thoughts coherently, clearly, and concisely is basic to good thinking skills. Many students arrive at college unable to write well. The quality of thinking is improved by the discipline required to state facts and judgments well. Many students are afraid to write down their thoughts, because they feel that writing is too revealing. Writing is important for the improvement of thinking because it can be reviewed using the UIS to evaluate the quality of the thinking reflected in the writing (Figure 2-3). These standards are discussed in greater detail later in the chapter. You may also refer back to Table 2–2.

One technique for improving the quality of your thinking through writing is to summarize, in your own words, the main idea in a reading assignment. Next, use that main idea in relation to a client care problem from the material you are studying. Then, put the writing away until the next day and reread it. Can you understand it? Submit it to a friend for critique. Can your friend understand what you meant to say? How could you improve what you have written? Improving your writing skills may not seem like fun, but it is an effective and vital process for improving the quality of your own thinking.

Critical Speaking

Perhaps the most neglected skill is disciplined speaking. We do not hear many examples of clear, logical, accurate spoken communication. Oral communication is different from written communication. It is usually more spontaneous and must be carefully presented because, unless recorded, it is present only for the moment. Ambiguous statements are misleading. Personal biases influence what the other person hears. Practicing in a small group and soliciting feedback from the listeners can help a student assess and improve this skill.

STANDARDS FOR CRITICAL THINKING

The simple definition of critical thinking used in the preceding section includes the provision that the assessment of your own thinking relies on the use of universal standards for quality thinking. As you begin to develop and apply critical thinking to nursing, the first requirement is to become familiar with these standards. The Spectrum of Universal Intellectual Standards developed by The Center for Critical Thinking is used in this discussion because it provides a valid and

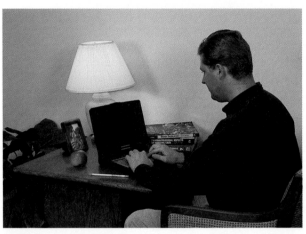

Figure 2-3 Effective writing skills are integral to critical thinking.

reliable measure for the quality of thinking. Whether you are reading the assigned material from a textbook, listening to an oral presentation, writing a paper, answering test questions, or presenting ideas in oral form, the following standards should be applied.

Clarity vs. Lack of Clarity

Fundamental to quality thinking is the ability to think clearly. Thinking clearly means that you can place the facts and ideas of course content into a logical and coherent framework. The measure for the degree to which this is true is the degree to which you can state these relationships orally or in writing so that others can understand your position. One tactic for increasing your clarity of thought is to pay particular attention to the exact meaning of the words encountered. The year that you spend in the practical/vocational nursing program is filled with many new terms and concepts. Time spent in practicing the proper use of these terms and in applying concepts appropriately will result in improved clarity of thought and increased retention of content. You can use small study groups to challenge one another to write and speak clearly as you review content together.

A review of the words used in the preceding paragraph may illustrate how the meaning of words can be misunderstood. For example, think about the word *clarity*. When you look up this word in a dictionary, you find that there are several shades of meaning. Look up the word for yourself and decide which of the definitions applies to the use of clarity in describing a standard for critical thinking.

Think about some expressions you use every day. Would someone who is from another part of the country understand them? An example is the use of the term *this evening,* which is common in some parts of the country. If someone told you that she would visit you "this evening," when would you expect her? In some places, the person might arrive in the early afternoon; in other places, at night. When speaking to clients, families, and other health team members, the nurse must be sure that the words used clearly express the intended message. When reading or listening, do not assume that you understand a term. Take the time to verify the meaning.

Precision vs. Imprecision

Sometimes, we have a "ballpark" mentality. That is, we learn enough about a subject to be "in the ballpark," but not enough to hit a home run. The result is a general idea of the meaning of a fact or idea, but not enough understanding to apply it or to use the information for problem-solving or promoting communication of an idea to someone else. You may be making this mistake if you find yourself saying something like this: "I knew that, but on the test, it was stated differently." Precision of thought means that the meaning of a concept is clearly understood in terms of its relationship to other concepts and to its practical implications, so that the thought is exact, accurate, and definite (Paul & Willsen, 1993).

Specificity vs. Vagueness

Specificity means that the student can be concrete or exact in stating or applying a fact. An example of vagueness, which can be commonly ascribed to nursing students, occurs during the use of the planning phase of the nursing process when students do not write concrete nursing interventions. For example, a student may state that the nursing action will "provide support to the client and his family." It is difficult to explain exactly what this statement means, either in general or in relation to this client and this nurse. Appropriate planning involves deciding on definite, well-stated nursing diagnoses, goals, and nursing actions. The use of the nursing process requires that the student learn the degree of specificity required for each nursing situation. State or itemize the nursing actions to be performed.

Accuracy vs. Inaccuracy

Accuracy means being correct and within the proper parameters. Nursing students can readily understand the need for accurate calculation of a drug dose or accurate measurement of blood pressure. In the same way, the collection and interpretation of data must be accurate. Accuracy usually implies the use of some measuring instrument. In the case of blood pressure, this is easy to see. In the case of accuracy in thinking, it may be harder to conceptualize. An example would be when the nurse uses the term *hypertension* to mean someone who is anxious and hyperactive instead of the actual meaning, an elevation of blood pressure above the accepted normal maximum. When dealing with more abstract concepts, accuracy of interpretation and understanding are equally important. Students can

improve the accuracy of their thinking by trying to write new information in their own words and having another student interpret the meaning. Inaccurate information will become evident.

Accurate recording of findings during client care is essential to quality care. Accurate understanding of the concepts underlying each part of your nursing course, plus understanding how each part of your nursing course relates to any given client, will enable you to be more accurate in your thinking.

There are degrees of accuracy. For example, you might measure a client's temperature using a thermometer that can measure to the 0.01 degree, but this degree of accuracy may be unnecessary. On the other hand, when figuring a pediatric dosage, a difference of 0.01 can be important. One of your challenges is to increase your awareness of the degree of accuracy required in given nursing situations.

Relevance vs. Irrelevance

Relevance refers to needed information as opposed to information that is not needed at the moment. Students must be able to separate the two; otherwise, they may spend time arguing for a position that does not matter. For instance, students may get sidetracked from the purpose of an exercise by failing to limit their responses to the central issue or heart of the question or problem to be solved. It is also important to be able to recognize when sufficient relevant information is not available. An example of failing to recognize relevant information might be ignoring a client's comment that his rash began the day after starting a new medication. On the other hand, the nurse may assume that a client is depressed about being in the hospital and so may fail to ask him why he seems sad.

During the study process, you can ask yourself how a particular concept is relevant to the application of the nursing process to client care. **Justify** (prove or show to be valid) your ideas to yourself and to another student.

Consistency vs. Inconsistency

Consistency means using principles and concepts appropriately for related applications. For instance, if you are using a particular nursing diagnosis based on accepted indicators, it should be applied when those indicators are present and should not be used when the indicators are not present. Failure to follow this standard results in inconsistent use of the nursing diagnosis.

Consistency can also refer to recognizing and using basic concepts appropriately whenever they apply. For example, knowing the basic actions of epinephrine will enable you to predict client responses to the administration of the drug. It will also help you understand that the client has the same response when an increased secretion of epinephrine is released by the client's kidneys.

Logical vs. Illogical

To be logical means to build one idea upon another so that the conclusion is based on a sequence of steps. Each step should be reasonable and related to the step before it and the step after it. Many symptoms that clients exhibit can be understood logically based on your knowledge of normal physiology and the changes produced by the client's given disease or malady. The successful student will make more efficient use of study time by identifying the logical basis of the material being presented.

The author of a nursing textbook uses nursing logic to organize the content of the book. You must use your own logic to grasp the meaning of the material. Do this by discovering the logic of the author. In this way you will begin to think within the logic of nursing.

Depth vs. Superficiality

Busy students may be tempted to rely on the specific learning objectives and the teacher's pretest review as indicators of the amount of material they must master. This, however, may result in only a superficial understanding of basic processes and principles. Students can improve their ability to recognize the depth to which they must explore concepts and ideas. There is no easy way to do this, but knowing that different material requires different depth of study can assist the student. With time, these decisions will be easier to make. Your instructor and the learning aids within your textbook are useful guides. The more you use them, the better you will become at identifying relevant information and the appropriate depth of knowledge required to make good clinical decisions.

Completeness vs. Incompleteness

During the assessment phase of client care it is important that the nurse know when the client database is sufficient. Proper nursing care is based on identification of priority needs. The nurse will provide care only for those problems that have been identified. Although the physician orders treatments related to the medical diagnosis, these orders are not meant to direct all required care. Nursing care is essential to client well-being. Incomplete information or analysis of client needs will result in inappropriate or inadequate nursing care. Of course, your ability to identify and prioritize client care problems depends on the completeness of your knowledge base. This standard is related to accuracy. An incomplete database leads to inaccurate conclusions.

Significance vs. Triviality

When making decisions or sorting out information it is important for the nurse to identify information that is necessary for good decision making. Being able to recognize irrelevant facts or data that are not helpful for the problem at hand is an important skill. It is easy for a student to view all the material in a textbook as equally significant. Learning to identify significant (important) concepts will minimize the chances of your being distracted by trivial material.

Adequacy vs. Inadequacy

In solving problems or exploring a subject, adequacy refers to the degree to which the available information is sufficient for the purpose and the amount of time and effort spent on the matter. When making clinical decisions, the nurse must be able to recognize when there is sufficient information upon which to base a decision. Premature closure of the process or the inability to decide because of fear that there is not enough information are equally detrimental to quality thinking.

As you study each chapter you will be given information that will help you identify the basic information required to care for each client. Knowing that good client care decisions are based on good preparation by the nurse can help you fit information into the logic of nursing.

Fairness vs. Bias

You, along with other students, come to the educational setting with a set of beliefs, opinions, and points of view. People are predisposed to believe that what they think is true must be true. The improvement of the quality of your thinking depends on your ability to identify the biases present in your thinking and the biases present in the thinking of others. Commitment to fairness will lead a person to challenge conclusions that are based on personal bias. A nursing example would be the assessment of a person in pain. Each individual has learned a way to respond to pain: Some become quiet, some complain loudly, some are stoic, and some are emotional. When a nurse who has a stoic response to pain assesses a person who has an emotional response to pain, it is possible that the nurse will allow personal values to influence the assessment. This can lead to stereotyping a client as a "cry baby," with the result being that the nurse provides inadequate pain control for the client.

REASONING AND PROBLEM-SOLVING

Reasoning has been defined as the process of figuring things out by using critical thinking skills. Although reasoning involves thinking, all thinking is not reasoning. A human being is thinking when daydreaming, jumping to conclusions, stereotyping, or deciding to listen to music. None of these activities can be called reasoning. In order to use reasoning, to figure things out, or to problem-solve, the student must become

Table 2–4 THE ELEMENTS OF THOUGHT IN REASONING

1. All reasoning has a PURPOSE.
   - Take time to state your purpose clearly
   - Distinguish your purpose from related purposes
   - Check periodically to be sure you are still on target
   - Choose significant and realistic purposes
2. All reasoning is an attempt TO FIGURE SOMETHING OUT, TO SETTLE SOME QUESTION, TO SOLVE SOME PROBLEM.
   - Take time to clearly and simply state the question at issue
   - Express the question in several ways to clarify its meaning and scope
   - Break the question into subquestions
   - Identify whether it is a factual question, a preference question, or a question that requires reasoning
3. All reasoning is based on ASSUMPTIONS.
   - Clearly identify your assumptions and check for their probable validity
   - Check the consistency of your assumptions
   - Reexamine the question at issue when assumptions prove insupportable
4. All reasoning is done from some POINT OF VIEW.
   - Identify your own point of view and its limitations
   - Seek other points of view and identify their strengths as well as their weaknesses
   - Strive to be fairminded in evaluating all points of view
5. All reasoning is based on DATA AND INFORMATION.
   - Restrict your claims to those supported by sufficient data
   - Lay out the evidence clearly
   - Search for information against your position and explain its relevance
6. All reasoning is expressed through, and shaped by, CONCEPTS.
   - Identify each concept that is needed to explore the problem, and precisely define it
   - Explain the choice of important concepts and the implications of each
   - Define when concepts are used vaguely or inappropriately
7. All reasoning contains INFERENCES by which we draw CONCLUSIONS and give meaning to data.
   - Tie inferences tightly and directly from evidence to conclusions
   - Seek inferences that are deep, consistent, and logical
   - Identify the relative strength of each of your inferences
8. All reasoning leads somewhere and has IMPLICATIONS AND CONSEQUENCES.
   - Trace out a variety of implications and consequences that stem from your reasoning
   - Search for negative as well as positive consequences
   - Anticipate unusual or unexpected consequences from various points of view

Courtesy of the Foundation for Critical Thinking, Dillon Beach, CA.

familiar with the components of reasoning. These elements are purpose, the question at issue, assumptions, point of view, data and information, concepts, inferences and conclusions, and implications and consequences (Paul & Willsen, 1993). Table 2–4 illustrates the elements of thought in reasoning.

Purpose

All reasoning is directed toward some specific purpose. This is one way whereby reasoning is different from daydreaming. In the case of the nursing student, the purpose of reasoning is to effectively solve client care problems. During your formal education process, you will use reasoning to discover the logic of the practice of nursing.

The Question at Issue

The reasoning process has as its purpose the solution to some problem. This problem must be clearly defined. At the beginning of each study period, you must be able to state clearly the particular problems presented by this particular material. In the clinical setting, good clinical judgment begins with the clear statement of the problems presented by each client. One purpose of the nursing process is to identify client problems in a sufficiently clear and simple manner to enable appropriate responses by the nurse.

Assumptions

Assumptions are those ideas or things that are taken for granted. In the process of reasoning, you must be aware of the assumptions that are made in contrast to the facts that are known. Assumptions are accepted as being true without examination. Assuming certain things may be helpful in problem-solving, but an attempt should be made to recognize the assumptions. An example of an assumption is that nursing makes a difference in the outcome of a client's illness. It is evident that this is a necessary assumption for the nurse to make in order to engage in problem-solving related to client care needs; but it is also important for the nurse to examine this assumption from time to time. One of the issues in nursing today is the question of what nurses do and what preparation is necessary.

It is important to remember that assumptions that have proven reliable can help in decision making. It is just as true that faulty assumptions may cause you to draw faulty conclusions and may lead to poor problem-solving. Learn to recognize your own assumptions and those of others. Never be afraid to challenge your own assumptions or to ask others to clarify the assumptions they are using.

Point of View

Each person reasons using his own logic. Logic consists of previous experience, the quality of thinking already acquired, available information, and many other factors. These factors work together to give each person a unique way of thinking and a unique perspective. This unique perspective determines the individual's point of view. This can be conceptualized by thinking about what a person can see from a small window as compared to a view of the same landscape from an airplane. Each person will see things differently. They may both see a house but each person's view of the house may differ. In the same way, the individual's point of view determines what facts and information will be noticed, the relative importance assigned to each bit of information, and even the acceptable solutions to the problem. You must take the time to recognize your own point of view and to affirm the right of others to have their own points of view (Figure 2-4).

Data and Information

Data and information are the basic materials of reasoning. These are needed in order to define the problem under consideration and to find the solution. During the nursing education program, you may often feel overwhelmed by the quantity of data and information that is presented to you. The result may be that you attempt to practice rote memorization. If data and information are seen as the evidence for reasoning and for problem-solving, however, the process will be more than an exercise in memory. There is a logical relationship between the ideas and facts that compose the content of the nursing course. This logic can be discovered by reasoning. Once the logic is found, the

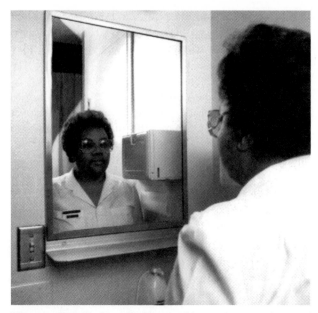

Figure 2-4 To be effective problem-solvers and critical thinkers, nurses must first take a good look at their own ideas and beliefs.

information can be used for problem-solving. Be sure to also look for evidence against your position.

Concepts

The evidence given in support of a conclusion consists of one or more statements relating the conclusion to the problem and to the supporting facts. Reasons must be logically related to the information; in other words, the conclusion cannot be based on something apart from the reasoning process. The concepts (such as pain, adaptation, and so on) that support the nursing process must be part of the evidence supporting a nursing judgment.

Inferences and Conclusions

Reasoning requires interpretation of facts and information. The interpretation must be justifiable in light of the relevant facts. It must be supported by logical connections to the problem and to appropriate data and information. Such interpretation can be called a judgment or inference. Too many times, students state opinions as judgments or inferences. This occurs when interpretations are based on personal preferences rather than on the information that is pertinent to the solution of the problem and on accepted authoritative information.

Properly drawing judgments or inferences is basic to thinking well. An inference results from the following kind of thinking: "Because that is true, then this must be true." For example, you have learned that when the body's temperature goes above normal, the body's metabolic rate increases. You also know that increased metabolism requires more oxygen for the tissues. One way more oxygen can be delivered to the tissues is to increase the heart rate. From these facts, you can infer that an elevated body temperature may result in an increased heart rate.

The product of reasoning is a conclusion in regard to the problem. The conclusion is the answer to the question that began the process. The conclusion must be logical and must answer the question. It must be based on the proper information and be logically related to the question.

Implications and Consequences

As an outcome of the reasoning process, more than one solution will usually be apparent. At this point, it will be necessary to examine the implications of each solution. This may require thinking about the ease with which a solution can be applied, the ability of a person to carry out the required actions, or the risks involved.

The outcomes of a particular approach to a problem under consideration are important. Consequences can result from action or inaction. Responsible problem-solving requires that all known consequences be acknowledged. Of course, it is not possible to predict all consequences; but the possible outcomes should be examined as completely as possible.

TRAITS OF A DISCIPLINED THINKER

The presentation in this chapter of some of the requirements of critical thinking will not make anyone think critically. By incorporating the idea that thinking about the quality of your own thinking in relation to UIS is a desirable goal, you can improve your own thinking. Improved thinking is not something that can

PROFESSIONAL TIP

Critical Thinking
Critical thinking is far more than an academic exercise. As a nurse, you are responsible for helping clients achieve and maintain their optimal level of health. To help sharpen your critical thinking skills, get in the habit of asking yourself questions such as "Why is this procedure being done?", "What are its benefits?", and "Do I see alternatives that might result in better client outcomes?" Do this several times a day while caring for clients. Training yourself to think critically about all client care and interactions will help you to become a more skilled and compassionate professional.

be acquired in a day or two. It is like any high-level skill; it takes time, effort, and disciplined practice. The result is well worth it, however. Consistent efforts to improve your thinking can result in the acquisition of the traits of an educated person (Paul & Willsen, 1993). These traits, or habitual ways of thinking, can be recognized by others and can enable a person to compete successfully in the high-tech world.

Reason

The educated person will be reasonable. This simply means that the person values reasoning in himself and in others. This person will not be interested in placing blame or dodging responsibility. There will be a commitment to problem-solving and to cooperative efforts aimed at logically solving the problems encountered in the workplace.

Humility

Another quality that results from consistent efforts to practice disciplined thinking is intellectual humility. To be intellectually humble means that an individual is aware of how much he does not know. There will be a willingness to examine conclusions and beliefs based on new evidence. There will be respect for the thoughts and ideas of others and a sense of continually learning and improving one's own thinking.

Courage

The thinking person will be intellectually courageous. One of the characteristics of this trait is a willingness to take unpopular positions based on reasoning. Conclusions and beliefs that direct activities will thus be the result of disciplined thinking, rather than the opinions of the group.

Integrity

Integrity refers to the constancy of one's actions, meaning that, based on reasoning, the same standards are applied consistently and are not changed to suit circumstances or personal prejudices. The result is a person whose behavior is in harmony with his thinking.

Perseverance

The thinking person will be capable of intellectual perseverance, meaning a willingness to undertake the challenge of completing hard intellectual tasks. Not giving up, pursuing a solution until its conclusion, and maintaining the quality of thinking are the qualities related to this trait.

Fairmindedness

The fairminded person considers all viewpoints without referring to feelings or vested interests, adheres to intellectual standards, and is impartial.

CASE STUDY

At this point in subsequent chapters, you will be given a client scenario or case study. This activity is designed to give you an opportunity to apply the knowledge and skills you have gained. This means that you will be expected to use critical thinking skills as you explore selected nursing situations. For this chapter, the scenario is to be written by you and about you.

1. Review the four basic skills of critical thinking: reading, writing, listening, and speaking.

2. Identify specifically the precise skills you want to improve. Write in your own words what you want to accomplish in terms of positive skills you will possess when you have implemented your plan and accomplished your goal. This means that you will identify both specific performance measures for your reading, writing, speaking, and listening skills, and time frames for points at which you will evaluate your performance. For example, if you set a goal of being able to identify the main points of an assigned reading, how would you measure that? In comparison with others in your study group? By your test performance? Write down your evaluation criteria and the time frames for evaluation.

3. When you have clearly stated in writing which basic skills you will work on, review the material in this chapter or from other resources to identify possible ways to work on those skills. Choose the most appropriate methods for you. Write down your plan. Be precise and specific.

4. Your next step is to actually put your plan into action by doing what you have planned to do.

5. Evaluate your actions to see whether they have resulted in the desired outcome. In order to perform a valid evaluation, you must evaluate your performance based on the evaluation criteria and goals you outlined in number 2.

6. Realize that you must know yourself well. If the processes of critical thinking and reasoning are new to you, select only one or two things on which to work. If you feel more adventurous, use the suggested process to explore your thinking in relation to the universal standards of thought and to the traits of a thoughtful person. Assess your problem-solving style in relation to the elements of thought in reasoning.

CRITICAL THINKING AND THE NURSING PROCESS

The purpose of the nursing education program is to help you develop the logic of nursing. Another way to state this is to say that you will learn to think like a nurse. The method that nurses have adoped to implement the practice of nursing is called the nursing process. The nursing process is an application of the problem-solving process to the practice of nursing. A form of the problem-solving process is part of every scientific or human service discipline. The use of the nursing process requires critical thinking. If you can find the relationship between the content of the textbooks and the logic of nursing you will find the study of nursing to be an exciting and challenging process. Use of the nursing process will thus become the means by which the quality of your thinking is improved. The use of reasoning will enhance your use of the nursing process.

SUMMARY

- Critical thinking is a disciplined way of thinking that the nursing student can begin to develop. The effective use of the nursing process depends on the ability to think well.

- There are many ways to define critical thinking. Essential components of any definition should emphasize self-assessment of the quality of one's own thinking according to standards of excellence and careful use of the elements of reasoning.

- Four basic intellectual skills are essential to quality thinking: critical reading, critical listening, critical writing, and critical speaking.

- The spectrum of Universal Intellectual Standards (UIS) can be the measure of competence in each of the basic skills.

- Reasoning is the process of applying critical thinking to some problem so as to find an answer or to figure something out. Therefore, reasoning has a purpose. The process of reasoning requires that attention be paid to the elements of thought in reasoning and to the UIS.

- When students begin to be aware of their own thinking and begin to assume responsibility for it, they will begin to use their own logic to discover the logic of nursing. The result will be better learning and the ability to make high-quality decisions related to client care.

- Consistent attention to improving the quality of thinking will produce the traits of an educated nurse. The student will become intellectually reasonable, humble, and courageous and will possess intellectual integrity and perseverance.

Review Questions

1. A branch of learning or field of study is called a:
   a. career.
   b. movement.
   c. principle.
   d. discipline.

2. Fundamental to quality thinking is the ability to think:
   a. clearly.
   b. effectively.
   c. quantitatively.
   d. with ambiguity.

3. The person who is concrete or exact when stating or applying a fact is practicing the standard for critical thinking called:
   a. accuracy.
   b. precision.
   c. consistency.
   d. specificity.

4. The person who has the ability to separate needed information from information not needed at the present time is practicing the standard for critical thinking called:
   a. logic.
   b. relevance.
   c. adequacy.
   d. significance.

5. Ideas or things that are taken for granted are called:
   a. evidences.
   b. inferences.
   c. assumptions.
   d. implications.

6. The person who is willing to take an unpopular position based on reasoning is said to have:
   a. courage.
   b. humility.
   c. integrity.
   d. perseverance.

Critical Thinking Questions

1. Of the four basic skills of critical thinking, which one are you able to do best? Why? How do you know?

2. How do you take responsibility for your own thinking?

WEB FLASH!

- Search the web for sites dealing with critical thinking. What date is the oldest entry? What date is the newest entry?
- Search the web using the names of the major nursing organizations such as National Federation of Licensed Practical Nurses (NFLPN), National Association of Practical Nurse Education and Service, Inc. (NAPNES), and the National League for Nursing (NLN). Do they have web sites that include pages that might offer information on critical thinking?

STUDENT NURSE SKILLS FOR SUCCESS

CHAPTER 3

MAKING THE CONNECTION

Refer to the following chapters to increase your understanding of student nurse skills for success:

- **Chapter 2, Critical Thinking**
- **Chapter 11, Client Teaching**
- **Chapter 16, Stress, Adaptation, and Anxiety**

LEARNING OBJECTIVES

Upon completion of this chapter, you should be able to:
- *Define key terms.*
- *Outline strategies for developing a positive attitude toward the learner role.*
- *Identify strategies for developing proficiency in basic skills.*
- *Identify learning-style methods that can be incorporated for effective study.*
- *Design a time-management plan.*
- *Design a personal study plan.*
- *Identify strategies for improving test-taking outcomes.*
- *Complete a stress-reduction exercise using guided imagery.*

KEY TERMS

ability	learning style
anxiety	metacognition
attitude	mnemonics
attribute	perfectionism
encoding	procrastination
learning	time management
learning disability	

INTRODUCTION

Learning is defined as the act or process of acquiring knowledge and/or skill in a particular subject. An individual never stops learning. This is especially true in the field of nursing and health care. The amount of information within the health care domain has expanded exponentially in just the past several years. Consider, for example, the advances in drug therapies, complementary/alternative therapies, and genetics. By graduation, some of the information learned in the beginning of the program will have been displaced by new information and discoveries. We are living in the information age and have constant access to thousands of pieces of information through various media, including television and the Internet. Knowledge is never static. Learning, defined as the act of acquiring knowledge, is also not static, but, rather, is a lifelong process.

Individuals seek knowledge to effect some type of change. As a student, you are seeking knowledge to learn skills and to prepare yourself for a career in nursing. Referring to yourself as a learner implies that you are an active participant in the learning process, as opposed to a passive recipient of information. You bring to this new adventure yourself, your past experiences, your abilities, and your motivation to master the knowledge necessary to reach your goals. You have already learned much in your lifetime and are ready to continue the process. It is important that you take some time to think about the competencies needed for the role of learner. It is equally important that you realize that *you* are in charge of developing the competencies that will enable you to learn.

The learning you are seeking will afford you the knowledge and skills necessary to become a nurse and, thus, to demonstrate your ability to competently provide care to clients who seek your professional talents. Nursing education is different from many other college majors in the turnaround time allowed for learning. Few other disciplines require the student to apply on Thursday that which was acquired on Monday. Nursing students must acquire a greater depth of understanding

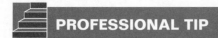
in a shorter amount of time; to achieve this, basic learning processes will need to be well developed.

This chapter addresses *how* you learn rather than *what* you learn. It focuses on competencies necessary to master the learning process: attitude, basic skills, learning style, time management, study strategies, critical thinking, and test-taking strategies. Assessing which habits you already practice and which ones you have yet to incorporate, internalize, and utilize will assist you in improving your process of learning. As you do so, your potential for attaining your goals will increase.

DEVELOP A POSITIVE ATTITUDE

Attitude is defined as a manner, feeling, or position toward a person or thing. In order to effect change in your behavior, you must first develop a positive attitude about this experience you are about to begin. You are in charge of setting yourself up for success. This is your opportunity to acquire the knowledge and skills that will make it possible for you to reach the goal of becoming a licensed practical/vocational nurse. You must develop a positive attitude toward yourself as a person and a learner, as well as a genuine desire to learn. To maintain this attitude late at night when you are struggling over the names of the latest drugs and writing client assessments, you must be convinced that you have the capability to complete your task, that some intrinsic factor will be able to support you in the pursuit of your goal. This positive self-attitude sustains the question "Why am I doing this?" Among the strategies you can practice to help you build a positive attitude are the following:

- Create positive self-images, and visualize yourself attaining your goals.
- Recognize your abilities.
- Identify realistic expectations.

Create Positive Self-Images

To begin to create a positive self-image, you must know those attributes that are unique to you. An **attribute** is a characteristic, either positive or negative, that belongs to you. For instance, some positive attributes that are typical to nurses including caring and compassion. Attributes are sometimes referred to as

My attribute chart	
Positive Attributes	Negative Attributes

Figure 3-1 Attribute Chart

strengths and weaknesses. Whatever you call them, you must actively engage in listing and recalling these qualities about yourself. Using a chart like the one presented in Figure 3-1, list as many words describing your attributes as you can. List both positive and negative qualities.

Which side has more entries? Did you start with the negative list? It is unfortunate that sometimes we can recall the negatives faster than the positives. We often speak about ourselves in negative terms, which creates negative self-images. For example, you may recall thinking some of the following: "I wish I were thinner . . . ," "I hope I can do this, I'm not very good at math." Neither of these statements draws a positive image of the speaker. You may need to lose 10 pounds, or improve your math skills, but these are not the total measure of your attributes. If they are the only qualities you recall, they might become the overall image you see of yourself. Regardless of where you started, you must concentrate on the positive side of the chart. You must actively recall your positive side at least as often as you recount the things that could be improved.

Begin to speak of yourself in positive terms and accept compliments from yourself! You will be building the sustenance to get through the rough parts of the new role you have taken on. When an assignment is particularly difficult you can refocus from "I hope I can do this. I have never been good at math" to "I can read and follow the chapter instructions on how to complete the problems." This simple restatement can sometimes make the difference in whether we succeed or fail at our attempts to acquire new knowledge.

The list does not have to stop at just the words you write today. Continue to practice and do periodic self-assessments. You will add more and more words to the positive side and begin to complement yourself more often. When things go awry you will be able to draw on these positive attributes and know that you have these strengths.

Recognize Your Abilities

Recognizing your abilities is also an attitude builder. **Ability** can be defined as competence in an activity. An ability is something you can learn; competency is proficiency in a task. Your degree of competence as a nurse will depend on such factors as prior exposure, motivation, how often and with whom you practice, expectations of those things that you should be doing, and a willingness to laugh at attempts and learn from mistakes.

You have abilities and skills that you perform well. To acquire these things took courage, discipline, and hard work. Recalling these abilities and the ways you developed competency in them not only adds to your positive self-image, but showcases your strengths. Begin to practice recalling your abilities by completing the exercise described in Figure 3-2. Under each of the columns (A and B), write an ending to each statement and place it in the big box. Next, list all of the skills you need to be able to be "really good" at that task. Write these skills in the smaller boxes. Do not worry if you cannot fill all the small boxes or if you run out of boxes.

As an example for column A, maybe you wrote, "I am really good at cooking." Following are some skills you could have included in the smaller boxes:

- *Arithmetic:* You must have an understanding of fractions and the relationships of parts to the whole.
- *Reading:* You must comprehend the words in the recipe in order to follow all the steps.
- *Prioritizing:* You must know with what to start in order to have all of the food ready at the same time.

- *Risk taker:* You may worry about whether your guests will like your dish, but you persist, confident in your ability to turn the raw ingredients into a delicious meal.

Now look at column B, using math as an example. Mathematics is an ability you must develop in order to safely administer medications to your clients. If you view this skill only as something to avoid, you start out with a negative attitude toward an ability you will need. You are creating a negative image of yourself completing this task. Instead, look to your past experiences for your strengths; you may realize that you already possess much of the mathematical knowledge you need to correctly compute medication dosages. Realizing this puts a positive slant on this ability.

Now you must develop mathematical competency. Begin by asking yourself which skills are needed to perform mathematical operations. You must pay attention to details, understand the way parts relate to the whole, and have solid skills in arithmetic (addition, subtraction, division, and multiplication). Mathematics requires you to choose appropriate formulas to solve a variety of real-world problems. For example, to give the correct dose of medication to your client, you must know the correct formula to use for the calculation. This is a real-world problem for which you must both choose the correct formula and understand it. You must then accurately perform the arithmetic operations.

Identify Realistic Expectations

As mentioned earlier, developing a positive self-image is of primary importance to learning. Your expectations regarding how you will perform in the role as a learner will affect your attitude toward both yourself and learning. You have an expectation about the way you will progress through this program. Ideally, you

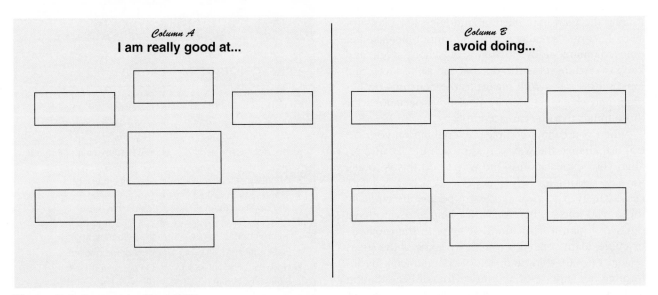

Figure 3-2 Recognizing Your Abilities

will attend all classes, pass all exams, and graduate. Further, your current life responsibilities will cooperate with and support this plan. You will likely, however, encounter at least some obstacles. When you hit that first "speed bump" to your plan, your ability to look at the reality of your expectations will be important in regaining a positive focus. Consider the following example:

> Marissa is a 25-year-old enrolled full time in a nursing program for the fall. She did well in high school and has already attended a college part time prior to this program. Marissa expects that she will get grades in the B and A range, as she did in prior course work. She works full time and has a 4-year-old daughter. When the class schedule is published, the times conflict with one of the days that she works. This will cause her to be 20 minutes late to work on that day. She has not shared with her employer that she is attending school. She has child care for her daughter, but the need to arrive at the clinical site at 7 A.M. means that she must rearrange her child care and that she will be 30 minutes late for clinical on Fridays. She does not tell her instructors of her time constraints for child care. She has always needed quiet time for study and is a morning person. Marissa finds her reading assignments take twice as long as she had planned. With all her other responsibilities, her only time for study is after her daughter goes to bed. She has a family that lives close by, but she does not like to burden them with baby-sitting. She has always found a way to do things on her own in the past.

Marissa is a capable person, but her expectation of being able to control all the various facets of her life in perfect harmony is unrealistic. Maintaining a positive attitude while in the midst of the stress of completing all the tasks at hand is difficult if not impossible, and the plan is often abandoned. In Marissa's case, abandoning the plan may mean abandoning her plans for school. Marissa's reality is that she cannot increase her time commitment by 30 hours of school work and keep everything else she does at the same level. She must set priorities with regard to the demands on her time, and she must identify realistic expectations for those things that she can accomplish.

When you cannot complete everything on your "to do" list, change the way you approach the list and realign your expectations. One way to do this is to ask for help. Asking for help is not a weakness, it is a success strategy. The most successful people are typically those who know when to ask for help and who have devised a plan to structure that help. In the previous example, Marissa needed to remove some of the stress related to both work and school commitments by informing her supervisor and instructors of her situation and asking for their help in guiding her to manage her

many demands. Help may mean something as simple as talking to your instructors so that they know you must leave on Thursdays at 3 P.M., due to work commitments. Present a proactive plan of how you will get the notes and make up the time and then ask them to accommodate you.

If you do not set realistic expectations for yourself, you may fall victim to a positive attitude's biggest enemy, perfectionism. **Perfectionism** is not synonymous with excellence, but rather is an overwhelming expectation of being able to get everything done. This is setting yourself up for failure, as it is a standard no one can live up to. Table 3–1 suggests some behaviors of perfectionists versus those of pursuers of excellence. Which list describes you most accurately? Remember to strive to be as realistic with your expectations as possible; be patient with yourself and ask for help when needed.

DEVELOP YOUR BASIC SKILLS

Dirkx and Prenger (1997) list the following skills as basic for success in academics and life: reading, arithmetic and mathematics, writing, listening, and speaking. They further describe each of the skills in terms of characteristics that provide a sense of what is expected from the learner in each area (Table 3–2).

When you consider these characteristics, the basic skills do not seem so basic but, rather, take on a new importance. Look at the list and make a quick note of your strengths and weaknesses. You must have a strong foundation in these basic skills to advance your knowledge beyond the level of memorization. You

Table 3–1 BEHAVIORS OF PERFECTIONISTS AND PURSUERS OF EXCELLENCE

PERFECTIONISTS	PURSUERS OF EXCELLENCE
• Reach for impossible goals	• Enjoy meeting high standards within reach
• Value themselves for what they do	• Value themselves for who they are
• Get depressed and give up	• Experience disappointment but keep going
• Are devastated by failure	• Learn from failure
• Remember mistakes and dwell on them	• Correct mistakes, then learn from them
• Can only live with being number one	• Are pleased with knowing they did their best
• Hate criticism	• Welcome criticism
• Have to win to maintain high self-esteem	• Do not have to win to maintain high self-esteem

SKILL	BASIC COMPETENCY
Table 3–2 **BASIC SKILL COMPETENCY LIST**	
Reading	Locate, understand, and interpret written information in prose and documents, including manuals, graphs, and schedules, to perform tasks; learn from a text by determining the main idea or essential message; identify relevant details, facts, and specifications; infer or locate the meaning of unknown or technical vocabulary; judge the accuracy, appropriateness, style, and plausibility of reports, proposals, or theories from other writers
Arithmetic and mathematics	Perform basic computations; use basic numerical concepts such as whole numbers and percentages (fractions, decimals) in practical situations; approach practical problems by choosing appropriately from a variety of mathematical techniques
Writing	Communicate thoughts, ideas, information, and messages; record information completely and accurately; compose and create documents and use language, style, organization, and format appropriate to the subject matter, purpose, and audience; include supporting documentation; attend to detail and check, edit, and revise for correct information, appropriate emphasis, form, grammar, spelling, and punctuation
Listening	Receive, attend to, interpret, and respond to verbal messages and other cues, such as body language, in ways that are appropriate to the purpose in order to comprehend, learn, evaluate critically, appreciate, or support the speaker
Speaking	Organize ideas and communicate oral messages appropriate to listeners and situations; use verbal language and other cues such as body language appropriate in style, tone, and level of complexity to the audience and occasion; speak clearly and communicate a message; understand and respond to listener feedback and ask questions when needed

Adapted from Planning and Implementing Instruction for Adults *(pp. 133–134), by J. Dirkx and S. Prenger, 1997, San Francisco: Jossey-Bass. Copyright 1997 by Jossey-Bass.*

must advance your knowledge level from memorization to comprehension and application. If you are struggling with these basic skills, you will have difficulty advancing. Developing these skills is basic to the habits of successful learners.

Reading

Ninety percent of your program is in written format. To study effectively, you must be highly adept in the basic skill of reading. Among the several strategies you can effectively implement in your reading and study plan to improve this skill are vocabulary building, comprehension, and reading level. Your basic skill of reading encompasses vocabulary building, which includes the skill of identification and understanding of both English and medical terminology. Investing in quality medical and English dictionaries is a good step to understanding both these languages. Another strategy is simply to take the time when reading to look up the words you do not know (Figure 3-3).

The primary reason for building a strong medical vocabulary is that words are the tools for thinking about and understanding your world, and you are entering the new world of nursing: You must therefore take the time to learn its language. Developing the habit of vocabulary building takes time initially, but as you persist in practicing this skill, your comprehension of the material will increase.

Comprehension goes beyond rote memorization. One sign of true comprehension is the ability to summarize the writer's message. When you summarize, you must recite the material in your own words (Sotiriou & Phillips, 1999). Unless you understand the words you have read, you will not be able to advance your level of knowledge from rote memorization to comprehension. When you are actively reading your nursing textbook and you realize that you are not understanding what you have read, you may find it helpful to use one, some, or all of the five strategies outlined in Table 3–3.

Reading level is another element of your reading skills. Reading level is not related to what you can understand, but, rather, refers to the length of the words and the sentences used in a text to explain, describe, and convey information. It does not have anything to do with your intelligence, but it has a great deal to do with the length of time it takes you to read.

Arithmetic and Mathematics

The next skill you must develop competency in is that of arithemtic and mathematics. You will be responsible for correctly calculating dosages and safely

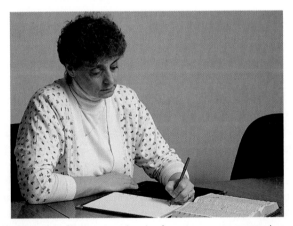

Figure 3-3 Keep a notebook of new terms to expand your vocabulary. Review your notebook and try to use the words in practice daily.

Table 3–3 STRATEGIES TO IMPROVE COMPREHENSION	
STRATEGY	**EXPLANATION**
Reread	Do this after reading one section of the text, or even after one paragraph.
Define new words	Write the definitions of each new word in the margin of your text and then reread the paragraph. Use a small notebook to build your own glossary. Make your own flash-cards for further study.
Visualize	Create mental pictures of the material you are reading. You may even want to draw a simple stick figure, and as you continue to read, adjust the picture.
Research	Many times the reason you are unable to comprehend the material presented is that you have insufficient background in the subject. A solution may be to consult another text that is specific to that knowledge base. Use a dictionary, anatomy and physiology text, general subject text (like a psychology text) or a nursing journal to increase your background knowledge in a subject area (Meltzer & Marcus-Palau, 1997)
Summarize	Use your own words to "tell" yourself what you just read and how this connects to what you are going to be doing. Ask yourself, "Why might I need to know this material?"

tency in mathematics and a commitment to improvement is essential to your practice in the profession.

Writing

In your role as a student and as a professional, you will need writing skills. Contrary to popular opinion, the influx of the computer into health care has not removed the need for this skill (Figure 3-4). You will be writing client assessments, transfer summaries, discharge summaries, and client-teaching plans, as well as contributing to development of policies and, possibly, even publishing your experiences in a journal. The skill of writing can be practiced and improved. Follow the steps outlined in Table 3–4 as a checklist for your writing assignments.

Listening

The old saying "I know you can hear me, but are you listening?" can be applied to all of us. You must be listening, understanding, and processing information, as opposed to just hearing, when you are in class, as well as when you begin working with clients. When listening during any lecture or demonstration, you receive, interpret, and respond to verbal messages and other cues such as body language. You are attempting to both comprehend the information and evaluate the

administering medications to your clients. You must therefore be able to recognize whether your calculations are correct and, upon looking at the amount on a medication order, estimate whether your answer is logical and correct. In nursing, your mastery of mathematical basic skills cannot be overemphasized. Consider the following excerpt from a study of medication errors done in 1998 at a tertiary care teaching hospital; this excerpt underscores the importance of mathematical competency among nurses.

> Forty-two percent of dosage errors were considered to put the patient at risk for a serious or severe, preventable adverse outcome. Errors in decimal point placement, mathematical calculation, or expression of dosage regime accounted for 59.5% of the dosage errors. The dosage equation was wrong in 29.5% (Lesar, 1998).

Give yourself a reality check on your competency in mathematics and commit to improving those areas where you are weakest. You may want to investigate a resource such as the learning services center at your school, enlist the assistance of a tutor, or use a programmed-learning text to refresh your skills. There are also numerous texts written to assist nursing students in developing these essential skills. Consider also using computer-assisted instruction (CAI) programs or self-paced study modules to hone these skills. Whatever means you use, an honest assessment of your compe-

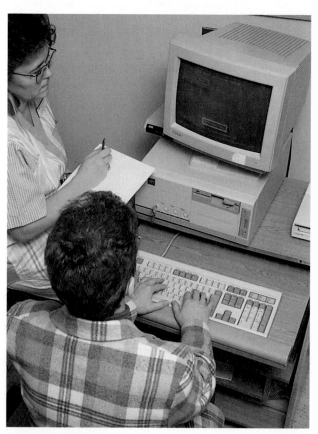

Figure 3-4 Although computers are being used more and more in health care, they do not replace the need for competent writing skills.

Table 3–4 STEPS TO CLEAR WRITING

STEP	EXPLANATION
Prewrite	Select a subject, collect details about that subject, and develop your writing plan
Establish a writing plan	Answer the following questions in outline form: • *What* are you writing (essay, test, questionnaire, dialogue)? • *Why* are you writing (to persuade, describe, explain, and narrate)? • *For whom* are you writing (peers, instructors, colleagues)? • *How* are you writing (alone, with a classmate, in a group, on computer)? • *Where* are you writing (on the bus, in the library, at the computer lab)? • *When* will you be writing (consider the time frame for this writing project)?
Write first draft	Organize your writing plan ideas into phrases, sentences, and paragraphs as appropriate to the task, content, and audience. Obtain feedback from your intended audience as to the accuracy, relevance, and understandability of your materials
Revise	Make changes to improve your writing so it conveys your main idea and purpose
Edit	Examine critically for errors in spelling, punctuation, grammar, or style

Adapted from Learning Strategies for Allied Health Students, *by S. Palau and M. Meltzer, 1998, Philadelphia: W. B. Saunders. Copyright 1998 by W. B. Saunders.*

speaker. You may need to polish up on ways that you can improve listening and evaluation skills to make the most of your class time. Class time is a time for listening. Listening effectively can make efficient use of this time to increase your comprehension of the content.

Among the many strategies that can be used to improve listening skills are the following:

- *Being interested in the subject.* Make a connection with the reason you are going to this lecture. What is the connection between the information and your need for the information? Have you prescanned the information and come with questions about the subject that tie in to how you will use the information presented?
- *Being open to the information.* When you hear a topic and immediately react with your instinct, you often miss the point and some aspect of the presentation you did not consider before. Listening does not automatically mean you will change your mind on topics, but it will allow you to evaluate and incorporate those aspects that are beneficial to you.
- *Not being critical of the speaker.* Focus on the message, not the messenger. The speaker is not there as a member of a theatrical company to entertain you. The speaker's role is to impart information. It is up

to you to concentrate on the information that you need to know and apply it properly.

- *Concentrating on the information.* Be present to the lecture. If you find yourself falling asleep, do muscle flexes or breathe deeply to try to stay alert and aware. Imagine test questions that might be asked on the information.
- *Evaluating the information.* Not every word is critical. Relate the information to what you know, where you may use it, and whether you agree with what is said. If you have difficulty with what is being said, use the next strategy to maintain your concentration.
- *Writing down questions as you listen.* This allows you to follow the speaker to the end of her thoughts. Many of your questions may be answered. If not, you have them written down and can refer later to the list. This promotes concentration on the information presented. You will not be distracted trying to remember questions you wanted to ask.

Speaking

Learning to speak or present in front of a group is one of the most-feared activities of many students. Yet as a nurse, you have entered one of the most "speaking"-oriented professions. You will communicate daily with your clients, their families, instructors, peers, ancillary staff members, and the multiple members of the health care team. Learning to do this well will free you from worry about doing it and allow you to use this skill to your advantage in your classes as well as in the professional environment.

Most of the fear of speaking in public arises from our fear of appearing the fool. Many students will not ask questions during a lecture specifically because they believe themselves incapable of speaking clearly and identifying exactly the information they need. We have all heard the saying, "There is no stupid question"; we must believe it. You must develop the confidence to speak up when you have a question; consider the potential consequences to your clients should you fail to clarify a medical order or question a procedure that is unclear.

The following strategies may help when you want to ask a question:

- *Understand why you are asking the question.* Instead of saying, "I don't understand," say, "I was with you on the physiology of the kidney until you traveled into the Bowman's capsule. Can you connect this particular part of the kidney with osmosis for me?" This puts you and the speaker in a positive light; you have not attacked the speaker's explanation, and you acknowledge your skill in listening. You are communicating what you need and asking the speaker to help by connecting the two concepts for you.
- *Know when to ask the question.* Writing down those topics on which you need further information may

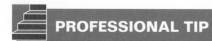

Speaking

Thorough preparation is an important strategy for speaking about anything. Formulating multiple examples is one way of increasing your comfort level with the given information. For example, if you are asked to explain the way the pancreas produces insulin, you might draw the organ and indicate where the islets of Langerhans are. Or you may use a lock and key to explain the way insulin works to open the channels for glucose to enter the cells. You may trace a cracker as it travels through the body from teeth to cells and indicate just where and when insulin is utilized. Regardless of the specifics, creating multiple examples will assist you in thoroughly learning a topic and therefore creating a feeling of comfort about your knowledge of the subject.

help you decide the correct time to ask a question. If the instructor begins by saying, "Today we will be speaking about pharmacokinetics," and you do not understand the word, stopping her before she has a chance to define the word may not be the most effective strategy. If instead you write down, "What does pharmacokinetics mean?" and listen for the meaning of that word in the context of the lecture, you will most likely hear clues as to the word's meaning. The instructor will use other words, such as *absorption, distribution, metabolism,* and *excretion* to describe what happens to a drug as it goes through the body. When an appropriate time in the presentation comes, review those things that have been said and clarify: "So, Prof. Z., am I correct when I say that pharmacokinetics has to do with the movement of drugs through all the systems of the body?" You will get your answer and your instructor will know from your question that you have been listening.

You must speak clearly and articulate those things you need daily as you attend classes; listen to your instructors; listen to your clients; and transmit information to instructors, colleagues, support staff, doctors, and allied health care team members. Practice both the skills of listening and speaking equally and keep asking questions.

DEVELOP YOUR LEARNING STYLE

The term **learning style** refers to the ways you best receive, process, and assimilate information (knowledge) about a particular subject. In your life as a stu-

dent, you have probably had both of the following experiences.

You attend class with Professor A for Course 100. The professor arranges the room casually in small groupings and breaks up class time to alternate short lectures with small group work. There is time for a hands-on demonstration of the principle along with actual work-related items used as examples. Professor A allows for student–teacher interchange of ideas and gives credence to experiences of the students during the class discussions. You leave the class exhilarated and with ideas, aware that this content connects with your desired outcome. You plan a review of the notes with a fellow student you met in your class group. You continue to prepare throughout the course and prior to the final, on which you get a B.

The next day you attend Course 200 with Professor B. The room is arranged in rows. Professor B puts up the class outline on the overhead, lectures for 40 minutes, then allows 10 minutes at the end for questions. If you hand him a written question, he will answer it during the next class. You dread his boring presentation and wish that Professor B was more like Professor A. You really do not know anyone in the class with whom to study, you cannot understand the text, and your grades are in the low C to D range. You know you need this class for your major. You try to do your part, but you just can't "get into it."

Think about Professor A, who presents information in a variety of methods—short lecture, small group, hands-on demonstration. As a student, you can grasp the information from whichever method appeals to you. You come away feeling connected to the subject and your classmates and want to continue learning about the subject. You are rewarded for your efforts through the academic grade system.

Now consider Professor B, who knows just as much about the subject as does Professor A, but who presents it using only one method—lecture. Lecture is not your preferred learning style, and your ability to clarify your understanding through questions is limited by the class format. Your outcomes on tests are less rewarding, and you begin to avoid putting time into studying the subject all together. You end up thinking that you really do not do well in that subject and consider changing your major.

The difference in the outcomes of the two examples lies in the perceived role of the learner. In these examples, the student relied heavily on the *teacher's* ability to present material in the student's preferred learning style. Remember that *you* are in charge of your learning. Teacher presentations vary in ways that may not appeal to your primary learning style, but you can still learn the information. You must take charge of

Learning Disabilities

According to the National Center for Learning Disabilities, Inc. (NCLD, 1999), 15% to 20% of the population have some form of learning disability. **Learning disability** is a generic term that refers to a heterogeneous group of disorders manifested as significant difficulties in the acquisition and use of listening, speaking, reading, writing, reasoning, or mathematical abilities.

If you think that having a learning disability will prohibit your success, you are incorrect; you must, however, understand your different abilities. You must know those types of accommodations that will enhance your learning capabilities, and you must be comfortable asking for those things that you need. Accommodations in postsecondary programs are mandated by the federal government, however the onus to disclose, provide documentation, and request accommodations is on the student. Accommodations are determined on a case-by-case basis. Reasonable accommodations in the classroom may be as simple as having the instructor wear a microphone, being able to use a tape recorder or note taker, or requesting textbook tapes. In the clinical area, all reasonable accommodations are made within the confines of client safety and essential skills needed to participate in a program of study for nursing. A quiet work area and ear protectors may provide quiet for students who are hypersensitive to background noise. Using a computer for writing assignments, note taking in class, and studying may assist students who have difficulty writing. Getting a tutor skilled at working with students with learning disabilities may be another intervention to consider.

Whatever you suspect your needs to be, getting professional testing to ascertain whether you have a disability and to determine any specific accommodations you will need is crucial. Seek the assistance of your instructors, student service personnel, learning center personnel, or call the special education coordinator at the nearest high school. These resources will help you locate an accredited testing agency to provide you with further resources and documentation.

developing your abilities, increasing your awareness of your preferred learning styles, and implementing some simple strategies to enhance those styles. As you increase your skills in your preferred methods and strengthen those in your weaker ones, you will change your outcomes.

Classification of Learning Styles

Learning styles are cognitive (mental) functions. They refer to the ways you perceive, remember, think, and solve problems: Their focus is *how* you learn as opposed to *what* you learn. Your preference for one style over another can be argued to be both genetic and developmental. Regardless, your awareness of the ways you best learn will affect your learning outcomes.

Learning styles are classified in many different ways. One classification method focuses on the route by which students best perceive and remember information: visual, auditory, or kinesthetic. These divisions are not mutually exclusive; we possess all three, and we use all of them to garner our information. Visual learners make up approximately 65% of the population, auditory learners approximately 30%, and kinesthetic learners approximately 5% (Mind Tools, 1998). To do a quick self-assessment, read the descriptions of the different styles in Figure 3-5 and note the one(s) that come closest to describing the way you prefer to receive information.

You may have selected two or three styles from Figure 3-5, because we sometimes use one style over another in certain learning situations. If all of the noted styles were "close," you may want to rank them to gain

☐ *Visual* learners think in pictures. It does not matter whether they are hearing the information, reading the information, or feeling the information. They take in the information through the senses and store it as visual images. When visual learners want to recall information, they "play the movie" in their brain. Visual learners also relate best to information they have seen written down in texts, in their own notes, in diagrams, and in pictures. A statement such as "I see," or "I get the picture" reflects the style of the visual learner.

☐ *Auditory* learners learn best by hearing and listening. They do not make mental pictures but filter information through listening and repeating skills. They relate best to the spoken word. They may not take notes in class, but rather may ask to tape the lecture. These learners prefer classroom discussion and oral presentations over writing assignments. Speech patterns represent exactly how the auditory learner thinks, "I hear you," "That clicks," "That sounds right," "That rings a bell".

☐ *Kinesthetic* learners learn by touch, movement, imitation, and practice. These learners will process and remember information well if they can touch or feel that which they are studying. These students are easily distracted during lectures, do not think in pictures, and can appear slow in understanding didactic material as it is being presented. They may have to go away and process (manipulate) material by rewriting the notes in a condensed format. These learners like to speak about learning in terms of their feelings, saying things like, "I feel" or "I'd like to get a better handle on this information."

Figure 3-5 Division of Learning Styles (*Adapted from Center for New Discoveries in Learning, Personal Learning Style Inventory, 1998*)

a better understanding of your overall learning style. All of us have the capacity to learn in all three modes. You naturally gravitate to one over the others based on which style has lead to your greatest learning successes.

Another way to classify learning styles is according to brain-hemisphere dominance. The left hemisphere of the brain is associated with analytical activities, such as logic, structure, speech, reasoning, numbers, verbal expression, verification of data, and analysis of parts of the whole. The right side is associated with creativity and synthesizing parts to form a whole idea. The right side is also considered the more emotional side and links to insight, intuition, daydreams, visualization, music, rhythm, and color visualization.

We need both sides of the brain to function and learn. Numerous studies demonstrated that individuals with left-brain dominance are primarily auditory learners and those with right brain dominance are primarily visual. Additional studies show that right-brain–dominant learners process, recall, and retain more from information presented in computer-assisted instructional programs, whereas left-brain–dominant learners derive more success from a lecture format. To overlook or use one style to the exclusion of the other is using only part of your overall potential learning ability.

Strategies for Learning

By determining your preferred learning style you will be able to adopt strategies to enhance that style when you study. You want to effectively move the required information into long-term memory and increase your knowledge level from memorization to comprehension and, finally, to application. To accomplish this you must know which strategies work with which learning styles. Refer to Table 3–5 and note all of the strategies listed that you consistently use in your study routine. Start with the style you previously ascertained to be your preferred learning style.

Are there strategies listed under your preferred style that you currently do not use? To enhance your acquisition of material, begin to incorporate these into your study plan. Are these strategies listed under any of the other styles that you could use when the material you are learning is especially difficult for you?

One way to incorporate more than one learning style into your study program is to employ a CAI program. Many texts now come with an accompanying disk designed to enhance learning style. Such disks may contain the total text along with testing materials, exercises that accompany the text, and/or resource material for the text. For example, several medical terminology packages come as program-instruction texts with disks and provide audio pronunciation in the computer programs. The student can read the text, manipulate the information on the computer, and hear the correct pronunciation.

To begin to incorporate new learning styles related to the way you receive and recall information, review the list in Table 3–6 and think about ways to add the study strategies to your study plan. You will notice that the three basic learning styles (visual, auditory, and kinesthetic) are expanded on in this list.

When faced with a particularly difficult passage or concept, incorporate more that one style and one strategy to process the information. The more action you put into your learning methods, the more effective your time and outcomes will be.

DEVELOP A TIME-MANAGEMENT PLAN

Somewhere in your decision-making process to go to school, you decided you would have the time to do so. You now must make that a reality by actively engaging in a time-management plan. **Time management** is a system to help meet goals through problem solving. Practicing time-management strategies will not eliminate the need to perform tasks you do not like, but it will make doing so more manageable. Active application of time-management strategies will make a difference in what you can accomplish in the time you have.

Table 3–5 SAMPLE LEARNING STRATEGIES

VISUAL LEARNER	AUDITORY LEARNER	KINESTHETIC LEARNER
Takes notes in class	Reads aloud	Takes notes and rewrites them to condense
Writes notes in margin of book	Reads into a tape recorder and plays it back to self	Expresses self with hands, even while reading
Looks for reference books with pictures, graphs, and charts	Discusses ideas about class content with others	Handles visual aids during class
Draws own illustrations	Requests explanations of illustrations	Requests to do a demonstration

Table 3–6 ADDITIONAL LEARNING STYLES AND STRATEGIES

STYLE	STUDY TECHNIQUES
Linguistic (word smart: uses words as cues, likes poems)	Speaks out loud, uses audiotapes of text information, uses workbooks, makes up **mnemonics** (words or phrases used to aid memory)
Logical/math (number smart: looks for patterns, enjoys science)	Needs to have a connection for information; uses charts, diagrams, note taking; may use mapping rather than straight words to see connections
Spatial (picture smart: visualizes, good at puzzles)	Draws diagrams; uses flash cards; chooses books with pictures, charts, and diagrams rather than total text, workbooks with pictures; uses highlighters in multiple colors to indicate special things and help information take hold in mind
Body/kinesthetic (body smart: rides a bike, walks, moves, loves the outdoors)	Tapes lectures, walks and listens, watches a video while on the treadmill, goes to a unit to "see" the information, goes to the library to get information, drives and listens to taped lectures or notes (allotted time takes on importance)
Music (music smart: listens to/ loves music, plays an instrument)	Makes up songs and rhymes, uses audio tapes of information or makes up own, listens to music while studying
Interpersonal (people smart: talks things though, likes to chat over coffee)	"Teaches" the material to somebody, studies in a group, runs material by mentor or coworkers
Intrapersonal (self smart: uses quiet time to process, a hobby person)	Uses examples from own experience to apply information, may process material from audio tape while doing a hobby

Adapted from Learning Out of the Box, "Tuning in to Your Unique Cluster of Intelligences," *by K. H. Matthews, 1997, Fall, 22–27,* The Next Step Magazine.

Strategies for time management include the following:

- Analyzing your time commitments
- Knowing yourself
- Clarifying your goals
- Setting priorities and identifying one or two valued goals to achieve
- Disciplining yourself to adhere to the plan through changes and until the goal is reached

Analyze Time Commitments

To analyze your time commitments, start by listing them. You should provide yourself with both a big-picture plan and a daily plan. Creating a year-at-a-glance calendar that lists all of your important time commitments can provide a quick illustration of the way the months ahead will be used. Start by putting in your graduation date in red capital letters. This will give you an instant visual reminder of your current goal. Next, using a pencil, insert all important dates including holidays, birthdays, work, and organizational obligations. Remember to also include activities for those in your household that will require your participation, such as carpooling, special school programs, after-school activities, and child care. Use your academic program calendar as the source for the dates classes, as well as vacations, begin and end, financial aid forms and tuition payments are due, and the like. Use your individual class schedules as the sources for dates of exams, special review or clinical days, field trips, or any other time commitments that you must meet in order to

complete the courses. This exercise will give you a big-picture view of your time commitments and will also point out any conflicts.

Conflicts are not impossible obstacles. Knowing about them in advance will allow you to take steps now to prioritize and reschedule. When prioritizing, think about delegating some tasks to other people. Do not always solve a conflict by removing those tasks you enjoy or that will renew you. Taking care of yourself during this time will be very important. Never give up the time you need to refresh and renew, even if it is just a hot bath, a brisk 15-minute walk, or a dinner out with family and friends. Place yourself near the top of the priority list to complete your goal.

Each learner's big-picture map will differ. The struggle is to mesh your map with your other relationships and keep yourself toward the top of the list. One strategy is to prominently display your big-picture calendar in an area where all of the members of your household can see it—including and especially you. Everyone will then have the opportunity to see that they are on the list and that they contribute to helping you reach your goal.

The next step is daily planning. Using a week-at-a-glance planner helps illustrate more concrete expectations of those things you plan to do and the amount of time you actually have (Figure 3-6). You should include time to sleep, eat, drive, work, attend class, and study.

You may find that you must rearrange your schedule. This does not mean continuing to do all of the things you have listed but just on different days; rather, it means choosing two valued goals on which to work.

	Monday	Tuesday	Wednesday	Thursday	Friday	Saturday	Sunday
7 AM	Work	Carpool	Carpool	Carpool	Clinical	House Chores	
9 AM	Work	Class	Class	Class		House	Sunday school
11 AM	Work	Class	Class	Class		Chores	Church
1 PM	Work	Class	Class	Class			
3 PM	Work				Work	Work	
5 PM	Carpool Dinner				Work	Work	
7 PM					Work	Work	

Figure 3-6 Week-at-a-Glance Calendar

One goal must be to be a learner. The other will be unique to you. This does not mean that you replace all other goals with these two valued goals. Rather, it means that these goals must take precedence when choosing ways to use your time. If you choose child care and learner as your most valued goals, you could refine them even further to complement each other. For example, you may opt to keep driving the carpool, but negotiate to drive every morning, because doing so will afford you 2 hours to study prior to class. You may then have to make child care arrangements for after school, which might mean asking your neighbor

PROFESSIONAL TIP

Time Wasters

Are you a time waster? We all sometimes behave in ways that sabotage the best of plans. Following are some examples of time wasters along with some strategies for helping you reclaim those wasted hours.

1. *Clutter:* Wisdom holds that you can save 1 hour each day by just clearing your work area of clutter and keeping it clean. This time can be put to good use in the form of study. Organize your study area so that when you arrive it is ready for work, and take a few minutes at the end of your session to prepare your area for the next session.

2. *Interruptions:* Intrusions into your study or work hours (from either people or things) can be real time wasters. Try the following:

   - Learn to say, "no." You do not have to agree to every request. Learn to pick your involvements carefully and according to those which are most important to you reaching your goals.
   - Put your answering machine on, and turn the phone's ringer off. Delegate a time to listen and respond to messages after studying.
   - Open your mail over the garbage can. Respond, delegate, or throw it out.

   - Organize your papers. For instance, have a folder for each child's paper/notes. Keep your class notebooks, your calendar, and phone lists in one three-ring binder, so you have all your essentials together.

3. *Procrastination:* This refers to intentionally putting off or delaying something that should be done. **Procrastination** is a time waster because it does not afford effective use of time. Time management is not necessarily finishing everything at one sitting, but, rather, scheduling time to return to the task until you complete it; whereas procrastination is intentionally delaying the task without good cause or a plan to complete it in a time-efficient manner. Breaking the task down into manageable segments and rewards will encourage you to return to it again and again until it is complete.

4. *Perfectionism:* Very often we do not stick to a plan because it does not give us results immediately or does not give the results we expected. Perfectionism affects your time-management plan by prohibiting you from accepting anything less than perfection; it also damages your positive attitude of yourself by setting unrealistic expectations. Focus on your positive accomplishments, look for ways to improve, accept your failures, and build on your experiences.

or contracting with an after-school program. You may also have to set aside 1 hour each evening to get everything laid out for the next day, a task you might ask someone else in the household to do each night so that you can gain an extra hour of study time. That extra hour, in turn, might mean that you dedicate Saturdays for nothing but family commitments. Regardless of the way you choose to solve such problems, the solutions must be designed to help you reach your goals.

Know Yourself

To develop your system you must know yourself. You must be honest with yourself about your work habits and preferences. Consider the time of day when you are at your intellectual best. Is it early in the morning, or do you come alive at 10 P.M.? You must be able to focus and concentrate when you are studying. Deciding you are going to carpool in the morning to get to school early to study will not be effective if you cannot concentrate until after noon. If this is the case, it would be better to do the more mechanical and less intellectually demanding tasks, such as the shopping or laundry, in the 2 hours before class. Are you a person who is more left-brain oriented (logical, orderly, structured, and plays by the rules)? Then writing out lists of tasks and crossing them off may be your time-management strategy to stay on track. Perhaps you are a more right-brain personality (creative, resists rules, has own sense of time)? Scheduling your task within a specific time frame that has a time-sensitive goal/reward at the end may assist you to use your available time more effectively.

Clarify the Goal

Without setting goals, we cannot know whether we are making any progress. Goals are like grocery lists. Think about when you go to the store without a list. You may purchase many items, but when you get home you often discover that, you did not get all the things you needed. If the next time you go to the store, you make a list, however, you will likely get all the items you want.

Just like the grocery list, goals must be written down. They must be based on reality and broken down into manageable parts. Say your goal is to provide study time each week that will allow you to be successful in each unit exam of your program. This time will comprise the time you need to prepare and review material, prepare for clinical assignments, view information in the library, and practice new skills in the lab. As a rule, you will need 1 to 2 hours of study time for each hour you spend in class. If you are in class 12 hours per week, you will thus need to find 24 more hours to study; and if you are in clinical 6 hours 3 days per week for a total of 18 hours, you will need to fit in 36 hours of study. As a rough estimate, this would mean 12 class hours plus 24 study hours plus 18

clinical hours plus 36 preparation hours for a total of 90 hours per week (30 class hours plus 60 study hours) for the ideal study week and 30 hours (class attendance only) for a week without any study. So now you know what amount of time you are aiming for. You can now take this goal of 60 study hours per week and compare it to your written schedule and calendar to determine how to best arrange the demands on your time in order to meet your goals.

Set Priorities

Another part of setting goals is prioritizing tasks into general categories. Look at your daily calendar and list the general categories. Some examples might be as follows:

- Work
- Study
- Personal (eating, sleeping)
- Household chores (shopping, budget)
- Transportation (self, others)
- Supervising children
- Decision making (planning, outside organizational responsibility, time for self, time for spouse, friends, and children)

Next, rank these general categories in order of priority, keeping in mind that not everything is a primary priority. If you uncover conflicts, try to further clarify which items take top priority.

Another way to prioritize is to group tasks according to the time frame in which you wish them to be accomplished. To do this, divide a sheet of paper into three parts. Label the first part column A, the second, column B, and the third, column C. Under column A, write "I must work on these tasks now." This list includes your priority tasks that need immediate attention. Under column B write "I can do these after A is done." Under column C write "I can delay, eliminate, or delegate these until after B is done" (Figure 3-7).

If you placed your entire list under column A, go back to your original two goals—one of which includes your new role as learner—and rethink your list. You must prioritize your activities in order to reach your goal. *You cannot be all things at all times to all people.* You also must know how to work smarter, not longer or harder, to remain focused on the priority task.

Discipline Yourself

The hardest strategy to commit to may be the last one. The idea that you must actively engage in using the plan sounds simple. In practice, the plan will not always work. When this happens, you may be tempted to abandon the plan instead of changing it. If the plan is not working, you must ascertain the reasons. Maybe you lack resources, have not scheduled enough time, or need to revisit and re-evaluate your goal. Build time

A	B	C
I must work on these tasks now	I can do these after A is done	I can delay, eliminate, or delegate until after B is done
school/study	*supervise children*	*organization*
child care		*shopping*
self-care		
work		

Figure 3-7 Prioritizing Tasks

to plan into your weekly schedule. If you really want to use a time-management system, your ability to go back to the plan and revise it will be very important.

DEVELOP A STUDY STRATEGY

Developing a study plan involves more than just buying a textbook and reading it. Several strategies that will assist you to study more efficiently and effectively follow.

Set Up the Environment

Where and when you study are as important as how. The fact that you assign a specific behavior to your study space will set you up for success. The space should fit your style. Do you like everything organized in neat spaces, or do you just need it near you? What type of lighting, seating, or noise level will assist or detract from your concentration? Consider your preferred learning style when setting up your study space (Figure 3-8). If you are a kinesethic learner, you may want to put motion into your space by, for instance, using a treadmill in your study plan. You may want to spend a percentage of your study time sitting to read and take notes and then switch to walking or running on the treadmill to recite and reflect on the material. You will be increasing comprehension and making connections, all while walking 2 miles! Regardless of the way you arrange your space, take into consideration the type of learner you are and your biological and personality preferences.

Gather Your Resources

Your resources should all be easily accessible from your study space. In some homes, the kitchen table serves as the study space. If your study space serves more than one function, as would the kitchen table, consider keeping your study resources in a milk crate or box so they are portable yet readily at hand when needed.

Gathering your resources is your start to building a library of textbooks, which will serve you throughout your program. These resources become a reference library for you when you study. Some general resources to keep on hand include the following:

- A recent edition of an unabridged dictionary
- A medical dictionary
- An anatomy and physiology text

Additional resources you will need as you progress through your program may include texts on pharmacology, nutrition, and the nursing process. Depending on your personal knowledge base, you may need further resources in the foundation sciences—biology, psychology, and sociology. These areas serve as the knowledge base for your future profession.

Keeping your learning style in mind, consider purchasing accompanying workbooks or other study aids that come with the text and research CAI or videotapes available in your nursing program library. Using varied and multiple resources enhances your knowledge base and will increase your comprehension of the con-

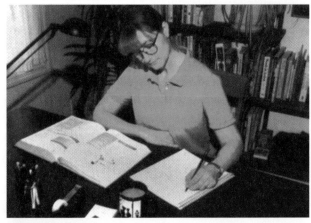

Figure 3-8 Create a study space that reflects your learning style. Ensure that all the resources you need to study are close at hand. *(Photo courtesy of Tom Stock)*

tent. You must go beyond memorization, beyond amassing facts, to comprehension of this knowledge base in order to answer the questions on the exams. Keep in mind that you are studying for the program examination, the National Council Licensure Examination (NCLEX-PN), and, ultimately, to apply your knowledge base to provide safe, effective care to your clients.

Remember to use journals as resources. The articles and related client situations can assist you in understanding the application of content to the clinical area. Your ultimate goal is to apply your content information to client care. Consider getting a subscription to your nursing journal, *The Journal of Practical Nursing*. Nursing organizations such as the National Federation of Licensed Practical Nursing are also valuable resources, and many have web sites, which you can visit.

Whatever resources you ultimately choose, gathering them and having your resources readily at hand are simple strategies that will make the time you have allotted for study more efficient and effective.

Minimize Interruptions

Interruptions to your study time decrease the actual time you can focus on the material and affect your concentration. Interruptions may also become your procrastination "triggers." If you allow your study time to be constantly interrupted, you will soon be doing something other than studying. At the very least, these interruptions minimize your efficient use of time. When you plan your time to study, do not set yourself up for interruptions. Look realistically at your time schedule and do not schedule your study time around the household's "naturally" busy times of the day—typically mornings, mealtimes, early evenings, and bedtimes.

This is where you put the strategies listed in the section on time management to work. If you have set aside a time and a space for study, make it known that you are not to be interrupted unless there is an emergency. Hang a sign on the door that reads, "Think, before you knock." Planning on studying in 1 or 1½ hour blocks is also a way to cut down on interruptions. This is a reasonable time period for you to put the world on hold in order to accomplish your task.

Get to Know the Textbook

Your textbook is not intended to be read like the latest mystery novel, from beginning to end in one sitting. It has both directions on the way to use it (introduction, preface) and built-in references (glossary, appendix, summary questions). It is arranged in sections, each dealing with a major topic, and then subdivided into the parts (chapters) that make up the sum of that topic. Getting to know your textbook and its resources and the author's approach to writing may constitute the first part of your study plan. Having this information gives you some insight into the way the material has been grouped and connected.

Another author may have written the book in totally stand-alone chapters and may encourage students to review the table of contents and start anywhere they feel they need to. Self-instruction modules or texts in math often give students instructions to first take all of the post-tests in the chapters and as long as a certain score is reached, to go on. This is a means of giving students credit for knowledge already learned and facilitating recall of knowledge in preparation for new learning.

Take a look at various parts of this text. How is the information organized? What built-in references can assist you? Consider the cues given about the way to use this text to help you organize the big picture.

Set Up the Study Plan

Each time you enter your study "space," your study plan should be with you. You should have a plan or a specific goal for that time. Each time you enter the space, bring a positive attitude toward reaching that goal. Your nursing course outline will drive your study plan. You will have a certain amount of material to cover in a specific time span. You first must know those things that are expected of you. Your course outline, curriculum, and instructors will give you this information.

As an example, consider a unit on vital signs, which is assigned to be completed in 1 week. The components of the unit include understanding the theory base about vital signs as well as learning the psychomotor skills involved in actually measuring these indicators. You are expected to acquire the knowledge by reading the chapter in the text, attending the lecture and demonstration, and practicing in the lab. You will be tested on your ability to apply your knowledge through a pencil-and-paper test and a redemonstration of your psychomotor skills. Now that you know the information you must cover, the sources of the information, and the way you will be tested, you can map out a study plan. Consider the following steps:

1. *Preview the material to be studied.* Your assigned reading from the text on the content of the unit may be contained in one chapter or may span several chapters. Always preview the assigned chapter(s). Often, the student reads only the pages assigned, thinking that this is the most efficient way to study. By not spending the 5 or 10 minutes to preview the entire chapter, the connections between the content may be lost. Previewing can be done very quickly by scanning the chapter headings, art, and tables.
2. *Consider the chapter heading.* The material about vital signs may be contained in a chapter labeled "Baseline Assessment" or "Measurement of Baseline Values" or "Physiologic Functions of the Body." All of these give you a cue as to what you are about to study.

3. *Read the objectives for the chapter.* The objectives list those things you should be able to do when you are finished learning the content of the chapter.

4. *Scan the vocabulary section and the end-of-chapter summary and questions.* Read the key terms and the summary and questions at the chapter's end. Doing so gives you an overview of the scope of the reading you will need to do and should take no more than 5 to 10 minutes

5. *Set up your questions.* Beginning at the chapter objectives, write down those things you already know, questions about those things you must learn for each objective, and some additional resources that you think you should check. For example, in a chapter about vital signs, the initial page may look like the one in Figure 3-9. Jot down your current knowledge, your questions. The resources note relates to the reasons you are trying to learn this material. Connecting the material to your role in the profession is most important. You are now ready to read the chapter critically for the answers to your questions. You may uncover more and have more questions at the end; but you have a plan and can move on to the next step.

6. *Read and take notes.* Answer your questions and check your vocabulary knowledge as you read.

7. *Reread when necessary.* Remember your basic skills and concentration.

8. *Reflect on the connections you can make between the material and client care.* Identify the reasons the information is important and the way you will use it.

9. *Recite or create your individual style cues.* This is where you will put your individual unique learning styles to work. Make up songs. Create mnemonics. Design flash cards for items that must be memorized. Try to create a logical connection when recalling information.

10. *Review or summarize the information.* Answer the objectives. Use your own words to answer your initial questions. Do you have more questions? Must you consult a second resource to answer them?

11. *End the session with a critical thinking question.* What would the client look like if his temperature were 103°F? What other body systems would be affected? What nursing measures might I use to support the client with this level temperature (e.g., monitor the client's fluid intake and output because the body would be losing fluid as a result of the thermoregulation [sweating and evaporation that would reduce the temperature]), and why? Write these down in your notes. You will soon have a collection of "client scenarios" that you will be able to build on as you increase your knowledge base.

The Measurement of Vital Signs

At the completion of this chapter, you should be able to:

1. Describe the physiologic mechanisms controlling temperature, pulse, respiration, and blood pressure.

   Temp = ?, Pulse = heart, Respiration = lungs, Blood pressure = arteries need to find out about temp.

2. Identify the normal range for vital sign measurements.

   For adults? Children?

3. Select the appropriate equipment used to take vital signs.

   Thermometer, stethoscope, blood pressure cuff

4. Demonstrate the correct psychomotor technique used in measuring vital signs.

   I do this in the lab/get procedure from book or instructor? Ask in class.

5. Document the normal findings of the measurement of blood pressure.

   Temp = 98.6, p = 60-80, bp = 120/80
   I need to know this to be able to tell if the client is normal or having trouble.

Figure 3-9 Start with the chapter objectives and devise questions and answers to determine those things that you know and those things that you will need to give more attention.

The preceding steps require skill in five areas: reading, rereading, reflecting, reciting, and review. With each step, you are engaging in the process of encoding the material. **Encoding** is thought of as actually laying down tracks in the areas of your brain. Each time you read, reread, reflect, recite, and review, you increase the depth of the tract, and your ability to recall and utilize the information increases. You move the information from short-term to long-term memory, and you increase your level of knowledge. The more senses and action you put into your study plan, the more you are able to utilize the information.

You move your level of knowledge from the memorization of a group of facts to the comprehension of the facts in a logical, organized fashion that allows you to relate the information to clients to whom you will provide care. Each time you sit down to study, this should be your goal. You can preview, question, and quickly outline the major points in the chapters prior to class. Listen to the lecture and take notes. Approach

Mnemonics

Create your own mnemonics to group the steps of a procedure. A mnemonic is simply a method for helping your association and recall; it consists of a memorable word or phrase created from the letters of the list of items you are trying to recall. For example, to remember all of the areas to include when assessing a client to whom a cast has been applied (pulse, circulation, sensation, movement, and temperature), you might make up a silly sentence to help you remember, such as "*Paul Can Shine My Tuba.*" This type of statement will help you group these facts together (pulse, circulation, sensation, movement, temperature) and assist you in recalling them. You could sing this also. Do whatever you can to be active in moving material from short-term to long-term memory.

new material with the read, reread, reflect, recite, and review steps before moving on to the next topic.

Note Taking

Note taking is an action that connects you to the content of written material or a lecture presentation and will assist you in identifying the main ideas and their connection to the overall topic.

Keep materials for each of your classes or topics in a separate three-ring binder. Take notes on loose-leaf paper and write on one side only, as this allows you to arrange your preview notes and lecture notes chronologically. You can also insert handouts from the class in the appropriate order as you receive them. Using this method, you can also review notes against additional information you have from other resources to assist you when it is time to review for the examinations.

When you are taking notes from the text, read with a pencil in your hand to put yourself in the action mode. You will thus be ready to receive and process information. You may also take notes from text readings on your computer, which facilitates editing and rearranging material.

Prior to class, preview your chapter material and divide your paper, leaving a 3-inch border on the left side. From the assigned reading, identify the main topic to be covered, list the main section and the subheadings, and summarize the information in the left column. Then write your questions in this column. This prepares you for more active participation in the lecture; use the right column to take notes from the lecture.

Regardless of the way you choose to take notes, note taking while you study sets you up for connecting with the content. It positions you as an active participant in the learning process, and any time you increase your active participation in the learning process, you increase your learning.

When taking notes in class, listen attentively, lean forward, and concentrate on the information the speaker is imparting (Figure 3-10). Take notes on the following:

- The topic, as stated by the speaker; write it on the top of the page
- The main ideas and the details that support the topic
- The most important points, based on the speaker's organization and emphasis

Memory and Activity

Remember the following as a guide for a study plan when you want to learn new material:

People Remember	Learner Activity
10% of what they READ	Reading
20% of what they HEAR	Hearing the words
30% of what they SEE	Watching still pictures (charts, diagrams)
50% of what they SEE and HEAR	Watching moving pictures (video or a demonstration)
70% of what they SAY and WRITE	Giving a presentation/making up a story (case studies)
90% of what they SAY AS THEY PERFORM THE EXPERIENCE	Talking your way through a demonstration Teaching someone else

Adapted from Audiovisual Methods in Teaching *(p. 43), by E. Dale, 1954, New York: Dryden Press.*

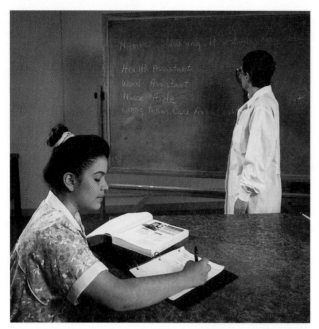

Figure 3-10 Note taking is an important component of increasing your comprehension of the material.

- Other students' questions and the responses from the speaker, which are often the very questions you had

Look for visual and auditory cues from the speaker, for example, if the speaker says, "This is important" or writes steps on the board. Do not form an opinion of what is being said until you have heard the entire lecture. As stated earlier, a good strategy is to write your questions as you think of them. They may be answered by the time the lecture is over.

The purpose of note taking during a lecture is not to create a transcript of the information imparted, but, rather, to record what you understand. The combination of attending lecture, listening, and note taking can provide you with much knowledge that you will not have to learn elsewhere. Previewing the material to be covered further contributes to this dynamic. When taking notes, consider the following guidelines to make your note taking efficient and effective:

PROFESSIONAL TIP

Attending Lectures

In general, the best strategies for getting the most from lectures are to:

- Get to class on time.
- Get a front row seat.
- Listen attentively with a pencil in your hand and take notes.

- Do not take notes with the intent of writing them over. This is a waste of time and, contrary to what you may expect, it does not improve recall. Making a note map of your notes is a more effective recall tool.
- If your handwriting is sloppy, print or use a laptop computer.
- Condense the amount of actual writing you do by using symbols and abbreviations and leaving out everything but necessary words. For instance, instead of writing "If the client's blood pressure reading is greater than 140 systolic and 90 diastolic, . . ." write "If BP > 140/90. . . ."
- Write definitions and mathematical formulas exactly as you heard them in lecture.
- In mathematics and science lab courses, write the process step by step exactly as explained. Indicate which formulas are used with which problems, for example

  "Use ratio/proportion for word problems."

- Pick an abbreviation system and stick to it.
- Review the notes as soon as possible after class. Many studies have demonstrated that even a brief review of notes after class increases retention of the material by 50%.

Prepare for Exams

The final plus of having a study plan is the ability to review for exams. Reviewing for exams is not studying all of the material over from the beginning. You will already have studied the subject matter you are going to cover on the exam; now, you are reviewing and recalling it through a series of exercises designed to increase your comprehension and facilitate application. Most nursing examinations are written at the comprehension or recall level. The NCLEX-PN is written at the application level. On this exam you will not see many questions about naming where the pulse points are (comprehension, recall), for instance. You will instead find questions about which of the pulse points of the body are most appropriate for assessing an infant (application). Making decisions about which fact or groups of principles you have learned will be the basis for most nursing examination questions.

Depending on the curriculum, you may have examinations every week or every month, a weekly quiz, a midterm, and a final. Regardless, you will know the schedule, and you must set aside review time for preparation. If you are to have weekly quizzes, you must build a time for review into your daily study plan. One way to do so is to set aside the last 30 minutes of each study session for review. Take each objective of your course outline and, without looking at your notes or text, turn them into questions and then answer them. If you are weak in one area, refer to your notes and devise a technique for recall, such as the use of flash cards, rhythms, mnemonics, pictures, or graphic drawings. Work through each of the objectives for the content that will be covered.

If your examinations are by unit, you must divide the material up over the time you will need to cover it, leaving at least 2 days for review and recall prior to the examination. Each of these review sessions will also serve as preparation for both your final examination and the NCLEX-PN. As you are successful in each of your examinations and continue to see further connections in your clinical application, your depth as well as breadth of content mastery will increase.

PRACTICE THINKING CRITICALLY

Most of this chapter thus far has been devoted to presenting strategies for the effective and efficient acquisition of knowledge. Your ultimate goal is to be able to use this knowledge to provide safe client care. To do so, you must go beyond the initial stage of simply acquiring information. In delivering nursing care, facts alone do not constitute a sufficient knowledge base for making sound decisions about client care. You must internalize these facts and be able to manipulate them when presented with new situations.

Your progress in this cognitive arena will be evaluated by testing. Practicing thinking critically will enhance your ability to increase your level of knowledge

You must think about *how* you think. Thinking is a process: It is the way you move information from one point to another to get something accomplished. Have you ever been asked, "How did you arrive at that conclusion?" Your explanation was an example of your thinking process. This process of examining how we think is called **metacognition** (from *meta,* meaning "among" plus *cognition,* meaning "the process of knowing").

Consider all the problem solving you have done in your life. How did you arrive at your decisions? Why did you make the choices you did? Given more information, would you have made different decisions? Have you made decisions you regretted?

To make sound decisions, you must consider the knowledge you have and choose that which is relevant given the unique parameters of the given situation. Each client situation is unique. Your text and instructors present information about nursing practice within what is called *predictable parameters,* but clients are anything but predictable.

In considering which actions you may need to take in a new situation, you must consider past experience and principles of care, postulate possible outcomes from a variety of interventions, and seek additional information from colleagues, clients, and resource materials. This process is called *thinking critically,* and it is

what you will be expected to do with the knowledge you are acquiring.

How do you foster this type of thinking and knowledge advancement as you are studying? The following strategies used during your study process will help develop your critical thinking skills.

1. *Recall the facts.* Remind yourself of those things you already know about the targeted topic. (***Example:*** The cardiovascular system is made up of the heart, the arteries, and the veins; it carries the blood to the cells.)
2. *Group facts into a pattern and organize the data.* (***Example:*** The heart is the center of this system. The arteries carry blood from the heart to the cells, the veins carry blood from the cells to the heart. The blood's function is to transport nutrients and oxygen to the cells and to take waste and carbon dioxide from the cells.)
3. *Associate this information with an experience or an action.* (***Example:*** The cardiovascular system is like a plumbing system, with the heart as the main pumping station, the arteries as the carriers of the hot water, and the veins as the carriers of the cold water.)
4. *Practice "what if" scenarios.* Imagine a person in your life and analyze the facts that you have learned in light of this person. Confirm whether the facts are applicable. If not, what was significant in this situation to alter your conclusion? What action might you take? (***Example:*** What happens when the pump doesn't work [as in Uncle Joe's pacemaker]? What causes this? What runs the heart's electrical system? What else can cause the main pump to stop working—no food [nutrients] or no oxygen? Where does the heart get its oxygen? How does this affect Joe's lifestyle? How could I tell whether a person has a pacemaker? What would I do if the pacemaker stopped?)
5. *Discuss these questions with peers and your instructor.* Conferring with others increases your experience and the variety of ways you look at a problem and promotes increased comprehension of the subject.
6. *Postulate new solutions.* Allow yourself to consider all possible solutions without assigning merit. There is no need to label an idea as "good" or "bad" before the idea has even been discussed. Often, such flashes of insight come when we are daydreaming, on the verge of sleep, or as we awaken. Our mind is free to roam and process during these times.

The last strategy will involve taking some risk, but students who take that risk quickly develop a thick skin and are the most likely to contribute innovatively to the clinical practice as a result of their thinking process. Chapter 2 on critical thinking provides much more information on this particular process, but the subject bears inclusion here. Practice this habit as you study, and never stop asking, "Why?" and "What about this?"

DEVELOP TEST-TAKING SKILLS

Testing is not studying; however, the skills you need for testing are similar to those needed for studying. The task involved in taking a test is not to pass it; to pass the test is the *outcome*. You cannot achieve the outcome if you do not know the task. The task is to read the question, understand what the question is asking, and make a decision about a correct response.

To hone your test-taking behaviors, you must first perform a personal analysis with regard to your attitudes, preparation methods, and behaviors related to a testing situation. Only after you have identified these variables can you initiate strategies to improve your outcomes.

Attitude and Expectations

If you are like most students, you may feel quite anxious about taking a test. You may think of each test as the final chance to show your worth. Or you may consider receiving less than an A on an examination as being the same as failing. Neither of these is a reasonable expectation for testing. Testing is a useful tool for both measuring your level of knowledge and showing what you still need to learn. Have you ever considered that receiving a grade of C on an examination usually indicates that you know 75% of all of the knowledge that was tested? And the knowledge on any given test does not represent all the knowledge you possess. Your attitude toward testing is very important if you are to improve your outcome. Maintaining a reasonable expectation regarding both the purpose of the test as well as the meaning of your grade is often a key factor in improving your test performance.

Preparation

In analyzing your preparation for test taking, you must critically examine your study habits. Review the section in this chapter on a study strategies and consider whether you are on task when it comes to your study habits. There may be some areas where you can improve. If you know of an area of weakness, make a conscious effort to develop this part of your preparation. Be reasonable in your expectations and do not expect to see results overnight. Building your study habits takes time and persistence. Persevere and your outcome on tests will improve.

Next, consider the way you review for an examination. Do you cram the night before, or are you consistently planning for questions in your study plan and adding time for review of material prior to the exami-

nation? One strategy is to use the technique of note mapping to help you organize the material into manageable parts. Taking each part and developing a more detailed one-page outline that you can take with you to review for 15 to 20 minutes at a time is another method to try. Another suggestion is to change your study place and times. Instead of 1-hour sessions, break your review sessions into 30-minute recall sessions. You must draw an imaginary line between studying and reviewing. Studying is the learning of new knowledge; reviewing comprises recall, organization, and summary of information.

Do not study only just prior to the test. This represents poor technique. What are the odds that prior to the examination you would hit upon just the right information that would be on the test in just the exact form that you would see it on the test? Approaching preparation in this manner serves only to put a few facts into short-term memory. Better to spend the time before the examination relaxing with a good book or good friends or at the spa or gym. You must be confident and rested and come to the testing area with that "good" feeling that results from doing something you like.

Consider the rest you get the night prior to the examination. Physical stamina is needed for concentration. If you cram for a test by "pulling an all-nighter," you are setting yourself up for possible errors on the examination. Be reasonable, revisit your study plan, and get adequate rest.

Next, consider whether you have enough energy to take the test. You can eat what you want, but eat. The cells of the brain require glucose to function; this glucose is supplied in the calories you consume. Try not to increase caffeine intake immediately prior to a test, as doing so may make you jittery.

Finally, ask yourself whether surrounding yourself with positive people helps keep you focused, or whether talking to students prior to a test only makes you more anxious. If the latter is the case, you should arrive with just enough time to walk into the testing room and you should not speak to anyone.

Minimize Anxiety

Anxiety is the physiologic response of the autonomic nervous system to a perceived stressful situation. As the situation becomes more stressful, the body's response increases. This affects the ability to process information and make rational choices. People are often not good at identifying what they are feeling and are often unaware of the degree to which stress affects the ability to take tests.

You must develop a plan to deal with anxiety. Anxiety about our performance is always with us. Past experience with testing often contributes to the development of test anxiety. If our expectation regarding our performance on a test is not mirrored in the grade

PROFESSIONAL TIP

The 30-Second Vacation

For those of you who need an "anxiety buster," consider a "30-second vacation." The 30-second vacation is based on a guided imagery technique that is used often in the client care arena. This technique takes practice. Start by doing the following:

Sit in a comfortable spot where you will not be disturbed, close your eyes, and think of an event or a place that evokes a feeling of calmness (not necessarily happiness). This is an event or place that made you feel like everything was right with the world and with you. It can be from any time in your life.

It may take some time to settle on the right event or place. Relax and take a few minutes now and think.

Once you have it, don't tell anyone! This is your secret place, your place of peace, and when you go there, no one can find you.

Once you have selected this event or place, start to give it "life." To do this, you must begin to recall this event or place regularly. Practice doing so at the beginning of your study sessions, when you are stuck in traffic, when you are at the dentist, when you have something difficult to do, at the beginning of your test-taking exercises, or at the beginning of your real tests.

Each time you recall your event or place, give it more "life." Recall the time of day, the setting, the colors of that day. Was it raining, was it sunny, was it snowing? If it was raining, was it a summer rain or an autumn rain? Recall what you were wearing and what colors you had on. Were you alone or with others? Were you eating something? What did the food smell like?

we receive, our confidence in our ability is shaken, and we approach the whole experience with more and more anxiety.

To deal with anxiety, consciously develop an activity to counter the feeling that anxiety evokes. Some people listen to music, pace, or do deep breathing to combat feelings of stress and anxiety. All of these are good strategies, even if all of them cannot be done *while you are actually taking the test*.

Improve Test-Taking Skills

How do you improve your test-taking skills? You practice, practice, practice and analyze, analyze, analyze. Consider the following:

Treat every wrong answer as a treasure. Examine it and discover the secret of why you got it wrong

This is the only way to know which errors you are making. From this point forward, always request to review your examinations, and track your incorrect responses using the analysis worksheet presented in Figure 3-11. Initially when you review your tests, do not concern yourself with the content of the questions. Simply write the number of the question in the row that indicates the reason you got that question incorrect. You will also notice that there is a heavy black line before the last row of the worksheet. The first four rows represent what are known as *mechanical errors;* these can be eliminated by developing positive habits and revising current practices. You will notice after 3 or 4 quizzes that a pattern starts to emerge. Imagine

that you just took a 100-question test and received a score of 60/100. You then use the worksheet to categorize your incorrect responses.

Of the 40 incorrect answers you provided, you see that 10 of them fell in "did not read carefully," 2 in "did not know the vocabulary," 7 in "inferred additional data," 4 in "identified priorities incorrectly," and 7 in "did not know the material." If you could eliminate the bad habits that resulted in the first 23 errors, this would improve your test score immediately. Your grade would be 83/100. More importantly, tests would truly represent only what you did not know, not areas where bad habits resulted in poor test scores.

After you have identified your error patterns, you can work on developing the counter habits that will eliminate them. Work first on the one that is the most glaring.

Read Carefully

Reading carefully is a test-taking behavior that must be practiced. The section on study strategies noted the value of scanning in looking for important words when you read. When you are reading a test question, however, you must *never* scan. Many students choose incorrect responses because they miss key words, scan the question for familiar terms, infer what the question is, or misinterpret words they read too quickly. Incorrect responses resulting from any of these actions represent poor reading habits rather than a substandard knowledge base. The following exercise will help improve your reading habits.

Test Question Analysis Worksheet

Reason for Incorrect Response	Test 1 Date	Test 2 Date	Test 3 Date	Test 4 Date	Test 5 Date	Test 6 Date	Test 7 Date	Test 8 Date
Did not read carefully (missed details, missed key words)								
Did not know the vocabulary (medical terminology, English vocabulary)								
Inferred additional data (made assumptions, "read into the question")								
Identified priorities incorrectly (placed events in wrong order)								
Did not know the material								

Figure 3-11 Test Question Analysis Worksheet

Exercise for Improving Your Literal Reading Skills

You will need

- A timer (stove/egg).
- An NCLEX-PN review text or any comparable question and answer book. It is important that you have the answers and the rationales for each answer in a review text.
- Two sheets of paper: one to take the test on and one to make your analysis worksheet.
- Pencil or pen.
- Dictionary.

1. Pick a time and a place where there will be no interruptions for 20 minutes. You may neither speak to anyone nor get up to use any other resources. You are taking a test.
2. Randomly pick a page of the review book and choose five questions from that page. It does not matter whether you have studied the content in your program.
3. Set the timer for 5 minutes.
4. Start the test. Read each question out loud.
   a. If you read "over" a word, stop reading, make a mark next to that word, and begin again from the beginning.
   b. If you mispronounce a word, stop reading, make a mark next to that word, and begin again from the beginning.
   c. If you do not know the meaning of a word (English or medical), stop and look it up.

5. At the end of the question, restate what is being asked of you.
6. Read the choices, connect each to the question, and choose the most correct answer.
7. When the timer goes off, score your questions.
8. Analyze why you got questions correct or incorrect.
9. Repeat this exercise with five different questions three or four times a week.

The object of this exercise is not to finish all the questions, nor is it even to get all the answers right. Rather, the object is to consciously practice reading every word literally. Each time you do this exercise, you must treat it as a test—no food, no talking, no music, no interruptions. You must associate this type of reading with taking a test, so that each time you take a test, this literal reading habit is instinctual.

Know the Vocabulary

If vocabulary is your weak area, there is only one thing to do—learn the vocabulary. Look up the word (English and medical) in the appropriate dictionary, write the definition on the back of your analysis sheet, and review the definition during your next study session. Add additional time in your study plan for vocabulary building. Use additional modes of learning such as audio or flashcards to master your vocabulary skills.

Do Not Infer Additional Data

The more experiences you have in life, the easier it is to infer additional data in any given situation. You must realize, however, that for the moment, the only relevant information is the information on the test paper—no more, no less. Based on that information alone and the given choices, you must decide on the correct responses. You base your decision on those things you have learned about the topic, on standards of care, on the nursing process, and on your base of knowledge. If you read into the question, you have in essence rewritten it and may not choose the correct answer. One strategy for overcoming this habit is to recognize whenever you begin to interject information upon getting to the last word in a question. In any such instance, you must stop, take some physical action to call your attention to the fact that you are adding information, and clear your mind—take a breath, clear your throat, wear a rubber band and snap it! Then start over again, concentrating on reading the question literally.

Identify Priorities Correctly

When questions concern priorities, ask yourself which of the given choices would result in serious consequences if not done first. When you are being questioned about procedural tasks, ask which of the given choices must be done before the others.

Know the Material

Not knowing the material represents a lack of knowledge base. Write down the content area of each of the questions you miss, then go back and review the concept or facts in question. If the same content areas are problematic over several tests, seek additional assistance from your instructor. You need clarification regarding your understanding of both the information and the questions.

Behaviors in the Testing Room

Setting yourself up in the testing room for a positive experience can make a difference in your outcome. Be sure to practice the following behaviors:

1. *Get a good seat.* Unless your seat is assigned, sit in an area that is quiet, has good light, and where you can "zone in" on the test and "zone out" the rest of the room. If you are a student who gets anxious when you are the last one left in the room, pick a seat in the front row and farthest from the door and turn your seat slightly toward the wall. You will be less apt to notice as people leave.

2. *Set the mood.* As you wait for the test to be passed out, take your 30-second vacation. Adopt the most positive attitude possible. Identify the task ahead of you. Take a breath and repeat the following:

   "I have prepared. I am able to read the questions, process the information, and, from the choices given, make the best choice and move on."

3. *Read—do not scan.* You must read literally every word in the question. Every word counts!

4. *Read the question to determine the following:*
   - *Who is the question about?* This will affect your chosen answer. If you automatically assume that all of the questions relate to the nurse, you may miss a question that asks you to decide those things the father might say to demonstrate his understanding of the discharge instructions, for example.
   - *What is the question about?* You must determine to which part of the knowledge base the question refers. Is the question about the way to teach a 9-year-old juvenile diabetic to check his blood glucose? To answer this question, you must consider the learning style of the 9-year-old, his cognitive development and manual dexterity, and any significant others who should be involved in the session. The correct choice must support all of these principles.
   - *When is the question about?* The time frame of the question is also significant in terms of the client's continuum of care. Is this the acute session? Is this a client who has had diabetes for 20 years and is now developing pulmonary vascular disease? Is this a new mother with her first child or a new mother with her fifth? Are you in the assessment phase of the nursing process, are you in the planning stage, or are you evaluating the effects of a treatment or a drug?
   - *Where is the question about?* The focus of the nurse in the acute care institution is different from that of the nurse in the community clinic. This will affect your choice.

5. *Do not argue with the question.* Whether you agree with the question is irrelevant. The task is to read the question, put your mind to the question, and, given the choices offered, make your choice based on principles and the application of your knowledge base.

6. *Plan your time.* Do not spend an inordinate amount of time on one question. There are some things you will not know, and if you spend so much time on one question, you can sabotage your success on others. You can come back to any question, but you must be able to clear your mind of this question before moving on to tackle another. This is a good place for a 30-second vacation to put you back on task! If you cannot let a question "go," you will be unable to concentrate on the next few questions and, very likely, will get several questions in a row incorrect. It is best to read, choose, and move on.

7. *Do not panic.* When you come to a question that you can not immediately answer, do not panic. Use your 30-second vacation to counter your anxiety and facilitate your ability to process. Recite

again, "I have prepared, I am able to read, process, choose, and move on." Remember, the answer is on the paper.

SUMMARY

- Developing a positive attitude will enhance your learning experience.
- Strategies for developing a positive attitude include creating a positive self-image, recognizing your abilities, and identifying realistic expectations for meeting those goals.
- Nurses must develop competency in the basic skills of reading, arithmetic and mathematics, writing, listening, and speaking.
- It is important to build your vocabulary and comprehension of medical terminology to better enable you to meet your clients' learning needs.
- Should you suspect that you have a learning disability, it is important to identify the disability so that you can seek the right tools to help compensate for the disability.
- The most common learning styles are visual, auditory, and kinesthetic.
- Identifying your preference for a particular learning style will help you identify the strategies you need to be a successful student.
- Organizing your study space and decreasing interruptions will increase your efficiency and facilitate your sticking to your study plan.
- Several methods can be used to take notes. Note taking in lectures and from your text is a strategy to help you retain the information presented.
- Critical thinking is the ability to apply your knowledge base.
- Developing a strategy to minimize anxiety when taking tests will improve your performance.
- To successfully complete a test, read each question thoroughly, do not infer additional information, and identify priorities.

Review Questions

1. Ninety percent of your program is based on which basic skill?
   a. listening
   b. writing
   c. reading
   d. mathematics

2. What is a sign of true comprehension of material?
   a. the ability to repeat a paragraph word for word
   b. memorization of the material
   c. the ability to recite the material
   d. the ability to summarize the material using your own words

3. If you suspect you have a learning disability, it is important that you:
   a. ignore it; you will be able to work around it on your own.
   b. be tested to determine the assistance you will need to compensate for the disability.
   c. keep it to yourself; you will not be able to pass the program if you tell anyone about it.
   d. use it as an excuse to put less work into the program.

4. A kinesthetic learner:
   a. learns by using the senses and visual images.
   b. learns by movement and imitation.
   c. learns by hearing and listening.
   d. learns by example.

5. The best way to study is to:
   a. read only the assigned material.
   b. take notes in the lecture only.
   c. read, reread, reflect, recite, and review.
   d. read and attend lectures.

6. What is the best way to deal with any anxiety you may experience during a test?
   a. jogging
   b. listening to music
   c. practicing deep breathing and imagery
   d. asking for more time to take the test

Critical Thinking Questions

In the section on Practicing Thinking Critically, you were asked, "How did you arrive at that conclusion?" Recall the last fairly crucial decision you made and outline your thinking process.

WEB FLASH!

- Visit your professional association's web site and gather information on your profession.
- Visit one of the learning sites to take a learning-style assessment.

History and Nursing Organizations

Chapter 4
Nursing History, Education,
and Organizations

Chapter 5
The Health Care Delivery System

NURSING HISTORY, EDUCATION, AND ORGANIZATIONS

MAKING THE CONNECTION

Refer to the following chapters to increase your understanding of nursing history, education, and organizations:

- **Chapter 7, Ethical Responsibilities**
- **Chapter 30, Leadership/Work Transition**

LEARNING OBJECTIVES

Upon completion of this chapter, you should be able to:
- *Define key terms.*
- *Define nursing as an art and a science.*
- *Identify major historical and social events that have shaped current nursing practice.*
- *Describe Florence Nightingale's impact on current nursing practice.*
- *Discuss the contributions of early nursing leaders in the United States.*
- *Discuss the impact of selected landmark reports on nursing education and practice.*
- *Define the role of the RN.*
- *Define the role of the LP/VN.*
- *Describe select nursing organizations and their purposes and functions.*
- *Differentiate between program approval and program accreditation.*

KEY TERMS

accreditation	history
autonomy	morbidity
clinical	mortality
didactic	nursing
empowerment	primary care provider
health maintenance	primary health care
organization	staff development

INTRODUCTION

Nursing is an art and a science by which people are assisted in learning to care for themselves whenever possible and are cared for by others when they are unable to meet their own needs.

Nursing has evolved from an unstructured method of caring for the ill to a scientific profession. The result has been movement from the mystical beliefs of primitive times to a "high-tech, high-touch" era. Nursing combines art and science. By using scientific knowledge in a humane manner, nursing combines critical thinking skills with caring behaviors.

Nursing focuses not on illness but, rather, on the client's *response* to illness. Nursing promotes health and helps the client move to a higher level of wellness. This aspect of nursing also includes providing assistance to the client with a terminal illness with the goal of maintaining comfort and dignity in the final stage of life.

This chapter traces the evolution of nursing by exploring its rich heritage and the social forces that have affected its development. Nursing education and nursing organizations are also discussed.

HISTORICAL OVERVIEW

To understand the present status of nursing, it is necessary to have basic historical knowledge about nursing. By studying nursing history, the nurse is better able to understand such issues as **autonomy** (being self-directed), unity within the profession, supply and demand, salary, education, and current practice. **History** is a study of the past, including events, situations, and individuals. By learning from historical role models, nurses can enhance their abilities to create positive change in the present and set a course for the future.

Learning from the past is the major reason for studying history. Ignoring nursing's history can be detrimental to the future of the profession (Ogren, 1994). By applying the lessons gained from a historical review, nurses will continue to be a vital force in the next millennium.

The study of nursing history offers another advantage: learning how the profession has advanced from its beginnings. **Empowerment** is the process of enabling others to do for themselves. Only when nurses are empowered are they truly autonomous. Autonomy has historically been difficult for nurses to achieve. Empowerment and autonomy go together and are necessary if nursing is to bring about positive changes in health care today. Personal power comes to individuals who are clear about what they want from life and who see their work as essential to the contributions they wish to make.

Evolution of Nursing

Nursing has evolved alongside human civilization. While it is not possible to present a complete history of nursing and health care within the scope of this text, it is necessary for all nurses to have some understanding of their profession's heritage and of those pioneers who led the way on the path to modern nursing. Table 4–1 is a chronological listing of events in the evolution of nursing.

Primitive Times

Primitive humans may very well have derived early nursing care practices from observing the animal world. Many animals care for their sick and injured. For example, wild turkeys feed their young wild berries to ward off the chill of inclement weather, much as we use vitamin C (found in wild berries) today; the snipe (a small bird) has been observed splinting an injured leg with sticks and straw; and many animals eat grass

Table 4–1 HISTORICAL EVENTS INFLUENCING THE EVOLUTION OF NURSING

DATE	EVENT	DATE	EVENT
4000 B.C.	Primitive societies	1871	Founded: New York State Training School for Nurses, Brooklyn Maternity, Brooklyn, New York
2000 B.C.	Babylonia and Assyria		
800–600 B.C.	Health religions of India		
700 B.C.	Greece: source of modern medical science	1872	New England Hospital for Women's one-year program for nurses yields America's first trained nurse, Linda Richards
460 B.C.	Hippocrates	1873	Founded: first three Nightingale schools in United States: Bellevue (New York City), Connecticut, and Massachusetts General
3 B.C.	Ireland: pre-Christian nursing		
A.D. 390	Fabiola: first hospital founded		
390–407	Early Christianity, deaconesses	1881	Founded: American Red Cross, by Clara Barton
711	Field hospital with nursing, Spain		
1096–1291	Military Nursing Orders (Knights Hospitalers of St. John in Jerusalem)	1892	Founded: Ballard School at YWCA Brooklyn, NY; first practical nursing school
1100	Ambulatory clinics, Spain (Moslems)	1893	Founded: American Society of Superintendents of Training Schools for Nurses
1440	First Chairs of Medicine, Oxford and Cambridge	1899	Founded: International Council of Nurses (ICN)
1500–1752	Deterioration of hospitals and nursing, "dark ages of nursing"	1900	*American Journal of Nursing (AJN)* established
1633	Founded: Daughters of Charity	1903	New York: efforts fail to pass a nurse licensing law
1820	Florence Nightingale born		
1836	Kaiserswerth, Lutheran Order of Deaconesses reestablished		North Carolina: first state nurse registration law passes
1841	Founded: Nursing Sisters of the Holy Cross		Founded: Army Nurse Corps
1848	Women's Rights Convention, Seneca Falls, New York	1907	Thompson Practical Nursing School in Brattleboro, VT established
1854–1856	Crimean War	1910	Flexner report
1859	Nightingale's *Notes on Nursing* published in England	1911	Founded: American Nurses Association (ANA), formerly the Associated Alumnae
1860	Founded: first Nightingale School of Nursing, St. Thomas Hospital, London	1912	Founded: National League of Nursing Education, formerly the Superintendents' Society
1861–1865	Civil War, United States	1914	Mississippi becomes first state to license practical nurses
1861	Dorothea Dix appointed Superintendent of the Female Nurses of the Army		

continues

Table 4–1 HISTORICAL EVENTS INFLUENCING THE EVOLUTION OF NURSING *continued*

DATE	EVENT	DATE	EVENT
1917	Smith-Hughes Act passes (provided federal funds for practical nursing programs in vocational schools)	1955	Practical nursing established under (Title III) Health Amendment Act
1918	Household Nursing Association School of Attendant Nursing in Boston, MA, established		All states pass licensure laws affecting practical/vocational nursing
1920s	First prepaid medical plan established, Pacific Northwest	1959	National Association of Practical Nurse Education (NAPNE) changes name to National Association for Practical Nurse Education and Service (NAPNES)
	Hospitals offer a prepaid plan	1960s	Established: Medicare and Medicaid
	Baylor Plan (prototype of Blue Cross) established	1961	National League for Nursing establishes a Council for Practical Nursing Programs
1921	Women get the right to vote		Surgeon General's Consultant Group
1923	Goldmark Report: Nursing and Nursing Education in the United States	1965	First nurse practitioner program, pediatric
1935	Social Security Act passes		ANA position paper on entry into practice
1941	Founded: Association of Practical Nursing Schools	1966	Educational opportunity grants for nurses
1942	Association of Practical Nursing Schools becomes National Association of Practical Nurse Education (NAPNE)	1970	Secretary's commission to study extended roles for nurses
	Practical nursing curriculum planned and advocated across United States	1973	Health Maintenance Organization Act
1944	U.S. Department of Vocational Education commissions intensive study to differentiate tasks of the practical nurse	1977	Rural Health Clinic Service Act
		1980	Omnibus Budget Reconciliation Act (OBRA)
1945	New York only state to have mandatory licensure law for practical nurses	1982	Budget cut to Health Maintenance Organization Act
1948	Brown Report: Future of Nursing		Tax Equity Fiscal Responsibility Act (TEFRA)
1949	Founded: National Federation of Licensed Practical Nurses (NFLPN)	1983	Institute of Medicine Committee on Nursing and Nursing Education study
1952	National League of Nursing Education changes name to National League for Nursing (NLN)	1987	Secretary's Commission on Nursing
		1990s	Health care reform
		1996	Certification Examination for Practical and Vocational Nurses in Long-term Care
		1997	Established: NLN Accrediting Commission (NLNAC)

Adapted from Fundamentals of Nursing: Standards & Practice, *by S. DeLaune and P. Ladner, 1998, Albany, NY: Delmar. Copyright 1998 by Delmar. Adapted with permission.*

as an emetic when they have stomach problems. Early humans were closely associated with the animals.

Early Civilizations

The evolution of nursing dates back to 4000 B.C. to primitive societies wherein mother–nurses worked with priests. In 2000 B.C., the use of wet nurses is recorded in Babylonia and Assyria.

Ancient Greece

The ancient Greeks built temples to honor Hygiea, the goddess of health. These temples were more like health spas than hospitals in that they were religious institutions governed by priests. Priestesses (who were not nurses) attended to those housed in the temples. The nursing that was done by women was performed in the home.

Hippocrates, a Greek physician born in 460 B.C., is considered the father of medicine. He used a system of physical assessment, observation, and record keeping in his care of the sick. Hippocrates wrote about many aspects of medicine, including pathology, anatomy, physiology, diagnosis, prognosis, mental illness, gynecology, obstetrics, surgery, client-centered care, bedside observation, hygiene, and professional ethics. Case histories that he wrote are still used as examples today. He emphasized the importance of caring for the client and thus laid a foundation for nursing. The Hippocratic Oath, based on his principles, is still taken by physicians today.

Roman Empire

Hospitals were first established in the Eastern Roman Empire (Byzantine Empire). St. Jerome was responsible, through one of his disciples, Fabiola, for introducing hospitals in the West. Western hospitals were primarily religious and charitable institutions housed in monasteries and convents. The caregivers had no formal training in therapeutic modalities and volunteered their time to nurse the sick (Bullough & Bullough, 1993).

Middle Ages

During the medieval era, hospitals in large Byzantine cities were staffed primarily by paid male assistants and male nurses. These hospitals were established as almshouses, and care of the sick was only secondary (Bullough & Bullough, 1993).

Medical practices in Western Europe remained basically unchanged until the 11th and 12th centuries, when formal medical education for physicians was required in a university setting. Although there were not enough physicians to care for all the sick, other caregivers were not required to receive any formal education or training. The dominant caregivers in the Byzantine setting were men; however, this was not true in the rural parts of the Eastern Roman Empire and in the West. In these societies, nursing was viewed as a natural nurturing job for women.

Renaissance

During the Renaissance (A.D. 1400–1550), interest in the arts and sciences emerged. This was also the time of many geographic explorations by Europeans. As a result, the world literally expanded.

Because of renewed interest in science, universities were established, but no formal nursing schools were founded. Because of social status and customs, women were not encouraged to leave their homes; they instead continued to fulfill the traditional role of nurturer/caregiver in the home.

Enlightenment and the Industrial Revolution

With the beginning of the Industrial Revolution came technology that led to a proliferation of factories. Conditions for the factory workers were deplorable. Long hours, grueling work, and unsafe conditions prevailed in the workplace. The health of laborers received little, if any, attention.

Medical schools were founded, including the Royal College of Surgeons in London in 1800. In France, men who were barbers also functioned as surgeons by performing procedures such as leeching, giving enemas, and extracting teeth.

At the end of the 18th century, there were no standards for nurses who worked in hospitals. In the early to mid-1800s, nursing was considered unseemly for women, even though some hospitals (almshouses) relied on women to make beds, scrub floors, and bathe the poor. Most nursing care was still performed in the home by female relatives of the ill.

Religious Influences

The strong influence of religions on the development of nursing started in India in 800–600 B.C. and flourished in Greece and Ireland in 3 B.C. via male nurse–priests.

In 1836, Theodor Fleidner, a pastor in Kaiserswerth, Germany, revived the Lutheran Order of Deaconesses to care for the sick in a hospital he had founded. He established the first real school of nursing to educate the deaconesses in the care of the sick. These deaconesses of Kaiserswerth became famous because they were the only ones formally trained in nursing. Pastor Fleidner had a profound influence on nursing through Florence Nightingale, who received her nurse's training at the Kaiserswerth Institute.

The Catholic Church established religious orders that were devoted to caring for the sick and poor. Secular nursing was not an acceptable option for women. Only nurses who functioned within a religious order received social approval. Social conditions and the need for nurses in the mid-19th century, however, set the stage for the reforms instituted by Florence Nightingale (discussed following).

The order of the Nursing Sisters of the Holy Cross was founded in LeMans, France, by Father Bassil Moreau in 1841. Also in 1841, a Father Sorin brought four sisters to Notre Dame in South Bend, Indiana. In 1844, these sisters established St. Mary's Academy in Bertrand, Michigan. In 1855, the school was moved to Notre Dame and became known as Saint Mary's College, which later had a strong influence on the emerging role of women (Wall, 1993).

Florence Nightingale

Florence Nightingale (1820–1910) is considered the founder of modern nursing. She grew up in a wealthy, upper-class family in England during the mid-1800s. Unlike other young women of her era, Nightingale received a thorough education, including studies in Greek, Latin, history, mathematics, and philosophy. She had always been interested in relieving suffering and caring for the sick. Social mores of the time made it impossible for her to consider caring for others because she was not a member of a religious order. After receiving encouragement from a family visitor, Dr. Samuel Gridley Howe, however, she became a nurse over the objections of society and her family.

After completing the 3-month course of study at Kaiserswerth Institute, Nightingale became active in reforming health care. Britain's war in the Crimea presented her with the opportunity to volunteer with 38 other nurses to serve in the battle-site hospital (Figure 4-1). The physicians in charge relegated the nurses to nonclient care duties. Florence Nightingale persisted in advocating cleanliness, good nutrition, and fresh air. When battle casualties mounted, the nurses were presented with the chance to prove their worth. They worked around the clock, caring for the wounded, carrying oil lamps to light their way in the darkness. The symbol of the oil lamp is still used today in nursing and is responsible for Florence Nightingale being called the "Lady With The Lamp." The implementation

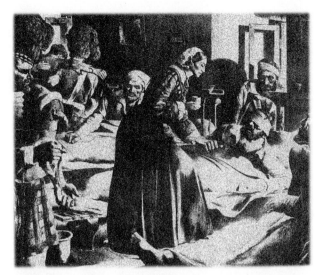

Figure 4-1 Florence Nightingale in the Crimea *(Photo courtesy of Parke, Davis & Company, a division of Warner-Lambert Company)*

of her principles in the areas of nursing practice and environmental modifications resulted in reduced **morbidity** (illness) and **mortality** (death) rates during the war.

Nightingale worked to further develop the public's awareness of the need for educated nurses and forged the future of nursing education as a result of her experiences in training nurses to care for British soldiers. She established the Nightingale Training School of Nurses at St. Thomas' Hospital in London. This was the first school for nurses that provided both theory-based knowledge and clinical skill building. She revolutionalized not only the public's perception of nursing but also the method for educating nurses. Some of Nightingale's novel beliefs about nursing and nursing education were the need for:

- A holistic framework inclusive of illness and health;
- A theoretical basis for nursing practice;
- A liberal education as a foundation of nursing practice;
- An environment that promotes healing; and
- A body of nursing knowledge distinct from medical knowledge (Macrae, 1995).

Nightingale introduced many other concepts that, although unique in her time, are still used today. Specifically, she advocated (1) a systematic method of assessing clients; (2) individualizing care on the basis of the client's needs and preferences; and (3) maintaining confidentiality.

Nightingale also recognized the influence of environmental factors on health. She advocated that nurses provide clean surroundings and fresh air and light to improve the quality of care (Nightingale, 1969). Nightingale believed that nurses should be formally educated and should function as client advocates (Se-

landers, 1993). She is credited with being the originator of modern nursing because many of these beliefs and concepts are still advocated in nursing schools today.

Nursing and the Civil War

America's need for nurses increased dramatically during the Civil War (1861–1865). The Sisters of the Holy Cross were the first to respond to the need for nurses during this war. Answering a request from Indiana's governor, 12 sisters started caring for wounded soldiers. By the end of the war, 80 sisters had cared for soldiers in Illinois, Missouri, Kentucky, and Tennessee (Wall, 1993).

During the Civil War, nursing care was provided by the Sisters of Mercy, Daughters of Charity, Dominican Sisters, and the Franciscan Sisters of the Poor. These sisters were influenced by the roles assigned to women during the 19th century. Although they were submissive to authority, they were willing to take risks when human rights were threatened (Wall, 1993). Other women also volunteered to care for the soldiers of both the Union and Confederate armies (Figure 4-2). These women performed various duties, including the implementation of sanitary conditions in field hospitals.

Dorothea Dix (1802–1887), a New England schoolteacher, was appointed Superintendent of the Female Nurses of the Army in 1861; no woman had ever before been appointed to an administrative position by the federal government. As a result of her recruitment efforts, more than 2,000 women cared for the sick in the Union Army. After the Civil War, Dix concentrated her energies on reforming treatment of the mentally ill (Johnson, 1997).

Clara Barton (1821–1912) volunteered her nursing services during the Civil War and, in 1881, organized the Red Cross in the United States.

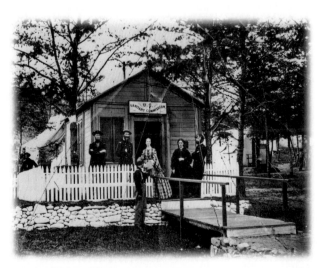

Figure 4-2 During the Civil War, women were instrumental in the effort to minimize the risk of spreading contagious diseases among wounded soldiers. *(Photo courtesy of Corbis-Bettmann)*

The Women's Movement

In 1848, the Women's Rights Convention in Seneca Falls, New York, signaled the beginnings of social unrest. Women were not considered equal to men, society did not value education for women, and women did not have the right to vote. With suffrage, not only were the rights of women advocated, but the nursing profession itself advanced. By the mid-1900s, more women were being accepted into colleges and universities, even though only limited numbers of university-based nursing programs were available.

Nursing Pioneers and Leaders

Modern nursing was forged by the contributions of many outstanding nurses through the years. The establishment of public health nursing, the provision of rural health care services, and the advancement of nursing education occurred as a result of the work of nurse pioneers and leaders, some of whom are discussed following. Note that the term *trained nurse* was used historically as the predecessor of *registered nurse*.

Lillian Wald

Lillian Wald (1867–1940) spent her life providing nursing care to the indigent population. In 1893, as the first community health nurse, she founded public health nursing with the establishment of the Henry Street Settlement Service (Figure 4-3) in New York City (Silverstein, 1994). Wald was a tireless reformer who:

- Improved housing conditions in tenement districts;
- Supported education for the mentally challenged;
- Advocated passage of more lenient immigration regulations; and
- Initiated change of child labor laws and founded the Children's Bureau of the U.S. Department of Labor.

In addition to initiating public health nursing, Wald also established a school of nursing.

Isabel Hampton Robb

Isabel Hampton Robb (1860–1910) founded several nursing organizations, including the Superintendents' Society in 1893 and the Nurses' Associated Alumnae of the United States and Canada in 1896 (Figure 4-4). She recognized the necessity of nurse participation in professional organizations to establish unity on positions and issues across the profession. She was instrumental in establishing both the American Nurses Association (ANA) and the National League of Nursing Education, the predecessor of the National League for Nursing (NLN). Robb was also an early supporter of the rights of nursing students. She called for shorter working hours and emphasized the role of the nursing student as learner instead of employee.

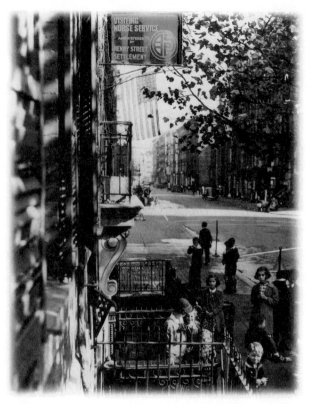

Figure 4-3 Nurses at the Henry Street Settlement in New York City *(Photo courtesy of Visiting Nurses Service of New York)*

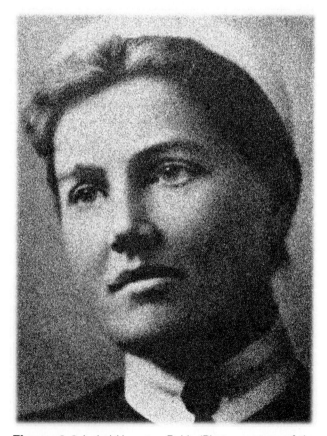

Figure 4-4 Isabel Hampton Robb *(Photo courtesy of the American Nurses Association)*

Adelaide Nutting

Adelaide Nutting (1858–1947) was a nursing educator, historian, and scholar. She actively campaigned for the education of nurses in university settings and was the first nurse to be appointed to a university professorship.

Lavinia Dock

An influential leader in nursing education was Lavinia Dock (1858–1956), who graduated from Bellevue Training School for Nurses in 1886. Early in her nursing practice, she worked at the Henry Street Settlement House in New York City, providing visiting nursing services to the indigent. She wrote one of the first nursing textbooks, *Materia Medica for Nurses.* Dock wrote many other books and was the first editor of the *American Journal of Nursing* (*AJN*).

Mary Breckenridge

In 1925, Mary Breckenridge (1881–1965) introduced a system of delivering health care to rural America. This decentralized system for primary nursing care services in the Kentucky Appalachian Mountains, called the Frontier Nursing Service, lowered the childbirth mortality rate in Leslie County, Kentucky, from the highest in the nation to below the national average.

Mamie Hale

In 1942, Mamie Hale was hired by the Arkansas Health Department to upgrade the educational programs for midwives (Figure 4-5). Hale, a graduate of Tuskegee School of Nurse–Midwifery, gained the support of granny midwives, public health nurses, and obstetricians. Through education, Hale decreased superstition and illiteracy among those functioning as midwives. Hale's efforts resulted in improved mortality rates for both mothers and infants (Bell, 1993).

Mary Mahoney

America's first African American professional nurse, Mary Mahoney (1845–1926), was a noted nursing leader who encouraged a respect for cultural diversity. Today, the ANA bestows the Mary Mahoney Award in recognition of individuals who make significant contributions toward improving relationships among multicultural groups.

Linda Richards

In 1873, the first diploma from an American training school for nurses was awarded to Linda Richards (1841–1930). Richards established numerous hospital-based training schools for nurses. She also introduced the practice of keeping nurses' notes and physicians' orders as part of medical records, and began the practice of nurses' wearing uniforms. As the first Superintendent of Nurses at Massachusetts General Hospital, she demonstrated that trained nurses gave better care than those without formal nursing education.

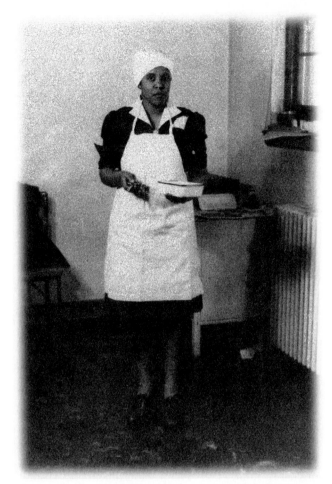

Figure 4-5 Mamie Hale *(Photo courtesy of Historical Research Center, University of Arkansas for Medical Sciences Library, Little Rock, RG 515, Box 47)*

PRACTICAL NURSING PIONEER SCHOOLS

Women who cared for others, but who had no formal education, often called themselves "practical nurses." Formal education for practical nursing began in the 1890s. The first schools were Ballard School, Thompson Practical Nursing School, and Household Nursing Association School of Attendant Nursing.

Ballard School

In 1892, the Ballard School, funded by Lucinda Ballard, was opened in New York City by the YWCA. It offered several courses for women, one of which was practical nursing. The 3-month course in simple nursing care focused on the care of infants, children, elders, and disabled persons in their own homes. The course included cooking, nutrition, basic science, and basic nursing procedures. When the YWCA was reorganized in 1949, the school closed.

Thompson Practical Nursing School

Thomas Thompson of Brattleboro, Vermont, left money in his will to help women who were making shirts for the army and were receiving only one dollar per dozen. His executor, Richard Bradley, saw the need for nursing service and, in 1907, established a practical nursing school in Brattleboro. It is still operating today and is accredited by the NLN.

Household Nursing School

In 1918, a group of women in Boston were concerned about providing nursing care for people who were sick at home. After talking with Richard Bradley, they opened the Household Nursing Association School of Attendant Nursing. The name was later changed to Shepard-Gill School of Practical Nursing. It closed in 1984.

NURSING IN THE 20TH CENTURY

The beginning of the 20th century brought about changes that have influenced contemporary nursing. Several landmark reports about medical and nursing education, as well as some contemporary reports, are discussed following. The establishment of visiting nurse associations and their use of protocols are also discussed.

Flexner Report

In 1910, Abraham Flexner, supported by a Carnegie grant, visited the 155 medical schools in the United States and Canada. The goal of the resulting Flexner report, which was based on his findings, was to impose accountability for medical education. Flexner's study resulted in the following changes: closure of inadequate medical schools, consolidation of schools with limited resources, creation of nonprofit status for remaining schools, and establishment of medical education in university settings that was based on standards and strong economic resources.

Seeing the value and impact of the Flexner report on medical education, Adelaide Nutting, together with colleagues from the Superintendents' Society, presented a proposal to the Carnegie Foundation in 1911 to study nursing education. Although the foundation never allocated monies to study nursing education, it did support educational studies in other disciplines such as law, dentistry, and teaching.

Although the efforts of Nutting and other nursing leaders went unheeded, in 1906 Richard Olding Beard successfully established a 3-year diploma school of nursing at the University of Minnesota under the College of Medicine.

Early Insurance Plans

At the turn of the 20th century, there were more than 4,000 hospitals and 1,000 schools of nursing. It was at this time that the concepts of third-party payments and prepaid health insurance were instituted. Third-party payment refers to payment made by someone other than the recipient of health care (usually an insurance company) for the health care services provided. Prepaid medical plans were started in lumber and mining camps of the Pacific Northwest, where employers contracted for medical services, for which they paid a monthly fee. This led to the establishment of the Bureau of Medical Services, where the employer contracted for medical services and the subscriber selected one of the physicians in the bureau.

Lillian Wald suggested the establishment of a national health insurance plan when she was the first president of the National Organization for Public Health Nursing.

Blue Cross and Blue Shield

The Depression provided the main impetus for the growth of insurance plans. The philosophy in the United States of health care for all further contributed to the growth of insurance plans. In 1920, American hospitals offered a prepaid hospital plan; this, in turn, led to the Baylor Plan, which eventually became the prototype of Blue Cross.

The American Hospital Association pioneered the development of an insurance company to provide benefits to subscribers who were hospitalized. Blue Shield was developed by the American Medical Association to provide reimbursement for medical services provided to subscribers. In 1933 the American Hospital Association endorsed Blue Cross, and in 1938 the American Medical Association endorsed Blue Shield.

The federal government became more involved in health care delivery in 1935 with the passage of the Social Security Act, which provided for (among other things) benefits for elderly persons, child welfare, and federal funding for training health care personnel. During World War II, the U.S. government extended the benefits for military personnel to include health care for veterans and their dependents.

Visiting Nurses Associations

In 1901, at the suggestion of Lillian Wald, the Metropolitan Life Insurance Company, which provided visiting nursing services to its policyholders, entered into an agreement with the Henry Street Settlement. Wald worked with Metropolitan to expand the services of the Henry Street Settlement to other cities; thus, one form of managed care began.

Nurses providing care in the home environment experienced greater autonomy of practice than did hospital-based nurses (Figure 4-6). This led to conflicts with some physicians regarding the scope of medical

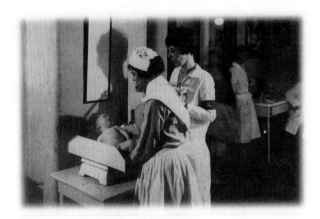

Figure 4-6 A Baby Being Weighed by a Student Nurse and a Junior League Volunteer in 1929 *(Photo courtesy of Touro Infirmary Archives, New Orleans, LA)*

practice versus that of nursing practice. Some physicians thought nurses were taking over their practice, whereas other physicians encouraged nurses to do whatever was necessary to care for the sick at home.

In 1912, in an effort to provide direction to home health staff nurses, the Chicago Visiting Nurse Association developed a list of standing orders for nurses to follow in providing home care. These orders were to direct the nursing care of clients when the nurse did not have specific orders from a physician. Thus, the groundwork for nursing protocols was established.

Landmark Reports in Nursing Education

During the first half of the 20th century, a number of reports were issued concerning nursing education and practice. Three of these reports, the Goldmark, the Brown, and the Institute of Research and Service in Nursing Education, are discussed following.

Goldmark Report

In 1918, Adelaide Nutting (relentless in her efforts to document the need for nursing education reform) approached the Rockefeller Foundation for support. Funding was provided, and, in 1919, the Committee for the Study of Nursing Education was established to investigate the training of public health nurses. Josephine Goldmark, a social worker, served as the secretary to the committee.

As secretary, Goldmark developed the methodology of data collection and analysis for a small sampling of the 1,800 schools of nursing in existence. The study of 23 of the best nursing schools across the nation represented a cross sample of schools—small and large, public and private.

The Goldmark report, entitled Nursing and Nursing Education in the United States, was published in 1923. Goldmark identified the major weakness of the hospital-

based training programs as that of putting the needs of the institution (service delivery) before the needs of the student (education). Nursing tradition and the apprenticeship form of education reinforced putting the needs of the client before the learning needs of the student.

Some major inadequacies in nursing education as identified by the study were limited resources, low admission standards, lack of supervision, poorly trained instructors, and failure to correlate clinical practice with theory. The report concluded that for nursing to be on equal footing with other disciplines, nursing education should occur in the university setting.

Brown Report

In 1948, Esther Lucille Brown, a social anthropologist, published *Nursing for the Future and Nursing Reconsidered: A Study for Change*. Several recommendations were put forth in this study, including the need for nurses to demonstrate greater professional competence by moving nursing education from the hospital to the university setting.

Although published 20 years after the Goldmark report, the Brown report identified many of the same problems in diploma education; for instance, nursing students were still being used for service by the hospitals, and inadequate resources and authoritarianism in hospitals still prevailed in nursing education.

Brown recognized that the university setting would provide the proper intellectual climate for educating the professional nurse. Visionary nurse educators were securing libraries, laboratories, and clinical facilities as necessary learning resources. Professional endeavors such as research and publication were being implemented by nurse leaders.

Institute of Research and Service in Nursing Education Report

The 1950s addressed different aspects of nursing. Post World War II, a deficit in the supply of nurses coincided with an increased demand for nursing services. Hospital closures were one result of the nursing shortage. Some contributing factors to the scarce supply of nurses were the low esteem of nursing as a profession, long hours combined with a heavy workload, and low salaries.

The Institute of Research and Service in Nursing Education Report resulted in the establishment of practical nursing under Title III of the Health Amendment Act of 1955. This led to a proliferation of practical nursing schools in the United States.

Other Health Care Initiatives

In the 1960s, health care services were provided to the elderly and the indigent populations with the federal programs of Medicare and Medicaid.

This era also saw passage of the Nurse Training Act (1964), which provided federal funds to expand enrollments in schools of nursing. Federal funds were used to construct nursing schools, and student loans and scholarships were made available to nursing students.

The Health Maintenance Organization Act of 1973 provided an alternative to the private health insurance industry. **Health maintenance organizations** (HMOs) are prepaid health plans that provide primary health care services for a predetermined fee. Because fees are set in advance of services being rendered, HMOs provide cost-effective services. **Primary health care** refers to the client's point of entry into the health care system and includes assessment, diagnosis, treatment, coordination of care, education, preventive services, and surveillance.

The National Commission for Manpower Study, released in 1977, resulted in amendments to the House of Representatives 2504 of Title XVIII of the Social Security Act, which provided payment for rural health clinic services. Through the efforts of Anne Zimmerman, former President of the ANA, the bill was amended to substitute the term **primary care providers** (health care providers whom a client sees first for health care) for *physician extenders,* thereby, allowing nurse practitioners to be paid directly for their services. This represented the first time that nurses could be directly reimbursed for care they rendered.

Costs and Quality Controls

During the 1970s, the cost-control systems of various federal health programs were inadequate because of the rapid escalation of health care expenditures. Consequently, the Tax Equity Fiscal Responsibility Act (TEFRA) of 1982 was created in response to the $287 billion spent on health care in 1981. At the same time that the federal government was trying to control costs with TEFRA and prospective payment legislation, concern was also growing regarding the quality of health care.

Although business and industry embraced quality control systems in the 1940s and 1950s, the health care industry failed to see the need for such controls until the 1980s. The Joint Commission on Accreditation of Healthcare Organizations' (JCAHO) agenda for change in the late 1980s emphasized monitoring quality for outcomes rather than process, thus advocating change from a static quality assurance system to dynamic quality improvement. The JCAHO (1996) views quality of care as an ongoing process of continuously looking for ways to improve the care provided.

Health Care Reform

With an ever-increasing number (over 60 million) of Americans being uninsured or underinsured, health care access and costs have become a major focus of attention in the 1990s (Edelman & Mandle, 1998). Children are especially at risk for having their health care neglected, with one in five children in the United States being uninsured (Baker, 1994).

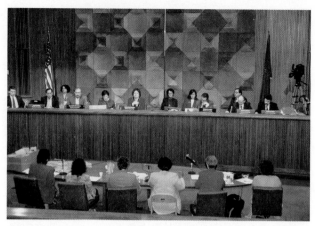

Figure 4-7 Nurses Making a Presentation Before a State Legislature *(Photo courtesy of the New York State Nurses Association)*

Nursing as a profession has made great strides in effecting federal and state health care legislation (Figure 4-7). Hospitals are moving away from the controlling, bureaucratic entities they once were and instead are more often being characterized by an environment of shared governance, where nurses have a voice in both administrative and clinical decision making. Nurses are serving as case managers and are working in collaboration with physicians and other health care providers.

Nurses are working to obtain prescriptive privileges for all advanced practitioners. Differentiated practice models are being developed and should settle the issue of educational preparation for entry into practice. The foundation has been laid for nursing to move forward with alternate client care delivery models that will allow access to care at a reasonable cost.

Health care providers are managing their organizations as does industry, focusing on quality management systems and competitive measures to market their services, and on information systems to facilitate data collection and cost efficiency.

NURSING EDUCATION

Educational programs that prepare graduates to take a licensing examination must be approved by a state board of nursing. Boards approve entry level programs to ensure the safe practice of nursing by setting minimum educational requirements and guaranteeing that the graduate of the program is an eligible candidate to take a licensing examination. In the United States, candidates must pass the National Council Licensure Examination (NCLEX) to obtain a license to practice nursing.

Types of Programs

Two types of entry level nursing programs are available in the United States: licensed practical or vocational nurse (LPN or LVN) and registered nurse (RN).

An entry level educational program is one that prepares graduates to take a licensing examination. Graduates of the licensed practical/vocational programs take the NCLEX for practical nurses (NCLEX-PN), and graduates of registered nurse programs take the NCLEX for registered nurses (NCLEX-RN).

Postgraduate programs prepare nurses to practice in various roles as advanced practice registered nurses (APRNs). Individual states have varying statutory provisions for APRNs.

Licensed Practical/Vocational Nursing

Licensed practical nurses (LPNs) or licensed vocational nurses (LVNs, as they are called in Texas and California), work under the supervision of an RN or other licensed provider such as a physician or dentist. The LP/VN, like the RN, was first trained in hospitals. The Smith Hughes Act passed by Congress in 1917 gave impetus to the formation of vocational-school–based practical nursing programs. In 1998, there were 1,205 practical/vocational nursing programs in the United States producing 38,732 graduates (NLN, 2000b).

Programs are state approved and in some cases also have accreditation by the NLN. **Accreditation** is a process by which a voluntary, nongovernmental agency or organization appraises and grants accredited status to institutions and/or programs or services that meet predetermined structure, process, and outcome criteria. These educational programs are generally 1 year in length and provide both **didactic** (systematic presentation of information) and **clinical** (observing and caring for living clients) experience. The education is focused on basic nursing skills and direct client care. Although the majority of clinical experience is in hospitals, long-term care facilities, physicians' offices, home health agencies, and ambulatory care facilities are also used.

Admission generally requires a high school diploma or General Education Development (GED) certificate. Schools may require a preentrance examination that assesses such skills as math, reading, and writing.

Once licensed, the LP/VN is prepared to work in structured settings such as hospitals, long-term care, home health, medical office, and ambulatory care facilities. Just as the RN has been delegated duties previously considered the domain of the physician, the LP/VN has been assigned duties once considered the domain of the RN. Many hospitals offer programs that provide levels of advancement for the LP/VN.

The National Federation of Licensed Practical Nurses, Inc. has written standards of nursing practice for the LP/VN. They are listed in Table 4–2.

Registered Nursing

Registered nurses are graduates of state-approved and, in many cases, NLN-accredited programs. They are typically prepared for entry into practice in one of three ways: associate degree nursing programs, hospital diploma programs, or baccalaureate degree nursing programs.

Associate Degree Programs Associate degree programs are typically 2 years in length and are offered through community colleges but may also be offered as options at 4-year–degree-granting universities. The graduate receives an Associate Degree in Nursing (ADN). In 1998, there were 899 associate degree programs producing 50,394 graduates (NLN, 2000b). This represents 59% of nurse graduates that year. Traditionally, program content reflected basic skill preparation and emphasized clinical practice in the hospital setting. Because of the decreasing demand for hospital beds, however, students are now likely to spend a higher number of clinical hours in community-based institutions (e.g., ambulatory settings, schools, and clinics).

Diploma Programs Diploma nursing programs are typically 3 years in length and are offered by hospitals. Most diploma programs are now affiliated with colleges or universities that grant college credit for select courses. Graduates of these programs receive a diploma as opposed to a college degree.

Program content prepares the graduate in basic nursing skills particularly suitable for hospitalized clients. In 1994, however, the majority of diploma schools reported using community-based settings such as physicians' offices, clinics, visiting nurse services, and health departments as training sites (NLN, 1998).

Although prominent in the early history of nursing education, the 93 diploma nursing programs in 1998 produced 3,443 graduates (NLN, 2000b). This represents 4% of nursing graduates that year. However, 24% of RNs working in 1996 were initially educated in diploma programs (U.S. Department of Health and Human Services [USDHHS], 1996).

Baccalaureate Degree Programs Baccalaureate degree programs, typically 4 years in length, are offered through colleges and universities. The graduate receives a Bachelor of Science in Nursing (BSN). These programs emphasize more preparation for practice in nonhospital settings, broader scientific content, and systematic problem-solving tools for autonomous and collaborative practice. In 1998, 549 baccalaureate programs produced 31,010 nursing graduates (NLN, 2000b). This represents 37% of the nursing graduates that year.

Staff Development and Continuing Education

Once a nurse is in practice, both staff development and continuing education are used to maintain the needed knowledge and skills for contemporary practice. **Staff development** typically occurs in the setting of employment and is described as the delivery of instruction to assist the nurse to achieve the goals of the employer. It is guided by the accreditation standards of

Table 4–2 NURSING PRACTICE STANDARDS FOR THE LICENSED PRACTICAL/ VOCATIONAL NURSE

Education

The licensed practical/vocational nurse:

1. Shall complete a formal education program in practical nursing approved by the appropriate nursing authority in a state.
2. Shall successfully pass the National Council Licensure Examination for Practical Nurses.
3. Shall participate in initial orientation within the employing institution.

Legal/Ethical Status

The licensed practical/vocational nurse:

1. Shall hold a current license to practice nursing as an LP/VN in accordance with the law of the state wherein employed.
2. Shall know the scope of nursing practice authorized by the Nursing Practice Act in the state wherein employed.
3. Shall have a personal commitment to fulfill the legal responsibilities inherent in good nursing practice.
4. Shall take responsible actions in situations wherein there is unprofessional conduct by a peer or other health care provider.
5. Shall recognize and commit to meet the ethical and moral obligations of the practice of nursing.
6. Shall not accept or perform professional responsibilities that the individual knows (s)he is not competent to perform.

Practice

The licensed practical/vocational nurse:

1. Shall accept assigned responsibilities as an accountable member of the health care team.
2. Shall function within the limits of educational preparation and experience, as related to the assigned duties.
3. Shall function with other members of the health care team in promoting and maintaining health, preventing disease and disability, caring for and rehabilitating individuals who are experiencing an altered health state, and contributing to the ultimate quality of life until death.
4. Shall know and utilize the nursing process in planning, implementing, and evaluating health services and nursing care for the individual patient or group.
   a. Planning: The planning of nursing includes:
      1) Assessment of health status of the individual patient, the family, and community groups
      2) Analysis of the information gained from assessment
      3) Identification of health goals
   b. Implementation: The plan for nursing care is put into practice to achieve the stated goals and includes:
      1) Observing, recording, and reporting significant changes that require intervention or different goals

   2) Applying nursing knowledge and skills to promote and maintain health, to prevent disease and disability, and to optimize functional capabilities of an individual patient
   3) Assisting the patient and family with activities of daily living and encouraging self-care as appropriate
   4) Carrying out therapeutic regimens and protocols prescribed by an RN, physician, or other persons authorized by state law.
   c. Evaluation: The plan for nursing care and its implementations are evaluated to measure the progress toward the stated goals and will include appropriate persons and/or groups to determine:
      1) The relevancy of current goals in relation to the progress of the individual patient
      2) The involvement of the recipients of care in the evaluation process
      3) The quality of the nursing action in the implementation of the plan
      4) A reordering of priorities or new goal setting in the care plan
5. Shall participate in peer review and other evaluation processes.
6. Shall participate in the development of policies concerning the health and nursing needs of society and in the roles and functions of the LP/VN.

Continuing Education

The licensed practical/vocational nurse:

1. Shall be responsible for maintaining the highest possible level of professional competence at all times.
2. Shall periodically reassess career goals and select continuing education activities that will help to achieve these goals.
3. Shall take advantage of continuing education opportunities that will lead to personal growth and professional development.
4. Shall seek and participate in continuing education activities that are approved for credit by appropriate organizations, such as the NFLPN.

Specialized Nursing Practice

The licensed practical/vocational nurse:

1. Shall have had at least one year's experience in nursing at the staff level.
2. Shall present personal qualifications that are indicative of potential abilities for practice in the chosen specialized nursing area.
3. Shall present evidence of completion of a program or course that is approved by an appropriate agency to provide the knowledge and skills necessary for effective nurisng services in the specialized field.
4. Shall meet all of the standards of practice as set forth in this document.

Reprinted with permission of the National Federation of Licensed Practical Nurses, Inc.

the JCAHO and ANA's *Standards for Nursing Staff Development* (ANA, 1990).

Orientation is an important organizational tool for recruitment and retention. Orientation sessions typically occur at the initiation of employment and whenever positions and roles change. The sessions include information unique to the institution of employment, such as philosophy, goals, policies and procedures, role expectations, facilities, resources and special services, and assessment and development of competency with equipment and supplies used in the work setting (ANA,1990).

In-service education occurs after orientation and supports the nurse in acquiring, maintaining, and increasing skills to fulfill assigned responsibilities.

Nurses are responsible for their own continuing education. Continuing education offers both personal and professional growth to the nurse and constitutes an essential dimension of lifelong learning. In some states, license renewal depends on acquiring continuing education units (CEUs) according to the board of nursing's rules. Lifelong learning is essential to career development and competency achievement in nursing practice.

Trends in Nursing Education

Trends in nursing education reflect issues in nursing, nursing education, delivery of care, and the public's health. At the heart of many of these trends are two fundamental issues: competency development and delivery of care.

Competency Development

Debate concerning multiple education levels for entry level nursing practice will continue. The focus on basic competency demonstration by all entry level graduates regardless of educational level is likely to gain much greater support from nursing because it allows for both consensus about the outcome (competency) and diversity (innovation) about the process of achieving the competency. Competency development in nursing education is stimulating many changes in nursing education.

Delivery of Care

The demand for nursing care will continue to be driven by a larger aging population that makes use of long-term care and home health services. Other changes will include: expansion of primary and preventive care to focus on health promotion and wellness; an increased use of ambulatory care services because they are less expensive; increased complexity of health care delivery which requires well-educated nurses; and increased demand to provide health services such as prenatal care, well child clinics, adolescent clinics, and neighbor care clinics, to underserved populations (such as inner city residents).

Managed care arrangements are the delivery systems of the future. They emphasize wellness, disease prevention, and health promotion. What a natural fit for nursing practice! Nursing has long been aware that health behaviors, genetics, the environment, and biological factors all contribute to health. As additional contributing factors of disease point to health behaviors and preventive interventions, nursing education must provide a strong scientific base in health-seeking and health behavior frameworks that can prevent premature morbidity and mortality. The Healthy People 2010 objectives (Table 4–3) will be accomplished only through the intervention of nursing in collaboration with other disciplines.

NURSING ORGANIZATIONS

Nursing organizations exist for LP/VNs and RNs. Some organizations also welcome as members those who are interested in nursing but who are not nurses. There are also many specialty nursing organizations. Table 4–4 provides pertinent information about the various general nursing organizations.

American Nurses Association

The ANA represents registered nurses through its constituent state organizations. The ANA fosters high standards of nursing practice, promotes the economic and general welfare of nurses in the workplace, projects a positive and realistic view of nursing, and lobbies Congress and regulatory agencies on health care issues affecting nurses and the public (ANA, 1998).

National Association of Practical Nurse Education and Service, Inc.

Originally called the Association of Practical Nurse Schools, this organization was dedicated exclusively to practical nursing. The multidisciplinary membership planned the first standard curriculum for practical nursing. The name was changed to National Association of Practical Nurse Education (NAPNE) in 1942. In 1945, they established an accrediting service for practical/vocational nursing schools. This service has been discontinued for some years. In 1959, the name was changed to National Association of Practical Nurse Education and Service (NAPNES, 1998).

National Federation of Licensed Practical Nurses, Inc.

The National Federation of Licensed Practical Nurses (NFLPN) was founded in 1949 by a group of LPNs who recognized that to gain status and recognition in the health field and to have a channel through

Table 4–3 HEALTHY PEOPLE 2010: GOALS, FOCUS AREAS, AND LEADING HEALTH INDICATORS

Goals
- Increase quality and years of healthy life
- Eliminate health disparities

Focus Areas
- Access to quality health services
- Arthritis, osteoporosis, and chronic back conditions
- Cancer
- Chronic kidney disease
- Diabetes
- Disability and secondary conditions
- Educational and community-based programs
- Environmental health
- Family planning
- Food safety
- Health communication
- Heart disease and stroke
- HIV
- Immunization and infectious diseases
- Injury and violence prevention
- Maternal, infant, and child health
- Medical product safety
- Mental health and mental disorders

- Nutrition and overweight
- Occupational safety and health
- Oral health
- Physical activity and fitness
- Public health infrastructure
- Respiratory diseases
- Sexually transmitted diseases
- Substance abuse
- Tobacco use
- Vision and hearing

Leading Health Indicators
- Physical activity
- Overweight and obesity
- Tobacco use
- Substance abuse
- Responsible sexual behavior
- Mental health
- Injury and violence
- Environmental quality
- Immunizations
- Access to health care

Data from Healthy People 2010: The Prevention Agenda (2000) [On-line]. Available: http://www.health.gov/healthypeople/prevagenda/

Table 4–4 SELECTED NURSING ORGANIZATIONS

ORGANIZATION	DESCRIPTION
American Nurses Association (ANA)	Established: 1911 Purpose: To work for the improvement of health standards and availability of health care service for all people, foster high standards for nursing, stimulate and promote the professional development of nurses, and advance their economic and general welfare. Activities: • Establish standards for nursing practice • Establish a professional code of ethics • Develop educational standards • Promote nursing research • Oversee a credentialing system • Influence legislation affecting health care • Protect the economic and general welfare of registered nurses • Assist with the professional development of nurses (i.e., by providing continuing education programs) Membership: • Registered nurses only • Federation of state nurses' associations • Individual, by joining respective state nurses' association Publications: • *American Journal of Nursing* • *American Nurse*

continues

Table 4–4 SELECTED NURSING ORGANIZATIONS *continued*

ORGANIZATION	DESCRIPTION
National Association for Practical Nurse Education and Service, Inc. (NAPNES)	Established: 1941 Purpose: To improve the quality, education, and recognition of nursing schools and LP/VNs in the United States Activities: • Provide workshops, seminars, and continuing-education programs • Evaluate and certify continuing-education programs of others • Provide individual student professional liability insurance program • Inform legislatures and public on LP/VN issues • Authorize those who pass the Certification Examination for Practical and Vocational Nurses in Long-term Care (CEPN-LTC) to use the initials *CLTC* Membership: • LP/VNs • RNs, physicians, and caregivers in all fields • Practical/vocational nursing students Publications: • *Journal of Practical Nursing* • *NAPNES Forum*
National Federation of Licensed Practical Nurses, Inc. (NFLPN)	Established: 1949 Purpose: • Provide leadership for LP/VNs • Foster high standards of practical/vocational nursing education and practice • Encourage continuing education • Achieve recognition for LP/VNs • Advocate effective utilization of LP/VNs • Interpret role and function of LP/VNs • Represent practical/vocational nursing • Serve as central source of information on practical/vocational nursing education and practice Activities: • Promote continuing education of LP/VNs; evaluate programs for CEU credit • Establish principles of ethics • Offer members an opportunity to participate in activities of the organization • Keep members informed on matters of interest and concern • Offer members best type of low-cost insurance • Represent and speak for LP/VNs in Congress • Encourage fellowship among LP/VNs • Develop mutual understanding and good will among members, other allied health groups, and the general public Membership: • Three-tier concept of local, state, and national enrollment • LP/VNs • Practical/vocational nursing students • Affiliate (person who has an interest in the work of NFLPN but is neither an LP/VN nor an LP/VN student) Publication: • *Practical Nursing Today*
National League for Nursing (NLN)	Established: 1952 Purpose: To identify the nursing needs of society and to foster programs designed to meet these needs Activities: • Accredit (through voluntary participation from schools) nursing education programs • Conduct surveys to collect data on education programs

continues

Table 4–4 SELECTED NURSING ORGANIZATIONS *continued*

ORGANIZATION	DESCRIPTION

National League for Nursing (NLN) (*continued*)	• Provide continuing-education programs
	• Offer testing services, including:
	   Achievement tests for use in nursing schools
	   Preadmission testing for potential nursing students
	Membership:
	• Open to any individual or agency interested in improving nursing services or nursing education
	• Composed of both nurses and non-nurses
	Publication:
	• *Nursing & Health Care Perspectives*

National Council of State Boards of Nursing, Inc. (NCSBN)	Established: 1978 Purpose: Provide an organization through which boards of nursing act and counsel together on matters that are of common interest and concern affecting the public health, safety, and welfare, including the development of licensing examinations in nursing Activities: • Develop and administer licensure examinations for registered nurse and licensed practical/vocational nurse candidates • Conduct job analyses that provide data required to support the NCLEX examinations and the test development process • Maintain a national disciplinary data bank • Monitor and analyze issues and trends in public policy, nursing practice, and nursing education that impact nursing regulation • Serve as the national clearinghouse of information on nursing regulation • Offer educational conferences and regional meetings Membership: • Boards of nursing in the 50 states, the District of Columbia, and five United States territories Publications: • *Issues* • *NCLEX-RN Program Reports* • *NCLEX-PN Program Reports*

Data from About ANA *(On-line), by American Nurses Association, 1999, Available: http://www.ana.org/about/summary/ 99hodact.htm;* History of NAPNES, *by National Association for Practical Nurse Education and Service, Inc., 1998, Silver Spring, MD: Author; All About NFLPN (On-line), by National Federation of Licensed Practical Nurses, 2000, Available: http://www.nflpn. org/allaboutnflpn.htm; Bylaws, by National League for Nursing, 1995, New York: Author; About NLN (On-line), by National League for Nursing, 2000a, Available: http://www.nln.org/info-default.htm; About the National Council (On-line), by National Council of State Boards of Nursing, Inc., 1999, Available: http://www.ncsbn.org/files/aboutnc/*

which they could officially speak and act for themselves, they needed an organization of their own. Since 1991, affiliate membership (lacking the rights to vote and hold office) has been available to anyone who is interested in the work of NFLPN but who is neither a practicing LP/VN nor an LP/VN student. The NFLPN is the official organization for LP/VNs (NFLPN, 2000).

National League for Nursing

The National League of Nursing Education changed its bylaws in 1952 to become the NLN. Because of the growth of practical/vocational nursing programs, the NLN established a Department of Practical Nursing Programs (now called Council of Practical Nursing Programs, [CPNP]) in 1961. The NLN offers accreditation services to all nursing programs through an independent subsidiary called the National League for Nursing Accrediting Commission (NLNAC) (National League for Nursing History, 1997).

National Council of State Boards of Nursing

The National Council of State Boards of Nursing (NCSBN) was established in 1978 to assist member boards, collectively and individually, to promote safe

PROFESSIONAL TIP

Professional Memberships

Every nurse should become involved in a nursing organization. Membership means more political clout for passing legislation to improve health care for all citizens and to improve the profession of nursing.

Nursing students must stay abreast of current issues and meet with local nursing leaders to discuss health care reform, alternative health care delivery models, and other issues. Then as graduates, they will be able to share this information with both the public and legislators.

and effective nursing practice in the interest of protecting public health and welfare. They have developed the NCLEX-PN and NCLEX-RN to test the entry level nursing competence of candidates for licensure as LP/VNs and RNs (National Council of State Boards of Nursing, 1999).

In 1996, they began the administration of the first large-scale, national certification examination available to LP/VNs. It is named the Certification Examination for Practical and Vocational Nurses in Long-Term Care (CEPN-LTC™). Those who pass the examination are certified in long-term care and are authorized by NAPNES to use the initials *CLTC* to signify their new status (National Council of State Boards of Nursing, 1996).

THE FUTURE OF NURSING

History is being made daily for nurses and other health care providers as the citizens of this country decide which way to move with health care reform initiatives. Pressing issues for nursing (e.g., third-party reimbursement and prescriptive privileges for advanced practitioners) will be determined by legislative outcomes. Nurses can make the most of this time of transformation, a time driven by societal needs (Mason & Leavitt, 1995).

SUMMARY

- Nursing is an art and a science whereby people are assisted in learning to care for themselves whenever possible and are cared for when they are unable to meet their own needs.
- By studying nursing history, the nurse is better able to understand such issues as autonomy, unity within the profession, supply and demand, salary, education, and current practice, and can thus promote the empowerment of nurses.

- Nursing's early history was heavily influenced by religious organizations and the need for nurses to care for soldiers during wartime.
- Florence Nightingale forged the future of nursing practice and education as a result of her experiences in training nurses to care for soldiers.
- Early American leaders, the professional organizations, and the landmark reports of nursing determined the infrastructure of current nursing practice.
- Influential nursing leaders such as Lillian Wald, Isabel Hampton Robb, Adelaide Nutting, and Lavinia Dock were instrumental in the advancement of nursing education and practice.
- Other nursing leaders such as Mary Breckenridge, Mary Mahoney, and Linda Richards made important contributions to both nursing education and practice.
- In 1923, the Goldmark Report concluded that for nursing to be on equal footing with other disciplines, nursing education should occur in the university setting.
- The Brown Report (1948) addressed the need for nurses to demonstrate greater professional competence by moving nursing education to the university setting.
- The Health Maintenance Organization Act of 1973 provided an alternative to the private health insurance industry.
- Title III of the Health Amendment Act of 1955 resulted in the establishment of practical nursing.
- Types of programs that currently prepare nurses for entry level practice are practical/vocational, diploma, associate degree, and baccalaureate degree.

Review Questions

1. The founder of modern nursing is considered to be:
   a. Lillian Wald.
   b. Dorothea Dix.
   c. Florence Nightingale.
   d. The Nursing Sisters of the Holy Cross.

2. The founder of the American Red Cross is:
   a. Lavinia Dock.
   b. Clara Barton.
   c. Linda Richards.
   d. Adelaide Nutting.

3. The first practical nursing school was:
   a. Ballard School.
   b. Thompson Practical Nursing School.
   c. Bellevue Training School for Nurses.
   d. Household Nursing Association School of Attendant Nursing.

4. Practical nursing was established under:

   a. Bureau of Medical Services, 1908.
   b. Health Maintenance Organization Act of 1973.
   c. Title III of the Health Amendment Act of 1955.
   d. Nursing and Nursing Education in the United States, 1923.

5. Staff development includes:

   a. recruitment.
   b. license renewal.
   c. continuing education.
   d. orientation and in-service.

6. The nursing organization that accredits schools of nursing is:

   a. ANA.
   b. NLN.
   c. NFLPN.
   d. NAPNES.

7. The National Council of State Boards of Nursing began administering a national certification examination available to the LP/VN. It is for:

   a. licensure.
   b. acute care.
   c. accreditation.
   d. long-term care.

8. The major recommendation of both the Goldmark and Brown reports was to:

   a. recruit more people into the nursing profession.

b. compensate nurses with higher salaries and more comprehensive benefits.
c. place nursing education within institutions of higher learning.
d. increase the amount of clinical practice in nursing education programs.

Critical Thinking Questions

1. Think of some lessons you have learned from the past. Can you identify some life experiences that have been excellent teachers? List two lessons gained from these experiences or situations.

2. Florence Nightingale has been described as being strong minded and assertive. In what ways would it be helpful for you to develop such characteristics?

 WEB FLASH!

- Search for nursing history, nursing education, and nursing organizations on the web. How many resources do you find for each topic?
- What type of information is provided about the nursing organizations? Is it enough to make a decision about becoming a member of an organization?

THE HEALTH CARE DELIVERY SYSTEM

MAKING THE CONNECTION

Refer to the following chapters to increase your understanding of the health care delivery system:

- **Chapter 6, Legal Responsibilities**
- **Chapter 7, Ethical Responsibilities**
- **Chapter 15, Wellness Concepts**

LEARNING OBJECTIVES

Upon completion of this chapter, you should be able to:
- *Define key terms.*
- *Describe the types of services in the U.S. health care delivery system.*
- *Discuss the various health care settings through which health care services are delivered.*
- *Identify the members of the health care team and their respective roles.*
- *Describe the differences among financial programs for health care services and reimbursement.*
- *Explain the factors that influence health care delivery.*
- *Identify the challenges to providing care.*
- *Discuss nursing's role in meeting the challenges within the health care system.*
- *Describe the emerging trends and issues for the health care delivery system.*

KEY TERMS

capitated rate	preferred provider
comorbidity	organization
exclusive provider	prescriptive authority
organization	primary care
fee-for-service	primary care provider
health care delivery	primary health care
system	prospective payment
health maintenance	secondary care
organization	single-payer system
managed care	single point of entry
medical model	tertiary care

INTRODUCTION

A **health care delivery system** is a mechanism for providing services that meet the health-related needs of individuals. The U.S. health care delivery system is currently experiencing dramatic change. Health care institutions that once flourished economically are now searching for ways to survive. Health care providers are seeking cost-effective ways to deliver an ever-increasing range of services to consumers. Consumers are demanding greater accessibility to quality health care services that are also affordable. The increase in consumerism is fueled by the Internet, regulatory changes, the rising popularity of nontraditional therapies, and frustration of clients and their families feeling they have been mistreated by the system (Haugh, 1999).

Nursing is a major component of the U.S. health care delivery system. Consequently, nurses must understand the changes occurring within this system, as well as nursing's role in shaping those changes. This chapter explores the types of health care services available, the various settings where those services are offered, and the members of the health care team. The economics of health care and the challenges within the health care delivery system are also addressed, as is nursing's role in meeting those challenges.

TYPES OF HEALTH CARE SERVICES

Health care services can be classified into three levels: primary, secondary, and tertiary. The complexity of care varies according to the individual's need, the provider's expertise, and the delivery setting. Table 5–1 provides an overview of the types of care. The trend is toward holistic care, that is, care of the entire person

Table 5–1 TYPES OF HEALTH CARE SERVICES

TYPE OF CARE	DESCRIPTION	EXAMPLES
Primary	*Goal:* To decrease the risk to a client (individual or community) for disease or dysfunction *Explanation:* General health promotion Protection against specific illnesses	Teaching Lifestyle modification for health (e.g., smoking cessation, nutrition counseling) Referrals Immunization Promotion of a safe environment (e.g., sanitation, protection from toxic agents)
Secondary	*Goal:* To alleviate disease and prevent further disability *Explanation:* Early detection and intervention	Screenings Acute care Various therapies Surgery
Tertiary	*Goal:* To minimize effects and permanent disability associated with chronic or irreversible conditions *Explanation:* Restorative and rehabilitative activities to attain optimal level of functioning	Education and retraining Provision of direct care Environmental intervention (e.g., advising on necessity of wheelchair accessibility for a person who has experienced a cardiovascular accident [stroke])

including physiological, psychological, social, intellectual, and spiritual aspects.

Primary Care

The major purposes of **primary care** are to promote wellness and prevent illness or disability. Care is coordinated by the office of the primary care provider, usually a family practice physician, pediatrician, internal medicine physician, or family nurse practitioner. Traditionally, the U.S. health care system focused on illness treatment rather than wellness promotion. Within the past two decades, however, focus has shifted to health-promoting behaviors such as regular exercise, reducing fat in the diet, reducing air pollution, and monitoring cholesterol level. Illness prevention activities may be directed toward the individual, the family, or the community.

Under the traditional **medical model**, our health care delivery system was not a *health* care system at all, but, rather, an *illness* care system. Services have traditionally been directed toward caring for an individual after disease or disability has developed rather than emphasizing preventive aspects of care (Pruitt & Campbell, 1994). Today, however, there is more of an emphasis on the holistic promotion of wellness and on the preventive aspects of care.

Secondary Care

Services within the realm of **secondary care**—diagnosis and treatment—occur after the client exhibits symptoms of illness. Acute treatment centers (hospitals) still constitute the predominant site for the delivery of these health care services. However, there is a growing movement to provide diagnostic and therapeutic services in locations that are more easily accessed by the population. These are often satellite care centers of a major hospital, where holistic care is promoted.

Tertiary Care

Restoring an individual to the state of health that existed before the development of an illness is the purpose of **tertiary** (rehabilitative) **care**. In situations where the person is unable to regain previous functional abilities, the goal of rehabilitation is to attain the optimal level of health possible, for example, a client regaining partial use of an arm after experiencing a stroke. Restorative care is holistic in that the physiological, psychological, social, and spiritual aspects of the person are all addressed in the provision of care.

HEALTH CARE DELIVERY SYSTEM

The U.S. health care delivery system is complex, involving myriad providers, consumers, settings, personnel, and services.

Providers/Consumers

Health care services in the United States are delivered by public (including official and voluntary), public/private, and private sectors. Consumers are the individuals who receive the health care services.

Public Sector

Public agencies are financed with tax monies; thus, these agencies are accountable to the public. The public sector includes official (or governmental) agencies and voluntary agencies. Figure 5-1 shows the hierarchy of the official agencies in the public sector of health care delivery.

At the national level, the U.S. Department of Health and Human Services (USDHHS) is administratively responsible for health care services delivered to the public. The U.S. Public Health Service (USPHS) is the major agency that oversees the actual delivery of care services. Table 5–2 lists the USPHS agencies and their purposes. The Veterans Administration (VA) has hospitals and clinics that provide services to veterans of the armed services. These services are also financed with tax monies.

Each state varies in the provision of public health services. Generally, a state department of health coordinates the activities of local health units.

At the local level, services provided include immunizations, maternal–child care, and activities directed toward controlling chronic diseases.

Voluntary agencies also constitute an important part of the public sector of the health care delivery system. These not-for-profit agencies (e.g., the National Federation of Licensed Practical Nurses [NFLPN], the American Nurses Association [ANA], the National League for

Table 5–2 AGENCIES OF THE U.S. PUBLIC HEALTH SERVICE	
AGENCY	**PURPOSE**
Health Resources and Services Administration (HRSA)	Provide health-related information Administer programs concerned with health care for the homeless; people with human immunodeficiency virus (HIV) and acquired immuno-deficiency syndrome (AIDS); organ transplants; rural health care; and employee occupational health
Food and Drug Administration (FDA)	Protect the public from unsafe drugs, food, and cosmetics
Centers for Disease Control and Prevention (CDC)	Study and prevent the transmission of communicable diseases
National Institutes of Health (NIH)	Conduct research and education related to specific illnesses
Alcohol, Drug Abuse, and Mental Health Administration (ADAMHA)	Serve as clearinghouse for information on substance abuse and mental health issues
Agency for Toxic Substances and Disease Registry (ATSDR)	Maintain registry of certain diseases Provide information on toxic agents Conduct mortality and morbidity studies on defined population groups
Indian Health Service (IHS)	Provide health care services to Native Americans, including health promotion, disease prevention, alcoholism prevention, substance abuse prevention, suicide prevention, nutrition, maternal–child health
Agency for Health Care Policy and Research (AHCPR)	Serve as primary source of federal support for research related to quality of health care delivery

Nursing [NLN], and the American Medical Association [AMA]) can exert significant legislative influence. Other voluntary agencies, such as the American Cancer Society and the American Heart Association, provide educational resources to the general public and to health care providers, such as dietary suggestions along with corresponding recipes. Voluntary agencies are funded in a variety of ways including individual contributions, corporate philanthropy, and membership dues.

Public/Private Sector

A blending of the public and private sectors in many areas of health care has gradually occurred following the inception of Medicare and the diagnosis-related groups (DRGs), discussed in an upcoming section. Federal regulations guide both the care provided to clients in private nonprofit and for-profit agencies by private physicians and the reimbursement to both the agencies and the physicians.

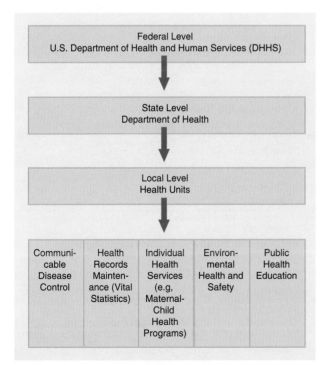

Figure 5-1 The Public Sector of Health Care Delivery (*From Fundamentals of Nursing: Standards & Practice, by S. DeLaune and P. Ladner, 1998, Albany, NY: Delmar. Copyright 1998 by Delmar. Reprinted with permission.*)

Private Sector

The private sector of the health care delivery system is composed primarily of independent health care agencies and providers who are reimbursed on a **fee-for-service** basis (the recipient directly pays the provider for services as they are provided). Fee-for-service clients may have private insurance or use their own financial resources to pay the provider for services rendered.

Settings

The variety of settings where health care is delivered and the roles of nurses in these settings are presented in Table 5–3.

Table 5–3 HEALTH CARE SETTINGS

SETTING	SERVICES PROVIDED	NURSE'S ROLE
Hospital	Diagnosis and treatment of illnesses (acute and chronic) Acute inpatient services Ambulatory care services Critical (intensive) care Rehabilitative care Surgical interventions Diagnostic procedures	Serves as caregiver Educates clients Provides ongoing assessment Coordinates care and collaborates with other health care providers Maintains client safety Initiates discharge planning Can specialize in a variety of areas: • Obstetrics • Nursery • Cardiology • Obstetrics • Critical care • Oncology • Dialysis • Orthopedics • Emergency • Pediatrics • Geriatrics • Psychiatry • Infection control • Rehabilitation • Neurology • Surgery
Extended-care (long-term care) facilities (e.g., nursing homes, skilled nursing facilities)	Intermediate and long-term care for people who have chronic illnesses and are unable to care for themselves Restorative care until client is ready for discharge home	Provides care directed toward meeting basic needs (e.g., nutrition, hydration, comfort, elimination) Provides teaching and counseling Plans and coordinates care Administers medications, treatments, and other therapeutic modalities
Home health care agencies	Wide range of services, including curative and rehabilitative	Provides skilled nursing care Coordinates health-promotion activities (e.g., education)
Hospices	Care of individuals who have terminal illnesses Improving the quality of life until death	Promotes comfort measures Provides pain control Supports grieving families Educates family/client
Out-patient settings (clinics, physician's offices, ambulatory treatment centers)	Treatment of illness (acute and chronic) Diagnostic testing Simple surgical procedures	*Traditional role:* Checks vital signs Assists with diagnostic tests Prepares client for examination *Expanded role:* Provides teaching and counseling Performs physical (or mental status) examination In some settings, advanced practice registered nurses (APRNs) act as primary care providers
Schools (school-based clinics [SBCs])	Federally funded to provide physical and mental health services in middle and high schools	Coordinates health-promotion and disease prevention activities Treats minor illnesses Provides health education *continues*

Table 5–3 HEALTH CARE SETTINGS *continued*

SETTING	SERVICES PROVIDED	NURSE'S ROLE
Industrial clinics	Maintain health and safety of workers	Coordinates health-promotion activities Provides education for safety Provides urgent care as needed Maintains health records Conducts ongoing screenings Provides preventive services (e.g., tuberculosis testing)
Managed care organizations	Reimbursement for health care services	Serves as case manager Uses triage to determine the most appropriate intervention for various clients
Community nursing centers	Direct access to professional services	Treats client's responses to health problems Promotes health and wellness
Rural primary care hospitals (RPCHs)	Stabilize clients until they are physiologically able to be transferred to more-skilled facilities	Performs assessments and provides emergency care

Personnel and Services

Many personnel and services exist within the various health care settings. Large hospitals provide the greatest number of services. Other health care settings may provide some but not all of these same services. The service departments most commonly found in the various settings include nursing units, specialized client care units, diagnostic departments, therapy departments, and support services.

Nursing Units

Nursing units are composed of client rooms, where most nursing care is provided. Units often serve one particular type of client such as cardiac, orthopedic, diabetic, surgical, pediatric, or obstetric. The nurse responsible for the unit may be called by several different titles, such as unit coordinator, nurse manager, or head nurse. Registered nurses (RNs), licensed practical/vocational nurses (LP/VNs), and nursing assistants provide the nursing care.

Specialized Client Care Units

Specialized units provide nursing care for specific needs of the clients. The LP/VN may work in these areas depending on experience, education, the size and location of the hospital, and the number of RNs available. Examples of specialized units include the following:

- Emergency department (ED): provides care to clients involved in all types of accidents and those confronted with medical emergencies such as heart attack or stroke
- Intensive care unit (ICU): provides care to critically ill clients until they are stabilized and can be managed with routine nursing interventions on a regular nursing unit
- Coronary care unit (CCU): provides care to clients who have had a heart attack or who have had heart surgery such as coronary artery bypass or valve replacement
- Mental health unit: provides care to clients who are having difficulty with relationships, coping with everyday demands, or dealing with a crisis
- Psychiatric unit: provides care to clients diagnosed as having mental illness
- Rehabilitation unit: provides care to clients who must learn to regain the highest level of self-care possible following injury, accident, or illness such as heart attack or stroke
- Dialysis unit: provides care to clients who need dialysis because of renal failure
- Hospice unit: provides both care to clients who are dying and support to their families; may be a unit in a hospital or a freestanding unit
- Outpatient unit: provides care to clients when admission to the hospital is unnecessary
- Home care: provides care to clients in their homes when professional supervision and/or minimal care is required; has been added to many hospitals to provide continuity of care
- Client education unit: provides teaching to clients, either individually or in groups, about specific client conditions or other health-related issues

Surgical Units

Care of the client just before, during, and after surgery is performed by the operating room (OR) and recovery room (RR) personnel. In addition to the main surgical unit, many hospitals also have a day surgery/ambulatory surgery unit. Clients come in a couple of hours before their scheduled surgeries and leave when recovered from the anesthesia. Total length of stay is shorter than 24 hours.

Diagnostic Departments

Diagnostic departments provide specialized tests that assist the physician in making a diagnosis for the client.

Clinical Laboratory Clinical laboratory personnel examine specimens of tissues, feces, and body fluids such as blood, sputum, urine, amniotic fluid, and spinal fluid. Testing assesses values of normal components as well as abnormal components of these specimens.

Radiology Department X-ray studies are performed in the radiology department, sometimes called nuclear medicine. This department also performs computed tomography (CT) scans, mammography, ultrasound, arteriograms, venograms, echocardiograms, and magnetic resonance imaging (MRI).

Other Diagnostic Services Other diagnostic services may include the following:

- Sleep center: provides observation, testing, and monitoring of clients as they sleep, to identify sleep-related problems
- Electroencephalography (EEG): records brain waves and ascertains electrical activity in the brain
- Electrocardiogram (ECG): records electrical activity in the heart
- Electromyogram (EMG): records electrical activity in body muscles

Therapy Departments

The function of the various therapy departments is to provide specialized treatments and/or rehabilitation services to clients to improve functional level in a specific area. Most hospitals have respiratory therapy and physical therapy departments. Some large teaching hospitals also have occupational therapy and speech therapy departments.

Support Services

Support services meet various other needs in providing care to clients.

Pharmacists mix and dispense medications to the various client care units. Nurses then administer the medications to the clients.

Dietitians supervise food preparation for all clients. They specifically choose the foods and calculate the amounts for special diets and provide client teaching for those clients on special diets.

Social workers help clients deal with psychosocial problems, providing assistance in areas such as housing, finances, and referrals to support groups.

Chaplains provide individual counseling to clients and support to families and assist clients in meeting spiritual needs.

The admission department handles the admission process by preparing necessary paperwork and ensuring that the ordered preadmission laboratory testing and x-rays are performed.

The business office oversees insurance and financial affairs upon client discharge from the health care agency.

Medical records, also called health information systems, maintains and stores all medical records for every client ever cared for by the health care agency.

Housekeeping and maintenance keep the physical facilities and equipment clean, in good repair, and in proper working order.

HEALTH CARE TEAM

Health care services are delivered by a multidisciplinary team (Figure 5-2). Table 5–4 lists the various health care team members, their educational requirements, and their roles. Because nurses work with the other team members on an ongoing basis, it is necessary to understand the role of each team member.

The nurse fulfills a variety of roles in assisting clients to meet their needs. Table 5–5 defines the most common roles of nurses. Nurses function in independent, interdependent, and dependent roles. In the independent role, the nurse requires no direction or order from another health care professional, for example, in deciding that a client's edematous arm should be elevated. In the interdependent role, the nurse works in collaboration with other health care professionals,

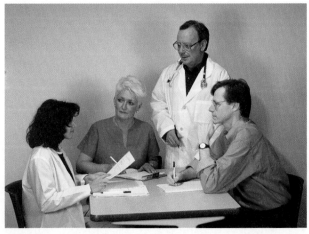

Figure 5-2 Members of the health care team work together for the benefit of the client.

Table 5–4 HEALTH CARE TEAM MEMBERS

TEAM MEMBER	EDUCATION	FUNCTION/ROLE
Nurse (LP/VN, RN, and APRN)	LP/VN: 1 year RN: 2 to 4 years APRN (Advanced Practice Registered Nurse): 1 to 3 years post-RN	Emphasizes health (wellness) promotion With a holistic approach, assists clients in coping with illness or disability by providing nursing care, health and health care education, and discharge planning Formulates nursing diagnoses to guide plan of care Addresses the needs of the client (individual, family, or community) Assists physician Functions may vary by state and specialization
Physician (medical doctor [MD])	8+ years	Formulates medical diagnoses and prescribes therapeutic modalities Performs medical procedures (e.g., surgery) May specialize in a variety of areas (e.g., gynecology/obstetrics, oncology, surgery)
Physician's assistant (PA)	2 years (plus a master's degree for PA licensure, required in many states)	Provides medical services under the supervision of a physician
Registered pharmacist (RPh)	5 to 6 years	Prepares and dispenses drugs for therapeutic use May be involved in client education
Dentist (both doctor of dental surgery [DDS] and doctor of dental medicine [DMD])	8+ years	Diagnoses and treats conditions affecting the mouth, teeth, and gums Performs preventive measures to promote dental health
Registered dietitian (RD)	4+ years	Plans diets to meet special needs of clients Promotes health and prevents disease through education and counseling May supervise preparation of meals
Social worker (SW)	4 years	Assists clients with psychosocial problems (e.g., financial, housing, marital) May assist with discharge planning Makes referrals to support groups
Respiratory therapist (RT)	2 years	Administers pulmonary function tests Performs therapeutic measures to assist with respiration (e.g., oxygen administration, ventilation) Provides various treatments for respiratory illnesses and conditions
Physical therapist (PT)	4 years	Works with clients experiencing musculoskeletal problems Assesses client's strength and mobility Performs therapeutic measures (e.g., range of motion, massage, application of heat and cold) Teaches new skills (e.g., crutch walking)
Occupational therapist (OT)	4 years	Works with clients who have functional impairment to teach skills for activities of daily living
Speech therapist	4 years	Assists clients who have speech impairments to speak understandably or to learn another method of communication
Chaplain	8 years	Assists clients in meeting spiritual needs Provides individual counseling Provides support to families Conducts religious services

Table 5-5 NURSING ROLES

ROLE	DESCRIPTION
Caregiver: LP/VN and RN	Traditional and most essential role Functions as nurturer Provides direct care Is supportive Demonstrates clinical proficiency Promotes comfort of client
Teacher: LP/VN and RN	Provides information Serves as counselor Seeks to empower clients in self-care Encourages compliance with prescribed therapy Promotes healthy lifestyles Interprets information
Advocate: LP/VN and RN	Protects the client Provides explanations in client's language Acts as change agent Supports client's decisions
Manager: LP/VN and RN	Makes decisions Coordinates activities of others Allocates resources Evaluates care and personnel Serves as a leader Takes initiative
Expert: RN	Advanced practice clinician Conducts research Teaches in schools of nursing Develops theory Contributes to professional literature Provides testimony at governmental hearings and in court
Case manager: RN	Tracks client's progress through the health care system Coordinates care to ensure continuity
Team member: LP/VN and RN	Collaborates with others Possesses excellent communication skills

for example, in a client care conference where several members of the health care team together plan ways to meet the client's needs. In the dependent role, the nurse requires direction from a physician or dentist, for example, medications must be ordered by a physician or dentist before a nurse may administer them to the client. The degree of autonomy nurses experience is related to client needs, nurse expertise, and practice setting.

ECONOMICS OF HEALTH CARE

The reform movement in health care has been motivated primarily by costs. Control of costs has shifted from the health care providers to the insurers, with the result being increasing constraints on reimbursement. For years, the predominant method of covering health care costs was fee for service, and there was little, if any, incentive for cost-effective delivery of care (Chamberlain, Chen, Osuna, & Yamamoto, 1995). All that is changing.

The U.S. health care system has a diverse financial base, composed of both private and public funding. As a result, administrative costs for health care reimbursement are higher in this country than in countries with a **single-payer system** (a model wherein the government is the only entity to reimburse health care costs, such as in Canada). The level of U.S. health care expenditures is higher than that of any other nation, and previous cost-containment measures have been ineffective in slowing the growth in expenditures (Schieber, Poullier, & Greenwald, 1997). Despite the enormous expenditure of public funds, the United States has not found a way to provide health care coverage for all citizens. Figure 5-3 shows the sources of the nation's health dollars in 1998.

Private Insurance

The system for financing health care services in the United States is based on the private insurance model. Private insurance companies constitute one of the largest sectors of the health care system. Currently, more than 1,000 private insurance companies exist

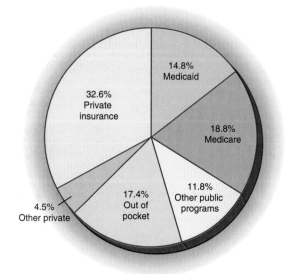

Figure 5-3 Source of the Nation's Health Dollar in 1998. (*Health Care Financing Administration, 2000.*)

(Feldstein, 1999). Payment rates to health care providers vary among insurance companies.

In the United States, insured individuals pay substantial monthly premiums for insurance coverage having high deductibles for health care services. For many, these costs may prove barriers to procuring necessary insurance coverage and health services. In addition, insurers will no longer pay for services that *they* deem unnecessary, effectively taking client care decisions out of the hands of physicians. The quality of care provided is now being monitored not only by providers (physicians), but by third-party payers (insurance companies) and, ever increasingly, by consumers.

Managed Care

Managed care is a system of providing and monitoring care wherein access, cost, and quality are controlled before or during delivery of services. The goal of managed care is the delivery of services in the most cost-efficient manner possible. Managed care organizations combine the financing and delivery of health care services. Managed care seeks to control costs by monitoring delivery of services and restricting access to expensive procedures and providers.

Managed care was designed to provide coordinated services with an emphasis on prevention and primary care (ANA, 1995). The rationale behind managed care is to give consumers preventive services delivered by a **primary care provider** (a health care provider whom a client sees first for health care; typically, a family practitioner, internist, or pediatrician). The primary care provider is responsible for managing or coordinating all care of a client when illness makes referrals necessary. This is supposed to result in less expensive interventions.

Managed care has been in existence for years; however, it is only within the past 20 years that it has enjoyed national prominence (Society for Ambulatory Care Professionals, 1994). The Health Maintenance Organization Act (passed in 1973) implemented two mandates. First, federal grants and loans were made available to **health maintenance organizations** (HMOs) (prepaid health plans that provide primary health care services for a preset fee and that focus on cost-effective treatment measures) that complied with strict federal regulations as opposed to the less-restrictive state requirements. Second, large employers were required to provide to employees an HMO as an option for health care coverage (Society for Ambulatory Care Professionals, 1994). From their inception, HMOs have constituted a viable alternative to the traditional fee-for-service system.

Managed care is not a place but, rather, an organizational structure with several variations. One such variation is the HMO, which is both provider and insurer. Other variations are **preferred provider organiza-**

Table 5–6 COMPARISON OF INDEPENDENT PRACTICE AND MANAGED CARE	
TYPE	**DESCRIPTION**
Independent Practice	Fee for service or salary
	Functions within socially prescribed boundaries (professional ethics)
	Free choice of provider
	Disease-oriented philosophy
Managed Care	
Health maintenance organizations (HMOs)	Provide services to a group of enrolled persons
	Preset and prepaid fees
	Limited to certain providers
Preferred provider organizations (PPOs)	Networks of providers that give discounts to sponsoring organization
	Members' choice of physician not mandated, but lesser reimbursement if physician is outside of the network
Exclusive provider organizations (EPOs)	No benefit if member is treated outside of the network
	Usually regulated by state insurance laws

tions (PPOs), wherein members must use providers within the system in order to obtain full reimbursement but may use other providers for lesser reimbursement, and **exclusive provider organizations** (EPOs) wherein care must be delivered by the providers in the plan in order for clients to receive any reimbursement. In the past decade, there has been a great shift on the part of the population from private insurance to HMOs and PPOs (Feldstein, 1999). Table 5–6 compares independent practice and managed care organizational structures.

Health Maintenance Organizations

Health maintenance organizations often maintain primary health care sites (although not necessarily) and commonly employ provider professionals. They use **capitated rates** (preset flat fees based on membership in, not services provided by, the HMO), assume the risk of clients who are heavy users, and exert control over the use of services. Health maintenance organizations have been noted for using advanced practice registered nurses (APRNs) as primary care providers and using precertification programs to limit unnecessary hospitalization. Further, HMOs emphasize client education for health promotion and self-care.

Another common feature of HMOs is the practice of **single point of entry** (entry into the health care system through a point designated by the plan), through which primary care is delivered. **Primary health care** is the client's point of entry into the health care system and includes assessment, diagnosis, treatment, coordination of care, education, preventive services, and surveillance. It comprises the spectrum of services provided by a family practitioner (nurse or physician) in an ambulatory setting. Primary care providers (PCPs) serve as "gatekeepers" to the health care system, in that they determine which, if any, referrals to specialists are needed by the client. To reduce costs, HMOs purposely limit direct access to specialists. Managed care plans assume a significant portion of the risk of providing health care and, consequently, encourage prudent use by both consumers and providers. In 1976, there were 175 HMOs in the United States; by 1995 there were 591 (Feldstein, 1999).

Preferred Provider Organizations

The most common managed care systems are PPOs. A PPO represents a contractual relationship between hospitals, providers, insurers, employers, and third-party payers to form a network wherein providers negotiate with group purchasers to provide health services for a defined population at a predetermined price (Feldstein, 1999). Care received within the network is associated with the highest reimbursement; care received outside the network is associated with lower reimbursement, with the client paying the difference. Preferred provider organizations have been very popular in the United States. In fact, the number of PPOs has increased from fewer than 10 in 1981 to over 700 in 1994 (Feldstein, 1999).

Exclusive Provider Organizations

Exclusive provider organizations create a network of providers (such as physicians and hospitals) and offer the incentive of consumer services for little or no copayment if the network providers are used exclusively. If a member receives treatment outside of the network, no benefit is paid. For instance, a member who becomes ill and receives treatment while visiting relatives in another state would receive no benefits for the treatment.

Federal Government Insurance Plans

The federal government became a third-party payer for health care services with the advent of Medicare and Medicaid in 1965. The Health Care Financing Administration (HCFA) is a federal agency that regulates Medicare, Medicaid, and Children's Health Insurance Program (CHIP) expenditures. There are many public programs for the financing of health care, with Medicare and Medicaid being the predominant ones. Medicare is the federally funded program that provides health care coverage for elderly persons and disabled persons. Medicaid pro-

vides health care coverage for the poor. Children's Health Insurance Program is a partnership between the federal and state governments to cover previously uninsured children.

With the ultimate goal of curtailing spending for hospitalized Medicare recipients, the federal government created diagnosis-related groups (DRGs) to categorize the average cost of care for each diagnosis. A prospective payment system was then created based on the DRGs. **Prospective payment** is a predetermined rate paid for each episode of hospitalization based on the client's age and principal diagnosis and on the presence or absence of surgery and **comorbidity** (simultaneous existence of more than one disease process in an individual). Hospitals are reimbursed the predetermined amount regardless of the actual cost of providing services to the client. The prospective payment system, originally designed for Medicare, has been adopted by other agencies and insurance companies.

Medicare

When Medicare was established in 1965, it was intended to protect individuals over the age of 65 years from exorbitant health care costs. In 1972, Medicare was modified to also cover permanently disabled individuals and those with end-stage renal disease. Because many individuals over the age of 65 do not have employee-paid insurance, public funds cover the majority of health care services for elderly persons (USD-HHS, 1993).

Medicaid

Medicaid is the largest third-party payer of nursing home health care expenditures (Feldstein, 1999). Medicaid is a shared venture between the federal and state governments. Each state has latitude in determining who is "medically indigent" and, thus, qualifies for pub-

 PROFESSIONAL TIP

Impact of Prospective Payment System and DRGs

- Decreased length of client stay in hospitals
- More emphasis on preventive care
- Increased concern about consumer's (client's) response to care
- An increased number of critically ill clients in hospitals
- Clients sicker upon discharge from hospital
- An increase in outpatient care
- Client and family more responsible for care
- Greater need for home health care
- Mergers or closures of hospitals because of inordinate competition

lic monies. Minimal services covered by Medicaid are defined by the federal government and include inpatient and outpatient hospital services, physician services, laboratory services (including x-ray), and rural health clinic services. States may elect to cover other services, such as dental, vision, and prescription drug.

Children's Health Insurance Program

Children's Health Insurance Program was created in 1997 as part of the Balanced Budget Act. The program is designed to provide health care to uninsured children, many of whom are members of working families that earn too little to afford private insurance on their own but earn too much to be eligible for Medicaid.

FACTORS INFLUENCING HEALTH CARE

Despite cost-containment efforts (such as DRGs, established by the federal government, and managed care, established by the insurers), the U.S. health care system still has problems with issues of cost, access, and quality. These issues are important for nurses to understand and are integral to any effort toward health reform.

Cost

Cost has been a driving force for change in the health care system as evidenced by the strength and numbers of managed care plans, increased use of outpatient treatment, and shortened hospital stays. These market forces (to maximize profits by minimizing costs) are dominating the current changes in the health care system.

The cost of providing health care has risen dramatically during the past 15 years. The U.S. government spends more on health care per person than does any other country (O'Neil, 1993). The increasing consumption of federal funds for health care means that resources are being moved from other areas of need, such as education, housing, and social services (Grace, 1997). Figure 5-4 illustrates health care expenditures.

The most cost-efficient programs in terms of administration are Medicare and Medicaid (HCFA, 1998). It should be noted that the administration of these programs is subcontracted to private agencies and organizations. In contrast, some private plans, particularly small business plans, use over 40 cents of each dollar for administration. The cost of employee health care benefits is thus an expensive commitment for small businesses.

Three major factors increase the cost of health care: (1) an oversupply of specialized providers (fees are raised to maintain provider income in light of fewer clients); (2) a surplus of hospital beds (empty beds are a cost liability); and (3) the passive role assumed by

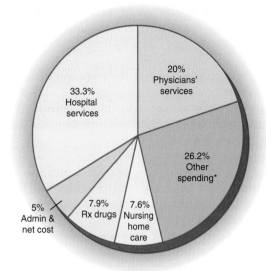

Figure 5-4 Health Care Expenditures in 1997. *Note:* Other spending included dental services, other professional services, home health, durable medical products, OTC medicines and sundries, public health, research, and construction. (*Health Care Financing Administration, 2000.*)

most consumers (when someone else pays the bill, consumers typically are less concerned about cost) (Feldstein, 1999). Other factors that contribute to the high cost of health care are the aging population, the increased number of people with chronic illnesses, the increase in health-related lawsuits and the associated unnecessary use of services (e.g., additional diagnostic testing), and advanced technology that has allowed more people to survive formerly fatal illnesses even though those people require extensive and lifelong care.

Access

Related to the issue of cost is that of access to health care services, which carries serious implications for the functioning of the health care system. As a result of high costs, health care for many people is crisis oriented and fragmented. Numerous people in the United States are unable to gain access to health care services because of inadequate or no insurance; thus, illness among these people may progress to an acute stage before intervention is sought. Services used by individuals during acute illnesses are typically provided by emergency departments. Emergency room and acute care services are expensive when compared to early intervention and preventive measures.

Only a small portion of the medically indigent are covered by Medicare. In addition, many individuals are underinsured. These people are neither poor nor old but, rather, are middle-class unemployed Americans or those who have jobs lacking adequate health care benefits. In addition to poverty and unemployment, other factors can hinder a person's ability to obtain insurance and/or health care services, including the following:

- Lack of insurance provision by employer because of prohibitive costs
- High costs of obtaining individual insurance
- Certain preexisting conditions making it difficult to obtain insurance
- Cultural barriers
- Shortages of health care providers in some geographic areas (especially rural or inner city areas)
- Limited access to ancillary services (e.g., child care and transportation)
- Status as single-parent or two-income family, making it difficult for parents to take time from work to transport children to health care providers

Quality

It is estimated that 30% to 40% of diagnostic and medical procedures performed in this country are unnecessary (Lee, Soffel, & Luft, 1997). This inappropriate use of resources can be traced to several factors, including:

- The litigious environment and resultant tendency toward defensive practice (e.g., ordering all possible tests instead of only those that the provider deems truly necessary).
- The widely held American belief that more is better.
- Lack of access to and continuity of services and the subsequent misuse of acute care services.

The greatest number of health care dollars are expended in the last days of life, with 40% of in-hospital days and 35% of prescription medications being used

 CULTURAL CONSIDERATIONS

Barriers to Health Care Services
Certain cultural beliefs and values may prevent individuals from seeking health care. These may include the following:

- Belief in divine healing
- Refusal of care on holy days
- Belief that the individual taking the ill person to a health care facility is responsible for the ill person for the rest of that person's life after recovery
- Belief that illness is a result of sins committed in previous life
- View of prayer as a tool for deliverance from illness
- Belief that illness is God's punishment

by elderly persons. Twelve percent of the U.S. population is aged 65 years or older and uses 33% of health care expenditures (Rowe, 1996).

In an attempt to provide universal access to services in a cost-effective manner, quality may be sacrificed. For example, hospitals that are reducing the numbers of nurses ("downsizing") risk endangering quality. Safety and quality are frequently compromised by the inappropriate substitution of unqualified personnel for LP/VNs and RNs in direct care of clients. Cross-training of staff, increased use of unlicensed personnel, and reductions in full-time positions for nurses are affecting the type of care delivered in hospitals. Any movement toward reform must focus on providing quality nursing care to all consumers.

CHALLENGES WITHIN THE HEALTH CARE SYSTEM

The major challenges facing the U.S. health care delivery system—which also happen to impact the control of costs—include the public's disillusionment with providers; providers' and consumers' loss of control over health care decisions; decreased use of hospitals and the accompanying negative impact on quality of care; changing practice settings; ethical issues; and vulnerable populations.

Disillusionment with Providers

Greed and waste have been identified as major problems of the U.S. health care system (Maraldo, 1997). Whether these problems are caused by defensive practice, consumer demand, or professional economics is irrelevant to the public. Success in reform depends on starting where the public expects reform should begin: eliminating the greed of providers and the waste in the health care system. Further, people in the United States have become suspicious of health care providers. The high level of esteem in which medicine has traditionally been held has eroded over the past few years. Consumers, increasingly tired of paying the high cost of care, are questioning medical practices and fees (Zerwekh & Claborn, 1997). However, the public is not disillusioned with nurses (Kellogg Foundation, 1994). As reported in the *American Journal of Nursing* (AJN), a November 1999 Gallup poll reported that almost three-quarters of those surveyed rated the honesty and ethics of nurses as "high" or "very high" (Health Care News, 2000). Nursing received higher ratings than any other profession including other health care professionals. Nurse Week and Sigma Theta Tau International commissioned another survey. It revealed that 92% of the public trust health information provided by registered nurses. This positive perception of nurses will be important as patterns of reform are established.

Positive Perception of Nurses

Several studies (ANA, 1993a; Kellogg Foundation, 1994) verify the public's trust in nurses. The public sees nurses as part of the solution, not the problem, and believes that if nurses were allowed to use their skills, they would significantly enhance quality and reduce costs. One survey (ANA, 1993a) inquired about consumer receptivity to nurses' taking on expanded responsibilities. Respondents supported **prescriptive authority** (legal recognition of the ability to prescribe medications) for RNs and endorsed the role of nurses in performing physical examinations and managing minor acute illnesses. Nurses should expand their focus on holistic care and spend as much time as possible on prevention of illness and wellness issues.

Loss of Control

Providers feel they have lost control over the care they provide to their clients. Increasingly, the insurance companies or the managed care organizations decide which care can and which care cannot be provided to the client.

Consumers express feeling terrorized by the health care delivery system. They feel they have lost personal control over their health care. Many stay in their current jobs because of their health care benefits or give up employment mobility out of fear of being denied a new policy because of preexisting conditions.

Decreased Hospital Use

In the early 20th century, hospitals focused on providing care to those who had no caregivers in the family or community. The focus of these early institutions was care as opposed to cure (Grace, 1997). The focus of hospitals changed in the mid-1940s as a result of technological changes and the passage by Congress in 1946 of the Hill–Burton Act, which provided funding for the renovation and construction of hospitals. One unanticipated outcome of this act was a substantial oversupply of hospital beds. Health care costs escalated because of the need to keep the hospital beds occupied: Everyone was put in the hospital, for everything from a complete physical examination, to specific diagnostic testing, to acute care or surgery.

From 1945 to 1982, the demand for hospital beds steadily increased. After 1982, however, a steady decline in the number of hospital admissions and the average length of stay occurred (Grace, 1997). In 1995, there were 23.7% fewer inpatient days than in 1985 (Feldstein, 1999). Many small hospitals have had to close their doors because they could no longer compete with the large hospitals.

Currently, hospitals continue to be the nucleus of the health care delivery system in the United States. Hospitals account for the largest proportion of expenditures and employ the majority of health care workers. Hospitals have fewer clients today because of the trend toward rapid discharge and a greater number of procedures being performed in outpatient settings. The clients who are hospitalized require more nursing care because of greater complexity of needs and severity of illness. Additional factors that have contributed to the decreased hospital population include:

- Shorter length of stays,
- Greater availability of outpatient facilities,
- Technological advances,
- An increased number of services available in outpatient settings, and
- Expectations/demands of third-party payers.

As a result of the changes in reimbursement practices, hospitals are restructuring (also referred to as redesigning and reengineering). Examples of restructuring activities include mergers with larger institutions; development of integrated systems that provide a full range of services focusing on continuity of care, such as preadmission, outpatient, acute inpatient, long-term inpatient, and home care; and the substitution of multiskilled workers for nurses.

Changing Practice Settings

Most nurses currently practice in hospitals and will continue to do so in the future (Aiken, 1995). The increasing presence of severely ill clients requires that nurses who work in hospitals possess technical expertise, critical thinking skills, and interpersonal competence. Outside the hospital setting, there is an ever-increasing need for nurses in different areas of practice. Home health services, in particular, will need to continue expanding in order to meet the growing needs of the steadily increasing elderly population (Hull, 1997). Social and political changes are affecting nurses by creating the need for expanded services and settings. Because of these changes, demand for nursing care fluctuates: For example, nursing employment outside the hospital continues to increase. More nurses will be needed in the future because:

- The growing elderly population will require more health care services.
- The number of people admitted to nursing homes is steadily growing.
- The number of homeless individuals, who are most often denied access to health care, is increasing rapidly.

As initial reform occurs, some nurses may be displaced from their current jobs. But overall, many more jobs will be created by the demand for greater access to health care services. Some examples of areas where larger numbers of nurses will be required are primary care, public health, extended care, and home care.

COMMUNITY/HOME HEALTH CARE

Cost of Home Health Care

- Since the advent of Medicare and Medicaid, home health care has grown rapidly. Because it is much less costly to provide home care, clients are sent home to recuperate.
- Expenditures for health care in the home are greatly increasing.

Ethical Issues

The United States is struggling with a major ethical conflict of cost containment versus compassionate care. According to Hicks and Boles (1997), no country, regardless of wealth, can provide all citizens with every health care service they desire or need. Today, the U.S. health care delivery system is faced with the dilemma of citizens' needs being greater than available resources. Thus, some difficult choices must be made to determine which needs will be met and which will remain unmet.

The national mentality, reflected in the expectation that everything must be done to save a dying person, has created an enormous drain on the health care resources of the United States and represents one example of an ethical issue related to health care. As decisions are made regarding how scarce resources are to be allocated, there will be much debate about the ethics involved. The appropriateness of futile life-sustaining measures—those that only keep the client in a vegetative state—must be addressed (Rowe, 1996). Nurses must strongly advocate for just and ethical distribution of resources as health care reform progresses.

Vulnerable Populations

Meeting the health care needs of underserved populations is especially challenging. Groups that may be unable to gain access to health care services include children, rural residents, people with AIDS, and the homeless and others living in poverty. An increase in poverty further strains hospitals because Medicaid is no longer adequate to meet the needs of the medically indigent.

Our current health care system neglects the overall needs of children. Children are more likely than adults to be uninsured or underinsured. Children who are covered by health insurance have a greater degree of well-being.

Many parents have their children immunized only when the children are ready to start school, because immunization is a requirement for entry into the public school system. Preventive health care should be encouraged and made available to children of all ages,

with an emphasis on early immunization. The ANA and a coalition of allied nursing associations are working together in an attempt to immunize all children in the United States.

Traditionally, rural areas have had fewer health care providers and facilities that are easily accessible than have their urban counterparts. Approximately 45% of those over the age of 65 years live in rural areas (Vrabec, 1995). Because people in rural areas tend to work for small businesses or be self-employed, many of them have no health insurance.

As of December 1997, 641,086 people in the United States have been diagnosed with AIDS, and estimates suggest that 650,000 to 900,000 persons in the United States are now living with HIV (CDC, 1998). It is estimated that at least 40,000 new infections occur each year (CDC, 1998). The most rapid spread of the disease is occurring among women, children, and intravenous drug users and their sexual partners. Women who have AIDS have a higher mortality rate than do men, and decreased access to health care may be one contributing factor (Tlusty, 1994). Although the cost of this epidemic is unmeasurable in terms of human suffering, approximately $10.5 billion was spent on care of people with AIDS in 1994 alone (Hull, 1997). Not only will additional funding be necessary, but outpatient care settings (such as hospices, home care, and

LIFE CYCLE CONSIDERATIONS

Health Care for Children

- Approximately one-third of the 71,731,000 children under age 18 who live in poverty are under 6 years of age (U.S. Census Bureau, 2000).
- Seven million of the 11 million children who are uninsured could have health care coverage today (RWJF, 2000).
- Six out of 10 parents whose children may qualify for Medicaid or State Children's Health Insurance Program (SCHIP) do not believe these programs apply to them (RWJF, 2000).
- Belief that their children do not qualify is highest in households where both parents work or when annual income is $25,000 or more (RWJF, 2000).
- By 1996, 90% or more of toddlers had received the most critical doses of vaccines for children by age 2 (CDC, 2000).
- Nine percent fewer poor children complete the full series of immunizatons (National Academies, 2000).
- Each day 11,000 babies are born who will need immunizations (National Academies, 2000).
- Federal funds supporting the immunization network are shrinking (CDC, 2000).

clinics) must be expanded to care for those affected by this epidemic.

The homeless and others living in poverty are often mobile, having no permanent address. They may not know which services are available to them or how to access the system except through inner city hospitals. This creates a significant financial burden on these health care agencies. Illegal aliens, because of fears of being arrested and deported, may enter emergency departments under false identities and in acute distress, receive treatment, and then disappear.

NURSING'S RESPONSE TO HEALTH CARE CHALLENGES

As the United States continues to look for ways to address the issue of health care reform, the implications for nursing will continue to increase. Some nurses feel threatened by impending changes, whereas others are excited about the possibility of transforming the health care system into something better. The nursing profession has responded to the myriad challenges in health care delivery by proposing a plan for reform.

Nursing's Agenda for Health Care Reform

In 1991, in response to the problems of high cost, limited access, and eroding quality that were affecting the U.S. health care system, the nursing community created a public policy agenda that is currently endorsed by more than 70 organizations. *Nursing's Agenda for Health Care Reform* (ANA, 1991) provides a valid framework for change in health care policies and establishes nursing's legislative program, through which these changes can be implemented. Table 5–7 lists the major tenets of this agenda. A cornerstone of nursing's proposal is the delivery of health care services in envi-

LIFE CYCLE CONSIDERATIONS

Rural Elders

Health care barriers experienced by elderly persons living in rural areas include the following:

- Inadequate financing of rural health care facilities. Medicare's lower reimbursement rates for rural hospitals than for urban hospitals has been a contributing factor to the closure of some hospitals in rural communities.
- Decreased availability of health care providers.
- Greater geographic distances that must be traveled in order to obtain services.

Table 5–7 NURSING'S AGENDA FOR HEALTH CARE REFORM

Nursing's agenda for health care reform includes several basic tenets, including the following:

- All citizens and residents of the United States must have equitable access to essential health care services.
- Primary health care services must play a very basic and prominent role in service delivery.
- Consumers must be the central focus of the health care system. Assessment of health care needs must be the determining factor in the ultimate structuring and delivery of programs and services.
- Consumers must be guaranteed direct access to a full range of qualified health care providers who offer their services in a variety of delivery arrangements at sites that are accessible, convenient, and familiar to the consumer.
- Consumers must assume more responsibility for their own care and become better informed about the range of providers and potential options for services.
- Health care services must be restructured to create a better balance between the prevailing orientation toward illness and cure and a new commitment to wellness and care.
- The health care system must ensure that appropriate, effective care is delivered through efficient use of resources.
- A standardized package of essential health care services must be provided and financed through an integration of public and private sources.
- Mechanisms must be implemented to protect against catastrophic costs and impoverishment.

From Nursing's Agenda for Health Care Reform, *by American Nurses Association, 1991, Kansas City, MO: Author.*

ronments that are easily accessible, familiar, and consumer friendly. Another essential part of nursing's agenda is the empowerment of consumers in the area of self-care. This goal has enormous implications for nurses as health educators and for the use of incentives for increasing personal accountability for one's own health status. A study in Maryland shows that universal coverage is feasible and will also save a substantial amount of money (Health Care News, 2000). A one-payment system with lower administrative costs accounts for the monetary savings.

Standards of Care

Another approach to the challenges of the health care delivery system has been the move toward standardization of care. In December 1990, the Agency for Health Care Policy and Research (AHCPR) was established with the specific charge of achieving consensus within the medical/health care community regarding the usual treatment of high-volume and expensive disease conditions that differ in therapeutic management despite substantial research. More simply put, there is significant variation in the diagnosis and treatment of certain illnesses and diseases. The medical justification for such variance has been that every client is an individual and that the choice of treatment is a private decision involving client and physician. Prostatic hypertrophy (enlarged prostate gland) and breast cancer are examples of high-volume diagnoses that have been studied by the AHCPR but for which appropriate diagnostic tests and treatments of choice have not yet been conclusively determined. The AHCPR aims to identify the standards of treatment to which the health care community can be held. Currently, 18 AHCPR-published guidelines are available to the public and should be integral to nursing practice.

Advanced Practice

The advanced practice of nursing has evolved as nursing has become more complex and specialized. Since the late 1960s, nurse practitioners (NPs), clinical nurse specialists (CNSs), certified nurse midwives (CNMs), and other advanced practice registered nurses (APRNs) have provided primary health care services to individuals, many of whom would have otherwise had inadequate or no access to services (Boyd, Lowes, Guglielmo, & Slomski, 2000). The APRN possesses advanced skills and in-depth knowledge in specific areas of practice (Stafford & Appleyard, 1997). Although there are differences among various advanced practice roles, all APRNs are experts who work with clients to prevent disease and promote health.

There are more than 80,000 APRNs in the United States (Boyd et al., 2000). Nurses in advanced practice are also moving toward independent practice. Data suggest that APRNs can independently diagnose and resolve over 80% of the primary health care problems of the American public (ANA, 1993a). The NP facilitates access to and continuity of care and provides high-quality care (Boyd et al., 2000). Advanced practice registered nurses prescribe less-expensive diagnostic tests, the length of their visits is comparable to that of physicians', and they charge less for services because of the comparatively lower cost of professional liability insurance (Boyd et al., 2000). Despite repeated proof of the cost efficiency and therapeutic effectiveness of APRNs, obstacles to this role for nurses persist. In a recent Division of Nursing report on APRNs, the single most formidable obstacle to practice is that most people are unaware of what APRNs offer.

Recent progress has been made on the access issues that constrain APRNs. Reimbursement is now available to some segments of the advanced practice community in every federal entitlement program (HCFA, 1998).

Currently, all states award APRNs some type of prescriptive authority (Pearson, 2000). In 10 states, this authority is complete and unrestricted, is unassociated with physician oversight, and includes all classes of drugs (Pearson, 2000). The ANA (through the JCAHO and the HCFA) began the groundwork for professional staff privileges for APRNs in its revision of the official definitions of professional staff that include a broad range of providers.

Public vs. Private Programs

The combination of public sector and private sector health care resources seems to be beneficial for U.S. residents. The competition between the two sectors has encouraged quality and progress. Each setting offers benefits as well as drawbacks to health care recipients.

The nursing profession supports an integration of public and private sector programs and resources. Public dollars are required to help the poor and those who do not receive health care benefits through the workplace. Actual services should be available through a variety of public and private sources. To safeguard the health care system from becoming a two-tiered process based on personal resources, both the poor and nonpoor and the privileged and nonprivileged must be enrolled in the same programs.

Finally, the basic required package of services must be defined in the same way in each state and required as the minimum for both public and private sector programs. Minimal national standards should be set, but local planning and implementation should be promoted.

The states' rights philosophy prevalent in the United States creates an obstacle to national standards, which are necessary for several areas of assurance. Some coast-to-coast consistency in the cost of services, with room for local adjustments, is needed.

Public Health

During the past several years, public health has perceptibly eroded. Public health includes services such as immunizations, prenatal care, environmental concerns (conditions that may affect health), and analysis of the prevailing disease patterns in a community. Current public health problems include:

- Appearance of new fatal diseases (e.g., AIDS and the Ebola virus),
- Emergence of drug-resistant strains of tuberculosis, and
- Presence of toxic environmental conditions.

Community Health

Parris and Hines (1995) recommend a commitment to a community-based approach to reforming the system of health care delivery. Community-based care focuses on prevention and primary care. Successful movement toward a healthy and empowered consumer requires access to community-based primary health care. Nursing has a rich heritage of providing such community

Table 5–8 TRENDS AFFECTING DELIVERY OF HEALTH CARE SERVICES

- Aging of the U.S. population
- Increasing diversity in the U.S. population
- Increased number of single-parent families and of children living in poverty
- Continued growth in outpatient settings and a greater demand for primary care providers
- Advances in technology with resultant ability to perform more services in outpatient settings (including the home)
- More states using managed care models to deliver services to the medically indigent
- Incentives for individuals who participate in preventive activities
- Federal funding of health care provider education focusing on service to underserved populations and areas
- The system as a union of both public and private sector resources and services
- Managed care dominating as the context for service delivery
- Continued focus on quality improvement

services, as evidenced by the work of pioneers such as Lillian Wald and Mary Breckenridge.

TRENDS AND ISSUES

As current trends continue, the delivery of health care services will continue to change. Table 5–8 lists factors that will continue to shape reform of the health care delivery system.

As health care reform occurs, some professions will experience opportunities for growth whereas others

LIFE CYCLE CONSIDERATIONS

Meeting the Needs of Elderly Clients

In 1992, the HCFA funded community nursing organizations (CNOs) to help meet the needs of elderly persons in four communities. These four projects yielded the following results:

- A high degree of client satisfaction
- Decreased Medicare expenditures associated with home care
- Use of less-expensive equipment
- Decreased emergency department costs (ANA, 1995)

will experience layoffs (O'Neil, 1993). The challenge is to improve the nation's delivery of health care services by positioning nursing to preserve its integrity and to guarantee its preferred future. Nurses must be at the forefront of change.

SUMMARY

- The three levels of health care services can be categorized as primary, secondary, and tertiary.
- Health care services are delivered and financed by the public (official, voluntary, and nonprofit agencies), public/private, and private (hospitals, extended-care facilities, home health care agencies, hospices, outpatient settings, schools, industrial clinics, managed care organizations, community nursing centers, and rural hospitals) sectors.
- The health care team is composed of nurses, nurse practitioners, physicians, physician's assistants, pharmacists, dentists, dietitians, social workers, therapists, and chaplains.
- Managed care organizations seek to control health care costs by monitoring the delivery of services and restricting access to costly procedures and providers.
- Managed care plans include health maintenance organizations, preferred provider organizations, and exclusive provider organizations.
- The primary federal government insurance plans are Medicare, the program that provides health care coverage for elderly persons and disabled persons, and Medicaid, the jointly administered program that provides health care services for the poor.
- To achieve equity for all Americans, health care reform must address the three critical issues of cost, access, and quality of health care services.
- The challenges that the health care delivery system must overcome are the public's disillusionment with providers; the public's loss of control over health care decisions; the decreased use of hospitals and the related impact on quality of care; the change in practice settings; ethical issues, and the health care needs of vulnerable populations.
- *Nursing's Agenda for Health Care Reform* outlines nursing's proposals for easing the current problems in health care delivery.
- The Agency of Health Care Policy and Research aims to identify therapeutic standards to which the health care community can be held.
- A primary goal of the nursing profession within the areas of public health, community health, and long-term care is to provide health care services that emphasize prevention and primary health care for clients in these settings and thus help reduce costs and increase the quality of health care.

Review Questions

1. When the goal of a health care service is to decrease the risk to clients for a disease or dysfunction, the type of care is called:
   a. primary.
   b. tertiary.
   c. exclusive.
   d. secondary.

2. Identified members of the health care team include:
   a. nurses, pharmacists, chaplains.
   b. nurses, physicians, ward clerks.
   c. therapists, housekeeping personnel, dietitians.
   d. dentists, social workers, maintenance personnel.

3. The primary federal government insurance plan(s) is (are):
   a. Medicaid and welfare.
   b. Medicaid and Social Security.
   c. Medicaid and diagnosis-related groups.
   d. Medicare and Children's Health Insurance Program.

4. Cost, access, and quality of health care services are the three critical issues that must be addressed by:
   a. schools.
   b. hospitals.
   c. health care reform.
   d. managed care plans.

5. The nursing role that protects the client and supports the client's decisions is:
   a. teacher.
   b. advocate.
   c. caregiver.
   d. team member.

6. The major health care problem for children is:
   a. living in poverty.
   b. having no transportation.
   c. receiving substandard health care.
   d. not receiving immunizations as infants.

Critical Thinking Questions

1. The U.S. health care system is first in technological advances, biomedical research, and state-of-the-art clinical equipment and facilities. Yet, even given these advantages, many consider the system to be in crisis. From your perspective, is the health care system in a state of strength or weakness? Why or why not?

2. What factors do you think have contributed to a positive perception of nurses? A negative perception? What can you do specifically to promote positive images of nurses among the public?

3. Think about the ethical ramifications of determining medically necessary therapeutics. Is rationing of scarce resources the answer to our health care dilemma?

 WEB FLASH!

- Search the Internet for information regarding Oregon's plan for allocating resources. What are the main points of the plan?
- Research health care reform on the web. What is its status? What are the future plans for health care reform?

Legal and Ethical Issues

Chapter 6
Legal Responsibilities

Chapter 7
Ethical Responsibilities

LEGAL RESPONSIBILITIES

MAKING THE CONNECTION

Refer to the following chapters to increase your understanding of legal responsibilities:

- **Chapter 7, Ethical Responsibilities**
- **Chapter 17, Loss, Grief, and Death**

LEARNING OBJECTIVES

Upon completion of this chapter, you should be able to:
- *Define key terms.*
- *Describe the difference between public law and civil law.*
- *State the purpose and identify various sources of standards of practice.*
- *Discuss the difference between intentional and unintentional torts.*
- *Discuss the importance of accurate documentation.*
- *Discuss ways that informed consent relates to nursing practice.*
- *Discuss the concept of advance directives.*
- *State the purpose and correct utilization of an incident report.*
- *Discuss ways the nurse can reduce personal liability.*
- *State the benefits of having one's own malpractice insurance policy.*
- *List steps to be taken when suspecting a colleague of being impaired by drugs or alcohol.*

KEY TERMS

administrative law	incident report
advance directive	informed consent
assault	law
battery	liability
civil law	libel
confidential	living will
constitutional law	malpractice
contract law	misdemeanor
criminal law	negligence
defamation	nursing practice act
durable power of attorney for health care	peer assistance programs
expressed contract	privacy
false imprisonment	public law
felony	restraint
formal contract	slander
fraud	standards of practice
Good Samaritan law	statutory law
impaired nurse	tort
implied contract	tort law

INTRODUCTION

Nursing, which embodies a concern for the client in every aspect of life, encompasses a great responsibility—one that requires knowledge, skill, care, and commitment. As society advances and technology changes, the issues that affect nursing practice also change. We continue to recognize the importance of informed consent, the right to decide what is best for one's self, and belief in the client's bill of rights. However, difficult issues, such as living wills, advance directives, do-not-resuscitate (DNR) orders, and impaired nurses, now confront the profession of nursing. Nurses in the past did not have to contend with these controversial topics. Today's nurse must be informed on these and other issues. This chapter provides a general overview of many legal concepts that affect nursing.

BASIC LEGAL CONCEPTS

Because it is useful to have working definitions of some basic legal concepts before applying them to a health care setting, a discussion of pertinent legal concepts follows.

Definition of Law

Laws are rules of conduct that guide interactions among people. Laws are binding, enforceable, and necessary so that people can live and work together. If laws are broken, a penalty is incurred.

The word **law** is derived from an Anglo-Saxon term meaning "that which is laid down or fixed." The two types of law are **public law**, which deals with the individual's relationship to the state, and **civil law**, which deals with relationships among individuals.

Sources of Law

The four sources of public law at the federal and state levels are constitutional, statutory, administrative, and criminal. The three sources of civil law at the federal and state levels are contracts, torts, and protective/reporting laws.

Public Law

Constitutional law, set forth in the U.S. and state constitutions, defines and limits the powers of government. **Statutory law** is enacted by legislative bodies. State boards and professional practice acts, such as nursing practice acts, are created and governed under statutory laws.

Administrative law (regulatory law) is developed by those persons appointed to governmental administrative agencies. These persons are entrusted with enforcing the statutory laws passed by the legislature. Administrative law gives state boards of nursing the power to make rules and regulations governing nursing as set forth in the nursing practice acts. In these administrative rules, nursing boards identify the specific processes for educational programs; licensure; grounds for disciplinary proceedings; and the establishment of fees for services and for penalties rendered by the board.

Criminal law, the most common example of public law, addresses acts or offenses against the safety or welfare of the public. Under criminal law, there are two types of crime: **felony** (a crime of a serious nature that is usually punishable by imprisonment at a state penitentiary or by death, or a crime in violation of federal statute and involving punishment of more than 1 year incarceration) and **misdemeanor** (offense that is less serious than a felony and may be punishable by a fine or a sentence to a local prison for less than 1 year). Table 6–1 outlines the types of public law.

Civil Law

Civil law addresses crimes against a person or persons in such legal matters as contracts, torts, and protective/reporting law (Table 6–2). Most cases of malpractice fall under the civil law of torts (Flight, 1998).

Contract law is the enforcement of agreements among private individuals. There are three essential elements in a legal contract:

- Promise(s) between two or more legally competent individuals that state what each individual must do or not do
- Mutual understanding of the terms and obligations the contract imposes on each individual
- Compensation for lawful actions performed

The terms of a contract may be agreed on orally or in writing. However, a **formal** (written) **contract**

Table 6–1 TYPES OF PUBLIC LAW

TYPE	FEDERAL	STATE
Constitutional law	U.S. Constitution Civil Rights Act	State Constitutions Law
Statutory law	None	State boards and professional practice acts such as nursing practice acts
Administrative law	Food, Drug, and Cosmetic Act Social Security Act National Labor Relations Act	Rules and regulations governing nursing as set by state boards of nursing
Criminal law	Controlled Substance Act Kidnapping	Criminal codes (defining murder, manslaughter, criminal negligence, rape, fraud, illegal possession of drugs, theft, assault, and battery)

Adapted from Fundamentals of Nursing: Standards & Practice, *by S. DeLaune and P. Ladner, 1998, Albany, NY: Delmar. Copyright 1998 by Delmar. Adapted with permission.*

Table 6–2 TYPES OF CIVIL LAW

TYPE	FEDERAL	STATE
Contract law	None	Employment contracts Business contracts with clients Contracts with allied groups Uniform Commercial Code
Torts	Federal Torts Claims Act	State Torts Claims Act (allows claims against the state) Negligence (common law claim) Malpractice statutes (professional liability) Assault Battery False Imprisonment Invasion of privacy Defamation (libel and slander) Fraud
Protective/ reporting laws	Child Abuse Prevention and Treatment Act Privacy Act of 1974	Age of consent statutes (medical treatment, drugs, sexually transmitted disease) Privileged Communication Statute Abortion statute Good Samaritan Law Abuse statutes (child, elderly, domestic violence) Involuntary Hospitalization Act Living will legislation

Adapted from Fundamentals of Nursing: Standards & Practice, *by S. DeLaune and P. Ladner, 1998, Albany, NY: Delmar. Copyright 1998 by Delmar. Adapted with permission.*

cannot be changed legally by an oral agreement. An **expressed contract** gives, in writing, the conditions and terms of the contract. An **implied contract** recognizes a relationship between parties for services.

In accord with U.S. Contract Law, the nurse is legally required to:

- Adhere to the employer's policies and standards unless they conflict with federal or state law,
- Fulfill the terms of contracted service with the employer, and
- Respect the rights and responsibilities of other health care providers, especially in areas that promote continuity of client care.

Along with these legal responsibilities, the nurse has a right to expect:

- Adequate and qualified assistance in providing care,
- Reasonable and prudent conduct from the client,
- Compensation from the employer for services rendered,
- A safe work environment with the necessary resources to render services, and
- Prudent, reasonable conduct from other health care providers.

A **tort** is a civil wrong committed by a person against another person or property (Zerwekh & Claborn, 1997). **Tort law** is the enforcement of duties and rights among individuals independent of contractual agreements.

The protective/reporting law may be considered criminal law, depending on the state classification. Two examples of protective law are The Americans with Disabilities Act (ADA) and the Good Samaritan Laws.

The ADA was passed by the U.S. Congress in 1990. It prohibits discrimination in employment, public services, and public accommodations on the basis of disability. The ADA defines a disability as a physical or mental impairment that substantially limits one or more of the major life activities. Disabilities that may be covered by the ADA include the following:

- Mental impairments
  Learning disabilities
  Psychiatric disorders
  Organic brain syndrome
  Retardation
- Physical impairments
  Addiction
  Cancer

Cerebral palsy
Diabetes
Epilepsy
Heart disease
Human immunodeficiency virus (HIV, sympto-
matic or asymptomatic)
Multiple sclerosis
Muscular dystrophy
Orthopedic, visual, speech, and hearing impair-
ments
Tuberculosis

All fifty states and the District of Columbia have enacted **Good Samaritan** laws which protect health care
providers by ensuring immunity from civil **liability**
(obligation one has incurred or might incur through
any act or failure to act) when care is provided at the
scene of an emergency and the caregiver does not intentionally or recklessly cause the client injury (Brown,
1999).

The Good Samaritan law applies only in emergency
situations, usually those outside the hospital setting. It
stipulates that the health care worker must not be acting for an employer or receive compensation for care
given. There is also a federal Good Samaritan law that
protects health care providers who voluntarily give
care to a person in distress during an airplane flight
(Brown, 1999).

In most states, health care professionals are not required to stop at the scene of accidents. If they do
stop, however, they are held to higher standards than
is a lay person. Health care professionals are expected
to use their specialized body of knowledge when providing care. They are expected to act as would most
other professionals with the same background and education.

PROFESSIONAL TIP

Good Samaritan Laws

Good Samaritan laws vary in coverage from state
to state and may be amended periodically by legislation. It is the responsibility of caregivers to know
the law for their respective jurisdictions (Brown,
1999).

NURSING PRACTICE AND THE LAW

Nursing practice falls under both public law and
civil law. In most states, nurses are bound by rules and
regulations stipulated by the **nursing practice act** as
determined by the legislature. For licensed practical/
vocational nurses (LP/VNs), four states—Texas, Cali-

PROFESSIONAL TIP

Nursing Practice Act/Title Act
- Nursing practice acts state those things that the
  nurse can and cannot do.
- Title acts state who can be called an LP/VN.

fornia, Tennessee, and South Dakota—have title acts
as opposed to practice acts.

Public laws are designed to protect the public. If
these laws are broken, the nurse can be punished by
paying a fine, losing her license, or being incarcerated.
An example would be a nurse guilty of diverting drugs,
which is considered a crime against the state. The offending nurse could lose her license to practice and
could be sent to jail.

Civil laws deal with problems that occur between a
nurse and the client. For example, if a nurse catheter-
izes a client and perforates the bladder, the client may
bring a civil suit against the nurse. No law affecting the
population as a whole has been broken, but the client
has sustained injury. This is a problem between individuals—the nurse and the client or the nurse, the
client, and the nurse's employer. The client may receive
compensation for injuries, but no jail time is incurred
by the nurse.

Multistate nursing practice has become more common with the increasing presence of telehealth, trans-
porting of clients across state lines, and being employed
by staffing companies that operate in several states
(Ventura, 1999b). Many states are considering a licensure system facilitating interstate nursing practice.

Standards of Practice

The state boards of nursing have been assigned the
responsibility of determining and regulating nursing
practice. The boards indicate what nursing is and is
not, defines registered nursing and practical nursing,
and sets educational guidelines for each program.

The state boards of nursing also stipulate who may
practice nursing in their respective states (licensure).
The related criteria usually involve graduating from a
state-approved or state-accredited program, passing
the National Council Licensure Exam (NCLEX), and
meeting certain moral and legal standards. The boards
have the authority to bring disciplinary action against a
nurse for violation of its rules and regulations. Disciplinary action can include suspension or revocation of a
nurse's license and/or a fine.

Under the auspices of the nursing practice acts,
guidelines have been developed to direct nursing care.
These guidelines are called **standards of practice** or
standards of care.

Standards of practice are derived from a variety of sources. As stated, they are usually defined by the board of nursing and described in the nursing practice act. However, professional organizations such as the American Nurses Association (ANA) for the registered nurse (RN) and the National Federation of Licensed Practical Nurses (NFLPN) for the LP/VN also develop standards of practice. Books on nursing care planning, especially for specialized areas, are additional resources for the development of practice standards.

Policy and procedure manuals also represent standards of practice. Each facility, based on a rigorous review process, has identified specific ways of performing procedures such as passing medications, inserting catheters, and collecting specimens. The nurse employed by the facility is expected to follow the guidelines as laid out by the policy and procedure manuals. For situations not covered in the policy and procedure manuals, the nurse is expected to exercise good judgment in the planning and providing of client care. In other words, the nurse is expected to act in a reasonable and prudent manner.

Liability

What is meant by reasonable and prudent? In the case of nursing, it means that the nurse is expected to act as would other nurses at the same professional level and with the same amount of education or experience. If most nurses would respond to a particular situation in a certain way, and the nurse in question does so also, the nurse would be acting in a reasonable and prudent manner. However, if most nurses would respond differently than the nurse in question, the nurse would not be behaving in a reasonable and prudent manner and can be held liable or responsible for damages. Liability is determined by whether the nurse adhered to the standards of practice.

Legal Issues in Practice

Many aspects relating to nursing practice and areas of nursing are subject to liability, including physician's orders, floating, inadequate staffing, critical care, and pediatric care.

Physician's Orders

The physician is in charge of directing the client's care, and nurses are to carry out the physician's orders for care, unless the nurse believes that the orders are in error or would be harmful to the client. In this case, the physician must be contacted to confirm and/or clarify the orders. If the nurse still believes the orders to be inappropriate, she should immediately contact the nursing supervisor and put in writing why the orders are not being carried out. A nurse who carries out an erroneous or inappropriate order may be held liable for harm experienced by the client. *Nurses are responsible for their actions regardless of who told them to perform those actions.*

Floating

Nurses sometimes are asked to "float" to an unfamiliar nursing unit. The supervisor should be informed about a float nurse's lack of experience in caring for the type of clients on the new nursing unit. The nurse should be given an orientation to the new unit and will be held to the same standards of care as are the nurses who regularly work on that unit.

Inadequate Staffing

The Joint Commission on Accreditation of Healthcare Organizations (JCAHO) has established guidelines for determining the number of staff needed for any given situation (staffing ratios) (JCAHO, 1995). When there are not enough nurses to meet the staffing ratio and provide competent care, substandard care may result, placing clients at physical risk and the nurse and institution at legal risk. The nurse in this situation should provide nursing administration with a written account of the situation. *A nurse who leaves an inadequately staffed unit could be charged with client abandonment.*

Critical Care

Because the monitors used in critical care units are not infallible, constant observation and assessment of the clients are required. This makes a one-to-one or a one-to-two nurse–client ratio imperative. Furthermore, equipment must be checked regularly, and on a schedule, by the biomedical department.

Pediatric Care

Legislation in each state requires that suspected child abuse or neglect be reported. Legal immunity is provided to the person who makes a report in good faith. When suspected child abuse or neglect is not reported by health care providers, legal action, civil or criminal, may be filed against them.

NURSE–CLIENT RELATIONSHIP

A variety of situations can develop between a nurse and a client that may require legal intervention. The following is a discussion of the types of torts that may arise.

Torts

When a case is brought against a nurse, it is usually a civil action that falls under tort law. Torts can be intentional or unintentional (Table 6–3). The person who commits an intentional tort violates the civil rights of another individual knowingly and willfully. Examples of intentional torts are assault and battery, defamation (libel and slander), fraud, false imprisonment, and

Table 6–3 SELECTED TORTS: DEFINITIONS AND EXAMPLES

TYPE OF TORT	DEFINITION	EXAMPLE
Intentional		
Assault and battery	Threaten or attempt to touch another person. Unconsented touching.	Nurse who unjustifiably forces a treatment against the client's will and in the absence of consent
False imprisonment	Unwarranted restriction of the freedom of an individual.	Nurse who uses the restraints on a client who is of sound mind and is not in danger of inflicting injury on self or another
Quasi-intentional		
Invasion of privacy	All individuals have the right to privacy and may bring charges against any person who violates this right.	Nurse who either discloses information about a client that is considered private or photographs a client without consent
Defamation (libel and slander)	Verbal (slander) or written (libel) remarks that may cause the loss of an individual's reputation.	Nurse who makes a statement that could either ruin the client's reputation or cause the client to lose his or her job
Unintentional		
Negligence	Failure to use such care as a reasonably prudent person would use under similar circumstances, which leads to harm.	Nurse who loses client's property Nurse who makes a medication error Nurse who burns a client via the improper use of equipment Nurse who fails to observe and/or report a change in the client's condition. Nurse who inaccurately counts sponges in the operating room
Malpractice	Failure of a professional to use such care as a reasonably prudent member of the profession would use under similar circumstances, which leads to harm.	Nurse who makes an inaccurate nursing diagnosis and implements the wrong treatment Nurse who does not follow physician's orders Nurse who does not question physician's clearly erroneous order

invasion of privacy. Unintentional torts are those actions that cause harm to the client and that result from carelessness or negligence on the part of the nurse. If found liable, the nurse generally must pay monetary damages. Prison terms are rare.

Intentional Torts

Assault and battery, defamation, fraud, false imprisonment, and invasion of privacy are types of intentional torts.

Assault and Battery Assault and battery, though frequently used together, are actually two separate terms. **Assault** is the threat to do something that may cause harm or be unpleasant to another person. **Battery** is the unauthorized or unwanted touching of one person by another.

Fear and intimidation are the key elements in assault. The person assaulted must believe that the threat made can and will be carried out, for example, a client who is confined to a wheelchair and told, "If you do not finish your meal, you are going to sit there all night." The client complies because he believes the health care worker will leave him to sit for an uncom-

CULTURAL CONSIDERATIONS

Assault and Battery Charges

To prevent assault and battery charges:

- Respect the client's cultural values, beliefs, and practices with regard to "touching."
- African Americans sometimes view touching another person's hair as offensive.
- Asian Americans usually do not touch others during conversations. Touching someone on the head is considered disrespectful because the head is considered sacred.
- European Americans employ handshakes for formal greetings.
- Hispanic Americans are very tactile and may embrace and shake hands when greeting one another.
- Native Americans prohibit touching a dead body. This may leave the offender open to charges of assault.

fortable period of time. The worker is in a position to carry out this threat, and the client knows it.

The key factor regarding battery is consent. People have the right to be free of unwanted handling of their person. Striking a client is battery. Performing a procedure without the client's consent is battery. Forcing a person to take medication they do not want is battery. Any unwanted touching, regardless of outcome, can be construed as battery.

Defamation Defamation is the use of words to harm or injure the personal or professional reputation of another person. If the words are written down, they constitute **libel**. If the information is communicated verbally to a third party, it constitutes **slander**.

Nurses must be discreet as to the ways that they characterize clients, peers, and other health care professionals. Negative or derogatory comments that are untrue leave the nurse no defense against charges of defamation. If comments are true, the relevance of the information is important. The most common examples of this tort are giving out inaccurate or inappropriate information from the medical record; discussing clients, families, or visitors in public areas; or speaking negatively about coworkers (Zerwekh & Claborn, 1997).

Fraud Fraud is a wrong that results from a deliberate deception intended to produce unlawful gain. Common forms of fraud in health care include illegal billing and deceit in obtaining or attempting to obtain a nursing license (Flight, 1998).

False Imprisonment False imprisonment refers to making the client wrongfully believe that she cannot leave a place. The most common example of this tort is telling a client not to leave the hospital until the bill is paid (Zerwekh & Claborn, 1997). Any mechanism used to confine a client or to restrict movement can be considered a restraint and a form of false imprisonment. This includes threats, locked doors, physical restraints such as wrist or vest restraints, side rails, geriatric chairs, and psychotropic drugs.

Nurses may find themselves in a quandary in situations where a client chooses to leave the health care facility, and no discharge order has been written. It is possible that the health care problem has not been resolved, and the nurse feels that it is not in the best interest of the client to leave. If the client is of sound mind, however, he has the right to make this decision, regardless of what others think is best. Detaining the individual could result in charges of false imprisonment.

Documentation is very important in these situations. The nurse should document the client's reasons for leaving the facility and include any teaching or interventions related to the situation. Facility policy usually requires that the client sign a form indicating that he is leaving against medical advice (AMA), which releases the facility of any liability. If the client is angry and refuses to sign the AMA form, the client's refusal should be documented, and the nursing supervisor and the client's physician should be notified.

As indicated, any device used to restrict movement is called a **restraint**. To safeguard against possible charges of false imprisonment, the nurse should carefully assess the situation and include the client or significant other in the care planning process. If it is determined that a restraint is needed, the purpose and use of the restraint should be explained, including the way the restraint fits into the plan of care, the length of time the restraint may be necessary, and the expected outcome. The planning session should be documented in the client's medical record.

Documentation must show that the client:

- Was assessed every 15 minutes (JCAHO, 2000),
- Was toileted,
- Received food and water, and
- Had position changes.

In acute care settings, restraints can usually be applied temporarily as a nursing measure for client safety; however, in most states, a physician's order must be immediately obtained. In long-term care settings, a physician's order is required prior to utilizing any restraints.

Invasion of Privacy Privacy includes the right to be left alone, to choose care based on personal beliefs, to govern body integrity, and to choose when and how sensitive information is shared (Badzek & Gross, 1999). People are entitled to **confidential** (nondisclosure of information) health care. All information gleaned from working with a client or from his medical records must be kept confidential. Therefore, a client's health status may not be discussed with a third party, unless either the client is present and has given verbal permission or permission has been obtained in writing. This does not apply to nurses' discussing a client's health status with other health care workers involved in the care of the client.

Invasion of privacy occurs when a person's private affairs become public knowledge without the person's permission. Photographing a client without his consent is an invasion of privacy. Failing to pull curtains to shield the client when performing personal or intimate care also constitutes an invasion of privacy.

A common mistake made by health care personnel is discussing clients in public areas. It is difficult to gauge who may overhear when comments are made while sitting in the cafeteria or waiting for the elevator (Figure 6-1). The results can be detrimental if the client is embarrassed by this loss of privacy: The client's job or family situation may be compromised, depending on the nature of the information. For example, news of an abortion, positive HIV status, or venereal disease may be socially damaging to some clients. Clients or their health care status should never be discussed in public areas or with those persons not directly involved in the care of the client.

All clients have the right to be free of unwanted public exposure. Permission should be obtained before

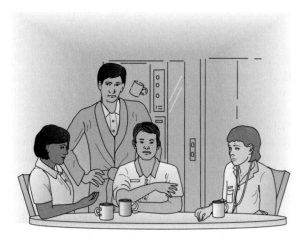

Figure 6-1 The nurse should not discuss clients, families, or coworkers in public areas.

going through a client's belongings. Doors should be kept closed and curtains pulled when providing personal care. People not involved in the performance of a procedure should not be invited to watch unless the client has given permission. Clients cannot be photographed or videotaped without their permission and a release form must be signed. Confidentiality should not be breached by using a client's full name on care plans, case studies, or other assignments that a student may have during clinical experience; only initials should be used. This helps protect the client's privacy should the papers be lost. The client's chart and other materials should not be left lying around, making a client's private information public knowledge.

Unintentional Torts

Negligence and malpractice are considered to be unintentional torts.

Negligence Negligence is a general term referring to negligent or careless acts on the part of an individual who is not exercising reasonable or prudent judgment. All nurses, including student nurses, are expected to use good judgment when providing client care. This means, for instance, that side rails should not be left down on confused clients' beds, and sedated clients should not be allowed to smoke unattended. To prevent falls, puddles and spills are cleaned up immediately, rather than waiting for housekeeping to take care of the matter. Any person, with or without the specialized knowledge required for nursing, could make these determinations. Should a nurse fail to protect a client in such a situation or in one requiring similar judgments, the nurse could be found negligent.

Malpractice Negligent acts on the part of a professional can be termed **malpractice**, or professional negligence. More specifically, malpractice relates to the conduct of a person while acting in a professional capacity.

Negligent or careless acts on the part of a nurse result from not meeting the standards of care, in other words, from not doing what a reasonable and prudent nurse would do under similar circumstances. A nurse can be charged with malpractice for acts committed or acts omitted. Failure to properly assess a client or to act on assessment information are examples of omission. Giving a client the wrong medication because of improper identification procedures (not checking the armband) or improper setup (not using the medication administration record) are acts of commission.

Malpractice can include attempting a procedure with which the nurse is unfamiliar, or improperly performing a procedure that results in client injury. Malpractice differs from negligence in that anyone can be accused of negligence; only professionals can be accused of malpractice.

Several factors must hold true for a nurse to be found guilty of malpractice (professional negligence):

- The nurse owed a special duty to the client; in other words, a nurse–client relationship existed.
- The nurse failed to meet the standards of care. Policy, procedure, or standards of care were not followed.
- The injury occurred as a result of the nurse's action or inaction, a direct cause and effect.
- Damage such as physical or emotional pain, suffering, monetary losses, or medical expenses must be proved. If there is not damage, the plaintiff is not entitled to an award (Lee, 2000).

The prudent nurse is protected by adhering to facility policy and procedure and attempting to meet the standards of care at all times. The case study discussed in Figure 6-2 illustrates some of the difficulties in distinguishing between malpractice and negligence.

Legal Risk

Nurses today are more likely to have problems for violating statutes, that is, laws and regulations, than to be sued for malpractice (Infante, 2000). Two common sources of statutory liability are federal antifraud laws and state reporting requirements. Statutory liability may lead to criminal charges rather than just civil penalties (Infante, 2000). The best protection against statutory liability is to learn about the federal and state laws and regulations that apply to the nurse's particular practice setting. A good resource is the facility's risk manager.

Federal Antifraud Laws

The federal government has:

- Expanded the list of activities that constitute fraud,
- Imposed new criminal sanctions on violators, and
- Increased the budget for investigating and prosecuting these activities.

Case Study: Standard of Care—Malpractice or Ordinary Negligence?

Facts: A 75-year-old client fell and fractured a hip while in the hospital. The client had been medicated with castor oil and a sleeping pill, and the nurse failed to raise the side rails on the bed. During the night, the client got out of bed to go to the bathroom and fell, fracturing the hip. The client sued, alleging that the nurse had been negligent in failing to raise the side rails and in failing to tell the client that a bedpan would be brought to the client when needed.

Holding: The nurse's conduct constituted negligence. Unlike a malpractice action, no expert testimony was necessary to establish the applicable standard of care. The duty to raise side rails on a bed and to instruct the client to use the call button beside the bed if assistance were needed did not involve the failure to render professional nursing or medical services requiring special skills. The jury, therefore, could evaluate the nurse's conduct under the standard of "the reasonably prudent person," rather than "the reasonably prudent nurse."

Norris v. Rowan Memorial Hospital, North Carolina Court of Appeals 1974

Comment: This case points out the difficulties even courts have in drawing the line between ordinary negligence and malpractice. Cases involving a nurse's failure to raise bed rails are decided under the standard of ordinary negligence as often as they are decided under the standard of professional malpractice.

Figure 6-2 Case Study: Standard of Care—Malpractice or Ordinary Negligence?

Infante (2000) lists as examples of fraudulent activities the following:

- Billing for services either unnecessary or not provided,
- Falsifying care plans,
- Forging physician's signature,
- Filing false cost reports, and
- Falsifying or omitting information about a client's condition to obtain reimbursement.

State Reporting Requirements

Nurses are required to report cases of suspected child abuse or neglect in every state (Infante, 2000). Most states also require nurses to report cases of suspected elder abuse and neglect (Morris, 1998). Infante (2000) identifies some criminal acts that must be reported. Many states require that:

- Police are notified of known or suspected cases of rape.
- Reports of gunshot or stab wounds are made.

Some states require that clients who have taken narcotics or who have a blood alcohol level higher than the legal limit for driving be reported (Ventura, 1999c).

These laws are not only for the general public but also for health care providers. If a suspected abuser is a health care provider, many states require that the event be reported to the agency that licenses that professional (Morris, 1998). Also, many states require nurses to report *any* provider who acts unprofessionally or is incompetent (Infante, 2000).

Professional Discipline

More than 5,000 nurses (RNs and LP/VNs) are annually disciplined for professional misconduct in the U.S. (LaDuke, 2000). That is, the nurses are found to have violated existing laws or regulations that govern a nurse's practice. LaDuke (2000) suggests that a nurse:

- Should *immediately* seek representation by an attorney specializing in professional misconduct and discipline if under investigation
- Is not obligated to talk to *any* investigator without an attorney present
- Know and understand the applicable state nursing practice act and established standards of care
- Look closely at the disciplinary process and ask questions to promote understanding

Sanctions

Boards of nursing determine and issue sanctions for nurses found to have demonstrated professional misconduct. Money damages are not generally awarded to consumers. A sample of sanctions from which boards of nursing may choose, includes:

- Warn, censure, or reprimand the licenses,
- Impose a fine,
- Place on probation or set a condition of licensure,
- Limit the license or credential,
- Suspend the license or credential,
- Revoke the license or credential, or
- Dismiss the complaint.

Disciplinary Data Banks

The National Council of State Boards of Nursing (NCSBN) maintains a Disciplinary Data Bank (DDB), as do many other professional organizations. The purpose of these data banks is to facilitate the communication of information about the unsafe practice of practitioners. In 1990, Congress created the National Practitioner Data Bank (NPDB) to improve the quality of health care by encouraging the identification and discipline of health care professionals who engage in incompetent and unsafe behavior.

Documentation

The source of information regarding the client's clinical history is the medical record, or the chart. The chart should accurately reflect diagnosis, treatment, testing, clinical course, nursing assessment, and intervention. According to the law, "If it was not charted, it was not done." If a chart ever winds up in court, this is the standard the jury applies when trying to determine what happened and who is at fault.

The nurse should not chart medications before they are given or treatments before they are completed. Either constitutes a direct violation of the standards of practice for documentation and medication administration. The standard of practice is that medications are documented *after* they are administered. All client care, including treatments, is documented after being provided.

Documentation must be accurate and objective. The nurse should describe what is seen and done. Nurses' notes should reflect facts, not inferences or opinions, about the client. Furthermore, it is not enough to chart nursing assessment or identified problems. The nurse must complete the task by documenting any actions taken, including nursing interventions and physician's orders implemented.

Entries must be neat, legible, spelled correctly, written clearly, and signed or initialed. It is illegal to go back and change a chart. If an error in charting is made, a line should be drawn through the incorrect entry and the nurse should initial it. Blacking out entries or using correction fluid is not acceptable, as this renders the original entry illegible. Sloppy, misspelled charting might discredit excellent nursing care.

Figures 6-3 and 6-4 reflect situations where nurses identified client problems. In Figure 6-3, documentation was incomplete. In the situation presented in Figure 6-4, the nurses clearly identified the problem, the client's response, and the actions taken.

INFORMED CONSENT

Informed consent refers to a competent client's ability to make health care decisions based on full disclosure of the benefits, risks, potential consequences of a recommended treatment plan, and alternate treatments, including no treatment and the client's agreement to the treatment as indicated by the client's signing a consent form. This detailed explanation, provided by the physician, allows the client to make intelligent decisions about treatment options. The issue of informed consent deals with the right of the client to determine what happens to his or her person. Consent to treatment also helps protect the health care worker from unwarranted charges of battery.

Individuals who are declared incompetent are assigned a guardian or someone who has power of attorney to make heath care decisions and give consent for treatment.

Nurses must obtain consent for nursing procedures. Each client, on admission, signs a general care consent form. The nurse is obligated to explain what is to be done to the client and to receive at least implied consent, as indicated by lack of objection on the part of the client. It is the physician's responsibility to obtain consent for medical or surgical treatment. The disclosure about the risks and benefits of treatment generally takes place at a time when the nurse is not present, often in the physician's office. It is usually on the basis of this discussion that the client decides whether to accept the treatment recommendation and sign the con-

---

Incomplete Documentation: Mrs. Drew

Mrs. Drew, 85 years old, was a resident on a transitional care unit. She lost 15 pounds over a 3-month period. When her chart was reviewed, the auditor targeted the weight loss as a problem. She examined the chart to discover what the nurses did to try to correct this situation.

The nurses had carefully documented the percentages Mrs. Drew had eaten at each meal, her lack of appetite, and the pattern of weight loss. They thought they had covered all bases. They were wrong.

The auditor referred to the standards of practice on weight loss in long-term care facilities. She questioned, "Did the nurses follow the guidelines?" No interventions were charted, so it was presumed that nothing was done.

In fact, the nurses had called the dietitian to see this client several times to discuss her food preferences and a calorie count was initiated. Student nurses assigned to Mrs. Drew sat with her at mealtimes to encourage her to eat. The nurses had spoken with the doctor and Mrs. Drew's family about their concern over her lack of appetite and loss of weight. However, none of this was charted. There was no proof, other than the dietitian's entries, that any attempt had been made to intervene in this client's nutritional deficit.

Figure 6-3 Incomplete Documentation: Mrs. Drew

Complete Documentation: Roberta Wilson

Roberta Wilson is a 44-year-old woman with a history of diabetes mellitus controlled by diet. She was admitted 2 days ago forabdominal pain. Ms. Wilson has been designated nothing by mouth (NPO) since midnight for an ultrasound scheduled at 9:30 AM The doctor instructed that she was to remain NPO until seen by a consultant. Her 11 AM accucheck revealed a blood sugar of 44. She was experiencing no symptoms of hypoglycemia.

What needed to be done and what needed to be documented to protect everyone involved? Hospital protocol stipulated giving 4 ounces of Coke for blood sugars less than 60, then repeating the accucheck in approximately 30 minutes. The nurses contacted the physician to cancel the NPO order, then administered the Coke. Roberta's blood sugar at 11:40 AM was 93. She was served an 1,800 calorie ADA (American Dietetic Association) diet for lunch.

What was charted?

2/08/00	11:10 AM	Accucheck 44. Client's skin is warm and dry, denies nausea, tremors, or confusion. States she feels "fine." Physician notified of low blood sugar and client condition. Orders received to discontinue NPO status and resume previous orders.
2/08/00	11:15 AM	4 ounces of Coke given.
2/08/00	11:40 AM	Blood sugar 93. Served 1,800 calorie ADA diet for lunch. Blood sugar to be repeated at 4 PM.

Figure 6-4 Complete Documentation: Roberta Wilson

---

sent form. Confusion arises, however, because nurses are often delegated the duty of collecting the signature for invasive procedures such as surgery, cardiac catheterization, and other diagnostic procedures. Student nurses should neither ask the client to sign a consent form, nor witness a consent form.

When a nurse has a client sign a consent form, the nurse is verifying the following three things:

- The client's signature is authentic.
- The client has the mental capacity to understand what was discussed with the physician.
- The client was not coerced into signing the form.

CLIENT TEACHING

Informed Consent

Consent may be withdrawn, either verbally or in writing, at any time.

PROFESSIONAL TIP

Consent in Emergencies

- Consent is implied when immediate action is necessary to save a life or to prevent permanent physical harm. Written consent is waived.
- After the emergency is over, consent must be obtained for further care.

If the nurse is unsure about the client's understanding or if the client still has questions, the client should not sign the form. The nurse should document the client's lack of understanding and contact the physician. Further clarification is needed, and it must come from the physician.

Clients over the age of 18 years may give consent for their own health care. Parents or guardians give consent for minor children. In most states, however, minors who are married, live on their own, become pregnant, or require treatment for sexually transmitted diseases, mental illness, or substance abuse may give consent for themselves.

Complex situations occur when minors refuse treatments to which parents have consented, or parents refuse consent or treatment that has been deemed medically necessary for their minor children. The court has had to intervene in such cases. In situations such as these, the child may be made a ward of the court and the decision-making capacity temporarily taken away from the parents. An example would be the child of Jehovah's Witnesses who needs a blood transfusion but whose parents refuse treatment on the basis of religious beliefs.

Invasive procedures or those that may have serious consequences, such as surgery, cardiac catheterization, or HIV testing, require written consent. Figure 6-5 illustrates a typical consent form used to obtain client permission for the performance of invasive medical, surgical, or diagnostic procedures. Consent for procedures that are not invasive can be either given verbally or implied. The client implies consent when he cooperates with the procedure offered. For example, if the orderly says, "Mr. Jones, I am here to take you for your

PROFESSIONAL TIP

Consent in Special Situations

- If a client is unable to consent and the family is too far away, consent may be received over the telephone, according to agency policy (usually, two persons must hear the consent being given).
- A client who has already received preoperative or preprocedure medication is not competent to sign a consent. When this situation arises, the surgery or procedure may have to be postponed.
- For blood transfusions, some facilities require that a denial form be signed if the client indicates *No* on the consent form.

CLIENT TEACHING

Advance Directives

- Advance directives should be discussed with the family and physician so that everyone understands the client's wishes, and conflicts are less likely to occur at a later time.
- An advance directive may be changed by the client as long as the client is competent.

chest x-ray," and Mr. Jones gets into the wheelchair, consent is implied by Mr. Jones' cooperation.

ADVANCE DIRECTIVES

An **advance directive** is a written instruction for health care that is recognized under state law and is related to the provision of such care when the individual is incapacitated. Advance directives emphasize the right of the client to self-determination. They are instructions about health care preferences regarding life-sustaining measures. These instructions may indicate who may make health care decisions for the client should he become unable to do so for himself. In essence, they express the client's wishes about the kinds of medical treatment wanted and not wanted.

A client of sound mind retains the right to make all health care decisions and even reverse previous decisions. Should a situation arise when the person becomes incapable of making decisions, however, advance directives serve as a guide to family members concerning those kinds of treatment that should or should not be allowed. Advance directives permit those involved in the decision-making process to know what the client prefers. Although these instructions are best put in writing, this is not always done. Sometimes, health care preferences are shared verbally with family members or friends. Such verbal instructions can be interpreted differently by different people, creating difficulty for all involved—the physician, the health care facility, and the family. Thus, it is best to get this information in writing. When an advance directive indicates that the client does not wish to have cardiopulmonary resuscitation (CPR) performed in the event of cardiac arrest, the physician must write a DNR order, also referred to as a "No Code."

All health care facilities that receive Medicare or Medicaid monies are required to offer the opportunity to execute advance directives to all competent clients on admission. The client should also be told about the purpose and availability of a living will and durable power of attorney for health care (discussed following). If desired, assistance in completing these documents should be offered to the client. In addition, the medical record must show that the client was offered the opportunity to complete these documents. The documentation must indicate decisions made or not made at that time. Clients cannot be coerced into signing advance directives, nor can they be discriminated against should they choose not to sign an advance directive.

Facility policies vary as to who provides the information on advance directives. Many health care facilities assign this responsibility to the admissions office or social services; others have the nurses do it. Regardless of which department is assigned this task, the nurse is frequently called on to assist the client in understanding this information.

Before discussing advance directives with a client, the nurse must be familiar with the Patient Self-Determination Act of 1990. In the role of client advocate, the nurse explains the different types of advance directives to the client and family members. Terms such as *palliative care, supportive care, comfort measures,* or *nutrition and hydration* may not be understood by the client. The nurse can define those concepts more clearly and emphasize that the client has the right to choose what he believes is best for himself.

The nurse may suggest that the client discuss personal preferences with the physician and family members. When the client does so, problems may be prevented later. If the wishes of the family are different from those of the client, the health care team is caught in the middle, the concern being that the family may bring a lawsuit against the facility and the physician. The advance directive serves as a guide from the client. The facility's ethics committee may also be involved. The nurse should emphasize that these advance directives only go into effect should the individual become incompetent, have a terminal illness, or when death is imminent.

TO THE PATIENT: You have the right as a patient to be informed about your condition and the recommended surgical, medical, or diagnostic procedure to be used so that you may make the decision whether or not to undergo the procedure after knowing the risks and hazards involved. This disclosure is not meant to scare or alarm you, but is simply an effort to make you better informed so you may give or withhold your consent to the procedure. Any questions or concerns you may have with respect to the proposed procedure, its risks, complications, or benefits should be directed to your treating physician.

I (we) voluntarily request Dr. _____ as my physician, and such associates, technical assistants and other health care providers as they may deem necessary to treat my condition, which has been explained to me as: _____

I (we) understand that the following surgical, medical, and/or diagnostic procedures are planned for me, and I (we) voluntarily consent and authorize these procedures: _____

I (we) understand that my physician may discover other or different conditions which require additional or different procedures than those planned. I (we) authorize my physician, and such associates, technical assistants, and other health care providers, to perform such procedures which are advisable in their professional judgment.

I (we) [DO] [DO NOT] consent to the use of blood and blood products as deemed necessary.

I (we) understand that no warrant or guarantee has been made to me as a result or cure.

Just as there may be risks and hazards in continuing my present condition without treatment, there are also risks and hazards related to the performance of the surgical, medical, and/or diagnostic procedures planned for me. I (we) realize that common to surgical, medical, and/or diagnostic procedures is the potential for infection, blood clots in veins and lungs, hemorrhage, allergic reactions, and even death. I (we) realize that the following risks and hazards may occur in connection with this particular procedure:

(Additional Consent Information On Back.)

INITIAL: _____

CHRISTUS SPOHN HEALTH SYSTEM

DISCLOSURE AND CONSENT
MEDICAL AND SURGICAL PROCEDURES
PATIENT CARE SERVICES

2704980   NEW: 05/82
                 REVISED: 10/99

3025

I (we) understand that anesthesia involves additional risks and hazards, but I (we) request the use of anesthetics for the relief and protection from pain during the planned and additional procedures. I (we) realize the anesthesia may have to be changed, possibly without explanation to me (us).

I (we) understand that certain complications may result from the use of any anesthetic, including respiratory problems, drug reaction, paralysis, brain damage, or even death. Other risks and hazards which may result from the use of general anesthetics range from minor discomfort to injury to vocal cords, teeth, or eyes. I (we) understand that other risks and hazards resulting from spinal or epidural anesthetics include headache, chronic pain, remote possibility of nerve injury, hematoma, infection, septic and aseptic meningitis, nausea, vomiting, itching, and urinary retention.

I (we) consent to the photographing of the operations or procedures to be performed, including appropriate portions of the body, for medical, scientific, or educational purposes, provided my identity is not revealed by descriptive texts accompanying the picture.

I (we) consent to the disposition by hospital authorities of any tissues or parts which may be removed.

I (we) have been given the opportunity to ask questions about my conditions, alternative forms of anesthesia and treatment, risks of non-treatment, the procedures to be used, and the risks and hazards involved, and I (we) believe that I (we) have sufficient information to give this informed consent.

My physician has discussed the alternatives, risks and benefits, of the proposed procedures. I (we) certify that this form has been fully explained to me; that I (we) have read it or have had it read to me; that the blank spaces have been filled in, and that I (we) understand its contents.

_____
PHYSICIAN'S SIGNATURE

DATE: _____ TIME: _____ A.M./P.M.

_____
Witness (Signature of witness/print name of witness)

_____
Patient/Other Legally Responsible Person
(Minor patient and parent/guardian signature)

Figure 6-5 Disclosure and Consent—Medical and Surgical Procedures (*Courtesy Christus Spohn Health System, Corpus Christi, TX*)

Durable Power of Attorney

A **durable power of attorney for health care** (DPAHC) is a legal document designating who may make health care decisions for a client when that client is no longer capable of decision making. This health care representative is appointed by the client and is expected to act in the best interests of the client. This appointment can be revoked any time the competent client chooses.

For example, if a client lapses into a coma and the prognosis is poor, the health care representative or the person appointed DPAHC can either give consent for certain types of treatment or withhold consent for treatment, even if the lack of treatment results in the client's death. It is expected that the health care representative has discussed treatment preferences with the client and thus knows the client's wishes. The DPAHC is activated only when the client is no longer competent to make health care decisions.

The person who has power of attorney or the authority to make decisions for a client in some areas does not necessarily have the same authority regarding health care issues. The granting of the right to make health care decisions has to be specified in the power of attorney agreement, or a DPAHC must be signed (Figure 6-6). Because of a possible conflict of interest, the health care representative may be different from the individual assigned the power of attorney.

A person who stands to benefit from the client's estate cannot be appointed health care representative. If a decision to terminate life support would benefit the designee financially, for instance, a conflict of interest would exist. This person could have the right to make decisions about the client in matters not pertaining to health care, however.

Living Will

A **living will** is a legal document that allows a person to state preferences about the use of life-sustaining measures should she be unable to make her wishes known. These preferences can be expressed either with a living will or a Life-Prolonging Procedure Declaration. These documents allow the client to specify, in advance, those life-sustaining measures that are to be done or not done.

The living will states that certain life-prolonging treatments are not to be used and that the individual prefers to die naturally. Food, fluids, and comfort measures are continued, and the person is not abandoned. However, artificial means of sustaining life, such as ventilators or feeding tubes, are not to be used.

Although not all states currently recognize living wills, the client's requests should be given due weight when making health care decisions. The nurse must be knowledgeable about living will legislation in her state. A sample living will is shown in Figure 6-7.

The Life-Prolonging Procedure Declaration indicates that the person wants all possible procedures done to delay the dying process (Figure 6-8). This can include the use of ventilators and any other methods to keep the person alive by artificial means.

Where a form for a living will, durable power of attorney, and/or health care representative is provided by statute, it should be utilized, because health care providers are familiar with it. However, variations of the forms, if all the required elements are included, may also be legal.

INCIDENT REPORTS

An **incident report** is a risk management tool used to describe and report any unusual event that occurs to a client, visitor, or staff member. It is used to help the facility identify or track problem areas and alert the legal department to possible lawsuits. An incident report is not meant to be a punitive device, although it is often perceived in that manner.

Incident reports are completed to document such events as falls, medication errors, forgotten treatment, injuries—anything that happens out of the ordinary. Another name for an incident report is a variance report or an occurrence report. The following three examples illustrate the types of occurrences that should be documented in an incident report.

- Mrs. Duncan had blood drawn for various laboratory tests. It was later discovered that the laboratory work had been ordered on Mrs. Falson, not Mrs. Duncan. The requisition had been stamped with the wrong name.
- Mrs. Barnes was given Lasix 20 mg po at 9 AM. When reviewing the physician's orders, the evening nurse discovered that Losec 20 mg had been ordered. Mrs. Barnes received the wrong medication.
- Mrs. Gomez was visiting her daughter, who had just given birth to the family's first grandchild. While walking down the hall, Mrs. Gomez slipped and fell, injuring her right hip.

All of the previous examples are incidents or variances that may typically occur in health care settings. For each situation, an incident report must be completed and channeled to the risk management department. Under the auspices of risk management, a subgroup comprising representatives from various departments, such as nursing administration, dietary services, environmental safety, and others, reviews the incident report. This group tries to identify those factors, if any, that contributed to the incident. Examples of questions asked include "Can the causal factors be eliminated or reduced?" "Does the possibility of a lawsuit exist as a result of the incident?" and "What can be done to prevent this incident from occurring again?"

Part I. Durable Power of Attorney for Health Care

- If you do NOT wish to name an agent to make health care decisions for you, write your initials in the box

[Initials]

This form has been prepared to comply with the "Durable Power of Attorney for Health Care Act" of Missouri.

1. Selection of agent. I appoint:
Name:_____
Address:_____
_____
Telephone:_____
as my Agent.

> It is suggested that only one Agent be named. However, if more than one Agent is named, anyone may act individually unless you specify otherwise.

2. Alternate Agents. Only an Agent named by me may act under this Durable Power of Attorney. If my Agent resigns or is not able or available to make health care decisions for me, or if an Agent named by me is divorced from me or is my spouse and legally separated from me, I appoint the person(s) named below (in the order named if more than one):

First Alternate Agent	Second Alternate Agent
Name:_____	Name:_____
Address:_____	Address:_____
_____	_____
Telephone:_____	Telephone:_____

> This is a Durable Power of Attorney, and the authority of my Agent shall not terminate if I become disabled or incapacitated.

Part II. Health Care Directive

- If you DO NOT WISH to make a health care directive, write your initials in the box to the right, and go to Part III.

[Initials]

I make this HEALTH CARE DIRECTIVE ("Directive") to exercise my right to determine the course of my health care and to provide clear and convincing proof of my wishes and instructions about my treatment.

If I am persistently unconscious or there is no reasonable expectation of my recovery from a seriously incapacitating or terminal illness or condition, I direct that all of the life-prolonging procedures which I have initialed below be withheld or withdrawn.

I want the following life-prolonging procedures to be withheld or withdrawn:

> - artificially supplied nutrition and hydration (including tube feeding of food and water) . . . . [Initials]

- surgery or other invasive procedures. . . . . [Initials]
- heart-lung resuscitation (CPR) . . . . [Initials]
- antibiotic. . . . . [Initials]
- dialysis. . . . . [Initials]
- mechanical ventilator (respirator). . . . . [Initials]
- chemotherapy. . . . . [Initials]
- radiation therapy. . . . . [Initials]
- all other "life-prolonging" medical or surgical procedures that are merely intended to keep me alive without reasonable hope of improving my condition or curing my illness or injury. . . . . [Initials]

However, if my physician believes that any life-prolonging procedure may lead to significant recovery, I direct my physician to try the treatment for a reasonable period of time. If it does not improve my condition, I direct the treatment be withdrawn even if it shortens my life. I also direct that I be given medical treatment to relieve pain or to provide comfort, even if such treatment might shorten my life, suppress my appetite or my breathing, or be habit forming.

IF I HAVE NOT DESIGNATED AN AGENT IN THE DURABLE POWER OF ATTORNEY, THIS DOCUMENT IS MEANT TO BE IN FULL FORCE AND EFFECT AS MY HEALTH CARE DIRECTIVE.

Part I. Durable Power of Attorney for Health Care (Continued)

3. Effective date and durability. This Durable Power of Attorney is effective when two physicians decide and certify that I am incapacitated and unable to make and communicate a health care decision.

- If you want ONE physician, instead of TWO, to decide whether you are incapacitated, write your initials in the box to the right.

[Initials]

4. Agent's powers. I grant to my Agent full authority to:

A. Give consent to, prohibit, or withdraw any type of health care, medical care, treatment, or procedure, even if my death may result;

- If you wish to AUTHORIZE your Agent to direct a health care provider to withhold or withdraw artificially supplied nutrition and hydration (including tube feeding of food and water), write your initials in the box to the right.

[Initials]

- If you DO NOT WISH TO AUTHORIZE your Agent to direct a health care provider to withhold or withdraw artificially supplied nutrition and hydration (including tube feeding of food and water), write your initials in the box to the right.

[Initials]

B. Make all necessary arrangements for health care services on my behalf, and to hire and fire medical personnel responsible for my care;

C. Move me into or out of any health care facility (even if against medical advice) to obtain compliance with the decisions of my Agent; and

D. Take any other action necessary to do what I authorize here, including (but not limited to) granting any waiver or release from liability required by any health care provider, and taking any legal action at the expense of my estate to enforce this Durable Power of Attorney.

5. Agent's Financial Liability and Compensation. My Agent acting under this Durable Power of Attorney will incur no personal financial liability. My Agent shall not be entitled to compensation for services performed under this Durable Power of Attorney, but my Agent shall be entitled to reimbursement for all reasonable expenses incurred as a result of carrying out any provision hereof.

Part III. General Provisions Included in the Directive and Durable Power of Attorney

YOU MUST SIGN THIS DOCUMENT IN THE PRESENCE OF TWO WITNESSES.
IN WITNESS WHEREOF, I have executed this document this_____day of
_____, year_____.

_____
Signature

Print name _____
Address _____

The person who signed this document is of sound mind and voluntarily signed this document in our presence. Each of the undersigned witnesses is at least eighteen years of age.

Signature_____   Signature_____
Print name _____   Print name _____
Address _____   Address _____

> ONLY REQUIRED FOR PART I — DURABLE POWER OF ATTORNEY

STATE OF MISSOURI   )
) as
_____OF_____   )

On this _____day of_____, year_____, before me personally appeared to me known to be the person described in and who executed the foregoing instrument and acknowledged that he/she executed the same as his/her free act and deed.

IN WITNESS WHEREOF, I have hereunto set my hand and affixed my official seal in the County of _____, State of Missouri, the day and year first above written.

_____
Notary Public

My Commision Expires:

Figure 6-6 Durable Power of Attorney for Health Care and Health Care Directive *(Reprinted with permission of the Missouri Bar)*

Sample Living Will

Declaration made this _____ day of _____, year_____.

I, _____, willfully and voluntarily make known my desire that my dying not be artificially prolonged under the circumstances set forth below, and I do hereby declare:

If at any time I have a terminal condition and if my attending or treating physician and another consulting physician have determined that there is no medical probability of my recovery from such condition, I direct that life-prolonging procedures be withheld or withdrawn when the application of such procedures would serve only to prolong artificially the process of dying, and that I be permitted to die naturally with only the administration of medication or the performance of any medical procedure deemed necessary to provide me with comfort care or to alleviate pain.

It is my intention that this declaration be honored by my family and physician as the final expression of my legal right to refuse medical or surgical treatment and to accept the consequences for such refusal.

In the event that I have been determined to be unable to provide express and informed consent regarding the withholding, withdrawal, or continuation of life-prolonging procedures, I wish to designate, as my surrogate to carry out the provisions of this declaration:

Name: _____
Address: _____
_____ Zip Code: _____
Phone: _____

I wish to designate the following person as my alternate surrogate, to carry out the provisions of this declaration should my surrogate be unwilling or unable to act on my behalf:

Name: _____
Address: _____
_____ Zip Code: _____
Phone: _____

Additional instructions (optional):

I understand the full importance of this declaration, and I am emotionally and mentally competant to make this declaration.
Signed: _____

Witness 1:
    Signed: _____
    Address: _____

Witness 2:
    Signed: _____
    Address: _____

Figure 6-7 Sample Living Will *(Reprinted by permission of Choice in Dying, 200 Varick Street, New York, NY 10014)*

CAYLOR-NICKEL MEDICAL CENTER   Date of Birth   Clinic #

LIFE PROLONGING PROCEDURES
DECLARATION

Patient
Name:

Declaration made this _____ day of _____ (month, year).

I _____, being at least eighteen (18) years old and of sound mind, willfully and voluntarily make known my desires that if at any time I have an incurable injury, disease, or illness determined to be a terminal condition, I request the use of life-prolonging procedures that would extend my life. This includes appropriate nutrition and hydration and the administration of medication and the performance of all other medical procedures necessary to extend my life, to provide me with comfort care, or to alleviate pain.

Other instructions:

In the absence of my ability to give directions regarding the use of life-prolonging procedures, it is my intention that this declaration be honored by my family and physician as the final expression of my legal right to request medical or surgical treatment and as acceptance of the consequences of the request.

I understand the full impact of this declaration.

Signed _____

City, County, and State of Residence

The declarant has been personally known to me, and I believe (him/her) to be of sound mind. I did not sign the declarant's signature above for or at the direction of the declarant. I am not a parent, spouse, or child of the declarant. I am not entitled to any part of the declarant's estate and/or financially responsible for the declarant's medical care. I am competent and at least eighteen (18) years old.

Witness _____ Date_____

Witness _____ Date_____

Forward to social service department

Figure 6-8 Life-Prolonging Procedures Declaration *(Courtesy Caylor-Nickel Medical Center)*

Incident reports are filed by the person who was responsible for, who witnessed, or who discovered the incident. The report should state what was observed, as opposed to what is supposed. It should be factual and concise. In the third example given previously, if the nurse did not witness the actual fall, the correctly worded report would read: "Mrs. Gomez found lying on floor outside room 222. Several puddles of liquid found under and around her; paper cup lying nearby." An incorrect, presumptuous, and potentially damaging report might read: "Mrs. Gomez tripped and fell outside room 222. She slipped in a puddle of water." Mrs. Gomez may have spilled the cup of water she was carrying during the fall. However, this second note implies that Mrs. Gomez slipped in water that was already on the floor, thus implicating the facility.

Incident reports should include a description of the care given to the client or individual, and the name of the physician who was notified. The incident should be charted in the client's medical record, but the incident report should not be referred to in any way. Although the incident report is not a part of the medical record, the details described in the medical record and in the incident report should be the same.

When completing an incident report, the nurse should be sure to include the date and time of the incident as well as assessments and interventions. The time that family members and physicians were notified should also be included. The nurse should refer to nursing administration policy and procedure regarding follow-up documentation.

PROFESSIONAL LIABILITY

Many nurses believe they do not need their own malpractice or liability insurance. They assume the coverage provided by their employer is adequate. This may be a misconception.

Nurses claim to be competent and knowledgeable health care providers. The health care consumer has heard this message and thus holds the nurse accountable for her actions. As a result, nurses are named as defendants in malpractice suits. Under the doctrine of *Respondeat Superior,* employers are responsible for the actions of their employees. However, this responsibility stops when the employee leaves work. Also, if the nurse violates policy and the employer is forced to pay damages, the employer has the right to sue the nurse to recover losses.

Having a professional liability policy provides the nurse with an attorney, someone who will represent that nurse in court. An attorney representing the facility or a group of employees will be most concerned about the employer; the needs of an individual nurse will be secondary. The decision to settle a case or pursue a particular course of action may be based on the needs of the employer. The individual nurse is better represented in court by private counsel.

Frequently, family members and friends ask a nurse for advice or assistance in health care matters. This advice is sought because of the nurse's knowledge, experience, and role. Should the family members or friends later take issue with the results of the advice or treatment given by a nurse, they might bring a suit against the nurse.

Despite the fact that no money was exchanged for information or services, the nurse is still accountable for the advice given. If the situation ends up in court, the nurse needs legal representation. Legal representation is costly as can be judgments against the nurse. A professional liability insurance policy protects the nurse by providing legal representation and paying the judgments.

There are two basic types of liability protection: the claims made policy and the occurrence policy. The claims made policy protects the nurse against claims made during the time the policy is in effect. If a claim is made after the policy has been terminated, the nurse is not covered. Occurrence policies protect the nurse against events that took place during the period of time the policy was active, even if a claim is filed after the policy is terminated. Occurrence policies seem to offer better protection for the nurse.

Opinions differ as to whether nurses should carry individual liability insurance. Some attorneys and health care professionals believe this practice encourages lawsuits. Nurses must compare the cost and the benefits of having professional liability insurance against the cost of potential legal fees and loss of personal assets. When securing liability insurance, the nurse should validate the company's reputation. Most nursing organizations offer group professional liability insurance.

IMPAIRED NURSE

One of the more sensitive issues in the nursing profession today is the subject of the impaired nurse. By definition, an **impaired nurse** is a nurse who is habitually intemperate or is addicted to the use of alcohol or habit-forming drugs. Although job performance may not be immediately compromised, substance abuse does eventually interfere with clinical judgment and performance. Because of the high level of job-related stress and the accessibility of drugs, the chemical dependency rate among nurses is greater than that among the general public.

In cases of impaired health care workers, the primary concern is client care. In the role of client advocate, a nurse cannot let loyalties to co-workers interfere with duty to the client. It is difficult reporting a coworker. No one wants to be a "squealer." In many states, however, the board of nursing requires nurses to report impaired coworkers. Nurses suspected of being under the influence of drugs or alcohol must be reported to the proper authority at the place of employment. The second consideration is getting help for the impaired nurse and taking action to correct the problem.

A nurse who suspects a coworker of diverting drugs or abusing alcohol should:

1. Document the dates, times, and observed behavior. Specific and descriptive accounts of what was observed are critical. For example:

    > January 3, 2001. P.P. working 3–11 shift. Client A and Client B verbalized unrelieved postoperative pain. Documentation by P.P. stated both clients were comfortable after administration of Demerol 75 mg IM. Narcotic count at shift change satisfactory.

    > January 4, 2001. Client C and Client D verbalized unrelieved pain. Documentation by P.P. indicated both clients stated pain was relieved after administration of Demerol 100 mg IM. Narcotic count at shift change okay.

    > January 5, 2001. Narcotic count showed 1 Demerol 100-mg syringe listed as broken and 1 Demerol 75-mg syringe listed as wasted, "client changed her mind." P.P. signed the narcotic sheet.

or

> March 1–2, 2001. S.L. working the night shift. Strong odor of alcohol on his breath.

> March 3, 2001. S.L. observed walking with unsteady gait, speech is slurred, strong odor of alcohol on breath.

2. Go to the supervisor and report concerns. Providing a copy of the documentation about the suspicious incidents is helpful. The supervisor will take responsibility for confronting the suspected employee. Intoxication requires immediate removal from the clinical area. In other situations, the supervisor will devise a plan before confronting the nurse.

3. Refrain from approaching or confronting the coworker. The impaired coworker may become defensive and deny the problem or make threats. Also, once aware that someone is suspicious, the nurse may become more secretive, making detection less likely. Frequently, the nurse will quit one facility and go to another, repeating the same pattern.

Some employers offer an employee assistance program to rehabilitate the impaired nurse. In addition, most states have **peer assistance programs** (rehabilitation programs designed to provide an impaired nurse with referrals, professional and peer counseling support groups, and assistance and monitoring for reentry into nursing). These peer assistance programs operate under the auspices of the state nurses association and in conjunction with the board of nursing. The goals of assistance programs are to protect the public from impaired nurses, provide the needed assistance to the impaired nurse, assist the nurse to reenter nursing, and monitor the nurse's compliance. With the help of the peer counselor, the impaired nurse develops a contract for treatment. Compliance is monitored, and confidentiality is ensured. Successful completion of the program allows the nurse to return to the practice setting.

Participation in employer and peer assistance programs is optional. If the nurse chooses not to cooperate, however, employment may be terminated, and sanctions by the board of nursing may follow, including revocation of the license to practice.

CASE STUDY

Mr. Jones is admitted for congestive heart failure. He is 66 years old, newly diagnosed, and acutely ill at this time. A student LP/VN is assisting the RN with the admission. The student notes that Mr. Jones has a living will. Later, she asks the RN, "Will you have to contact the doctor regarding a No Code status for Mr. Jones? He's got a living will, so he doesn't want anything done."

1. List factors that the nurse should explain to assist the student in understanding the concept of a living will.

2. Describe how a cardiac arrest might affect this situation.

Mr. Jones' wife speaks privately with the RN, stating, "I want everything possible done to save my husband. I don't care what it takes."

3. Describe how Mrs. Jones' statements may or may not affect the living will requests that Mr. Jones has made.

4. Delineate how the nurse might respond in this situation.

When Mr. Jones refuses a recommended treatment option, Mrs. Jones disagrees and tells the doctor to go ahead with the recommended treatment plan.

5. How does the Patient Self-Determination Act affect Mr. Jones' refusal of treatment?

6. List the parameters that allow Mrs. Jones to consent to or refuse treatment for her husband.

Jamal Wilkins came to the hospital for outpatient diagnostic testing. Passing an open door, he saw his high school principal, Mr. Jones, lying in a bed. A respiratory therapist was giving Mr. Jones a treatment, and there seemed to be tubes and bags hanging everywhere. Alarmed, Jamal went to the nurse's station seeking information. He pointed to Mr. Jones' name and room number, which were listed on the board, and began asking questions.

7. Discuss ways to calm Jamal's fears without violating Mr. Jones' right to privacy.

8. Identify those ways that this client's privacy has already been violated.

SUMMARY

- Laws are rules that guide personal interaction. They are derived from several sources and can be classified as public or civil.
- Within most states, the nursing practice act indicates the scope of practice for nurses. Standards have been developed to guide nursing practice.
- The nurse should be familiar with client rights. Care should be taken not to falsely imprison a client or violate the client's right to privacy.
- The client's chart is a legal document and should accurately reflect client status and care. Entries should be neat and timely.
- Informed consent is more than just signing a form. It requires an understanding of the risks, benefits, and alternatives to treatment.
- Whether to purchase malpractice insurance is a personal decision. However, having one's own policy provides both coverage off the job and individual legal counsel.
- Impaired nurses are everyone's concern. Dates and times of inappropriate behaviors should be documented and reported to the immediate supervisor.
- Incident reports are a risk management tool. They are not meant to be used for punitive purposes.
- Advance directives are instructions about health care preferences. They both protect the rights of the client and guide the family through difficult decisions.

Review Questions

1. Standards of practice are:
    a. different for each school of nursing.
    b. guidelines to direct nursing care.
    c. not legally binding.
    d. specific criteria on how to perform procedures.

2. Immunity for nurses giving care in emergency situations is provided under the:
    a. Care and Good Faith Act of 1937.
    b. Good Samaritan Law.
    c. state nursing practice act.
    d. Patient Self-Determination Act.

3. Select the situation that violates client privacy.
    a. copying information from the chart for a case study
    b. discussing client status with clinical instructor
    c. shutting the door and closing the curtain during a procedure
    d. talking in the cafeteria about an interesting client

4. To make the best use of time in the clinical area, the nurse should:
    a. chart events as they happen.
    b. chart in a block at the end of the shift.
    c. have a coworker who is not busy chart for her.
    d. sign off all meds at the beginning of the shift.

5. The responsibility for informed consent rests with the:
    a. nurse.
    b. client.
    c. physician.
    d. unit clerk.

6. Informed consent occurs when the:
    a. nurse discusses the surgical procedure with the client.
    b. client gives consent verbally.
    c. client understands the risks, benefits, and alternatives to treatment.
    d. client signs the consent form.

7. If a coworker is suspected of diverting drugs, the nurse should:
    a. approach the coworker and tell him what she thinks.
    b. document dates, times, and observed behavior and report same to the supervisor.
    c. say nothing; it is none of her business.
    d. tell coworkers what she thinks so that they can help watch for suspicious behavior.

8. Advance directives:
    a. are binding only if written.
    b. cannot be changed once they are notarized.
    c. guide family members through difficult decisions.
    d. prevent clients from determining the course of their health care.

9. The health care representative or durable power of attorney for health care:
    a. is appointed by hospital administrators to make medical decisions for the client.
    b. can give or withhold consent for treatment.
    c. is contacted to override the decisions the client makes for himself.
    d. is the client's physician or health care provider.

10. Which of the following situations reflects inappropriate use of an incident report?
    a. Mrs. Khamel falls in the hall while visiting her daughter.

b. A student nurse gives Losec instead of Lasix.

c. The safety committee reviews incident reports regarding falls on the 3–11 shift on A-wing.

d. An instructor, frustrated with a disorganized student nurse, fills out an incident report because the student gave a 9 AM medication at 9:25.

Critical Thinking Questions

1. How would you explain advance directives to your family?

2. How would you know whether a client gave informed consent?

WEB FLASH!

- What organizations or professional journals could you search to obtain information on nursing and legal issues?
- Search the web sites of certain law schools, such as Harvard or the University of Texas, for information pertaining to nurses or health care.
- What resources are available on the web for nurses needing legal advice?
- Search for information about the Good Samaritan law, malpractice, and professional liability insurance.

ETHICAL RESPONSIBILITIES

MAKING THE CONNECTION

Refer to the following chapters to increase your understanding of ethical responsibilities:

- **Chapter 2, Critical Thinking**
- **Chapter 6, Legal Responsibilities**
- **Chapter 12, Cultural Diversity and Nursing**

LEARNING OBJECTIVES

Upon completion of this chapter, you should be able to:
- *Define key terms.*
- *Explain the relationship among the concepts of ethics, morality, and law.*
- *Discuss the ethical theories of teleology and deontology.*
- *Describe the major ethical principles that have an impact on health care.*
- *Explain the link between ethics and values and the process involved in reconciling the potential conflicts between them.*
- *Relate the ethical codes developed by the National Federation of Licensed Practical Nurses and the International Council of Nurses to daily nursing practice.*
- *Identify the rights of the client as established by the American Hospital Association.*
- *Apply the steps identified in the framework for ethical decision making to issues such as euthanasia, refusal of treatment, and scarcity of resources.*
- *Discuss the roles of the nurse as client advocate and whistleblower in the delivery of ethical nursing care.*

KEY TERMS

active euthanasia	fidelity
assisted suicide	justice
autonomy	material principle of
beneficence	justice
bioethics	nonmaleficence
categorical imperative	passive euthanasia
client advocate	teleology
deontology	utility
ethical dilemma	value system
ethical principle	values
ethical reasoning	values clarification
ethics	veracity
euthanasia	whistleblowing

INTRODUCTION

Every day, nurses encounter situations wherein they must make decisions based on the determination of right and wrong. How do they make such decisions? Whose values determine the rightness of an action?

The delivery of ethical health care is becoming an increasingly difficult and confusing issue in contemporary society. Nurses are committed to respecting their clients' rights in terms of providing health care and treatment. This desire to maintain clients' rights, however, often conflicts with professional duties and institutional policies. Nurses must thus learn to balance these potentially conflicting perspectives so as to achieve the primary objective—the care of the client.

In considering the situations presented throughout this chapter, one must realize that there are no absolute right answers. Dealing with the gray areas (ambiguities) causes much discomfort for many nurses. Because clients and nurses are humans, no two situations, no matter how similar, can ever be exactly alike. This chapter explores the concept of ethics, including ethical principles and theories; ethics and values; ethical codes; the client's rights; ethical dilemmas; ethical decision making; and the application of ethical guidelines to nursing practice.

CONCEPT OF ETHICS

Ethics is the branch of philosophy concerned with determining right from wrong on the basis of a body of knowledge rather than on just the basis of opinions. Ethics deals with one's responsibilities (duties and obligations) as defined by logical argument. Ethics is *not* a religious dogma. Ethics looks at human behavior—which things people do under which types of circumstances. But ethics is not merely philosophical in nature; ethical persons put their beliefs into action.

Ethics in Health Care

The application of general ethical principles to health care is referred to as **bioethics**. Ethics affects every area of health care, including direct care of clients, allocation of finances, and utilization of staff. As Aroskar (1994) states:

> Ethics encompasses the whole of life: our conduct and behavior toward ourselves, toward others, and toward the environment. Ethics in nursing and health care is not just about terrible dilemmas at the beginning or end of life. Most human activity involves an ethical dimension even if it is not recognized or articulated.

Ethics does not provide easy answers, but it can help provide structure by raising questions that ultimately lead to answers.

Ethical practice is gaining ever-increasing importance in health care today. Several factors contribute to the increased need to provide health care in an ethical manner. Some of these factors are:

- An increasingly technological society. The nature of advanced technology creates situations involving complicated issues that never had to be considered before. As a result of technological advances:

  Many newborns are surviving at earlier gestational ages, and many of them have serious health problems.
  People are living much longer than ever before.
  Organ transplants and the use of bionic body parts are becoming more common.

- The changing fabric of our society. Family structure is moving from extended families to nuclear families, single-parent families, and nonrelated groups living together as families.

- Clients are becoming more knowledgeable about both their health and health-related interventions. As consumer demand for information increases, health care providers must adapt quickly. The result is a focus on the consumer-driven system.

Every day, nurses face situations wherein they must make decisions that transcend technical and professional concerns. These situations may or may not be life threatening. Such situations raise complex problems that cannot be answered completely with technical knowledge and professional expertise. The way that nurses relate to clients, families, and other health care providers is the true demonstration of ethical behavior.

ETHICAL PRINCIPLES

Ethical principles are codes that direct or govern actions. They are widely accepted and generally based on the humane aspects of society. Ethical decisions are principled, that is, they reflect what is best for the client and society. Table 7–1 summarizes the major ethical principles. Each principle is discussed in detail in the following paragraphs.

By applying ethical principles, the nurse can become more systematic in solving ethical conflicts. Ethical principles can be used as guidelines in analyzing dilemmas; they can also serve as justification (rationale) for the resolution of ethical problems. It should be emphasized that these principles are not absolute; there can be exceptions to each principle in any given situation.

Autonomy

The principle of **autonomy** refers to the individual's right to choose and the individual's ability to act on that choice. The individuality of each person is respected. This respect for personal liberty is a dominant value in U.S. society.

Nurses must respect the client's right to decide and must protect those clients who are unable to decide for themselves. Although the legal definition of competency varies among states, the ethical principle of autonomy reflects the belief that every competent person has the right to determine his own course of action. The right to free choice thus rests on the client's competency to decide.

Table 7–1 OVERVIEW OF ETHICAL PRINCIPLES	
PRINCIPLE	**EXPLANATION**
Autonomy	Respect for an individual's right to self-determination; respect for individual liberty
Nonmaleficence	The obligation to do or cause no harm to another
Beneficence	The duty to do good to others and to maintain a balance between benefits and harms
Justice	The equitable distribution of potential benefits and risks
Veracity	The obligation to tell the truth
Fidelity	The duty to do what one has promised

PROFESSIONAL TIP

Autonomy

- Competent clients have a right to self-determination, even if their decisions may result in self-harm.
- Probably one of the most difficult things for nurses to accept is that clients are ultimately responsible for themselves; they will do what they want to do.

Informed consent is based on the client's right to decide for herself. Upholding autonomy means that the nurse accepts the client's choices, even those choices that are not in the client's best interests or those choices that conflict with the nurse's values. Following are examples of autonomous behavior on the part of the client that can impair recovery or treatment:

- Smoking after a diagnosis of emphysema or lung cancer
- Refusing to take medication
- Continuing to drink alcohol after being diagnosed with cirrhosis of the liver
- Refusing to receive a blood transfusion because of religious beliefs

Nonmaleficence

Nonmaleficence is the obligation to cause no harm to others. Harm can take many forms: physiological, psychological, social, financial, and/or spiritual. Nonmaleficence refers to both intentional harm and the risk of harm. The principle of nonmaleficence

COMMUNITY/HOME HEALTH CARE

Client Autonomy

With the increased acuity level of clients cared for in the home setting, home health nurses face ever-increasing ethical challenges.

> Clients who are being cared for at home have more control over their decisions and actions than those who are institutionalized. . . . Client autonomy becomes a much stronger influence in the outcome of care than it does in institutional settings, because the provider has less control over what the client does on a day-to-day basis at home. . . . [Home health care] represents a power reversal in which the client's autonomy takes on greater significance. (Kristoff, Sellin, & Miller, 1994)

Table 7–2 VOCATIONAL NURSE'S PLEDGE

God being my Witness and Judge and the Light whereby my life is patterned, do solemnly pledge myself to keep the following vows:

I shall endeavor in all ways so to live and to conduct myself, at home and abroad, that my vocation shall be uplifted in the eyes of all people.

I shall help to elevate the standards of my vocation by doing my work, where ever I may be, at least a little better on each tomorrow than I was able to do it on each today.

I shall put the welfare of my patients above all else.

I shall not engage in idle talk about other vocational nurses, professional nurses, or doctors, for we are united in our care of the patient and gossip destroys unity.

So let me live that I may be of service to Him Who "so loved the world that He gave His only begotten Son that whosoever believeth in Him should not perish but have everlasting life."

Author unknown: Used for over 30 years by the Department of Vocational Nurse Education, Del Mar College, Corpus Christi, TX.

helps guide decisions about treatment approaches; the relevant question is "Will this treatment modality cause more harm or more good to the client?" Determining whether technology is harmful to the client is not always a clear-cut process. Factors to consider when choosing a treatment include:

- A reasonable prospect of benefit, and
- Lack of excessive expense, pain, or other inconvenience.

Nonmaleficence requires that the nurse act thoughtfully and carefully, weighing the potential risks and benefits of research or treatment. It is sometimes easier to weigh the risk than to measure the benefit. Further, it is possible to violate this principle without acting maliciously and without ever being aware of the harm, making the principle of nonmaleficence closely related to the concept of negligence. When upholding the principle of nonmaleficence, the nurse practices according to professional and legal standards of care.

Nonmaleficence is considered a fundamental duty of health care providers. The Vocational Nurses's Pledge (Table 7–2), The Practical Nurse's Pledge (Table 7–3), and the Nightingale Pledge (Table 7–4) all profess the same basic philosophy of nursing care. Some clinical examples of nonmaleficence are:

- Preventing medication errors (including drug interactions),
- Being aware of potential risks of treatment modalities, and
- Removing hazards (e.g., obstructions that might cause a fall).

Table 7–4 NIGHTINGALE PLEDGE

I solemnly pledge myself before God and in the presence of this assembly: To pass my life in purity and to practice my profession faithfully.

I will abstain from whatever is deleterious and mischievous, and will not take or knowingly administer any harmful drug.

I will do all in my power to maintain and elevate the standards of my profession, and will hold in confidence all personal matters committed to my keeping, and all family affairs coming to my knowledge in the practice of my profession.

With loyalty will I endeavor to aid the physician in his work, and devote myself to the welfare of those committed to my care.

Table 7–3 PRACTICAL NURSE'S PLEDGE

Before God and those assembled here, I solemnly pledge:

To adhere to the code of ethics of the nursing profession.

To cooperate faithfully with the other members of the nursing team and to carry out faithfully and to the best of my ability the instructions of the physician or the nurse who may be assigned to supervise my work.

I will not do anything evil or malicious and I will not knowingly give any harmful drug or assist in malpractice.

I will not reveal any confidential information that may come to my knowledge in the course of my work.

And I pledge myself to do all in my power to raise the standards and the prestige of practical nursing.

May my life be devoted to service, and to the high ideals of the nursing profession.

Reprinted with permission of the National Association for Practical Nurse Education and Services Inc., Silver Spring, MD.

Beneficence

Beneficence is the duty to promote good and to prevent harm. Beneficence is often viewed as the core of nursing practice. The nurse serves as a client advocate and promotes the rights of the client. The nurse nurtures the client and incorporates the desires of the client into the plan of care. Sometimes, it is difficult to determine what is "good," especially when doing good causes the client discomfort. For example, a client who has been in a serious car accident may resist performing painful range-of-motion exercises and become angry at the nurse for insisting. The nurse understands the long-term value of performing the exercises, yet understands the client's physical and psychological pain.

Justice

The principle of **justice** is based on the concept of fairness extended to each individual. The major health-related issues of justice involve the way people are treated and the way resources are distributed. Justice considers action from the point of view of the least fortunate in society. As a result of equal and similar treatment of people, benefits and burdens are equally distributed. The distribution of scarce resources is commonly decided according to individual need (Davis & Aroskar, 1997).

The ethical principle of justice requires that all people be treated equally unless there is a justification for unequal treatment. The **material principle of justice** is the rationale for determining those times when there can be unequal allocation of scarce resources. This concept specifies that resources be allocated:

- Equally,
- According to need,
- According to individual effort,
- According to the individual's merit (ability), and
- According to the individual's contribution to society (DeLaune & Ladner, 1998).

An example of the application of the material principle of justice (according to the individual's contribution to society) is the Veterans Affairs (VA) Medical Centers. Only individuals who gave to their country by serving in the military are eligible to receive health care through the VA in ambulatory, acute care, and psychiatric facilities.

In health care institutions, the principle of justice is being strenuously tested on the issue of allocating one important resource: nursing personnel. Many institutions and agencies are downsizing their professional staff as a cost-containment measure. As a result, some health care facilities are so poorly staffed or have such a high ratio of underqualified personnel providing care, that quality of care is being severely compromised (Schildmeier, 1997).

Veracity

Veracity means truthfulness (neither lying nor deceiving others). Deception can take many forms: intentional lying, nondisclosure of information, or partial disclosure of information. Veracity often is difficult to achieve. It may not be hard to tell the truth, but it can be very hard to decide how much truth to tell. Exceptions to truth-telling are sometimes upheld by the principle of nonmaleficence, when the truth does greater harm than good. The act of giving placebo medications is an example of when telling the truth does greater harm than good.

Fidelity

The concept of **fidelity** (which is the ethical foundation of nurse–client relationships) means faithfulness and keeping promises.

Clients have an ethical right to expect nurses to act in their best interests. As nurses function in the role of **client advocate** (a person who speaks up for or acts on behalf of the client), they are upholding the principle of fidelity. Fidelity is demonstrated when nurses:

- Represent the client's viewpoint to other members of the health care team,
- Avoid letting their own personal values influence their advocacy for clients, and
- Support the client's decision, even when it conflicts with their own preferences or choices.

Within the nurse–client relationship, nurses should be loyal to their responsibilities, keep promises, maintain privacy, and meet resonable expectations of clients. Nurses also have a duty to be faithful to themselves. Conflict between commitments can complicate matters for the nurse, who may question who is owed fidelity. Although maintaining client centeredness may help clarify this question, it may not resolve the conflict. For example, if the mother of a frightened teenage girl tried to pressure the nurse into revealing the results of the daughter's pregnancy test after the daughter had already requested that her mother not be told, although the nurse may believe that the mother has the girl's best interests at heart, the nurse must protect the client's right to privacy.

ETHICAL THEORIES

Ethical theories were debated by ancient philosophers such as Plato and Aristotle, and the debate continues today. Whereas ethical theories can be used as a way to analyze ethical problems, no theory in and of itself can provide the "correct" answer to any single ethical conflict. Common ethical theories include teleology, deontology, situational theory, and caring-based theory.

Teleology

Teleology is an ethical theory that states that the value of a situation is determined by its consequences. Thus, the outcome of an action—not the action itself—is the criterion for determining the goodness of that action. An example would be immunizations—receiving an injection is not "good," but preventing the illness is.

This theory (also called the consequentialist theory) was advocated by the philosopher John Stuart Mill. The principle of **utility** is a basic concept of teleology; utility states that an act must result in the greatest degree of good for the greatest number of people involved in a given situation. "Good" refers to positive benefit. Thus, any act can be ethical if it delivers positive results. Concepts considered inherently good for all members of a society include health, strength, truth, freedom, security, and peace (Edge & Groves, 1999). Every alternative is assessed for its potential outcomes, both positive and negative. The selected action is the one that results in the most benefits and the least

CULTURAL CONSIDERATIONS

Smoke-Free Facilities
- Declaring health care facilities "smoke free" results in the most benefit and least harm for everyone.
- The minority group of smokers and the individual's right to smoke are ignored.

amount of harm for all those involved. A major disadvantage is that minority and individual rights may be ignored for the benefit of the masses.

Safety: Immunizations
- The outcome of immunizations is the prevention of given illnesses in the individual and, thus, the prevention of the spread of those illnesses to the community.
- The greatest good for the greatest number of persons is achieved with immunizations.

Deontology

Deontology is an ethical theory that considers the intrinsic significance of an act itself as the criterion for determination of good. That is, in determining the ethics of a situation, a person must consider not the consequences of the act, but the motives of the individual performing the act. This theory (also called formalism) was postulated by the philosopher Immanuel Kant. Kant established the concept of the **categorical imperative**, which states that a person should act only if the action is based on a principle that is universal (that is, everyone would act in the same way in a similar situation). The categorical imperative also mandates that a person should never be treated as a means to an end. Adherence to this concept may pose an ethical problem for health care researchers, who sometimes might be willing to risk the well-being of a person participating in an experimental procedure for the sake of finding, for example, a drug that will save many victims from suffering.

Situational Theory

The situational theory holds that there are no set rules, norms, or majority-focused results. Each situation must be considered individually, with an emphasis on the uniqueness of the situation and a respect for the person involved. Decisions made in one situation cannot be generalized to another situation (Pappas, 1997).

Caring-Based Theory

Caring-based theory is founded on the premise that people do not make ethical decisions based on princi-

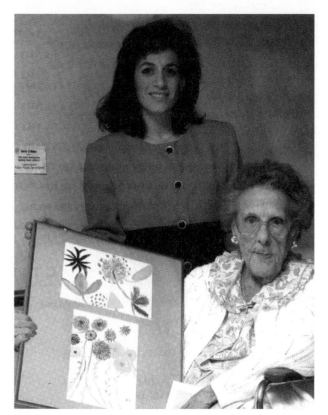

Figure 7-1 Caring-based theory is expressed by this nurse, who is supporting the client through caring.

ples. Decisions are made with respect to relationships, caring, communication, a desire not to hurt others, and responsiveness. Caring-based theory focuses on emotions, feelings, and attitudes (Figure 7-1). This theory is sometimes referred to as the "voice of care" and is contrasted with the "voice of justice." Justice and caring are not considered mutually exclusive and can, in fact, be complementary (Beare & Myers, 1998).

ETHICS AND VALUES

The close relationship between ethics and values both illuminates and complicates the nurse's approach toward balancing the ethical principles of the health care profession with those of the client. Nurses must examine their own value systems to ascertain the best approach in managing the care of clients whose values may be different from their own. In order to practice ethically, nurses must understand their own values. **Values** are different from principles, in that they influence the development of beliefs and attitudes rather than behaviors, although they might, and usually do, indirectly influence behaviors. A **value system** is an individual's collection of inner beliefs that guides the way the person acts and helps determine the choices the person makes in life. Although nearly nothing in life is value free, the impact of values on decisions and resultant behaviors is often not considered. Values are

similar to the act of breathing; one does not think about them until a problem arises.

Nurses often care for clients whose value systems conflict with their own. "Rarely do diagnostic and treatment decisions occur without reference to values" (Gordon, Murphy, Candee, & Hiltunen, 1994). For example, a client with a value system of "grin and bear it" may be insulted by a nurse's attempts to offer pain medications. In order to ascertain those things that are meaningful to the client, the nurse must have an understanding of the client's value system (Figure 7-2). Furthermore, nurses must be aware of their own values, especially when they conflict with the values of clients.

Values Clarification

Values clarification is the process of analyzing one's own values to better understand those things that are truly important. Through values clarification, nurses can increase self-awareness and become better able to care for clients whose values differ from their own. In their classic work *Values and Teaching*, Raths, Harmin, and Simon (1978) formulated a theory of values clarification and proposed a three-step process of valuing, as follows:

- Choosing: Beliefs are chosen freely (that is, without coercion) from among alternatives. The choosing step involves analysis of the consequences of the various alternatives.
- Prizing: The beliefs that are selected are cherished (that is, prized).
- Acting: The selected beliefs are demonstrated consistently through behavior.

Nurses must understand that values are individual rather than universal and that, therefore, the nurse

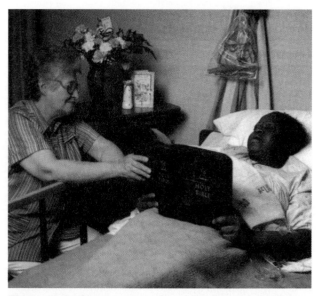

Figure 7-2 Clients' values determine those things that are meaningful to them.

PROFESSIONAL TIP

Values Clarification

It is the nurse's responsibility to make known to the supervisor any personal values that may influence or interfere with client care. For instance, a nurse who believes abortions should not be performed would find a conflict in working on a unit where abortions are performed. The nurse with this belief should make her values known to the employer before employment so that an assignment to that unit would not be made.

should not try to impose personal values on clients. The provision of ethical nursing care is directly related to one's values. For example, the nurse who strongly values the sanctity of life may experience an ethical conflict when caring for a terminally ill client who refuses treatment that may extend life for a short time.

ETHICAL CODES

One hallmark of a profession is the determination of ethical behavior for its members. Several nursing or-ganizations have developed codes as guidelines for ethical conduct. The Code for Licensed Practical/Vocational Nurses, developed by the National Federation of Licensed Practical Nurses (NFLPN), is presented in Table 7–5. This code, adopted by NFLPN in 1961 and revised in 1979 and in 1991, provides a motivation for establishing, maintaining, and elevating professional standards. Each LP/VN, upon entering the profession, inherits the responsibility to adhere to the standards of ethical practice and conduct as set forth in this code.

The Code for Nurses (Table 7–6) was developed by the International Council of Nurses (ICN). The American Nurses Association (ANA) has also established a code for the ethical conduct of registered nurses. Although a code of ethics, which provides broad principles for determining and evaluating nursing care, is not legally binding, most state boards of nursing have authority to reprimand nurses for unprofessional conduct that results from violation of the ethical code.

THE CLIENT'S RIGHTS

The concept of rights is often misused, overused, and abused. Our society tends to take rights for granted. Rights and obligations are culturally defined. The dominant culture in the United States, however, holds the ethnocentric perspective that our rights and values are shared globally.

Clients have certain rights that apply regardless of the setting for delivery of care. These rights include, but are not limited to, the right to:

- Make decisions regarding their care (Figure 7-3),
- Be actively involved in the treatment process, and
- Be treated with dignity and respect (Figure 7-4).

When clients are admitted to short-term acute care agencies or extended care facilities, they are also entitled to certain rights. In 1972, the American Hospital

---

Table 7–5 THE CODE FOR LICENSED PRACTICAL/VOCATIONAL NURSES

1. Know the scope of maximum utilization of the LP/VN as specified by the nursing practice act and function within this scope.

2. Safeguard the confidential information acquired from any source about the patient.

3. Provide health care to all patients regardless of race, creed, cultural background, disease, or lifestyle.

4. Refuse to give endorsement to the sale and promotion of commercial products or services.

5. Uphold the highest standards in personal appearance, language, dress, and demeanor.

6. Stay informed about issues affecting the practice of nursing and delivery of health care and, where appropriate, participate in government and policy decisions.

7. Accept the responsibility for safe nursing by keeping oneself mentally and physically fit and educationally prepared to practice.

8. Accept responsibility for membership in NFLPN and participate in its efforts to maintain the established standards of nursing practice and employment policies which lead to quality patient care.

From Nursing Practice Standards for the Licensed Practical/ Vocational Nurse, *by National Federation of Licensed Practical Nurses, Inc. (NFLPN), 1996, Garner, NC: Author. Copyright 1996 by Author. Reprinted with permission.*

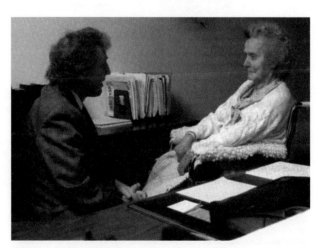

Figure 7-3 Clients have the right to information that will enable them to make decisions regarding their care.

Table 7–6 INTERNATIONAL COUNCIL OF NURSES CODE FOR NURSES

The fundamental responsibility of the nurse is fourfold: to promote health, to prevent illness, to restore health, and to alleviate suffering.

The need for nursing is universal. Inherent in nursing is respect for life, dignity, and rights of man. It is unrestricted by considerations of nationality, race, creed, color, age, sex, politics, or social status.

Nurses render health services to the individual, the family, and the community and coordinate their services with those of related groups.

Nurses and People

The nurse's primary responsibility is to those people who require nursing care.

The nurse, in providing care, promotes an environment in which the values, customs, and spiritual beliefs of the individual are respected.

The nurse holds in confidence personal information and uses judgment in sharing this information.

Nurses and Practice

The nurse carries personal responsibility for nursing practice and for maintaining competence by continual learning. The nurse maintains the highest standards of nursing care possible within the reality of a specific situation.

The nurse uses judgment in relation to individual competence when accepting and delegating responsibilities.

The nurse, when acting in a professional capacity, should at all times maintain standards of personal conduct that reflect credit upon the profession.

Nurses and Society

The nurse shares with other citizens the responsibility for initiating and supporting action to meet the health and social needs of the public.

Nurses and Coworkers

The nurse sustains cooperative relationships with coworkers in nursing and other fields. The nurse takes appropriate action to safeguard the individual when his care is endangered by a coworker or any other person.

Nurses and the Profession

The nurse plays the major role in determining and implementing desirable standards of nursing practice and nursing education.

The nurse is active in developing a core of professional knowledge.

The nurse, acting through the professional organization, participates in establishing and maintaining equitable social and economic working conditions in nursing.

From ICN Code for Nurses: Ethical Concepts Applied to Nursing, by International Council of Nurses (ICN), 1973, Geneva, Switzerland: Imprimeries Populaires. Copyright 1973 by ICN. Reprinted with permission.

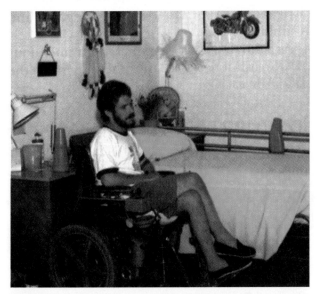

Figure 7-4 Clients have the right to dignity and respect and may keep personal articles in their rooms.

Association (AHA) established *A Patient's Bill of Rights*, which outlines the rights and responsibilities of clients receiving care in hospitals (Table 7–7). This document, revised in 1992, increases health care providers' awareness of the need to treat clients in an ethical manner and encourages all health care providers to protect the rights of clients.

ETHICAL DILEMMAS

An **ethical dilemma** occurs when there is a conflict between two or more ethical principles—when there is no "correct" decision. Ethical dilemmas are situations of conflicting requirements; something ought to be done and ought not to be done at the same time. When an ethical dilemma occurs, the nurse must make a choice between two alternatives that are equally unsatisfactory. Ethical analysis is not an exact science. In some cases, even after a dilemma seems to have

COMMUNITY/HOME HEALTH CARE

The Client's Rights

The client's rights as outlined in Table 7–7 must be respected regardless of the setting for delivery of care. For care delivered in the home environment, for instance, the home health care nurse should discuss the client's rights with the client during the initial assessment (Figure 7-5).

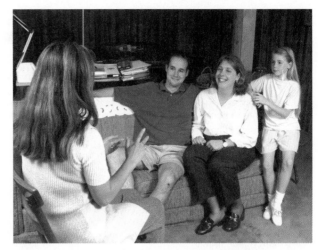

Figure 7-5 A home health nurse explains a client's rights.

Table 7–7 A PATIENT'S BILL OF RIGHTS

Introduction

Effective health care requires collaboration between patients and physicians and other health care professionals. Open and honest communication, respect for personal and professional values, and sensitivity to differences are integral to optimal patient care. As the setting for the provision of health services, hospitals must provide a foundation for understanding and respecting the rights and responsibilities of patients, their families, physicians, and other caregivers. Hospitals must ensure a health care ethic that respects the role of patients in decision making about treatment choices and other aspects of their care. Hospitals must be sensitive to cultural, racial, linguistic, religious, age, gender, and other differences as well as the needs of persons with disabilities.

The American Hospital Association presents *A Patient's Bill of Rights* with the expectation that it will contribute to more effective patient care and be supported by the hospital on behalf of the institution, its medical staff, employees, and patients. The American Hospital Association encourages health care institutions to tailor this bill of rights to their patient community by translating and/or simplifying the language of this bill of rights as may be necessary to ensure that patients and their families understand their rights and responsibilities.

Bill of Rights*

1. The patient has the right to considerate and respectful care.

2. The patient has the right to and is encouraged to obtain from physicians and other direct caregivers relevant, current, and understandable information concerning diagnosis, treatment, and prognosis. Except in emergencies when the patient lacks decision-making capacity and the need for treatment is urgent, the patient is entitled to the opportunity to discuss and request information related to the specific procedures and/or treatments, the risks involved, the possible length of recuperation, and the medically reasonable alternatives and their accompanying risks and benefits. Patients have the right to know the identity of physicians, nurses, and others involved in their care, as well as when those involved are students, residents, or other trainees. The patient also has the right to know the immediate and long-term financial implications of treatment choices, insofar as they are known.

3. The patient has the right to make decisions about the plan of care prior to and during the course of treatment and to refuse a recommended treatment or plan of care to the extent permitted by law and hospital policy and to be informed of the medical consequences of this action. In case of such refusal, the patient is entitled to other appropriate care and services that the hospital provides or transfer to another hospital. The hospital should notify patients of any policy that might affect patient choice within the institution.

4. The patient has the right to have an advance directive (such as a living will, health care proxy, or durable power of attorney for health care) concerning treatment or designating a surrogate decision maker with the expectation that the hospital will honor the intent of that directive to the extent permitted by law and hospital policy. Health care institutions must advise patients of their rights under state law and hospital policy to make informed medical choices, ask if the patient has an advance directive, and include that information in patient records. The patient has the right to timely information about hospital policy that may limit its ability to implement fully a legally valid advance directive.

5. The patient has the right to every consideration of privacy. Case discussion, consultation, examination, and treatment should be conducted so as to protect each patient's privacy.

6. The patient has the right to expect that all communications and records pertaining to his/her care will be treated as confidential by the hospital, except in cases such as suspected abuse and public health hazards when reporting is permitted or required by law. The patient has the right to expect that the hospital will emphasize the confidentiality of this information when it releases it to any other parties entitled to review information in these records.

7. The patient has the right to review the records pertaining to his/her medical care and to have the information explained or interpreted as necessary, except when restricted by law.

8. The patient has the right to expect that, within its capacity and policies, a hospital will make reasonable response to the request of a patient for appropriate and medically indicated care and services. The hospital must provide evaluation, service, and/or referral as indicated by the urgency of the case. When medically appropriate and legally permissible, or when a patient has so requested, a patient may be transferred to another facility. The institution to which the patient *continues*

Table 7-7 A PATIENT'S BILL OF RIGHTS *continued*

is to be transferred must first have accepted the patient for transfer. The patient must also have the benefit of complete information and explanation concerning the need for, risks, benefits, and alternatives to such a transfer.

9. The patient has the right to ask and be informed of the existence of business relationships among the hospital, educational institutions, other health care providers, or payers that may influence the patient's treatment and care. The patient has the right to obtain information as to the existence of any professional relationships among individuals, by name, who are treating him.

10. The patient has the right to consent to or decline to participate in proposed research studies or human experimentation affecting care and treatment or requiring direct patient involvement, and to have those studies fully explained prior to consent. A patient who declines to participate in research or experimentation is entitled to the most effective care that the hospital can otherwise provide.

11. The patient has the right to expect reasonable continuity of care when appropriate and to be informed by physicians and other caregivers of available and realistic patient care options when hospital care is no longer appropriate

12. The patient has the right to be informed of hospital policies and practices that relate to patient care, treatment, and responsibilities. The patient has the right to be informed of available resources for resolving disputes, grievances, and conflicts, such as ethics committees, patient representatives, or other mechanisms available in the institution. The patient has the right to be informed of the hospital's charges for services and available payment methods.

The collaborative nature of health care requires that patients, or their families/surrogates, participate in their care. The effectiveness of care and patient satisfaction with the course of treatment depend, in part, on the patient's fulfilling certain responsibilities. Patients are responsible for providing information about past illnesses, hospitalizations, medications, and other matters related to health status. To participate effectively in decision making, patients must be encouraged to take responsibility for requesting additional information or clarification about their health status or treatment when they do not fully understand information and instructions. Patients are also responsible for ensuring that the health care institution has a copy of their written advance directive if they have one. Patients are responsible for informing their physicians and other caregivers if they anticipate problems in following prescribed treatment.

Patients should also be aware of the hospital's obligation to be reasonably efficient and equitable in providing care to other patients and the community. The hospital's rules and regulations are designed to help the hospital meet this obligation. Patients and their families are responsible for making reasonable accommodations to the needs of the hospital, other patients, medical staff, and hospital employees. Patients are responsible for providing necessary information for insurance claims and for working with the hospital to make payment arrangements, when necessary.

A person's health depends on much more than health care services. Patients are responsible for recognizing the impact of their lifestyle on their personal health.

Conclusion

Hospitals have many functions to perform, including the enhancement of health status, health promotion, and the prevention and treatment of injury and disease; the immediate and ongoing care and rehabilitation of patients; the education of health professionals, patients, and the community; and research. All these activities must be conducted with an overriding concern for the values and dignity of patients.

*These rights can be exercised on the patient's behalf by a designated surrogate or proxy decision maker if the patient lacks decision-making capacity, is legally incompetent, or is a minor.

A Patient's Bill of Rights *was first adopted by the American Hospital Association (AHA) in 1973. This revision was approved by the AHA Board of Trustees on October 21, 1992. Copyright 1992 by the American Hospital Association, 840 North Lake Shore Drive, Chicago, IL 60611. Printed in the U.S.A. All rights reserved. Reprinted with permission of the American Hospital Association.*

---

been resolved, questions remain. This ambiguity makes it emotionally painful for the persons involved. Three areas where ethical dilemmas are possible are euthanasia, refusal of treatment, and scarcity of resources.

Euthanasia

Most people hope to experience a peaceful, gentle death when their "time comes." The word *euthanasia* comes from the Greek word *euthanatos*, which literally means "good, or gentle, death." In current times, **euthanasia** refers to intentional action or lack of action that causes the merciful death of someone suffering from a terminal illness or incurable condition.

Active euthanasia refers to taking deliberate action that will hasten the client's death, such as removing a client who is in a vegetative state from a respirator. In contrast, **passive euthanasia** means cooperating with the client's dying process. Passive euthanasia is "a decision made not to prolong life. . . . It is the omission of an action that would prolong the dying process" (Sumodi, 1995). An example is not putting in a feeding tube to provide nourishment when the client cannot or will no longer eat.

Assisted suicide is a form of active euthanasia whereby another person provides a client with the means to end his own life. Recently, physician-assisted suicide has been the topic of much controversy. Nurses have differing opinions regarding assisted suicide. Some look on it as a violation of the ethical principles on which the practice of nursing is based: autonomy, nonmaleficence, beneficence, justice, veracity, and fidelity. Other nurses may see assisted suicide as an ethical dilemma; they agree that it violates some ethical principles but question whether it violates others. For example, in answer to the question "Does assisted suicide violate the principle of autonomy?" one might argue that it is *refusal* to assist a suicide that violates a client's autonomy. Regardless of a nurse's personal viewpoint, assisted suicide is still illegal.

Refusal of Treatment

The client's right to refuse treatment is based on the principle of autonomy. In fairness, the client can refuse treatment only after the treatment methods and their consequences have been explained. A client's rights to refuse treatment and to die challenge the values of most health care providers.

> Honoring the refusal of treatments that a patient does not desire, that are disproportionately burdensome to the patient, or that will not benefit the patient is ethically and legally permissible (Curtin, 1995).

One possible ethical dilemma in this area relates to the use of ventilators for clients who would otherwise die. Medical technology makes it possible for these clients to continue breathing as long as they are connected to the machine. But one might ask "What are the emotional, physical, psychological, and fiscal costs?" and "What is the quality of a life prolonged by technology?"

Scarcity of Resources

With the current emphasis on containing health care costs, the use of expensive services is being closely examined. The use of specialists, organ transplants, and distribution of services are being influenced by social and political forces. For example, the length of stay in a hospital and the number of office visits allowable for individual clients are already predetermined by many third-party payers. In addition to economics, the availability of goods (such as organs) is contributing to a scarcity of resources.

In many situations, clients wait extended periods before receiving donated organs. The allocation of scarce resources is emerging as a major ethical dilemma: Who should receive the benefit of such a scarce and precious resource as a living organ? How should the determination be made? Currently, the selection of organ recipients is based on objective criteria such as organ availability, donor/recipient match, the degree of the recipient's need, and the recipient's willingness to commit to a lifetime of drug therapy and follow-up care. But should only objective criteria be used in determining who receives a donated organ, or should moral judgments also be made?

ETHICAL DECISION MAKING

Nurses must understand the basis on which they make their decisions. **Ethical reasoning** is the process of thinking through what one ought to do in an orderly, systematic manner based on principles. Ethical decisions cannot be made in a scattered, unorganized manner based entirely on intuition or emotions. Ethical decision making is a rational way of making decisions in nursing practice. It is used in situations where either the right decision is not clear or conflicts

of rights and duties exist. A framework for resolving ethical dilemmas follows.

Framework for Ethical Decision Making

"After a moral conflict has been formulated, the nurse must differentiate the relevant parts of the conflict and resolve it" (Gordon et al., 1994). When making an ethical decision, the nurse must consider the following relevant questions:

- Which theories are involved?
- Which principles are involved?
- Who will be affected?
- What will be the consequences of the alternatives (ethical options)?

To resolve ethical dilemmas, the nurse must be able to make decisions in a systematic fashion. Figure 7-6 illustrates a method for making ethical judgments.

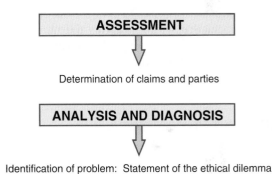

ASSESSMENT

Determination of claims and parties

ANALYSIS AND DIAGNOSIS

Identification of problem: Statement of the ethical dilemma

PLANNING

Consideration of priorities of claims;
Generation of alternatives for resolving the dilemma;
Consideration of the consequences of alternatives

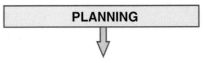

IMPLEMENTATION

Carrying out selected moral actions

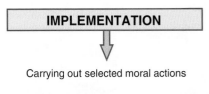

EVALUATION

Evaluation of the outcome of moral actions;
"Were the actions ethical?"
"What were the consequences?"

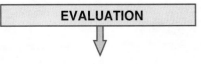

Figure 7-6 Ethical Decision-Making Model (*Adapted from Fundamentals of Nursing: Standards & Practice, by S. DeLaune and P. Ladner, 1998, Albany, NY: Delmar. Copyright 1998 by Delmar. Adapted with permission.*)

The first step of ethical analysis is to gather relevant data in order to identify the ethical problem and to determine which type of ethical problem exists: Do principles conflict with principles? Do actions conflict with actions? Do actions conflict with principles? What are the claims?

Next, all the people involved (the parties) must be considered. What are their rights, responsibilities, duties, and decision-making abilities? Who is the most appropriate person to make the decision? Whose problem is it? It is important to identify several possible alternatives and predict the outcome of each. Then, and only then, can a course of action be selected—one that, it is hoped, ends in resolution of the problem. The final step of ethical decision making is evaluation of the resolution process.

ETHICS AND NURSING

As professionals, nurses are accountable for protecting the rights and interests of the client. Consequently, sound nursing practice involves making ethical decisions. Ethics affects nurses in every health care setting, and each practice setting presents the nurse with its own set of ethical concerns. Whatever the setting, nurses must balance their ethical responsibilities to each client as an individual with their professional obligations. Often, there is an inherent conflict.

Ethics Committees

The provision of ethical health care requires both self-examination on the part of the care provider and dialogue among health care providers. Many health care agencies now recognize the need for a systematic manner for discussing ethical concerns (Figure 7-7). Multidisciplinary committees (also referred to as institutional ethics committees) constitute one arena for dialogue regarding ethical dilemmas. In addition to serving as a forum where ethical issues are discussed, ethics committees can lead to the establishment of policies and procedures for the prevention and resolution of dilemmas.

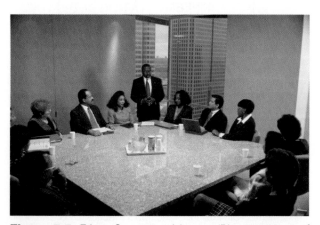

Figure 7-7 Ethics Committee Meeting *(Photo courtesy of Photodisc)*

PROFESSIONAL TIP

Providing Ethical Care

- Initiate dialogue concerning the client's wishes. Do more listening than talking. (For example, the following is a question you might ask to help determine the client's wishes: "If your heart stopped, would you want us to try to start it again?")
- Assess the client's understanding of the illness and the available treatment options.
- Allow time for the client to explore values and to communicate.
- Facilitate communication of the client's desires to family and other health care providers.

Nurse as Client Advocate

When acting as a client advocate, the nurse's first step is to develop a meaningful relationship with the client. The nurse is then able to make decisions with the client based on the strength of the relationship. The nurse's primary ethical responsibility is to protect clients' rights to make their own decisions.

> Nurses have an ethical obligation to do everything possible to prevent anyone from taking advantage of vulnerable patients—or clouding objectivity so that the patients' best interests fade from sight. (Haddad, 1995)

Nurse as Whistleblower

The term **whistleblowing** refers to calling public attention to the unethical, illegal, or incompetent actions of others. Whistleblowing is based on the ethical principles of veracity and nonmaleficence. As professionals, nurses are expected to monitor coworkers' abilities to perform their duties safely. Although nurses are expected to "blow the whistle" on incompetent health care providers, many are reluctant to do so because there are inherent risks in whistleblowing. Haddad (1999b) identifies some of the questions a person should consider before reporting unethical or incompetent behavior:

- Has the behavior in question created or is it likely to create serious harm?
- Have I gathered all appropriate information, and am I competent to judge this behavior?
- Do others confirm my information and judgment?
- Have all internal resources been exhausted to resolve the problem?
- Is it likely that past wrongdoing will be corrected or future damage prevented after the problem is reported?

CASE STUDY

Janice is a 45-year-old woman who is pregnant with her fourth child. The pregnancy was unplanned and distressed Janice and her husband at first, but now they have accepted it and look forward to the delivery of their child. Janice has been receiving prenatal care from her family practice physician since her second month of pregnancy. She is now in her seventh month.

During her sixth month of pregnancy, the physician ordered laboratory tests, and the results indicated a fetal abnormality. The physician requested to perform further diagnostic testing on the fetus during the seventh month. Janice and her husband refused further fetal testing. Although the physician explained the importance of the testing, the couple continued to refuse it.

After the couple left the office, the physician turned to the nurse and stated, "Since they will not follow my suggestions, write them a letter and tell them I am terminating our relationship. Tell her to see a specialist." No arrangements for a referral were made for Janice by the doctor, who feared that the high-risk delivery predisposed him to a lawsuit.

The following questions are related to the case study.

1. Based on the information presented, what are the primary ethical issues?
2. What are your personal values in relation to the situation?
3. What course of action would you recommend for the nurse and why? What ethical principles would guide you?
4. To what extent, in your opinion, is Janice noncompliant?
5. Was the medical intervention adequate? Is the nurse in the position to judge medical care?
6. What is the nurse's responsibility to ensure follow-up care?

- Is the harm created by whistleblowing likely to be less than the harm done by the behavior in question?

The False Claims Act (FCA) encourages whistleblowers to report evidence of fraud against the federal government (Polston, 1999).

Federal law and state laws (to varying degrees) provide protection, such as privacy, to whistleblowers. Unfortunately, however, the inclination to protect one's coworkers and the fear of reprisal may deter a nurse from fulfilling the ethical obligation to report substandard behaviors.

SUMMARY

- Ethics is the branch of philosophy concerned with the distinction of right from wrong on the basis of a body of knowledge rather than on just opinions. It is the study of the rightness of conduct.
- Ethics examines human behavior—those things that people do under a given set of circumstances.
- There is a connection between acts that are legal and acts that are ethical. Professional nursing actions are both legal and ethical.
- Teleology is an ethical theory that states that the value of a situation is determined by its consequences.

- Deontology is an ethical theory that considers the intrinsic significance of an act itself as the criterion for determination of good.
- Ethical decisions are based on principles such as autonomy, nonmaleficence, beneficence, justice, veracity, and fidelity.
- Because ethics and values are so closely associated, nurses must explore their own values in order to acknowledge the value systems of their clients.
- Ethical codes that have been developed by nursing organizations such as the NFLPN, the ICN, and the ANA establish guidelines for the ethical conduct of nurses with clients, coworkers, society, and the nursing profession.
- The Patient's Bill of Rights is designed to guarantee ethical care of clients in terms of their decision making about treatment choices and other aspects of their care.
- Nurses must apply the process of ethical reasoning to resolve ethical dilemmas wherein conflict exists between principles and duties.
- The roles of client advocate and whistleblower enable nurses to protect their clients' rights and ensure the ethical and competent actions of their peers within the nursing profession.

Review Questions

1. Nurses would use the Code for Licensed Practical/Vocational Nurses to:
   a. solve an ethical dilemma.
   b. develop a nursing care plan.
   c. seek an answer to a client care problem.
   d. understand the professional expectations required of them.

2. Values influence the nurse–client relationship because:
   a. the client's values take precedence over the nurse's values.
   b. every individual has a personal value system that helps determine actions.
   c. the nurse must help the client clarify his values in order to ensure effective nursing care.
   d. the nurse cannot effectively care for a client who has values that differ from those of the nurse.

3. Values clarification is a useful exercise for the nurse to perform because it helps the nurse:
   a. make ethically sound decisions.
   b. stay informed of new developments.
   c. avoid conflicts with clients and coworkers.
   d. establish policies about proper and improper client care.

4. An ethical dilemma is a:
   a. choice to be made between right and wrong.
   b. problem with two equally unsatisfactory solutions.
   c. series of problems that the nurse encounters in each client care situation.
   d. problem the nurse cannot solve without the intervention of a physician.

5. Active euthanasia means a person:
   a. helps a client to die.
   b. has an advance directive.
   c. limits the amount of care.
   d. chooses to stop pain therapy.

Critical Thinking Questions

1. A client delivers a baby with multiple congenital defects. The prognosis is poor, with the infant not being expected to live longer than 12 months at most. The mother says, "We can't afford to pay for the baby's care." Who should determine the degree of intervention? Should the cost of care be the foremost basis for the decision?

2. An 80-year-old woman is in a persistent vegetative state as a result of a cardiovascular accident. She has always talked about "someday" signing a living will requesting that heroic measures not be taken, but her family wants "everything to be done that can be done." Whose wishes should prevail? What ethical principles would come into play in this decision process?

 WEB FLASH!

- What organizations or professional journals can you locate for information on nursing and ethical issues?
- What resources and references can you find when you search under health care ethics as related to organ donation, euthanasia, scarcity of resources, or refusal of treatment?

Communication

Chapter 8
Communication

Chapter 9
Nursing Process

Chapter 10
Documentation

Chapter 11
Client Teaching

COMMUNICATION

MAKING THE CONNECTION

Refer to the following chapters to increase your understanding of communication:

- **Chapter 2, Critical Thinking**
- **Chapter 6, Legal Responsibilities**
- **Chapter 12, Cultural Diversity and Nursing**
- **Chapter 17, Loss, Grief, and Death**
- **Chapter 25, Assessment**

LEARNING OBJECTIVES

Upon completion of this chapter, you should be able to:
- *Define key terms.*
- *Describe the process of communication and factors that influence it.*
- *Differentiate between verbal and nonverbal communication.*
- *Utilize therapeutic communication.*
- *Understand the psychosocial aspects of communication.*
- *Demonstrate proper telephone communication.*
- *Communicate effectively with clients and families.*
- *Demonstrate communicating with special clients who are visually impaired, hearing impaired, speech impaired, unconscious, and non-English speaking.*
- *Communicate effectively with terminally ill clients and their families.*
- *Communicate effectively with other members of the health care team.*

KEY TERMS

active listening	listening
aphasia	nonverbal communication
communication	professional boundaries
congruent	proxemics
dysarthria	rapport
dysphasia	telemedicine
empathy	therapeutic communication
feedback	verbal communication
hearing	

INTRODUCTION

Why study communication? Students in a nursing program have generally had a minimum of 17 years of communicating. Have you ever told another person a story and then heard the story repeated by someone else? Or have you ever played the game "telephone," where a message is whispered from one person to another and the last one states the message out loud? In both situations, when you hear the story or message again, it typically has changed from the original. When communicating with a client, family, or another member of the health care team, it is important that the message be sent and received accurately.

This chapter addresses the process of communication; methods of communicating, including verbal and nonverbal communication and factors that influence communication, such as age, culture, education, language, attention, emotions, and surroundings. Techniques that promote effective (therapeutic) communication are also described, as are barriers to communication, and examples of both are presented. Also explored are psychosocial aspects of communication, such as style, gestures, meaning of time, meaning of space, cultural values, and political correctness, and their importance to the health care system. Finally, communication with the client, family, and health care team as well as self-communication is discussed.

PROCESS OF COMMUNICATION

The simplest definition of **communication** is the sending and receiving of a message. The six aspects of communication are: sender, message, channel, receiver, feedback, and influences.

Sender

The sender of a message is the person who has a thought, idea, or emotion to convey to another person. Messages stem from a person's need to relate to others, to create meanings, and to understand various situations.

Message

The message is the thought, idea, or emotion one person sends to another person. It is a stimulus produced by the sender and responded to by the receiver.

Channel

The person sending the message must decide how to send the message. The channel, or medium, through which a message is transmitted may be auditory, visual, or kinesthetic.

The auditory channel involves the verbal (speaking) method for the sender and the **hearing** (act or power of perceiving sounds) and/or **listening** (interpreting sounds heard and attaching meaning to them) modes of transmission for the receiver.

The visual channel involves the verbal (writing) and/or nonverbal methods for the sender and the sight, reading, observation, and perception modes of transmission for the receiver.

The kinesthetic channel involves touch for the sender and experience of sensation for the receiver (Table 8–1).

Receiver

The physiological component involves the processes of hearing, seeing, and the reception of the touch stimulus. The psychological processes may enhance or impede the receiving of messages. For example, anxiety may cause an individual to experience alterations in hearing, sight, or feeling.

The cognitive aspect is the "thinking" part of receiving. It involves interpreting stimuli and converting them into meaning.

Feedback

Feedback is a response from the receiver that enables the sender to verify that the message sent was the message received. If this is not the case, additional messages are sent and received until an understanding of the primary message is reached between the sender and receiver.

Influences

Both the sender and receiver are influenced by their education, culture, emotions, and perceptions and by the situation within which they find themselves. These elements are collectively referred to as a person's frame of reference. Sometimes these influences help communication, and sometimes they hinder communication. Figure 8-1 shows the process of communication and the influences on the sender and receiver.

Table 8–1 COMMUNICATION CHANNELS

CHANNEL	MODE OF TRANSMISSION	OUTCOME	EXAMPLE
Auditory (verbal)	• Hearing	Receiving an auditory stimulus	Hearing the client say, "I feel fine"
	• Listening	Interpreting sounds heard and attaching meaning to them	Hearing loud moaning in a client's room, the nurse enters the room to check whether the client is in pain
Visual (nonverbal or verbal)	• Sight	Receiving a visual stimulus	Watching the rise and fall of a client's chest while counting respirations
	• Reading		Reading the client's record
	• Observation	Interpreting a visual stimulus by making note of accompanying sounds	Making note of sounds of labored breathing while counting respirations and concluding that breathing is abnormal
	• Perception	Assigning meaning to a visual event	Diagnosing an alteration in oxygenation related to respiratory distress
Kinesthetic (tactile or nonverbal)	• Procedural touch	Performing nursing procedures and techniques	Giving the client a bed bath
	• Caring touch	Conveying emotional support	Holding the client's hand

Adapted from Fundamentals of Nursing: Standards & Practice, *by S. DeLaune and P. Ladner, 1998, Albany, NY: Delmar. Copyright 1998 by Delmar. Adapted with permission.*

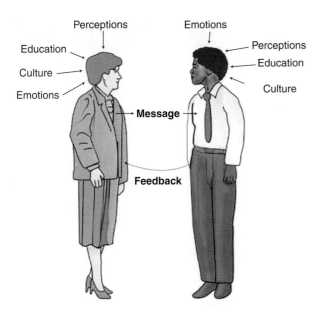

Education — Perceptions — Emotions
Culture — Perceptions
Emotions — Education
Culture
Message
Feedback

Figure 8-1 Process of Communication

METHODS OF COMMUNICATING

There are two methods of communicating: verbally and nonverbally. Which is better? The answer is neither, or more accurately, it depends on what the sender is trying to communicate. Seldom is a spoken message sent without some accompanying nonverbal aspects. Some experts believe that nonverbal communication is more honest than is verbal communication because it usually is conveyed unconsciously by the sender.

Verbal Communication

Verbal communication is the use of words, either spoken or written, to send a message. Methods of verbal communication include speaking, listening, writing, and reading.

Speaking/Listening

Most commonly, speaking is thought of as verbal communication. The receiver of a spoken message must listen. Speaking and listening must both occur in order for there to be communication. Have you ever sent a spoken message to someone in the same room with you and received nonmeaningful, senseless feedback from that person, or no feedback at all? More than likely, the other person was only hearing the message but not listening.

Communication experts say that people speak at a rate of 125 to 150 words per minute (WPM) but hear at a rate of 400 to 800 WPM. This extra time allows for distractions. Listeners are generally distracted because they are not concentrating on what is being said. Listening is one of the most difficult skills to learn and execute well.

Writing/Reading

The other mode of verbal communication is writing. The receiver of the written message must read the words. The reader must understand the words and attach meaning to them. With a written message, immediate feedback is generally not available. Therefore, great care should be taken to ensure clarity when composing a written message. Charting is a good example. The physician may read the chart after the caregivers who did the charting go off duty, allowing little chance for immediate feedback. In such an instance, if a chart read that a client was "uncooperative," for example, the physician would have little idea exactly what the caregiver meant. An entry of "refused to eat lunch, refused to get out of bed and sit in chair," however, is far more exact, illustrating the clarity in writing that is essential to good communication.

Nonverbal Communication

Nonverbal communication, sometimes called body language, is the sending of a message without using words. There are many ways we communicate without words, including gestures, facial expressions, posture and gait, tone of voice, touch, eye contact, body position, and physical appearance.

Nonverbal communication is generally unconscious—part learned behavior and part instinct. Because there is little conscious control involved in nonverbal communication, feelings are generally most honestly expressed nonverbally.

Clients seem to believe and are particularly sensitive to nonverbal messages. Nurses must thus make an effort to be aware of the nonverbal messages they may be sending to clients. For example, consider those aspects of nursing care that are not pleasant but must be done. Think how the client would feel if a nurse were to register an expression of disgust or revulsion on her face when changing a surgical dressing.

Nurses must also be sensitive to the client's nonverbal messages. Many clients do not want to bother "busy" nurses. Such clients may say they are fine or do not need anything when this is in fact not the case. An astute nurse, however, will observe nonverbal signs such as stiff posture, clenched fists, or a frowning facial expression and know that something is not right. Further assessment would then be undertaken to determine why the client is sending such nonverbal clues.

Gestures

Gestures are often referred to as "talking with hands." Gestures may be used to help clarify a verbal message, to emphasize an idea, to hold other's attention, or to relieve stress. Fingertapping, fidgeting, or ring twisting generally indicates tension, nervousness, or impatience. Shaking a fist indicates anger, whereas pointing may be used to clarify directions.

Facial Expressions

Although some people have very expressive faces, others do not. A big smile is easily interpreted as indicating happiness. Eyebrows can be very expressive, showing surprise, worry, thoughtfulness, or displeasure. The manner in which the forehead is wrinkled also sends a message.

Nurses must be very aware of their own facial expressions, especially when caring for a client under "unpleasant" conditions, such as when a client is vomiting or suffering from bowel incontinence. An expression of displeasure manifested as a "curled up" nose or disgust is easily identified by the client. The client, often already embarrassed at requiring such care, is likely to feel even worse should the nurse's facial expressions indicate anything but caring, concern, and empathy.

Posture and Gait

Good posture, with the head held up, and a purposeful gait are usually interpreted as meaning self-confidence, competence, and a positive self-image. Stooped shoulders, a downward-held head, and a shuffling gait generally convey low self-esteem, depression, and lack of confidence.

Tone of Voice

Tone of voice has been estimated to convey 23% of the context of a message. When the same words are said in different tones of voice, they can have very different meanings. Tone of voice might be pleasant, sincere, sorrowful, sarcastic, joyful, or angry.

Touch

Touch is a simple yet powerful form of nonverbal communication that even a newborn infant can understand. Touch can communicate caring, understanding, encouragement, warmth, reassurance, or affection. Of course, touch can also communicate anger, displeasure, or a lack or caring and understanding. Sometimes touch can hurt or be harmful to the person being touched.

While some people are natural "touchers," others are not. The use of touch can be learned, however. Many nursing tasks involve touching the client. If the nurse is uncomfortable touching a client, the touch along with other nonverbal communication such as facial expression, posture, eye contact, and tone of voice will all convey the nurse's discomfort. Most clients accept touch as an integral part of nursing care when it is done appropriately and professionally.

Eye Contact

Eyes, it is said, mirror the soul. Have you ever seen joy, sadness, pain, or laughter in someone's eyes? It is very difficult to control these messages of the eyes.

Eye contact is generally interpreted as indicating interest and attention, whereas lack of eye contact is thought to indicate avoidance, disinterest, or discomfort.

CULTURAL CONSIDERATIONS

Eye Contact
In some cultures it is considered rude or disrespectful to make direct eye contact.

Body Position

Body position is often a good indicator of a person's attitude. For example, crossed arms generally indicate withdrawal, although the person could just be cold. Open body positions, with the arms held freely at the sides, are usually taken to mean a receptive attitude.

Physical Appearance

A person's physical appearance says a great deal about that person. A clean, neat, appropriately dressed individual conveys a positive self-image, knowledge, and competence. A dirty, sloppy, or inappropriately dressed person conveys the message of "I don't care how I look," with the potential implication of "maybe I am not too knowledgeable or competent," or "I am sloppy in what I do."

It is very important for every nurse to be clean, neat, and professionally dressed. Clients and families understand the nonverbal message that appearance conveys. Appearance does influence communication.

INFLUENCES ON COMMUNICATION

Communication involves more than just the sending and receiving of verbal and nonverbal messages. How a person sends or receives a message is influenced by such factors as age, education, emotions, culture, and language. Attention to the message and the surroundings are other influences. These factors must be taken into account for accurate communication to take place.

Age

Factors related to age affect communication. For instance, communicating with a child is different from communicating with an adult and is dependent on the age of the child. Nonverbal communication, particularly touch, and facial expression can be understood by infants. Before learning to understand words, a child can interpret tone of voice and gestures. Preschool children respond well to communication involving toys or play situations. They should be allowed some choices, but no more than two alternatives should be offered. As the child's vocabulary increases, more verbal communication can take place.

Elderly persons may have some degree of hearing loss or a slowed response time. The nurse should face the elderly client when speaking and allow time for a response. The client should be addressed as "Mr." or "Ms." unless he or she asks to be called by his or her first name. Elderly clients should be treated with respect and not talked to as if they were children; they are individuals with special needs (Figure 8-2).

Education

Education is another strong influence on communication. The more educated a person, the greater the vocabulary of that person. Highly educated persons are generally able to discuss and understand concepts and abstract ideas, whereas less educated persons generally communicate in a more literal and less abstract way.

Emotions

A person's emotional state greatly influences how messages are sent or received. Someone who is very anxious or upset, for example, may not hear what is said or may interpret the message differently than the sender intended. This same person typically speaks in an abrupt manner, loudly, and in harsh tones. The depressed person, on the other hand, typically says very little, speaking only one or two words or in very short sentences.

Culture

Each culture has its own standards of communication, especially with regard to nonverbal behavior. In the United States, for example, eye contact is considered a sign of openness and honesty. Those of Spanish heritage, however, believe eye contact to be disrespectful. Similarly, in many parts of Europe, a kiss on the cheek between two men is accepted. People from other parts of the world, however, may look suspiciously on this behavior.

Language

Language certainly influences communication. Speaking the same language assists people in understanding each other, although regional accents or dialects of a language can inhibit communication and understanding. When verbal communication comes to a standstill, nonverbal communication is often employed to assist. Any nurse who works in an area where there is a predominate second language should learn a few words or phrases in that language to help put clients at ease and to facilitate their understanding.

Attention

The amount of attention each individual focuses on a given communication greatly affects the outcome. In selective listening, the receiver hears only what he

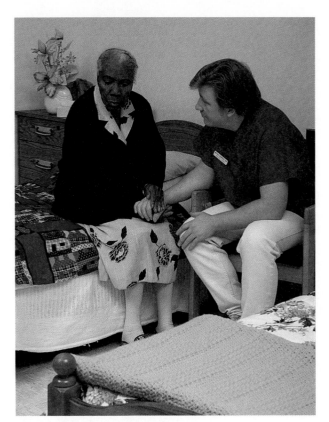

Figure 8-2 When addressing elderly clients, face them directly and allow adequate response time. A warm touch on the hand or arm will communicate caring and respect.

wants or expects to hear. Pain or discomfort, physical or mental, may result in preoccupation, limiting the attention given to the communication.

Surroundings

Most people do not want to talk about the intimate details of their health care concerns in public (Figure 8-3). Thus, privacy should be provided. If the client occupies a room alone, the nurse should close the room door; if the client shares a room, the nurse should take the client to a conference room or to another private place, if possible, to discuss personal information.

The nurse should respect the client's current "home" (e.g., the hospital room) as she would any person's home, knocking on the door before entering the room, not sitting on the bed without permission, and asking before moving any personal articles that are in the way. These simple courtesies show respect for the client as a person. When the client feels respected, communication is enhanced.

CONGRUENCY OF MESSAGES

It is important that verbal and nonverbal communications be **congruent**, or in agreement. Saying, "I really appreciate what you just did," in a happy tone of voice while smiling is congruent and clear; saying the

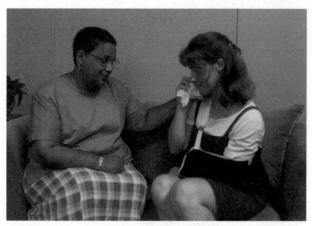

Figure 8-3 Provide privacy when discussing personal or intimate health concerns with clients.

same words in a disgusted tone of voice while frowning is incongruent and, thus, potentially unclear. The receiver may not know whether the sender is genuinely pleased with what was done or is displeased and being sarcastic. Messages such as these can confuse the receiver, who then may require feedback in order to correctly interpret the message.

It is important for the nurse to watch for congruency between verbal and nonverbal messages and to ask for clarification when incongruity exists.

LISTENING/OBSERVING

Listening and observing are two of the most valuable skills a nurse can have. These two skills are used to gather the subjective and objective data for the nursing assessment. Because the nursing diagnoses and nursing interventions are based on the assessment, it is imperative that the assessment be accurate.

The term **active listening** has been used to describe this behavior of listening and observing; it reflects the process of hearing spoken words and noting nonverbal behavior. It takes energy and concentration. The nurse who is at eye level with the client, who leans slightly forward toward the client, and who makes eye contact is showing undivided attention to the client and will be able to listen and observe more accurately. Responses from the nurse such as "go on," "tell me more," "yes," "what else?" or "mmhm" both encourage the client to continue and communicate that the nurse is really listening.

THERAPEUTIC COMMUNICATION

Therapeutic communication, sometimes called effective communication, is purposeful and goal di-

rected, creating a beneficial outcome for the client. One person is the helper (nurse) and the other is being helped (client). The focus of the conversation is the client, the client's needs, or the client's problems, not the needs or problems of the nurse.

Goals of Therapeutic Communication

There are several goals or purposes of therapeutic communication. One or more of these goals guide every therapeutic communication in the nurse–client relationship. The goals are to obtain or provide information, develop trust, show caring, and explore feelings.

Obtain or Provide Information

The nurse obtains information from the client about general health and specific health problems. It is with this information that the nurse can make an accurate assessment and plan of care.

The nurse provides information to the client from admission to discharge, beginning with the orientation of a new client to the hospital policies and routines. Information provision continues throughout the hospital stay as the nurse explains procedures, treatments, and tests; teaches the client self-care; clarifies instruction from other health care workers; and answers client questions. The discharge instructions constitute the final stage of information provision.

Develop Trust

Client and nurse are generally strangers at the time of their first meeting. The nurse must work to establish trust with each client. Answering questions honestly, responding to call lights promptly, and following through are examples of ways to build trust. Trust develops faster when caring is shown. Mutual trust established between client and nurse is termed **rapport**.

Show Caring

Fluffing a pillow or offering a drink of water without being asked are two ways to show caring. Taking time to always greet the client by name and knocking on the room door before entering are other ways.

Explore Feelings

Once rapport is established, the nurse can encourage the client to explore feelings. Generally, most clients are anxious about illness. Some fear the results of diagnostic tests, and some are anxious about the hospital environment. Many clients do not want to admit they are anxious or fearful. By using therapeutic communication techniques, the nurse is often able to help the client talk about feelings and reduce anxiety. Sometimes, a clarifying statement is all that is needed to alleviate fear or anxiety. Other times, allowing the client to talk about the fear or anxiety reduces that fear or anxiety.

Behaviors/Attitudes to Enhance Communication

Some behaviors and attitudes enhance therapeutic communication. These include self-disclosure, caring, genuineness, warmth, active listening, empathy, and acceptance and respect.

Self-Disclosure

Self-disclosure means sharing something about yourself such as thoughts, expectations, feelings, or ideas. It does not mean sharing your personal problems. When the nurse shares something, such as future goals in nursing, it shows that the client is trusted with that knowledge. The more the client feels trusted, the more the client will trust the nurse and therapeutic communication is enhanced.

Caring

Caring is not only a goal of therapeutic communication but also an attitude that enhances communication. Caring is the foundation of a nurse–client relationship. A caring attitude is easily identified by the client. Make the client feel important. Table 8–2 gives some examples of ways to show caring.

Keller and Baker (2000) identify four steps to help communicate a caring attitude to clients.

Table 8–2 WAYS TO SHOW CARING

ACTIVITY	STATEMENTS TO USE WITH ACTIVITY
Cover the client with a blanket.	"It feels chilly in here. Perhaps this blanket will help."
Assist the client to dress.	"I noticed you're having a little trouble getting your robe on. Perhaps I can help."
Serve a tray to the client.	"It's time to eat. I hope you're hungry because it really looks good."
Offer assistance.	"Here, let me help you. Perhaps together we can arrange these flowers."
When leaving the room.	"Is there anything more I can do for you before I go?" or "I'm leaving now, but I'll be back in 20 minutes."
Move the client up in bed.	"You look so uncomfortable. Let me move you up in bed."
Make the client's bed.	"Now you have a nice fresh bed."
Regulate environmental temperature.	"It seems very warm in here. Perhaps if I turn the air conditioner up, it will help."
Turn the client in bed.	"Changing position really makes a difference, doesn't it?"
Straighten a pillow.	"Let me straighten your pillow for you."

Adapted from Mental Health Concepts *(4th ed.), by C. Waughfield, 1998, Albany, NY: Delmar. Copyright 1998 by Delmar. Adapted with permission.*

- *Connect with the client.* Make eye contact; be at eye level when speaking to client; address client by last name.
- *Appreciate the client's situation.* Listen carefully; focus on what client is saying; acknowledge client's point of view; express concern.
- *Respond to client needs.* Clarify what is being asked; respond in ordinary language; let client know what to expect.
- *Empower the client.* Find out what client knows about condition and acknowledge opinions; work as partner to develop plan of care; allow choices as appropriate; encourage questions.

Genuineness

Effective communication must be genuine. The nurse must be himself. It means being honest about one's feelings. Sometimes it is "ok" to cry with a client.

It means being truthful and never attempting to answer a question when the answer is not known. The nurse should admit not knowing but offer to find the answer and then do so.

Being genuine builds trust. However, the nurse must use good judgment when expressing negative thoughts or confronting a client, family member, or another health care worker.

Warmth

Warmth makes the client feel welcomed, relaxed, and unjudged. It is expressed predominantly by nonverbal communication. A smile helps the client feel relaxed.

Touch is an important method to show warmth, but it must be used appropriately. Society dictates the type of touching that is appropriate in different situations. Holding a client's hand or putting a hand on the shoulder can greatly enhance communication by providing a connection between the nurse and the client. Touch may not always be welcomed by the client.

Active Listening

As the words imply, listening is an active process requiring energy and concentration. It involves listening to the words spoken as well as being aware of nonverbal messages. The nurse listens to both the words spoken and the nonverbal messages.

Active listening requires responses from the listener. This indicates that the nurse is really listening to the client. It is important for the nurse to concentrate on the interaction at hand and not let other thoughts become a distraction (Figure 8-4).

Empathy

Empathy is the capacity to understand another person's feelings or perception of a situation. It is an objective awareness of, or a sensitivity to, another person's feelings and thoughts. Although the nurse does

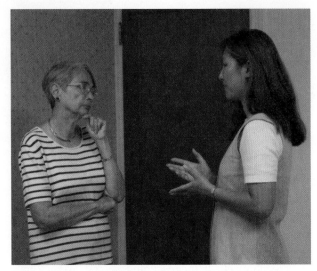

Figure 8-4 Active listening, concentrating on the interaction with the client, enhances communication.

not share the thoughts and feelings of the client, with empathy the nurse is able to understand and accept the thoughts and feelings of the client. Sympathy and empathy are not the same. In sympathy, the nurse becomes involved in the feelings and thoughts of the client, which are generally related to a loss.

Acceptance and Respect

Accepting clients as individuals with beliefs and values of their own is an attitude that enhances communication. The nurse must be nonjudgmental, that is, accepting of the client at face value. It is acceptable to privately disagree with the client's values and beliefs, but the nurse must accept that the client has different values and beliefs.

The nurse shows acceptance by not expressing differing values or beliefs and by simply accepting the statements or complaints of clients. Clients may then feel free to communicate and cooperate in their care.

Respect follows acceptance. Accepting clients in a nonjudgmental way leads to understanding them as unique individuals. Acceptance and respect on the part of the nurse let clients know that they can be themselves; they can then feel that they will still receive the best quality care, even though they have different values and beliefs than the nurse. The nurse also shows respect by introducing himself and addressing the client by name (preceded by "Mr.," "Mrs.," or "Ms.").

Techniques of Therapeutic Communication

Certain techniques promote therapeutic communication. These techniques should be learned and incorporated into the nurse's manner of communicating.

Clarifying/validating

Clarifying or validating are used when the nurse is not sure of the meaning of a message. Clarifying is the technique used to understand verbal messages. For example:

"Do you mean . . . ?"

Validating is used to establish truth or accuracy. It is used for nonverbal as well as verbal messages. Examples are as follows:

"Are you saying that you did not get your medication today?"

"You are holding your side. Are you having pain there?"

Open Questions

Open questions encourage clients to express their own thoughts and feelings. *How, when, where,* and *what* are words with which to begin an open question. Open questions cannot typically be answered with "yes" or "no" or with just one or two words. For example:

"How has this medication affected your vision?"

"What did the doctor tell you about going home?"

Indirect Statements

An indirect statement calls for a response from the client. Because it is a statement and not a question, the client does not feel quizzed. Indirect statements allow the client to determine the direction of the conversation, thus helping the client maintain a feeling of independence. Examples of indirect statements are as follows:

"Tell me about your physical therapy today."

"You were telling me about. . . ."

Reflecting

Reflecting is repeating all or part of a message back to the sender. Often, reflecting focuses on feelings and helps the sender "hear" the message from the receiver. This allows the sender a chance to clarify the message and shows that the listener is trying to understand the message. Reflecting can be a very useful technique if not overused. Examples include the following:

Client: "I'm really nervous about my surgery tomorrow. My friend got an infection after her surgery. I'm very frightened."

Nurse: "You are anxious about your surgery and afraid of getting an infection?"

Paraphrasing

Paraphrasing is restating the message in the receiver's own words. This lets the sender know how the receiver interpreted the message. Clarification can then be done if necessary. The sender is aware that the receiver is listening and trying to understand the message. For example:

Nurse: "You are afraid that you might have complications from your surgery?"

Summarizing

Summarizing in a sentence or two the major points of a conversation lets the sender know what was heard. The sender can then add more information or clarify what was originally heard. An example might be as follows:

"Let me see, we have discussed. . . ."

Focusing

Keeping communication focused on the topic being discussed can sometimes be difficult. Clients may wander off to other topics, or the topic may shift to the nurse. It is important to keep the focus on the client and not the nurse. For example the nurse could say:

"We can discuss that in a minute, right now I'd like to discuss. . . ."

"A minute ago you mentioned that you'd had an upset stomach after taking your medication. Tell me more about that."

Silence

Silence is one of the most difficult techniques to use. In the dominant U.S. culture, most people are uncomfortable with silence and feel the urge to fill the gap by saying something. Silence can be a valuable therapeutic technique, however, allowing the client time to gather thoughts or check emotions. Silence also gives the nurse a chance to decide how best to continue the interaction. If the nurse employs behaviors to enhance communication during the silence, the client will often verbalize thoughts or feelings.

Barriers to Communication

Employing behaviors and attitudes to enhance communication will be of little use if the nurse also employs barriers to communication. Although the communication process is sensitive, it should not be threatening. The purpose in learning about those things that block communication is to enable the nurse to identify them and avoid using them. Many mistakes can be corrected when identified. A simple "I'm sorry, I shouldn't have said that" will often take care of the situation. Practice helps sharpen communication skills. The most common barriers are discussed following.

Closed Questions

Questions that can be answered with "yes" or "no" or with only one or two words are considered closed.

After the one- or two-word answer, communication is usually ended; there is no other avenue for the communication to follow. This type of question is appropriate in certain circumstances, however, such as when taking a health history or in an emergency. Examples of closed questions are as follows:

"Is the pain gone?"

"Did you sleep well?"

Clichés

Clichés are overused, trite phrases that are almost meaningless. They are impersonal and often used when individuals are at a loss for anything better to say. They are used without thinking of the impact on the other person, and often seem disrespectful of the client's individual circumstances. Examples include the following:

"Hang in there, tomorrow is another day."

"It could be worse."

False Reassurance

False reassurance is often used in an effort to cheer up the client regardless of the facts, giving false hope about the outcome of a situation. False reassurance can be especially traumatic to a terminally ill client who may be desperate to believe assurances even if they are not founded in reality. An example of false reassurance is as follows:

"Don't worry, I'm sure everything will be fine."

Judgmental Responses

Judgmental responses are based on the nurse's personal value system and imply right or wrong. Such responses allow no room for further discussion. For example:

"You shouldn't feel that way."

Agreeing/Disagreeing or Approving/Disapproving

Whether the nurse is agreeing/approving or disagreeing/disapproving, offering an opinion implies that one belief is right and the other wrong. Clients are thus prevented from sharing their feelings and may feel pressured to express the same values and opinions as the nurse. One example is as follows:

"I wouldn't do it that way."

Giving Advice

Giving advice involves offering personal rather than professional opinion. When the nurse does this, the client's responsibility for making decisions is diminished. Furthermore, some clients may end up feeling unable to make their own choices and may therefore become more dependent on the nurse. One example might be:

"I think you should. . . ."

Stereotyping

Stereotyping occurs when individual differences are ignored and a person is automatically put into a specific category. The stereotype may have either a positive or negative connotation. For example:

"Someone your age shouldn't worry about that."

"Boys aren't supposed to cry."

Belittling

Belittling conveys to a person that his thoughts or feelings really have no value, that it is silly to think or feel a certain way, or that he is no different from other individuals in similar circumstances. Examples include the following:

"Many people have it much worse."

"Yes, everyone feels like that."

Defending

Defending is a response to a feeling of being directly or indirectly threatened. The nurse may make statements in defense of self, another nurse, a doctor, or the health care facility. Defending implies that the client is not permitted to criticize or express feelings. This may be one of the most difficult communication barriers to overcome. No one likes to be criticized or to hear coworkers criticized. A natural first response is to defend why something was said, done, or not done. An example of defending is as follows:

"No one on this unit would say that."

Requesting an Explanation

It can be very intimidating for a client when a nurse asks for an explanation of behaviors, feelings, or thoughts. Often, the client does not know the "why." The usual results are increased anxiety and an end to communication. Examples are as follows:

"Why did you do that?"

"Why do you feel that way?"

Changing the Subject

An abrupt change of subject by the nurse generally indicates to the client that the nurse is uncomfortable or anxious about the topic under discussion. It often is used to avoid listening to a client's fear, distress, or problems and is interpreted by the client as a lack of interest.

Client: "I don't think I'll ever get well."

Nurse: "Isn't it a beautiful day?"

PSYCHOSOCIAL ASPECTS OF COMMUNICATION

The psychosocial aspects of communication include: style, gestures, meaning of time, meaning of space, cultural values, and political correctness. These aspects are based on individuality and culture and will influence the nurse–client relationship. It is important to understand these aspects and how they vary in different persons and cultures.

PROFESSIONAL TIP

When Clients Block Communication
In instances when clients block communication, keep the following things in mind:

- The client may not wish to discuss the topic introduced by the nurse or may not wish to talk at all. Everyone needs time alone to think.
- Accept and respect the client's desires to not communicate at a particular time.
- Let the client know that you are ready to listen whenever she is ready to talk.

PROFESSIONAL TIP

Understanding Communication Barriers
Take measures to become aware of communication barriers. For instance, join a classmate in pointing out the barriers that each of you use, then discuss how you each feel when confronted with these communication barriers.

Style

Each person has a style of communication that reflects the personality and self-concept of that person. According to Jack (1997), style can be divided into three common types: passive, aggressive, and assertive. It is important to remember that a person's style of communication is learned and reinforced over the years. The fact that communication style is learned indicates it can change.

When a person becomes a client in the health care system, fear and anxiety may change the person's style of communication causing the client's communication style to become passive or aggressive.

Passive

The person who uses the passive style of communication does not stand up for himself, is not able to share feelings or needs with others, has difficulty asking for help, and feels hurt and angry at others for taking advantage of him. This person uses apologetic words; has a weak, soft voice; makes little eye contact; and is often fidgety. The person with a passive style of communication will often go along with others without expressing a personal desire for an alternate plan of action. The client who has a passive style of communication is generally very compliant, asks for nothing, and gets little attention.

Aggressive

The person who uses the aggressive style of communication puts his own feelings, rights, and needs first and communicates them in a haughty or angry way. The voice is often demanding, and the eyes expressionless. Such a person also has an attitude of superiority, works to control or manipulate others, and shows no concern for anyone else's feelings.

Assertive

The person who uses the assertive style of communication stands up for himself without violating the basic rights of others. He expresses true feelings in an honest, direct manner and does not allow others to take advantage of him. His voice is firm and confident, and he makes appropriate eye contact. Such a person also respects the rights, needs, and feelings of others;

CULTURAL CONSIDERATIONS

Gestures

The meaning of gestures is not universal. For instances, in many places, a small circle made with the thumb and forefinger means "okay." This is not true in Japan and France, however, where this gesture means "money" and "zero," respectively. And in Brazil and Turkey, this gesture is a symbol for female genitalia and is considered an insult.

takes responsibility for the consequences of his actions; and behaves in a manner that enhances self-respect.

A person using the assertive style of communication effectively lets others know his thoughts, feelings, and needs. He also listens to and acknowledges the other person's thoughts, feelings, and needs. If the thoughts, feelings, or needs of the persons communicating are in conflict, a compromise acceptable to both can usually be worked out.

Gestures

Gestures are movements of the hands and arms. Some gestures are known globally, such as applause to indicate approval. Some gestures, however, have entirely different meanings in various countries. The nurse must be sensitive to cultural variances and exercise good judgment when caring for clients of different backgrounds and heritages.

Meaning of Time

In the United States, great emphasis is placed on time and schedules. Being on time is very important. Time is precious. The clock tells us what we are to do and where we are to be every hour of the day and night. A person is considered dependable when scheduled appointments are kept.

People of some cultures know a day has passed only because the sun has risen, set, and is rising again. In fact, some cultures do not even have an instrument for telling time. They have different ways of perceiving and dividing time. Scheduling in such cultures may mean "when they get around to doing it."

PROFESSIONAL TIP

Being Assertive

"I" messages—I think . . . , I expect . . . , I feel . . . , I need . . .—are excellent ways to begin practicing assertive communication. Such messages indicate ownership of the thought, feeling, or need—a fact with which no one can argue.

PROFESSIONAL TIP

Time Orientation

Be sensitive to the fact that clients of different cultural backgrounds may value time differently than you do. Do not jump to conclusions that the client who is always late is lazy or inconsiderate of schedules.

Meaning of Space

Edward T. Hall (1959) has for many years studied **proxemics**, the study of space between people and its effect on interpersonal behavior. Hall says that humans, like other animals, are territorial. Some examples of human territoriality include the following: On a beach, people mark territory with a towel or blanket; in waiting rooms, people mark space with a jacket, hat, luggage, or newspaper; in a classroom, students generally sit in the same place and expect others to respect that space.

How close do you like to be to another person? Generally, this distance varies with the person and the situation. Age, gender of those interacting, and cultural values all influence the distance at which one person is comfortable with another person. Hall (1959) categorizes these comfort zones as intimate, personal, social, and public space.

- Intimate—touch to 18 inches; usually limited to family and close friends; necessary when performing most nursing procedures.
- Personal—18 inches to 4 feet; used with friends and coworkers; effective for many nurse–client interactions involving interviewing or data gathering.
- Social—4 to 12 feet; preferred distance with casual acquaintances.
- Public—12 feet or more; generally used with strangers in public places.

The distances associated with the comfort zones vary from person to person. Some people are comfortable being quite close in space to the person with whom they are interacting. Others prefer a greater distance. Nurses must always be aware of the client's comfort level with regard to space (Figure 8-5).

Much of nursing care involves touching the client, yet on admission, the nurse and client generally do not know each other. Thus, in a very short span of time, the nurse moves from the client's public space to the client's intimate space when giving care. Care given competently and professionally will help the client feel comfortable when the nurse occupies the client's intimate space.

Cultural Values

It is important that the nurse be familiar with the cultural values of the people in the nurse's region of employment, especially when those values differ from the values of the dominant culture. For example, optimal health for all is the focus of the dominant U.S. culture. In some cultures, however, health is not a major concern, and little financial or political effort is dedicated to health. Likewise, individualism is stressed in our culture. In many other cultures, however, the social group, not the individual, is the primary focus.

As another example, consider that a number of cultural groups have learned to enjoy what they have and do not feel the need to keep working for some goal or material object. This contrasts with the dominant U.S. culture, where persons must work hard, achieve, and keep busy in order to be considered successful. Finally, in the dominant U.S. culture, cleanliness is closely related to optimal health and is a dominant value. Few cultural groups emphasize cleanliness in the way the U.S. culture does, however. In fact, many have no problem with being dirty, and some even see it as a positive value.

Political Correctness

To be politically correct in communication means to use language that shows sensitivity to those who are different from oneself. It is intended to help eliminate prejudice by avoiding the use of language that offends. Politically correct language is designed to replace terms that suggest inferior status for members of minority groups and terms that exclude women, older people, and those with handicaps. Racist and bigoted language perpetuates prejudice and false ideas and often leads to violence.

Importance to Health Care System

It is important for nurses to understand the psychosocial aspects of communication and be aware of them with regard to individual clients. Communication is more effective when these aspects are taken into consideration.

Effective communication has a positive influence on a client's well-being. Furthermore, clients often judge nurses' competence by their communication skills. Good communication skills also result in increased client satisfaction, and increased client satisfaction leads to increased compliance with the therapeutic regimen.

Communication, then, is a key factor in the client's perception and evaluation of the health care services provided.

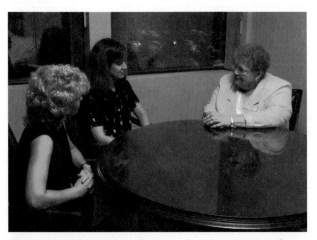

Figure 8-5 A distance of up to 4 feet is appropriate for interviewing and data gathering.

PROFESSIONAL BOUNDARIES

All communication with clients must take place within **professional boundaries** (the limits of the professional relationship that allow for a safe, therapeutic connection between the professional and the client). The nurse must abstain from obtaining personal gain at the expense of the client, and refrain from inappropriate involvement in the client's personal relationships.

NURSE–CLIENT COMMUNICATION

One of the most important aspects of nursing care is communication. Whether the nurse is gathering admission information, taking a health history, teaching, or implementing care, good communication skills are essential.

Nurses have both an ethical and moral responsibility to use any information gathered from the client in the client's best interest. Information that affects the health status or care of the client should be shared with other members of the health care team. All information concerning a client is confidential and should never be discussed in elevators, the cafeteria, the hallways, or other public places outside the health care facility.

Formal/Informal Communication

Formal communication is purposeful and is employed in a structured situation such as information gathering on admission or scheduled teaching sessions (Figure 8-6). Specific items are covered in a planned sequence. In this way, more information can be given or received in the shortest amount of time.

Informal communication does not follow a structured approach, though it often reveals information that is pertinent to the client's care. For instance, a client may comment that the tape holding her bandage in place is irritating to her skin. This would lead the nurse to assess the wound area and take action to correct the problem. This interaction, although not planned or structured, was nonetheless helpful in ensuring quality nursing care.

Social Communication

Social communication is the everyday conversations held with family, friends, and acquaintances. Topics are generally those of interest to both parties and reflect the social relationship of those involved. Both parties share information, thoughts, and feelings. When getting acquainted with clients, social communication provides a way to learn about each other and to begin a nurse–client relationship.

Although social communication is not considered therapeutic communication, it is part of nurse–client communication. Because it is nonthreatening, social communication puts the client at ease; it also allows the nurse to get to know the client and what is important to the client. Clients often interpret social communication as expressions of caring on the part of the nurse—that is, the nurse cares enough about the client to spend some time communicating on a person-to-person level rather than on a nurse-to-client level.

Interactions

Nurse–client interactions and relationships progress through three phases. The amount of time spent on each phase depends on the purpose of the interaction.

Introduction Phase

The beginning of any interaction is usually fairly short. The client is greeted by name, and the nurse introduces himself and defines his role. Expectations of the interaction are clarified, and mutual goals are set. A good format might be:

> "Good morning, Mrs. Jamal. My name is Paul Farrell. I am a student practical (vocational) nurse and I will be caring for you today and tomorrow. I would like to teach you some breathing and coughing exercises that you will be asked to do after your surgery tomorrow."

Working Phase

The working phase generally constitutes the major portion of any interaction. It is used to accomplish the goal or objective defined in the introduction. The nurse should always ask for feedback to ensure understanding on the part of the client. In the previously presented scenario, the client's demonstrating the breathing and coughing exercises and verbalizing why the exercises are necessary would indicate understanding.

Termination Phase

The final phase of any interaction is the termination phase. Seldom do nurses have unlimited time to spend with one client, and there are several ways for the

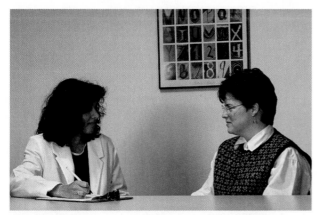

Figure 8-6 Formal Interaction, Admission Interview

nurse to indicate the end of an interaction. The nurse may ask whether the client has any questions about the topic discussed. Summarizing the topic is another good way for the nurse to indicate closure.

Factors Affecting Nurse–Client Communication

As mentioned previously, factors such as age, education, emotions, culture, language, attention, and surroundings, affect both parties in a communication. In nurse–client communications, additional factors relating to both the nurse and client also come into play. The nurse must be sensitive to these factors and to personal biases in order to provide appropriate nursing care.

Nurse

Many personal factors pertaining to the nurse can influence nurse–client communication. Past experiences as a nurse, state of health, home situation, workload, and staff relations can all impact the thinking, concentration, attitude, and emotions of the nurse. These in turn influence how the nurse sends and receives messages. Self-awareness is very important for the nurse when communicating.

Client

Factors related to the client that must be considered include: social factors, religion, family situation, visual ability, hearing ability, speech ability, level of consciousness, language proficiency, and state of illness.

Social Factors Some health concerns are easy to discuss because they are socially acceptable, such as having the gallbladder or appendix removed or having the flu. It may be more difficult, however, to communicate with a woman who is having a breast removed. The symbolic meaning of the breast may make its removal hard for the client to accept and may influence how she relates to others. A person with a sexually transmitted disease or one who is HIV positive may be very reluctant to discuss any aspect of the illness.

Religion Members of some religions seek healing through faith and not through conventional medical services. Others will not receive blood transfusions when an accident or disaster places these individuals in the health care system. When religious beliefs conflict with those of the health care team, communication can be difficult.

A client may have a priest, minister, or rabbi visit. Privacy for such visits should be provided if at all possible.

Family Situation Illness often unites family members around the client. If the family has not been close to or supportive of the client before the illness, communication between the family and client may be strained. Such stress may be noticed in the course of nurse–client interactions. If so, the nurse must be careful not to discuss aspects of the client's condition or treatment in front of family members. In fact, it is best to ask family members to step out of the room when any nursing care is being given. This applies whether assessing the client, providing physical care, or gathering information. The client's right to privacy and confidentiality is thus maintained.

Sometimes the client expresses a desire for a specific person to remain in the room. Unless contraindicated, this is usually allowed.

Visual Ability Communicating with clients who are visually impaired may not seem to be a challenge at first. However, because the nonverbal part of any message, such as facial expressions, gestures, and other body language, is missed, an important part of every message is lost to the client.

Persons who are visually impaired generally speak only when spoken to. Their speech may be loud if they are not sure where the other person is. Silence makes them uncomfortable if they are not sure of another person's presence in the room.

The nurse must include an explanation of "hospital sounds" when orienting a new client who cannot see.

LIFE CYCLE CONSIDERATIONS

Older Client
- Assess for sensory disturbances.
- Face the client when speaking.
- Have patience, response may be slow.
- Show respect and be considerate of the older client's personal dignity.

Children
- Be at eye level with the child.
- Use vocabulary appropriate for the child's level of development.

PROFESSIONAL TIP

Caring for the Client Who Is Visually Impaired
- Look directly at the client when speaking.
- Use a normal tone and volume of voice.
- Advise the client when you are entering or leaving the room.
- Orient the person to the immediate environment; use clock hours to indicate positions of items in relation to the client.
- Ask for permission before touching the client.

Adapted from Health Assessment & Physical Examination, 2nd ed., *by M. E. Z. Estes, 2002, Albany, NY: Delmar. Copyright 2002 by Delmar. Adapted with permission.*

The room must be described in detail and the client guided around the room if possible. It is important for nurses to always speak and identify themselves when entering the room. As with any client, all procedures should be explained. Each step of the procedure as well as any touching should be described before it is initiated. As with any client, the nurse should always inform the client who is visually impaired before touching so as not to startle him.

Hearing Ability Many persons who are hearing impaired can communicate by sign language, but few hearing persons can understand or use sign language. If the person who is hearing impaired is able to read, writing may be the easiest method of communication. Many persons who are hearing impaired have learned, at least to some degree, to speechread, formerly known as lipread. Communicating with a client who is hearing impaired requires time and patience.

The nurse should face the client and speak slowly and deliberately using slightly exaggerated word formation. Gesturing can also be very effective. Check to see whether the client has a hearing aid and, if so, encourage its use during the communication.

The frustration of trying to communicate can make the client who is hearing impaired stubborn or even hostile. Such frustration generally stems more from trying to understand others rather than from trying to be understood. Touching the client's arm when entering the room lets the client know that someone is there and helps prevent feelings of paranoia.

Speech Ability **Dysphasia**, the impairment of speech, and **aphasia**, the absence of speech, both can result from a brain lesion, although they are most com-

monly seen as the result of a stroke. Other neurological diseases such as Parkinson's disease may also cause dysphasia. A dysfunction of the muscles used for speech is termed **dysarthria**, which makes a person's speech difficult, slow, and hard to understand. Dysphasia, aphasia, and dysarthria create communication problems.

The person with dysphasia has difficulty both putting thoughts and feelings into words and sending messages. It should be noted, however, that seldom does the person with dysphasia have difficulty receiving and interpreting messages; thus, explanations should be given before doing anything. If the client can write, a magic slate or paper and pencil can be used for communication. A picture board, word board, or letter board may also be employed, as can a computer, assuming that one is available and that the client is able to use a computer. A person with any of these speech impairments may feel frustrated and helpless. Establishing some method of communication for the client provides hope and maintains self-esteem while at the same time minimizing or preventing feelings of depression, anger, and hostility.

Level of Consciousness True communication cannot be accomplished with unconscious or comatose clients. It should be remembered, however, that unconscious or comatose clients can hear even though they cannot respond. Caregivers should speak to these clients just as they would to alert clients. Always greet the client by name, identify yourself, and explain why you are in the room (i.e., what you are going to do). Then let the client know when you are leaving and, if possible, when you will return. Although one-sided, this interaction is important to the client.

Language Proficiency The client's ability to communicate effectively through the spoken language also influences the nurse–client interaction. Clients who do not speak English are generally from another culture. It is important to learn about the other culture, especially about the values and beliefs. Doing so will help prevent the nurse from violating those values and beliefs.

If a family member speaks English, that person could be used as an interpreter, as shown in Figure 8-7. Sometimes another health care worker on the nursing unit may speak the same language as does the client. As long as it does not interfere with his or her work, this person could also be used as an interpreter.

Pictures or a two-language dictionary are often helpful. If the other language is prevalent in the community, the nurse should learn some phrases in the language that are useful in client assessment and in care. Remember, gestures and other nonverbal communication send messages without the use of language.

Stage of Illness The stage of a client's illness may influence the client's desire to communicate with the nurse. Clients in the early stages of illness may be

PROFESSIONAL TIP

Caring for the Client Who Is Hearing Impaired

- Check to see whether the client wears a hearing aid. Be sure it is in working order and turned on.
- Make every effort to move the client to a setting with minimal background noise.
- Always face the client.
- Speak in a normal tone and at a normal pace.
- Determine whether the client uses sign language. If signing is used, enlist the assistance of an interpreter.
- Pay particular attention to nonverbal cues of the client and to your own nonverbal behavior.
- Provide a pen and paper to facilitate communication, if necessary.

Adapted from Health Assessment & Physical Examination *(2nd ed.), by M. E. Z. Estes, 2002, Albany, NY: Delmar. Copyright 2002 by Delmar. Adapted with permission.*

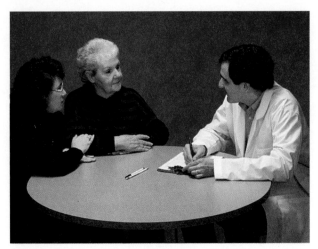

Figure 8-7 A family member interprets communications with a non-English-speaking client.

eager to learn all they can about the illness or may express anger and resentment at their current state of health.

Terminally ill clients may pose special challenges for the nurse. Most terminally ill clients know they are dying and are concerned about those whom they love. It is thus important for the nurse to have the client identify those persons the client considers to be "family." Family and nurses often struggle with the proper way to speak with those who are dying; no one can escape death, but many people do not want to discuss it. Death is often considered a defeat by health care workers and therefore is not a prime subject for discussion. It is important to remember that listening and silence are both part of communication.

PROFESSIONAL TIP

Objectivity
The nurse must remain objective and nonjudgmental when the client's idea of family is different from the nurse's idea of family.

CULTURAL CONSIDERATIONS

Family Interaction Patterns
- In some families the male members make all the decisions.
- In some families, decisions are made jointly, with all members (or all adults) participating.
- In some families, unrelated persons such as godparents or special friends are involved in decision making.

Anytime a client initiates a conversation regarding death the nurse must be willing to participate. Too often nurses hesitate to communicate with the terminally ill for fear of saying the wrong thing. When the client wants to talk, a good listener is needed. Let the client guide the conversation. Try not to give advice, just listen and accept what the client says. This may be very difficult to do.

The nurse and the family must work together to understand the ways that the terminally ill client communicates. It can take persistence and insight to identify and decipher some messages. "Listening" to the client's gestures and facial expressions helps facilitate understanding of messages.

COMMUNICATING WITH THE HEALTH CARE TEAM

Providing care to clients is a team effort. For the team to work efficiently and effectively and to provide continuous quality care to clients, effective communication is necessary. This communication may be oral or written, individual or group, or even on computer.

Oral Communication

Oral communication among the health care team is necessary for the appropriate planned care of the client and for the efficient and effective functioning of the nursing unit. In order to provide continuity of care, all persons who provide direct care to clients must communicate orally with each other concerning that care.

Nurse–Nurse

Nurse–nurse communications can be either peer–peer or superior–subordinate communication. Peer–peer communication takes place many times every day. If each nurse uses effective communication with peers as well as clients, the unit will run more efficiently, and client care will be more effective. Superior–subordinate communication often directs the client care to be performed by the subordinate. The way this communication is handled affects both the attitude of the subordinate and the client care given.

Nurse–Nursing Assistant

The nurse is responsible for informing the nursing assistants of their duties. Taking time to answer questions and providing reasons for specific activities requested helps establish a relationship of trust and mutual respect.

An experienced nursing assistant can be of considerable assistance to the new graduate (whether an RN or LP/VN). Nursing assistants are often much more comfortable and confident in providing bedside care. They often have creative solutions to problems and should be included in planning care.

Nurse–Student Nurse

Student nurses must communicate not only with the clinical instructor but also with the staff nurses. How well the staff nurses interact with student nurses depends on how the staff nurses were treated as students and on the experiences the staff nurses have had with other student nurses. Student nurses are involved in the clinical facility for specific learning experiences selected by the instructor and related to classroom topics. They must have time to review client records, observe others performing procedures, and communicate with and care for their clients. Students are limited in their nursing activities depending on how far they have progressed through the nursing curriculum. Because staff nurses retain responsibility for the care of clients even when clients are assigned to students, communication between student nurses and staff nurses is essential. Generally, a complementary relationship develops between nursing students and staff nurses.

Nurse–Physician

Nursing education and expertise have evolved over the years to a professional level. Nurses are responsible for their own actions even when under the direction of a physician.

When the term *nursing diagnosis* was introduced, many physicians had difficulty understanding how nurses could make a diagnosis. Whereas medical diagnoses focus on disease conditions, nursing diagnoses focus on human needs. Nurses must communicate openly and honestly with physicians, demonstrating their competence in assessments, nursing skills, and provision of quality care.

Nurse–Other Health Professionals

Communication with professionals in other departments should always be on a peer basis. Clarification of goals for each client and of ways to meet those goals should be the focus of communication. Listening to those in other departments and establishing mutual respect for each other's area of expertise provides the client with top quality care.

Group Communication

Client care conferences may be scheduled regularly or whenever the need arises. Some conferences may be solely for the staff of a particular nursing unit; others may include members of other departments. In either case, only those persons directly involved with the care of the client should be invited (Figure 8-8).

The conference leader should establish the objectives of the conference and make all necessary arrangements. A conference room or other private place should be used as a meeting site. One person should be designated to record the discussion. If the conference is about a specific client, only facts should be documented on the client's chart. If the topic is general

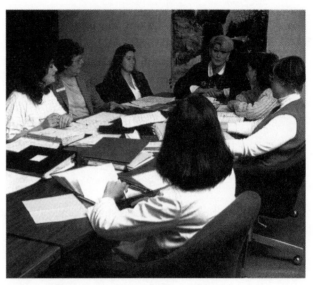

Figure 8-8 Nurses work together to plan client care.

and not related to a specific client, only a record of the discussion is needed.

Telephone

When a student nurse is the only person available to answer a telephone call, the call should be answered with the name of the department or floor and the student's full name and position (i.e., student nurse). The caller should then be informed that an appropriate person will be found to take the call. If a message must be taken, the student nurse should write it down and read it back to the caller and ask for the caller's name and for the caller to spell out his or her name. The nurse must never give out any information about clients.

Written Communication

Most written communication relates to the client's chart. All aspects of a client's care are recorded on that client's chart.

Requisitions to x-ray or to physical or respiratory therapy and requests for laboratory services for a client are all forms of written communication. The reports resulting from these requests become part of the client's chart.

One type of written communication not pertaining to a specific client is the interdepartmental memo requesting equipment, supplies, maintenance, or housekeeping. Such documents are necessary to keep the nursing unit functioning efficiently and effectively.

Electronic Communication

Computers are being used extensively in the business offices of health care agencies and have been so for years. The introduction of computers into the departments of direct client care has been slower, however. Nonetheless, in many places, computers are used by client care departments to send requisitions to other

COMMUNITY/HOME HEALTH CARE

Use of Telemedicine
- From the office, a home health nurse can watch a client at home change a dressing or self-administer insulin.
- During a video consult, a home health nurse might assist by manipulating the peripherals or actually performing a physical assessment.

PROFESSIONAL TIP

Telemedicine Confidentiality
- Avoid sending or receiving client data by e-mail unless the computer has encryption capabilities.
- During a two-way video consultation, inform the client of any other people who are present in the room, but off camera. Try to ensure that only those persons who must know about the client's condition are present (Granade, 1997).

departments and to receive test results. Some hospital pharmacies use computer programs that show safe dosages and drug interactions. There are also programs to aid physicians in diagnosing and treating some conditions. With the expanding use of computers in health care and the corresponding potential for increased use, it is important for all health care workers to have some knowledge about computers.

Although the computerized patient record (CPR) as envisioned by the Institute of Medicine (IOM) is not yet available in the United States, parts of the CPR have been implemented. The IOM defines the CPR as an "electronic record that resides in a system specifically designed to support users through availability of complete and accurate data, practitioner reminders and alerts, clinical decision support systems, links to bodies of medical knowledge and other aids." This moves the client record from simply tracking client care to serving as a resource for health care delivery (Zolot, 1999).

Before there is widespread use of the CPR, many questions must be be answered, including: How can changes to the data entered be prevented? How will charting errors be corrected? What happens when the computers are down? How will security be maintained? What are the legal implications of electronic or digital signatures? According to Zolot (1999), all client records must be confidential, accurate, secure, and protected from unauthorized access and disclosure, regardless of the form.

Telemedicine

The Telemedicine Research Center (1997) defines **telemedicine**, also called telehealth, as the use of communications technology to transmit health information from one location to another. Included is the transmission of radiographic (teleradiology) and pathologic (telepathology) images, telemetry, and telephone triage.

The use of two-way video allows the client and health care provider to see, hear, and talk to each other. A stethoscope or otoscope (called peripherals) can be included in the hookup so that the sounds and visual images can be transmitted (Granade, 1997). This allows physician specialists in large medical centers to examine a client many miles away.

California and Arizona have both passed legislation requiring providers to obtain written and verbal informed consent before providing any nonemergency care via telemedicine. Oklahoma is also considering such legislation (Granade, 1997).

Nurses should document all activities, assessment findings, information provided by the client, and any instructions given to the client. All data transmissions (e.g., telemetry printouts or videotapes) should be stored in the client's record. Most telemedicine laws require that existing confidentiality rules be maintained.

COMMUNICATING WITH YOURSELF

Whether they admit it or not, people talk to themselves every day. Oftentimes, such communication takes the form of thoughts rather than spoken words. What people say to themselves influences their personalities and, therefore, how they interact with others. Sherman (1994) describes self-talk as positive or negative.

Positive Self-Talk

Practicing positive self-talk is the key to positive self-esteem. Send positive thoughts to yourself about yourself. Better yet, say the thoughts out loud. Thinking, saying, and hearing positive statements about oneself reinforces positive self-esteem. Remind yourself of your good attributes and accomplishments. When you have had a difficult day, whether in the classroom or clinical area, pat yourself on the back for what you did accomplish. Each day verbally tell yourself what you learned or what good care you gave to your client(s).

Positive self-talk reinforces the desire to succeed. Memories of successes can serve as positive influences, especially when things are not going well and frustration sets in.

Positive affirmation is a positive thought or idea on which a person consciously focuses to produce a desired result. Positive affirmation can be used to change negative inner messages to positive messages. Instead

CASE STUDY

Martha, a 25-year-old Mexican American female, is admitted for severe abdominal pain. Martha clings to her mother's arm when the nurse asks the mother to leave the room during the admission procedure. The mother asks to stay in the room. The nurse looks at Martha, who smiles but says nothing.

Consider the following:

1. What do you think may be causing Martha to cling to her mother?
2. What can the nurse do to communicate with Martha?
3. What subjective and objective data should the nurse gather?

---

of saying, "I don't know if I can pass this test," for instance, say, "I know I can pass this test." Of course, positive affirmation is not a substitute for studying and preparing for the test. Positive affirmation merely serves to modify your attitude about the test—or about any other situation.

Negative Self-Talk

Whenever you say to yourself, "I can't do . . . ," you are decreasing your self-esteem with the negative self-talk. Negative self-talk may originate within you, or you may be replaying things that others have said about you. Negative self-talk is self-destructive. Your self-image is lowered by your own criticism, and you begin to see yourself as a failure.

SUMMARY

- Communication is influenced by age, education, emotions, culture, language, attention, and surroundings.
- Nonverbal messages are generally more accurate in communicating a person's feelings.
- Verbal and nonverbal messages must be congruent for clear communication to take place.
- Techniques of therapeutic communication should be practiced and incorporated into the nurse's communication.
- Barriers to communication should be identified and avoided when communicating.
- People have four comfort zones of closeness: intimate, personal, social, and public.
- Therapeutic communication is purposeful and goal directed.
- Psychosocial aspects of communication may aid or hinder communication.
- Almost every nurse–client interaction should involve therapeutic communication.

- Nurse–client communication is influenced by both the nurse and the client.
- The nurse is often a role model for the family in terms of communicating with the terminally ill client.
- Accurate communication among the health care team is necessary for continuity of care.

Review Questions

1. Mr. George is looking out the window, with his back to the door. A nurse opens the door and says, "You will not be able to eat or drink after supper because of tests tomorrow." Then the nurse leaves. Did communication take place?

    a. No, there was no feedback.
    b. No, there was no eye contact.
    c. Yes, Mr. George had to hear the message.
    d. Yes, there was a sender, receiver, and message.

2. What is the best way to communicate?

    a. verbally.
    b. nonverbally.
    c. it depends on what the message is.
    d. verbally and nonverbally together.

3. Initial client assessment related to communication would include:

    a. vital signs.
    b. visual ability.
    c. ambulatory ability.
    d. complete health history.

4. When performing a nursing procedure on a client, the nurse should:

    a. only listen to what the client says.
    b. be aware of her own nonverbal messages.
    c. always have someone witness the procedure.

    d. tell the client how fortunate he is to be the nurse's client.

5. The nurse is aware that most nursing procedures are performed in which spatial comfort zone?

    a. public
    b. social
    c. personal
    d. intimate

6. Which of the following are all examples of verbal communication?

    a. singing, dancing, smiling
    b. reading, writing, listening
    c. shaking hands, reading, grimacing
    d. whispering, making eye contact, answering

7. When a client says, "I'm not sure how I'll handle all this;" which response of the nurse represents clarification?

    a. "Handle all this?"
    b. "Well, you can ask your sister to help."
    c. "Oh, you'll be able to handle things. You're an intelligent person."
    d. "I'm not sure I understand what it is you're concerned about being able to handle."

8. The statement "I'm sure you'll feel much, much better after your surgery" is an example of:

    a. advice.
    b. false reassurance.
    c. a judgment.
    d. excessive emotionalism.

9. That phase of an interview during which goals and objectives are identified is called the:

    a. working phase.
    b. interview phase.
    c. termination phase.
    d. introduction phase.

10. The most effective technique the nurse can use to facilitate communication is:

    a. giving.
    b. focusing.
    c. listening.
    d. questioning.

11. Which of the following represents the best way for a nurse to show caring?

    a. constantly staying with the client
    b. doing everything for the client
    c. assisting the client in learning self-care
    d. relaying to the physician everything the client says

12. A terminally ill client denies there is anything wrong and talks constantly about going back to work. The nurse should:

    a. listen but not comment.
    b. acknowledge the client's hopes and wishes.
    c. advise the client that it will be impossible to return to work.
    d. assist the client in planning when to return to work.

13. The nurse uses therapeutic communication with the client to:

    a. cure the client of fear.
    b. discuss personal problems.
    c. obtain or provide information.
    d. relieve the client of all concerns.

14. The nurse is aware that communication among members of the health care team is necessary because it:

    a. provides for continuity of care.
    b. identifies who provides better care.
    c. allows team members to become friends.
    d. promotes competition between departments.

15. Mrs. Banc tells the nurse that she would rather die than have radiation. To whom should the nurse report this communication?

    a. the physician only.
    b. everyone on the nursing unit.
    c. the physician and charge nurse.
    d. no one; the communication is confidential.

Critical Thinking Questions

1. How can you communicate with an unconscious adult?

2. Which barriers to communication do you use? How can you change?

⚡ WEB FLASH!

- Search for information on the web about the Telemedicine Research Center. What are the latest reports?
- How much information about telemedicine is available on the Internet?
- What current information can you obtain about computerized client records?

NURSING PROCESS

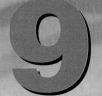

MAKING THE CONNECTION

Refer to the following chapters to increase your understanding of the nursing process:

- **Chapter 1, Holistic Care**
- **Chapter 8, Communication**
- **Chapter 10, Documentation**

- **Chapter 25, Health Assessment**
- **Chapter 30, Leadership/Work Transition**

LEARNING OBJECTIVES

Upon completion of this chapter, you should be able to:
- *Define key terms.*
- *Describe the components of the assessment step of the nursing process.*
- *Describe the four types of nursing diagnoses.*
- *List the tasks involved in the planning and outcome identification step of the nursing process.*
- *Discuss the types of skills that nurses must possess in order to perform the nursing interventions during the implementation step of the nursing process.*
- *Identify factors that may influence evaluation.*
- *Explain the way that critical thinking is related to the nursing process.*
- *Relate the nursing process to the problem-solving method.*
- *Describe the nursing process as a tool for promoting multidisciplinary collaboration.*

KEY TERMS

actual nursing diagnosis	critical pathway
analysis	data clustering
assessment	defining characteristic
assessment model	delegation
assumption	dependent nursing intervention
bias	discharge planning
comprehensive assessment	etiology
	evaluation

expected outcome	objective data
focused assessment	ongoing assessment
goal	ongoing planning
health history	planning
implementation	primary source
independent nursing intervention	process
	protocol
initial planning	risk nursing diagnosis
interdependent nursing intervention	secondary source
	short-term goal
long-term goal	specific order
medical diagnosis	standing order
nursing audit	subjective data
nursing care plan	synthesis
nursing diagnosis	wellness nursing diagnosis
nursing intervention	
nursing process	

INTRODUCTION

The nursing process is a systematic method of providing care to clients. Use of the nursing process allows nurses to communicate their roles in planning and executing client-centered activities to clients, their families, and other health care professionals. It is a process that encourages orderly thought, analysis, and planning when working with clients to decide those things that need to be done. The nursing process consists of five steps: assessment, diagnosis, planning and outcome identification, implementation, and evaluation.

This chapter presents information about both the historical development of the nursing process and the elements that compose each step of the process. A discussion on the way the nurse uses critical thinking in each step of the nursing process is included. The relationship of the nursing process to problem solving, decision making, and collaboration is also discussed.

HISTORICAL PERSPECTIVE

Lydia Hall first referred to nursing as a "process" in a 1955 journal article, yet the term *nursing process* was not widely used until the late 1960s (Edelman & Mandle, 1998). Referring to the nursing process as a series of steps, Johnson (1959), Orlando (1961), and Wiedenbach (1963) further developed this description of nursing. At that time, the nursing process involved only three steps: assessment, planning, and evaluation. In their 1967 book *The Nursing Process,* Yura and Walsh identified four steps in the nursing process:

- Assessing
- Planning
- Implementing
- Evaluating

Fry (1953) first used the term *nursing diagnosis,* but it was not until 1974, after the first meeting of the group now called the North American Nursing Diagnosis Association (NANDA), that nursing diagnosis was added as a separate and distinct step in the nursing process. Prior to this, nursing diagnosis had been included as a natural conclusion to the first step, assessment. Currently, the steps in the nursing process are:

- Assessment
- Diagnosis
- Planning and outcome identification
- Implementation
- Evaluation

OVERVIEW OF THE NURSING PROCESS

A **process** is a series of steps or acts that lead to accomplishment of some goal or purpose. According to Bevis, "processes have three characteristics: (1) inherent purpose, (2) internal organization, and (3) infinite creativity" (1989). These characteristics can be applied to the nursing process. The **nursing process** is a systematic method of providing care to clients. The purpose is to provide client care that is individualized, holistic, effective, and efficient. Although the steps of the nursing process build on each other, they are not linear. Each step overlaps with the previous and subsequent steps (Figure 9-1).

The nursing process is dynamic and requires creativity in its application. Although the steps remain the same in each client situation, the application and results will differ. The nursing process is designed to be used with clients throughout the life span and in any care setting. It is also a basic organizing system for the National Council Licensure Examination for both practical/vocational nurses (NCLEX-PN) and registered nurses (NCLEX-RN).

Assessment

Assessment is the first step in the nursing process and includes systematic collection, verification, organization, interpretation, and documentation of data. It is a very important step because the completeness and correctness of the information obtained in this step are directly related to the accuracy of the steps that follow. Assessment involves several steps:

- Collecting data from a variety of sources
- Validating the data
- Organizing the data
- Interpreting the data
- Documenting the data

Purpose of Assessment

The purpose of assessment is to establish a database concerning a client's physical, psychosocial, and emotional health in order to identify health-promoting behaviors as well as actual and/or potential health problems. Through assessment, the nurse ascertains the client's functional abilities and the absence or presence of dysfunction. The client's normal activities of daily living and lifestyle patterns are also assessed. Identification of the client's strengths provides the nurse and other members of the treatment team information about the skills, abilities, and behaviors the client has available to promote the treatment and recovery process. The assessment phase also offers an opportunity for the nurse to form a therapeutic interpersonal relationship with the client. During assess-

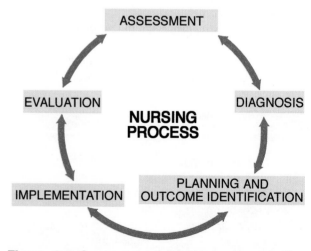

Figure 9-1 Components of the Nursing Process *(From Fundamentals of Nursing: Standards & Practice, by S. DeLaune and P. Ladner, 1998, Albany, NY: Delmar. Copyright 1998 by Delmar. Reprinted with permission.)*

PROFESSIONAL TIP

The Nursing Process

- Rather than being linear, the nursing process involves overlapping steps.
- The steps are explained one after the other for ease of understanding, but in actual practice, there may not be a definite beginning or ending to each step.
- Work in one step may begin before work in the preceding step is completed.

ment, the client is provided an opportunity to discuss health care concerns and goals with the nurse.

Types of Assessment

The type and scope of information needed for assessment are usually determined by the health care setting and needs of the client. Three types of assessment are comprehensive, focused, and ongoing. Although a comprehensive assessment is most desirable in initially determining a client's need for nursing care, time limitations or special circumstances may dictate the need for abbreviated data collection, as represented by the focused assessment. The assessment database can then be expanded after the initial focused assessment, and data should be updated through ongoing assessment.

Comprehensive Assessment A **comprehensive assessment** provides baseline client data including a complete health history and current needs assessment. It is usually completed upon admission to a health care agency. This database provides a baseline against which changes in the client's health status can be measured and should include assessment of physical and psychosocial aspects of the client's health; the client's perception of health; the presence of health risk factors; and the client's coping patterns.

COMMUNITY/HOME HEALTH CARE

Ongoing Assessment

- In the home, ongoing assessment may involve specific questions to elicit specific information.
- Clients are more comfortable and feel in charge in their own homes as opposed to a health care facility.
- The client may have a tendency to spend a lot of time telling stories about past medical problems and treatment, as opposed to providing information relevant to the situation at hand (Humphrey, 1998).

Focused Assessment A **focused assessment** is an assessment that is limited in scope in order to focus on a particular need or health care concern or on potential health care risks. Focused assessments are not as detailed as comprehensive assessments and are often used in health care agencies where short stays are anticipated (e.g., outpatient surgery centers and emergency departments), in specialty areas such as labor and delivery, in mental health settings, or for the purpose of screening for specific problems or risk factors (e.g., well-child clinics).

Ongoing Assessment Systematic follow-up is required when problems are identified during a comprehensive or focused assessment. An **ongoing assessment** is an assessment that includes systematic monitoring and observation related to specific problems. This type of assessment allows the nurse to broaden the database or to confirm the validity of the data obtained during the initial assessment. Ongoing assessment is particularly important when problems have been identified and a plan of care has been implemented to address these problems. Systematic monitoring and observation allow the nurse to determine the response to nursing interventions and to identify any emerging problems.

Sources of Data

Although data are collected from a variety of sources, the client should be considered the **primary source** of data (the major provider of information about a client). As much information as possible should be gathered from the client, using both interview techniques and physical examination skills. Sources of data other than the client are considered **secondary sources** and include family members, other health care providers, and medical records.

Types of Data

Two types of information are collected through assessment: subjective and objective. **Subjective data** are data from the client's (sometimes family's) point of view and include feelings, perceptions, and concerns. The primary method of collecting subjective data (also called symptoms) is the interview. The **health history**, a review of the client's functional health patterns prior to the current contact with the health care agency, provides much of the subjective data.

PROFESSIONAL TIP

Clients Who Were Adopted

Keep in mind that clients who were adopted will have varying degrees of knowledge about their biological parents. Sensitivity to this issue is critical in gaining client trust during the interview process.

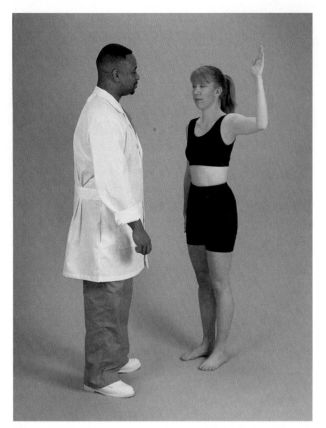

Figure 9-2 The nurse is gathering objective data through assessment of the client's ability to perform range-of-motion (ROM) activity.

Table 9–1 TYPES OF DATA

DATA

A client, age 47, has come to the clinic after "passing out" twice in the last 2 days. She tells the nurse that she becomes "lightheaded" after almost any type of activity. She has experienced some nausea since yesterday and vomited after eating breakfast this morning. She also tells the nurse that she is very nervous about these occurrences because she remembers her mother having similar symptoms when the mother suffered from a brain disorder. The nurse observes that the client's gait is unsteady and skin pale. The client also has large bruises on her right arm and on the right side of her face, which she states occurred when she fell.

TYPE OF DATA

Subjective	Objective
Report of fainting	Vomiting
Complaint of dizziness	Unsteady gait
Nausea	Pale skin
Verbalization of anxiety	Bruises on right side of face
Self-reported fall	and right arm

From Fundamentals of Nursing: Standards & Practice, *by S. DeLaune and P. Ladner, 1998, Albany, NY: Delmar. Copyright 1998 by Delmar. Reprinted with permission.*

Objective data (also called signs) are observable and measurable data that are obtained through both standard assessment techniques performed during the physical examination (Figure 9-2) and the results of laboratory and diagnostic testing. Table 9–1 provides examples of both subjective and objective data.

Validating the Data

Objective data may add to or validate subjective data. A critical step in data collection, validation prevents omissions, misunderstandings, and incorrect inferences and conclusions (Figure 9-3). This process is particularly important if data sources are considered unreliable. For example, if a client is confused or unable to communicate, or if two sources provide conflicting data, it is necessary to seek further information or clarification. Findings should also be compared with norms. Any grossly abnormal findings should be rechecked and confirmed.

Organizing the Data

Collected data must be organized so as to be useful to the health care professional collecting the data and to others involved in the client's care. After being organized into categories, the data are clustered into groups of related pieces. **Data clustering** is the process of putting data together in order to identify areas of the

client's problems and strengths. Many health care agencies use an admission assessment format, which assists the nurse in collecting and organizing data.

An **assessment model** is a framework that provides a systematic method for organizing data. A few of the many assessment models available to nurses are described following.

Hierarchy of Needs Maslow's hierarchy of needs proposes that an individual's basic needs (physiological) must be met before higher-level needs can be met. Use of a hierarchy of needs model requires initial

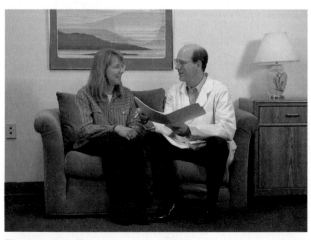

Figure 9-3 This nurse is validating information collected from the client during assessment.

assessment of all physiological needs followed by assessment of higher-level needs.

Body Systems Model The body systems model organizes data collection according to organ and tissue function in the various body systems (e.g., cardiovascular, respiratory, gastrointestinal). This method is sometimes referred to as the "medical model," because it is frequently used by physicians to investigate the presence or absence of disease.

Functional Health Patterns Gordon's Functional Health Patterns (Gordon, 1997) provides a systematic framework for data collection that focuses on 11 functional health patterns. These functional health pattern areas allow the gathering and clustering of information about a client's usual patterns and any recent changes in order to ascertain whether the client's response is functional or dysfunctional. For example, the activity–exercise pattern is assessed for a client who recently experienced a stroke. Data collection would be focused on mobility and exercise patterns prior to the stroke, current muscle strength and joint mobility, and the effect of any changes on the client's lifestyle and functional ability. The 11 patterns are as follows:

- Health perception/health management pattern
- Nutritional/metabolic pattern
- Elimination pattern
- Activity/exercise pattern
- Cognitive/perceptual pattern
- Sleep/rest pattern
- Self-perception/self-concept pattern
- Role/relationship pattern
- Sexuality/reproductive pattern
- Coping/stress-tolerance pattern
- Value/belief pattern (Gordon, 1997)

Theory of Self-Care The theory of self-care, developed by Orem (1995), is based on a client's ability to perform self-care activities. Self-care is learned behavior and deliberate action in response to need. It includes activities that an individual performs to maintain health. A major focus of this theory is the appraisal of the client's ability to meet self-care needs and the identification of existing self-care deficits. Because this theory focuses on deficits in care, it primarily addresses illness states. The self-care requisites are as follows:

- Maintenance of a sufficient intake of air
- Maintenance of a sufficient intake of water
- Maintenance of a sufficient intake of food
- Provision of care associated with elimination processes and excrements
- Maintenance of a balance between activity and rest
- Maintenance of a balance between solitude and social interaction
- Prevention of hazards to human life, human functioning, and human well-being

- Promotion of human functioning and development within social groups in accord with human potential, known human limitations, and the human desire to be normal (Orem, 1995)

Interpreting the Data

After data have been collected, the nurse can begin to develop impressions or inferences about the meaning of the data. Organizing data in clusters helps the nurse to recognize patterns of response or behavior. When data are placed in clusters, the nurse can:

- Distinguish between relevant and irrelevant data,
- Determine whether and where there are gaps in the data, and
- Identify patterns of cause and effect.

Documenting the Data

Assessment data must be recorded and reported. The nurse must make a judgment about which data are to be immediately reported to the head nurse and/or physician and which data need only be recorded at that time. Data that reflect a significant deviation from the normal (for example, rapid heart rate with irregular rhythm, severe difficulty in breathing, or a high level of anxiety) would need to be reported as well as recorded. Examples of data that need only to be recorded at the time include a report that prescribed medication has relieved a headache and a determination that an abdominal dressing is dry and intact.

Accurate and complete recording of assessment data is essential for communicating information to other health care team members. In addition, documentation is the basis for determining quality of care and should include appropriate data to support identified problems.

Diagnosis

The second step in the nursing process involves further **analysis** (breaking down the whole into parts that can be examined) and **synthesis** (putting data together in a new way) of the data that have been collected. Formulation of the list of nursing diagnoses is the outcome of this process. According to NANDA, a **nursing diagnosis**

> is a clinical judgment about individual, family, or community responses to actual or potential health problems/life processes. A nursing diagnosis provides the basis for selection of nursing interventions to achieve outcomes for which the nurse is accountable. (NANDA, 2001)

The nursing diagnoses developed during this phase of the nursing process provide the basis for client care delivered through the remaining steps.

Clients receive both medical and nursing diagnoses.

Table 9–2 compares the two categories of diagnoses. It is important to have a clear understanding of the nature of a nursing diagnosis as compared to a **medical diagnosis** (clinical judgment by the physician that identifies or determines a specific disease, condition, or pathological state). Table 9–3 compares selected nursing and medical diagnoses.

The nurse uses critical-thinking and decision-making skills in developing nursing diagnoses. This process is facilitated by asking questions such as:

- Are there problems here?
- If so, what are the specific problems?
- What are some possible causes of the problems?
- Is there a situation involving risk factors?
- What are the risk factors?
- Can a problem develop if preventive measures are not taken?
- If so, under what circumstances?
- Has the client indicated a desire for a higher level of wellness in a particular area of function?
- What are the client's strengths?
- What data are available to answer these questions?
- Are more data needed to answer the question?
- If so, what are some possible sources of the data that are needed?

Components of a Nursing Diagnosis

Several formats have been used to structure nursing diagnosis statements. Two formats that are frequently seen in the nursing literature are the two-part statement and the three-part statement. The two-part statement is NANDA approved and is used by most nurses mainly because of its brief and precise format. The three-part statement is usually required of nursing students and is preferred by those nurses desiring to strengthen the diagnostic statement by including specific manifestations. Refer to the appendices for the NANDA-approved nursing diagnoses.

Two-Part Statement The first component, the actual nursing diagnosis, is a problem statement or diagnostic label that describes the client's response to an actual or potential health problem or a wellness condition.

The second component of a two-part nursing diagnosis statement is the etiology. The **etiology** is the related cause or contributor to the problem and is identified in the complete NANDA diagnosis description. The diagnostic label and etiology are linked by the term *related to* (R/T). Because the NANDA list of nursing diagnoses is constantly evolving, there may be times when no etiology is provided. In such cases, the nurse should attempt to describe likely contributing factors to the client's condition. Examples of a two-part nursing diagnosis statement are *Disturbed Body Image R/T loss of left lower extremity* and *Activity Intolerance R/T decreased oxygen-carrying capacity of cells.*

Three-Part Statement The nursing diagnosis can also be expressed as a three-part statement. As in the two-part statement, the first two components are the diagnostic label and the etiology. The third component consists of **defining characteristics** (collected

Table 9–2 COMPARISON OF MEDICAL AND NURSING DIAGNOSES

MEDICAL DIAGNOSIS	NURSING DIAGNOSIS
Identifies conditions the physician is licensed and qualified to treat	Identifies situations the nurse is licensed and qualified to treat
Focuses on the illness, injury, or disease process	Focuses on the client's responses to actual or potential health problems or life processes
Remains constant until a cure is effected	Changes as the client's response and/or the health problem changes
EXAMPLE: Breast cancer	EXAMPLE: *Deficient Knowledge, Powerlessness, Anticipatory Grieving, Disturbed Body Image, Ineffective Coping.*

Adapted from Fundamentals of Nursing: Standards & Practice, *by S. DeLaune and P. Ladner, 1998, Albany, NY: Delmar. Copyright 1998 by Delmar. Adapted with permission.*

Table 9–3 COMPARISON OF SELECT NURSING AND MEDICAL DIAGNOSES

NURSING DIAGNOSIS	MEDICAL DIAGNOSIS
Ineffective Breathing Pattern	Chronic obstructive pulmonary disease
Activity Intolerance	Cerebrovascular accident
Pain	Appendectomy
Disturbed Body Image	Amputation
Risk for Imbalanced Body Temperature	Strep throat

Adapted from Fundamentals of Nursing: Standards & Practice, *by S. DeLaune and P. Ladner, 1998, Albany, NY: Delmar. Copyright 1998 by Delmar. Adapted with permission.*

Benefits of Nursing Diagnosis
- Nursing diagnosis is unique in that it focuses on a client's *response* to a health problem rather than on the problem itself, and it provides a structure through which nursing care can be delivered.
- Nursing diagnosis provides a means for effective communication.
- Holistic client, family, and community-focused care are facilitated with the use of nursing diagnosis.

Nursing Diagnosis
- The nursing diagnosis must be developed from the data, never the other way around.
- Do not try to fit a client to a nursing diagnosis; rather, select the appropriate diagnosis from the data cues presented by the client. Failure to do so may result in errors in developing a nursing diagnosis.

data, also known as signs and symptoms, subjective and objective data, or clinical manifestations). The third part is joined to the first two components with the connecting phrase *as evidenced by* (AEB). An example of a three-part nursing diagnosis statement is *Ineffective Breathing Pattern R/T pain AEB respiratory rate less than 11 and use of accessory muscles.*

Writing the Nursing Diagnosis Statement

The nursing diagnosis selected from the NANDA list becomes the diagnostic label, the first part of the diagnosis statement. Etiologies are also chosen from the NANDA descriptions. The appropriate etiology is selected and joined to the first part of the statement with the "related to" phrase. Table 9–4 compares selected NANDA-approved diagnoses in two- and three-part formats.

Types of Nursing Diagnoses

Analysis of the collected data leads the nurse to make a diagnosis in one of three categories:

- An **actual nursing diagnosis** indicates that a problem exists; it is composed of the diagnostic label, related factors, and signs and symptoms. An example of an actual diagnosis is *Impaired Skin Integrity R/T prolonged pressure on bony prominence AEB Stage II pressure ulcer over coccyx, 3 cm in diameter.*
- A **risk nursing diagnosis** (potential problem) indicates that a problem does not yet exist, but that special risk factors are present. A risk diagnosis is composed of the phrase *Risk for* followed by the diagnostic label and a list of the specific risk factors. An example of a risk diagnosis is *Risk for Impaired Skin Integrity; risk factors include physical immobilization AEB inability to turn self from side to side in bed.*
- A **wellness nursing diagnosis** indicates the client's expression of a desire to attain a higher level

Table 9–4 **EXAMPLES OF NURSING DIAGNOSES EXPRESSED IN TWO- AND THREE-PART STATEMENTS**	
TWO-PART STATEMENT	**THREE-PART STATEMENT**
Feeding Self-Care Deficit R/T decreased strength and endurance	*Feeding Self-Care Deficit R/T decreased strength and endurance AEB inability to maintain fork in hand from plate to mouth*
Anxiety R/T change in role functioning	*Anxiety R/T change in role functioning AEB insomnia, poor eye contact, and quivering voice*
Ineffective Airway Clearance R/T fatigue	*Ineffective Airway Clearance R/T fatigue AEB dyspnea at rest*
Deficient Knowledge (Insulin Injection Technique) R/T misinterpretation of information	*Deficient Knowledge (Insulin Injection Technique) R/T misinterpretation of information AEB inaccurate return demonstration of self-injection*
Spiritual Distress R/T separation from religious ties	*Spiritual Distress R/T separation from religious ties AEB crying and withdrawal*

Adapted from Fundamentals of Nursing: Standards & Practice, *by S. DeLaune and P. Ladner, 1998, Albany, NY: Delmar. Copyright 1998 by Delmar. Adapted with permission.*

of wellness in some area of function. It is composed of the phrase *Potential for Enhanced* followed by the diagnostic label. For example, a couple expecting their first child asks the nurse for suggestions on books to read and classes to attend so that they can be well prepared for their child. The nurse would make a wellness diagnosis of *Readiness for Enhanced Family Coping.*

Examples of the three types of diagnoses are shown in Table 9–5.

After formulation, the nursing diagnoses should be discussed with the client, if possible. If this is not possible, the diagnoses may be discussed with family members. Finally, the list of nursing diagnoses is recorded on the client's record. After this list has been developed and recorded, the remainder of the client's care plan can be completed. The list of nursing diagnoses is not static. It is dynamic, changing as more data are collected and as client goals and client responses to interventions are evaluated.

Planning and Outcome Identification

Planning combines with outcome identification to comprise the third step of the nursing process and includes both the formulation of guidelines that establish the proposed course of nursing action in the resolution of nursing diagnoses and the development of the client's plan of care. After the nursing diagnoses have been developed and the client's strengths have been identified, planning can begin.

The planning of nursing care occurs in three phases: initial, ongoing, and discharge. Each type of planning contributes to the coordination of the client's comprehensive plan of care. **Initial planning** involves development of a preliminary plan of care by the nurse who performs the admission assessment and gathers the comprehensive admission assessment data. Because of progressively shorter lengths of hospitalization, initial planning is important in addressing each problem and in correlating nursing care to hasten resolution of these problems. **Ongoing planning** entails continuous updating of the client's plan of care. As new information about the client is gathered and evaluated, revisions may be generated and the initial plan of care

further individualized to the client. **Discharge planning** involves critical anticipation and planning for the client's needs after discharge.

The planning phase involves several tasks:

- Prioritizing the list of nursing diagnoses
- Identifying and writing client-centered long- and short-term goals and outcomes (outcome identification)
- Developing specific nursing interventions
- Recording the entire nursing care plan in the client's record

Prioritizing the Nursing Diagnoses

Prioritizing the nursing diagnoses involves making decisions about which diagnoses are the most important and therefore require attention first. One of the most common methods of selecting priorities is to consider Maslow's hierarchy of needs, which leads the nurse to consider a life-threatening diagnosis more urgent than a non–life-threatening diagnosis. After basic physiological needs (e.g., respiration, nutrition, temperature, hydration, and elimination) are met to some degree, the nurse would then consider needs on the next level of the hierarchy (e.g., safe environment, stable living condition, affection, and self-worth) and so on up the hierarchy until all of the client's nursing diagnoses have been prioritized. Table 9–6 illustrates this process.

Identifying Outcomes

Outcome identification includes establishing goals and expected outcomes, which together provide guidelines for individualized nursing interventions and establish evaluation criteria to measure the effectiveness of the nursing care plan.

Goals A **goal** is an aim, intent, or end. Goals are broad statements that describe the intended or desired

---

Table 9–5 **TYPES OF NURSING DIAGNOSES**	
NURSING DIAGNOSIS	**EXAMPLE**
Actual diagnosis	*Deficient Fluid Volume R/T nausea and vomiting AEB dry skin and mucous membranes and decreased oral intake of fluids*
Risk diagnosis	*Risk for Infection R/T presence of invasive lines (intravenous line and indwelling bladder catheter)*
Wellness diagnosis	*Readiness for Enhanced Spiritual Well-Being*

Table 9–6 **PRIORITIZING NURSING DIAGNOSES**		
NURSING DIAGNOSIS	**MASLOW'S HIERARCHY OF NEEDS**	**PRIORITY**
Anxiety R/T hospitalization	Safety and security	Moderate
Ineffective Coping R/T situational crisis	Self-esteem	Low
Ineffective Airway Clearance R/T excessive secretions	Physiological	High

change in the client's condition or behavior. Client-centered goals are established in collaboration with the client whenever possible. Goal statements refer to the diagnostic label (or problem statement) of the nursing diagnosis. If the client or significant others are unable to participate in goal development, the nurse assumes that responsibility until the client is able to participate. Client-centered goals ensure that nursing care is individualized and focused on the client.

A **short-term goal** is an objective statement that outlines the desired resolution of the nursing diagnosis over a short period of time, usually a few hours or days (less than a week). Short-term goals focus on the etiology component of the nursing diagnosis. A **long-term goal** is an objective statement that outlines the desired resolution of the nursing diagnosis over a longer period of time, usually weeks or months. Long-term goals focus on the problem component of the nursing diagnosis. Table 9–7 provides examples of short-term and long-term goals.

Expected Outcomes After the goals have been established, the expected outcomes can be identified based on those goals. An **expected outcome** is a detailed, specific statement that describes the methods through which the goal will be achieved and includes aspects such as direct nursing care, client teaching, and continuity of care. Outcomes must be measurable, time limited, and realistic. Several expected outcomes may be required for each goal (Table 9–8). After goals and expected outcomes have been established, nursing interventions are formulated to enable the client to reach the goals.

Developing Specific Nursing Interventions

A **nursing intervention** is an action performed by the nurse that helps the client achieve the results specified by the goals and expected outcomes. Nursing interventions refer directly to the related factors in the actual or wellness nursing diagnoses and to the risk factors in risk nursing diagnoses. If the nursing interventions can remove or reduce the related factors and the risk factors, the problem can be resolved or prevented.

For each nursing diagnosis, there may be a number of nursing interventions. Nursing interventions are individualized and are stated in specific terms. Examples of nursing interventions are as follows:

- Assist client to turn, cough, and deep breathe q 2 h beginning at 0800, 2/10
- Teach nipple care when breastfeeding at 1000, 2/11
- Weigh client at each visit

After interventions have been formulated for each diagnosis, they are recorded on the client's care plan. As is true with other steps in the nursing process, the list of interventions is not static. As the nurse interacts with the client, assesses responses to interventions, and evaluates those responses, interventions may change.

Categories of Nursing Interventions

Nursing interventions are classified into one of three categories: independent, interdependent, or dependent. **Independent nursing interventions** are nursing actions that are initiated by the nurse and do not require direction or an order from another health care professional. In many states, the nursing practice act allows independent nursing interventions with regard to activities such as daily living, health education, health promotion, and counseling. An example of an independent nursing intervention is the nurse's elevating a client's edematous extremity.

Table 9–7 SHORT- AND LONG-TERM GOALS

Nursing Diagnosis: *Pain related to rheumatoid arthritis*

Short-term Goals (Focused on Etiology)	Long-term Goal (Focused on Problem)
Verbalizes the presence of pain	Verbalizes comfort
Identifies factors that influence the pain experience	
Client or significant other administers pain medication appropriately	

From Fundamentals of Nursing: Standards & Practice, by S. DeLaune and P. Ladner, 1998, Albany, NY: Delmar. Copyright 1998 by Delmar. Reprinted with permission.

Table 9–8 GOAL WITH EXPECTED OUTCOMES

Nursing Diagnosis: *Disturbed Sleep Pattern R/T sensory alterations: internal (illness) and external (social cues)*

Goal	Expected Outcomes
Client will sleep uninterrupted for 6 hours.	• When ready for bed, client will request back massage for relaxation. • By the next visit, client will have set limits for visits from family and significant others.

Nursing Diagnosis: *Ineffective Tissue Perfusion (Peripheral) R/T interruption of venous flow*

Goal	Expected Outcomes
Client will have palpable peripheral pulses in 1 week.	• Client will identify three factors to improve peripheral circulation within 2 days. • Client's feet will be warm to touch within 2 weeks.

Interdependent nursing interventions are those actions that are implemented in a collaborative manner by the nurse in conjunction with other health care professionals. A client care conference with an interdisciplinary health care team results in interdependent nursing interventions. For example, the nurse may assist a client to perform an exercise taught by the physical therapist.

Dependent nursing interventions are those actions that require an order from a physician or another health care professional. An example of a dependent intervention is administration of a medication. Although this intervention requires specific nursing knowledge and responsibilities, it is not within the realm of legal practice for licensed practical/vocational nurses (LP/VNs) to prescribe medications. When administering medications, the nurse is responsible for knowing the classification, pharmacological action, normal dosage, adverse effects, contraindications, and nursing implications of the drug. Therefore, dependent nursing interventions, like all nursing actions, must be guided by appropriate knowledge and judgment.

Recording the Nursing Care Plan

The **nursing care plan** is a written guide that organizes data about a client's care into a formal statement of the strategies that will be implemented to help the client achieve optimal health. Nursing care plans usually include components such as assessment, nursing diagnoses, goals and expected outcomes, and nursing interventions. The nurse begins the nursing care plan on the day of admission and continually updates and individualizes the client's plan of care until discharge.

There are several types of care plans including student-oriented, standardized, institutional, and computerized care plans. The student-oriented care plan promotes learning of problem-solving skills, the nursing process, verbal and written communication skills, and organizational skills. This comprehensive care plan offers great depth for teaching the process of planning care and usually includes a scientific rationale for each intervention. Although educational programs vary, the student-oriented care plan usually begins with assessment and proceeds in a sequential manner until it concludes with the evaluation of the care plan.

The standardized care plan is a preplanned, preprinted guide for the nursing care of client groups with common needs. This type of care plan generally follows the nursing process format. The nurse may use standardized care plans when a client has predictable, commonly occurring problems. Individualization may be accomplished by the inclusion of additional handwritten notes regarding unusual problems.

Institutional nursing care plans are concise documents that become a part of the client's medical record after discharge. The Kardex nursing care plan is an example of this type of care plan and is frequently used.

The institutional nursing care plan may simply include the nursing diagnoses, nursing interventions, and evaluation. In addition, the Kardex nursing care plan may be expanded to include assessment, nursing diagnoses, goals, implementation, and evaluation. Figure 9-4 provides an example of an institutional care plan.

Computers are used for creating and storing nursing care plans and can generate both standardized and individualized nursing care plans. The nurse selects appropriate diagnoses from a menu suggested by the computer, which then lists possible goals and nursing interventions. The nurse has the option of reading the client's plan of care from the computer screen or printing an updated working copy. Figure 9-5 is an example of a computerized nursing care plan.

Implementation

The fourth step in the nursing process is implementation. **Implementation** involves the execution of the nursing care plan derived during the planning phase. It consists of performing nursing activities (interventions) that have been planned to meet the goals set with the client. It also involves the **delegation** (process of transferring a select nursing task to a licensed individual who is competent to perform that specific task) of some nursing interventions to staff members or to assistive personnel capable of competently performing the task. The nurse remains accountable for appropriate delegation and supervision of care provided by these individuals.

Requirements for Effective Implementation

Implementation involves many skills. The nurse must continue to assess the client's condition before, during, and after each nursing intervention. Assessment prior to intervention implementation provides the nurse with baseline data. Assessment during and after intervention implementation allows the nurse to detect positive or negative responses the client may have to the intervention. If negative responses occur during the intervention, the nurse must take appropriate action. If positive responses occur, the nurse adds this information to the database for use in evaluating the efficacy of the intervention.

The nurse must also possess psychomotor skills, interpersonal skills, and cognitive skills to perform the nursing interventions that have been planned. The nurse uses psychomotor skills to safely and effectively perform nursing activities. Nurses must be able to both handle medical equipment with a high degree of competency and perform such skills as giving injections, changing dressings, and helping the client perform range-of-motion (ROM) exercises.

Interpersonal skills are necessary as the nurse interacts with the client and the family to collect data, provide information in teaching sessions, and offer support

NURSING DIAGNOSIS	NURSING INTERVENTIONS	EVALUATION
Ineffective breathing pattern R/T operative site/incisional pain.	1. Auscultate breath sounds q̄ 4h. & PRN 2. Assist Pt. to TCDB q̄ 2h while awake.	1. Lungs clear on auscultation. 2. "It doesn't hurt as much to cough today."
Risk for infection R/T surgical incision & indwelling catheter	Assess for S/S of infection q̄ 4h.	T-100.2°, incision site warm & pink, non-edematous. "It really hurts under the bandage."

Figure 9-4 Handwritten Institutional Care Plan *(From* Fundamentals of Nursing: Standards & Practice, *by S. DeLaune and P. Ladner, 1998, Albany, NY: Delmar. Copyright 1998 by Delmar. Reprinted with permission.)*

in times of anxiety. The nurse–client relationship is established and maintained through the use of therapeutic communication. Interaction between and among members of the health care team promotes collaboration and enhances the holistic care of the client.

Cognitive skills enable the nurse to make appropriate observations, understand the rationale for the activities performed, ask the appropriate questions, and make decisions about those things that need to be done. Critical thinking is an important element within the cognitive domain because it helps the nurse analyze data, organize observations, and apply prior knowledge and experiences to current client situations.

Types of Nursing Interventions

Nursing interventions are written as orders in the care plan and may be nurse initiated, physician initiated, or derived from collaboration with other health care professionals. Interventions can be implemented on the basis of specific orders, standing orders, or protocols.

A **specific order** is an order written in a client's medical record or nursing care plan by a physician or nurse especially for that individual client; it is not used for any other client.

A **standing order** is a standardized intervention written, approved, and signed by a physician that is

Client Name: Margaret Jones
Age: 55　　　**Temp:** 98.8　　　**BP:** 150/90　　　**Pulse:** 90　　　**Sex:** F

Disease/Disorder/Condition: Diabetes

Client Health History

Mrs. Jones was diagnosed 2 years ago with type 2 (non-insulin-dependent) diabetes and takes metformin (Glucophage) 500 mg b.i.d (twice a day) with meals. She is being seen in the clinic for her 6-month visit. She says, "I hardly have the energy to get up and dress in the morning. I am thirsty all day and awaken several times during the night, having to go to the bathroom." She does not work outside the home and has not been involved in community activities for the past five years since her youngest child graduated from high school. Her daily routine involves cooking for her husband and brother, reading, and watching the TV for 6-8 hours. She says, "I eat because I have nothing else to do." She is concerned about her eating habits and her recent weight gain.

Assessment Findings

Weight, 177 lb.　　　Weight gain, 8 lb.
Height, 5'4"　　　Sedentary lifestyle
Triceps skinfold, 28mm　　　Eats in response to boredom
Elevated blood glucose

Nursing Diagnosis: Imbalanced Nutrition: More than Body Requirements

Goals: Mrs. Jones will:
1. Come to clinic weekly for 4 weeks.
2. Modify eating habits to decrease amount of intake.
3. Lose 2 lb./month.
4. Participate in some exercise.
5. Begin involvement outside of home.

continues

Figure 9-5 Computer-Generated Nursing Care Plan

Intervention	Rationale
1. Conduct a dietary history, using open-ended statements to assist the client in exploring psychological factors that may contribute to eating.	1. Nonjudgmental approach to acquiring information will encourage client trust and honesty.
2. Encourage client to modify eating habits to decrease amount of intake (smaller servings, taking small bites and chewing each bite 12 times, putting the fork on the plate between bites, drinking water with meals, eating only at mealtime, chewing sugar-free gum when watching TV).	2. Healthy eating habits and tips on recognizing fullness during a meal will help the client eat to satisfy hunger, not boredom.
3. Assess client's motivation to lose weight.	3. Having client's support for care plan will influence success.
4. Discuss risk factors and symptoms (thirst and urination) of diabetes.	4. Client understanding of her disease may increase motivation to manage it.
5. Instruct client to maintain a daily dietary intake log; time of meals and snacks, type and amount of foods eaten.	5. Helps client recognize her eating patterns and note healthy and unhealthy behaviors.
6. Provide with dietary materials, review the Food Pyramid and Diabetic Exchange List; plan with client a 1600-kilocalorie per day diet for a week, taking into consideration food preferences.	6. Ensures client has information necessary to plan healthy meals within recommended guidelines.
7. Review with client age-appropriate exercises; emphasize need for daily walking.	7. Changing sedentary lifestyle will increase self-esteem, burn calories, and increase energy level
8. Review with client community and church interests outside the home, unrelated to cooking and eating.	8. Helps client focus on activities not involving food to decrease boredom and to increase self-esteem.
9. Schedule return visit with nurse in one week; Monitor progress and assess plan of care.	9. Close monitoring and follow-up will allow modification of plan of care as required to meet client needs.

Evaluation/Outcome

1. Client made return clinic appointment; noted phone number of nurse and dietitian to answer questions; agreed to 1800-kilocalorie meal plan for one week.

2. On return visit, the client reported drinking more water with meals, chewing her food slowly, and chewing gum while watching TV.

3. On return visit, the client was found to have lost 1.8 lbs.

4. On return visit, the client indicated that she now walks to the store 4-5 times a week (40 minutes round trip).

5. The client reported on return visit that she is now volunteering 2 hours 3 times a week at the church's child care center.

Format from Delmar's Electronic Care Plan Maker, *by Susan Sheehy, 1998, Albany, NY: Delmar. Content from* Fundamentals of Nursing: Standards & Practice *by S. DeLaune and P. Ladner, 1998, Albany, NY: Delmar. Copyright 1998 by Delmar.*

Figure 9-5 *continued*

kept on file within health care agencies to be used in predictable situations or in circumstances requiring immediate attention. Nurses can implement standing orders in these situations after assessing the client and identifying the primary or emerging problem. An example of a physician-initiated standing order on an inpatient unit would be specification of certain medications to be administered for a common headache.

A **protocol** is a series of standing orders or procedures that should be followed under certain specific conditions. The protocol defines those interventions that are permissible and those circumstances under

which the nurse is allowed to implement the measures. Health care agencies or individual physicians frequently have standing orders or protocols for client preparation for diagnostic tests or for immediate interventions in life-threatening circumstances. These protocols prevent needless duplication of effort with regard to writing the same orders repeatedly for different clients, often saving valuable time in critical situations.

Documenting and Reporting Interventions

The implementation step also involves documenta-

COMMUNITY/HOME HEALTH CARE

Standing Orders
Nurses in home health care agencies may have standing orders for administering certain medications or ordering laboratory tests when indicated.

tion and reporting. Data to be recorded include the client's condition prior to the intervention, the specific intervention performed, the client's response to the intervention, and client outcomes. This documentation not only constitutes a legal record, but also allows for valuable communication among other health care team members for purposes of ensuring continuity of care and evaluating progress toward expected outcomes. In addition, written documentation provides data necessary for reimbursement for services.

Verbal interaction among health care providers is also essential for communicating current information about clients. Communication between nurses generally occurs at the change of shift, when the responsibility for care changes from one nurse to another. Nursing students must communicate relevant information to the nurse responsible for their clients when they leave the unit. Information that should be shared in the verbal report includes:

- Those activities completed and those yet to be completed,
- Status of current relevant problems,
- Any abnormalities or changes in assessment,
- Results of treatments, and
- Diagnostic tests scheduled or completed (and results).

All communication—both written and verbal—must be objective, descriptive, and complete. All communication must include observations rather than opinions and be stated or written to convey an accurate picture of the client's condition. Thorough and detailed communication of implementation activities is fundamental to ensuring that client care and progress toward goals can be adequately evaluated.

Evaluation

Evaluation, the fifth step in the nursing process, involves determining whether the client goals have been met, partially met, or not met. If a goal has been met, the nurse must then decide whether nursing activities should cease or continue in order for status to be maintained. If a goal has been partially met or not met, the nurse must reassess the situation. Data are collected to determine both the reasons the goal has not been achieved and the necessary modifications to the plan of

care. Among a number of possible reasons that goals are not met or are only partially met are the following:

- The initial assessment data were incomplete.
- The goals and expected outcomes were not realistic.
- The time frame was too optimistic.
- The goals and/or the nursing interventions planned were not appropriate for the client or situation.

Evaluation is a fluid process that is dependent on all the other components of the nursing process. As shown in Figure 9-6, evaluation affects, and is affected by, assessment, diagnosis, planning and outcome identification, and implementation of nursing care. Table 9–9 shows the way evaluation is woven into every phase of the nursing process. Ongoing evaluation is essential if the nursing process is to be implemented appropriately. As Alfaro-LeFevre (1998) states:

When we evaluate early, checking whether our information is accurate, complete, and up-to-date, we're able to make corrections *early*. We avoid making decisions based on outdated, inaccurate, or incomplete information. Early evaluation enhances our ability to act safely and effectively. It improves our *efficiency* by helping us stay focused on priorities and avoid wasting time continuing useless actions.

Nursing Audit

A **nursing audit** is the process of collecting and analyzing data to evaluate the effectiveness of nursing interventions. A nursing audit can focus on implementation of the nursing process, on client outcomes, or on both in order to evaluate the quality of care provided. Health care facilities each have an ongoing nursing audit committee to evaluate the quality of care given. Nursing audits examine data related to:

- Safety measures,
- Treatment interventions and client responses to those interventions,

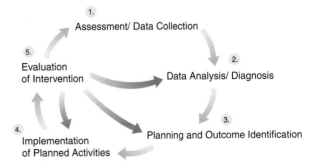

Figure 9-6 Relationship of Evaluation to the Nursing Process *(From* Fundamentals of Nursing: Standards & Practice, *by S. DeLaune and P. Ladner, 1998, Albany, NY: Delmar. Copyright 1998 by Delmar. Reprinted with permission.)*

COMMUNITY/HOME HEALTH CARE

Effectiveness of Care

When evaluating the effectiveness of care, the home health care nurse can use the following questions to examine client achievement of expected outcomes:

- Were the goals realistic in terms of client abilities and time frame?
- Were there external variables (for example, housing problems, impaired family dynamics) that prevented goal achievement?
- Did the family have the resources (for example, transportation) to assist in meeting the goals?
- Was the care coordinated with other providers to facilitate efficient delivery of care?

- Preestablished outcomes used as a basis for interventions,
- Discharge planning,
- Client teaching, and
- Adequacy of staffing patterns.

THE NURSING PROCESS AND CRITICAL THINKING

A number of skills are required of nurses in their use of the nursing process as a framework for providing client care. One important skill is critical thinking. Critical thinkers ask questions, evaluate evidence, identify assumptions, examine alternatives, and seek to understand various points of view.

Critical thinking is a skill that can be learned, just as other skills are learned. The skill of critical thinking is important and useful in all aspects of a person's life and is an especially vital tool for the nurse with regard to the nursing process. Critical thinkers develop a questioning attitude and delve into situations in order to seek possible explanations for what is happening. Examples of questions that the nurse as critical thinker might ask at each step in the nursing process are listed in Table 9–10.

Assumptions are those beliefs or attitudes that one takes for granted in a situation that requires action or resolution; they are the things that one accepts as "givens." Assumptions are the implicit views one uses to filter and make sense of everyday experiences. Cause-and-effect relationships are understood within the context of these assumptions. Assumptions both are related to one's point of view and influence the way one looks at things.

Bias is a mental inclination or leaning. It can manifest in two ways. According to one interpretation of bias, a person's point of view causes that person to be more observant about certain things. According to an-

Table 9–9   INTERACTION BETWEEN EVALUATION AND THE OTHER PHASES OF THE NURSING PROCESS

NURSING PROCESS PHASE	EVALUATION FOCUS
Assessment	Data collection was thorough and complete.
	Data were collected from multiple, varied sources.
	Data were relevant to client needs.
	Appropriate methods were used to obtain data.
	A systematic, organized method was used in collecting data.
Diagnosis	Nursing diagnoses were client centered, accurate, and relevant.
	Each nursing diagnosis was complete.
	Nursing diagnoses were comprehensive.
	Diagnoses were based on the collected data.
	Nursing diagnoses guided planning and implementation of care.
Planning and Outcome Identification	Outcomes were realistic and achievable.
	Nursing diagnoses were prioritized.
	Expected outcomes were relevant to nursing diagnoses.
	Resources (including team members) were used efficiently.
	Nursing plans were documented.
Implementation	Team members followed the plan of care.
	Necessary resources were available.
	Nursing actions assisted client in meeting expected outcomes.
	Client achieved expected outcomes.
	Care plan was revised according to the client's needs.
	Documentation reflected the client's status, including responses to nursing interventions.

Adapted from Fundamentals of Nursing: Standards & Practice, *by S. DeLaune and P. Ladner, 1998, Albany, NY: Delmar. Copyright 1998 by Delmar. Adapted with permission.*

other interpretation of bias, a person is blind to or unwilling to consider weaknesses in his own point of view. Critical thinkers attempt to be aware of both interpretations of bias and avoid the latter.

THE NURSING PROCESS AND PROBLEM SOLVING

The steps in the nursing process and in problem solving are similar. People use problem solving in their

Table 9–10	EXAMPLES OF CRITICAL THINKING QUESTIONS FOR USE WITH THE NURSING PROCESS

NURSING PROCESS STEP	CRITICAL-THINKING QUESTION
Assessment	Are the data complete? What other data do I need? What are some possible sources of those data? What assumptions or biases do I have in this situation? What is the client's point of view? Are there other points of view?
Diagnosis	What do these data mean? What else could be happening? Are there any gaps in the data? How are these data similar, and how are they different? What assumptions or biases do I have in this situation? Have my assumptions affected my interpretation of the data? If so, in what way?
Planning and outcome identification	What are the goals for this client? How are my goals related to what the client wants to accomplish? What are the expected outcomes for this client? What interventions are to be used? Who is the best-qualified person to perform these interventions? How much involvement can the client and family or significant others have at this time? How much involvement does the client wish to have at this time?
Implementation	What is the client's current status? What are the most critical steps in this intervention? How must I alter the intervention to best meet this client's needs and maintain principles of safety? What is the client's response during and after the intervention? Is there a need to alter the intervention in any way? If so, why and how?
Evaluation	Were the interventions successful in assisting the client to achieve the desired goals? How could things have been done differently? What data do I need to make new decisions? Where will I get the data? Were there assumptions, biases, or points of view that I missed that affected the outcomes? What can be done about these assumptions, biases, or points of view?

From Fundamentals of Nursing: Standards & Practice, *by S. DeLaune and P. Ladner, 1998, Albany, NY: Delmar. Copyright 1998 by Delmar. Reprinted with permission.*

sometimes based on guesses. Conversely, the nursing process, which is used by nurses to identify and make decisions about client needs, is a systematic and scientifically based process that requires the use of many cognitive and psychomotor skills. Table 9–11 compares the nursing process and the problem-solving method.

THE NURSING PROCESS AND DECISION MAKING

Nurses make decisions every day. It is important that those decisions be the best decisions possible, that they be based on reliable information, and that they be made with as much critical thought as possible. Nurses make decisions at each step of the nursing process. Through a process of problem solving, one arrives at the point at which decisions can be made. The nursing process is the specific problem-solving method used by nurses to arrive at the point at which decisions about client care can be made.

Because the nursing process is a dynamic, circular, and fluid process, decisions must be made at many points as the nurse implements the various steps. Each of these decisions, resulting from critical thought and problem-solving strategies, leads to the determination of appropriate nursing interventions for the client.

THE NURSING PROCESS AND HOLISTIC CARE

Nurses bring to each client situation a broad knowledge base. The theoretical base of nursing knowledge comes from many different fields, including the natural sciences, behavioral sciences, social sciences, arts and

Table 9–11	COMPARISON OF THE PROBLEM-SOLVING METHOD AND THE NURSING PROCESS

PROBLEM-SOLVING METHOD	NURSING PROCESS
Identify the problem	Assessment
Gather information	Assessment
Name the problem	Diagnosis
Develop a plan	Planning and outcome identification
Activate the plan	Implementation
Evaluate results	Evaluation

From Fundamentals of Nursing: Standards & Practice, *by S. DeLaune and P. Ladner, 1998, Albany, NY: Delmar. Copyright 1998 by Delmar. Reprinted with permission.*

daily lives. With the problem-solving method, problems are identified, information is gathered, a specific problem is named, a plan for solving the problem is developed, the plan is put into action, and results of the plan are evaluated. Problem solving, however, is frequently based on incomplete data, and plans are humanities, and nursing science. This broad knowledge base allows the nurse to interact with the client from a holistic viewpoint. Each nurse–client interaction adds to the client database and allows for individualized planning and care. The nursing process assists the nurse in determining client responses to situations, and critical-thinking and decision-making skills allow the nurse to prioritize client needs and decide which person can best meet certain client needs. Referral and collaboration among nurses and other health care professionals contribute to optimal achievement of client goals.

In some settings, the traditional nursing care plan formulated solely by nurses has been replaced by plans that are developed by a multidisciplinary team and referred to as critical pathways. **Critical pathways** are comprehensive, standard plans of care for specific case situations. Included in these plans are nursing interventions, medical interventions, interventions from other team members, specific client outcomes, and time lines for those outcomes. Because the nurse has a broad base of knowledge, the nurse is often the person who manages the care of the client through these critical pathways.

SUMMARY

- The nursing process is an organized method of planning and delivering nursing care. It is composed of five steps: assessment, diagnosis, planning and outcome identification, implementation, and evaluation.
- The nurse uses the process of assessment to establish a database about the client, to form an interpersonal relationship with the client, and to provide the client with an opportunity to discuss health care concerns.

- The second step in the nursing process involves further analysis and synthesis of the data and results in a list of nursing diagnoses.
- Nursing diagnoses contribute to a clearer conceptualization of knowledge unique to nursing, improved communication among nurses and other health care professionals, and promotion of individualized client care.
- The types of nursing diagnoses are actual, risk, and wellness.
- Planning and outcome identification, the third step in the nursing process, involves prioritizing nursing diagnoses, identifying and writing goals and client outcomes, developing nursing interventions, and recording the plan of care in the client's record.
- The nursing care plan documents health care needs, coordinates nursing care, promotes continuity of care, encourages communication among health care team members, and promotes quality nursing care.
- The implementation step of the nursing process is directed toward meeting client needs, resulting in health promotion, prevention of illness, illness management, or health restoration.
- Interventions can be nurse initiated, physician initiated, or collaborative in origin and, thus, are considered independent, dependent, or interdependent.
- Evaluation, the fifth step in the nursing process, measures the effectiveness of nursing interventions by the examination of the goals and expected outcomes, which provide direction for the plan of care and serve as standards against which the client's progress is measured.
- Critical-thinking, problem-solving, and decision-making skills are important in the use of the nursing process.

CASE STUDY

Mr. Jona is a client on your unit. A 70-year-old widower, he was admitted 2 days ago with a broken left hip. While bowling with his church bowling league, Mr. Jona tripped, fell, fractured his hip, and sprained his right wrist. He recently retired from an administrative position with a large company and moved to Florida from his home in Iowa. He has two children: one son who lives in Shumak, Washington, and a daughter who lives in Ono, New York. Mr. Jona lives alone in a one-bedroom apartment approximately 10 blocks from the hospital. In 4 days, Mr. Jona will be discharged and referred to the home health division for follow-up care.

The following questions will guide your development of a nursing care plan for the case study.

1. What assessments must be done with regard to Mr. Jona's going home?
2. Which three nursing diagnoses may apply to Mr. Jona?
3. What goals and outcomes may be appropriate for Mr. Jona?
4. What nursing interventions may be appropriate to meet the goals?

Review Questions

1. Mrs. Rose was admitted to your unit 2 hours ago. The following data are recorded on her chart. Which data are objective?

   a. temperature 102°F
   b. nausea
   c. headache
   d. pain in abdomen

2. Which of the following statements would describe the nursing process?

   a. It is a linear, static procedure.
   b. It is a circular, dynamic process.
   c. It is a hierarchy of steps to plan client care.
   d. It is a long, detailed form to be filled out for each client.

3. The nursing care plan includes:

   a. collected documentation of all team members providing care for the client.
   b. physician orders, demographic data, and medication administration and rationales.
   c. client's nursing diagnoses, goals, expected outcomes, and the nursing interventions.
   d. client assessment data, medical treatment regimen and rationales, and diagnostic test results and significance.

4. When establishing priorities for a client's plan of nursing care, the nurse should rank life-threatening diagnoses as the highest priorities and which as the lowest priorities?

   a. safety-related needs
   b. client needs regarding referral agencies
   c. the client's social, love, and belonging needs
   d. needs of family members and friends who are involved in plan of care

5. What are the essential components of an expected outcome?

   a. nursing diagnosis, interventions, and expected client behavior
   b. target date, nursing action, measurement criteria, and desired client behavior
   c. nursing client behavior, target date, and conditions under which the behavior occurs
   d. client behavior, measurement criteria, conditions under which the behavior occurs, and target date

6. Which guideline is most appropriate when developing nursing interventions?

   a. Make intervention statements specific to ensure continuity of care.
   b. Choose actions that a nurse can perform without leaving the unit or consulting with medical staff.
   c. Make sure that nursing care activities receive priority over other aspects of the treatment regimen.
   d. Write interventions in general terms to allow maximum flexibility and creativity in delivering nursing care.

Critical Thinking Questions

1. How are goals and outcomes different?

2. Differentiate between the three categories of nursing interventions: independent, interdependent, and dependent.

WEB FLASH!

- Can you find specific sites or resources dealing with the nursing process?
- Do the resources listed for this chapter also have web sites? What types of information do they provide?
- What resources on the Internet are available for nurses needing assistance with the nursing process or nursing diagnosis?

DOCUMENTATION

MAKING THE CONNECTION

Refer to the following chapters to increase your understanding of documentation:

- **Chapter 6, Legal Responsibilities**
- **Chapter 8, Communication**
- **Chapter 9, Nursing Process**

LEARNING OBJECTIVES

Upon completion of this chapter, you should be able to:
- *Define key terms.*
- *Explain the purposes of documentation in health care.*
- *Discuss the principles of effective documentation.*
- *Describe various methods of documentation.*
- *Recount various types of documentation records.*
- *Delineate the latest advances in computerized documentation.*

KEY TERMS

charting by exception (CBE)
critical pathway
documentation
focus charting
incident report
Kardex
narrative charting
Nursing Intervention Classification (NIC)
Nursing Outcome Classification (NOC)
Nursing Minimum Data Set (NMDS)
PIE charting
point-of-care charting
problem-oriented medical record
SOAP charting
source-oriented charting
variation
walking rounds

INTRODUCTION

Throughout the development of modern nursing, multiple documentation systems have emerged in response to changes in health care delivery. Systems of recording and reporting data pertinent to the care of clients have evolved primarily in response to the demand that health care practitioners be held to societal norms, professional standards of practice, legal and regulatory standards, and institutional policies and standards.

As with all facets of health care, advanced technology has affected the expectations for documentation. Activities in the areas of quality improvement and cost containment have also increased the demands on health care practitioners to create efficient documentation systems. Efficiency is measured in terms of time, thoroughness, and the quality of the observations being recorded. The documentation systems used today reflect the specific needs and preferences of the numerous health care agencies. Select systems and their ramifications are discussed in this chapter.

DOCUMENTATION AS COMMUNICATION

Communication is a dynamic, continuous, and multidimensional process for sharing information as determined by standards or policies. Reporting and recording are the major communication techniques used by health care providers in directing client-based decision making and continuity of care. The medical record serves as a legal document for recording all client activities initiated by all health care practitioners.

Documentation Defined

Documentation is defined as written evidence of:

- The interactions between and among health professionals, clients, their families, and health care organizations;
- The administration of tests, procedures, treatments, and client education; and
- The results of, or client's response to, diagnostic tests and interventions (Eggland & Heinemann, 1994).

Documentation provides written records that reflect client care provided on the basis of assessment data and the client's response to interventions.

In implementing the nursing process, nurses rely on the documentation tools of client charts and other documents that facilitate a logical sequencing of events. All the tools used by nurses to record their nursing care should form a system. Systematic documentation is critical because it presents the care administered by nurses in a logical fashion, as follows:

- Assessment data, obtained through interview, observation, and physical examination, identify the client's specific alteration and lay the foundation for the nursing care plan.
- The identified alteration in functional health pattern directs the formulation of a nursing diagnosis.
- The nursing diagnoses trigger the client's expected outcomes (both short- and long-term goals) and accompanying supportive nursing interventions—the planning and implementation phases.
- The effectiveness of the nursing interventions in achieving the client's expected outcomes becomes the criterion for evaluation, determining the need for subsequent reassessment and revision of the plan of care (Eggland & Heinemann, 1994; Iyer & Camp, 1999).

The system becomes a vehicle for expressing each phase of the nursing process. Nurses rely on systems that provide thorough, accurate charting reflective of the nurse's decision-making ability and the client's plan of care. The nurse's critical-thinking skills, judgments, and evaluations must be clearly communicated through proper documentation.

Purposes of Health Care Documentation

Professional responsibility and accountability are two primary reasons for documentation. Other reasons to document include communication; education; research; satisfaction of legal and practice standards; and reimbursement. The professional responsibility of all health care practitioners, documentation provides written evidence of the practitioner's accountability to the client, the institution, the profession, and society.

Communication

Documentation is a communication method that confirms the care provided to the client and clearly outlines all important information regarding the client. Thorough documentation provides:

- Accurate data needed to plan the client's care and to ensure continuity of care;
- A method of communication among the health care team members responsible for the client's care;
- Written evidence of those things done for the client, the client's response, and any revisions made in the plan of care;
- Evidence of compliance with professional practice standards (e.g., those of the American Nurses Association [ANA]);
- Evidence of compliance with accreditation criteria (e.g., those of the Joint Commission on Accreditation of Healthcare Organizations [JCAHO]);
- A resource for review, audit, reimbursement, education, and research; and
- A written legal record to protect the client, institution, and practitioner.

The client's medical record contains documents for record keeping. The type of document that constitutes the medical record in a given health care institution is determined by that institution. Throughout this chapter, various types of medical record documents are referenced. Table 10–1 outlines the content of these documents.

Education

The documentation contained in the client's medical record is used for the purpose of education. Health care students can use the medical record as a tool to learn about disease processes, complications, medical and nursing diagnoses, and interventions. The results from physical examinations and laboratory and diagnostic testing provide valuable information regarding specific diagnoses and interventions.

Nursing students can enhance their critical-thinking skills by examining the records in chronological order, analyzing the results, and following the health care team's plan of care, including the way it was developed, implemented, and evaluated. Students and all health care professionals must be aware of confidentiality issues before reading any client's chart; these issues are discussed later in the chapter.

Research

Researchers rely heavily on the client's medical record as a clinical data source to determine whether clients meet the research criteria for a study. Documentation also can direct the need for research. For example, if documentation demonstrates an increased infection rate in association with intravenous catheters,

Table 10–1 MEDICAL RECORD DOCUMENTS

DOCUMENT	INFORMATION
Face sheet	Lists biographical data (name, date of birth, address, phone number, Social Security number, marital status, employment, race, gender, religion, closest relative); insurance coverage, allergies, attending physician, admitting medical diagnosis, assigned diagnosis-related group (DRG), statement of whether the client has an advance directive
Consent form	Admit: gives the institution and physician the permission to treat Surgery: explains the reason for the operation in lay terms; the risks for complications; and the client's level of understanding Blood transfusion: grants permission to administer blood or blood products Various others: grant permission to participate in research, have photograph taken, know HIV status
Medical history and physical examination	Details results of the client's initial history and physical assessment as performed by the physician
Physician's order sheet	Outlines medical orders to admit; to treat; to discharge
Physician's progress notes	Delineates physician's evaluation of the client's response to treatment; may also contain the progress recording of other practitioners, e.g., dietary or social services
Consultation sheet	Initiated by the physician to request the evaluation or services of other practitioners
Diagnostic results	Contains the results from laboratory and diagnostic tests, e.g., x-ray, hematology
Nursing admit assessment	Records data obtained from the interview and physical assessment conducted by the nurse
Nursing plan of care	Contains the treatment plan, e.g., nursing diagnosis or a problem list, initiation of standards of care, or protocols
Graphic sheet	Lists data related to vital signs and weight
Flow sheet	Contains all routine interventions that can be indicated via a check mark or other simple code; allows for a quick comparison of measurements
Nurse's progress notes	Details additional data that do not duplicate information on the flow sheet, e.g., client's achievement of expected outcome, revision of the plan of care
Medication administration record (MAR)	Contains all medication information for routine and prn (as needed) drugs: date, time, dose, route, site (for injections)
Client education record	Records both the nurses' educational efforts directed toward the client, family, or other caregiver and the learner's response
Health care team record	Serves as the treatment and progress record for nonmedical and nonnursing practitioners (e.g., respiratory, physical therapy, dietary) when the physician's progress notes are not used by those practitioners
Critical pathway	A multidisciplinary form for each day of anticipated hospitalization; identifies the interventions and achievement of client outcomes; in the progress notes, explains the practitioner's initial implementation and the variances from the norm
Discharge plan and summary	A multidisciplinary form used before discharge from a health care facility; contains a brief summary of care rendered and of discharge instructions (e.g., food–drug interactions, referrals or follow-up appointments)
Advance directive or living will	Federal law requires that health care providers discuss with the client the use of advance directives, a living will, or a durable power of attorney. Most states recognize the living will as a legal document. If the client has advance directives, they are reviewed at the time of admission and placed in the medical record.

Adapted from Fundamentals of Nursing: Standards & Practice, *by S. DeLaune and P. Ladner, 1998, Albany, NY: Delmar. Copyright 1998 by Delmar. Adapted with permission.*

researchers can identify and study the variables that may be associated with the increased infection rate.

Legal and Practice Standards

"Failure to document appropriately is a key factor in clinical mishaps and a pivotal issue in many malpractice cases" (Springhouse, 1999). The client's medical record is a legal document, and in the case of a lawsuit, it is the record that serves as the description of exactly what happened to a client. In 80% to 85% of malpractice lawsuits involving client care, the medical record is the determining factor in providing proof of significant events (Iyer & Camp, 1999). The legal issues of documentation require:

- Legible and neat writing,
- Proper use of spelling and grammar,
- Use of authorized abbreviations, and
- Factual and time-sequenced descriptive notations.

To focus attention on the importance of communicating and documenting all information, Fiesta (1991) cites *Ramsey v. Physician Memorial Hospital*. An emergency room nurse failed to communicate to the physician that the mother of two pediatric clients had found a tick on one of the two children. One of the children later died from Rocky Mountain spotted fever. The physician had questioned the health team about ticks because of the children's elevated temperature, but was told nothing. The court dismissed the hospital from liability, but the appeal court held the hospital liable because the nurse had failed to communicate to the physician the information obtained from the mother about the tick.

The nurse is responsible for documenting on the chart both that the physician was notified and the significant information that was orally communicated. If the physician does not respond in a way that indicates an understanding of the urgency of the information, the nurse must document the physician's response and notify the supervisor of the situation. Nurses are responsible for the care the client receives and can be held liable if appropriate interventions are not imple-

PROFESSIONAL TIP

The Importance of Communication

Important information obtained from an assessment and warranting immediate intervention should not only be documented in the medical record but also communicated orally to those other practitioners involved in the client's care. The element of time must direct decision making when critical information is obtained.

PROFESSIONAL TIP

Consent from Sedated Clients

Sedated clients should never be requested or allowed to sign an informed consent. Because the client may not be capable of understanding the nature of and risks associated with the procedure, the consent will be invalid, and the nurse and institution will be at legal risk. Instead, either wait for the client to be competent and free of sedation (usually 4 hours after administration of the last medication that alters the level of consciousness) or have a legally acceptable family member brought into the decision.

mented in a timely manner when information is available that would dictate otherwise.

Informed Consent Informed consent is a competent client's ability to make health care decisions based on full disclosure of the benefits, risks, and potential consequences of a recommended treatment plan and of alternative treatments, including no treatment, and the client's agreement to the treatment as indicated by the client's signing a consent form. Although the physician who is to perform the procedure is responsible for obtaining the client's informed consent, the nurse is often the person who actually has the client sign the form.

Advance Directives An advance directive (i.e., living will and durable power of attorney for health care) is written instructions about an individual's health care preferences regarding life-sustaining measures that guides family members and health care professionals as to those treatment options that should or should not be considered in the event that the individual is unable to decide for herself. This effectively allows clients, while competent, to participate in end-of-life decisions and to choose the types of life-sustaining procedures they wish to be performed.

State Nursing Practice Acts In an attempt to recognize and control the practice of nursing, nursing practice acts, on a state-by-state basis, establish guidelines to ensure safe practice and to demonstrate accountability to society. The standards of care, as set forth in the practice acts, are based on the phases of the nursing process and require compliance as evidenced in documentation. Nurses should be familiar with the practice act of the state in which they work.

Joint Commission on Accreditation of Healthcare Organizations The JCAHO surveys health care facilities to measure compliance with its standards for safe health care provision. Although facilities voluntarily submit to this accreditation process, reimbursement eligibility for Medicare, Medicaid, and private funding is dependent on JCAHO accreditation.

The JCAHO no longer requires that health care organizations have traditional nursing care plans, but documentation of an individualized plan of care must be evident for each client (JCAHO, 1998). The JCAHO's standards require:

- The involvement of the client or family in the development of the plan, which must be documented in the medical record, and
- Interdisciplinary planning and implementation of all aspects of care.

The use of interdisciplinary tools has proved an effective approach to documenting client and family education for agencies not yet using critical pathways (discussed later in the chapter). By complying with JCAHO's client and family teaching standards, one medical center, through the use of an interdisciplinary record, increased its education documentation rate from 30% to 84% (Tucker, 1995).

During the accreditation survey (or process), the reviewer looks for evidence of an organized and systematic method of monitoring and evaluating client care as reflected through documentation in the medical record. Documenting the steps of the nursing process ensures compliance with JCAHO's plan of care requirements.

Reimbursement

Peer review organizations (PROs), consisting of physicians and nurses, are required by the federal government to monitor and evaluate the quality and appropriateness of care provided. Medical record documentation is the mechanism for the PRO review, which evaluates the intensity of services and the severity of illness on the basis of a comparison of sample medical records from different facilities against specific screening criteria.

The federal enactment of the diagnosis-related group (DRG) classification system changed the health care provider reimbursement process from a cost-per-case to a prospective payment system (PPS). With PPS, the medical record must provide documentation that supports the DRG and the appropriateness of care. Nursing documentation must also show evidence of client and family education and discharge planning.

From a hospital's perspective, when information in the medical record demonstrates compliance with Medicare and Medicaid standards, the reimbursement is maximized. If nurses fail to document the equipment or procedures used daily (e.g., feeding pump; daily weight, intake and output; intravenous therapy; drug additives), reimbursement to the facility can be denied.

Another federal law, the Comprehensive Omnibus Budget Reconciliation Act (COBRA), allows employees to temporarily carry their employer-provided health insurance benefits for 90 days after termination, reduc-

COMMUNITY/HOME HEALTH CARE

Documentation

Home health agencies also keep documents: physician's orders, history and physical form, home care team records, and nursing records (initial assessment form, plan of care, problem list for daily progress notes, client teaching activities, and discharge summary). Home health care providers are required to comply with state and federal regulations that affect health care, documentation, and reimbursement.

tion in the work hours, or retirement. The law requires that for any COBRA client receiving care in an emergency room, the client's condition must be stabilized before the client can be transferred to another facility. If the client's condition is not stable, the institution cannot initiate a transfer.

Facilities in violation of COBRA laws are fined and stand to lose their eligibility for Medicare and Medicaid funding. Compliance with this law is evaluated through medical record review. The documentation concerning client transfers must include:

- Chronology of the event,
- Measures taken or treatment implemented,
- The client's response to treatment, and
- Results of measures taken to prevent the client's condition from deteriorating.

PRINCIPLES OF EFFECTIVE DOCUMENTATION

Documentation requirements differ depending on the health care facility (hospital, nursing home, home health agency), the setting within the facility (e.g., emergency room, perioperative unit, medical–surgical unit), and the specific client population (e.g., obstetric, pediatric, geriatric). Regardless of the client care administered, the documentation of that care must reflect the nursing process. General documentation guidelines are listed in Table 10–2.

PROFESSIONAL TIP

Chart Following the Nursing Process

Charting in accordance with the nursing process ensures thorough documentation in compliance with nursing practice acts and with reimbursement and accreditation criteria.

Table 10-2 GENERAL DOCUMENTATION GUIDELINES

- Ensure that you have the correct client record or chart and that the client's name and identifying information are on every page of the record.
- Document as soon as the client encounter is concluded to ensure accurate recall of data (follow institutional guidelines on frequency of charting).
- Date and time each entry.
- Sign each entry with your full legal name and with your professional credentials, or per your institutional policy.
- Do not leave space between entries.
- If an error is made while documenting, use a single line to cross out the error, then date, time, and sign the correction (follow institutional policy); avoid erasing, crossing out, or using correction fluid (Figure 10-1).
- Never change another person's entry, even if it is incorrect.
- The first entry of the shift should be made early (e.g., at 7:30 A.M. for the 7–3 shift, as opposed to 11:30 A.M. or 12 P.M.). Chart at least every 2 hours, or per institutional policy.
- Use quotation marks to indicate direct client responses (e.g., "I feel lousy").
- Document in chronological order; if chronological order is not used, state why.
- Write legibly.
- Use a permanent-ink pen (black is usually preferable because it photocopies well).
- Document in a complete but concise manner by using phrases and abbreviations as appropriate.
- Document all telephone calls that you make or receive that are related to a client's case.

Adapted from Health Assessment & Physical Examination *(2nd ed.), by M. E. Z. Estes, 2002, Albany, NY: Delmar. Copyright 2002 by Delmar. Adapted with permission.*

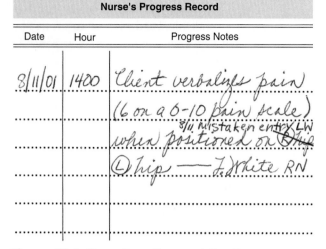

Figure 10-1 Correcting a Documentation Error

Nursing notes must be logical, focused, and relevant to care, and the outcomes must represent each phase in the nursing process (Simmons & Meadors, 1995; Thompson, 1995). Nursing documentation based on the nursing process facilitates effective care because client needs can be traced from assessment, through identification of the problems, to the care plan, implementation, and evaluation. A brief outline of the elements of the nursing process as they relate to documentation follows:

- *Assessment*: Assessment data related to an actual or potential health care need are summarized without duplication. With reassessment, any new findings or any changes in the client's condition (e.g., increased pain) are highlighted.
- *Nursing diagnosis*: NANDA terminology to identify the client's problem or need.
- *Planning and outcome identification*: The expected outcomes and goals of client care, as discussed with

the client and communicated to members of the multidisciplinary team, should be documented on the care plan or critical pathway rather than in the progress notes.

- *Implementation:* After an intervention has been performed, observations, treatments, teaching, and related clinical judgments should be documented on the flow sheet and progress notes. Client teaching should include learning needs, teaching plan content, methods of teaching, who was taught, and the client's response.
- *Evaluation:* The effectiveness of the interventions in terms of the expected outcomes is evaluated and documented: progress toward goals; client response to tests, treatments, and nursing interventions; client and family response to teaching and significant events; questions, statements, or complaints voiced by the client or family.
- *Revisions of planned care:* The reasons for the revisions along with the supporting evidence and client agreement are documented.

Elements of Effective Documentation

Several factors are important in producing effective documentation. To ensure effective documentation, nurses should:

- Use a common vocabulary,
- Write legibly and neatly,
- Use only authorized abbreviations and symbols,
- Employ factual and time-sequenced organization, and
- Document accurately and completely, including any errors that occurred.

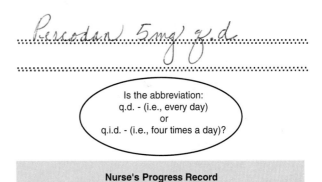

PROFESSIONAL TIP

Abbreviations

Avoid abbreviations that can be misunderstood (Figure 10-2). For example, what does the abbreviation *Pt* mean? Does it refer to the patient, prothrombin time, physical therapy, or part-time? Refer to your institution's approved abbreviations listing.

The following discussion of effective charting refers to all nursing documents, such as flow sheet, progress notes, etc. An entry should be made in nursing documents when:

- The client's condition changes,
- The client's response to an intervention or expected outcome is measured, or
- The client or family voices a complaint.

Use of Common Vocabulary

During the past decade, nurse researchers have observed inadequacies in the clinical record that prevent data collection and comparison among large groups of clients. One such inadequacy relates to the vocabulary used. Documented clinical data cannot be correlated without a common vocabulary for addressing client outcomes related to specific nursing interventions (McCloskey & Bulechek, 1994). Nursing practice reflects the use of multiple terms for nursing interventions, thus preventing cross-institutional comparisons of nursing care. Current efforts to establish a taxonomy for nursing interventions determined by specific nursing diagnoses will both enhance the quality of documentation and support the efforts of researchers. Use of a common vocabulary will also improve intrateam communication and lessen the chance of misunderstandings.

Legibility

Whatever is charted must be easily readable, without any chance of error in interpretation due to poor penmanship.

Abbreviations and Symbols

Facilities usually have a list of abbreviations and symbols that is approved by the Medical Records Committee for use in documenting information in the client's record. The nurse should always refer to the facility's approved listing (see Appendix C).

Organization

Every entry should start with the date and time. Charting should be done in chronological order: assess-

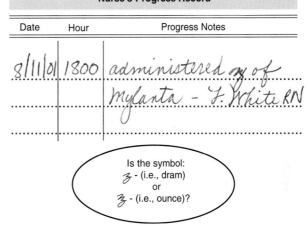

Figure 10-2 Misleading Abbreviation and Symbol

ment data, observation, intervention, and evaluation (Figure 10-3). The nurse should comply with the time frame indicated in the facility's guidelines for documentation, for example, the frequency of charting observations for a client with restraints or the time frame within which the admit assessment must be completed.

Charting should be done in a timely fashion to prevent omission of pertinent data. It is never good practice to wait until the end of the shift to chart on all clients. Should a client's condition suddenly deteriorate and documentation has not been performed during the shift, the nurse may forget to record a pertinent piece of information that may later become a legal issue. To prevent errors, the nurse should chart medications immediately after administration. The nurse should also sign her name after each entry.

When the nurse forgets to document significant data, it is appropriate and advisable to include these data at a later date (Fiesta, 1991). Examples of situations possibly necessitating late entries include the following:

- The chart was not available (e.g., the chart was with the client in special procedures lab).
- Entries had to be added after notes were completed.
- Information was documented on the wrong record.

As with other aspects of documentation, the nurse should follow the facility's policy for charting a late

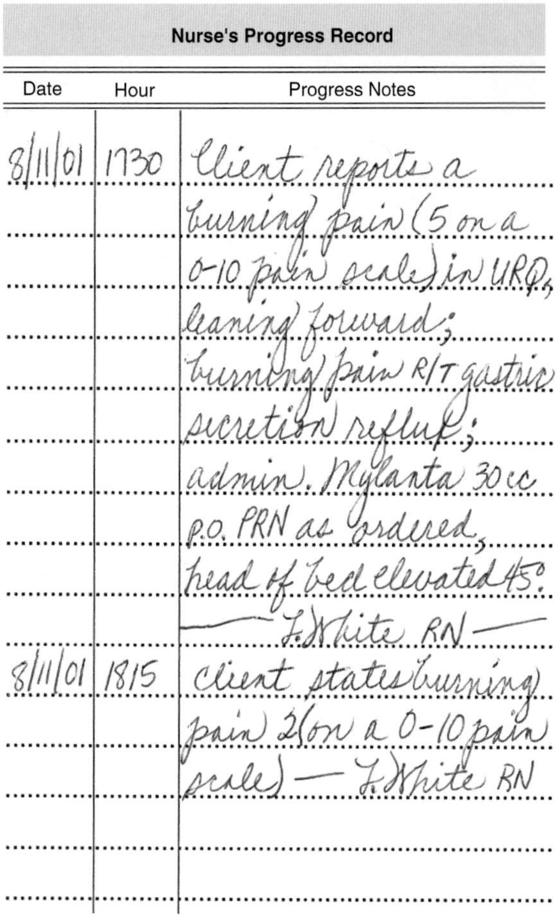

Nurse's Progress Record

Date	Hour	Progress Notes
8/11/01	1730	Client reports a burning pain (5 on a 0-10 pain scale) in URQ, leaning forward; burning pain R/T gastric secretion reflux; admin. Mylanta 30 cc P.O. PRN as ordered, head of bed elevated 45°. —— J. White RN ——
8/11/01	1815	Client states burning pain 2 (on a 0-10 pain scale) — J. White RN

Figure 10-3 Charting a prn Medication

entry. Common practice is to enter the date and time and to notate "Late entry" to indicate that the entry is out of sequence. Then the date and time the entry should have been made is recorded in the body of the entry, as shown in Figure 10-4.

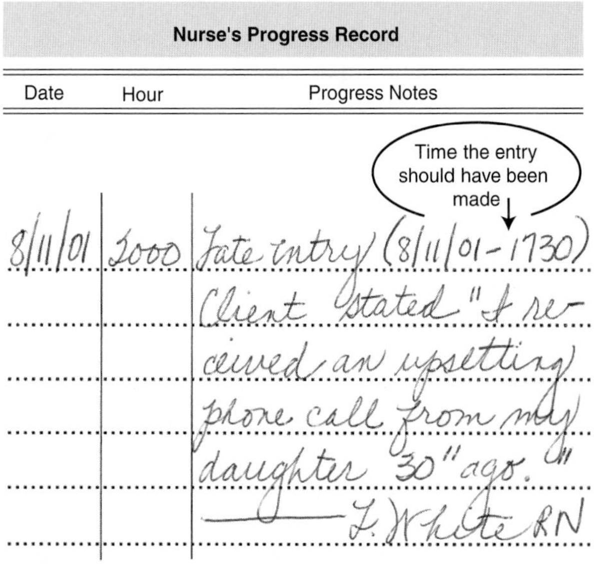

Nurse's Progress Record

Date	Hour	Progress Notes
8/11/01	2000	Time the entry should have been made ↓ Late entry (8/11/01 - 1730) Client stated "I received an upsetting phone call from my daughter 30" ago." J. White RN

Figure 10-4 Charting a Late Entry

Accuracy

"Accuracy is crucial if the documentation is to be useful either clinically or for research" (Hayes, Norris, Martin, & Androwich, 1994). Factual, descriptive terms must be used to chart exactly those things that were observed or done. For example, an entry reading "wound is 2.5 cm by 1.0 cm" is more accurate than is "wound appears the same." Likewise, "foul-smelling, yellowish drainage completely soaked two 4 × 4s in 20 minutes" is clearly more accurate than "large amount of drainage."

Correct spelling and grammar and complete sentences (following institutional policy) should be used. The nurse should differentiate who did what, for example, "Dr. Diaz inserted a triple-lumen, 20-gauge catheter into the right subclavian vein." To maintain continuity of care, the nurse should read the notes recorded by nurses on previous shifts and document the client's current status in the areas previously documented.

Documenting a Medication Error

Facilities require nurses to report medication errors on incident reports (discussed later in this chapter). The medication given in error should appear on the MAR and in the nurses' progress notes. It should be remembered that the purpose of the medical record is to report any care or treatment the client receives, including any errors made. However, no mention is made of an incident report being completed.

When a medication error occurs, the following should be done (Grane, 1995):

- The medication should be charted on the MAR to prevent other caregivers from giving the client additional doses of the same drug, doses of similar drugs, or doses of drugs that may be contraindicated.
- The error should be documented in the nurses' notes as follows: name and dosage of the medication; time it was given; client's response to the medication; name of the practitioner who was notified of the error; time of the notification; nursing interventions or medical treatment to counteract the error; and client's response to treatment.

METHODS OF DOCUMENTATION

Documentation must reflect the complexity of care and must embody accuracy, completeness, and evidence of professional practice. The clinical standards (structure, outcome, process, and evaluation) are used to develop a system that complies with legal, accreditation, and professional practice requirements of documentation.

Among the many methods used for documentation are the following:

- Narrative charting
- Source-oriented charting
- Problem-oriented charting
- PIE charting
- Focus charting
- Charting by exception
- Computerized documentation
- Critical pathways

Narrative Charting

Narrative charting, the traditional method of nursing documentation, takes the form of a story written in paragraphs and describing the client's status, interventions and treatments, and the client's response to treatments. Before the advent of flow sheets, this was the only method for documenting care.

Narrative documentation is easy to use in emergency situations, wherein a simple, chronological order is needed. With this type of documentation, however, subjectivity is a common problem, and analysis and critical decision making on the part of the nurse tend to be lacking. Narrative charting is now being replaced by other formats because:

- The flow of care is disorganized. It is difficult to show a relationship between data and critical-thinking skills. Each nurse writes in a unique style, making continuity of care difficult to identify.
- It fails to reflect the nursing process. The focus is on tasks rather than on assessment data or progress toward achievement of outcomes.
- It is time-consuming. Because the paragraphs are free flowing, it takes more time both to accurately record information and to read information recorded by others.
- The information is difficult to retrieve, and because the same problems may not be addressed from shift to shift, it is difficult to track the client's progress.

Source-Oriented Charting

Source-oriented charting is described as a narrative recording by each member (source) of the health care team on separate records. Because each discipline uses a separate record, care is often fragmented, and communication between disciplines is time-consuming. Source-oriented charting has similar advantages and disadvantages to narrative charting, because both methods take an unstructured approach to documenting in the progress notes.

Problem-Oriented Charting

Problem-oriented medical record (POMR) focuses on the client's problem and employs a structured, logical format called **SOAP charting**:

- S: subjective data (what the client states)
- O: objective data (what is observed/inspected)
- A: assessment (conclusion reached on the basis of data)
- P: plan (actions to be taken)

SOAPIE and SOAPIER refer to formats that add the following:

- I: implementation
- E: evaluation
- R: revision

Figure 10-5 shows an example of SOAPIE charting. Some physicians use this format when writing progress notes.

There are four critical components of POMR/POR:

- Database (assessment data)
- Problem list (client's problems labeled as acute, chronic, active, or inactive)
- Initial plan (outline of goals, expected outcomes, and learning needs)
- Progress notes (charting based on the SOAP, SOAPIE, or SOAPIER format)

PIE Charting

After SOAP charting gained popularity, the problem, intervention, evaluation **(PIE) charting** system evolved to streamline documentation. The key components of this system are assessment flow sheets, nurses' progress notes, and an integrated plan of care. Figure 10-6 shows an example of PIE charting. This system eliminates the traditional care plan by incorporating an ongoing plan of care (problem, intervention, evaluation) into the daily documentation.

Focus Charting

Focus charting is a documentation method that uses a column format to chart data, action, and response (DAR) (Smith, 2000). The column format of focus charting is used within the progress notes to distinguish the entry from other recordings in the narrative notes, as shown in Figure 10-7.

Charting by Exception

Charting by exception (CBE) is a documentation method that requires the nurse to document only deviations from preestablished norms. The CBE system has three key components:

- Flow sheets: highlight significant findings and define assessment parameters and findings
- Reference documentation: related to the standards of nursing practice
- Bedside accessibility: related to the documentation forms (Burke & Murphy, 1995)

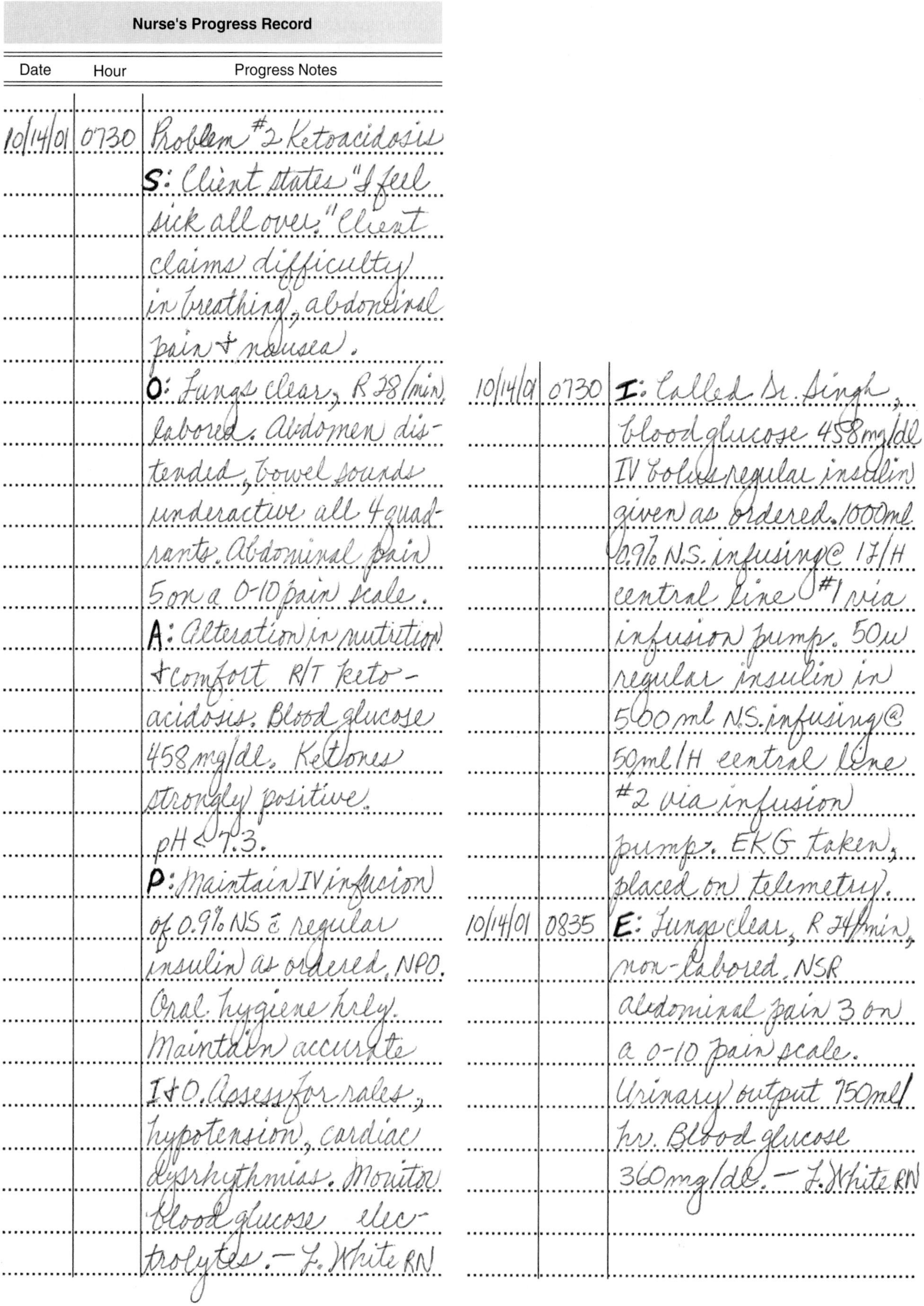

Nurse's Progress Record		
Date	Hour	Progress Notes

10/14/01 | 0730 | Problem #2 Ketoacidosis

S: Client states "I feel sick all over." Client claims difficulty in breathing, abdominal pain + nausea.

O: Lungs clear, R 28/min, labored. Abdomen distended, bowel sounds underactive all 4 quadrants. Abdominal pain 5 on a 0-10 pain scale.

A: Alteration in nutrition + comfort R/T ketoacidosis. Blood glucose 458 mg/dl, Ketones strongly positive. pH < 7.3.

P: Maintain IV infusion of 0.9% NS c̄ regular insulin as ordered, NPO. Oral hygiene hrly. Maintain accurate I&O. Assess for rales, hypotension, cardiac dysrhythmias. Monitor blood glucose electrolytes. — F. White RN

10/14/01 | 0730 | **I:** Called Dr. Singh, blood glucose 458 mg/dl IV bolus regular insulin given as ordered. 1000ml 0.9% N.S. infusing @ 1?/H central line #1 via infusion pump. 50u regular insulin in 500 ml N.S. infusing @ 50ml/H central line #2 via infusion pump. EKG taken, placed on telemetry.

10/14/01 | 0835 | **E:** Lungs clear, R 24/min, non-labored. NSR abdominal pain 3 on a 0-10 pain scale. Urinary output 750ml hr. Blood glucose 360 mg/dl. — F. White RN

Figure 10-5 Sample SOAPIE Charting

Nurse's Progress Record		
Date	Hour	Progress Notes
10/14/01	0730	**P:** altered nutrition R/T ketoacidosis. Blood glucose 458mg/dl. ketones strongly positive, pH 7.2. **I:** called Dr. Singh, blood glucose 458mg/dl IV bolus regular insulin given as ordered. 1000ml 0.9% N.S. infusing @ 1U/H central line #1 via infusion pump. 50u regular insulin in 500 ml N.S. infusing @ 50ml/H, central line #2 via infusion pump. EKG taken, placed on telemetry.
10/14/01	0835	**E:** Lungs clear, R 24/min nonlabored NSR, abdominal pain 3 on a 0-10 pain scale. Urinary output 750 ml/H (0730-0830) Blood sugar 360mg/dl. — T. White RN —

Figure 10-6 Sample PIE Charting

Computerized Documentation

In response to the large demand for clinical, administrative, and regulatory information in today's health care system, nurse leaders are working to develop computerized records. The resultant nursing information systems (NIS) will complement existing hospital information systems (HIS). These NIS will collect, store, process, retrieve, display, and communicate timely information. Health care facilities work in collaboration with producers of computer software to design medical record documents that complement existing documentation systems.

Computerized documentation enhances the systematic approach to client care with standardized protocols, teaching documents, data management, and communication. The practical advantages to staff nurses are as follows:

- Decreased documentation time: Data entry needs to be done only once; the system eliminates duplication of effort. For example, a physician's medication order goes immediately to the pharmacy, eliminating the need to transcribe and transmit orders; the pharmacy receives the order and the client's MAR is immediately updated.
- Increased legibility and accuracy: A computer printout is easy to read and legible. Accuracy is achieved through standardized documents that prompt the nurse for information, making the charting more complete, thorough, concise, and organized. For example, the fall-prevention standard is automatically initiated for all high-risk clients. Bedside terminals allow for client care data to be entered in a timely fashion.
- Clear, decisive, and concise key words: Standardized nursing terminology provides for consistency in key words (e.g., "alert") and eliminates ambiguous phraseology (e.g., "appears to be").
- Statistical analysis of data.
- Enhanced implementation of the nursing process: Documentation tools provide an individualized plan of care (admission and nursing history data, diagnoses, goals, measurable outcomes, and interventions, inclusive of client teaching).
- Enhanced decision making: Quick electronic access to other data, such as laboratory results, facilitates correlation of that data with the nurses' assessment data. If a trend is developing (e.g., decreasing levels of oxygenation), the nurse will recognize it quickly.
- Multidisciplinary networking: Information is quickly coordinated and integrated by other departments; all departments have access to the data.

Disadvantages associated with computerized documentation include high installation cost, which limits the number of terminals at nursing stations; slow processing speed at peak usage times; and downtime

(time for routine servicing or sudden unexpected failure). Further, practitioners are often reluctant to change from the familiar "pen-and-paper" methods to high-tech electronic systems.

A series of legal issues has emerged in relation to computerized documentation: problems in protecting client confidentiality; sharing of access codes (passwords); determining who should have access to the clinical database and how it should be used. Computerized software can be designed to record all transactions, thus permitting the identification of all staff members who request sensitive information.

			Nurse's Progress Record		

Date	Hour	Focus	Progress Notes
10/14/01	0730	Altered nutrition R/T ketoacidosis	**D:** Client experiencing labored breathing, abdominal pain, 5 on a 0-10 pain scale, & nausea. Blood sugar 458 mg/dl; ketones strongly positive; pH 7.2. T 99.8, R 28, P 110, B/P 100/56. **A:** Auscultation reveals lungs clear + underactive bowel sounds in all 4 quadrants. Abdomen distended. Dr. Singh notified of blood glucose, ketones, & pH. IV bolus of regular insulin given as ordered. IVs infusing as ordered through central lines c̄ infusion pumps. STAT EKG done, telemetry, NPO, oral hygiene admin., measuring I & O. L. White RN —
10/14/01	0830		**R:** Within 1 H (0730-0830) blood glucose 360 mg/dl R 24 non-labored. Urinary output 750 ml/H. Client identifies abdominal pain as 3 on a 0-10 pain scale. — L. White RN —

Figure 10-7 Sample Focus Charting

Point-of-Care Charting

Point-of-care charting is a computerized documentation system that allows health care providers to gain immediate access to client information. The system allows for the input and retrieval of client data at the bedside through a handheld portable computer.

The advantages of point-of-care charting relate to the efficiency of the computer system. Because this documentation method allows health care providers to record client data at the point of care, it:

- Controls operating costs,
- Complements existing information systems,
- Eliminates redundant data entry,
- Allows the provider more one-on-one time for client care, and
- Provides crucial client information to all health care providers in a timely fashion.

Point-of-care computerized documentation also facilitates the transition to a managed-care system (an integrated health care team) by focusing on the continuum of care. Each health care practitioner is provided with all pertinent client data to ensure continuity of care without duplication. One final advantage of point-of-care charting is that it fosters compliance with accreditation and regulatory standards.

Disadvantages include all of the problems inherent in computerized storage of records, such as maintaining confidentiality, controlling who has access to which data, and correcting errors.

Critical Pathway

A **critical pathway** (or critical path) is a comprehensive, standard plan of care for specific case situations. The pathway is monitored to ensure that interventions are performed on time and that client outcomes are achieved on time.

Variations, sometimes referred to as variances, are goals not met or interventions not performed according to the established time frame. The nurse documents on a variance form why a goal is not met or an intervention is not performed (Klenner, 2000).

Critical pathways allow for the efficient use of time and increase the quality of care by having the expected outcomes identified on the plan. When clients have more than two diagnoses or variations, however, documentation becomes complicated because of limited space. This situation requires additional documentation forms to complement the pathway, such as intervention flow sheets and nurses' notes.

FORMS FOR RECORDING DATA

There are several types of forms used in record keeping: Kardex, flow sheets, nurses' progress notes, and discharge summaries. All of these forms are designed to facilitate record keeping, minimize duplication of effort, and ensure quick and easy access to information.

Kardex

A **Kardex** is a summary worksheet reference of basic client care information that traditionally is not part of the medical record. A concise client data source, Kardex is used as a reference throughout the shift and during change-of-shift reports. Kardexes come in various sizes, shapes, and types, including computer-generated. The Kardex is designed to complement the care delivery setting and usually contains the following information:

- Client data: name, age, marital status, religious preference, physician, family contact with phone number
- Medical diagnoses: listed by priority
- Nursing diagnoses: listed by priority
- Allergies
- Medical orders: diet, medications, intravenous (IV) therapy, treatments, diagnostic tests and procedures (inclusive of dates and results), consultations, DNR (do-not-resuscitate) order (when appropriate)
- Activities permitted: functional limitations, assistance needed in activities of daily living, and safety precautions

Flow Sheets

Flow sheets have vertical or horizontal columns for recording dates and times and related assessment and intervention information, making it easy to track changes in the client's condition. Client teaching, use of special equipment, and IV therapy are other aspects of the flow sheet. Because flow sheets have small spaces for recording, these forms usually contain legends that identify the approved abbreviations for charting data (Figure 10-8). It is important to fill out flow sheets completely because blank spaces imply that an intervention was not completed, attempted, or recognized.

Because they decrease the redundancy of charting in the nurses' progress notes, flow sheets are used as supplements to most documentation systems. They do

 COMMUNITY/HOME HEALTH CARE

Home Health Kardex

In addition to the usual information, the home health Kardex contains information related to family contacts, practitioners (physician), other services, and emergency referrals.

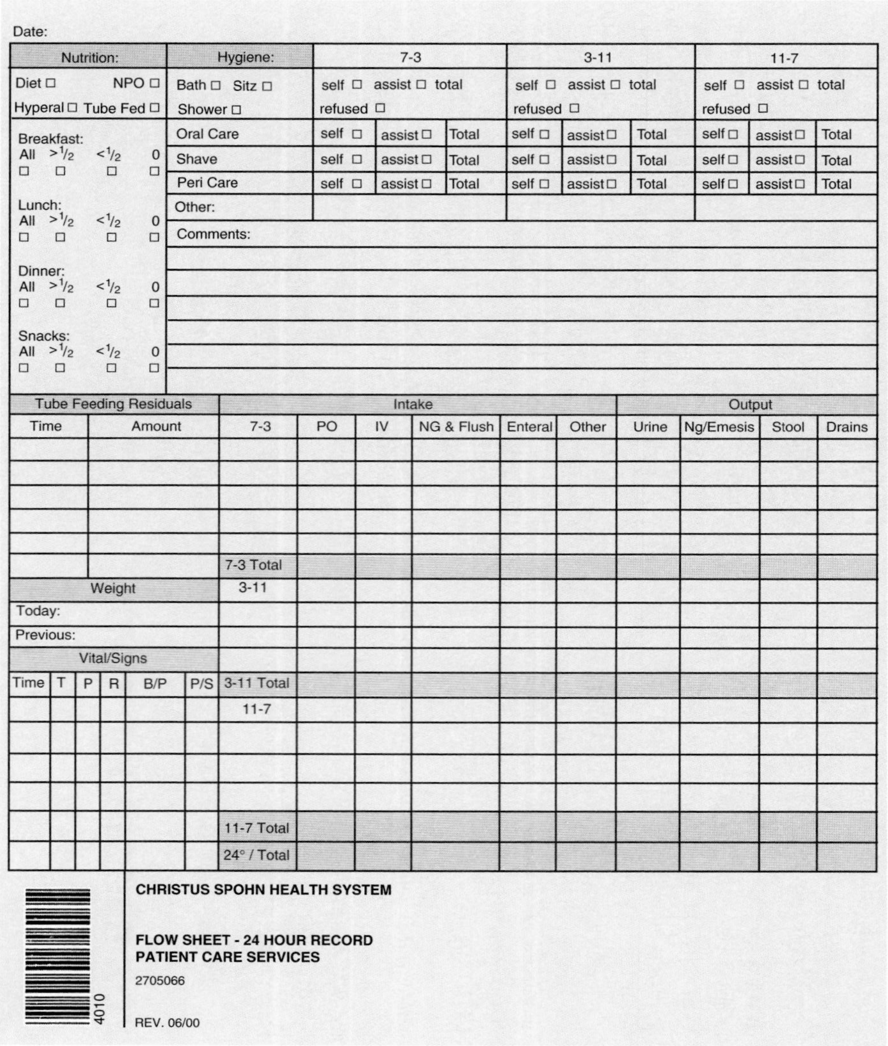

The assessment form (Figure 10-8) includes sections for Nutrition, Hygiene, and assessment areas organized by the three shifts (7-3, 3-11, 11-7).

Nutrition section:
Diet □ NPO □
Hyperal □ Tube Fed □

Breakfast:
All □ >1/2 □ <1/2 □ 0 □
Lunch:
All □ >1/2 □ <1/2 □ 0 □
Dinner:
All □ >1/2 □ <1/2 □ 0 □
Snacks:
All □ >1/2 □ <1/2 □ 0 □

Hygiene:
Bath □ Sitz □
Shower □

Oral Care
Shave
Peri Care
Other:
Comments:

Intake / Output table

Tube Feeding Residuals

Time	Amount	7-3									

Intake: NG & Flush | IV | PO | Enteral | Other
Output: Urine | Ng/Emesis | Stool | Drains

7-3 Total
11-7 Total
24° Total

Weight
Today:
Previous:

Vital Signs
Time | T | P | R | B/P | P/S | 3-11 Total
11-7

CHRISTUS SPOHN HEALTH SYSTEM
FLOW SHEET - 24 HOUR RECORD
PATIENT CARE SERVICES
2705066
REV. 06/00
4010

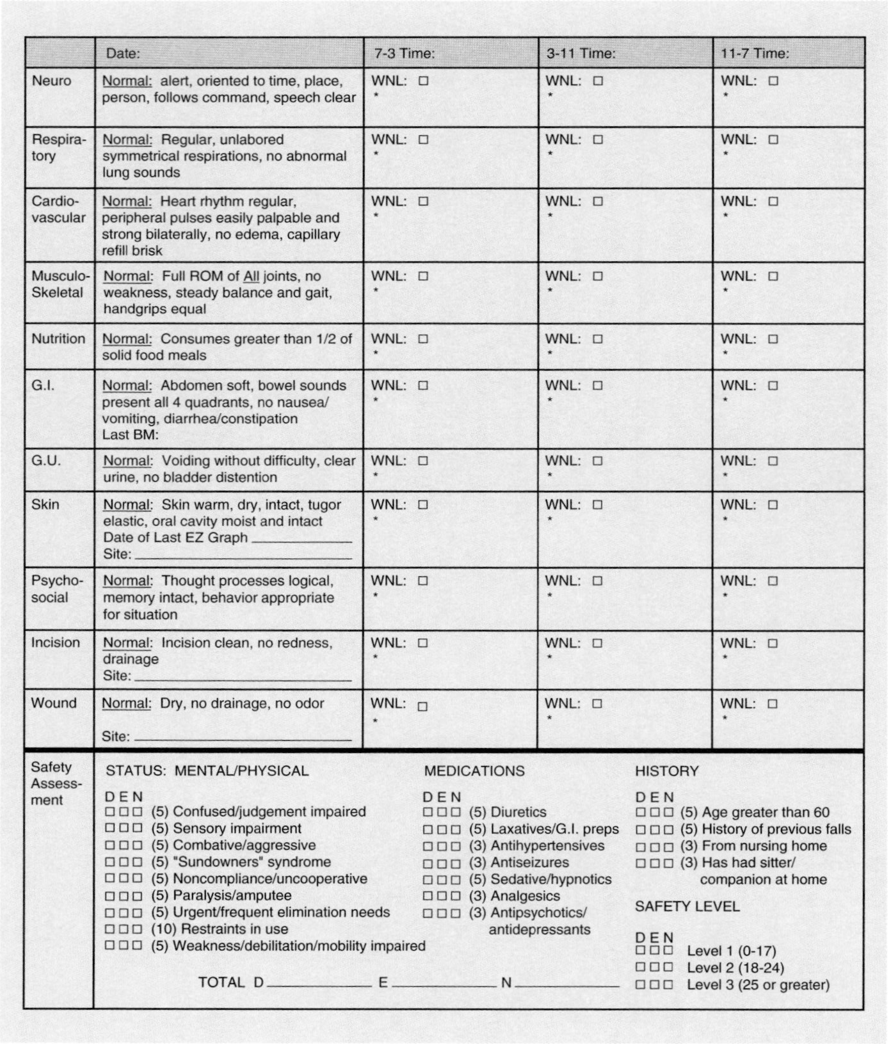

Assessment side (by shift: 7-3 Time, 3-11 Time, 11-7 Time; WNL: □ *)

Date:

Neuro — Normal: alert, oriented to time, place, person, follows command, speech clear

Respiratory — Normal: Regular, unlabored symmetrical respirations, no abnormal lung sounds

Cardiovascular — Normal: Heart rhythm regular, peripheral pulses easily palpable and strong bilaterally, no edema, capillary refill brisk

Musculo-Skeletal — Normal: Full ROM of All joints, no weakness, steady balance and gait, handgrips equal

Nutrition — Normal: Consumes greater than 1/2 of solid food meals

G.I. — Normal: Abdomen soft, bowel sounds present all 4 quadrants, no nausea/vomiting, diarrhea/constipation
Last BM:

G.U. — Normal: Voiding without difficulty, clear urine, no bladder distention

Skin — Normal: Skin warm, dry, intact, tugor elastic, oral cavity moist and intact
Date of Last EZ Graph ____
Site:

Psycho-social — Normal: Thought processes logical, memory intact, behavior appropriate for situation

Incision — Normal: Incision clean, no redness, drainage
Site:

Wound — Normal: Dry, no drainage, no odor
Site:

Safety Assessment

STATUS: MENTAL/PHYSICAL
D E N
□ □ □ (5) Confused/judgement impaired
□ □ □ (5) Sensory impairment
□ □ □ (5) Combative/aggressive
□ □ □ (5) "Sundowners" syndrome
□ □ □ (5) Noncompliance/uncooperative
□ □ □ (5) Paralysis/amputee
□ □ □ (5) Urgent/frequent elimination needs
□ □ □ (10) Restraints in use
□ □ □ (5) Weakness/debilitation/mobility impaired

MEDICATIONS
D E N
□ □ □ (5) Diuretics
□ □ □ (5) Laxatives/G.I. preps
□ □ □ (5) Antihypertensives
□ □ □ (3) Antiseizures
□ □ □ (5) Sedative/hypnotics
□ □ □ (3) Analgesics
□ □ □ (3) Antipsychotics/antidepressants

TOTAL D ____ E ____ N ____

HISTORY
D E N
□ □ □ (5) Age greater than 60
□ □ □ (5) History of previous falls
□ □ □ (3) From nursing home
□ □ □ (3) Has had sitter/companion at home

SAFETY LEVEL
D E N
□ □ □ Level 1 (0-17)
□ □ □ Level 2 (18-24)
□ □ □ Level 3 (25 or greater)

Figure 10-8 Assessment and Intervention Flow Sheet (*Courtesy of Christus Spohn Health System, Corpus Christi, TX*) (*continues*)

EDUCATION REASSESSMENT

Have the Education needs of the patient changed in past 24 hours?	☐ Yes	☐ No
Is the patient scheduled for any new test or procedure today?	☐ Yes	☐ No
Explanation given?	☐ Yes	☐ No
Patient/significant other verbalizes understanding:	☐ Yes	☐ No

Patient desires/requires education on: ____________

Have Discharge Planning needs changed in past 24 hours? If yes, send consult to Social Services and document changes below.	☐ Yes	☐ No

ALL EDUCATION MUST BE DOCUMENTED ON THE MULTIDISCIPLINARY EDUCATION FORM

TIME	PROBLEM #	PROGRESS NOTES

TIME	PROBLEM #	PROGRESS NOTES

PLAN OF CARE VERIFICATION	____________ RN	________ Time

IV SITE ASSESSMENT		7-3 Time:	3-11 Time:	11-7 Time:
Normal: IV Patent; No redness, drainage or edema	Site #1: Start Date:	WNL: ☐ *	WNL: ☐ *	WNL: ☐ *
# of IVAC's in use ___	Site #2: Start Date:	WNL: ☐ *	WNL: ☐ *	WNL: ☐ *

IV Site Care per hospital standard ☐ Time: *

IV Tubing Change per hospital standard ☐ Time: *

IV Start:	Time	Attempts	Site	Needle Size	S	U
					☐	☐
					☐	☐
Site prep per Standard ☐					☐	☐

INITIALS	SIGNATURE	INITIALS	SIGNATURE

Figure 10-8 Assessment and Intervention Flow Sheet

not, however, replace the progress notes. Nurses still must document observations, client responses and teaching, detailed interventions, and other significant data in the progress notes.

Nurses' Progress Notes

Nurses' progress notes are used to document the client's condition, problems, and complaints; interventions; the client's response to interventions; and achievement of outcomes. Progress notes comprise the following elements: nurses' notes, MAR, personal care flow sheets, teaching records, intake and output forms, vital sign records, and specialty forms (e.g., diabetic flow sheet or neurologic assessment form) (Eggland & Heinemann, 1994). Progress notes can be either completely narrative or incorporated into a standardized flow sheet to complement SOAP(IE), PIE, focus charting, and other documentation systems.

Discharge Summary

The discharge summary highlights the client's illness and course of care. When a narrative discharge summary is entered into the progress notes, it includes:

- The client's status at admission and discharge;
- A brief summary of the client's care;
- Intervention and education outcomes;
- Resolved problems and continuing care needs for unresolved problems, inclusive of referrals; and
- Client instructions regarding medications, diet, food–drug interactions, activity, treatments, follow-up, and other special needs.

Many facilities have a documentation form that itemizes discharge and client instructions. The form has a duplicate copy for the client, with the original being placed in the medical record. Figure 10-9 shows the common elements of this tool.

Follow-up to be seen in: ______ (Dr. Name/Clinic) office on ______ (date/time)
Follow-up to be seen in: ______ (Dr. Name/Clinic) office on ______ (date/time)
Follow-up to be seen in: ______ (Dr. Name/Clinic) office on ______ (date/time)
DIET: ______ Diet instructions given to patient ______ (period of time/date)

ACTIVITY: ______ Services: ○ Home Health ○ Hospice ○ DME
Treatments/Self Care ______ Other (Specify): ______
Drug Nutrient Interactions ______ Return to: ______ for
○ PT ○ OT ○ RT ○ Other ______

MEDICATIONS	DOSAGE	FREQUENCY	MEDICATIONS	DOSAGE	FREQUENCY

MEDICATION/PAIN CONTROL INSTRUCTIONS:
1. Take your medication according to M.D. instructions.
2. Never stop taking your medication without speaking to your M.D.
3. Refill your medication when you have 7 days worth left.
4. Notify your M.D. if your pain medication needs adjusting; you are having uncontrolled pain or you are having difficulty with side effects.

___ Preprinted Instructions Given to Patient/Family Other Instructions: ______

CHRISTUS Spohn associates trust we have met your needs while in the hospital. Shortly after discharge, you will receive a patient survey. It is our hope that you will circle high scores of 5s when you take a few moments to complete and mail the survey. I understand and am able to implement continuing care needs at home as explained to me. ______ (Patient/Family Signature)

Admission Date: ______ Discharge Date: ______ Via: ______ Escorted By: ______
Time: ______ Destination: ______

PATIENT DISCHARGE STATUS

1. Vital Signs ______
2. Elimination–Date of last BM ______
GU ______
3. Neuro ______
4. Cardiac ______
5. Resp ______
6. Skin/Wound/Incisions ______
7. Vascular Access Removed ______
8. Pain Free: No, But Controlled by Pain Medication ___
Yes, at time of Discharge ______
9. Other ______

Own medications from home returned to patient/family ___ Yes ___ No ___ N/A
Prescriptions given to patient/family ___ Yes ___ No ___ N/A
Valuables returned to patient/family ___ Yes ___ No ___ N/A

Original to chart, copy to Patient/Family
Signature/Title Discharge Nurse: ______ Date: ______

1045
CHRISTUS Spohn Health System
DISCHARGE INFORMATION RECORD
PATIENT CARE SERVICES
2704965 REV: 05/00 FM7

Figure 10-9 Discharge Summary *(Courtesy of Christus Spohn Health System, Corpus Christi, TX)*

TRENDS IN DOCUMENTATION

Computerized charting has become one of the most widespread trends in nursing documentation. However, computerized nursing documentation can demonstrate the quality, effectiveness, and value of the services nurses provide only if standardized databases are developed that will ensure accuracy and precision in the information. At the 1991 conference of the National Center for Nursing Research of the National Institutes of Health, the need was identified for databases that would permit analysis of the effectiveness and costs of specific interventions in achieving desired outcomes for clients with a variety of nursing diagnoses (Ozbolt, Fruchtnight, & Hayden, 1994). The recommendations arising from this conference supported the need to define and develop standard terminology for nursing data, nursing diagnoses, nursing interventions, and nursing outcomes.

Nursing Minimum Data Set

In 1985, Werley and Lang convened an invitational working conference at the University of Wisconsin—Milwaukee to identify the elements that should be included in a **nursing minimum data set** (NMDS). These are the elements that should be contained in clinical records and abstracted for studies on the effectiveness and costs of nursing care (Werley & Lang, 1988). The sixteen identified elements were grouped into the following three categories:

- Demographics: personal identification, date of birth, gender, race and ethnicity, and residence
- Service: unique facility or service agency number, episode admission or encounter date, discharge or termination date, disposition of client, expected payer, unique health record number of client, and unique number of principal registered nurse provider
- Nursing care: nursing diagnosis, nursing intervention, nursing outcome, and intensity of nursing care (Werley & Lang, 1988)

Several challenges are inherent in the development of the four nursing care categories: diagnoses, interventions, outcomes, and intensity (Hayes et al., 1994). For example, automated information systems must be capable of supporting cost-effective nursing practice through efficient, comprehensive documentation. Further, basic to standardizing databases is the consistent use of a taxonomy that promotes validity and reliability. The NMDS, however, does not specify for any of the four elements a taxonomy such as NANDA (2001) nursing diagnoses, Nursing Interventions Classification (NIC) (NIC, 1995), or acuity ratings. Nursing must achieve consensus of terminology in order for clinical data to be included in nursing care elements of a NMDS.

Nursing Diagnoses

A nursing diagnosis is a clinical judgment about individual, family, or community responses to actual or potential health problems or life processes (NANDA, 2001). The American Nurses Association (ANA) endorsed NANDA to develop a classification for nursing diagnoses. There are 155 approved nursing diagnoses classified into 13 domains. Each diagnosis has a label, definition, major and minor defining characteristics, and related factors. The diagnoses identify client states which can then be used to select interventions that are intended to achieve the desired outcomes. In 1992, the NANDA terms were accepted into the Unified Medical Language System (UMLS). The UMLS was begun in 1986 by the National Library of Medicine as a way to help health professionals and researchers retrieve and integrate electronic biomedical information from a variety of sources (National Library of Medicine, 2000).

Nursing Intervention Classification

The **Nursing Intervention Classification (NIC)** is a comprehensive standardized language for nursing interventions organized in a three-level taxonomy (McCloskey & Bulechek, 1995). This taxonomy attempts to sort, label, and describe interventions used by nurses for various diagnostic categories. Initiated by a research team (Iowa Intervention Project, 1993) at the University of Iowa in 1987, the three-level taxonomy now comprises 7 domains, 30 classes, and almost 500 interventions. The seven domains are:

- Physiological: basic
- Physiological: complex
- Behavioral
- Safety
- Family
- Health system
- Community

Each nursing intervention has a label, a definition, and a set of activities to carry out the interventions. *Activities are not interventions and should not be labeled as such in nursing information systems* (McCloskey & Bulechek, 2000).

 COMMUNITY/HOME HEALTH CARE

Taxonomy of Nursing Interventions

Grobe and colleagues at the University of Texas at Austin have been developing a lexicon and taxonomy of nursing interventions taken from home care records (Grobe, 1992).

Although continuing to evolve, this classification system already provides assistance in choosing interventions based on nursing diagnoses or problems. The NIC interventions have been incorporated into health care data sets and the computerized client medical record. The ANA has recognized NIC as one of the first nursing languages to be included in the *National Library of Medicine's Metathesaurus,* one of four knowledge sources for the UMLS (McCloskey & Bulechek, 1995).

Nursing Outcomes Classification

A nursing outcome is defined as the resolution status of the nursing diagnosis according to the NMDS (Ozbolt et al., 1994). The Iowa Outcomes Project being conducted at the University of Iowa has developed a taxonomy of client outcomes for nursing care, called **Nursing Outcomes Classification (NOC)**. This classification system comprises 260 outcomes grouped into 29 classes and 7 domains (Johnson, Maas, & Moorhead, 2000).

The seven domains are:

- Functional health
- Physiologic health
- Psychosocial health
- Health knowledge and behavior
- Perceived health
- Family health
- Community health

Each NOC outcome has four parts: the outcome label, the outcome definition, a list of indicators for measurement, a five-point measurement scale, and a list of references (Aquilino & Keenan, 2000). The ANA has recognized NOC as a standardized language and it is included in the National Library of Medicine's Metathesaurus for a Unified Medical Language (NCVHS, 1999).

REPORTING

Reporting is the verbal communication of data regarding the client's health status, needs, treatments, outcomes, and responses (Eggland & Heinemann, 1994). A report must summarize the current critical information pertinent to clinical decision making and continuity of care. As with recording, reporting is based on the nursing process, standards of care, and legal and ethical principles. The nursing process provides structure for an organized report, a challenge inherent in verbal communications. In order to verbally communicate an efficient and well-organized report, the nurse must consider the following questions:

- What must be said?
- Why must it be said?
- How must it be said?
- What are the expected outcomes?

PROFESSIONAL TIP

Information for Shift Report

1. Client name, room and bed, age, and gender
2. Physician, admission date and diagnosis, and any surgery
3. Diagnostic tests or treatments performed in the past 24 hours; results, if available
4. General status, any significant change in condition
5. New or changed physician's orders
6. Nursing diagnoses and suggested nursing orders
7. Evaluation of nursing interventions
8. Intravenous fluid amounts, last prn medication
9. Concerns about the client

Considering these aspects of reporting before communicating the information provides for a concise, organized report.

Another critical element in reporting is listening. Reports require participation from everyone present. When receiving a report, the nurse must focus behaviors to enhance listening skills: The nurse eliminates distractions, puts thoughts and concerns aside, concentrates on those things being said, and does not anticipate the presenter's next statements. The reporting process is an integral component of developing effective interpersonal and intrapersonal relationships that promote continuity of client care. Regardless of the type of communication, planned presentation of client data is key to accurate, concise, effective reporting. Summary reports, walking rounds, telephone reports and orders, and incident reports are all types of reporting.

Summary Reports

Summary reports outline information pertinent to the client's needs as identified by the nursing process. Summary reports commonly occur either at the change of shift when a new caregiver is involved or when the client is transferred to another area. A summary, or end-of-shift, report should include the following information in the order indicated:

1. Background data obtained from client interactions and assessment of the client's functional health patterns
2. Primary medical and nursing diagnoses and priority problems
3. Identified client risks
4. Recent changes in condition or in treatments (e.g., new medications, elevated temperature)
5. Effective interventions or treatments of priority problems, inclusive of laboratory and diagnostic results (e.g., client's response to pain medication)

6. Progress toward expected outcomes (priority problems, teaching, or discharge planning)
7. Adjustments in the plan of care
8. Client or family complaints

This logical and time-sequenced format follows the nursing process and thus provides structure and organization to the data. In order to provide continuity of care, the new caregiver must receive an accurate, concise report about those things that have happened during the previous shift. Client and family complaints relative to each client should be addressed last, because these situations usually generate questions and discussion.

Walking Rounds

Walking rounds can take the form of nursing rounds, physician–nurse rounds, or multidisciplinary rounds. **Walking rounds** is a reporting method used when the members of the care team walk to each client's room and discuss care and progress with each other and with the client, as shown in Figure 10-10.

Nursing rounds are used most frequently by charge nurses as their method of report. During the rounds, the oncoming nurse is introduced to the client and the off-going nurse discusses with the client and the on-coming nurse any changes in the plan of care. Although more time-consuming than the end-of-shift report, walking rounds give the nurses and the client the opportunity to evaluate the effectiveness of care together.

Nursing rounds are also used as a teaching method. The instructor introduces the client to the student, and together they discuss the client's care. The instructor can also use this time to appraise the student's observation, communication, and decision-making skills.

Nurse–physician rounds involve the physician and either the staff nurse or the charge nurse. These rounds usually occur daily and provide the nurse, the physician, and the client the opportunity to evaluate the effectiveness of care.

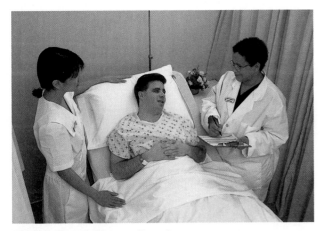

Figure 10-10 Nursing Rounds

Multidisciplinary rounds, which involve all disciplines, usually occur less frequently than the other types of rounds; primarily because it is difficult to schedule caregivers from all the disciplines for rounds. Multidisciplinary rounds are done most commonly in place of or to supplement case conferences and to discuss discharge planning. Multidisciplinary rounds support the concept of critical pathways and are seen most frequently in facilities that use pathways.

Telephone Reports and Orders

Telephone communications are another way nurses report transfers, communicate referrals, obtain client data, solve problems, and inform a client's family members regarding a change in the client's condition. Nurses are expected to demonstrate phone courtesy and professionalism when initiating and receiving telephone reports.

When initiating a phone call, the nurse should organize the information to be reported or received. For example, the nurse should:

• Ensure all lab results are back; if they are not, the nurse should identify in advance those that are missing and should phone the lab or check the computer to ascertain whether other results are available. If phoning the lab, the nurse should spell the client's name and provide the client's medical record number to minimize the chances of receiving results for the wrong client. The nurse should write down those tests that have been performed and the results.

• Review her notes and have the client's assessment data readily available, especially any significant data related to abnormal results. If the nurse has not assessed the client, this should be done before telephoning the practitioner; otherwise, the practitioner might ask questions that the nurse is unable to answer.

• Inform the charge nurse or someone else at the nurses' station of plans to place the call, so as to minimize the chances of being interrupted while on the phone.

When placing the call, the nurse should state the reason for the call, for example, "I am calling Dr. Wojtal regarding the blood sugar results for Mrs. Beacon." The nurse should be brief, listen carefully, and repeat the test results and any orders the physician gives over the phone.

The date and time the phone call was placed, the client data reported by the nurse, the name of the person with whom the nurse spoke, and whether an order was obtained should be recorded accurately in the medical record. Rather than charting, "Physician notified, no orders obtained," The nurse should chart, "Dr. Wojtal notified by phone, blood sugar 260 mg (drawn by the lab at 1300), orders received and recorded on the physician order sheet." Telephone orders should be charted and the nurses' progress notes updated as soon as possible after the phone call to prevent another caregiver from posting an entry before the telephone orders have been posted.

Figure 10-11 demonstrates the way to write a telephone order on the physician's order sheet: the entry is dated and timed; the order as given by the physician is recorded; and the order is signed beginning with t.o. (telephone order), the physician's name is written, and the nurse's name is signed. If another nurse witnesses the phone order, that nurse's signature should follow the first nurse's signature.

The physician must countersign the order within a time frame specified by the facility's policy. Fax machines have decreased the need for lengthy or complicated telephone orders, both saving time and minimizing errors. The physician should be phoned to confirm the physician's identity as the initiator of the fax orders. The physician must countersign the fax orders according to agency policy.

Incident Reports

Incident reports, or occurrence reports, are used to document any unusual occurrence or accident in the delivery of client care, such as falls or medication errors. Incident reports are not a means of punishing the caregiver; rather, ethical practice requires that the nurse file an incident report to protect the client.

Incident reports are not merely an internal device for the facility; they are required by federal, national, and state accrediting agencies. For legal reasons, nurses are often advised not to document the filing of an incident report in the nurses' notes. As previously discussed, however, a medication error (Grane, 1995)

necessitates both an incident report and documentation in the nurses' notes to ensure that the client receives safe care.

The incident report serves two functions:

- It informs the facility's administration of the incident, thereby allowing risk management personnel to consider changes that might prevent similar occurrences in the future.
- It alerts the facility's insurance company to a potential claim and the need for further investigation.

Each person with firsthand knowledge of the occurrence should fill out and sign a separate report. Although the incident report format varies from one facility to another, the following key elements must be addressed when filing a report:

- The date, exact time, and place the nurse discovered the occurrence should be recorded.
- The person(s) involved in the occurrence, including witnesses, should be identified.
- The exact occurrences witnessed by the nurse must be accurately and objectively documented; for example, "Found the client sitting on the floor, client stated that . . . ," rather than "Client fell."
- The exact details of what happened and the consequences for the persons involved must be recorded in time sequence.
- The nurse's actions to provide care and the results of the nurse's assessment for injuries and client complaints should be recorded.
- The supervisor on duty should be notified and the time and name of the physician notified recorded; if telephone orders were received from the physician, these should be documented as previously discussed and the orders implemented.
- The nurse should not record personal opinions, judgments, conclusions, or assumptions about what occurred; point blame; or suggest ways to prevent similar occurrences.
- The incident report should be forwarded to the designated person as defined by the facility's policy.

Iyer and Camp (1999) suggest an additional safeguard for the nurse: writing a brief, accurate descrip-

Physician Order Sheet		
Date	Hour	Progress Notes
10/14/01	0845	Decrease IV infusion of 50u of regular insulin in 500ml of NS. to infuse @ 2u per hour.
		T.O. Dr. Singh / F. White RN

Figure 10-11 Documenting a Telephone Order

PROFESSIONAL TIP

Documenting an Incident Report

The incident should be factually documented in the nurse's notes, but the notes should not say "incident report filed."

tion of the incident and keeping it at home. Included in the description should be the details of the incident and the names of the people who were involved, especially if these people can substantiate the nurse's description. Lawsuits may take several years from the time of the incident until the time that the case goes to court; thus, personal notes will help the nurse accurately recall the incident. Because they may be read by the plaintiff's attorney, the nurse's notes should reflect the same elements as are included in an incident report.

Special attention should be given to documenting falls, because current research shows that client falls constitute 75% to 80% of all incident reports on clinical units (Springhouse, 1999). Client falls are the main reason nurses are sued (Iyer & Camp, 1999).

SUMMARY

- Documentation provides a system of written records that reflect client care provided on the basis of assessment data and the client's response to interventions.
- The medical record can be used by health care students as a teaching tool and is a main source of data for clinical research.
- Nurses are responsible for assessing and documenting that the client has an understanding of the treatment prior to the intervention.
- Accreditation and reimbursement agencies require accurate and thorough documentation of the nursing care rendered and the client's response to interventions.
- Effective documentation requires clear, concise, accurate recording of all client care and other significant events in an organized and chronological fashion representative of each phase of the nursing process.
- Client safety requires appropriate reporting and recording of medication errors and other occurrences, in compliance with the facility's policy.
- Narrative charting requires an organized, chronological presentation of the client's problems and responses to interventions.
- Problem-oriented charting provides structure when documenting the client's problems and responses in the nurses' progress notes.
- Computerized documentation saves time, increases legibility and accuracy, provides standardized nursing terminology, enhances the nursing process and decision-making skills, and supports continuity of care.
- Critical pathways are comprehensive, standard plans of care for specific cases. Variations are documented on the back.

- Incident reports are used to document any unusual occurrence in a health care facility.

Review Questions

1. Systematic documentation is critical because it:
   a. is done every hour.
   b. shows the care given by all health care providers.
   c. identifies the planning and implementation phases.
   d. presents in a logical fashion the care provided by nurses.

2. The two primary reasons for health care documentation are:
   a. education and research.
   b. research and reimbursement.
   c. accountability and responsibility.
   d. fulfillment of legal and practice standards.

3. The legal issues of documentation require the use of:
   a. black ink pens.
   b. legible, neat writing.
   c. short, descriptive phrases.
   d. hourly recording of client status.

4. The person responsible for obtaining a client's informed consent is the:
   a. physician.
   b. staff nurse.
   c. admissions clerk.
   d. nurse supervisor.

5. The person responsible for ensuring that the client understands the procedure or intervention and has signed the informed consent is the:
   a. nurse.
   b. physician.
   c. social worker.
   d. admission officer.

6. Documentation of the nursing care the client receives must:
   a. never have an error.
   b. be neatly spaced out.
   c. reflect the nursing process.
   d. be signed at the end of each shift.

7. A medication error is documented on the:
   a. graphic sheet.
   b. nursing plan of care.

c. health care team record.

d. medication administration record.

8. When a documentation error has been made, it should:

   a. be erased.

   b. be scratched out.

   c. have one line drawn through it.

   d. be whited out so as to keep the record neat.

Critical Thinking Questions

1. Of what value is a client's medical record in a court of law? How can it be used?

2. Why are there so many types of charting? Of what value is each?

WEB FLASH!

- Search the various methods of documentation; use search terms such as PIE, charting, and Kardex.
- Research what the Internet has to offer about computerized documentation.
- What can you find about NIC, NOC, and NMDS?

CLIENT TEACHING

Refer to the following chapters to increase your understanding of client teaching:

- **Chapter 6, Legal Responsibilities**
- **Chapter 8, Communication**
- **Chapter 9, Nursing Process**
- **Chapter 12, Cultural Diversity and Nursing**
- **Chapter 14, The Life Cycle**
- **Chapter 16, Stress, Adaptation, and Anxiety**

LEARNING OBJECTIVES

Upon completion of this chapter, you should be able to:
- *Define key terms.*
- *Explain the importance of client education in today's health care climate.*
- *Relate principles of adult education to client teaching.*
- *Identify common barriers to learning.*
- *Explain the ways that learning varies throughout the life cycle.*
- *Discuss the nurse's professional responsibilities related to teaching.*
- *Relate the teaching–learning process to the nursing process.*
- *Describe teaching strategies that make learning meaningful to clients.*

KEY TERMS

affective domain	psychomotor domain
auditory learner	readiness for learning
cognitive domain	self-efficacy
formal teaching	teaching
informal teaching	teaching–learning
kinesthetic learner	process
learning	teaching strategies
learning plateau	visual learner
learning style	

INTRODUCTION

Client education is an integral part of nursing care. It is the nurse's responsibility to help identify with the client the learning needs and resources that will restore and maintain that client's optimal level of functioning. This chapter offers an overview of the teaching and learning process, including barriers and responsibilities, and relates it to the nursing process.

THE TEACHING–LEARNING PROCESS

The **teaching–learning process** is a planned interaction that promotes behavioral change that is not a result of maturation or coincidence. **Teaching** is an active process wherein one individual shares information with another to facilitate learning and thereby promote behavioral changes. A teacher is someone who uses a variety of goal-directed activities to promote change by assisting the learner to absorb new information.

Learning is the process of assimilating information, resulting in behavior change. Knowledge is power. By sharing knowledge with clients, the nurse helps them achieve their maximum level of wellness. The teaching–learning process is familiar to nurses in that it mirrors the steps of the nursing process: assessment, identification of learning needs (nursing diagnosis), planning, implementation of teaching strategies, and evaluation of learner progress and teaching efficacy. These steps are discussed in greater detail later in this chapter.

According to Edelman and Mandle (1998), the goal of health education is to help individuals achieve optimal states of health through their own actions. Teaching, one of the most important nursing functions, addresses the client's need for information. Often, a knowledge deficit about the course of illness and/or self-care practices will hinder the client in recovering from illness or practicing health-promoting behaviors. The nurse's charge is to help bridge the gap between those things a client knows and those things a client needs to know to achieve optimal health.

Client teaching is done for a variety of reasons, including:

- Promotion of wellness
- Prevention of illness
- Restoration of health
- Facilitation of coping abilities

Client education focuses on the client's ability to practice healthy behaviors. The client's ability to care for self is enhanced by effective education. Client education has been credited with the following (Seley, 1994):

- Improved quality of care
- Shorter length of hospital stays
- Decreased chance of hospital readmission
- Greater compliance with prescribed treatment regimens

These benefits are enhanced through nurses' continued active participation as client educators.

Formal teaching is planned and goal directed, but informal teaching can occur in any setting at any time.

Formal Teaching

Formal teaching takes place at a specific time, in a specific place, and on a specific topic. It is planned and goal directed (Figure 11-1). The teacher prepares the information and/or activities related to the topic. Formal teaching may take place in a class setting with several learners, or it may be performed one-on-one. For example, many health care facilities provide formal classes related to diabetes. The same basic information is necessary for all clients with diabetes.

Informal Teaching

Informal teaching takes place any time, any place, and whenever a learning need is identified. In the course of providing nursing care, nurses have many opportunities for informal teaching, such as answering the clients' questions and explaining care being given to the client (Figure 11-2). Informal teaching may also occur in the midst of formal teaching. A comment or question from a learner in a formal setting may trigger some informal teaching in response. For example, during a class on diet for the diabetic client,

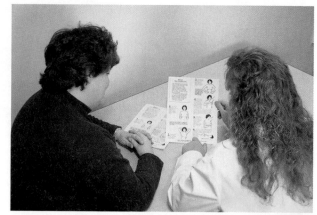

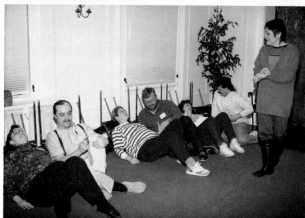

Figure 11-1 Nurses engage in formal teaching, with both individual and group clients. (*Second photo courtesy of Bellevue Woman's Hospital, Niskayuna, NY*)

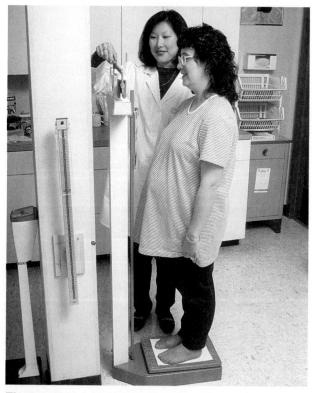

Figure 11-2 Informal teaching can occur during a routine procedure.

a question about dietary cholesterol may be asked. The response would be considered informal teaching because it was not the planned topic.

An understanding of learning domains, learning principles, learning styles, learning barriers, and teaching methods is also helpful. These topics are discussed below.

Learning Domains

In his classic work, Bloom (1977) identifies three areas or domains wherein learning occurs: the **cognitive domain**, which involves intellectual understanding; the **affective domain**, which involves attitudes, beliefs, and emotions; and the **psychomotor domain**, which involves the performance of motor skills. Each domain responds to and processes information in very different ways. Table 11–1 briefly outlines the three learning domains and provides clinical examples.

Nurses must be sensitive to all three learning domains when developing effective teaching plans and must use **teaching strategies**, or techniques to promote learning, that will tap into each of the domains. For instance, teaching a diabetic client why and how to measure the proper daily balance of insulin against the glucose level falls within the cognitive domain; helping the same client learn the way to self-administer insulin falls within the psychomotor domain; and encouraging the client to view diabetes as only one aspect of the individual falls within the affective domain.

Learning Principles

Certain fundamental learning principles can be used by nurses when teaching clients. Knowles, Holton, and Swanson (1998) cite four basic assumptions about adult learners, which are applicable to client education:

- *Assumption 1:* An individual's personality develops in an orderly fashion from dependence to independence. *Nursing application:* The nurse should plan teaching–learning activities that promote client participation, thus encouraging independence and increasing client control and self-care through empowerment.
- *Assumption 2:* Learning readiness is affected by developmental stage and sociocultural factors. *Nursing application:* The nurse should conduct a thorough psychosocial assessment before planning the teaching–learning activities.
- *Assumption 3:* An individual's previous learning experiences can be used as a foundation for further learning. *Nursing application:* The nurse should perform a complete assessment to ascertain what the client already knows and build on that knowledge base.
- *Assumption 4:* Immediacy reinforces learning. *Nursing application:* The nurse should provide opportu-

Table 11–1 LEARNING DOMAINS		
DOMAIN	**DEFINITION**	**EXAMPLE**
Cognitive	Learning that involves the acquisition of facts and data; used in problem solving and decision making	Client states the name and purpose of prescribed medications.
Affective	Learning that involves changing attitudes, emotions, and beliefs; used in making judgments	Client starts to accept the nature of the chronic illness.
Psychomotor	Learning that involves gaining motor skills; used in physical application of knowledge	Client gives self an injection.

From Fundamentals of Nursing: Standards & Practice, *by S. DeLaune and P. Ladner, 1998, Albany, NY: Delmar. Copyright 1998 by Delmar. Reprinted with permission.*

nities for immediate application of knowledge and skills and should incorporate feedback as a continuous part of each nurse–client interaction.

Learning principles include relevance, motivation, readiness, maturation, reinforcement, participation, organization, and repetition.

Relevance

The material to be learned must be meaningful to the client, easily understood by the client, and related to previously learned information. Individuals must believe that they need to learn the information before learning can occur. Does the client perceive relevance (meaningfulness) in the current information to be taught? If an individual sees the information as being personally valuable, the information is more likely to be learned. If the client does not view the content as relevant, however, learning is not likely to occur. Because relevance is individually determined, the nurse must assess the personal meaning of learning for each client.

Motivation

The psychologist Bandura (1977) purports that **self-efficacy** (one's belief that one will succeed in attempts to change behavior) has a profound influence on motivation. Clients should perceive value in the information. If clients feel they will not achieve the goals, they will lack motivation to try. To maximize motivation, the nurse must keep the teaching–learning goals realistic by breaking the content down into small, achievable

PROFESSIONAL TIP

Checking Literacy

"Lscean uyro sdhna. Seu yver dloc rweat."

The preceding is what some clients will see when given printed educational materials. Always avoid making assumptions about client literacy level and be sure to assess the client's ability to comprehend written materials. Check comprehension through return explanation of the written material.

steps. For example, the cardiac client must see value in information about exercise, such as that the heart will be strengthened and the client will have more energy.

Readiness

The client should be able and willing to learn. Readiness is closely related to growth and development. For example, the client must have the requisite cognitive and psychomotor skills for learning a particular task, and the client must comprehend the information. One indicator of learning readiness is the client's asking questions; another is the client's becoming involved in learning activities, such as actively participating in return demonstration of a dressing change. Some indicators of lack of client readiness are anxiety, avoidance, denial, lack of participation in discussion or demonstration, and lack of participation in self-care activities.

Maturation

The client should be developmentally able to learn and have requisite cognitive and psychomotor abilities. The nurse assesses the client for characteristics that will hinder or facilitate learning. One such characteristic is the client's developmental stage. The nurse must asess the client's developmental stage and not automatically assume, for instance, that a client who is 34 years old has mastered the developmental tasks of earlier stages.

Maturity level greatly influences the client's ability to learn information. Each developmental stage is characterized by unique skills and abilities that affect the

LIFE CYCLE CONSIDERATIONS

Ability to Learn

Remember that age is not always synonymous with developmental level; observation of behavior provides the clearest picture of developmental level.

response to various teaching tools. Developmental stage greatly determines the type of data to be taught, the method(s) to be used, the vocabulary to be used, and the location of teaching. In addition to developmental stage, the nurse should also evaluate the client's cognitive skills, problem-solving abilities, and attention span.

Reinforcement

Feedback provided to the learner should be positive and immediate in order to reinforce the client's motivation and readiness to learn. For example, the client who is learning to apply a sterile dressing to an open wound should be told during the application of the dressing that it is being done correctly (if it is) and should be praised upon completion for learning so quickly (or whatever is appropriate). If some aspect of the dressing application is lacking, the nurse must maintain a positive approach in guiding the client in correctly performing the application.

Participation

The client's active involvement in the learning process will promote and enhance learning. Client involvement is relatively easy to monitor when a psychomotor skill is to be learned, as the client is actively involved in practicing a physical skill. Learning that takes place in the cognitive or affective domain is also most effective when active involvement of the client is encouraged. For example, the client who is to be on a low-fat diet can be involved in learning to self-regulate with regard to diet by reading labels of foods and planning menus of low-fat meals.

Organization

The material to be learned should incorporate previously learned information and be presented in sequence from simple to complex and from familiar to unfamiliar. Again using the example of the client learning about a low-fat diet, the nurse should begin the teaching session by finding out what the client knows about the nutrient content of foods and should proceed to helping the client first learn to read food labels, then plan a meal, and then plan a menu for a day and a week, and so forth.

Repetition

Retention of material is reinforced with practice, repetition, and presentation of the same material in a variety of ways. The more often the learner hears or sees the material, the greater the chance that the material will be retained.

It is good to keep in mind that a **learning plateau**, or peak in the effectiveness of teaching and depth of learning, will occur in relation to the client's motivation, interest, and perception of relevance of the material. Frequent reinforcement of learning through immediate feedback and continual reassessment of effectiveness will enhance the value of the learning process for both the teacher and the learner. Making the information-acquisition process as user friendly as possible will also increase satisfaction and success. This can be done by organizing content from the simple to the complex and from the familiar to the new, making learning as creative and interesting as possible, and adopting a flexible approach to allow the learning process to be dynamic.

Learning Styles

Each individual has a unique way of processing information. The manner whereby an individual incorporates new data is called **learning style**. Some people learn by processing information visually (**visual learner**), others by listening to the words (**auditory learner**), and others by experiencing the information or by touching, feeling, or doing (**kinesthetic learner**). The nurse should use a variety of techniques, such as lecture, discussion, small-group work, role play, modeling, return demonstration, imitation, problem solving, games, and question-and-answer sessions, to match different learning styles of clients. A good way to discover learning style is for the nurse to ask the client, "What helps you to learn?" or "What kinds of things do you enjoy doing?" The nurse can then match teaching strategies with the client's learning style.

Barriers to the Teaching–Learning Process

The giving and receiving of information does not, in and of itself, guarantee that learning will occur. Several

PROFESSIONAL TIP

Common Beliefs about Learning

- Each individual has the capacity to learn, but learning ability varies among people and situations.
- The pace of learning varies from person to person.
- Learning is a continuous process, occurring throughout the life cycle.
- Learning can occur in formal and informal settings and interactions.
- Learning is an individualized process.
- Learning new information is based on previous knowledge and experiences.
- Motivation and readiness are necessary prerequisites for learning.
- Prompt feedback facilitates learning.

Table 11–2 LEARNING BARRIERS

EXTERNAL BARRIERS	INTERNAL BARRIERS
Environmental • Interruptions • Lack of privacy • Multiple stimuli	**Psychological** • Anxiety • Fear • Anger • Depression • Inability to comprehend
Sociocultural • Language • Value system • Educational background	**Physiological** • Pain • Fatigue • Sensory deprivation • Oxygen deprivation

From Fundamentals of Nursing: Standards & Practice, *by S. DeLaune and P. Ladner, 1998, Albany, NY: Delmar. Copyright 1998 by Delmar. Reprinted with permission.*

barriers can impede the teaching–learning process. In a nursing situation, the nurse, the client, or both may encounter one or more of these barriers. Learning barriers can be classified as either internal (psychological or physiological) or external (environmental or sociocultural). Examples of these barriers are listed in Table 11–2. To facilitate the learning process, the nurse must assess for the presence of learning barriers. Specific assessment information is presented later in this chapter.

Environmental Barriers

Both the nurse and client are subject to environmental barriers. As part of planning for a teaching session, the nurse should ensure necessary privacy and minimize interruptions and multiple stimuli.

Sociocultural Barriers

When language is a barrier to the teaching–learning process, several steps can be taken to ensure that learning does take place, such as using pictures, providing printed material in the appropriate language, or using an interpreter. Even when the nurse and client both speak the same language, a language barrier may exist when clichés, health care jargon, or value-laden terms are used. Furthermore, the meanings that the nurse and client attach to specific types of body language may differ depending on cultural influences. Nurses must be aware of their own value systems but focus client teaching within the client's value system. The educational background of the client must be kept in mind, and language should be tailored to the client's developmental level, without "talking down" to the client.

CULTURAL CONSIDERATIONS

Overcoming Sociocultural Barriers

- Use pictures whenever possible.
- Provide written material in the appropriate language.
- Use a culturally sensitive interpreter or a family member who understands health care terminology.
- Avoid the use of clichés, jargon, or value-laden terms.
- Learn about the client's cultural norms.
- Be aware of your own values.
- Tailor teaching (information and questions) to the client's ability to read and write.
- Have the client verbalize what has been understood from the teaching–learning session.

Psychological Barriers

Nurses may be anxious about client teaching. Knowing the client's learning needs should help alleviate some of this anxiety, as should adequate preparation related to content, environmental and sociocultural aspects, and developmental ability of the client. What little anxiety is left will likely serve to make the nurse more alert and sensitive.

Clients and families are often upset about the health situation they are experiencing. They may be anxious, fearful, angry, or depressed. In addition to the client's words, the nurse should pay attention to body language and behavior. If clients or family members are obviously angry, the nurse should recognize and acknowledge the anger by saying something like "You appear to be very angry about something. Tell me what you are feeling." Allowing clients and family members to express their emotions clears the air and allows learning to take place.

PROFESSIONAL TIP

Overcoming Psychological Barriers

- Recognize your own emotions related to client teaching.
- Prepare content of teaching and assess for environmental, sociocultural, psychological, and physiological barriers to learning.
- Acknowledge the client's emotions but do not respond in kind.

PROFESSIONAL TIP

Physiological Comfort and Learning

- Administer pain medication, as appropriate, before a teaching session to enable the client to concentrate on the information being presented.
- Plan teaching sessions when the client is not fatigued, as might be the case after a physical therapy session, for example.
- Ensure that the client is in a comfortable position and does not have to go to the bathroom.

Physiological Barriers

Physiological situation affects the client's ability to learn. The client who is struggling to breathe, for example, is unable to pay attention to any teaching. A teaching session should be planned for a time when the client is rested and free from pain.

Teaching Methods

Many different teaching methods can be used depending on the client's learning need and the applicable learning domain.

Teaching Methods Applicable in the Cognitive Domain

Effective methods for promoting cognitive learning include discussion, formal lecture, question-and-answer sessions, role play, and games/computer activities.

Discussion Discussions may involve the nurse and one or several clients who need to learn the same information. Active participation is promoted in the topic of discussion. Group discussions allow peer support.

Formal Lecture In formal lectures, the teacher presents the information to be learned, and learner participation is usually minimal.

Question-and-Answer Sessions Question-and-answer sessions can take two forms. In one, the client's concerns are addressed by the client asking the questions and the nurse providing answers. In the other the nurse assists the client in applying the knowledge learned by asking the client questions that the client then answers (Figure 11-3).

Role Play Role play provides the client an opportunity to apply knowledge in a safe, controlled environment. In role play, the nurse and client each assume a certain role in order to play out different potential scenarios. For instance, the nurse teaching a client sex education information intended for an adolescent may have the client assume the role of parent, while the

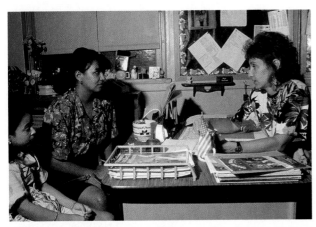

Figure 11-3 A Question-and-Answer Session with School Nurse, Mother, and Child

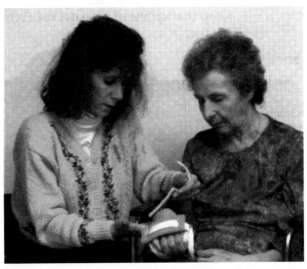

Figure 11-5 Demonstrating Application of a Splint

nurse assumes the role of the teenager. The two can then engage in practice discussion sessions to prepare the client for the actual parent–teen discussion.

Games/Computer Activities Games and computer activities can be used to teach clients at a level that is appropriate for them. These methods allow the client to use the new information in various situations and to have fun while learning.

Teaching Methods Applicable in the Affective Domain

Role play and discussion are both effective methods for stimulating affective learning.

Role Play Role play allows expression of feelings, attitudes, and values in a safe, controlled environment. The client can "try out" different attitudes and values.

Discussion One-on-one discussion between nurse and client is effective for personal or sensitive topics related to values, feelings, attitudes, and emotions (Figure 11-4).

Teaching Methods Applicable in the Psychomotor Domain

Demonstration, supervised practice, and return demonstration assist the client to learn psychomotor skills.

Demonstration In demonstration, the nurse presents in a step-by-step manner the skill or procedure to be learned, explaining what is being done and why. In this way, the client sees not only the equipment and the way it is used, but also the nurse's attitude and behaviors (Figure 11-5).

Supervised Practice In supervised practice, the client uses the equipment and performs the skill or procedure while the nurse watches. The nurse gives suggestions and corrects the client as the practice proceeds. Repetition can continue until the client feels confident in performing the skill or procedure.

Return Demonstration In return demonstration, the client performs the skill or procedure without any coaching from the nurse. Upon completion of the task, the nurse provides feedback and reinforcement to the client.

LEARNING THROUGHOUT THE LIFE CYCLE

One basic assumption underlies teaching effectiveness: *All people are capable of learning.* However, the ability to learn varies from person to person and from situation to situation. Further, learning needs and learning abilities change throughout life, and the client's chronological age and developmental stage greatly influence the ability to learn. The principles of learning discussed earlier in this chapter have relevance to learners of all ages. However, teaching approaches must be modified according to the client's developmental stage and level of understanding. Specific information

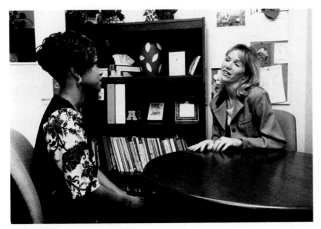

Figure 11-4 Sensitive topics are discussed in a one-on-one setting.

for children, adolescents, and older adults is described in the following sections.

Children

Readiness for learning (evidence of willingness to learn) varies during childhood depending on maturation level. Responding to knowledge deficits of young children requires that the nurse work closely with the child's caretaker. Including the family or caregiver in teaching is especially important when caring for young children.

Young children learn primarily through play. Incorporating play into teaching activities for children can therefore enhance learning (Figure 11-6). Puppets, toys, and coloring books can be effective teaching tools for the young child. Creativity is effective in encouraging the young child to be an active participant in the learning process.

Older children can also benefit from the use of art materials to express their emotions and their understanding of those things that are or will be happening to them. Using medical supplies (such as medicine cups or bandages), for example, the child may play at giving medicine to a doll or putting a bandage on the doll like the bandage that will be put on the child. While the child is involved in play, the nurse is both teaching the child what to expect regarding treatment procedures and alleviating anxiety.

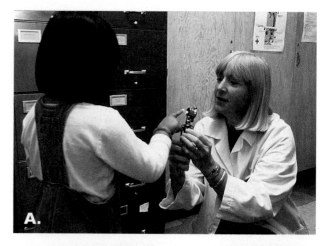

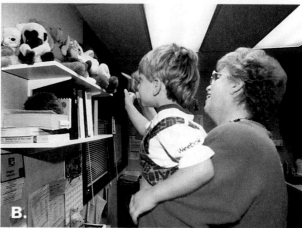

Figure 11-6 A. The nurse is at the child's level while the child learns about the instrument to be used in the examination; B. The nurse encourages a child to select a toy to help in teaching.

Adolescents

As individuals approach adolescence, they are better able to conceptualize relationships between things. Usually, reading and comprehension ability have advanced, and the adolescent can understand more complex information. Because one of the strongest influences on the adolescent is peer support, group meetings are often useful in teaching. The nurse can

LIFE CYCLE CONSIDERATIONS

Teaching Children
- Ensure that the child is comfortable.
- Encourage caregiver participation.
- Assess the child's learning readiness, motivation, and developmental level. Do not equate age with developmental level.
- Assess the child's psychological status.
- Determine self-care abilities of the child and caregiver.
- Use play, imitation, and role play to make learning fun and meaningful.
- Use different visual stimuli, such as books, chalkboards, and videos, to convey information and assess understanding.
- Use terms that are easily understood by the client and caregiver.
- Provide frequent repetition and reinforcement.
- Develop realistic goals that are consistent with developmental abilities.
- In planning teaching approaches, remember that the goals of educating children are to "prevent excessive anxiety, improve cooperation, and hasten the recovery process" (Biddinger, 1993).

CLIENT TEACHING

Do As I Do
- The adage "Do as I say, not as I do" goes against all wisdom. Individuals learn from examples set by role models.
- Adolescents are especially sensitive to discrepancies between an adult's words and actions.
- Encourage parents to model the behaviors they wish their children to develop.

often be a powerful teacher by acting as a role model. The accompanying display provides guidelines for teaching adolescents.

Older Adults

Aging is accompanied by many physiological changes. As a result of these changes, some older adults experience perceptual impairments such as vision and hearing impairments. The nurse must thus assess for perceptual changes and adjust teaching materials accordingly. For example, providing large-print written material and verifying that the client hears all instructions and directions are strategies helpful in teaching older clients. The accompanying display provides guidelines for teaching older adults.

PROFESSIONAL RESPONSIBILITIES RELATED TO TEACHING

Through teaching, the nurse empowers clients in their self-care abilities. Teaching is the tool for providing information to clients about specific disease processes, treatment methods, and health-promoting behaviors. Although each state has its own definition

LIFE CYCLE CONSIDERATIONS

Teaching Adolescents

- Show respect for adolescents by recognizing their struggle to gain the knowledge and experience of adulthood while breaking away from the grasp of childhood.
- Boost adolescents' confidence by requesting their input and opinions on health care matters.
- Encourage adolescents to explore their own feelings about self-concept and independence.
- Be sensitive to the peer pressure many adolescents face.
- Help adolescents identify and build on their positive qualities.
- Gear teaching to the adolescent's developmental level and use language that is clear yet appropriate to the health care setting.
- To encourage independent and informed decision making, engage adolescents in problem-solving activities.

LIFE CYCLE CONSIDERATIONS

Teaching Older Adults

- Ensure that the client is comfortable. Pain, fatigue, a full bladder, or hunger can impair learning.
- Assess the client's learning readiness, motivation, and developmental level. Do not equate age with developmental level.
- Assess the client's psychological status. Depression, severe anxiety, or denial can interfere with learning.
- Ascertain the client's self-care abilities.
- Use terms that are easily understood by the client. Avoid talking down to the client; a condescending, paternalistic manner impedes learning.
- Ascertain the time of day when the client is best able to concentrate.
- Present material slowly and use examples.
- Encourage client involvement and participation.
- Ask for feedback and employ active listening.
- Provide frequent feedback.
- Assess for perceptual impairments and individualize teaching strategies accordingly:

For memory-impaired clients:
- Use repetition
- Use a variety of cues (spoken words, written materials, pictures, and symbols)

For visually impaired clients:
- Provide large-print materials
- Provide magnifying glasses
- Be sure client is wearing prescription eyeglasses
- Provide adequate lighting and reduce glare

For hearing-impaired clients:
- Face the client directly when speaking
- Use short sentences and words that are easily understood
- Use signals to reinforce verbal information (point, gesture, and demonstrate)
- Eliminate distractions (noises or activities from the environment) as much as possible

Adapted from Principles and Practice of Adult Health Nursing, *by P. G. Beare & J. L. Myers 1998. St. Louis: Mosby; and from "Altered Patterns of Degenerative Origin," by S. C. Delaune, in* Mental Health and Psychiatric Nursing *[3rd ed.] by J. L. Davies [Ed.] 1991, Boston: Jones and Bartlett.*

of nursing practice, teaching is a required function of nurses in most states. Redman (1997) cites National League for Nursing documents dating back to 1918 as stating that "the nurse is essentially a teacher and an agent of health."

Providing client education is expected of all nurses. Freda (1997) is disturbed by reports that some nurses in the United States, however, are voluntarily giving up their client teaching responsibilities, mainly because of a perceived lack of time. She believes that if nurses give up their role as client educators in favor of spending that time performing additional tasks, nursing's worth to the health care system could greatly diminish. Client teaching requires the depth of information that only nurses possess; as such, it is one of the truly independent functions of nursing practice.

Client teaching is also mandated by several accrediting bodies including the Joint Commission for Accreditation of Healthcare Organizations (JCAHO, 1998). The American Hospital Association's *Patient's Bill of Rights* (1992) calls for the client's understanding of health status and treatment approaches. Informed consent for treatment procedures can be given only by clients who are well informed. The nurse assesses the client's level of understanding about treatment methods and corrects any knowledge deficits. The nurse often serves as an interpreter for the client—explaining in easily understood terms, clarifying, and referring.

Teaching supports behavioral changes that lead to positive adaptation by the client. Thus, teaching decreases the fear of change. Reducing anxiety and anticipatory stress is an important component of teaching.

Client teaching is an essential function of every nurse regardless of practice setting. All clients require information about disease prevention, growth and development, safety, first aid, nutrition, and hygiene. The client who is hospitalized needs information about his condition, the expected treatment, and the environment of the health care facility. By the time of discharge, clients must also have information about

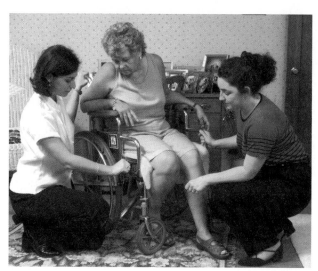

Figure 11-7 Nurse Teaches a Family Member to Provide Care

postdischarge care related to medications, dietary modifications, activity, complication prevention, and rehabilitation plans.

Clients who are recovering at home and their families also have significant learning needs. A primary role of the home health nurse is to teach the client about caring for himself at home. This often involves teaching family members ways to provide care (Figure 11-7). Home-based clients need information regarding their illness, accident, or injury. They also need to learn ways to achieve and maintain a maximum state of wellness. Accurate teaching plans for the home-based client and family are established by assessing multiple factors, some of which are listed in Table 11–3.

Self-Awareness

Several characteristics of nurses influence the outcome of the teaching–learning process. Nurse self-awareness with regard to the concepts discussed in the following sections is an all-important first step in teaching.

Knowledge Base

It is impossible for nurses to teach if they lack the knowledge or skills that are to be taught. Staying both current in knowledge and proficient in skills is the first step to maintaining efficacy and credibility as a teacher. Although it is impossible for one individual to be an expert in every area of nursing, knowing when to refer the client to others for teaching is an important critical-thinking skill.

Interpersonal Skills

Effective teaching is based on the nurse's ability to establish rapport with the client. The empathic nurse shows sensitivity to the client's needs and preferences. An atmosphere in which the client feels free to ask

 COMMUNITY/HOME HEALTH CARE

Client Teaching Considerations

- Preparation of the client and family for home care begins at the time of hospital admission, not at the time of discharge.
- The nurse's effective teaching is the link to thorough follow-up care in the home.
- Discharge planning requires consideration of current learning needs of clients and caregivers as well as potential needs after discharge.
- Teaching involves consideration of community resources and possible referral.

Table 11–3 FACTORS AFFECTING LEARNING NEEDS OF HOME HEALTH CLIENTS

FACTOR	EXAMPLE
Environmental	• Accessibility of home to the client with a physical disability • Need for and availability of equipment and supplies • Space to accommodate special needs of the client • Need for information about environmental cleanliness as it relates to health • Need for assistance with self-care activities
Economic	• Ability to purchase medications, equipment, and supplies • Available financial assistance
Support system	• Persons available to assist with caregiving • Caregiver's knowledge deficits regarding necessary care
Community resources	• Resources in the immediate area • Awareness of and access to support services • Available respite for the family

From Fundamentals of Nursing: Standards & Practice, *by S. DeLaune and P. Ladner, 1998, Albany, NY: Delmar. Copyright 1998 by Delmar. Reprinted with permission.*

questions promotes learning. Activities that help establish an environment conducive to learning include:

• Showing genuine interest in the client,
• Including the client in *every* step of the teaching–learning process,

PROFESSIONAL TIP

Medical Jargon and Teaching
• Consider the language used by most nurses; think of the terms nurses take for granted. When a client is asked to "void," for example, does the client understand what is meant?
• Think of the following frequently used terms that can easily be misunderstood by clients and families: *ambulate, defecate, dangle, NPO, vital signs,* and *contraindicated.*
• Listen to the language nurses use when communicating with clients.
• How can you communicate without using professional jargon?

• Employing a nonjudgmental approach, and
• Communicating at the client's level of understanding.

Documentation

The reasonable and prudent standard calls for nurses to document client education. From a legal perspective, if the nurse teaches the client and fails to document it, the educational activities never occurred. Documentation of teaching promotes continuity of care and facilitates accurate communication to other health care colleagues involved in the client's care.

Many different approaches can be used to document client teaching. Figure 11-8 is an example of a documentation form related to client teaching in an inpatient setting; Figure 11-9 is a sample form for documenting teaching in the home setting.

Because client education is a standard and essential component of nursing practice, each nurse must document the teaching interventions used and the client's response. Elements to be documented in all practice settings include:

• Content
• Teaching methods
• Learner(s) (e.g., client, family member, other caretaker)
• Client/family response to teaching activities

TEACHING–LEARNING AND THE NURSING PROCESS

The teaching–learning process and the nursing process are interdependent. Both are dynamic and comprise the same phases: assessment, diagnosis, planning, implementation, and evaluation. Figure 11-10 compares the nursing process and the teaching–learning process.

Assessment

The nurse should assess each learning situation for each client. Primary (client) and secondary (family or significant other) sources are used by nurses to assess learning needs. Communication with the client and family or significant others is the foundation of assessment related to learning. Several factors must be considered during assessment:

• Actual learning needs
• Potential learning needs
• Client strengths and limitations
• Previous experiences

Actual Learning Needs

Everyone who receives health care services has some need for learning. Client teaching may be indicated when a client:

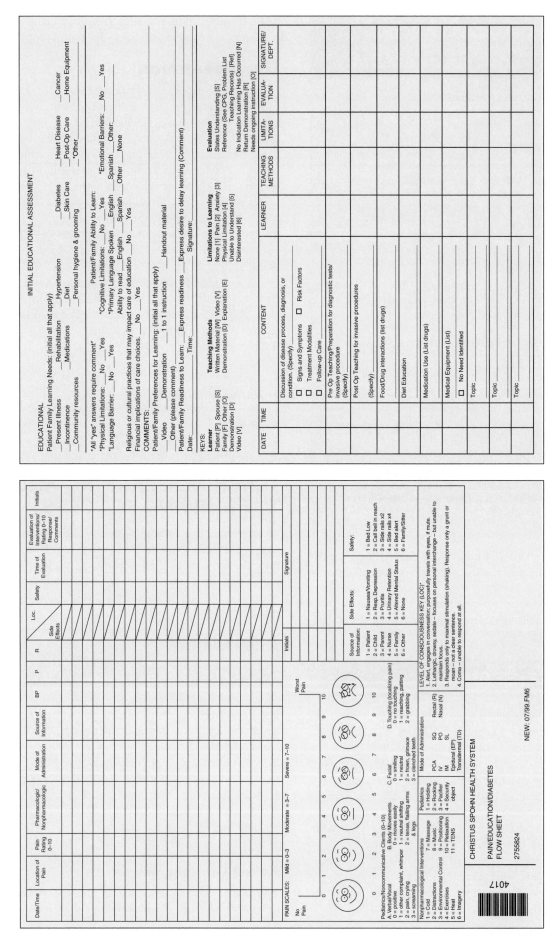

Figure 11-8 Documentation Form for Client Teaching: Inpatient Setting (*Courtesy of Christus Spohn Health System, Corpus Christi, TX*) (*continues*)

INJECTION SITE:
RA – Right Arm
LA – Left Arm
RT – Right Thigh
LT – Left Thigh
RG – Right Gluteal
LG – Left Gluteal
RQ – Right Abdominal Quadrant
LQ – Left Abdominal Quadrant

Initial/Signatures
1. _____
2. _____
3. _____
4. _____
5. _____
6. _____
7. _____

DIET: _____
8. _____
9. _____
10. _____
11. _____
12. _____
13. _____
14. _____
15. _____
16. _____
17. _____
18. _____
19. _____
20. _____
21. _____

For Documentation of Routine Blood Sugar Results i.e. BID, TID or AC and HS

DATE		AC Breakfast	AC Lunch	AC Dinner	AC HS Snack	COMMENTS	2 AM	Exp. Date of Resol.	Date Comp. Int.
	Bid Glu								
	Meter #								
	Insulin Admin.								
	Bid Glu								
	Meter #								
	Insulin Admin.								
	Bid Glu								
	Meter #								
	Insulin Admin.								
	Bid Glu								
	Meter #								
	Insulin Admin.								

Int.	#	Problem	Goal	Exp. Date of Resol.	Date Comp. Int.
		Alteration in Comfort	Comfort maintained		
		Injury Potential	Safety Maintained		
		Fever	Temp. within Normal Limits		
		Anxiety/Fear	Reduced Anxiety/Fear		
		Knowledge Deficit	Increased Understanding		
		Infection	Minimized/Absent Signs		
		Body Image Disturbance	Acknowledge Change		
		Fluid/Lyte Imbalance	Main. Fluid/Lyte Bal.		
		Impaired Gas Exchange	Main./Increase Gas Ex.		
		Ineffective Airway Clearance	Maintain Patient Airway		
		Ineffective Breathing Pattern	Maintain Patient Airway		
		Altered Tissue Perfusion	Optimal Tissue Perfusion		

Int.	#	Problem	Goal	Exp. Date of Resol.	Date Comp. Int.
		Impaired Skin Integrity	Regain Skin Integrity		
		Pot. For Skin Impairment	Skin Integrity Maintained		
		Activity Intolerance	Maintain/Increase Activity		
		Impaired Mobility	Imp. Function/Mobility		
		Self Care Deficit	Improve ADL's		
		Altered Thought Process	Reduced Disorientation		
		Impaired Communication	Improve Communication		
		Constipation	Bowel Elim. With WNL		
		Diarrhea	Bowel Elim. With WNL		
		Incontinence	Maintain Bowel Integrity		
		Impaired Swallowing/Chewing	Optimal Nutrition Status		
		Alteration in Nutrition	Optimal Nutrition Status		

Pain-Ed-Diabetes.FM6   09/16/99

DATE	TIME	CONTENT	LEARNER	TEACHING METHODS	LIMITATIONS	EVALUATION	SIGNATURE/DEPT.
		Rehabilitation (Describe)					
		PT _____ OT _____ Speech _____					
		Special Treatments (Describe)					
		Community Resources (Specify)					
		Diabetes Teaching ☐ DM Medication ☐ Insulin Adm. Techniques ☐ Diet Guidelines ☐ Hypoglycemia–Sx., Tx, Prev. ☐ Foot Care ☐ Sick Day Guidelines ☐ Referred to OP Diabetes Class					
		Explanation of safety program, level precautions, and wristband					
		Topic: Pain Management Information Sheet					
		Topic _____					
		Topic _____					
		Topic _____					
		Topic _____					
		Topic _____					
		Topic _____					
		Topic _____					
		Topic _____					

Figure 11-8 *(continued)*

RIVER REGION HOME HEALTH SERVICES, INC.
PSYCHIATRIC NURSE PROGRESS NOTE

PATIENT NAME _____ MR# _____ _____ IN _____ OUT _____

NURSE NAME _____ DAY _____ DATE _____

VSBP _____ T _____ P _____ R _____ WT _____ DIET _____

Nutritional Status _____   Heart/Lung Status _____

Neuro Oriented X _____ PEERL _____   Homebound Status _____

Physical Status _____

_____

Assess Degree of Existing Problem: (1) Mild, (2) Moderate, (3) Severe

Somatic Concern	_____	Emotional Withdrawal	_____	Anxiety	_____
Depressive Mood	_____	Hostility	_____	Uncooperativeness	_____
Blunted Affect	_____	Lack of Insight	_____	Delusions	_____
Suicidal Ideation	_____	Motivational Disability	_____	Hallucinations	_____
Impaired Memory	_____	Rx Non–Compliance	_____	Socialization	_____
Communication	_____	Mannerisms & Posturing	_____		
ADL's	_____	Unusual Thought Concern	_____		
Conceptual Disorganization	_____				

SN Assessment/Intervention/Teaching: _____

_____

_____

_____

Teaching: _____

_____

_____

_____

Feedback to Teaching: _____

_____

_____

_____

Changes: Meds/Plan of Care: _____

_____

Aide Supervision AS/PAS: _____

Reason HHA Needed: _____

Comments Regarding Care: _____

_____

HOME HEALTH ASSISTANT _____   PATIENT _____

Current Requisition in Home _____   Appearance _____   Dolpe _____

Completes Assignment _____   Bathed Completely _____

Rapport with Patient _____   Body Alignment _____

PT/FMY Satisfied _____

Room Tidy _____

Planning: Continue Same Plan _____   Personal Hygiene _____

Increase Visits _____

Decrease Visits _____

Discharge Planning _____

_____   _____

NURSE SIGNATURE   PATIENT OR CAREGIVER SIGNATURE

Figure 11-9 Documentation Form for Client Teaching: Home Health *(Courtesy of River Region Home Health Services, Inc., LA)*

TEACHING-LEARNING PROCESS

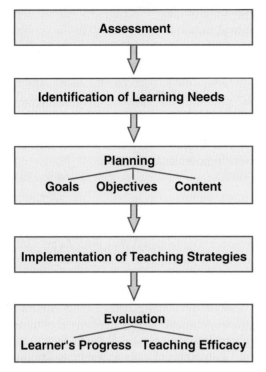

NURSING PROCESS

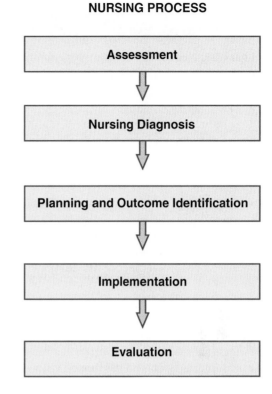

Figure 11-10 Comparison of Teaching–Learning Process and Nursing Process *(From* Fundamentals of Nursing: Standards & Practice, *by S. DeLaune and P. Ladner, 1998, Albany, NY: Delmar. Copyright 1998 by Delmar. Reprinted with permission.)*

- Expresses a need for information to make decisions,
- Needs new skills,
- Wants to make lifestyle modifications, or
- Is in an unfamiliar environment.

A crucial step in teaching is to determine the client's learning needs—those things the client needs to know and those things the client already knows. The nurse must evaluate the client's knowledge about the content to be taught. Previous knowledge can then be used as a foundation for new concepts. If the client is misinformed, the nurse must develop a remediation plan for learning. Determining the client's learning needs is accomplished in a variety of ways, including:

- Questioning the client directly,
- Observing client behaviors, and
- Interacting with the client's family or significant others.

It is imperative that the nurse first address the client's immediate need for knowledge by assessing the client's perception of learning needs and prioritizing those needs on the basis of client input and status. For example, preoperative clients must be taught deep breathing exercises and leg exercises before surgery so that they will be able to perform those exercises after

surgery and thereby prevent potential complications. After surgery, incision care to be performed at home can be taught. Comprehensive assessment is a mutual process between client and nurse. The client's opinion regarding the most pressing needs is a critical factor in prioritizing those needs.

Potential Learning Needs

The nurse also assesses for potential learning needs so that anticipatory planning can be done to avert a relapse in the recovery process and to maintain wellness. Following are two scenarios with related anticipatory learning needs noted:

- Mrs. Stone is pregnant for the first time. *Potential learning need:* Infant care.
- Mr. Carpenter has diabetes that is currently controlled by dietary modifications. He has just been told that he may have to take daily insulin in the future. *Potential learning need:* Self-administration of insulin.

Client Strengths and Limitations

Identification of the client's strengths and limitations provides a foundation for realistic expectations. An understanding of the client's strengths and weaknesses allows the nurse to plan successful teaching–learning

PROFESSIONAL TIP

Learning Needs Assessment

Questions to ask in assessing the client's learning needs include the following:

- Does the client express uncertainty over an up-coming procedure?
- Is the client able to tell you about medications, purposes, and side effects?
- Can the client describe necessary lifestyle modifications?
- Does the client correctly perform self-care activities?
- Is the client able to demonstrate necessary treatment procedures (e.g., colostomy irrigations, injections, blood glucose monitoring)?

CULTURAL CONSIDERATIONS

Learning and Culture

- Culture plays an important role in knowledge acquisition.
- Attitudes (which are derived from a cultural context) toward what is appropriate to learn and who should teach may require alterations in the nurse's approach.
- Sensitivity to cultural values affects every aspect of the teaching–learning process.

experiences. Determination of client strengths assists the nurse in selecting appropriate teaching methods. For example, a client who has limited vision should not be given pamphlets or other reading material in small print from which to learn the intended information.

Previous Experiences

The client has a knowledge base acquired through life experiences. Previous knowledge affects the client's attitudes about learning and the client's perception of the importance of the information to be learned. Previous knowledge is related to the client's type of educational experiences. A client who has had several experiences of hospitalization will have both a basis of knowledge and feelings (positive and negative) about those experiences. Current attitudes about this hospitalization will be influenced by prior hospital experiences.

Nursing Diagnosis

Several nursing diagnoses are pertinent to the learning process. When lack of knowledge is the primary learning need, the diagnosis of *Deficient Knowledge (specify)* is applicable. For example:

- A client who does not understand the way to use crutches for assisted ambulation may have the diagnosis of *Deficient Knowledge: Crutchwalking, R/T inexperience AEB multiple questions and hesitancy to walk*.
- A client who has had a colostomy and will be discharged soon may have a diagnosis of *Deficient Knowledge: Follow-up Care R/T colostomy care and maintenance AEB requests for information*.

Deficient Knowledge may also be a component of many other nursing diagnoses that encompass risk or

impaired behavior. For instance, *Risk for Infection* may relate to a client's compromised health status; this risk can be modified or reduced through certain physical and environmental changes and through proper client education. A client presenting with a diagnosis of a *Bathing/Hygiene Self-Care Deficit* may need both assistance in acquiring the physical supplies to remedy the deficit and instruction in techniques related to present physical and mental abilities.

Planning

Learning does not just happen by chance—it is planned. An important part of planning in the teaching–learning process is goal setting. The client and family or significant others must be involved in the setting of goals. Mutually determined goals promote learning. Specific learning goals should include the following elements:

- Measurable behavioral change
- Time frame
- Methods and intervals for evaluation

Teaching–learning goals must be realistic, that is, based on the abilities of the learner and the teacher.

Establishing teaching–learning goals involves setting priorities. One way to set priorities with regard to goals is to teach "need-to-know" content (that which is necessary for survival) before moving on to "nice-to-know" content. For example, Mrs. Stone, who is in her first trimester of pregnancy, must be taught guidelines for diet and exercise ("need-to-know" content); information about infant care ("nice-to-know" content at this time) can be given later in the pregnancy.

Planning, an ongoing phase of the teaching process, involves consideration of the following:

- Why teach?
- What should be taught?
- How should teaching be done?
- Who should teach and who should be taught?

- When should teaching occur?
- Where should teaching occur?

Why Teach?

Client need is *why* teaching is done. The client may realize the need for knowledge about a given subject and ask for information or ask questions about the subject. The nurse should recognize the client's need for knowledge even when the client does not recognize that need. For example, the nurse should recognize that a preoperative client needs to know how to do deep breathing exercises and leg exercises after surgery. The nurse should then plan teaching for that purpose.

What Should Be Taught?

Determination of *what* to teach is accomplished through comprehensive assessment. The content to be taught depends greatly on the client's knowledge base, readiness to learn, and current health status.

How Should Teaching Be Done?

Deciding *how* to teach involves ascertaining which teaching strategies are best given the content and the client's learning style and abilities. The nurse who is an effective teacher uses methods that capture the client's interest. Selection of teaching methods is often influenced by the teaching location. For example, videos can often be used effectively in inpatient settings; however, the same information may need to be presented with flipcharts or brochures in the home setting.

Who Should Teach and Who Should Be Taught?

Planning also means deciding *who* will teach the client. Although effective client education is the result of a multidisciplinary effort, the nurse is the coordinator of the health care team's teaching activities. Responsibility for planning a comprehensive teaching approach, from admission to postdischarge, rests with the nurse. Continuity of care is greatly affected by the teaching plan. The "who" part of planning also relates to who should be taught. The nurse must determine who in addition to the client (e.g., family members, significant others) must be taught about the illness and recovery process.

When Should Teaching Occur?

When to teach should be carefully considered. The nurse should recognize that every interaction with the client is an opportunity for teaching. Whenever a client asks a question, there is an opportunity for teaching. These windows of teaching opportunity must be used. Nothing destroys a client's motivation to learn more quickly than hearing comments such as "Ask your doctor that" or "We'll talk about that later. Right now, take your medicine." The best time for teaching is when the client is comfortable—physically and psychologically.

Where Should Teaching Occur?

Where teaching occurs must also be well planned. The location of teaching affects the quality of learning. Some factors to be considered in determining the location of teaching include provision of privacy and availability of equipment.

Implementation

Katz (1997) suggests several strategies to achieve successful client teaching, as outlined in the following sections.

Get and Keep the Client's Attention

The nurse should begin a teaching session by letting the client know what is going to be taught and why it is important to the client. The nurse can retain the client's interest by varying the tone of voice and using assorted teaching methods to present the material. Making the abstract concrete by using realistic examples from the client's experience is also effective in keeping the client's attention.

Stick to the Basics

Because the average adult can remember only five to seven points at a time, the nurse must be specific about what the client is to learn. Simple, everyday language should be used, and the most critical information should be presented first.

Use Time Wisely

The nurse can incorporate teaching into client care by providing information during each nurse–client interaction. Involving the client's family and friends,

PROFESSIONAL TIP

Guidelines for Effective Client Teaching
- Assess the client's knowledge and needs.
- Focus on the client's perceived needs.
- Relate material to the client's prior knowledge.
- Encourage the client's active participation.
- Provide opportunity for immediate application of knowledge or skill.
- Expect learning plateaus.
- Reinforce learning frequently.
- Provide immediate feedback to facilitate learning.
- Ensure a comfortable environment.
- Organize content from the simple to the complex, building on what the client already knows.
- Use a variety of teaching methods.
- Emphasize oral instructions with the written word and pictures.
- Maintain a flexible approach.
- Be creative.

allowing them to discuss the material with the client, is also helpful. The nurse should consider supplementing teaching with written material for the client and/or family to read; doing so provides time for the learners to review the material and then ask questions to clarify understanding.

Reinforce Information

Repetition creates habits; the nurse can take advantage of this by reviewing the material with the client and serving as a role model. For example, when teaching a client a procedure, the nurse must be sure to do it correctly each time and to avoid taking shortcuts. The nurse can reward the client by giving positive reinforcement such as a smile, a nod, or a few words of praise.

Evaluation

Evaluation of teaching–learning is a twofold process:

1. Determining what the client has learned
2. Assessing the nurse's teaching effectiveness

Evaluation of Learning

In performing the continual process of evaluating what the client has learned, the nurse must determine whether a behavior change has occurred, whether the behavior change is related to learning activities, whether further change is necessary, and whether continued behavior change will promote health. The following strategies can be used to evaluate client learning:

- Oral questioning
- Observation
- Return demonstration
- Written follow-up (e.g., questionnaires)

Evaluation of Teaching

A major purpose of evaluation is to assess the effectiveness of the teaching activities and to decide which modifications, if any, are necessary. When learning objectives are not met, reassessment is the basis for modifying teaching–learning activities. Evaluation is facilitated by the use of goals that are measurable and specific. Several activities can be used in evaluating teaching effectiveness:

- Feedback from the learner
- Feedback from colleagues
- Situational feedback
- Self-evaluation

SUMMARY

- Client education is designed to help individuals achieve optimal states of health.
- The teaching–learning process is a planned interaction that promotes behavioral change that is not a result of maturation or coincidence.

PROFESSIONAL TIP

Evaluation of Learning
- Did the client meet mutually established goals and objectives?
- Can the client demonstrate skills?
- Has the client's attitude changed?
- Can the client cope better with illness-imposed limitations?
- Does the family understand the health problem and know ways to help?

PROFESSIONAL TIP

Evaluation of Teacher Effectiveness
- Was content presented clearly and at the client's level of comprehension?
- Was the presentation (session) interesting?
- Did the nurse use a variety of teaching aids?
- Were the teaching aids appropriate for the client and the content?
- Was client participation encouraged?
- Was the nurse supportive?
- Did the nurse communicate an interest in the client and in the material?
- Did the nurse give frequent feedback and allow for immediate return demonstration?
- Were learning objectives stated in behavioral terms (i.e., easy to evaluate)?

- Teaching supports behavior change leading to positive adaptation.
- Learning is the process of assimilating information, resulting in behavioral change.
- Learning occurs in three domains: the cognitive (intellectual), the affective (emotional), and the psychomotor (motor skills).
- Learning readiness is affected by developmental and sociocultural factors and is present throughout the life span and at every developmental stage.
- Elements of documenting client education include the content taught, the teaching methods used, the person(s) taught, and the response of the learners.
- The teaching–learning process and the nursing process are interdependent, dynamic processes.
- Evaluation of the teaching–learning process involves two aspects: determination of what the client has learned and assessment of teacher efficacy.

CASE STUDY

Mr. Martinez, a 65-year-old widower from Mexico, recently moved in with his daughter and her family. He has just been diagnosed with diabetes. The physician orders dietary modifications. Mr. Martinez just sits and shakes his head, saying "I don't understand."

The following questions will guide your development of client teaching for Mr. Martinez.

1. What other data should be collected about Mr. Martinez?
2. Which domain(s) of learning should be considered?
3. What barriers to learning might be pertinent?
4. Identify a nursing diagnosis related to client teaching for Mr. Martinez.
5. Determine the *why, who, what, when, where,* and *how* of a teaching plan for Mr. Martinez.
6. What goals might be set with Mr. Martinez?
7. How will the effectiveness of teaching be evaluated?

Review Questions

1. Bloom identified three areas wherein learning occurs: the psychomotor domain, the affective domain, and the:

   a. attitude domain.
   b. cognitive domain.
   c. emotional domain.
   d. knowledge domain.

2. A clinical example of psychomotor learning is when a client:

   a. changes the dressing on a leg ulcer.
   b. states an acceptance of a chronic illness.
   c. states the name and purpose of a medication.
   d. chooses to change the type of exercise performed.

3. Kinesthetic learners learn by:

   a. doing.
   b. seeing.
   c. hearing.
   d. listening.

4. It is important for the nurse to be aware that learning needs:

   a. change daily.
   b. are the same for everyone.
   c. change throughout the life cycle.
   d. change as teaching approaches are modified.

5. Nurses are required to provide teaching by:

   a. all state nursing practice acts.
   b. the National League for Nursing.
   c. the American Hospital Association.
   d. the Joint Commission for Accreditation of Healthcare Organizations.

6. Because age is not synonymous with developmental level, the nurse, when preparing to teach a client, must:

   a. teach everyone the same way.
   b. set the goals for the client.
   c. observe the client's behavior.
   d. ask the client about self-efficacy.

Critical Thinking Questions

1. Is it ethical for a nurse to attempt to change a client's beliefs under the guise of teaching? Should a nurse "teach" a client the "right" attitude or belief?

2. Will knowledge acquisition alone result in learning (behavioral change)? Why? Why not?

WEB FLASH!

- Search the web for topics such as client teaching, teaching elders, teaching children, teaching adolescents. Can you find information specific to nursing?
- What organizations are available for help with teaching methods?
- What resources can you locate that provide teaching aids and materials?

UNIT
5
Cultural Aspects of Nursing

Chapter 12
Cultural Diversity and Nursing

Chapter 13
Complementary/Alternative Therapies

CULTURAL DIVERSITY AND NURSING

MAKING THE CONNECTION

Refer to the following chapters to increase your understanding of cultural diversity and nursing:

- **Chapter 7, Ethical Responsibilities**
- **Chapter 8, Communication**
- **Chapter 13, Complementary/Alternative Therapies**
- **Chapter 15, Wellness Concepts**
- **Chapter 26, Pain Management**

LEARNING OBJECTIVES

Upon completion of this chapter, you should be able to:
- *Define key terms.*
- *Describe the components and characteristics of culture.*
- *Describe the impact of cultural beliefs on health and illness.*
- *Compare and contrast diverse health beliefs of major cultural groups in the United States.*
- *Describe specific differences of cultural groups in relation to time and space.*
- *Identify nutritional preferences held by various cultural groups.*
- *Identify the general beliefs that account for the differences among religions.*
- *Describe the way that the nurse's religious beliefs or lack thereof can influence nursing care.*
- *Discuss the nurse's role in meeting the spiritual needs of the client and family.*
- *Analyze personal cultural beliefs and values.*
- *Perform a cultural assessment.*

INTRODUCTION

Every aspect of one's life—including attitudes, beliefs, and values—is influenced by one's culture. Behavior, including behavior affecting health, is culturally determined. As the population of the United States continues to diversify, recognition of cultural differences and their impact on health care becomes more critical. Nurses provide health care to culturally diverse client populations in a variety of settings. Knowledge of culturally relevant information is thus essential for delivery of competent nursing care. This chapter discusses the various concepts related to culture, the influence of culture on health, the relationships between culture and health beliefs, cultural aspects and the nursing process, and illnesses associated with ethnic groups.

CULTURE

Each individual is culturally unique. Behavior, self-perception, and judgment of others all depend on one's cultural perspective. To provide holistic care, the nurse needs a thorough understanding of concepts relating to culture.

KEY TERMS

acculturation
agnostic
atheist
cultural assimilation
cultural diversity
culture
dominant culture
ethnicity
ethnocentrism
minority group
oppression
race
religious support system
spiritual care
spiritual need
stereotyping
yin and yang

In society, **culture** refers to dynamic and integrated structures of knowledge, beliefs, behaviors, ideas, attitudes, values, habits, customs, languages, symbols, rituals, ceremonies, and practices that are unique to a particular group of people. This structure provides the group of people with a general design for living.

Individuals often acquire cultural beliefs unconsciously throughout the process of growth and maturation (Giger & Davidhizar, 1999). People are exposed to culture at an early age through the observance of traditions (established customary patterns of thought and behavior). Cultural beliefs, values, customs, and behaviors are transmitted from one generation to another through interaction, daily activities, and celebrations. For instance, the birth of a child is celebrated according to the family's cultural norms and customs, which may include prayers, blessings, special naming ceremonies, religious rites, and so forth. Grandparents, other elders, and parents all teach children cultural expectations and norms through role modeling, demonstration, and discussion (Figure 12-1).

CULTURAL CONSIDERATIONS

Sharing Culture

Cultural messages are transmitted in a variety of settings such as homes, schools, religious organizations, and communities. The various media, such as radio and television, are also powerful transmitters and shapers of culture.

Culture is not static nor is it uniform among all members within a given cultural group. Culture represents adaptive dynamic processes learned through life experiences. Diversity among and within cultural groups results from individual perspectives and practices. Consider, for example, the way that a family deals with a crisis. A crisis may cause a family that is part of a culture with a strong sense of responsibility to family and blood relatives to become closer; conversely, the same situation may cause a family that is from a culture that values independence and individuality to withdraw and create distance among its members. These reactions are rooted in the family's cultural background and heritage.

Ethnicity and Race

Ethnicity is a cultural group's perception of itself, or a group identity. Ethnicity is a sense of belongingness and a common social heritage that is passed from one generation to the next. Members of an ethnic group demonstrate their shared sense of identity through common customs and traits. Ethnic identity can be expressed in many ways, including dress; for instance, many African Americans display ethnic pride by choosing clothing that highlights their ethnic origin and shared heritage.

Race refers to a grouping of people based on biological similarities. Members of a racial group have similar physical characteristics such as blood group, facial features, and color of skin, hair, and eyes. There is often overlap between racial and ethnic groups because the cultural and biological commonalities support one another (Giger & Davidhizar, 1999). The similarities of people in racial and ethnic groups reinforce a sense of commonality and cohesiveness.

Cultural Diversity

Cultural diversity refers to the differences among people that result from racial, ethnic, and cultural variables. Within the United States a variety of rich cultural heritages exists. The vast potential of human resources with divergent viewpoints and behaviors enriches the sociopolitical climate. New and varied ideas, viewpoints, and problem-solving approaches and increased tolerance are all outcomes of a diverse population.

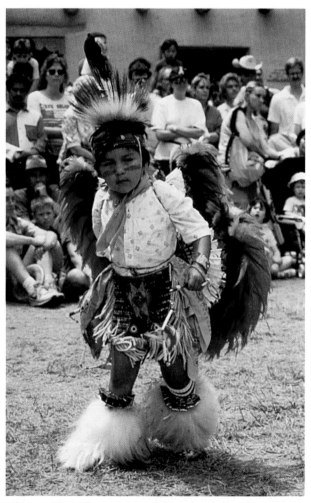

Figure 12-1 This child is celebrating his Native American heritage by participating in a traditional ceremony that has been passed down through the generations. (*Photo courtesy of Smithsonian Institution*)

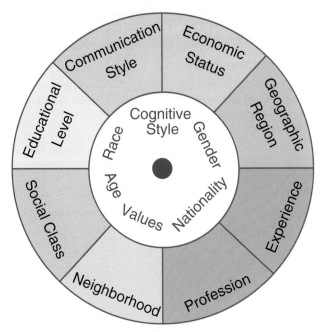

Figure 12-2 Areas of Cultural Diversity (*From* Fundamentals of Nursing: Standards & Practice, *by S. DeLaune and P. Ladner, 1998, Albany, NY: Delmar. Copyright 1998 by Delmar. Reprinted with permission.*)

There are also some disadvantages associated with living and working in such a culturally diverse society. Problems arise when differences across and within cultural groups are misunderstood. Misperception, confusion, and ignorance often accompany people's expectations of others. Figure 12-2 illustrates the many areas in which individuals may differ.

Members of some cultural groups have historically and globally experienced bias or prejudice in the forms of racism (discrimination based on race and biological differences), sexism (discrimination based on gender), and classism (prejudice based on perceived social class). These biases are perpetuated (consciously and unconsciously) by society. The basic underlying premise of these biases is that one way is better or "right," and every other way is inferior. **Ethnocentrism**, an assumption of cultural superiority and an inability to accept other cultures' ways of organizing reality, results in oppression. **Oppression** occurs when the rules, modes, and ideals of one group are imposed on another group. Oppression is based on cultural biases, which stem from values, beliefs, traditions, and cultural expectations.

Stereotyping is the belief that all people within the same racial, ethnic, or cultural group will act alike and share the same beliefs and attitudes. Stereotyping results in labeling people according to cultural preconceptions, thereby ignoring individual identity.

A **dominant culture** is the group whose values prevail within a given society. The dominant culture of the United States is that composed of white, middle-class Protestants of European ancestry. The European value orientation has greatly influenced U. S. culture, as illustrated by the following beliefs held by the dominant culture:

- Achievement and success
- Individualism, independence, and self-reliance
- Activity, work, and ownership
- Efficiency, practicality, and reliance on technology
- Material comfort
- Competition and achievement
- Youth and beauty

Frequently, these dominant values conflict with the values of minority groups. A **minority group** is a group of people that constitutes less than a numerical majority of the population. Because of their cultural, racial, ethnic, religious, or other characteristics, such groups are often labeled and treated differently from others in the society. Minority groups are usually considered to be less powerful than the dominant group (Giger & Davidhizar, 1999).

People assume the characteristics of the dominant culture through **acculturation**, which is the process of learning norms, beliefs, and behavioral expectations of a group. **Cultural assimilation** occurs when individuals from a minority group are absorbed by the dominant culture and take on the characteristics of the dominant culture.

Components of Culture

Stewart has identified five components of culture that organize the way people think about life (as cited in Lock, 1992).

- Activity: identifies how people organize and value work
- Social relations: explains the importance and structure of friendships, gender roles, and class
- Motivation: describes the value and methods of achievement
- Perception of the world: refers to the interpretation of life events and religious beliefs
- Perception of self and the individual: refers to personal identity, value, and respect for individuals

 CULTURAL CONSIDERATIONS

Individuality

Remember that each person is first and foremost an individual, and secondly a member of a cultural group. While similarities may exist within an ethnic or culture group, individual differences must also be respected.

This model is particularly helpful to the nurse who is planning care for a client from another ethnic group. Work, social relationships, success, religion, and self-identity influence both the definition cultural groups attribute to health and illness and the cultural group's response to health events. For example, if a culture values relationships more than work, the culture may sanction an extended period of illness and a lengthy time away from the employment site. However, if a culture measures achievement by output at work, illness may be interpreted in a negative manner. Members of the latter culture may deny illness and delay seeking appropriate health care.

Characteristics of Culture

Spradley and Allender (1996) have identified five characteristics shared by all cultures.

- Culture is learned. Patterns of behavior are acquired as children imitate adults and develop actions and attitudes acceptable by others in society.
- Culture is not inherited or innate, but, rather, culture is integrated throughout all the interrelated components. Activities, relationships, motivations, world views, and individuality are permeated with consistent patterns of behavior to form a cohesive whole.
- Culture is shared by everyone who belongs to the cultural group. Behavioral patterns are not individually defined, but, rather, are accepted and practiced by all.
- Culture is tacit (unspoken), in that acceptable behavior is understood by everyone in the cultural group, regardless of whether beliefs are written down or spoken. Cultural beliefs are commonly known and adopted.
- Culture is dynamic; it is constantly changing. Each generation experiences new ideas that may generate different standards for behavior.

CULTURAL INFLUENCES ON HEALTH CARE BELIEFS AND PRACTICES

It is common for cultural groups to have a body of knowledge and beliefs about health and disease. Cultural practices can positively and negatively affect health and disease distribution. In cultures where raw foods are not consumed, for instance, the incidence of shigellosis may be lower than cultures where consumption of raw meat and fish is common. On the other hand, cultural taboos against eating protein during pregnancy have a harmful or destructive effect on fetal development. Human responses to illness are defined by cultural values. Whether an individual seeks professional care when ill and complies with prescribed treatment depends on cultural values.

PROFESSIONAL TIP

Cultural Sensitivity

Nurses must be able to provide culturally appropriate care to a diverse population of clients. Cultural diversity presents special challenges for nurses who must provide care that is incongruent with personal beliefs and values. Nurses caring for clients who differ from themselves must remember to ascertain the client's perception of the event (illness), including the significance (meaning) that the client assigns the event. The nurse must honor individual differences and understand that culture influences the way clients are viewed and treated within health care settings.

Beliefs and patterns of behavior affect attitudes about various aspects of health. Beliefs about the definition of health; etiology (cause and origin of disease); health promotion and protection practices; and health practitioners and remedies are all influenced by cultural background. Clients tend to define wellness and illness in the context of their own culture (Estin, 1999).

Definition of Health

The most widely accepted definition of health, developed by the World Health Organization (WHO), purports that health is not only the absence of disease, but also complete physical, mental, and social wellness. While this definition of health is broad enough to be global, that which is understood to be physical, mental, and social wellness is culturally defined. Any deviation from that which is culturally understood to be normal health is considered illness. For example, a biological disease of immediate etiology might not be interpreted as an illness by some cultures; intestinal parasites are so common in some areas in Africa that the presence of ascaris in stools is considered normal. When the cultural group does not recognize certain behaviors or symptoms as illness, individuals are not likely to seek medical intervention when these symptoms appear. In such cases, disease conditions may persist untreated to an irreversible state.

Etiology

Peter Morley, a noted medical anthropologist, presents four views of the origin of disease: supernatural, nonsupernatural, immediate, and ultimate (Morley & Wallis, 1978). The supernatural view of disease traces disease to metaphysical forces such as witchcraft, sorcery, and voodoo. In this view, an individual might ascribe illness to evil spirits or to a curse by a powerful spiritual person. The nonsupernatural view holds that diseases have an accepted cause-and-effect relationship, even though that relationship may lack scientific rationale. For example, people of many cultures believe that colic in an infant is caused by breast milk rendered impure when a nursing mother has sexual relations. In such cultures, sexual relations are prohibited for nursing mothers. The immediate view of disease traces diseases to known pathogenic agents, such as chickenpox is caused by *Herpes varicella;* and the ultimate view describes determinates for diseases, such as smoking resulting in lung cancer. Most cultural groups support a multietiologic origin, borrowing from three or all four explanations for how and why diseases occur.

Health Promotion and Protection

Strategies for achieving and maintaining good health vary by cultural group. For example, the dominant U.S. culture has come to endorse a low-fat, high-fiber diet; regular exercise; and appropriate immunizations as means to promote and protect health. Other cultures may place greater value on meditation, prayer, and restored relationships, particularly those cultures wherein health protection and disease prevention are closely linked to beliefs about disease etiology. For example, preventing disease may require paying homage to ancestral spirits in order to avoid offending them and provoking their revenge through illness.

Practitioners and Remedies

Variety in health/illness care providers is a natural extension of culturally diverse concepts of etiology and definitions of health and illness. Alternative remedies and practitioners are characteristic of culturally diverse groups. When a scientific rationale for the etiology of disease is not accepted by a cultural group, standard medicine may not be accepted as treatment. In order to enhance client compliance with treatment regimens health care providers must make efforts to base therapy and prescribe treatments that respect culturally traditional remedies. Clients who trace disease etiology to a supernatural cause are more likely to seek interventions from spiritual leaders or traditional healers.

The folk medicine system categorizes illnesses as either natural or unnatural (Giger & Davidhizar, 1999). The classification of an illness determines the type of treatment and healer used. Because the folk medicine system (also referred to as alternative medicine) can present challenges to nurses caring for clients from diverse cultures, knowledge of basic beliefs about illness, factors contributing to illness, and home remedies is necessary.

Folk healers are knowledgeable about cultural norms and customs (Edelman & Mandle, 1998). Table 12–1 lists both the various healers within the five dominant cultural groups in the United States (European American, African American, Hispanic American, Asian American, and Native American) and the common folk healing practices within these cultures. Nurses must be able to relate care and treatment to the client's cultural context and incorporate informal caregivers, healers, and other members of the client's support system as allies in treatment.

Beliefs of Select Cultural Groups

While the population of the United States encompasses innumerable ethnic groups—European Americans, African Americans, Hispanic Americans, Asian Americans, and Native Americans together represent a majority. These groups form the basis for the following brief discussion of specific health beliefs influenced by culture.

European American

In 1990, Americans of European descent represented 75% of the U.S. population; this figure is expected to be only 53% by the year 2020, however (U.S. Department of Commerce, Bureau of the Census, 1999). The prevailing value system for many European Americans is based on what is referred to as the white, Anglo-Saxon, Protestant (WASP) ethic (Sue & Sue, 1999). This ethnic group traces its origins to the Caucasian Protestants who came to this country from Northern Europe over 200 years ago. Values that still dominate the Caucasian American middle-class ethic include independence, individuality, wealth, comfort, cleanliness, achievement, punctuality, hard work, aggression, assertiveness, rationality, orientation toward the future, and mastery of one's own fate (Andrews & Boyle, 1998; Edmission, 1997).

Traditionally, most Caucasian Americans have wanted to be recognized as individuals rather than as members of groups. Thus, Caucasian Americans, unlike members of many other cultures, tend to be competitive rather than cooperative with each other. Mainstream American culture also values the nuclear family and its traditions (Luckmann, 1999).

African American

The African American population currently represents the largest minority group in the United States (U.S. Department of Commerce, Bureau of the Census,

CULTURAL CONSIDERATIONS

Subculture

Many Caucasian Americans do not belong to the mainstream culture, but, instead, belong to ethnic subcultures that hold strong values of their own (e.g., Irish, Jewish, German, Italian, Norwegian, Appalachian, and Amish subcultures).

Table 12–1 FOLK MEDICINE: HEALERS AND PRACTICES

CULTURAL GROUP	TRADITIONAL HEALERS	HEALING PRACTICES
European American	• Nurse • Physician	• Exercise • Medications • Modified diets • Amulets • Religious healing rituals
African American	• Elderly women healers • "Community Mother" or "Granny" • "Root doctor" • Voodoo healer ("Mambo" or "oungan") • Spiritualist	• Herbs, roots, oils • Poultices • Religious healing through rituals (e.g., laying on of hands) • Talismans worn around the wrist or neck or carried in a pouch to ward off disease
Hispanic American	• Curandero • Espiritualista • Yerbero (herbalist) • Brujo (healer who uses witchcraft) • Sobadora • Santiguadora	• Hot and cold foods to treat some conditions • Herbal teas, such as manzanilla, to treat gastrointestinal problems, insomnia, and menstrual cramps • Prayers and religious medals • Massage • Azabache, a black stone, worn as a necklace or bracelet to ward off the "evil eye" • Among some Haitian mothers, the "three baths" ritual (bathing for the first 3 postpartum days in water boiled with special leaves)
Asian American	• Herbalist • Physician	• Hot and cold foods • Herbs, soups • Cupping, pinching, and rubbing • Meditation • Acupuncture • Acupressure • Application of tiger balm (a salve) to relieve muscular pains • Energy to restore balance between yin and yang
Native American	• Shaman • Medicine man/woman	• Plants and herbs • Medicine bundle or bag filled with herbs that have been blessed by a medicine man/woman during a healing ceremony • Sweet grass (herbs) burned to purify the ill person • Estafiate (dried leaves) boiled to produce a tea for treating stomach disorders • The Blessingway ceremony (a healing ritual conducted by the medicine man/woman) • In some Navajo tribes, sand paintings made by the medicine man/woman for diagnostic purposes

Data compiled from Cultural Diversity and Community Health Nursing Practice, by C. Degazon, in Community Health Nursing *(5th ed.), by M. Stanhope and J. Lancaster (Eds.), 2000, St. Louis: Mosby-Yearbook; Transcultural Nursing: Assessment and Interventions (3rd ed.), by J. Giger and R. Davidhizar, 1999, St. Louis, MO: Mosby-Yearbook; and Cultural Dimensions in Home Health Nursing, by D. Grossman, 1996, American Journal of Nursing, 96(7).*

1999). African American ancestors came to North America from various African countries and the Caribbean as either slaves or free immigrants. The different countries of origin as well as disparate educational levels, income, occupations, and religious beliefs explain the heterogeneous (different) cultural practices among African Americans today.

Some African American beliefs about health and illness are linked to either a supernatural or a nonsupernatural view of disease. In traditional African societies, disease may be viewed as caused by disharmony in relationships. Discord may occur between a client and ancestral spirits, evil spirits, or living relatives. For example, if, following a wedding, a man were to refuse to finish making bride-price payments to his in-laws and the man were subsequently to become ill, his illness may be attributed to the break in relations with his wife's family caused by his outstanding debt. Healing comes with restoration of harmony and may be achieved through prayer, meditation, or activities considered to be therapeutic, such as offering a gift, wearing a charm, or confessing a wrong.

Disease may also be viewed as sent by God or another higher power as a punishment for a serious infraction against Him or another person. Evil forces may be thought to account for illness in other cases. Treatments may be found in herbs and home remedies, consultation with a local healer, and prayer.

Hispanic American

Hispanic Americans constitute the second largest minority ethnic group in the United States. The majority of this group has origins in Mexico, Puerto Rico, and Cuba. Although the Spanish language is common to most Hispanics, cultural patterns vary due to the different countries of origin. In general, the Hispanic American belongs to a large extended-family system within which females are seen as subservient to males but as having a major role in family cohesiveness (Giger & Davidhizar, 1999).

The influence of religion on culture is particularly evident in Hispanic populations. Most Hispanic Americans have roots in Catholicism blended with traditional Indian beliefs. Illness may be viewed as having a natural cause, as "an act of God" as punishment for sin, or as the result of witchcraft or a curse by an enemy. Diseases may be traced to an imbalance between "wet" and "dry" or "hot" and "cold" forces. Treatment depends on the cause. Western medicine is appropriate for some diseases, whereas the native healer (curandera) may have to intervene for illnesses having supernatural causes. Treatment may consist of herbal potions, diets based on hot and cold foods, or religious ceremonies.

Asian American

Asian Americans have origins in the Pacific-rim countries: Korea, Vietnam, Laos, the Philippines, Cambodia, China, and Japan. Generalization of a specific Asian culture is not possible among peoples from such a diversity of countries; however, certain similarities exist. Asian cultures are typically patrilineal, that is, family relations are traced through males. Males are the heads of household, and decision-makers, and elders are respected. Only physical complaints are acceptable, and maintaining eye contact is considered disrespectful (Estin, 1999).

Asians hold to a yin (cold) and yang (hot) etiology of disease. **Yin and yang** are opposing forces that when in balance yield health (Figure 12-3). Illness occurs as a consequence of an imbalance in these forces.

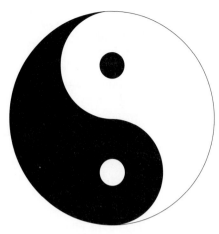

Figure 12-3 Yin and Yang

Foods are identified as either hot or cold and are used in treatment. For example, if yang is overpowering yin, hot foods are avoided until balance is restored. Illness may also be viewed as being caused by supernatural powers such as God, evil spirits, or ancestral spirits. In this situation, healing might be attained through prayer or treatment by a traditional healer. Many Asian Americans rely on herbal remedies, acupuncture, and cupping and burning, a treatment that draws blood to the skin's surface when a warmed cup is placed on the skin. In cupping, the inside and rim of a cup are heated with a candle flame. The rim of the cup is then applied directly to the client's skin, and, as the cup cools, blood is drawn to the surface of the skin, causing a bruised appearance. Cupping is used to draw out evil or illness in order to restore yin and yang. The nurse must be aware of these cultural practices so they are not viewed as abuse but, rather, as important cultural customs.

Native American

The fourth major minority ethnic group in the United States is Native Americans (U.S. Department of Commerce, Bureau of the Census, 1999). These peoples form a very diverse group, stemming from over 200 different tribes across the United States. Although many Native Americans have assumed Euro-American practices with regard to health, some still use traditional practices. Health is believed to result from a harmonious relationship with nature and the universe. Illness is frequently traced to a supernatural origin and discord with the forces of nature. Use of witchcraft can cause illness, and treatment may require exorcism of evil spirits. Prevention may be attained through prayer, charms, and fetishes (objects having power to protect or aid the owner). Remedies often include herbal drinks. "Medicine men" are persons thought to have supernatural powers of healing. Through prayers, rituals, ceremonies, and herbal drinks, health may be restored.

CULTURAL AND RACIAL INFLUENCES ON CLIENT CARE

Clients' cultural backgrounds and preferences influence the manner whereby they interact with other people and with the world around them. In an unfamiliar situation, such as admission to a health care setting, cultural differences may seem even greater, because in times of stress, most people hold tightly to that which is familiar in order to protect themselves from the unknown. The nurse can show caring in such a situation by acknowledging the expression of these differences and encouraging the client to retain what is familiar.

The influences of culture and race can be viewed through the phenomena of communication, space and time orientation, social organization, and biological variations.

Communication

Although language is common to all human beings, not everyone shares the same language. This cultural difference can lead to misunderstanding and frustration. The nurse must realize that a client who speaks a different language or with an accent, simply has a different means of expressing needs. When communication is restricted because of language differences, alternative methods of communication such as gestures and flash cards can be used.

The client's family may be able to assist when there is a block in communication. Family members can interpret procedures and instructions for the client and communicate the client's thoughts and questions to the nurse (Figure 12-4). If no family members are avail-

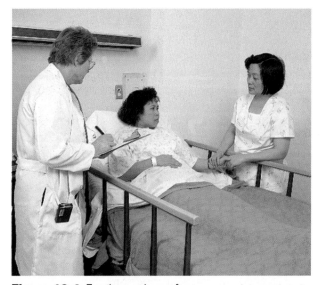

Figure 12-4 Family members often serve as interpreters to help clients who do not speak English understand procedures and instructions and to communicate the client's thoughts and questions to the nurse.

PROFESSIONAL TIP

Non-native Speakers
When interacting with someone who does not understand English well, many people will try to compensate for the lack of understanding by speaking loudly. Speaking slowly, distinctly, and in a normal volume are more effective measures to ensure communication.

able, the hospital social worker may be able to find an interpreter.

Orientation to Space and Time

Orientation with regard to space and to time represents two other culturally influenced variables that may affect a client's attitude toward care. Territoriality, or interpretation of personal space, is a pattern of behavior resulting from an individual's belief that certain spaces and objects belong to that person. The distance that a person prefers to maintain from another is determined by one's culture. In general, people of Arabic, Southern European, and African origin frequently sit or stand relatively close to each other (0 to 18 inches), whereas people from Asian, Northern European, and North American origin are more comfortable with a larger personal space (more than 18 inches).

Affection and caring behavior are not communicated by touch in some cultures. For instance, among Asians, adults seldom touch one another, and the head is believed to be sacred. The nurse should thus not touch an Asian client's head without permission to do so. When working with clients from cultures where personal touch is viewed negatively, the nurse should use the universal sign of caring: the smile.

People in U.S. society tend to be future oriented: They plan for the future, establish long-term goals, and, increasingly, are concerned with prevention of future illnesses. In daily life, they are oriented to time of day, constantly referring to clock time for everything from meal time to time of appointments with health care professionals as well as other obligations. The nurse must also be very attentive to time. Medications are given at scheduled times, and work begins and ends at specified times. Other groups that tend to be future oriented are Japanese, Jews, and Arabs. These groups tend to view time as a commodity for achieving future goals.

Not all cultural groups are future oriented, however. People of some cultures (e.g., Asians) may be oriented to the past. For Asians, this orientation is reflected in the roles that ancestor worship and Confucianism play in the present. Members of other cultural groups, such as Native Americans, tend to be present oriented. Many Native Americans do not own clocks, and they live one day at a time, showing little concern for the future (Giger & Davidhizer, 1999). Mexican Americans and African Americans often value relationships with people in the present more than in the future. African Americans tend to be present oriented in health care behaviors as well. They often express the fatalistic belief that "it's going to happen anyway, so why bother" and fail to seek medical attention until a disabling condition occurs. The African American culture often teaches flexible attention to schedules; whatever is happening currently is most important. Explanations about the necessity of time scheduling, for instance, the need for strict schedules for medication requiring therapeutic blood level maintenance, must be given to the client.

How does time orientation affect health care? An individual's orientation to time may affect promptness or attendance at health care appointments, compliance with self-medication schedules, and reporting the onset of illness or other health concerns. Clients might not see the necessity for preventive health care measures if they experience no difference in their health today when they follow a special diet or exercise programs. The nurse must both teach clients when timing is critical in health care situations and practice patience when working with people whose background differs from that of the dominant culture.

Social Organization

Social organization refers to the ways that cultural groups determine rules of acceptable behavior and roles of individual members. Examples of social organization include family structure, gender roles, and religion.

Family Structure

The definition of family has changed dramatically through the years (Doherty, 1992). Until 1920 the norm was the "institutional family," which was organized around economic production and the kinship network. Marriage was a functional, not a romantic, relationship. Family tradition and loyalty were more important than individual goals or romantic interests. The chief value was responsibility.

CULTURAL CONSIDERATIONS

Environmental Control

Environmental control refers to the relationships between people and nature and to a person's perceived ability to control activities of nature, such as factors causing illness. One's cultural background and heritage influence one's perception of environmental control.

PROFESSIONAL TIP

Families

Each individual defines family differently. These definitions are shaped by personal experience and observation of other families. You must remain objective and nonjudgmental when the client's family is different from your idea of family. Have the client identify family members, so you know exactly who the client considers to be family.

From 1920 to 1960, the norm was the "psychological family." Family affairs were more private and less tied to the extended kinship network. Family was based on personal satisfaction and fulfillment of the individual members in a nuclear, two-parent arrangement. The chief value was satisfaction.

The social changes of the 1960s, including gender equality and personal freedom, caused changes in the family. The increased divorce rate may have resulted from the sexual revolution and the attitude that the individual deserves more and owes less to the family.

Today, no single family arrangement has a monopoly. Many types of families have emerged and are accepted. The chief value is flexibility. Family no longer necessarily implies biological relation, but rather has come to mean members of a shared household who have similar values and participate in shared goals. Fawcett (1993) cites the following characteristics of family:

- Love and affection
- Caring and compassion
- A sense of belonging and connectedness
- A history and linkage to posterity
- Rituals of rejoicing
- A sense of place
- Acceptance of members, including shortcomings
- Honor of elders
- A system of earning and spending money
- A competent manner of parenting or caretaking
- Division of chores and labor

According to systems theory, families are considered to be interdependent, interacting individuals related by birth, marriage, or mutual consent (Sherman, 1994). Examples of families with varying lifestyles today are two-parent nuclear, single-parent, blended (through remarriage), extended (including grandparents), cohabitating (couple having never married), gay or lesbian, divorced, adoptive, multi-adult, and mixed or interracial families (Figure 12-5).

Gender Roles

Gender roles vary according to cultural context (Figure 12-6). For example, in families organized around a

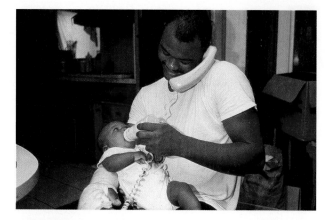

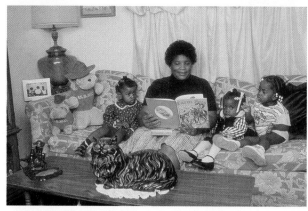

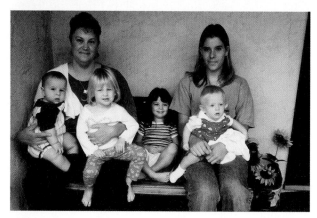

Figure 12-5 Families come in all shapes, sizes, and configurations.

COMMUNITY/HOME HEALTH CARE

Culturally Sensitive Care

To provide culturally sensitive care in the home:

- Remember that the setting for care is controlled by the client and family, not by the health care provider.
- Be sensitive to the fact that the nurse is often viewed as a guest by the client and family. Social chatter may be necessary to facilitate rapport.
- Be nonjudgmental about the condition of the home (e.g., presence of clutter and disarray).
- Show respect and consideration for the client. For example:
  - Wipe your feet before entering the home.
  - Ask permission to use the sink or bathroom to wash your hands.
  - Ask permission before moving the client's belongings and replace items after you have finished the task.
- Take advantage of the home environment to assess cultural values and norms. Clues to cultural values may include:
  - Decor and possessions on display in the home.
  - Assignment of family roles and tasks.
  - Types of interactions among family members.
  - Value placed on privacy.
  - Value placed on possessions.

patriarchal structure (with the man being the head of the household and chief authority figure), the husband/father is the dominant member. Such expectations are typically the cultural norm in Latino, Hispanic, and traditional Muslim families. The husband/father is the one who makes decisions regarding health care for all family members. Also, in such cultures, the wife is responsible for child care and household maintenance, whereas the father's role is to protect and support the family members (Grossman, 1996).

Religion

Anthropologists have identified the strength of the influence of religion on culture. In many cases, culture

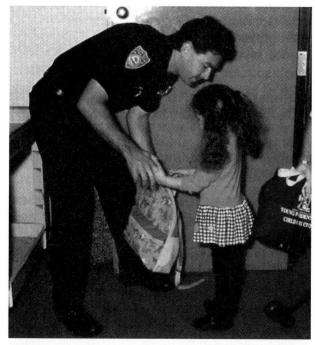

Figure 12-6 One example of changing gender roles is fathers assuming more responsibility in caring for children.

and tradition have been maintained and preserved through religious beliefs. Religion often includes the formal organizational structures for social behavior.

Spiritual and religious beliefs are important in many individuals' lives. These beliefs can influence lifestyle, attitudes, and feelings about life, pain, and death. Some organized religions specify practices about diet, birth control, and appropriate medical care. Spiritual beliefs often assume a greater significance at the time of illness than at any other time in a person's life. These beliefs help some people accept their own illnesses and help explain illness for others. Spiritual beliefs often help people plan for the future. Religion can both help people live fuller lives as well as strengthen or console people during suffering and in preparation for inevitable death. By providing meaning to life and death, religion can supply the client, the family, and the nurse with a sense of strength, security, and faith during a time of need.

Spiritual needs are identified as an individual's desire to find meaning and purpose in life, pain, and death. The spiritual realm is often considered a very private area. In order to provide holistic care, however, the nurse must pay attention to the spiritual dimension of each client, recognizing spiritual needs and assisting the client in meeting them (Figure 12-7).

Although spiritual needs are recognized by many nurses, **spiritual care** (recognition of spiritual needs and the assistance given toward meeting those needs) is often neglected. Spirituality is characterized as an individual's search to find meaning and purpose in life. The goal of spiritual nursing care is to enable clients to identify and utilize their spiritual beliefs as coping mechanisms when faced with a health crisis. Among the reasons that nurses fail to provide spiritual care are the following:

- They feel that spirituality is a private matter.
- They are uninformed about the religious beliefs of others.
- They have not identified their own spiritual beliefs.
- They view meeting the spiritual needs of the client as a family or clergy responsibility, not a nursing responsibility.

Spiritual nursing care is appropriate when the nurse cares about the client's emotional, physical, and psychosocial health. The nursing diagnosis, *Spiritual Distress*, can be apparent in a client who is unable to practice religious or spiritual rituals due to illness or confinement in a health care institution.

The **religious support system** is a group of ministers, priests, rabbis, nuns, mullahs, shamans, or laypersons who are able to meet clients' spiritual needs in the health care setting. The nurse has the responsibility of working with these individuals, including them in the client care team.

Nurses must be aware of the general philosophies of their clients' spiritual beliefs, and also be aware that some individuals do not believe in a higher being or practice a specific religion. **Agnostics** believe that the existence of God cannot be proved or disproved, whereas **atheists** do not believe in God or any other deity.

It is important to identify particular beliefs from various religions that can influence client care activities. Some of these beliefs concern holy day practices, dietary restrictions, birth, death, and organ donation.

Protestant Many separate denominations (over 1,200) constitute the group known as Protestant. Protestant groups include such denominations as Baptist, Episcopal, Lutheran, Methodist, Presbyterian, and Seventh Day Adventist. The majority worship on Sunday, and their primary written reference is the Holy Bible.

Baptist Baptists do not practice infant baptism. For them, baptism is a rite to be performed only after a believer reaches an age of understanding and confesses his acceptance of the saving work of Jesus Christ. Communion is a spiritual act and symbolizes the suffering, death, and resurrection of the Lord.

Episcopal Episcopalians have a number of sacraments including confession, anointing of the sick (Holy Unction), communion, and baptism. Holy Unction is most often given as a healing sacrament. Episcopalians believe that a dying infant should be baptized, and the nurse may perform the rite. The usual administration of these sacraments is by an Episcopal priest.

Lutheran Traditionally, Lutherans practice baptism of infants and adults by sprinkling. Emergency baptisms may be performed by any baptized Christian. The Lutheran churches recognize two sacraments, baptism and Holy Communion. Holy Communion is understood

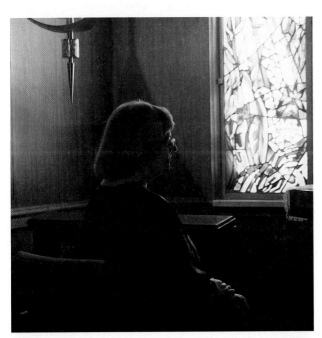

Figure 12-7 Spiritual needs often increase when individuals are sick.

as the body and the blood of the Lord and is often administered to those who are ill or awaiting surgery. Central to the Lutheran belief is the doctrine of "justification by faith." People are redeemed by God solely on the basis of God's grace, which they receive through faith or acceptance of what God has done for them.

Methodist Methodists practice both infant and adult baptism. They believe that religion is a matter of personal belief, and they use the conscience as a guide for living.

Presbyterian Presbyterians also practice communion, remembering the death of Jesus Christ for them and baptism. Salvation is believed to be a gift from God.

Seventh Day Adventist Seventh Day Adventists do not believe in infant baptism, but baptize individuals when they reach an age of accountability. They follow some dietary restrictions. Their Sabbath worship is observed from sunset on Friday to sunset on Saturday. They do not pursue their jobs or worldly pleasures during this time.

Roman Catholic Various rites known as Sacraments (sacred) are performed by the priest at appropriate times in the life of the Catholic. Sacraments that might be encountered in the health care setting are: baptism, the Eucharist (Communion), confession, and sacrament of the sick. Baptism, administered only once in the life of a Catholic, is believed to be absolutely necessary for salvation. A client preparing to take communion is normally asked to abstain from food or drink for an hour before the rite, although water and medications are allowed at any time. Confession is a rite for the forgiveness of sins. It is a very private matter and should be respected. The Sacrament of the Sick, in which the client is anointed with holy oil, was formerly known as the "last rites" given to someone near death.

Orthodox The Orthodox churches express their love of God through worship liturgies. It is important to the church that they remain faithful to the teachings of the ancient church. Holy Unction is practiced using oil to anoint the body for healing of bodily and spiritual infirmities. Baptism is also important; in life-threatening situations involving an unbaptized child an emergency baptism is performed.

Jehovah's Witness Jehovah's Witnesses are prohibited from receiving any blood or blood products, including plasma. They also will not eat anything containing blood. Blood volume expanders are permissible if they are not derivatives of blood. In some cases, children have been made wards of the court so that they could receive blood when a medical condition requiring blood transfusion was life-threatening. They have a special observance of the Lord's Supper.

Mormon (Church of Jesus Christ of the Latter Day Saints) Mormons do not believe in baptizing infants, but will baptize at the age of eight years. If necessary, baptism of the dead will be performed for adults. Mormons wear a special undergarment that has

special significance symbolizing dedication to God. This garment may be worn under the hospital gown.

Christian Science Christian Scientists generally believe that illness can be eliminated through prayer and spiritual understanding. Healing is considered an awakening to this belief. When a critically ill Christian Scientist client is admitted to a health care facility they may wish to have a Christian Science practitioner contacted to give treatment through prayer. Christian Scientists ordinarily do not use medicine, agree to surgical procedures, or accept blood transfusions.

American Indian Religions All life is sacred and all things are interconnected is the central belief of the various religions. Community importance is emphasized. The individual who is able to communicate with the spirits or the Great Spirit is the spiritual leader. There are no written religious books. Religious traditions are passed on orally and through participation in ceremonies and festivals. Illness may be the result of a sin or a spirit or god who is unhappy.

Judaism Judaism is both a religious faith and an ethnic identity. The religion is based on the five books of Moses called the Torah. Culture and religion are deeply interwoven in the Jewish faith. As a result, ritual, tradition, ceremony, religious and social laws, and the observance of holy days are major influences in the Jewish daily life.

There are three groups in Judaism: Orthodox, Conservative, and Reformed. All share the fundamental teachings of Judaism but vary in how strictly they follow the traditions. Orthodox Jews strictly observe all traditional practices. The Conservative group observes many of the traditional practices, and the Reformed group interprets traditions loosely.

The rabbi is the spiritual leader of the Jewish congregation and is the representative to be informed when a client of the Jewish faith requests it.

The Jewish Sabbath, the day of worship, begins at sunset on Friday and ends at sunset on Saturday.

Circumcision is a religious custom in Judaism that is performed on the male infant eight days after birth. It may be done by the pediatrician or by the Mohel who may be a rabbi.

Islam The religion of Muslims is Islam. They believe that Allah is the supreme deity and that Mohammed, the founder of Islam, is the chief prophet. The Muslim's holy day of worship extends from sunset on Thursday to sunset on Friday. Some Muslims may desire to pray to their god Allah five times a day (after dawn, at noon, at mid-afternoon, after sunset, and at night). If the client requests that he face Mecca, the holy city of Islam, a bed or chair may be positioned facing the southeast direction (if in the continental United States). The Muslim client may be wearing an article of writing from the Koran on a piece of string around his neck, arm, or waist. This should not be allowed to get wet or to be removed. Rules of cleanliness include eating with the right hand and cleansing self with the left hand after urinating or defecating. Medications or other materials should be handed to the Muslim client with the right hand so as not to offend them, as they consider the left hand dirty.

Some Islamic females prefer to be clothed from head to ankle. During the physical examination, they may prefer to undress one body part at a time. They may refuse to be cared for by male nurses or physicians.

Buddhism Buddhism is a general term that indicates a belief in Buddha, "the enlightened one." Nirvana, a state of greater inner freedom and spontaneity, is the goal of existence. When one achieves Nirvana, the mind has supreme peace, purity, and strength. Buddhism does not dictate any specific practices or sacraments. There are no religious restrictions for therapy or special holy days. Buddhists do not believe in healing through faith. The religious support system for the sick is the priest. The Buddhist believes in reincarnation. Figure 12-8 shows the inside of a Buddhist temple.

Hindu Hinduism has no common creeds or doctrines that bind Hindus together. The major distinguishing characteristic is the social caste system. The religion of Hinduism is founded on the Scripture called the Vedas. Brahma is the principal source of the universe and the center from which all things proceed and to which all things return. Reincarnation is a central belief in Hindu thought. The goal of existence is freedom from the cycle of rebirth and death and en-

trance into what the Hindus, like the Buddhists, call Nirvana. Hindu temples are dwelling places for deities to which people bring offerings. Some Hindus believe in faith healing; others believe that illness is God's way of punishing a person for sins.

Biological Variation

Biological variations distinguish one cultural or racial group from another. Common obvious biological variations include hair texture, skin color, thickness of lips, eye shape, and body structure (Degazon, 2000). Biological variations that are less obvious include enzymatic differences and susceptibility to disease (Andrews & Boyle, 1998; Giger & Davidhizar, 1999). Enzymatic differences account for diverse responses of some groups to dietary therapy and drugs (Table 12–2).

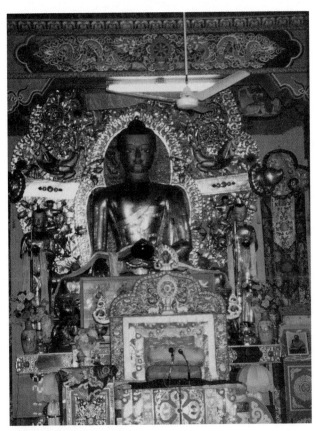

Figure 12-8 Inside of a Buddhist Temple. (*Photo courtesy of John White, Corpus Christi, TX.*)

Table 12–2 EFFECTS OF BIOLOGICAL VARIATIONS ON SELECT DRUGS	
CULTURAL GROUP	**EFFECT OF BIOLOGICAL VARIATION ON DRUG ACTION**
European American	• Due to liver enzyme difference, caffeine is metabolized and excreted faster than by people of other cultural groups.
African American	• Isoniazid (drug used to treat tuberculosis) is rapidly metabolized, thus becoming inactive quickly: occurs in approximately 60% of population. • An enzyme deficiency interferes with metabolism of primaquine (used to treat malaria); occurs in approximately 35% of population. • Antihypertensive drugs (e.g., propranolol) must be administered in higher doses to produce same effects as in European Americans.
Hispanic American	None noted
Asian American	• Isoniazid is rapidly metabolized, thus becoming inactive quickly; occurs in approximately 85% to 90% of population. • Rapid metabolism of alcohol results in excessive facial flushing and other vasomotor symptoms. • Chinese men need only approximately half as much propranolol (antihypertensive drug) to produce same effects as in European American men.
Native American	• Isoniazid is rapidly metabolized, thus becoming inactive quickly; occurs in approximately 60% to 90% of population. • Rapid metabolism of alcohol results in excessive facial flushing and other vasomotor symptoms.

Data from Transcultural Nursing: Assessment and Intervention *(3rd ed.), by J. Giger and R. Davidhizar, 1999, St. Louis: Mosby-Yearbook.*

CULTURAL ASPECTS AND THE NURSING PROCESS

Each individual comes from a cultural background that, in some way, influences behavior and attitudes about health and illness. Personal attitudes and behaviors determine not only the ways that clients interpret health events and utilize health care, but also the ways that nurses interpret health events and provide health care. The central role that culture plays in determining perception compels health care providers to evaluate their personal views about health and illness before examining those of clients from other cultural groups. Nurses must be able to recognize the way that culture affects the health care needs of clients and respond appropriately.

Assessment

Culturally sensitive nursing care begins with an examination of one's own culture and beliefs. It is followed by an assessment of the client's cultural beliefs and background.

PROFESSIONAL TIP

Culturally Diverse Coworkers

Many nursing units represent a mix of nationalities and cultures. While such a mix has the potential of improving nursing care, in practice it often leads to conflict and poor teamwork. The same cultural differences discussed in relation to clients may also be found among coworkers. Grensing-Pophal (1997) suggests five ways to successfully manage diversity in the workplace:

- Be aware of your own biases, and strive to avoid stereotyping others.
- Be aware of the way the things you do and say affect others.
- Help others to be more sensitive and help correct misconceptions.
- Learn to welcome different opinions and viewpoints.
- Be open to feedback.

Learn more about your coworkers and remember that respect for individual differences reflects acknowledgment of each person's uniqueness. Have a unit conference focusing on a cultural assessment of each other. Grossman and Taylor (1995) suggest having a potluck lunch, with everyone bringing a typical ethnic dish. Such strategies might also work well in a nursing program where various cultures are represented.

Personal Cultural Assessment

Spradley and Allender (1996) identify five areas to be examined in assessing one's own culture and the influence it may have on personal beliefs about health care.

- Influences from own ethnic/racial background
- Typical verbal and nonverbal communication patterns
- Cultural values and norms
- Religious beliefs and practices
- Health beliefs and practices

They suggest that the nurse should gather as much information as possible on each issue and then validate this information with one or two other persons from the same cultural group.

Client Cultural Assessment

Having examined one's own culture and the influences it may have had in developing personal beliefs about sickness and health, the next step to providing culturally appropriate care is to assess the client's cultural background (Figure 12-9). Data about various cultures may be collected from members of the culture to be studied, from others familiar with the culture, or from the local library.

Spradley and Allender (1996) identify six categories of information necessary for a comprehensive cultural assessment of the client. These categories may also be useful in organizing interviews with representatives from the culture.

- *Ethnic or racial background.* Where did the client group originate, and how does that influence the status and identity of group members?
- *Language and communication patterns.* What is the preferred language spoken, and what are the culturally based communication patterns?
- *Cultural values and norms.* What are the values, beliefs, and standards regarding such things as roles, education, family functions, child-rearing, work and leisure, aging, death and dying, and rites of passage?
- *Biocultural factors.* Are there physical or genetic traits unique to the ethnic or racial group that predispose group members to certain conditions or illnesses?
- *Religious beliefs and practices.* What are the group's religious beliefs, and how do they influence life events, roles, health, and illness?
- *Health beliefs and practices.* What are the group's beliefs and practices regarding prevention, causes, and treatment of illnesses?

Nursing Diagnosis

Any nursing diagnosis may be appropriate for a client of any cultural group. When cultural variables

Cultural Assessment Interview Guide

Name: _____

Nickname or other names or special meaning attributed to your name: _____

Primary language:

      When speaking _____

      When writing _____

Date of birth: _____

Place of birth: _____

Educational level or specialized training: _____

To which ethnic group do you belong? _____

To what extent do you identify with your cultural group? _____

Who is the spokesperson for your family? _____

Describe some of the customs or beliefs that you have about the following:

      Health _____

      Life _____

      Illness _____

      Death _____

How do you best learn information?

    ☐ Reading

    ☐ Having someone explain verbally

    ☐ Having someone demonstrate

Describe some of your family's dietary habits and your personal food preferences: _____

_____

Are there any foods forbidden from your diet for religious or cultural reasons? _____

_____

Describe your religious affiliation: _____

What role do your religious beliefs and practices play in your life during times of good health and bad health? _____

_____

On whom do you rely on for health care services or healing, and to what type of cultural health practices have you been exposed? _____

_____

Are there any sanctions or restrictions in your culture that the person taking care of you should know about? _____

_____

Describe your current living arrangements: _____

How do members of your family communicate with each other? _____

Describe your strengths: _____

Who /what is your primary source of information about your health? _____

Is there anything else that is important about your cultural beliefs that you want to tell me? _____

Figure 12-9 Cultural Assessment Interview Guide (*From* Fundamentals of Nursing: Standards & Practice, *by S. DeLaune and P. Ladner, 1998, Albany, NY: Delmar. Copyright 1998 by Delmar. Reprinted with permission.*)

are identified during assessment, the nurse should be as specific as possible when asking questions and determining appropriate nursing diagnoses, so that interventions can be individualized with respect to the client's cultural beliefs. For instance, *Decreased Cardiac Output* may be viewed by the nurse or physician as having a medical or physical cause, whereas the client may attribute the origin to an imbalance of yin and yang. Table 12–3 lists select nursing diagnoses that are most likely to have cultural implications.

Planning/Outcome Identification

Cultural variables must be taken into consideration when establishing goals and planning interventions. Care will be most effective when the client and family are active participants in planning care, and when cul-

Table 12–3 NURSING DIAGNOSES WITH CULTURAL IMPLICATIONS
Anxiety
Disturbed Body Image
Ineffective Breastfeeding
Impaired Verbal Communication
Compromised Family Coping
Ineffective Coping
Decisional Conflict (specify)
Fear
Anticipatory Grieving
Ineffective Health Maintenance
Health-Seeking Behaviors (specify)
Noncompliance
Imbalanced Nutrition: More Than Body Requirements
Pain
Ineffective Role Performance
Disturbed Sleep Pattern
Impaired Social Interaction
Spiritual Distress

CLIENT TEACHING

Culturally Sensitive Teaching Guidelines

When caring for clients from diverse cultures, consider the following guidelines for client teaching:

- Determine the client's cultural background.
- Evaluate the client's current knowledge base by asking the client to state what he knows about the specific topic.
- To identify the client's perception of need, ask the client and family what they need and want to learn.
- Observe the interaction between the client and family to determine family roles and authority figures. Ask the client whether the dominant family member should be included in teaching and care sessions.
- Use language easily understood by the client, avoiding jargon and complex medical terms.
- Clarify your verbal and nonverbal messages with the client.
- Have the client repeat the information. If feasible, have the client do a return demonstration of the material taught.

tural preferences are respected. Suggested goals to consider when cultural factors are involved include:

- Client will express health care needs to family and caregiver.
- Client will maintain cultural health practices as appropriate.
- Client and family will understand the effect that health care beliefs have on health status.

Implementation

Cultural aspects are always a factor in a nursing care plan, and effective communication and client education are important nursing responsibilities that can enhance cultural understanding and appreciation. Interventions should be carried out in a manner that will respect, to the degree possible, the preferences and desires of the client. When a client does not speak or understand the native language well, the nurse should arrange to have an interpreter present to explain procedures and tests.

Evaluation

Evaluation should include feedback from the client and family to determine their reaction to the interventions. Revisions to the plan of care should be made with client and family input, and alternative sources and resources brought in when needed to enhance communication and exchange of information. Nurses should also perform self-evaluations to identify their attitudes toward caring for clients from diverse cultures.

PROFESSIONAL TIP

Culturally Appropriate Care
- Respect clients for their different beliefs.
- Be sensitive to behaviors and practices different from your own and respond accordingly.
- Accommodate differences if they are not detrimental to health. For example, a client might believe that eating onions will resolve his respiratory infection. While eating onions may not be therapeutic, it is also not likely to negatively impact health.
- Listen for cues in the client's conversation that relay a unique ethnic belief about etiology, transmission, prevention, or some other aspect of disease. For example, a client might say, "I knew I would be sick today. I heard an owl last night."
- Use the occasion to teach positive health habits if the client's practices are deleterious to good health. For example, when asked about her diet, a pregnant woman might reply that she never eats meat or eggs while pregnant because she believes that gaining too much weight will increase her risk of a difficult delivery. Such a situation offers the nurse an opportunity to provide nutritional instruction.

SAMPLE NURSING CARE PLAN

THE FAMILY WITH INEFFECTIVE COPING

Mrs. Chang, a 74-year-old Asian American housewife, was admitted to the hospital with complaints of nausea and difficulty keeping food down related to treatment for recurrent breast cancer with bone metastasis. For the past few weeks, her appetite has been decreasing. She is able to drink some fluids.

Mrs. Chang's husband of 53 years remains at her bedside, as do their two grown daughters. Mrs. Chang insists that they remain at her bedside so that she does not have to bother the nurses for her basic care and insists that the oldest daughter bathe her and walk her to the bathroom. Mr. Chang leaves her bedside only to go home and shower; when he does so, both daughters remain with Mrs. Chang.

The nurses notice that Mr. Chang is looking exhausted and appears to have lost weight. The daughters have tried to relieve their father at night to allow him to go home and rest, but he insists on remaining at the hospital.

Although Mrs. Chang never voices discomfort, she has her husband and daughters constantly massaging her back and legs. She changes position slowly and grimaces with each movement. She does not verbalize to the nursing staff, but lets her family do the talking for her. She denies pain when questioned by the nurse, but she complains of pain to her family. She does not sleep well.

Mrs. Chang's treatment plan is supportive. The hospital staff has mentioned the idea of hospice care to the family. Mrs. Chang has stated that she wants to go home.

Nursing Diagnosis *Compromised Family Coping related to prolonged disease or disability progression that exhausts the supportive capacity of significant people as evidenced by Mr. Chang's looking exhausted.*

PLANNING/GOALS	NURSING INTERVENTIONS	RATIONALE	EVALUATION
Family will plan a specific rotation schedule to meet each other's needs for rest and support while caring for Mrs. Chang.	Provide empathy and support for the husband and daughters. Provide them with unlimited visitation, adequate space for members who stay overnight, and privacy.	The family is one of the most important factors in the life of the Asian American. A sense of obligation to intervene and assist is highly valued. Casual help from strangers is avoided.	Family is sharing bedside care responsibilities. Husband and eldest daughter remain at bedside during daytime hours. Youngest daughter rests at home during the day and exchanges places with the father and eldest sister at night. Mrs. Chang is agreeable.
	Assess family members for signs of fatigue or overexertion.	Asian Americans value self-control and self-sufficiency. To ask for help would mean loss of face and dignity.	
	Explore with husband and daughters other possible extended family members who would be willing and be accepted by Mrs. Chang to keep her company and give her support.	This family will not be able to keep up this vigil for an unknown period of time. Family obligations take precedence over individual desires.	

continues

PLANNING/GOALS	NURSING INTERVENTIONS	RATIONALE	EVALUATION
Client and family will maintain open communication.	Develop trusting and respectful relationships with Mrs. Chang and family members.	Asian Americans tend to be reserved with those whom they view as being in authority. The nurse should remember that this family needs to establish a caring, trusting relationship before they participate in self-disclosure.	Mr. Chang meets with both daughters to discuss their mother's plan of care. He includes the primary care nurse in the discussion.
	Encourage Mr. Chang to have family meetings as necessary to discuss realistic plans and expectations of other family members, using health care providers as needed.	Asians traditionally value authoritarian styles of leadership, where the father makes unilateral family decisions. Authority and communication come from the top down. Discouragement of verbal communication, avoidance of discussion of personal problems, and limited expression of emotion have been noted as common patterns in the traditional Asian family.	
	Encourage and assist family to explore outside resources to assist them in dealing with the crisis.	This family structure cannot maintain bedside attendance without help. The outside resource might take the form of extended family, sisters, brothers, nieces, or nephews of Mrs. Chang who live in the neighborhood.	
Family members will perform client care without compromising their own physical and emotional health.	Assess whether basic physical and emotional needs of Mrs. Chang and family members are being met.	The ideal pattern of communication in Asian society is silent communication. Stoic reactions to pain and other uncertain situations is common. Direct expression of negative feelings is unusual. The nurse will need to assess for nonverbal clues indicating the status of needs.	Mr. Chang and his daughters continue to provide the physical care for Mrs. Chang. Mr. Chang appears more rested and has gained back some weight. The daughters express gratefulness that their father is stronger and has taken on the leadership role.
	Monitor ability of family members to carry out treatment plan and provide safe care.	When care is provided by family members who are exhausted, safety is always an issue. The	

continues

PLANNING/GOALS	NURSING INTERVENTIONS	RATIONALE	EVALUATION
		nurse is ultimately responsible for the well-being of the client.	
	Teach coping strategies for managing tension and strain in the event of previous techniques losing their effectiveness.	Coping strategies to maintain healthy emotional and psychological health may be necessary. This is especially true for individuals from a culture that discourages placing individual needs or emotions ahead of those of the family.	

CASE STUDY

Maria Garcia brings her Catholic, 18-year-old sister, Rosa, to the hospital emergency room. Rosa has a high temperature and chills, is vomiting, and complains of right-lower-quadrant pain. Maria also brings her three children, ages 3, 2, and 1 year old, with her. Maria understands and speaks broken English, but Rosa is fluent in Spanish only. The nurse directs Maria to the waiting room with her children, then takes Rosa to the examination room. Rosa is examined by a male nurse, who promptly complains at the nurses' station about how uncooperative Rosa was during the physical examination. Rosa is admitted for inpatient care and is diagnosed with appendicitis requiring emergency surgery. Maria is left in the waiting room, unaware of the difficulty that the nursing staff has had in communicating with Rosa. Rosa is taken upstairs to her room to await her surgical preparation. Maria is notified that she can go upstairs for a few minutes but must then leave because her children do not meet the age requirement for visitor privileges. Maria finds Rosa weeping, nearly hysterical. The physician walks in and asks Maria why she waited so long to bring Rosa in for treatment. He informs her that Rosa's appendix was close to rupturing and that treatment should have been started 3 days ago, when her symptoms first began. Maria informs him that she had taken Rosa to the curandero, who had given her some herbal tea to drink. When that did not help, she had brought Rosa to the hospital.

The following questions will guide your development of a nursing care plan for the case study.

1. Why was communication among Maria, Rosa, and the health care professionals problematic?
2. What Mexican American cultural diversities were not addressed by the health care professionals?
3. What needs of Maria and Rosa are being ignored by the health care professionals?
4. What questions do you feel must be asked by the health care professionals to give them a better understanding of this situation?
5. Identify two individualized culturally sensitive nursing diagnoses and goals for Rosa.
6. Formulate pertinent nursing interventions for the diagnoses and goals identified in question 5.
7. List resources that the nurses could use to assist Rosa in her recovery.
8. List at least two successful client outcomes for Rosa.

SUMMARY

- Culture is composed of beliefs about activity, relations, motivation, perception of the world, and perception about self.
- Culture is learned, integrated, shared, unspoken, and dynamic.
- Beliefs about concepts of health, disease etiology, health promotion and protection, and practitioners and remedies are influenced by culture.
- Unlike opinions, preferences, and attitudes, which can change, cultural characteristics are deeply rooted and are thus difficult to change. Clients reflect their cultural and ethnic heritage every time they interact with the world around them.
- Culture is influenced by religion, which in turn affects beliefs and practices about health and illness.
- Spiritual and religious beliefs are important in many people's lives. They can influence lifestyle, attitudes, and feelings about illness and death.
- The nurse should not make assumptions about clients based on the client's religious and cultural affiliations. Individuality exists among all peoples.
- The focus of nursing care is to help the client maintain his own beliefs in the midst of a health care crisis and to use those personal beliefs to strengthen coping patterns.
- Understanding and encouraging client differences are important aspects of nursing.
- Response to health and illness varies depending on cultural origin.
- Culturally appropriate care begins with an understanding of one's own cultural beliefs.
- Client cultural assessment is a prerequisite to providing appropriate nursing care.

Review Questions

1. A mother is observed breastfeeding her 4-year-old son, who is a client in the pediatrics wing of the hospital. A nurse is overheard talking in the nursing station about the "weird" way the mother has continued to breastfeed a 4-year-old. She comments that the American way is the best. The nurse is guilty of:

   a. ethnocentrism.
   b. stereotyping.
   c. unusual break behavior.
   d. not insisting that the mother stop breastfeeding.

2. Which religious group teaches that physical healing comes exclusively through prayers and readings?

   a. Roman Catholic
   b. Jewish
   c. Christian Science
   d. Seventh Day Adventist

3. Which religious group observes the Sabbath from sunset Friday until sunset Saturday?

   a. Mormons
   b. Jews
   c. Presbyterians
   d. Muslims

4. A client of which religion would most likely refuse a blood transfusion, even if his life were in jeopardy?

   a. Hindu
   b. Jehovah's Witness
   c. Jew
   d. Mormon

5. The nursing diagnosis that might be used for a client who is hospitalized and has religious practices that conflict with hospital practice is:

   a. *Emotional Depression.*
   b. *Guilt and Misery.*
   c. *Spiritual Distress.*
   d. *Spiritual Manipulation.*

6. It is important for the nurse to know the client's religion in order to:

   a. chart it on his record.
   b. give holistic care.
   c. meet his physical needs.
   d. know how to pray for him.

7. Which of the following is a characteristic of culture?

   a. Culture is learned.
   b. Culture stays the same.
   c. Culture is biologically inherited.
   d. Culture is individually determined.

8. Which of the following is descriptive of Hispanic Americans?

   a. They are culturally homogeneous.
   b. Their culture is not based on religion.
   c. Illness may be viewed as a punishment from God.
   d. They always seek Western medical intervention.

9. When a client says to the nurse, "I need to pray with my pastor in order to get well," the most appropriate response from the nurse is:

   a. "The medicine you take will make you well."
   b. "When you are released from the hospital, you can go to church and pray."
   c. "May I call your pastor for you and ask him to visit you?"
   d. "Why do you think prayer will make you well?"

10. It is important to be aware of cultural aspects of health and disease because:

   a. some cultural groups are represented in greater numbers than others.
   b. cultural groups respond differently to illness.
   c. differences in care should not be based on culture.
   d. reimbursement is related to ethnicity.

Critical Thinking Questions

1. How does your culture influence your beliefs about health practices?

2. Suppose one of your clients practiced the custom of placing an amulet (religious icon and necklace) around a newborn's neck. You are concerned about the risk of strangulation this presents. How would you approach this client to discuss your concerns?

 WEB FLASH!

- Search "cultural diversity" on the web. What related topics do you find?
- Can you locate health-related web sites specific to European Americans, African Americans, Hispanic Americans, Asian Americans, and Native Americans?

COMPLEMENTARY/ ALTERNATIVE THERAPIES

LEARNING OBJECTIVES

Upon completion of this chapter, you should be able to:
- *Define key terms.*
- *Describe the historical influences on current complementary/alternative modalities.*
- *Discuss the connection between mind and body and the effect of this relationship on a person's health.*
- *Explain the concept of the nurse as an instrument of healing in holistic nursing practice.*
- *Identify the various mind-body, body-movement, energetic-touch healing, spiritual, nutritional, and other modalities that can be used as complementary therapies in client care.*
- *Discuss the use of complementary/alternative modalities.*

KEY TERMS

acupressure	healing touch
acupuncture	hypnosis
alternative therapy	imagery
antioxidant	instrument of healing
aromatherapy	meditation
biofeedback	neuropeptide
bodymind	neurotransmitter
centering	phytochemical
complementary therapy	psychoneuro- immunology
curing	shaman
energetic-touch therapy	shamanism
	therapeutic massage
free radical	therapeutic touch
healing	touch

INTRODUCTION

Western society tends to think of health and healing in terms of medical, surgical, and other technological interventions. However, in many other cultures—both past and present—healing has been promoted by faith, magic, ritual, and other nonmedical approaches.

The use of **complementary therapies** (therapies used *in conjunction with* conventional medical therapies) and **alternative therapies** (therapies used *instead of* conventional or mainstream medical modalities) is becoming more prevalent among the general public (NCCAM, 2000).

This chapter addresses complementary/alternative treatment methods that are currently being used in ho-

listic nursing practice. Nurses are encouraged to think critically before recommending or implementing any of these approaches. Whether they simply discuss complementary/alternative therapies with clients or perform these therapies, nurses should understand the ramifications.

Because more and more states are regulating complementary/alternative therapies, nurses must know the laws that govern these therapies in the states in which they work. Some states have outlawed certain therapies or consider them experimental procedures, whereas other states require licensure or certain educational standards before allowing practitioners to perform complementary/alternative therapies. Nurses who perform complementary/alternative therapies not in accordance with the laws of their respective states could have legal charges filed against them (Brooke, 1998).

Employer policy and the nurse's job description must also be checked to confirm that performing complementary/alternative therapies is within the nurse's scope of practice at that agency. Employer malpractice insurance policies typically do not cover situations where a client is injured as a result of a complementary/alternative therapy. The financial risk of any nurse who engages in complementary/alternative therapies will be lowered by having insurance that specifically covers those therapies.

HISTORICAL INFLUENCES ON CONTEMPORARY PRACTICES

For as long as history has been recorded, people have tried to cure ills and relieve pain. Early cave drawings depict healers practicing their art. Primitive healers attributed the cause of mysterious diseases to magic and superstition; as a result, religious beliefs and health practices became intertwined. Remedies and practices that are based in ancient traditions are being rediscovered and used by contemporary holistic healers. A brief look at ancient Greek, Far Eastern, Chinese, Indian, and Shamanistic practices will highlight their influences on modern complementary/alternative modalities.

Ancient Greece

In the ancient Greek culture, health was perceived as the maintenance of balance in all dimensions of life. In Greek mythology, Asclepius was the god of healing. Temples (called Ascleipions) were beautiful places for people (regardless of ability to pay) to rest, restore themselves, and worship. The elaborate healing system consisted of myths, symbols, and rites administered by rigorously trained priest-healers. Illnesses were treated by restoring balance to a person's life through music, art, baths, massage, laughter, herbs, and simple surgery (Keegan, 1994). Many of our current therapies such as massage, art therapy, and herbal therapy have origins in ancient Greek traditions.

The Far East

Healing systems from the Far East have traditionally integrated mind, body, and spirit into a system of balanced energy between the individual and the universe. The concept of a life force or life energy "has been recognized in many cultural traditions. . . . What is universally agreed on is that the more [life energy] you have, the more vital your mental and bodily processes" (Chopra, 1998). The origins of some energetic-touch therapies can be traced to the Far East.

China

The traditional Chinese healing system is based on the belief in the oneness of all things in nature. Life energy qi (pronounced "chi") flows through both the universe and the person, thus creating a wholeness among all things and people. Qi provides warmth, protection from illness, and vitality. Qi flows along an invisible system of meridians (pathways) that link the organs together and connect them to the external environment and, therefore, to the universe. Illness and injury can alter the flow of this energy. The energy flow can be influenced by stimulating points along the meridians.

Herbalism is an essential component of traditional Chinese healing practice. In seeking to promote balance, healers use herbs for dual purposes. For example, the herb dan qui relaxes the uterus when it is contracted (as in preterm labor) and tightens it if it is too relaxed (when normal labor needs to be enhanced). A complete discussion of the use of herbs in contemporary health practices appears later in this chapter.

Many contemporary Western health care providers are studying and now using traditional Chinese healing techniques. **Acupuncture**, one technique used in traditional Chinese medicine, is the application of heat and needles to various points on the body to alter the energy flow (Figure 13-1). The National Institutes of Health (NIH) (1997) acknowledged the efficacy of acupuncture in treating headaches, menstrual cramps, fibromyalgia, myofacial pain, osteoarthritis, low back pain, carpal tunnel syndrome, asthma, postoperative and chemotherapy-induced nausea and vomiting, and postoperative dental pain. They could not, however, determine a scientific basis for the circulation of qi.

India

Practiced for more than 4,000 years by the people of India, Ayurvedic medicine emphasizes prevention and a holistic approach to life (Keegan, 1994). The term *ayurveda* (meaning "the science of life") refers to

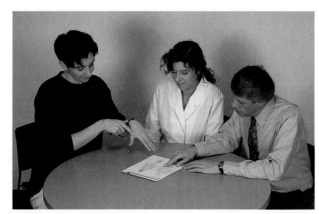

Figure 13-1 Acupuncturist, Nurse, and Client

India's traditional medicine and has an underlying spiritual basis. The life energy (prana) is transported through the body by a "wind" or vata. Vata regulates every type of movement.

Vata, Kapha, and Pitta are the three metabolic principles (doshas) that provide life to all living things (Chopra, 1998). Kapha is the energy responsible for body structure, and pitta is the transformative process between vata and kapha. Each person is born with a unique balance of the three doshas. One predominates, and that dosha determines body type, temperament, and susceptibility to certain illnesses.

In the Ayurvedic system, chakras are areas of energy concentration in the body. Like the Chinese pathways (or meridians), these areas can become stagnant and blocked, thus causing illness. Ayurvedic healers seek to activate chakra energy for self-healing.

Prevention of illness and restoration of health through inner search and spiritual growth are the primary goals in the Ayurvedic system. Union of the Divine and the Truth occurs through the physical and meditative practice of yoga. In contemporary practice, Ayurvedic intervention may consist of yoga, herbs, diet, and exercise; methods to cleanse the body, such as steam baths, cathartics, and detoxifying massage; and nasal purging.

Shamanistic Tradition

A need to understand and explain life processes (i.e., birth, health, illness, and death) is part of being human. In many cultures, both modern and ancient, ritualized practices have been used to keep peace with the great spirits, to harness their power, to promote power, and to prevent death.

Shamanism refers to the practice of entering altered states of consciousness with the intent of helping others. The **shaman** is a folk healer-priest who uses natural and supernatural forces to help others and who has an extensive knowledge of herbs, is skilled in many forms of healing, and serves as guardian of the spirits. Illness is considered to be the result of spirit loss; shamans have the power to heal by working with the spirits to encourage their full return to the individual. The shaman functions as both healer and priest and one who has access to the supernatural.

Seeking wisdom about the universe, establishing a relationship with the creator, and avoiding death are all feats accomplished through ritualized processes performed by the shaman. The shaman's practice incorporates special objects such as power animals, totems, and fetishes as well as ritual songs, dances, food, and clothing. Sleep deprivation, ritual chants, isolation, imagery, drumming, and hallucinogenic drugs may be used to create a trance-like state that is the vehicle through which the shaman contacts the spirit world. The contemporary practices of hypnosis and guided imagery have roots in Shamanistic traditions.

MODERN TRENDS

The public perception of complementary/alternative treatment methods has been changing over the past few decades. In the late 1960s and early 1970s, the "natural," "new age," and "self-help" movements began to attract followers, first among consumers and later among health care practitioners. During that time period, there was a growing trend toward rejection of traditional medicine because of its perceived invasiveness, painfulness, cost, and ineffectiveness. A rekindled interest in Eastern religions, lifestyle, and medicine has fueled the development of contemporary holistic, complementary/alternative modalities. Clients are seeking out complementary/alternative therapies because most such therapies are noninvasive, holistic, and, in many instances, less expensive than going to a physician (Keegan, 1998).

In 1992, the U.S. government established the Office of Alternative Medicine (OAM) at the National Institutes of Health and allocated $2 million to disseminate information about complementary and alternative medicine to practitioners and the public. Congress increased the OAM's budget to $20 million for fiscal year 1998 (National Institutes of Health, 1998).

Then in late 1998, Congress established the National Center for Complementary and Alternative Medicine (NCCAM), which replaced the Office of Alternative Medicine. Their budget for the fiscal year 2000 is $68.7 million (National Institutes of Health, 2000). The NCCAM has the added responsibility of conducting and supporting basic and applied research and research training on CAM. The NCCAM (2000) reports that more than 42% of the U.S. population in 1997 used some type of complementary/alternative therapy, spending more than $27 billion on these therapies.

Mind/Body Medicine and Research

The traditional medical model is founded on the belief that the mind, body, and spirit are separate entities. A relatively new field of science, however, called **psychoneuroimmunology** (PNI), is studying the complex relationship among the cognitive, affective, and physical aspects of humans. Psychoneuroimmunologists are investigating the way the brain transmits signals along the nerves to enhance the body's normal immune functioning. This research supports the idea that the human mind can alter physiology.

All body cells have receptor sites for **neuropeptides**, amino acids that are produced in the brain and other sites in the body and that act as chemical communicators. Neuropeptides are released when **neurotransmitters** (chemical substances produced by the body that facilitate nerve-impulse transmission) signal emotions in the brain. Pert, of the National Institutes of Health, wrote in 1986 that "the more we know about neuropeptides, the harder it is to think in the traditional terms of a mind and a body. It makes more sense to speak of a single integrated entity, a '*body-mind*'" (Pert, 1986).

Thus, it is possible for cells to be directly affected by emotions. In other words, people can affect their health by what they think and feel. There are many examples of terminally ill persons hanging on to life until the occurrence of a specific event such as a child coming to visit or a grandchild's graduation or marriage.

The intermeshed, complex system of psyche and body chemistry is now referred to as the **bodymind**, the inseparable connection and operation of thoughts, feelings, and physiological functions. According to psychologist Earnest Rossi (1993), because all body systems are interconnected, mental images can be converted into neurotransmitters in the autonomic nervous system, hormones in the endocrine system, and white blood cells in the immune system. These three systems (nervous, endocrine, and immune) are interactive, thus modulating the activity of each other (Rossi, 1993). This helps explain how some complementary/alternative therapies allow the calming influences of the parasympathetic system to take over during stress-inducing situations such as illness (Dossey, 1999).

Holism and Nursing Practice

The expansion of the holistic health movement has been based on the growing acceptance of the concept that body, mind, and spirit are interconnected. Nursing in its broadest sense (theory, concept, and practice) is truly holistic in nature. Holism encompasses consideration of the physiological, psychological, sociocultural, intellectual, and spiritual aspects of each individual. Holistic nursing can be described as the art and science of caring for the whole person, knowing that each person is unique in all expressions of self. This means that the nursing assessment must include eliciting information regarding client use of alternative/complementary therapies (Hodge & Ullrich, 1999).

As holistic caregivers, nurses may employ alternative/complementary techniques to promote clients' well-being. The focus of care in these practices is healing, as opposed to curing. The word **healing** is derived from the Anglo-Saxon word *hael,* meaning "to make whole, to move toward, or to become whole." It is important to establish that healing is not the same as **curing** (ridding one of disease), but is instead a process that activates the individual's forces from within. As a healing facilitator, the nurse enters into a relationship with the client and can assist the client by offering to be a guide, change agent, or **instrument of healing** (a means by which healing can be achieved, performed, or enhanced).

When the nurse serves as an instrument of healing, the objective is to help the client call forth inner re-

sources for healing. In order to accomplish this goal, nurses must develop the following attributes:

- Knowledge base: initially established in nursing school and then continuously expanded through lifelong learning
- Intentionality: having a conscious direction of goals, essential in helping the healer to focus
- Respect for differences: demonstrated by honoring clients' culturally based health beliefs
- Ability to model wellness: tending to one's own needs and attempting to stay as healthy and balanced as possible

COMPLEMENTARY/ ALTERNATIVE INTERVENTIONS

Many complementary/alternative interventions are used in holistic nursing practice. These interventions are categorized as mind/body, body-movement, energetic-touch, spiritual, nutritional/medicinal, and other methodologies (Table 13–1). Although different in technique, many of the complementary/alternative therapies have common ideological threads, as follows:

- The *whole system* must be considered if the *parts* of the individual are to be helped to function.
- The person is integrated and related to the surroundings.
- There exists some life force or energy that can be used in the healing process.
- Ritual, prescribed practice and skilled practitioners are integral parts of holistic healing interventions.

PROFESSIONAL TIP

Use of Complementary/Alternative Therapy

Practical ways for nurses to use complementary/ alternative therapies include:

- Having a nonjudgmental attitude about these therapies;
- Asking clients whether they use any nontraditional therapies and, if so, asking which therapies, why, and how the therapies have worked;
- Getting adequate instruction in these therapies before trying to administer them;
- Trying one or two basic therapies such as massage or guided imagery; and
- Discussing a therapy with the client *before* using it (Keegan, 1998).

Table 13–1 CATEGORIES OF COMPLEMENTARY/ALTERNATIVE INTERVENTIONS

MIND/BODY	BODY MOVEMENT	ENERGETIC TOUCH	SPIRITUAL	NUTRITIONAL/ MEDICINAL	OTHER
Meditation	Movement and exercise	Touch	Faith Healing	Phytochemicals and antioxidants	Aromatherapy
Relaxation	Yoga	Therapeutic massage	Healing Prayer	Macrobiotic diet	Humor
Imagery	Tai chi	Therapeutic touch	Shamanism:	Herbal therapy	Pet Therapy
Biofeedback	Chiropractic therapy	Healing touch	• Sand painting		Music therapy
Hypnosis		Acupressure	• Sweat lodges		
		Reflexology	• Drumming		

Adapted from Fundamentals of Nursing: Standards & Practice, *by S. DeLaune and P. Ladner, 1998, Albany, NY: Delmar. Copyright 1998 by Delmar. Adapted with permission.*

Mind/Body (Self-Regulatory) Techniques

Self-regulatory techniques are methods by which an individual can, independently or with assistance, consciously control some functions of the sympathetic nervous system (for example, heart rate, respiratory rate, and blood pressure). When the client is learning the way to perform these techniques, an assistant is involved; later, however, the client can perform them independently. Self-regulatory techniques include meditation, relaxation, imagery, biofeedback, and hypnosis.

Meditation

The practice of **meditation**, quieting the mind by focusing the attention, can bring about remarkable physiological changes. People who meditate strive for a sense of oneness within themselves and a sense of relatedness to a greater power and the universe.

A person can be guided into a meditative or relaxed state with breath coaching (assisting the client to become aware of or focus on breathing and thus slow it). Meditation has proved particularly beneficial for clients in labor. Nurses can teach this modality to clients by using verbal cues, counting the client's inhalations and exhalations, and showing the client the way to take slow, deep breaths. According to Borysenko and Borysenko (1994), some therapeutic benefits of meditation are:

- Stress relief
- Relaxation
- Reduced level of lactic acid
- Decreased oxygen consumption
- Slowed heart rate
- Decreased blood pressure
- Improved functioning of the immune system

Relaxation

In 1975, cardiologist Herbert Benson studied the effects of meditation on individuals. He then incorporated

 CLIENT TEACHING

Progressive Muscle Relaxation

After explaining the purpose and process of progressive muscle relaxation, instruct the client to:

- Assume a comfortable position in a quiet environment.
- Close eyes and keep them closed until the exercise is completed.
- Breathe in deeply to a count of 4.
- Hold breath for a count of 4.
- Breathe out to a count of 4.
- Continue to breathe slowly and deeply.
- Tense both feet until muscle tension is felt.
- Hold a gentle state of tension in both feet for a count of 3.

Caution the client to tighten the muscles only until the muscles are tensed, not to the point of pain.

- Slowly release the tension from the feet.
- Fully experience the difference between tension and relaxation.
- Repeat the previous three steps.
- Gently tense the muscles of both lower legs.
- Continue this procedure with all the muscle groups in a toe-to-head direction.
- After tensing and releasing all muscle groups, take in a few more deep relaxing breaths and scan your body for any areas that remain tense. Concentrate on tensing and relaxing the muscles in those areas.
- Breathe in deeply to a count of 4.
- Hold breath for a count of 4.
- Breathe out to a count of 4.
- Resume your usual breathing pattern.
- Slowly stretch and open your eyes.

To be effective, this procedure requires approximately 20 to 30 minutes. Like all other relaxation exercises, progressive muscle relaxation is most effective with repetition.

the basic elements of meditation into the therapeutic process he called the *relaxation response* (Benson, 1975). Benson employed the relaxation response with individuals experiencing high blood pressure and heart disease. Benson discovered that the techniques were more effective if individuals focused on an inspirational prayer or phrase. The basic elements of the relaxation response are:

- A quiet environment
- A comfortable position
- Focused attention
- A passive attitude
- Practice

One method for achieving relaxation is progressive muscle relaxation (PMR), which is the alternate tensing and relaxing of muscles. Clients are instructed to concentrate on a certain body area (the jaw, for instance), tense the muscles for a count of five, then relax the muscles for a count of five. This process is repeated for muscle groups over the entire body until the client has achieved a state of overall relaxation.

Nurses can use relaxation techniques in their work with clients to reduce pain and stress. Relaxation techniques are also an essential aspect of cognitive behavioral therapy when treating people with phobias, fear, and depression.

Imagery

Imagery is a technique of using the imagination to visualize a pleasant, soothing image. The practitioner encourages the client to use as many of the senses as possible in order to enhance the formation of vivid images. Table 13–2 presents examples of incorporating all five senses into imagery.

Nurses can create guided imagery for many clients who are capable of hearing and understanding the nurse's suggestions of meaningful and physiologically correct images. For example, a nurse can show a chart of the stages of bone healing to a client who has suffered a fracture and ask the client to imagine this sequential activity in his body.

Table 13–2	INCORPORATING ALL FIVE SENSES INTO IMAGERY
SENSE	**IMAGERY**
Visual	See the dark blue sky
Auditory	Hear the babbling brook
Kinesthetic	Feel yourself floating on a cloud
Gustatory	Taste the tartness of a freshly cut lemon
Olfactory	Smell the salt air at the ocean

CLIENT TEACHING

Guided Imagery

After explaining the purpose and process of guided imagery, instruct the client to:

- Assume a comfortable position in a quiet environment.
- Close your eyes and keep them closed until the exercise is completed.
- Breathe in deeply to a count of 4.
- Hold breath for a count of 4.
- Breathe out to a count of 4.
- Continue to breathe slowly and deeply.
- Think of your favorite place and prepare to take an imaginary journey there. Select a place in which you are relaxed and at peace.
- Picture in your mind's eye your favorite place. Look around you and see all the colors, the light and shadows, and all the pleasant sights.
- Listen to all the sounds. Pay attention to what you hear.
- Feel all the physical sensations . . . the temperature . . . the textures . . . the movement of the air.
- As you take in a deep breath, smell the aromas of your favorite place.
- Taste the foods and drinks you usually consume in your favorite place. Savor each taste fully.
- Focus all your attention totally on your favorite place.
- Breathe in deeply to a count of 4.
- Hold breath for a count of 4.
- Breathe out to a count of 4.
- Resume your usual breathing pattern.
- Slowly open your eyes and stretch, if desired.

This procedure works best when all five senses are used. Like all other relaxation exercises, guided imagery becomes more effective with repetition.

"The nurse using guided imagery can promote a sense of well-being in clients and help them change their perceptions about their disease, treatment, and healing ability" (Dossey, 1995). Studies have found that a combination of medication and guided imagery decreases physical tension, anxiety, and the adverse effects of chemotherapy (Keegan, 1998). In addition to being a tool for distraction when a person is confronting pain, discomfort, and fear, imagery is also a powerful mechanism for making decisions and for altering behaviors, as it allows the client to try out decisions and behaviors before actually implementing them. The power of the human imagination is limitless, and helping clients to use that power can be a rewarding role for the nurse.

Biofeedback

Biofeedback is a measurement of physiological responses that yields information about the relationship between the mind and the body and helps clients learn ways to manipulate those responses through mental activity. Biofeedback allows a person to see the effect of the mind on the body. While attached to sensitive devices that measure bodily responses such as skin temperature, blood pressure, galvanic skin resistance, and electrical activity in the muscles, the individual imagines stressful experiences. The individual's physiological responses are then measured and recorded, as are the individual's physiological responses to relaxation. The individual receives an interpretation of these responses and is taught methods for practicing relaxation to control reactions to stressful experiences.

Biofeedback is used as a restorative method in rehabilitation settings to help clients who have lost sensation and function as the result of illness or injury. Machines that can detect a person's internal bodily functions translate them into a form that the client can detect, such as a light or beep. After training with the machine, clients are able to alter their responses without the machine. Biofeedback also enhances relaxation in tense muscles, relieves tension headaches and backache, and reduces bruxism (grinding of the teeth) and the pain associated with temporomandibular joint syndrome (Association of Psychophysiology and Biofeedback, 1998). Temperature biofeedback is useful in training clients to purposefully warm their hands to treat Raynaud's disease (a circulatory disorder), to lower blood pressure, and to prevent or relieve migraine headaches.

Hypnosis

The practice of hypnosis was once overshadowed by mystery and misconception. Today, with our expanding knowledge of the human mind, hypnosis is becoming a more common nursing intervention (Zahourek & Larkin, 1995). Therapeutic **hypnosis** induces an altered state of consciousness or awareness resembling sleep and during which the person is more receptive to suggestion. Hypnosis also enhances the client's ability to form images.

Nurses wishing to use hypnosis in their practices must be aware of the guidelines concerning this modality with regard to the scope of practice as defined by their respective state boards of nursing. They also should receive advanced training in the art of hypnosis (Kolkmeier, 1999).

Body-Movement (Manipulation) Strategies

As the name implies, body-movement therapies employ techniques of moving or manipulating various body parts to achieve therapeutic outcomes. Modalities such as movement and exercise, yoga, tai chi, and chiropractic treatment are discussed in the following sections.

Movement and Exercise

Movement, as a therapeutic intervention and health-promoting activity, is associated with athletic exercise, dance, celebration, and healing rituals. Although the primary goal of exercise is fitness (muscle strength, flexibility, endurance, and cardiovascular and respiratory health), there are many other positive outcomes of exercise, such as feeling more energetic and sleeping better.

Nurses can help clients use movement as therapy in a variety of ways such as range of motion exercises, water exercises, physical therapy, and stretching exercises. Movement is an effective method through which people of all ages can improve their level of functioning. Exercise has also been documented to improve functional ability in people with arthritis (Budesheim, et al., 1994).

Yoga

Many cultures believe that particular forms of movement keep the body's life forces in correct balance and flow. Yoga and tai chi are examples of ancient ritual movements that enhance overall health including spiritual enlightenment and well-being. Both of these approaches require concentration and the use of symbolic movements.

A form of meditative exercise, yoga rejuvenates, promotes longevity and self-realization, and speeds the natural evolution of the person toward self-enlightenment. Traditional yoga has always been primarily concerned with healthy individuals and promoting health by maintaining the balance and flow of life forces.

Yoga therapy is an effort to integrate traditional yogic concepts and techniques with Western medical and psychological knowledge (Feuerstein, 1998). The focus of yoga therapy is to holistically treat various psychological or somatic dysfunctions ranging from back problems to emotional distress.

Both yoga and yoga therapy are based on the understanding that the human being is an integrated body/mind system that best functions in a state of dynamic

 LIFE CYCLE CONSIDERATIONS

Exercise and the Very Old
Those of very advanced ages (95 years and older) are achieving positive results from regular exercise and weight lifting, including increased physical strength and flexibility and improved mental status in areas such as memory and depression (Mills, 1994).

balance (Feuerstein, 1998). Studies regarding benefits of yoga practice have found that mentally challenged individuals become more aware of their bodies and enjoy improved coordination, while clients with osteoarthritis of the hands experience less pain (Keegan, 1998). Claims made by yoga authorities range from a beneficial effect on physical flexibility, muscle tone, and stamina to a reduction in obesity, back pain, hypertension, various respiratory diseases, anxiety, and memory loss (Feuerstein, 1998).

Tai Chi

Tai chi is based on the philosophy of the quest for harmony with nature and the universe through the laws of complementary (yin and yang) balance. When perfect harmony exists, everything functions effortlessly, spontaneously, perfectly, and in accordance with the laws of nature. If one moves to the right, then one must also move to the left. Tai chi consists of a series of sequential, dance-like movements connected in a smooth-flowing process. The movements, accompanied by deep breathing, improve flexibility, range of motion, muscle strength, and balance (Cerrato, 1999d).

People who regularly perform tai chi believe that it enhances stamina, agility, and balance and that it boosts energy and confers a sense of well-being. Tai chi has been shown to reduce blood pressure and the risk of falling in the elderly, and significantly reduced discomfort of clients with low back pain (Cerrato, 1999d).

Chiropractic Therapy

The major principle underlying chiropractic therapy is that the brain sends vital energy to every organ in the body via the nerves originating in the spinal column. Disease, body disharmony, or malfunction results from vertebral subluxation complex (spinal nerve stress). The body is rebalanced and realigned using chiropractic "spinal adjustment" techniques.

The goal of chiropractic care is to awaken the client's own natural healing ability by correcting any areas of vertebral subluxation complex. Vitality, strength, and health are thus promoted. Chiropractic Arts Center (1998) reports case histories of clients recovering from heart trouble, hyperactivity, fatigue, digestive problems, and many other conditions.

Stedman (1999) explains that chiropractic practitioners fall into one of two groups, the "straights" and the "mixers." The straights believe in the chiropractic therapy just described, despite the fact that no scientific evidence exists to support the claims. The mixers use spinal adjustments mainly to relieve back pain, neck stiffness, and headaches, conditions that have sometimes been shown to be alleviated by chiropractic therapy. Most mixers are willing to work closely with a client's medical doctor.

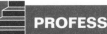

PROFESSIONAL TIP

Preparing for Chiropractic Therapy

As with any complementary/alternative intervention, nurses should encourage clients who are considering the use of chiropractic services to first undergo comprehensive health assessment to rule out any contraindications.

Chiropractic services have gained increasing acceptance in the United States. Chiropractors are licensed in all 50 states, and 41 states require insurance reimbursement for chiropractic services (Japsen, 1995).

Energetic-Touch Therapies

One category of complementary/alternative therapies that has been incorporated into nursing practice in the past 20 years is the **energetic-touch therapies**, techniques of using the hands to direct or redirect the flow of the body's energy fields and thus enhance balance within those fields. These modalities are effective interventions for many problems and can be used to restore harmony in all aspects of a person's health. Energetic-touch therapies can be used with persons of all ages and all stages of wellness and illness.

Energetic-touch therapies have their roots in traditional Chinese, ancient Eastern, and Native American philosophies. The fundamental concept is that individuals are composed of a life force, a source of energy that is not confined to physical skin boundaries. Figure 13-2 illustrates the energy field that extends beyond a person's physical body.

An individual's energy field consists of energy layers in constant flux. These energy layers can be diminished or otherwise adversely affected by any type of illness, trauma, or distress. The energy system can also be positively affected by the intentionally directed use of a practitioner's hands. The primary focus of the nurse using an energetic-touch therapy is "to restore the optimal flow of life energy through the field" (Cowens, 1996).

Many energetic-touch therapies are being used by nurses today. Touch, therapeutic massage, therapeutic touch, and healing touch are some examples. Other modalities include acupressure and reflexology, techniques that involve deep-tissue body work and require advanced training on the part of practitioners.

Touch

One of the most universal complementary/alternative modalities is touch. **Touch**, simply defined, is the means of perceiving or experiencing through tactile

Contraindications for Touch

It is important to know when *not* to touch.

- It may be difficult for persons who have been neglected, abused, or injured to accept touch therapy.
- Touching those who are distrustful or angry may escalate negative behaviors.
- Persons with burns or overly sensitive skin may not benefit from touch.

Touch has several important uses in nursing practice, in that it:

- Is an integral part of assessment;
- Promotes bonding between nurse and client (Figure 13-3);
- Is an important means of communication, especially when other senses are impaired;
- Assists in soothing, calming, and comforting; and
- Helps keep the client oriented.

Therapeutic Massage

Therapeutic massage is the application of pressure and motion by the hands with the intent of improving the recipient's well-being. It involves kneading, rubbing, and using friction.

Massage therapy is now recognized as a highly beneficial modality and is prescribed by a number of physicians. In addition, many states now have licensing requirements for massage practitioners.

Traditionally, back rubs have been administered by nurses to provide comfort to hospitalized clients. Massage techniques can be used with all age groups and are especially beneficial to those who are immobilized. A back rub or massage can achieve many results, including relaxation, increased circulation of the blood and lymph, and relief from musculoskeletal stiffness, pain, and spasm.

 Safety: Precautions for Massage
- Massage should be used with caution on people with heart disease, diabetes, hypertension, or kidney disease, because increased circulation may be harmful in the presence of these conditions.
- Massage should never be attempted in areas of circulatory abnormality, such as aneurysm, varicose veins, necrosis, phlebitis, or thrombus, or in areas of soft-tissue injury, open wounds, inflammation, joint or bone injury, dermatitis, recent surgery, or sciatica.

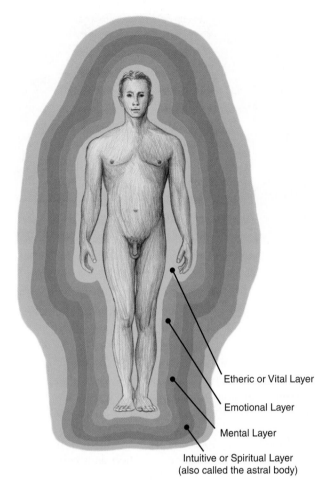

Etheric or Vital Layer

Emotional Layer

Mental Layer

Intuitive or Spiritual Layer
(also called the astral body)

Figure 13-2 Layers of the Human Energy Field Extending Beyond the Physical Boundaries

sensation. Although it was used in all ancient cultures and shamanistic traditions for healing, the advent of scientific medicine and Puritanism led many healers away from the purposeful use of touch. It should be noted that touch carries with it taboos and prescriptions that are culturally dictated. Some cultures are very comfortable with physical touch; others specify that touch may be used only in certain situations and within specified parameters.

Because touch involves personal contact, the nurse must be sure to convey positive intentions. When in doubt, the nurse should withhold touch until effective communication with the client has been established.

CULTURAL CONSIDERATIONS

Touch
- Ask permission before touching a client.
- Tell the client what is going to happen.
- The meaning of touch and the body areas acceptable to touch vary from culture to culture.

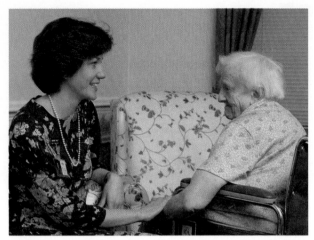

Figure 13-3 Touch promotes bonding between nurse and client.

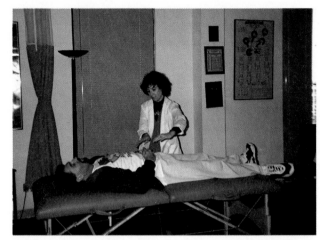

Figure 13-4 A Nurse Administering Therapeutic Touch to a Client

Therapeutic Touch

Therapeutic touch, which is based on ancient healing practices such as the laying on of hands, consists of assessing alterations in a person's energy field and using the hands to direct energy to achieve a balanced state. Therapeutic touch is based on four assumptions:

- A human being is an open energy system.
- Anatomically, a human being is bilaterally symmetrical.
- Illness is an imbalance in an individual's energy field.
- Human beings have natural abilities to transform and transcend their conditions of living (Krieger, 1993).

The therapeutic touch process is readily learned in workshops, can be done with hands either on or off the body, complements medical treatments, and has demonstrated reasonably consistent and reliable results (Figure 13-4). Table 13–3 outlines the five-phase process of therapeutic touch.

The relaxation response may be apparent in the client as quickly as 2 to 5 minutes after a therapeutic touch treatment has begun, and some clients may fall asleep or require less pain medication after a treatment. When done correctly, the practice of therapeutic touch can be mutually beneficial, energizing and increasing feelings of wellness in the practitioner as well as in the client (Mackey, 1995).

Research has documented the effectiveness of therapeutic touch in numerous areas. Therapeutic touch has been shown to accelerate wound healing of infections after cesarean section delivery (Wetzel, 1993); promote relaxation, increase energy, enhance a sense of well-being, and improve immunological functioning (Quinn, 1993); decrease anxiety in hospitalized psychiatric clients (Gagne & Toye, 1994); reduce postoperative pain, thereby decreasing the need for medication (Meehan, 1993); enhance the relaxation response, pain management, and immune function (Wilson, 1995); and alleviate generalized anxiety (Olsen & Sneed, 1995).

Healing Touch

Healing touch is an energy-based therapeutic modality that alters the energy field through the use of touch, thereby affecting physical, mental, emotional, and spiritual health (Keegan, 1999). Healing touch was developed in the 1980s by Janet Mentgen, a nurse. In 1990, healing touch was established as a certification program of the American Holistic Nurses' Association (AHNA). The curriculum includes varied techniques in general balancing of the body's energy field, relaxation, and specific problems such as headaches, spinal problems, and pain.

Healing touch can be administered in a few minutes or, ideally, in a session lasting one full hour (Mentgen, 1996). Implicit in this therapy is the need for follow-up or sequential treatments as well as discharge planning and referral to assist the client in adequately meeting goals.

In both therapeutic touch and healing touch, the practitioner uses **centering** (a process of bringing oneself to an inward focus of serenity) before initiating treatment. Centering is a valuable tool to use before performing any treatment or before any situation that may be stressful or difficult (such as a major school examination).

Shiatsu and Acupressure

Shiatsu, from the word meaning "finger pressure," is a Japanese form of acupressure. Both shiatsu and acupressure are based on the Chinese meridian theory, which states that the body is divided into meridian channels through which qi, or energy, flows. Cold, damp, fire, bacteria, or viruses may block the flow of qi, causing disease in the body. **Acupressure** is a technique of releasing blocked energy within an individual when specific points (Tsubas) along the meridians are

Table 13–3 PHASES OF THERAPEUTIC TOUCH

PHASE	DEFINITION	TECHNIQUES
Centering	• Bringing body, mind, and emotions to a quiet, focused state of consciousness • Being still • Being nonjudgmental	Become centered: • Controlled breathing, • Imagery, and • Meditation.
Assessment ("scanning")	• Using the hands to determine the nature of the client's energy field • Being attuned to sensory cues (e.g., warmth, coolness, static, pressure, tingling) to detect changes in the client's energy	• Hold the hands 2 to 6 inches from the client's energy field while moving the hands from the head to the feet in a rhythmic, symmetrical manner.
Unruffling ("clearing")	• Facilitating the symmetrical and rhythmic flow of energy through the field	• Use slightly more vigorous hand movements from midline while continuing to move in a rhythmic and symmetrical manner from the head to the feet.
Treatment ("balancing," "rebalancing," or "intervention")	• Projecting, directing, and modulating energy on the basis of the nature of the living energy field • Assisting to reestablish order in the system.	• Because each practitioner experiences the living energy field uniquely, the law of opposites serves as a guideline for intervening (e.g., if a pulling or drawing sensation is detected, energy is directed to the depleted area until it feels replenished). • Continue to assess, clear, and balance the field while remaining centered.
Evaluation	• Using professional, informed, and intuitive judgment to determine when to end the session	• Reassess the field. • Elicit feedback from the client. • Give the client an opportunity to rest and integrate the process.

The phases, although learned sequentially by beginners, are dynamic and often performed concurrently and repetitively by experienced practitioners.

Adapted from Therapeutic Touch: Teaching Guidelines: Beginner's Level Krieger/Kunz Method, *by Nurse Healers-Professional Associates, Inc., 1992, New York: Author.*

pressed or massaged by the practitioner's fingers, thumbs, and heel of the hands. When the blocked energy is freed, the disease subsides. The most commonly treated conditions include muscular pains, joint pains, depression, digestive disturbances, and respiratory disorders (Lanfranco, 1997). Contraindications include venous stasis, phlebitis, and traumatic and deep tissue injuries (Sutherland, 2000).

Shiatsu primarily focuses on health maintenance rather than on treatment of illness (Keegan, 1999); that is, it is used to make sure the qi is able to flow freely so that the individual does not become ill. When practicing shiatsu, nurses must be self-aware and grounded (focused on their inner energy). This focus enables the practitioner to concentrate completely on promoting the client's comfort.

Reflexology

Reflexology, rooted in ancient healing arts, is the art and science of enervating over 7,000 nerves in the feet believed to correspond to every muscle system or organ in the body (Worden, 1999). The fundamental concept of reflexology is that the body is divided into 10 equal, longitudinal zones that run the length of the body, from the top of the head to the tip of the toes. These 10 zones are correlated with the 10 fingers and toes. The foot is thus viewed as a microcosm of the entire body. Reflexology theory posits that illness manifests itself in calcium deposits and acids in the corresponding part of the person's foot. The pressing of specific points on the foot elicits an autonomic nervous system response or reflex. Reflexology induces an optimal state of relaxation, which is conducive to healing. It promotes health by relieving pressures and accumulation of toxins in the corresponding body part (Figure 13-5).

Reflexology can be used as a complementary method for managing chronic conditions such as asthma, sinus infections, migraines, irritable bowel syndrome, kidney stones, and constipation.

Spiritual Therapies

A state of wholeness or health is dependent on one's relationship not only to the physical and interpersonal environments, but also to the spiritual aspects of self. The idea that there is a relationship between

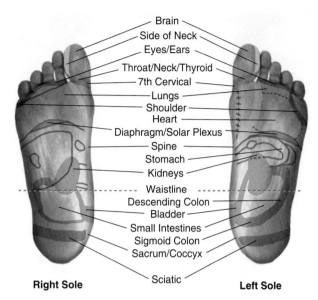

Figure 13-5 Foot Reflexology Charts *(Reproduced with permission from* Better Health with Foot Reflexology. *Copyright 1983 by Dwight C. Byers, Ingham Publishing, Inc., POB 12642, St. Petersburg, FL 33733-2642.)*

spirituality and health is not new. "From the earliest time of the shaman we have witnessed the mysterious spiritual element of healing . . . the connection of the healer with the divine" (Keegan, 1994).

The role of the spirit in healing is witnessed in all cultures. The inseparable link between the state of one's soul (life energy or spirit) and the state of one's health is accepted by many cultures. Scientists (especially psychoneuroimmunologists) are beginning to validate that individuals have inner mechanisms of healing. Many of the major religions have ideologies relating to health, illness, and healing.

Faith Healing

At the heart of spiritual or faith healing is the belief that practitioners must purify themselves and reach a state of unity with God or a Higher Power before faith healing can occur. This process, based on religious belief, is usually accomplished through prayer. During preparation for healing, the practitioner adapts a passive and receptive mood in order to be a channel for divine power. The ill person's belief enhances, but is not crucial to, the success of healing.

Healing Prayer

When individuals pray, they believe they are communicating directly with God or a Higher Power. Prayer is an integral part of a person's spiritual life and, as such, can affect well-being. Florence Nightingale recognized that prayer helps connect individuals to nature and the environment (Nightingale, 1969). Medical research is currently investigating the effects of prayer on physical health (Dossey, 1999).

A study conducted by Byrd and Sherrill (1995) investigated the effects of prayer on clients in critical care units. The results showed that clients who received standard medical treatment with the addition of intercessory prayers had fewer complications, required less medication, and improved faster than did clients in the control group, who received standard medical care and no prayers. Findings reported by Marwick (1995) showed that religious involvement may lead to improved physical health status.

Shamanism

Shamanism was discussed earlier in this chapter.

Nutritional/Medicinal Therapies

In the past 20 to 30 years, nutritional interventions for prevention and treatment of disease have generated increasing interest among consumers and health care providers. This section addresses the complementary/alternative nutritional and medicinal approaches.

Phytochemicals

Currently, certain foods are being studied for their medicinal value. **Phytochemicals** are nonnutritive, physiologically active compounds present in plants in very small amounts (Simons, 1997). *Phyto* is the Greek word for "plant." Therefore, phytochemicals are plant chemicals. These chemicals have several functions including storage of nutrients and provision of structure, aroma, flavor, and color. Phytochemicals protect against cancer and prevent heart disease, stroke, and cataracts. Phytochemicals are found in fruits and vegetables.

No single fruit or vegetable contains all phytochemicals. The consumption of a wide variety of fruits and vegetables provides the best supply. The major sources of phytochemicals are onions, garlic, leeks, chives, carrots, sweet potatoes, squash, pumpkin, cantaloupe, mango, papaya, tomatoes, citrus fruits, grapes, strawberries, raspberries, cherries, legumes, soybeans, tofu, and the cruciferous vegetables (broccoli, cauliflower, brussels sprouts, and cabbage). Nurses can use this information to encourage clients to eat more fruits and vegetables.

Antioxidants and Free Radicals

Antioxidants are substances that prevent or inhibit oxidation, a chemical process whereby a substance is joined to oxygen. In the body, antioxidants prevent tissue damage related to **free radicals**, which are unstable molecules that alter genetic codes and trigger the development of cancer growth in cells. Vitamins C and E, beta-carotene (which is converted to vitamin A in the body), and selenium are antioxidants. Antioxidants may prevent heart disease, some forms of cancer, and cataracts. Free radicals contribute to cardiovascular disease by oxidizing low-density lipoproteins (LDLs) and allowing cholesterol to adhere to vessel walls. Antioxidants help repair eye tissue damaged from sunlight and thus prevent cataract formation (Simons, 1997). Other vitamins, minerals, trace elements, and enzymes are being investigated for their possible therapeutic value. Phytosterols (plant sterols) are the active ingredients in the new lipid-lowering margarines. These inhibit absorption of dietary cholesterol and slow down the reabsorption of cholesterol secreted in bile (Cerrato, 1999a).

Macrobiotic Diet

In the 1960s, macrobiotic (from the Greek words *makro,* meaning "long," and *bios,* meaning "life") diets became popular because of a heightened interest in "natural" and more spiritual approaches to managing health and illness. The basis of macrobiotics is the Taoist concept of balance between opposites as achieved through food intake. Food has the qualities of *yin* (associated with death, cold, and darkness) and *yang* (associated with immortality, heat, and light). For example, tropical sweet foods are yin, and meat and eggs are yang. Overindulgence in either type causes difficulties; for example, too much yin food yields worry and resentment, whereas too much yang food leads to hostility and aggression. People need balance and, therefore, should consume foods that balance yin and yang.

Because brown rice and whole grains are categorized as balanced foods, they are major staples of a macrobiotic diet. The diet should be flexible and related to the season and should consist of foods indigenous to the area where the individual lives. Foods to be avoided include processed and treated foods, red meat, sugar, dairy products, eggs, and caffeine. The macrobiotic diet generally conforms to the recommendations of the American Dietary Association in terms of the guidelines for low-fat, low-cholesterol, high-fiber diets (Guinness, 1993).

Herbal Therapy

Herbal medicine has been a powerful tool in folk healing for centuries. Medicinal herbs have been catalogued for thousands of years and have probably been used in every culture. Many drugs commonly used today were, in an earlier time, tribal remedies derived from plants. Herbal medicine, also known as botanical medicine or phytotherapy, uses plant extracts for therapeutic outcomes.

Learning about herbal treatment is similar to learning pharmacology. Many holistic practitioners incorporate the use of herbs into their practices. Herbs work because of their chemical composition. Different herbs contain different compounds that can strengthen the immune system, alter the blood chemistry, or protect specific organs against disease. Table 13–4 lists medicinal values of commonly used herbs.

Others

S-adenosylmethionine (SAMe) is a modified amino acid produced naturally by the body; however, the level decreases with age. Controlled research has shown that SAMe may work at least as well as certain antidepressants and may benefit clients with osteoarthritis by assisting in cartilage repair (Cerrato & Rowell, 1999).

Omega-3 fatty acids, found in salmon, trout, sardines, walnuts, canola oil, and flax seeds help reduce the threat of cardiac arrhythmias. Research has also shown that the omega-3 fatty acids suppress inflammation of rheumatoid arthritis and may improve glucose control in Type 2 diabetes (Cerrato, 1999b).

Other Methodologies

The mind/body, body-movement, energetic-touch, spiritual, and nutritional/medicinal treatment modalities are not the only available complementary/alternative therapies. Others, such as aromatherapy, humor, pet therapy, music therapy, and play therapy, are also used by holistic practitioners.

Aromatherapy

Aromatherapy is defined as the therapeutic use of concentrated essences or essential oils that have been extracted from plants and flowers. When diluted in a carrier oil for massage or in warm water for inhalation, essences may be stimulating, uplifting, relaxing, or soothing. The following are some popular essential oils (Keville & Green, 1995):

- *Lavender* is said to have anti-inflammatory, antidepressant, and antibacterial effects.
- *Eucalyptus* is claimed to act as a decongestant, antimicrobial, and stimulant.

LIFE CYCLE CONSIDERATIONS

Macrobiotic Diets

Children and pregnant women should use the macrobiotic diet with caution. It may not have sufficient variety and, thus, be deficient in vitamin D and B_{12}.

PROFESSIONAL TIP

Use of Medicinal Plants

Nurses are cautioned against the casual use of plants to treat self or others. "Natural" substances can be harmful. In fact, if not processed properly, many plants (including some herbs) can be poisonous.

Table 13–4 MEDICINAL VALUE OF HERBS

HERB	MEDICINAL VALUE	HERB	MEDICINAL VALUE
Aloe vera	• Promotes wound healing • Soothes minor cuts, abrasions, and burns	Ginkgo	• Enhances cerebral blood flow • Helps lessen mild depression • Eases dementia • Combats impotence • Decreases peripheral vascular insufficiency • Relieves premenstrual syndrome symptoms • Decreases vascular fragility
Calendula	• Promotes healing of cuts, abrasions, minor burns, sunburn, acne, and athlete's foot • Soothes oral thrush (as a mouthwash) and vaginal thrush (as a douche)		
Celery	• Lowers cholesterol • Decreases dizziness • Relieves headache		
Chamomile	• Produces a calming effect • Relieves nausea • Eases tension headache	Peppermint	• Relieves headache • Eases sinus congestion • Reduces muscle spasms
Eucalpytus	• Acts as an antibacterial • Acts as a decongestant	Sage	• Acts as an antibacterial
Garlic	• Acts as an antimicrobial remedy for intestinal worms • Helps protect against and treat respiratory infections • Used as expectorant in cases of bronchitis or a cold	Saint John's Wort	• Relieves mild to moderate depression • Lessens severity of viral infections
Ginger	• Eases nausea (especially effective for motion sickness and morning sickness associated with pregnancy) • Stimulates circulation in feet and hands • Acts as expectorant • Helps relieve indigestion and flatulence • Relieves diarrhea	Thyme	• Acts as an antimicrobial • Helps relieve symptoms of common cold • Acts as an antispasmodic on bronchioles • Relieves cystitis • Acts as an antifungal (especially when applied as a lotion for athlete's foot) • Used as a mouthwash for oral thrush

Note: This information is not intended to serve as a guide for self-medication or the treatment of others. Consult a health care practitioner trained in the use of herbs before consuming or giving any herb for medicinal purposes.

From Herbs for Health, by S. Foster, 1995, The Herb Companion, 8(1), *Down to Earth: An Ancient Herb for a Modern Garden, by J. Long, 1995.* The Herb Companion, *8(1), 22; Eight Healing Herbs, 1995–1996, by M. Polunin and C. Robbins, 1995,* Holistic Health Directory, The Backyard Medicine Chest: An Herbal Primer, *by D. Schar, 1995, Washington, DC: Elliot & Clark;* Spontaneous Healing: How to Discover and Enhance Your Body's Natural Ability To Maintain and Heal Itself, *by A. Weil, 1996, New York: Alfred A. Knopf; and* Herbal Medicines, *by C. O'Neil, J. Avila, & C. W. Fetrow, (1999),* Nursing99, 29(4).

- *Chamomile* is believed to benefit the gastrointestinal tract, relieve allergies, and act as a sedative.
- *Marjoram* is purported to work as an antiseptic and anti-inflammatory agent and to relieve muscle spasms.

LIFE CYCLE CONSIDERATIONS

Essential Oils

Essential oils should be used with caution in elderly persons. These clients are usually more sensitive to essential oils than are adults and teenagers and thus require smaller amounts and less-concentrated forms of the essence.

- *Peppermint* is believed to improve digestion and act as an antiseptic and decongestant.
- *Rosemary* is said to stimulate the circulation.
- *Geranium* is thought to balance the mind and body.

Aromatherapists use concentrated oils derived from the roots, bark, or flowers of herbs and other plants to treat specific ailments. The aromas cause physiological, psychological, and pharmacological reactions (Trevelyan, 1993). Some essential oils have antibacterial properties and are found in a wide variety of pharmaceutical preparations. Essential oils should be used intelligently and with caution.

A clinical study reported by Wilkinson (1995) concluded that massage oil that incorporated the essential oil Roman chamomile reduced anxiety and improved the quality of life of cancer clients to a greater extent than did unscented oil. Another study found that postcardiac surgery clients receiving foot massages with neroli oil (from orange flowers) experienced greater and more lasting psychological benefits than did those receiving massages without neroli oil (Stevenson, 1994). Weiss and James (1997), however, report clients with allergic contact dermatitis to essential oils.

Some contraindications for aromatherapy are listed in Table 13–5.

 Safety: Aromatherapy
- Essential oils are very potent and should never be used in an undiluted form, be used near the eyes, or be ingested orally.
- Because some people are allergic to certain oils, a small skin-patch test should be done before generalized application.

Humor

Of all the complementary interventions addressed in this chapter, humor is the one that can be used most often by nurses to benefit clients. "Humor is probably one of the least understood, easiest to do, and most beneficial of the nonpharmacologic interventions" (Mornhinweg & Voignier, 1995). Therapeutic humor includes any intervention that promotes health and wellness by stimulating a playful discovery, expression, or appreciation of the absurdity or incongruity of life's situations (AATH, 2000).

To avoid giving offense, it is important to determine the client's perception of what is humorous. Whether a given situation is considered humorous or offensive will vary greatly from culture to culture and person to person. Good taste and common sense should serve as guides.

Nurses can use humor with clients in a variety of ways. A humor cart (portable cart or carrier filled with cartoon and joke books, magic tricks, and silly noses) is easy to use and allows clients to select their own humor tools for health. A "humor room" may be made available, where clients can watch comedy videos or play fun games with visitors or other clients.

Humor has many therapeutic outcomes. Norman Cousins, former chairman of the Task Force in Psychoneuroimmunology at the School of Medicine at UCLA, relates how he enhanced his recovery from an incurable connective tissue disorder, ankylosing

Table 13–5 AROMATHERAPY CONTRAINDICATIONS	
ESSENTIAL OIL	**CONTRAINDICATION**
Sweet fennel	Epilepsy
Rosemary, sage, thyme	Hypertension
Peppermint, rose, rosemary	First trimester of pregnancy
	Use only in well-diluted form in later stages of pregnancy
Arnica, basil, celery, sage, cypress, jasmine, juniper, marjoram, myrrh, sage, thyme	Pregnancy
Camomile, lavender	Use with care in pregnancies carrying the risk of bleeding or miscarriage

From "Aromatherapy," by J. Trevelyan, 1993, Nursing Times, 89(25), 39.

spondylitis, by the daily watching of films and movies that made him laugh (Cousins, 1979). Humor can be used effectively to relieve anxiety and promote relaxation, improve respiratory function, enhance immunological function, and decrease pain by stimulating the production of endorphins.

Animal-Assisted Therapy

The use of pets to enhance health status has a long history. In Britain in the 18th and 19th centuries, pets were used in institutions to give a sense of meaning and purpose to people institutionalized because of developmental delays (i.e., mental retardation). Pet therapy was also used during the Crimean War and World

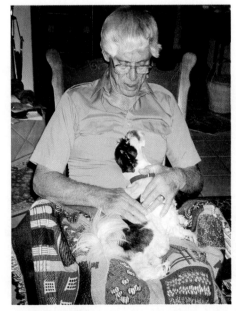

Figure 13-6 Pet therapy provides health benefits. *(Photo courtesy of John White, Corpus Christi, TX.)*

 PROFESSIONAL TIP

Use of Humor

Never do or say anything that gives clients the idea that you are laughing *at* them as opposed to *with* them (McGhee, 1998).

War II (Mornhinweg & Voignier, 1995). Animal-assisted therapy (AAT) is currently used as a complementary therapy for people in both acute and long-term care settings (Figure 13-6).

Dogs are the animals most often used in AAT. Cats are less predictable and many people are allergic to cat dander (Miller & Connor, 2000). Animal-assisted therapy has many applications including overcoming physical limitations, improving mood, lowering blood pressure, and improving socialization skills and self-esteem.

Music Therapy

Music enters the bodymind through the auditory sense. Therapeutic use of music consists of playing music to elicit positive changes in behavior, emotions, or physiological response. Music complements other treatment modalities and encourages clients to become active participants in their health care and recovery.

Music is a good adjunct to use with imagery, as it can enhance the relaxation response and, therefore, heighten images. Different types of music elicit different responses, but all music stimulates the neurotransmitters that evoke chemical changes in the bodymind (Achterberg, Dossey, & Kolkmeier, 1994). Music-thanatology is a holistic and palliative method of using music with dying clients (Schroeder-Shecker, 1994). It is used to help dissipate obstacles to the client's peaceful transition to death.

Music on audiocassette and heard via a tape player and headphones can be a very useful tool for clients who are immobilized, who must wait for diagnostic tests, or who are undergoing the perioperative experience (Figure 13-7). Some facilities allow clients to choose the type of music played while they undergo procedures such as cardiac catheterization. Clients may request that their music and tape player accompany them during surgery. Pleasurable sound and music can

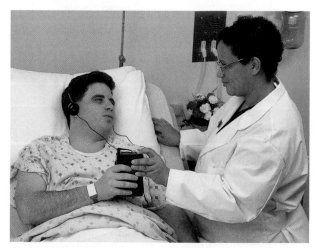

Figure 13-7 Music therapy helps client relax.

reduce stress, perception of pain, anxiety, and feelings of isolation. Music can also be especially useful in helping adolescent clients relax.

Play Therapy

Play therapy is especially useful with children. Toys are used to allow children to learn about what will be happening to them and to express their emotions and their current situations. Drawing and art work also provide a way for children to share their experiences. When language ability is reduced or not yet well developed, play therapy and drawings constitute a method for children to communicate their needs and feelings to care providers.

NURSING AND COMPLEMENTARY/ ALTERNATIVE APPROACHES

Some methods labeled by Western society as "alternative" (e.g., acupuncture) have already been validated by having been used successfully for centuries. Other complementary/alternative methods such as biofeedback have been proven through research. Still other complementary/alternative modalities such as therapeutic touch need further investigation and validation. Nurses play an important role in educating consumers about nontraditional interventions appropriate throughout the life cycle (Table 13–6) by providing information about the safety and efficacy of such methods. The following are terms frequently used to describe various treatment modalities:

- *Proven:* have been scientifically tested in clinical trials
- *Experimental:* are undergoing Food and Drug Administration (FDA) investigations to ascertain safety and efficacy
- *Untested:* have not been investigated by the FDA with regard to safety and efficacy
- *Folklore:* have been passed from one generation to another as remedies, many of which have therapeutic value

Table 13–6 CORRELATION OF SELECTED STAGES OF LIFE CYCLE WITH RECOMMENDED COMPLEMENTARY THERAPIES

STAGE OF LIFE CYCLE	RECOMMENDED COMPLEMENTARY THERAPIES	
Adolescents	All modalities discussed in this chapter, as appropriate to the condition	
Adults	All modalities discussed in this chapter, as appropriate to the condition	
Elders	• Massage (lighter pressure and other modifications for body's status) • Aromatherapy (with precautions) • Any other modalities discussed in this chapter, as appropriate to the condition and with precautions	
Terminally ill	• Massage • Reflexology • Energetic-touch therapies • Music-thanatology	• Prayer • Any other modalities discussed in this chapter, as appropriate to the condition and with precautions

Adapted from Fundamentals of Nursing: Standards & Practice, *by S. DeLaune and P. Ladner, 1998, Albany, NY: Delmar. Copyright 1998 by Delmar. Adapted with permission.*

• *Quackery:* have not proven effective, may result in harm to consumers, and are usually marketed with numerous unfounded promises (e.g., as "cure-all" products or therapies) (Brown, Cassileth, Lewis, & Renner, 1994)

According to Keegan (1998), research has documented the effectiveness of specific complementary/alternative therapies:

• Meditation combined with guided imagery decreases physical tension, anxiety, and the adverse effects of chemotherapy.
• Nutrition, exercise, and meditation—without the use of medication or surgery—can reverse coronary heart disease.
• Yoga can help mentally challenged individuals become more aware of their bodies and improve coordination.
• Yoga can help reduce pain in clients with osteoarthritis of the hands.

Numerous complementary/alternative interventions can be incorporated into nursing practice. As Frisch (1997) states:

While holistic nurses use many alternative and complementary approaches to care, it is not the alternative modality that makes us holistic; it is our presence, our caring, and our willingness to put the client first.

Putting the client first means individualizing every intervention on the basis of the client's unique needs. From the time before birth until the moment of death, people of all ages experience trauma, stress, and life challenges and have needs in all dimensions. Nurses are challenged to discover and meet those needs.

The power of the nurse's presence with any client should never be underestimated. Many of the complementary/alternative modalities require further study and advanced training. However, nursing students already have the ability to listen, to touch, and to care. Clients can benefit from intent, compassion, and something as simple as having another person present with them.

CASE STUDY

Mr. Vincent, who is receiving chemotherapy for colon cancer, tells the nurse that he is seeing both an aromatherapist to relieve his pain and nausea and a practitioner of healing touch to cure his cancer. He also says that he does not know whether he will come back for his next chemotherapy session because it makes him feel bad. The other therapies make him feel better.

Consider the following:

1. What should the nurse do with this information?
2. How should the nurse respond?
3. What assessments should the nurse make?
4. Identify a nursing diagnosis and goal for Mr. Vincent.
5. List three nursing interventions for this nursing diagnosis.
6. Identify sources for information about the therapies.

SUMMARY

- Ever-increasing numbers of health care consumers are using nontraditional treatment modalities.
- Psychoneuroimmunology is the study of the way that the body and mind are connected and the way that beliefs, thoughts, and emotions affect health.
- Holistic nursing practice encompasses consideration of each client as a unique and whole being with many aspects: physiological, psychological, sociocultural, intellectual, and spiritual.
- Healing is not curing but, rather, is regaining balance and finding harmony and wholeness as changes take place from within the individual.
- No one can heal another, but a nurse can act as a guide, support system, or instrument of healing for the client.
- Some of the mind/body modalities that nurses use are meditation, relaxation, imagery, biofeedback, and hypnosis.
- Body-movement modalities include movement and exercise and chiropractic therapy.
- Energetic-touch therapies can be used with persons of all ages and in various stages of illness and wellness.
- Energetic-touch therapies include therapeutic massage, therapeutic touch, healing touch, shiatsu, acupressure, and reflexology.
- Spiritual therapies such as faith healing, healing prayer, and laying on of the hands are helpful modalities to use in caring for clients.
- Nutritional/medicinal therapies include the use of antioxidants, macrobiotic diets, and herbal therapy.
- Other modalities such as aromatherapy, humor, pet therapy, music therapy, and play therapy are valuable adjuncts to conventional treatment.

Review Questions

1. Therapies that are used instead of mainstream medical practice are called:
   a. alternative therapies.
   b. contemporary therapies.
   c. complementary therapies.
   d. nontraditional therapies.

2. Therapies that are used in conjunction with conventional medical therapies are called:
   a. alternative therapies.
   b. contemporary therapies.
   c. complementary therapies.
   d. nontraditional therapies.

3. The National Center for Complementary and Alternative Medicine:
   a. investigates treatments shown to be effective.
   b. refers persons to practitioners of nontraditional therapies.
   c. monitors the number of people using nontraditional therapies.
   d. grants a license to those who practice nontraditional therapies.

4. Healing is:
   a. curing a disease.
   b. treating a disease.
   c. making a client well.
   d. a process that activates internal forces.

5. Imagery is a:
   a. balancing of life forces.
   b. relaxation technique using the five senses.

c. measurement of physiological responses when dreaming.

d. blocking of the body's energy fields with unhappy thoughts.

6. One of the most universal complementary/alternative modalities is:

a. touch.
b. massage.
c. nutrition.
d. faith healing.

7. Learning about herbal treatments can be compared to learning about:

a. hypnosis.
b. nutrition.
c. reflexology.
d. pharmacology.

8. Clients using animal-assisted therapy:

a. play with a cat.
b. have no other companions.
c. experience a decrease in blood pressure.
d. show an increase in physical limitations.

9. The complementary therapy recommended for all ages in the life cycle is:

a. massage.
b. hypnosis.
c. reflexology.
d. aromatherapy.

Critical Thinking Questions

1. Your close friend has AIDS and is experiencing a great deal of pain and discouragement. She wants to find alternative methods to ease the pain. She confides in you that she believes there may be a cure available at the holistic health center. How do you best help your friend in this situation? What do you advise?

2. A client asks the nurse to rub his foot in a particular spot because that is where his reflexologist rubs to relieve his abdominal pain. How should the nurse handle this situation?

WEB FLASH!

- Are there specific sites listed under complementary therapies or alternative therapies?
- Search the web for the organizations listed as resources for this chapter at the end of the book. What information do they provide?
- What resources (books, videos, discussion forums) are available through the Internet for clients interested in a specific complementary/alternative therapy?

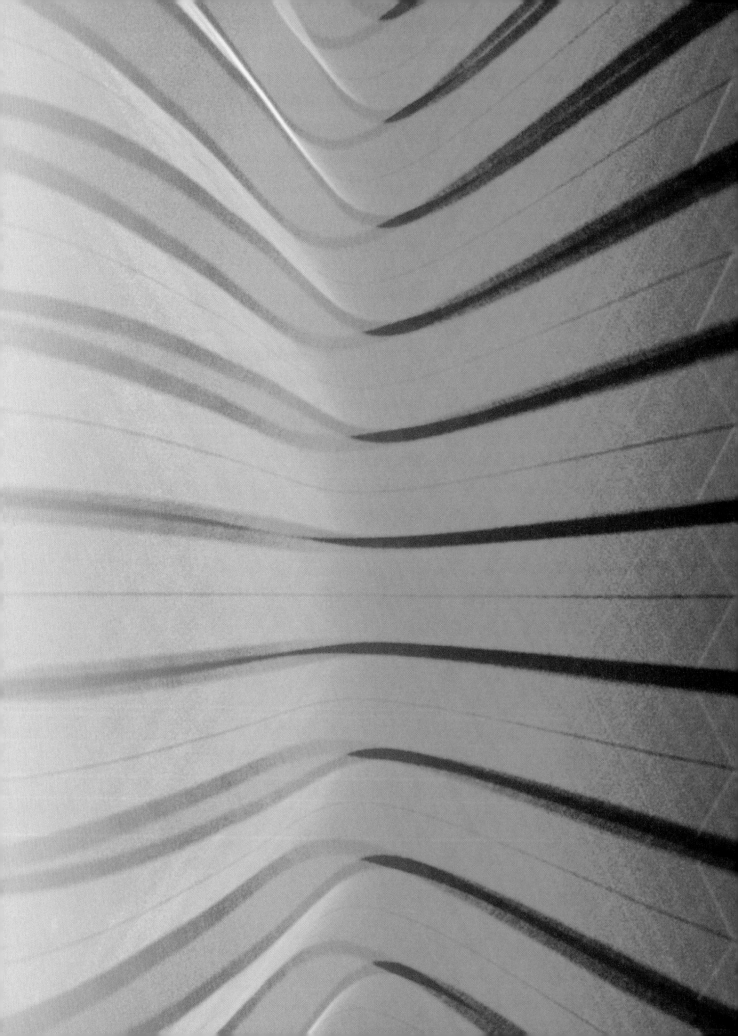

Unit 6
Human Development
Over the Life Span

Unit 7
Health Promotion

Unit 8
Infection Control

Unit 9
Homeostasis

THE LIFE CYCLE

LEARNING OBJECTIVES

Upon completion of this chapter, you should be able to:
- *Define key terms.*
- *Discuss the basic principles of growth and development.*
- *Identify the factors that influence growth and development.*
- *Compare the major developmental theories.*
- *Discuss the importance of development as a holistic framework for assessing and promoting health.*
- *Identify the critical milestones of each developmental stage.*
- *Describe the specific nursing interventions that are relevant to each developmental stage.*

KEY TERMS

accommodation	maturation
adaptation	menarche
adolescence	middle adulthood
anorexia nervosa	moral maturity
assimilation	neonatal period
bonding	obesity
bulimia nervosa	older adulthood
critical period	preadolescence
development	prenatal period
developmental task	preschool period
embryonic stage	puberty
fetal alcohol syndrome	school-age period
fetal stage	self-concept
germinal stage	spirituality
growth	teratogenic substance
infancy	toddler period
intrapsychic theory	young adulthood
learning	

INTRODUCTION

From conception to death, individuals are constantly changing. Physical growth, psychological development, emotional maturation, cognitive development, moral development, and spiritual growth occur throughout life. Progression through each developmental stage influences health status. A thorough understanding of developmental concepts is essential for professional quality nursing practice. This chapter presents the types of changes that occur in each stage of the life cycle.

BASIC CONCEPTS OF GROWTH AND DEVELOPMENT

Development occurs continuously through the life span. Adults continue to have transition periods during which growth and development occur.

Growth is the quantitative (measurable) changes in the physical size of the body and its parts, such as increases in cells, tissues, structures, and systems. Examples of growth are physical changes in height, weight, bone density, and dental structure. Even though growth is not a steady process through the life cycle, growth patterns can be predicted. The growth rate varies from periods of rapid increase to periods of slower increase within each individual. Rapid growth is most common in the prenatal, infant, and adolescent stages.

Development refers to behavioral changes in functional abilities and skills. Thus, developmental changes are qualitative, that is, not easily measured. **Maturation** is the process of becoming fully grown and developed and applies to both physiological and behavioral aspects of an individual. Maturation depends on biological growth, functional changes, and **learning** (assimilation of information with a resultant change in behavior). During each developmental stage of the life cycle, certain goals (**developmental tasks**) must be achieved. These developmental tasks set the stage for future learning.

The **critical period** is the time of the most rapid growth or development in a particular stage of the life cycle. During these critical periods, an individual is most vulnerable to stressors of any type.

Growth, development, maturation, and learning are interdependent processes. For learning to occur, the individual must be mature enough to grasp the concepts and make required behavioral changes. Physical growth is also a prerequisite for many types of learning; for example, a child must have the physical ability to control the anal sphincter before toilet training skills are learned. Likewise, cognitive maturation precedes learning.

Principles of Growth and Development

All persons have individual talents and abilities that contribute to their development as unique entities. Thus, *there are no absolute rules in predicting the exact rate of development for any given individual.* There are, however, a few general principles regarding the growth and development of all humans (Table 14–1).

Although evidence of specific skills varies with each person, the sequence of development is predictable. For example, not all infants roll over at the same age, but most roll over before they crawl.

Table 14–1 PRINCIPLES OF GROWTH AND DEVELOPMENT

PRINCIPLE	EXAMPLE
Development occurs in a *cephalocaudal* (head-to-toe) direction.	An infant raises his head before sitting up.
Development occurs in a *proximodistal* manner. Functions closer to the midline (proximal) of the body develop before functions farther away from the body's midline (distal).	The infant is able to move his arms before picking up objects with hands and fingers.
Development occurs in an orderly manner from *simple to complex* and from the *general to the specific*. Gross motor control is achieved before fine motor coordination.	An infant crawls before walking. A child holds a crayon with the entire hand before being able to grasp it between thumb and finger.
The pattern of growth and development is continuous, orderly, and predictable. However, growth and development do not proceed at a consistent rate.	Periods of rapid growth (similar to the growth spurts of adolescence) alternate with periods of slower growth (as seen in middle adulthood).
All individuals go through the same developmental processes; individual differences occur but the process is consistent.	At a certain age in normal development, all individuals will learn how to smile.
Every person proceeds through stages of growth and development at an individual rate.	A child who grows more slowly may be shorter than other children of the same age.
Every stage of development has specific characteristics.	An infant is dependent on others for physical and emotional survival. Adolescence is characterized by a search for identity.
Each stage of development has certain tasks to be achieved or acquired during that specific time. Tasks of one developmental stage become the foundation for tasks in subsequent stages.	An infant must master the psychological task of developing trust to mature as an adolescent who can establish a separate identity.
Some stages of growth and development are more critical than others.	The first trimester of pregnancy is a critical time for embryonic development. During this critical phase, the developing human is most vulnerable to damage from toxins (e.g., drugs, chemicals, viruses).

From Fundamentals of Nursing: Standards & Practice, *by S. DeLaune and P. Ladner, 1998, Albany, NY: Delmar. Copyright 1998 by Delmar. Reprinted with permission.*

Factors Influencing Growth and Development

Multiple factors such as heredity, life experiences, health status, and cultural expectations influence a person's growth and development. The interaction of these factors greatly influences how an individual responds to everyday situations; the choices a person makes regarding health behaviors are also greatly determined by these factors.

Heredity

A complex series of processes transmits genetic information from parents to children. The genetic composition of an individual determines physical characteristics such as skin color, hair texture, facial features, and body structure, as well as a predisposition to certain diseases (i.e., Tay-Sachs, sickle cell anemia). Heredity is a genetic blueprint from which an individual grows and develops; to a great extent, it determines the rate of physical and mental development.

Life Experiences

A person's experiences can also influence the rate of growth and development. For example, contrast the differences in physical growth rates between a child whose family can afford food, shelter, and health care and a child whose family has little, if any, resources. The child from an environment lacking in physical resources has a higher risk of experiencing physical and mental lags in growth and development.

Health Status

Individuals who experience wellness progress normally through the life cycle. Illness or disability can interfere with an individual's achievement of developmental milestones. Individuals with chronic conditions will often meet developmental milestones but will be delayed in doing so.

Cultural Expectations

Society expects people to master certain skills at each developmental period. The age at which an individual masters a particular task is determined in part by culture. For instance, cultures that discourage boys from showing tenderness and nurturance may well produce men who are reluctant or incapable of fully expressing these qualities.

 CULTURAL CONSIDERATIONS

Growth and Development

The time for mastery of such developmental tasks as speaking and toilet training is as dependent on cultural norms as it is on physiological development.

THEORETICAL PERSPECTIVES OF HUMAN DEVELOPMENT

Nurses must have a thorough understanding of human growth and development in order to provide individualized care. Remember that chronological age and developmental age are not synonymous. An overview of the major developmental theories follows. These theories are discussed more fully in the specific sections about each developmental period.

Physiological Dimension

Physiological growth (physical size and functioning) of an individual is influenced primarily by interaction of genetic predisposition, the central nervous system (CNS), the endocrine system, and maturation. The role of heredity in human development is complex and not yet fully understood. Genetics is the foundation for achievement of specific tasks. Factors such as the psychosocial environment and health status help individuals live up to their genetic potentials.

Psychosocial Dimension

The psychosocial dimension of growth and development consists of subjective feelings and interpersonal relationships. A favorable **self-concept** (perception of one's self, including body image, self-esteem, and ideal self) is perhaps the most important key to a person's success and happiness. Following are characteristics of an individual with a positive self-concept:

- Self-confidence
- Willingness to take risks
- Ability to receive criticism without becoming defensive
- Ability to adapt effectively to stressors
- Innovative problem-solving skills

People with a healthy self-concept believe in themselves. As a result, they set goals that can be achieved. The achievement then reinforces the positive belief about one's self. Figure 14-1 illustrates this positive cycle of self-fulfilling beliefs and actions.

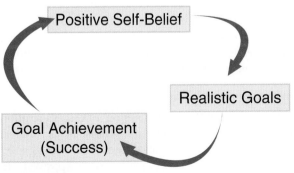

Figure 14-1 Self-Fulfilling Cycle in Positive Self-Concept

A person with a positive self-concept is likely to engage in health-promoting activities. For example, a person who values self is more likely to change unhealthy habits (such as smoking and sedentary lifestyle) to promote health. An individual with a negative or poor self-concept, on the other hand, is likely to have low self-esteem, a lack of confidence, and difficulty setting and achieving goals.

There are many and varied psychosocial theories that explain the development of self-concept. Following is a discussion of the intrapsychic and interpersonal theories of personality development.

Intrapsychic Theory

Intrapsychic (also called psychodynamic) **theory** focuses on an individual's unconscious processes. Feelings, needs, conflicts, and drives are considered to be motivators of behavior, learning, and development. Sigmund Freud, Erik Erikson, and Robert Havighurst are three of the major intrapsychic theorists.

Freud's theories, developed in the early 1930s, continue to influence current concepts related to human development. A basic belief of the Freudian model is that all behavior has some meaning. According to Freud (1961), to mature, a person must successfully travel through five stages of development (Table 14–2). In each stage, there is a conflict to be mastered; if the conflict is not resolved, the individual is halted, developing a fixation at that stage. Fixation implies either inadequate mastery of or failure to achieve a developmental task. A fixation in earlier stages inhibits healthy progression through subsequent stages.

Erikson (1968) expanded Freud's concept of developmental stages by theorizing that psychosocial development is a lifelong process that does not end with the cessation of adolescence. Erikson also emphasized the importance of societal expectations on development. According to Erikson, certain psychosocial tasks must be mastered at each developmental stage. Erikson's model proposes that psychosocial development is a series of conflicts that can have favorable or unfavorable outcomes. These conflicts occur in eight developmental stages of life, described in Table 14–3.

Havighurst (1972) theorizes six developmental stages of life, each with essential tasks to be achieved. Mastery of a task at one developmental stage is essential for mastery of tasks in subsequent stages. When a task at one stage is mastered, it is learned for life, independent of subsequent neurological change (which may occur with disease or injury). Table 14–4 presents Havighurst's developmental stages and the associated tasks.

Interpersonal Theory

Interpersonal theory focuses on a person's relationships with those around him. Harry Stack Sullivan (1953) theorizes that relationships with others influence how one's personality develops. Approval and disapproval from significant others shape the formation of one's personality. To form satisfying relationships with others, an individual must complete six stages of development, shown in Table 14–5.

Table 14–2 FREUD'S STAGES OF PSYCHOSEXUAL DEVELOPMENT		
STAGE	**AGE**	**DESCRIPTION**
Oral	Birth–18 months	Management of anxiety by using mouth and tongue.
Anal	18 months–3 years	Control of muscles, especially those controlling urination and defecation.
Phallic (Oedipal)	3 years–6 years	Awareness of gender and genitalia.
Latency	6 years–12 years	Exhibition of latent sexual development and energy.
Genital	12 years–adulthood	Emergence of sexual interests and development of relationships with potential sexual partners.

Data from Civilization and Its Discontents, *by S. Freud, 1961, New York: Norton. Copyright 1961 by Norton.*

Cognitive Dimension

The cognitive dimension is characterized by the intellectual process of knowing, which includes perception, memory, and judgment. It develops as an individual progresses through the life span. Intelligence is an adaptive process. Individuals use intelligence to adapt by changing the environment to meet their needs and by altering their responses to environmental stressors. The ability to change behavior in response to the demands of an ever-changing environment is characteristic of intelligent beings.

Jean Piaget (1963) studied the differences between children's thinking patterns at different ages and how intelligence is used to solve problems and answer questions. He theorized that children learn to think by playing. Four factors are catalysts to intellectual development:

- Maturation of the endocrine and nervous systems
- Action-centered experience that leads to discovery ("learning by doing")
- Social interaction with opportunities for receiving feedback
- A self-regulating mechanism that responds to environmental stimuli (Murray & Zentner, 1997)

Piaget and Inhelder (1969) enumerate four phases of intellectual development: sensorimotor, preoperational, concrete operations, and formal operations.

Table 14–3 ERIKSON'S STAGES OF PSYCHOSOCIAL DEVELOPMENT

STAGE	AGE	TASK TO BE ACHIEVED	IMPLICATIONS
Trust vs. mistrust	Birth–18 months	To develop a sense of trust in others.	To promote mastery, give consistent, affectionate care. Deficient, inconsistent care produces an unfavorable outcome at this stage.
Autonomy vs. shame and doubt	18 months–3 years	To learn self-control.	To facilitate the child's use of newly acquired skills of independence, provide support, praise, and encouragement. Shaming or insulting the child will lead to unnecessary dependence.
Initiative vs. guilt	3 years–6 years	To initiate spontaneous activities.	Give clear explanations for events and encourage creative activities. Threatening with punishment or labeling behavior as "bad" leads to development of guilt and fear of doing wrong.
Industry vs. inferiority	6 years–12 years	To develop necessary social skills.	To build confidence, recognize the child's accomplishments. Unrealistic expectations or excessively harsh criticism leads to a sense of inadequacy.
Identity vs. role confusion	12 years–20 years	To integrate childhood into a personal identity.	Help the adolescent make decisions. Encourage active participation in home events. Assist with planning for the future.
Intimacy vs. isolation	18 years–25 years	To develop commitments to others and to a life work (career).	Teach the young adult to establish realistic goals. Avoid ridiculing romances or job choices.
Generativity vs. stagnation	21 years–45 years	To establish a family and become productive.	Provide emotional support. Recognize individual accomplishments and provide appropriate praise.
Integrity vs. despair	45+ years	To view one's life as meaningful and fulfilling.	Explore positive aspects of one's life. Review contributions made by the individual.

Data from Childhood and Society, *by E. Erikson, 1968, New York: Norton. Copyright 1968 by Norton;* American Nursing Review of Psychiatric and Mental Health Nursing Certification, *by N. Randolph, 1998, Springhouse, PA: Springhouse. Copyright 1998 by Springhouse.*

Table 14–4 HAVIGHURST'S DEVELOPMENTAL STAGES AND TASKS

DEVELOPMENTAL STAGE	DEVELOPMENTAL TASKS	
Infancy and early childhood	Eat solid foods Walk Talk Control elimination of wastes Relate emotionally to others	Distinguish right from wrong through development of a conscience Learn gender differences and sexual modesty Achieve psychological stability Form simple concepts of social and physical reality
Middle childhood	Learn physical skills required for games Build healthy attitudes toward oneself Learn to socialize with peers Learn appropriate masculine or feminine roles Gain basic reading, writing, and mathematical skills	Develop concepts necessary for everyday living Formulate a conscience based on a value system Achieve personal independence Develop attitudes toward social groups and institutions
Adolescence	Establish more mature relationships with individuals of the same age and of both genders Achieve a masculine or feminine social role Accept own body Establish emotional independence from parents	Achieve assurance of economic independence Prepare for an occupation Prepare for marriage and establishment of a family Acquire skills necessary to fulfill civic responsibilities Develop a set of values that guides behavior

continues

Table 14–4 HAVIGHURST'S DEVELOPMENTAL STAGES AND TASKS *continued*

DEVELOPMENTAL STAGE	DEVELOPMENTAL TASKS	
Early adulthood	Select a partner Learn to live with a partner Start a family Manage a home	Establish self in a career/occupation Assume civic responsibility Become a part of a social group
Middle adulthood	Fulfill civic and social responsibilities Maintain standard of living appropriate to economic status Assist adolescent children to become responsible, happy adults	Relate to one's partner Adjust to physiological changes Adjust to aging parents
Later maturity	Adjust to physiological changes and alterations in health status Adjust to retirement and altered income Adjust to death of spouse	Develop affiliation with one's age group Meet civic and social responsibilities Establish satisfactory living arrangements

Data from Developmental Tasks and Education, *by R. J. Havighurst, 1972, New York: Longman. Copyright 1972 by Longman.*

Table 14–6 lists descriptions of these phases. Each phase is characterized by the ways that the child interprets and uses the environment. Approximate ages are indicated for each phase, although there is great variation among individuals.

The individual learns by interacting with the environment through three processes: assimilation, accommodation, and adaptation. **Assimilation** is the process of taking in new experiences or information. **Accommodation** allows for readjustment of the cognitive structure (mindset) to take in the new information thus increasing understanding. **Adaptation** refers to the changes that occur as a result of assimilation and accommodation (Murray & Zentner, 1997).

Moral Dimension

The moral dimension consists of a person's value system, which helps one differentiate right and wrong. **Moral maturity** (the ability to independently decide for oneself what is "right") is closely related to emotional and cognitive development. Lawrence Kohlberg (1977) established a framework for understanding how individuals determine a moral code to guide their behavior. Kohlberg's model states that a person's ability to make moral judgments and behave in a morally correct manner develops over a period of time.

According to Kohlberg, there are six stages of moral development, with each stage being built on the previous stage and becoming the foundation for successive stages. Moral development progresses in relationship to cognitive development. Individuals who are able to think at higher levels have the necessary reasoning skills on which to base moral decisions. Table 14–7 provides an overview of Kohlberg's stages of moral development. Kohlberg purports that although individuals move through the six stages in a sequential fashion; not everyone reaches the fifth and sixth stages in the development of personal morality (Kohlberg, 1977).

Table 14–5 SULLIVAN'S INTERPERSONAL MODEL OF PERSONALITY DEVELOPMENT

STAGE	AGE	DESCRIPTION
Infancy	Birth–18 months	Infant learns to rely on caregivers to meet needs and desires.
Childhood	18 months–6 years	Child begins learning to delay immediate need for gratification of needs and desires.
Juvenile	6 years–9 years	Child forms fulfilling peer relationships.
Preadolescence	9 years–12 years	Child relates successfully to peers of the same gender as the child.
Early adolescence	12 years–14 years	Adolescent learns to be independent and forms relationships with members of the opposite sex.
Late adolescence	14 years–21 years	Person establishes an intimate, long-lasting relationship with someone of the opposite sex.

Data from Interpersonal Theory of Psychiatry, *by H. S. Sullivan, 1953, New York: Norton. Copyright 1953 by Norton.*

Table 14–6 PIAGET'S PHASES OF COGNITIVE DEVELOPMENT

PHASE	AGE	DESCRIPTION
Sensorimotor	**Birth–2 years**	Sensory organs and muscles become more functional.
Stage 1: reflex use	Birth–1 month	Movements are primarily reflexive.
Stage 2: primary circular reaction	1 month–4 months	Perceptions center around one's body. Objects are perceived as extensions of the self.
Stage 3: secondary circular reaction	4 months–8 months	Becomes aware of external environment. Initiates acts to change the environment.
Stage 4: coordination of secondary schemata	8 months–12 months	Differentiates goals and goal-directed activities.
Stage 5: tertiary circular reaction	12 months–18 months	Experiments with methods to reach goals. Develops rituals that become significant.
Stage 6: invention of new means	18 months–24 months	Uses mental imagery to understand the environment. Uses fantasy ("make-believe").
Preoperational	**2 years–7 years**	Ability to think emerges.
Preconceptual stage	2 years–4 years	Thinking tends to be egocentric. Exhibits use of symbolism.
Intuitive stage	4 years–7 years	Unable to break down a whole into separate parts. Able to classify objects according to one trait.
Concrete Operations	**7 years–11 years**	Child learns to reason about events in here-and-now.
Formal Operations	**11+ years**	Child is able to see relationships and to reason in the abstract.

Data from The Origins of Intelligence in Children, *by J. Piaget, 1963, New York: Norton. Copyright 1963 by Norton.*

Table 14–7 KOHLBERG'S STAGES OF MORAL DEVELOPMENT

LEVEL AND STAGE	DESCRIPTION
Level I: Preconventional	Authority figures are obeyed.
(Birth–9 years)	Misbehavior is viewed in terms of damage done.
Stage 1: *punishment and obedience orientation*	A deed is perceived as "wrong" if one is punished; the activity is "right" if one is not punished.
Stage 2: *instrumental-relativist orientation*	"Right" is defined as that which is acceptable to and approved by the self. When actions satisfy one's needs, they are "right."
Level II: Conventional	Cordial interpersonal relationships are maintained.
(9 years–13 years)	Approval of others is sought through one's actions.
Stage 3: *interpersonal concordance*	Authority is respected.
Stage 4: *law and order orientation*	Individual feels "duty bound" to maintain social order. Behavior is "right" when it conforms to the rules.
Level III: Postconventional (13+ years)	Individual understands the morality of having democratically established laws.
Stage 5: *social contract orientation*	It is "wrong" to violate others' rights.
Stage 6: *universal ethics orientation*	The person understands the principles of human rights and personal conscience. Person believes that trust is basis for relationships.

Data from Recent Research in Moral Development, *by L. Kohlberg, 1977, New York: Holt, Rinehart, & Winston. Copyright 1977 by Holt, Rinehart, & Winston.*

Spiritual Dimension

The spiritual dimension is characterized by a sense of personal meaning. The term *spirit* is derived from the Latin word meaning breath, air, and wind. Thus, spirit refers to whatever gives life to a person. **Spirituality** refers to relationships with one's self, with others, and with a higher power or divine source. Spirituality does not refer to a specific religious affiliation; rather, it can be defined as the core of a person. Development of spirituality is an ongoing, lifelong process.

Fowler's theory of spiritual development was influenced by the works of Erikson, Piaget, and Kohlberg.

Fowler's theory is composed of a prestage and six distinct stages of faith development (Fowler, 1995). Although individuals vary in the age at which they experience each stage, the sequence of stages remains the same. Table 14–8 outlines Fowler's theory.

Although some clients seem to be unaware of their spiritual natures, each client has a personalized definition of spiritual self. Acknowledgment of a client's spirituality is essential to the practice of nursing. Caring for the whole being is the hallmark of a holistic nurse.

HOLISTIC FRAMEWORK FOR NURSING

Providing care to the whole person is a basic concept of nursing. Knowledge of growth and development concepts is essential for nurses because nursing interventions must be appropriate to each client's developmental stage. Nursing's holistic perspective recognizes the progression of individual development across the life span. Developmental progress, or lack thereof, in one dimension affects all other dimensions of life. Figure 14-2 shows the holistic nature of individuals.

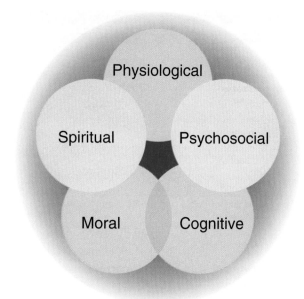

Figure 14-2 Holistic Nature of Human Beings

Growth and development theories are useful to nurses as assessment parameters. Alterations in expected patterns are indicators for early intervention. Examples of situations wherein knowledge of developmental milestones is essential for prompt identification of problems and comprehensive intervention include the following:

- The infant who does not sit, crawl, or walk at expected times
- The adolescent girl who has not experienced menarche by the expected time
- The adult who has failed to develop adequate problem-solving skills

STAGES OF THE LIFE CYCLE

For purposes of this discussion, eleven developmental stages are considered: prenatal, neonatal, infant, toddler, preschooler, school-age, preadolescent, adolescent, young adult, middle adult, and older adult. For each stage, the manifestations of growth and development in the physiological, psychosocial, cognitive, moral, and spiritual dimensions are discussed together with relevant nursing implications.

Prenatal Period

The **prenatal period** (the developmental stage beginning with conception and ending with birth) is a critical time in a human being's development and consists of three developmental phases: germinal, embryonic, and fetal. The **germinal stage** begins with conception and lasts approximately 10 to 14 days. This stage is characterized by rapid cell division and implantation of the fertilized egg in the uterine wall. In

Table 14–8 FOWLER'S STAGES OF FAITH		
STAGE	**AGE**	**CHARACTERISTICS**
Prestage: *undifferentiated faith*	Infant	Trust, hope, and love compete with environmental inconsistencies or threats of abandonment.
Stage 1: *intuitive-projective faith*	Toddler and preschooler	Imitates parental behaviors and attitudes about religion and spirituality. Has no real understanding of spiritual concepts.
Stage 2: *mythical-literal faith*	School-age child	Accepts existence of a deity. Religious and moral beliefs are symbolized by stories. Appreciates others' viewpoints. Accepts concept of reciprocal fairness.
Stage 3: *synthetic-conventional faith*	Adolescent	Questions values and religious beliefs in an attempt to form own identity.
Stage 4: *individuative-reflective faith*	Late adolescent and young adult	Assumes responsibility for own attitudes and beliefs.
Stage 5: *conjunctive faith*	Adult	Integrates other perspectives about faith into own definition of truth.
Stage 6: *universalizing faith*	Adult	Makes concepts of love and justice tangible.

Data from Stages of Faith: The Psychology of Human Development and the Quest for Meaning, *by J. W. Fowler, 1995, New York: Harper & Row. Copyright 1995 by Harper & Row;* Psychiatric–Mental Health Nursing: Adaptation and Growth *(4th ed.), by B. S. Johnson, 1997, Philadelphia: Lippincott. Copyright 1997 by Lippincott.*

this very early stage, the central nervous system (CNS) is already beginning to form.

The **embryonic stage** (weeks 2 to 8 after conception) is characterized by rapid cellular differentiation, growth, and development of the body systems. This critical period is when the embryo is most vulnerable to noxious stimuli, which may lead to a spontaneous abortion (i.e., miscarriage) (Murray & Zentner, 1997).

The **fetal stage** (the intrauterine developmental period from 8 weeks to birth) is characterized by rapid growth and differentiation of body systems and parts.

Nursing Implications

The pregnant woman needs physical examinations and screenings throughout pregnancy. Early prenatal care is essential for a positive pregnancy outcome.

Learning that one is pregnant can elicit many emotions including happiness, fear, sadness, excitement, and anxiety. Because emotions lead to alterations in biochemicals, the mother's emotional state can bring about biochemical changes in the fetus. By teaching pregnant women how to relax, the nurse can promote a supportive environment for the developing embryo and fetus.

Wellness Promotion The uterus is the primary environment affecting prenatal growth and development. Ideally, this environment nurtures positive growth of the embryo and fetus.

An ample supply of nutrients must be provided by the mother. For example, the rate of preterm and low birth weight infants among women who consume insufficient amounts of protein during pregnancy is high. Such infants are at risk for developmental alterations.

When teaching the pregnant woman about nutrition, the nurse must emphasize that vitamin supplements are not substitutes for adequate food intake. Other nursing interventions that promote prenatal health include:

- Screening (blood pressure, urine glucose, and albumin)
- Teaching (e.g., about nutritional guidelines)
- Counseling (e.g., providing guidance about bonding with the child and incorporating a child into the family unit)
- Promoting the use of alternative modalities to reduce stress
- Working with economically disadvantaged clients to obtain prenatal care

Safety Considerations The fetus is especially vulnerable to substances consumed by the mother. In addition to providing the fetus with wholesome nutrients, maternal blood can also transport deadly toxins.

Cigarettes contain several toxic substances, including nicotine, that cross the placental barrier and interfere with the transport of oxygen to the fetus. Such toxins often result in increased risk of premature birth, retarded growth, learning difficulties, and fetal death.

Use of alcohol during pregnancy can result in **fetal alcohol syndrome** (FAS), a condition wherein fetal development is impaired, as manifested by physical and intellectual problems. Typically, FAS infants are small, have facial abnormalities (such as thin upper lips and short, upturned noses), and may have some degree of brain damage (Levin, 1995). Alcohol consumption is most dangerous during the first 3 months of pregnancy, when the embryo's brain and other vital organs are developing. The effects of alcohol on the fetus are permanent. Fetal alcohol syndrome is considered to be the leading cause of mental retardation among infants, and the incidence continues to increase (Wong et al., 1999).

 Safety: Tobacco and Alcohol Use During Pregnancy
Total abstinence from cigarette smoking is advised during pregnancy. Because a "safe" amount of alcohol consumption has not been determined, caution all pregnant women to abstain from drinking alcohol.

There are many other teratogenic substances in addition to nicotine and alcohol. A **teratogenic substance** is any substance that can cross the placental barrier and impair normal growth and development. The Food and Drug Administration requires that all manufactured drugs list their potential for causing birth defects. The use of illegal drugs by pregnant women presents a very serious threat to the unborn. Substance abuse prevention programs are effective in preventing or reducing this threat.

Neonatal Period

The **neonatal period** (the first 28 days of life following birth) is a time of major adjustment to extrauterine life. The energies of the neonate (newborn) are focused on achieving equilibrium through stabilization of major body systems. Table 14–9 outlines neonatal development.

The neonate's activities, which are reflexive in nature, consist primarily of sucking, crying, eliminating, and sleeping. The neonate blinks in response to bright light and demonstrates the startle reflex in response to

 CLIENT TEACHING

Pregnancy and Medications

Teach pregnant women to check labels of *all* medicines for information about potential effects on the fetus. Encourage expectant mothers to call their practitioner with any questions about the safety of any drug taken during pregnancy.

Table 14–9 NEONATE: GROWTH AND DEVELOPMENT

DIMENSION	CHARACTERISTICS	NURSING IMPLICATIONS
Physiological	Circulatory function shifts from umbilical cord to heart.	Accurately assess neonate's cardiovascular status.
	Gas exchange (oxygen and carbon dioxide) is transferred from placenta to lungs.	Immediately after birth, hold the neonate with head lower than body to allow for drainage of fluids that may block respiratory passages.
	Seconds after birth, respiratory reflexes are activated.	If spontaneous respirations do not occur, resuscitate immediately.
	Neck and shoulder muscles are weak.	Carefully support the neonate's head.
	Temperature-regulating mechanism is immature.	To conserve heat: • Dry neonate immediately after birth and place in a warmed bassinet and • Place a stockinette cap on neonate's head.
	Ossification (process of cartilage changing to bone) is incomplete.	Protect the anterior fontanel on neonate's skull.
	Visual acuity is poor, and visual focus is generally rigid.	Instruct parents to be directly in front of the neonate (approximately 9 to 12 inches away from child's face) when communicating.
Motor	Reflexes direct the majority of movement.	Teach parents to recognize neonate's protective reflexes.
	The full-term neonate has some limited ability to hold the head erect and is able to lift the head slightly when lying prone.	Support neonate's neck and head when lifting.
Psychosocial	Crying is the neonate's method of communication. There is a reason for the cry.	Teach parents about the dynamics of crying so that they neither label the neonate as "fussy" nor develop the misconception that they are inadequate caregivers. Encourage parents to learn to discriminate crying patterns.
	The bonding process begins shortly after birth.	Teach parents the importance of interacting with the neonate during every contact (feeding, bathing, changing, cuddling).
Cognitive	Neonates learn through sensory experiences. Learning is enhanced by an environment that provides stimuli without bombarding the neonate. Learning occurs by repeated exposure to stimuli.	To promote learning, encourage parents to provide frequent sensory stimuli (touching, talking, looking the neonate in the eyes).

Data from Health Assessment: A Nursing Approach *(3rd ed.), by J. Fuller and J. Schaller-Ayers, 2000, Philadelphia: Lippincott Williams & Wilkins. Copyright 2000 by Lippincott Williams & Wilkins;* Health Assessment & Promotion Strategies through the Life Span *(6th ed.), by R. B. Murray and J. P. Zentner, 1997, East Norwalk, CT: Appleton & Lange. Copyright 1997 by Appleton & Lange;* Whaley & Wong's Nursing Care of Infants and Children *(6th ed.), by D. L. Wong, M. Hockenberry-Eaton, D. Wilson, M. L. Winkelstein, E. Ahmann, and P. DiVito-Thomas, 1999, St. Louis, MO: Mosby–Yearbook. Copyright 1999 by Mosby–Yearbook;* Fundamentals of Nursing: Standards & Practice, *by S. DeLaune and P. Ladner, 1998, Albany, NY: Delmar. Copyright 1998 by Delmar.*

loud noises. Neonatal reflexes play a major role in the ability to survive.

During the first month of life, the neonate progresses developmentally from a mass of reflexes to behavior that is more goal directed (purposeful). In addition to the major physiological adjustments necessitated by extrauterine life, the neonate also undergoes psychological adaptation.

The major psychological task of neonates is to adjust to the parental figure(s). **Bonding**, the formation of attachment between parent and child, begins at birth, when the neonate and parent make initial eye

contact. The quality of parent–neonate bonding lays the foundation for the trust necessary for the development of future interpersonal relationships.

Nursing Implications

A complete and thorough assessment of the neonate is performed immediately after delivery. Evaluation of the neonate's reflexes should be performed at the same time or as soon as the neonate is physiologically stable.

In the first few hours after birth, the nurse should encourage the parents to cuddle the newborn, explain the neonate's interactive abilities, and encourage mutual eye contact between neonate and parents by showing parents how to hold the child in a position facing them.

Wellness Promotion Teaching is among the most important nursing activities in promoting neonatal wellness. Other nursing interventions that promote neonatal wellness are as follows:

- Continually assessing the neonate's physiological status
- Providing a warm environment. (Neonates breathe more easily when they are warm.)
- Monitoring nutritional status. It is normal for neonates to lose weight (up to 10% of birth weight) during the first week of life.
- Providing a clean environment to protect neonates from infection; teaching parents that neonates need a clean environment, not a sterile one.
- Conducting screening tests; for example, the blood test for phenylketonuria (PKU), a genetic disorder that, if untreated, can lead to impaired intellectual functioning.
- Promoting *early* parent–neonate interaction.

Selection of a feeding method for the neonate is a major decision for parents. Breastfeeding is the option recommended by the American Academy of Pediatrics. However, some parents choose to use commercially prepared formula. For a comparison of feeding methods, see the discussion about nutrition for the infant in this chapter.

Safety Considerations Because neonates are totally dependent on others to meet their needs, safety is of primary concern when caring for neonates. Accidents are the primary cause of neonatal mortality (Fuller & Schaller-Ayers, 2000). One of the most important methods of neonatal accident prevention is to teach parents about the use of infant car seats. Under current federal law, neonates and infants must be secured in an approved infant car seat every time the child travels in a car.

 Safety: Car Seats
Never discharge a neonate from the birthing center or hospital unless an infant seat is available for the trip home.

In addition to accidents, infections pose a serious health risk to the neonate. Newborns should be isolated from anyone experiencing an infectious disease. Because the skin is the body's major defense against invasion by disease-producing microorganisms, it is essential that the neonate's skin integrity be maintained. Parents must be taught the importance of skin cleanliness. Diaper rash is a common skin problem for newborns and infants because of the ammonia found in urine. In wet diapers, ammonia can burn and irritate the skin, resulting in localized irritation, blisters, or fissures. In addition to prompt changing of wet diapers, bathing and use of protective creams or powder are useful in preventing skin breakdown.

Infancy

Infancy (the developmental stage from the end of the first month to the end of the first year of life) is a time of continued adaptation. During this stage, the infant experiences rapid physiological growth and psychosocial development (Figure 14-3). Table 14–10 provides an overview of infant development in the

 CLIENT TEACHING

Parents and Newborn
Parents need information about:

- Basic newborn needs (i.e., to be held, rocked, and talked to),
- Nutrition,
- Infection control (especially handwashing and hygienic diaper changing practices),
- Care of the umbilicus,
- Incorporating the newborn into the family unit, and
- Growth and development milestones in order to provide appropriate stimulation and have realistic expectations for their newborn.

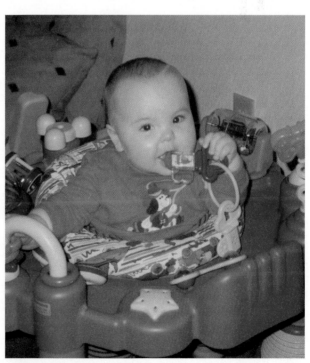

Figure 14-3 This child is exploring the world and is developing mastery of both the physiological and cognitive dimensions of development.

Table 14–10 INFANT: GROWTH AND DEVELOPMENT

DIMENSION	CHARACTERISTICS	NURSING IMPLICATIONS
Physiological	Physical growth is rapid. Birth weight usually triples by the end of the first year. Height increases by approximately 50%.	Inform parents of the developmental norms.
	Progressive maturation of all body systems occurs.	Encourage parents to have "well-baby" checkups as recommended.
	Body temperature stabilizes.	
	Heart rate slows (to approximately 80 to 130 beats per minute).	
	Blood pressure rises.	
	At approximately 4 to 6 months, eruption of teeth begins.	
	Brain grows rapidly (reaching approximately half the adult size).	
	Posterior fontanel closes at approximately 2 months.	Protect infant's skull.
	Eyes begin to focus.	
Motor	Physical maturation allows for development of motor skills.	Teach parents anticipated ages for motor skill development.
	Primitive reflexes are replaced by movement that is more voluntary and goal directed.	
	Motor skills develop rapidly:	
	• 6 months: rolls over voluntarily	
	• 6 to 7 months: crawls	
	• 8 months: sits alone	
	Grasping of objects, reflexive for the first 2 to 3 months, gradually becomes voluntary.	
Psychosocial	*Freud:* oral stage	Encourage parents to provide toys and objects for teething and sucking.
	Seeks immediate gratification of needs.	
	Receives pleasure and comfort through mouth, lips, and tongue.	
	Erikson: trust vs. mistrust stage	Encourage parents to feed in a prompt, consistent manner (feed on demand rather than a fixed schedule).
	A sense of self begins to develop.	
	Responds to caregiver's voice.	Other activities that promote trust are providing warmth, diapering, and comforting.
	Separation anxiety develops at approximately 6 months.	
	Havighurst: Developmental tasks include learning to eat solid food, crawl, walk, and talk.	Teach parents approximate ages that developmental milestones are expected to occur.
Cognitive	*Piaget:* sensorimotor stage	Encourage parents to provide a variety of sensory stimuli: visual, sensory, auditory, and tactile (e.g., colorful mobiles; musical toys; soft, plush animals; rubbing, patting, and stroking of the infant's skin).
	Infant learns by interacting with the environment.	
	Language development includes babbling, repetition, and imitation.	Tell caregivers to talk to the infant often. Encourage caregivers to name objects that are the focus of the infant's attention.
Moral	*Kohlberg:* preconventional stage	Teach parents that now is the time to start teaching (by role modeling) the difference between "right" and "wrong."
Spiritual	*Fowler:* stage of undifferentiated faith	Encourage caregivers to model the values they want the infant to learn.

Data from Health Assessment & Promotion Strategies through the Life Span *(6th ed.), by R. B. Murray and J. P. Zentner, 1997, East Norwalk, CT: Appleton & Lange. Copyright 1997 by Appleton & Lange;* Whaley & Wong's Nursing Care of Infants and Children *(6th ed.) by D. L. Wong, M. Hockenberry-Eaton, D. Wilson, M. L. Winkelstein, E. Ahmann, and P. DiVito-Thomas, 1999, St. Louis, MO: Mosby–Yearbook. Copyright 1999 by Mosby–Yearbook;* Fundamentals of Nursing: Standards & Practice, *by S. DeLaune and P. Ladner, 1998, Albany, NY: Delmar. Copyright 1998 by Delmar.*

physiological, motor, psychosocial, cognitive, moral, and spiritual dimensions.

Nursing Implications

The nurse providing care to an infant must focus on safety, prevention of infection, and teaching parents about incorporating the child into the family. Teaching parents and other caregivers about developmental milestones is also essential. Nursing care involves the provision of support, reassurance, and information to the parents.

Wellness Promotion Nurses promote infant wellness by teaching growth and development concepts to parents and other caregivers. Knowledge of the type of behavior to expect at certain times during infancy serves to both guide and reassure parents. Three specific areas about which parents need guidance from the nurse in caring for their infants are nutrition, protection from infection, and promotion of sleep.

A major factor influencing health maintenance of the infant is the provision of adequate nutrients delivered in a loving, consistent manner. Caregivers should be taught that the nutrients must be germ free and must provide the recommended amounts of carbohydrates, protein, calcium, iron, and vitamins. The American Academy of Pediatrics recommends that infants be breastfed for the first 12 months (Murray & Zentner, 1997). Nurses can teach parents about the benefits of breastfeeding, including that it:

- Offers immunologic benefits (e.g., it contains immunoglobulins, lymphocytes, and other bacteria growth retardants),
- Is more easily digested because it contains smaller curds than those found in cow's milk and formula, and
- Enhances absorption of fat and calcium.

In addition, breastmilk is readily available and economical. Furthermore, the act of breastfeeding promotes maternal–infant bonding (Wong et al., 1999).

Special formulas are available for infants who are hypersensitive to protein, who have PKU, and who experience fat malabsorption. Soy-based formulas have been developed for the infant who is lactose intolerant or allergic to regular formula. Infants who are formula

CULTURAL CONSIDERATIONS

Choice of Infant Feeding Method

There are some cultural sanctions against breastfeeding, and some cultures view bottle-feeding as a status symbol. Be sensitive to the client's cultural background and norms when discussing choice of infant feeding method. Nurses can also teach parents about the benefits of bottle-feeding.

CLIENT TEACHING

Bottle-Feeding

- Assume a comfortable position and place the baby in a semireclining position, cradled close to your body.
- Never prop a bottle in a baby's mouth because choking may result.
- Use care if heating bottles. Do not warm bottles in the microwave because the hot liquid can cause esophageal and oropharyngeal burns.
- Avoid using the bottle as a pacifier because this action may result in tooth decay and may set the stage for overeating in the future.

fed generally have greater deposits of subcutaneous fat (Murray & Zentner, 1997). Whole cow's milk is not recommended for infants under 1 year of age. Human milk and commercially prepared formula are more easily digested.

It is important for the nurse to provide accurate information about the types of feeding available and to support the parents' decision about the method chosen.

Solid foods are usually introduced at 3 to 4 months of age. Rice cereal is the first solid food of choice because it generates the fewest allergic responses (Murray & Zentner, 1997).

Infants are especially vulnerable to infections. Because the immune system is not fully matured, infections pose a great threat.

Infection Control: Handwashing and Infant Care

Handwashing is the most important action in preventing the transmission of microorganisms. This is especially true when caring for infants, whose immune systems are still immature.

Immunizations are of utmost importance in preventing infections. Nurses should advocate the administration of all necessary immunizations and should confirm those received by the infant. Refer to the appendices for a recommended schedule for immunizations.

Parents often need information about normal sleep patterns of infants and how those patterns change with maturation. Activities that promote sleep include:

- Providing a quiet room for the infant,
- Scheduling feedings and other care activities during periods of wakefulness rather than drowsiness,
- Developing sensitivity to the unique sleep and rest periods established by the infant,
- Providing comfort and security measures (e.g., rocking, singing), and
- Establishing routine times for sleep.

CLIENT TEACHING

Preventing Infant Accidents

- To prevent vehicular accidents: use infant seats and keep the infant out of the paths of automobiles and other vehicles.
- To prevent burns: keep the infant away from open heaters, furnaces, fireplaces, hot stoves, and matches.
- To protect from falls: keep crib rails up at all times, never leave the infant lying unattended on furniture, and use protective gates and barriers to block stairways.
- To prevent drowning: never leave the infant unattended near water (bathtubs, buckets, swimming pools).
- To prevent electrocution: when the infant begins to crawl, keep electrical cords out of the infant's reach and use plastic safety plugs to cover all electrical outlets.
- To prevent choking: closely monitor the infant who is exploring the environment. During this oral phase of development, the infant tends to test out the environment and seeks pleasure through the mouth. Aspiration accidents are common, with infants choking on objects such as buttons, coins, and food.

Safety Considerations Most infant injuries and deaths are related to motor vehicle accidents. The consistent and proper use of infant car seats is thus one of the most effective measures parents can take to ensure their infant's safety.

Safety: Aiding the Choking Infant
Never use the Heimlich maneuver on an infant who is choking. Instead, use alternating back blows and chest compressions to dislodge the object.

Toddler Period

The **toddler period** begins at 12 to 18 months of age, when a child begins to walk alone, and ends at approximately 3 years of age. The family is very important to the toddler in that the family promotes language development and teaches toileting skills. During this stage, the child becomes more independent and, when attempts to demonstrate autonomy are prevented, temper tantrums often result. This stage is thus often referred to as "the terrible twos." Parents must understand that the toddler's frequent use of the word *no* is an expression of developing autonomy.

Nurses can greatly influence the quality of parent–child interaction by teaching parents about develop-

mental concepts. This information helps parents form realistic expectations of the toddler's behavior. The use of firm limits applied consistently both helps the toddler learn and provides parameters for safe and socially acceptable behavior. Table 14–11 outlines the toddler's growth and development in the physiological, motor, psychosocial, cognitive, moral, and spiritual dimensions.

Nursing Implications

Nurses who work with toddlers must be sensitive to the fact that children of this age are likely to be anxious and fearful when in the presence of strangers. The establishment of rapport with the child will help alleviate stranger anxiety. Play is an effective tool for building rapport with children of this age.

When toddlers are hospitalized, whether for an extended time or only a day, fear and anxiety can make the experience a negative one. The major stressor related to hospitalization is separation from the parents. An unfamiliar environment also results in stress for the toddler. Nurses can help reduce stress in the hospitalized toddler by teaching both the child and the parents about procedures. Preprocedural teaching lessens anxiety.

Toddlers need regular health examinations, and immunizations remain an essential part of health care. Parents should be involved during examinations and immunizations. Parents can alleviate the toddler's stress by holding the child and talking in a calm manner when in the presence of the health care provider.

Wellness Promotion Teaching involves both toddlers and their parents. Play can be used to establish an effective relationship with the child. Play is a valuable process for toddlers in that it is the primary mechanism for learning and socialization. To facilitate teaching, the nurse should approach toddlers at eye level and use terminology they can understand.

Respiratory infections are common health threats to the toddler. Parasitic diseases are also fairly common.

PROFESSIONAL TIP

Health Care for Toddlers

- In a calm tone of voice, explain what is being done.
- Use play to alleviate anxiety (e.g., demonstrate a procedure on a teddy bear or doll; allow the child to manipulate equipment, such as a stethoscope, prior to using it on the child).
- Give short, simple directions.
- After a painful procedure, comfort the child (e.g., cuddle, rock).
- Encourage parents' active participation.

Table 14–11 TODDLER: GROWTH AND DEVELOPMENT

DIMENSION	CHARACTERISTICS	NURSING IMPLICATIONS
Physiological	Overall rate of growth slows. By 24 months of age, weight usually reaches four times that at birth. Brain grows rapidly. Bones in extremities grow in length. Physiological readiness for bowel and bladder control develops.	Instruct parents on need for vitamin D, calcium, and phosphorus. Recognize that "growing pains" are normal. Instruct parents of timing for toilet training and need for consistency and patience.
Motor	Child walks and runs. Child becomes more coordinated.	Tell parents to assess home environment for safety as toddler becomes more mobile.
Psychosocial	*Freud:* anal stage Receives pleasure from contraction and relaxation of sphincter muscles. *Erikson:* autonomy vs. shame and doubt stage *Havighurst:* Developmental tasks include: • Beginning to learn gender differences and • Learning to talk Toddler engages in parallel play (playing near other children but not necessarily interacting with them). A reemergence of separation anxiety often occurs. By age 3, most toddlers are able to tolerate being left with strangers.	Instruct parents to avoid overemphasis on toilet training. Teach parents to encourage toddler's attempts at independence (e.g., trying to feed and dress self). Explain that sexual curiosity is normal. Encourage parents to talk to child frequently. Provide opportunities for child to socialize with peers. Reassure child that parents will return.
Cognitive	*Piaget:* preoperational stage Child can follow simple directions. Child's thought processes are concrete. Child is able to anticipate future events. Child has short attention span. Child comprehends self as a separate entity. *Language:* At approximately 1 year of age, the child can make two-syllable sounds (e.g., ma-ma, da-da) At approximately 2 years, the child can form short sentences and has a vocabulary of approximately 900 words.	Instruct parents to give only one direction at a time. Use a calendar to show today's date and the number of days until a significant event. Teach caregivers importance of calling child by name. Instruct caregivers to talk to child frequently and to avoid the use of "baby talk."
Moral	*Kohlberg:* preconventional stage Child learns to distinguish right from wrong.	Teach parents to be consistent in setting limits. Emphasize the significance of modeling desired behavior to the child.
Spiritual	*Fowler:* intuitive-projective stage of faith	Instruct parents to provide simple answers to questions related to religion, God, and church. Instruct on the importance of incorporating religious rituals and ceremonies into daily life.

Data from Health Assessment & Promotion Strategies through the Life Span *(6th ed.), by R. B. Murray and J. P. Zentner, 1997, East Norwalk, CT: Appleton & Lange. Copyright 1997 by Appleton & Lange;* Whaley & Wong's Nursing Care of Infants and Children *(6th ed.) by D. L. Wong, M. Hockenberry-Eaton, D. Wilson, M. L. Winkelstein, E. Ahmann, and P. DiVito-Thomas, 1999, St. Louis, MO: Mosby–Yearbook. Copyright 1999 by Mosby–Yearbook;* Fundamentals of Nursing: Standards & Practice, *by S. DeLaune and P. Ladner, 1998, Albany, NY: Delmar. Copyright 1998 by Delmar.*

Teaching parents about preventive measures such as frequent handwashing with antibacterial soaps is thus the focus of wellness promotion. The nurse should also verify which immunizations are needed.

As the rate of growth slows during the toddler period, nutritional needs change. Toddlers need fewer calories than do infants. The required amounts of protein and fluids (Wong et al., 1999) also decrease; however, toddlers still need more protein than do older children. Because most toddlers become selective ("picky") about the foods they will eat, it is sometimes difficult to provide increased amounts of calcium and iron. The toddler should consume an average of 2 to 3 cups of milk per day to ensure adequate calcium

CLIENT TEACHING

Toddler Nutrition

- Avoid using food as a reward because doing so encourages overeating.
- Do not serve large helpings because doing so may overwhelm the child, possibly resulting in a refusal to eat.
- Expect sporadic eating patterns (e.g., the toddler eats a lot one day and very little the next, or the toddler enjoys one food for several days and then suddenly refuses to eat that food).
- Avoid power struggles related to meals. Trying to force a child to eat is counterproductive to establishing healthy eating habits.
- Establish a mealtime routine and follow it; rituals are comforting to toddlers.
- Provide nutritional snacks to meet dietary requirements.

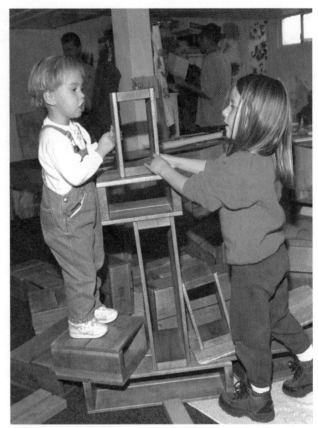

Figure 14-4 Toddlers enjoy playing with a variety of toys. Parents must be diligent in checking all toys for potential safety hazards—considering not only the toy itself but also the manner in which it is used—and must supervise toddler play at all times.

intake. The toddler who drinks more than a quart of milk per day, however, is at increased risk of developing anemia, because high milk consumption may limit the amount of other nutrients taken in (Wong et al., 1999). Nurses can play a key role in nutritional counseling for toddlers.

Safety Considerations Accidents (especially those involving automobiles) are the most frequent cause of disability and death among toddlers (Edelman & Mandle, 1998; Murray & Zentner, 1997). The information previously provided regarding use of car seats for neonates and infants also applies to toddlers.

Another common type of accident among toddlers involves toys. As children gain new skills, parents must reassess the safety of toys and of all environments where the toddler might play (Figure 14-4).

 Safety: Toys for Toddlers
Teach parents to inspect toys for the following:

- Age appropriateness
- Sharp pieces or corners
- Small parts that can be swallowed
- Poisonous paint (e.g., lead-based paint)
- Flammable or toxic materials

With their increased mobility and curiosity, toddlers are especially prone to accidental poisoning (Figure 14-5). Parents should thus child-proof the home and carefully observe the toddler.

Preschool Period

The developmental stage from ages 3 to 6 years is called the **preschool period**. During this stage, physical growth slows, and psychosocial and cognitive de-

velopment accelerate. Table 14–12 outlines preschool development in detail.

During this period of childhood, curiosity becomes pronounced, and the child is better able to communicate. The nurse should teach parents that the child's

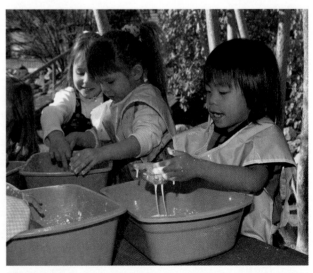

Figure 14-5 Parents must ensure that all materials a child plays with are safe, nontoxic, and nonflammable.

Table 14–12 PRESCHOOLER: GROWTH AND DEVELOPMENT

DIMENSION	CHARACTERISTICS	NURSING IMPLICATIONS
Physiological	Physical growth slows; average weight at age 5 years is 45 pounds. Head size approximates that of an adult. Deciduous teeth come in fully; these "baby teeth" start to fall out about age 6 and will be replaced by permanent teeth.	Can eat larger meals and a variety of foods.
Motor	Fine motor skills develop, e.g., ability to skip, throw a ball over hand, use scissors, tie shoelaces.	Emphasize providing a safe environment for play and exploration. Tell parents to praise attempted independent activities.
Psychosocial	*Freud:* phallic stage Oedipal conflict leads to development of superego (conscience). *Erikson:* initiative vs. guilt stage *Havighurst:* Developmental tasks include: • Learning gender differences and modesty, • Language development and basic ability to formulate concepts, • Emerging reading readiness, and • Distinguishing right from wrong	Inform parents that preschoolers learn self-control through interacting with others. Encourage parents to provide sex education information at the child's comprehension level. Encourage parents to read to child.
Cognitive	*Piaget:* preoperational stage Increased curiosity coupled with improved ability to use reason and logic lead to frequent questioning. Play becomes more reality based. As a result of increased ability to communicate, socialization with peers increases.	Tell parents that children of this age learn through frequent use of the word *why.*
Moral	*Kohlberg:* preconventional stage A conscience begins to develop. Child fears wrongdoing. Child seeks parental approval.	Encourage parents to teach the child basic values, ideally by modeling. Encourage parents to provide consistent praise and acceptance of child.
Spiritual	*Fowler:* intuitive-projective stage of faith Child is not yet able to understand spiritual concepts and imitates parental behaviors.	Remind parents that teaching by example is the best approach for a child of this age.

Data from Health Assessment & Promotion Strategies through the Life Span *(6th ed.), by R. B. Murray and J. P. Zentner, 1997, East Norwalk, CT: Appleton & Lange. Copyright 1997 by Appleton & Lange;* Whaley & Wong's Nursing Care of Infants and Children *(6th ed.) by D. L. Wong, M. Hockenberry-Eaton, D. Wilson, M. L. Winkelstein, E. Ahmann, and P. DiVito-Thomas, 1999, St. Louis, MO: Mosby–Yearbook. Copyright 1999 by Mosby–Yearbook;* Fundamentals of Nursing: Standards & Practice, by *S. DeLaune and P. Ladner, 1998, Albany, NY: Delmar. Copyright 1998 by Delmar.*

frequent use of the word *why* is necessary for normal cognitive and psychosocial development.

The child's world continues to expand outside the immediate home environment. Play is the mechanism used by the preschooler to both learn about and develop relationships.

Nursing Implications

Play is a tool that can be used by nurses to help reduce fear and anxiety in the preschooler. Through the use of play, preschoolers learn about the environment, incorporate socially defined expectations for behavior, and reduce tension (Figure 14-6).

Wellness Promotion When working with a preschooler, it is important for the nurse to communicate at the child's level of comprehension while at the same time not talking down to the child. The nurse should include the child in activities and decisions as much as possible. The preschool years are the optimal time for the child to begin showing an interest in

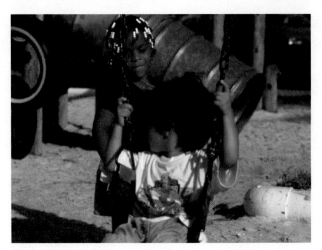

Figure 14-6 Play is an important vehicle for socialization among preschoolers.

health. In order to promote the development of life-long health-promoting lifestyles, the astute nurse capitalizes on this opportunity by making health education fun. A major wellness intervention for preschoolers is immunization. The nurse should thus verify at each checkup that immunizations are up to date.

Safety Considerations Accidents are the leading cause of death among young children. Cognitive immaturity coupled with an eagerness to explore the environment lead to the preschooler's risk for accidents. Children in this stage often act impulsively and cannot be expected to remember and follow all safety rules. To prevent accidents, parents must understand the importance of teaching young children the meaning of the word *no*.

Common accidents among preschoolers include automobile accidents, burns, falls, drowning, animal bites, and ingestion of poisonous substances.

The nurse should place emphasis on educating parents about protecting preschoolers from potential hazards. The safety practices developed by the preschooler will tend to be lifelong. Adults can best teach preschoolers about accident prevention through modeling. For example, parents who buckle their seatbelts every time they get into a car are not only protecting themselves, but are also teaching their children an important accident prevention measure.

School-Age Period

During the **school-age period** (the developmental stage from the ages of 6 to 10 years), physical changes occur at a slow, even, continuous pace. Table 14–13 gives an overview of growth and development of the school-age child.

The school-age child's world expands greatly. Participation in school activities, team sports, and play contributes to an enlarging social network. As children continue to mature, their play time becomes more structured and less spontaneous. Communication levels increase, and vocabulary expands greatly to accommodate the expression of needs, thoughts, and feelings.

As the school-age child's cognitive abilities expand, creativity is expressed in a variety of unique ways. Involvement in academic, sporting, and social activities stimulates the development of creativity and provides outlets for its expression.

Nursing Implications

The most common health problems among school-age children are accidents and minor illnesses such as upper respiratory infections. Health-promotion teaching is a major role of the nurse in caring for school-age children.

Wellness Promotion Lifestyles begin to be established during childhood; nurses can intervene to promote the development of healthy lifestyles among children in schools. Schools are an area where health-promotion behaviors can be taught in a cost-effective manner.

Safety Considerations Many accidents experienced by school-age children occur during play. Injuries related to the use of skates, skateboards, in-line skates, and bicycles are common.

 Safety: Accidents and Abductions
- Children must know the safety rules for use of riding toys (e.g., use of protective equipment, see Figure 14-7).
- Parents must frequently remind children of the danger of playing near traffic.
- Children must also be taught to use caution with regard to strangers because of the possibility of abduction.

 CLIENT TEACHING

Promoting Wellness
- Encourage healthy lifestyles (nonsedentary activities, nutritious meals)
- Have children immunized
- Teach children appropriate hygienic measures
- Schedule regular checkups with the primary health care provider
- Keep immunizations up to date
- Schedule dental checkups and encourage daily brushing and flossing
- Teach safety precautions
- Establish sleep patterns alternating with periods of activity
- Report any symptoms of illness immediately to the health care provider

Table 14–13 SCHOOL-AGE CHILD: GROWTH AND DEVELOPMENT

DIMENSION	CHARACTERISTICS	NURSING IMPLICATIONS
Physiological	Physical growth is steady (approximately 3 to 6 pounds and 2 to 3 inches per year).	Emphasize to parents the need for a balanced diet to sustain growth requirements.
	Due to changes in amount and distribution of fat, body has an overall slimmer shape.	
	Maturation of the CNS is nearly complete. By age 12, all permanent teeth (except second and third molars) are present.	Teach parents about the need for dental hygiene (daily brushing and flossing) and regularly scheduled visits to the dentist.
		Instruct to change toothbrushes every 3 months.
Motor	Motor control continues to develop.	Encourage participation in physical activities.
	Child becomes less dependent on parents for activities of daily living.	Provide praise for independent activities.
Psychosocial	*Freud:* latency stage	To develop a sense of confidence, encourage child to:
	Same-gender companions are preferred.	• Participate in both group and individual activities and
		• Become involved in a variety of activities
	Erikson: industry vs. inferiority stage	
	Child develops initiative and high self-esteem as manifested in school and sports.	Encourage parents to praise child's efforts.
	Child exhibits less dependency on family.	
	Havighurst: Developmental tasks include the ability to perform more complex motor functions (e.g., ride a bicycle, catch a ball).	
Cognitive	*Piaget:* concrete operations stage	
	Ability to cooperate with others and to see other points of view leads to more meaningful communication.	Encourage child to engage in group activities.
	Reasoning ability moves from intuitive to logical and rational.	
	Ability to think in the abstract is not fully developed.	Communicate at child's level of comprehension.
	Child develops the concept of time:	
	• Knows difference between past and present	
	• Begins to learn to tell time	
	• Better able to understand the process of aging	
	Child is able to order, categorize, and classify groups of objects as evidenced by increased interest in collections (e.g., coins, stamps, rocks).	
	Child sees relationships between objects.	
Moral	*Kohlberg:* conventional stage	Encourage parents to provide consistent limits.
	Child can understand what society deems as unacceptable behavior but cannot always choose between right and wrong without assistance.	Emphasize modeling appropriate behavior.
		Tell parents to praise appropriate behavior.
Spiritual	*Fowler:* mythical-literal stage	Encourage parents to discuss their beliefs.
	Child accepts existence of a diety.	Storytelling and use of parables can reinforce understanding of spiritual concepts.
	Beliefs are symbolized through stories.	

Data from Health Promotion throughout the Lifespan *(4th ed.), by C. L. Edelman and C. L. Mandle, 1998, St. Louis, MO: Mosby–Yearbook. Copyright 1998 by Mosby–Yearbook;* Health Assessment & Promotion Strategies through the Life Span *(6th ed.), by R. B. Murray and J. P. Zentner, 1997, East Norwalk, CT: Appleton & Lange. Copyright 1997 by Appleton & Lange;* Fundamentals of Nursing: Standards & Practice, *by S. DeLaune and P. Ladner, 1998, Albany, NY: Delmar. Copyright 1998 by Delmar.*

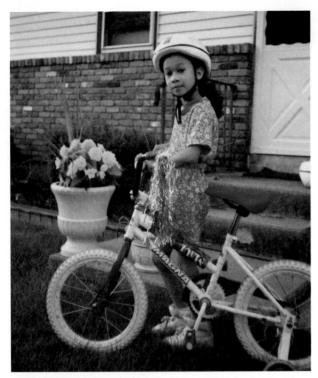

Figure 14-7 The use of equipment such as safety helmets helps protect school-age children from injury.

Preadolescence

Preadolescence (the developmental stage from the ages of 10 to 12 years) is marked by rapid physiological changes having psychological and social implications. The child begins to experience hormonal changes that will result in the onset of **puberty** (the emergence of secondary sex characteristics). Girls generally experience puberty at a younger age than do boys—approximately 9 to 10 years of age, as compared to 10 to 11 years of age for boys (Edelman & Mandle, 1998). Table 14–14 provides an overview of preadolescent development.

In girls, breast development begins between the ages of 10 and 11. Further breast development is stimulated by the release of estrogen, which occurs during puberty. Approximately 2 years after the appearance of breast buds, **menarche** (onset of the first menstrual period) occurs. The first menstrual periods are usually irregular, scant, and may or may not be accompanied by ovulation. The average age of menarche in the United States is 12.8 years. This number represents a gradual decline over the past century in average age of menarche; a decline probably due to improved general health status, particularly nutrition and sanitation (Wong et al., 1999).

The menstrual cycle is a complex blend of physiological and psychological changes that occur approximately every month. After approximately the first 6 to 12 months, a girl's cycle typically becomes established

in a regular pattern. Nurses must be aware that some girls may have received inadequate or incorrect information regarding the onset of menstruation. Client teaching should address the physiological changes, emotional changes, and hygienic practices and should emphasize that cyclical, hormone-induced changes are normal.

In preadolescent boys, the first signs of puberty are:

- Testicular enlargement,
- Penile enlargement,
- Thinning and reddening of the scrotum, and
- Pubic hair growth.

Nursing Implications

Sensitivity is essential in working with the preadolescent. To increase sensitivity, the nurse should use a nonjudgmental approach and attend to the preadolescent's body language.

Wellness Promotion The preadolescent needs information about nutrition, rest and activity, and the physiological changes being experienced. This client should be taught about the dramatic growth spurt, the sexual changes, and the psychosocial changes that characterize this life stage (Figure 14-8). By preparing the preadolescent for upcoming changes, the nurse promotes physical and emotional health. The nurse should also confirm that immunizations are current.

Safety Considerations The preadolescent is at risk for injury from sports and play activities. Another major health risk posed to many preadolescents is vio-

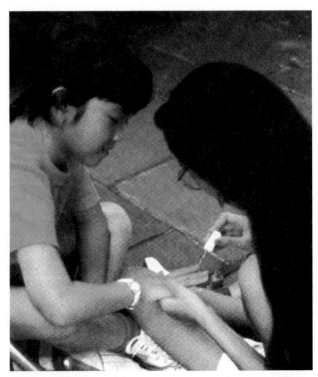

Figure 14-8 Preadolescence is a time of gender role discovery and increasing independence.

Table 14–14 PREADOLESCENT AND ADOLESCENT: GROWTH AND DEVELOPMENT

DIMENSION	CHARACTERISTICS	NURSING IMPLICATIONS
Physiological	*Physiological changes:* Physical growth accelerates and is accompanied by changes in body proportion. Extremities grow first, then trunk and hips. Growth in skull and facial bones results in changes in physical appearance.	Teach the child and parents about expected growth spurts. Provide reassurance that it is not uncommon for facial appearance to change in only a few months.
	Endocrine changes: Hypothalamus stimulates secretion of pituitary gonadotropins, leading to reproductive maturity. Both primary and secondary sex characteristics develop. Beginning of puberty is evidenced in girls by: • Breast development, • Pubic and axillary hair growth, • Menarche (onset of menses), and • Increases in height. Beginning of puberty is evidenced in boys by: • Genital development, • Growth of facial, pubic, and axillary hair, • Nocturnal ejaculations, • Height increases, and • Voice changes.	Provide support and information about sexual changes. Remember that the physiological changes are accompanied by psychological and social alterations.
	Musculoskeletal changes: Bones ossify. Muscle mass and strength increase. *Cardiovascular changes:* Heart increases in size and strength. Heart rate decreases to adult norms. Blood volume and blood pressure increase.	Encourage physical activities and intake of adequate amounts of calcium.
	Respiratory changes: Rate decreases to an average of 15 to 20 respirations per minute. Respiratory volume and vital capacity increase. Larynx, laryngeal cartilage, and vocal cords grow; voice pitch deepens.	Instruct about anticipated changes.
	Gastrointestinal changes: Spleen, liver, kidneys, and digestive tract enlarge but experience no functional changes. *Genitourinary changes:* Genitalia develop as described previously.	
	Dental changes: Last four molars erupt.	Emphasize importance of continued dental hygiene.
	Integumentary changes: Skin becomes thicker and tougher. Activation of sebaceous glands possibly leads to acne. Pubic hair appears.	Teach proper skin care: • Wash two to three times per day with soap and water • Avoid vigorous facial scrubbing • Avoid cosmetics with a fat or grease base • Use sunscreen and avoid prolonged exposure to sunlight • Provide support to preadolescents experiencing acne
Motor	The adolescent displays complete independence with regard to performing self-care activities.	Encourage parents to allow some freedom of choice and expression.

continues

Table 14–14 PREADOLESCENT AND ADOLESCENT: GROWTH AND DEVELOPMENT
continued

DIMENSION	CHARACTERISTICS	NURSING IMPLICATIONS
Psychosocial	*Freud:* genital stage *Erikson:* identity vs. role diffusion stage The major task is to develop a sense of identity. The adolescent develops a new body image. Intimacy with members of opposite gender is established. Peer group is the primary mechanism of support. The adolescent rebels against adult authority. *Havighurst:* achievement of personal independence Relationships established with others are characterized by increased maturity.	Offer support. Provide sex education. Inform parents that rebellion is a normal developmental experience. Encourage attempts to achieve independence while providing assistance and support as needed.
Cognitive	*Piaget:* formal operations stage Approach to thinking is logical, organized, and consistent. The adolescent thinks in terms of cause and effect. **Note:** Not all adolescents achieve this level of cognitive development. Some are capable of flights from reality. The adolescent tends to be extremely idealistic. Egocentric (self-centered) thinking is common, as is a view of self as omnipotent. The adolescent sees self as exceptional, special, and unique, and views self as being immune to problems.	Teach parents expected developmental changes in thinking patterns. Recognize that a false sense of immunity ("It can't happen to me" attitude) has an impact on health behaviors. Teach safety issues to preadolescents: • Safe sex practices • Safe driving practices (never mixing driving and use of alcohol)
Moral	*Kohlberg:* postconventional stage The adolescent tends to support the morality of law and order in determining right from wrong. Adolescents begin to question and discard the status quo and to choose different values. Moral maturity varies dependent on the context of the situation and the relationship. Peer pressure may override the adolescent's own moral reasoning.	Teach parents that questioning of values is normal. Teach preadolescent assertiveness skills to use in communicating with peers.
Spiritual	*Fowler:* synthetic-conventional stage The adolescent questions values and beliefs.	Inform parents that curiosity about other religious beliefs is normal.

Data from Health Promotion throughout the Lifespan *(4th ed.), by C. L. Edelman and C. L. Mandle, 1998, St. Louis, MO: Mosby–Yearbook. Copyright 1998 by Mosby–Yearbook;* American Nursing Review of Psychiatric and Mental Health Nursing Certification, *by N. Randolph, 1998, Springhouse, PA: Springhouse. Copyright 1998 by Springhouse;* Fundamentals of Nursing: Standards & Practice, *by S. DeLaune and P. Ladner, 1998, Albany, NY: Delmar. Copyright 1998 by Delmar.*

lence both in and away from the home. Education is a major preventive approach to violence and is a tool for helping break the intergenerational pattern of child abuse (Johnson, 1995).

Other areas to be emphasized in promoting preadolescent safety are substance abuse prevention, sex education, and development of healthy lifestyles.

Adolescence

Adolescence (the developmental stage from the ages of 13 to 20 years) begins with the onset of puberty. During adolescence, the individual undergoes the major transition from child to adult. Numerous physiological changes and rapid physical growth occur during this stage. The rapid changes that occur

![Professional Tip icon]

PROFESSIONAL TIP

Preadolescent–Nurse Relationship
To encourage the preadolescent to ask questions about any health-related concerns it is imperative that the nurse establish a trusting relationship with the preadolescent.

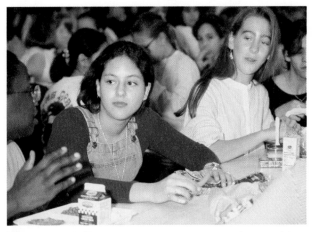

Figure 14-9 Peer group is very important during adolescence.

during adolescence are not only physical; many psychosocial adjustments must be made by the adolescent. Friendships become very important (Figure 14-9). Establishing a sense of personal identity takes up a great amount of the adolescent's psychic energy. Questions such as "Who am I?" and "What is *really* important?" are common ones among adolescents.

Most adolescents are greatly concerned about their appearance. This emphasis on physical attractiveness sometimes results in eating disorders, such as **anorexia nervosa** (self-imposed starvation that results in a 15% loss of body weight). It is projected that 1 out of every 10 girls in the United States will develop anorexia nervosa (AACAP, 1998a). Male adolescents are also affected by eating disorders, but at a much lower percentage than are girls. Other types of eating disorders common in adolescents are **bulimia nervosa** (episodic binge-eating followed by purging) and **obesity** (weight that is 20% or more above ideal body weight).

Nursing Implications

The nurse can support the adolescent by providing information about the numerous bodily changes experienced during this developmental stage. The nurse should encourage adolescents to share their health concerns with parents, but must honor the adolescent's choice to withhold sensitive information from parents. The confidentiality of the client as well as of those in relationship with the adolescent (such as sexual partners) must be protected.

Wellness Promotion The nurse promotes the adolescent's wellness primarily through teaching. Areas to be emphasized in health education of adolescents include hygiene, nutrition, sex education, developmental changes, and substance abuse prevention. Information is available from the American Academy of Pediatrics (AAP, 2000).

The nurse should teach adolescents about the physical changes they are undergoing. Health teaching is often done by school nurses, and nurse-managed clinics in schools represent one avenue for promoting wellness among adolescents (Figure 14-10). School-based clinics are rapidly increasing, allowing the possibility of delivering care to 23 million children and their

parents, the majority of whom are uninsured (Baker, 1994). *Nursing's Agenda for Health Care Reform* (American Nurses Association, 1990) calls for the delivery of primary health care services to individuals in convenient, familiar places. What better place to teach adolescents about health care than in the schools?

Safety Considerations As a group, today's adolescents are less healthy than were their parents at the same age (Roye, 1995). Unhealthy behaviors contribute to the three major causes of adolescent death: accidents,

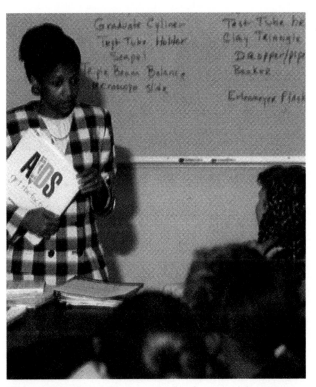

Figure 14-10 Wellness promotion for the adolescent may include in-school seminars by school nurses, such as this one on AIDS prevention.

PROFESSIONAL TIP

Working with Adolescents

- Use a nonjudgmental attitude to establish rapport when working with adolescents.
- Treat every adolescent in a respectful, dignified manner.
- Avoid using a condescending attitude when communicating with the adolescent.
- To form a collaborative partnership, treat the adolescent as an active participant in health care.
- Answer all questions honestly.
- Be especially sensitive to nonverbal clues. Adolescents are often too embarrassed to initiate discussion of their health-related concerns.
- Remember that the peer group is of major importance to the adolescent; thus, use group settings whenever possible to provide health education.
- Demonstrate acceptance of the adolescent even when limits must be established in the face of unhealthy or inappropriate behaviors.
- Questioning adult authority is a normal part of adolescent rebelliousness. Do *not* personalize such behavior. Nurses who do so become defensive and lose their interpersonal effectiveness and credibility with adolescents.

homicide, and suicide (Roye, 1995). The following factors increase the adolescent's risk for accidents:

- Impulsive behavior
- Sense of being invulnerable to accidents ("It can never happen to me!")
- Testing limits
- Rebelling against adult advice

As a result, many adolescents engage in unhealthy behaviors such as smoking, consuming alcohol and other drugs, reckless driving, violence, and unprotected sexual activity.

Many health problems in adolescents are related to sexual behaviors. For example, consider the following facts:

- Acquired immunodeficiency syndrome (AIDS) is the fifth leading cause of death (CDC, 1999a) of individuals between the ages of 24 and 54 years; many of these people were infected during their adolescent years.
- Adolescents between the ages of 15 and 19 years have the highest rates of hospitalization for treatment of sexually transmitted diseases (STDs).
- Every year, about 1 million teenagers become pregnant (CDC, 1999b).

The effect of teen pregnancy on families and communities is great. Social programs that provide resources for meeting the special needs of pregnant adolescents are decreasing. A result for many pregnant teens is becoming trapped in a cycle of school failure (or dropout), limited employment opportunities, and poverty. Adolescents who become pregnant experience developmental difficulties in that they must make adult decisions. Infants born to adolescent mothers are likely to experience health-related problems such as preterm birth and low birth weight.

The pregnant adolescent needs expert prenatal care, a supportive environment, and information. Client teaching must emphasize the prevention of STDs because the pregnancy itself is evidence of high-risk (i.e., unprotected) sexual activity.

Sexually transmitted diseases present a serious health threat to adolescents. Diseases such as genital herpes, chlamydia, syphilis, and gonorrhea are spread through sexual contact. The human immunodeficiency virus (HIV), which causes AIDS, is also transmitted through unprotected sexual activity.

Nurses must educate adolescents about methods for preventing the spread of STDs. Nurses who teach adolescent clients about safe sex practices must be especially sensitive to cultural influences on sexual activity.

A major health problem during adolescence is the high risk of suicide. The rate of suicide is higher among adolescent males than females. Often, suicide is perceived by the adolescent as the only alternative to an overwhelming situation. Suicidal behavior can be traced to low self-esteem, lack of maturity, and resultant impulsive behaviors.

When assessing for suicide potential, the nurse should always directly question adolescents about any plans for harming or killing themselves. Nurses should be aware of the following signs of suicide risk in adolescents:

- Change in eating and sleeping habits
- Writing suicide notes
- Discussion of suicide
- Aggressive behavior
- Substance abuse
- Loss of interest in pleasurable activities
- Preoccupation with death
- Neglect of personal hygiene
- The giving away of treasured objects
- Marked personality change
- Verbal cues (e.g., "You won't have to worry about me much longer.")
- Fatigue, headache, stomachache
- Social withdrawal

When teaching suicide prevention, the nurse should encourage *immediate* contact of a health care professional should someone exhibit any indicators of suicide risk. Most communities have a special telephone suicide-prevention line available.

Safety: Suicide Prevention
- Never leave the suicidal adolescent alone.
- Close observation is the best deterrent to suicide.

Another significant health problem for many adolescents is substance abuse. Use of alcohol or other drugs represents a common maladaptive attempt to cope with the stressors of adolescence. Indicators of substance abuse by adolescents include the following:

- Decline in academic performance
- Mood swings
- Changes in personality
- Fatigue
- Drowsiness
- Behaviors indicative of depression (e.g., appetite changes, insomnia, weight loss, apathy)

Nurses can play a key role in substance abuse prevention among adolescents. A comprehensive substance abuse prevention education program covers:

- Hazards of drug use
- Misuse of legal substances such as tobacco and alcohol
- Methods of boosting self-esteem
- Assertive communication skills (how to say "no" to peers)
- Adaptive coping mechanisms for dealing with stress

By providing such information, nurses can help adolescents make responsible, informed decisions before experimentation with drugs begins.

Young Adulthood

Physical growth stabilizes during **young adulthood** (the developmental stage from the ages of 21 years through approximately 40 years). The young adult continues to experience physical and emotional changes, but at a slower rate than does the adolescent. Table 14–15 outlines the development of young adults. Young adulthood is a time of transition from an adolescent to a person capable of assuming adult responsibilities and making adult decisions.

Table 14–15 YOUNG ADULT: GROWTH AND DEVELOPMENT

DIMENSION	CHARACTERISTICS	NURSING IMPLICATIONS
Physiological	*Physiological changes:* Physical growth stabilizes. Physical functioning is at an optimum and therefore less likely to be concerned with own health. Maturation of body systems is complete. *Cardiovascular changes:* Men are more likely to have an increased cholesterol level than are women. *Gastrointestinal changes:* After age 30, digestive juices decrease. *Dental changes:* By the mid-20s, dental maturity is achieved with the emergence of the last four molars ("wisdom teeth"). *Musculoskeletal changes:* At approximately age 25, skeletal growth is complete. *Reproductive changes:* System is completely matured. *Women:* Ages 20–30 are optimal years physically for reproduction. *Men:* Beginning at approximately age 24, male hormones slowly decrease (does not affect ability to reproduce).	Teach importance of health-promoting behaviors. Encourage development of healthy lifestyles.
Psychosocial	*Erikson:* intimacy vs. isolation stage Young adults engage in productive work. The young adult develops intimate relationships. *Havighurst:* The individual becomes part of a social group. The young adult selects a partner. The person assumes civic responsibility.	Emphasize need for social support as the person assumes new roles. Teach time management skills. Provide sex education information, including information on prevention of STDs. *continues*

Table 14–15 YOUNG ADULT: GROWTH AND DEVELOPMENT *continued*		
DIMENSION	**CHARACTERISTICS**	**NURSING IMPLICATIONS**
Cognitive	*Piaget:* formal operations stage	Encourage the development and use of appropriate judgment.
	Problem-solving abilities are realistic.	
	The young adult demonstrates less egocentricism.	
	Many young adults engage in formal educational activities.	
Moral	*Kohlberg:* postconventional stage	Assess the person's value system and respect the person's beliefs.
	Right and wrong are defined in terms of personal beliefs and principles.	
Spiritual	*Fowler:* individuative-reflective faith stage	Encourage client to use spiritual support system.
	The young adult assumes responsibility for own beliefs.	

Data from Adult Health Nursing *(3rd ed.),* by P. G. Beare and J. L. Myers, 1998, St. Louis, MO: Mosby–Yearbook. Copyright 1998 by Mosby–Yearbook; Health Promotion throughout the Lifespan *(4th ed.),* by C. L. Edelman, and C. L. Mandle, 1998, St. Louis, MO: Mosby–Yearbook. Copyright 1998 by Mosby–Yearbook; Fundamentals of Nursing: Standards & Practice, by S. DeLaune and P. Ladner, 1998, Albany, NY: Delmar. Copyright 1998 by Delmar.

Pregnancy, a time of transition and lifestyle adjustment, is experienced by many young adults. Throughout pregnancy, women experience changes in self-concept and may need reassurance that such changes are normal.

Nursing Implications

Young adulthood is usually the healthiest time in a person's life. Consequently, concern for health is low, and wellness is taken for granted by many young adults. Preventive measures for young adults have two primary components:

- Avoidance of accident, injury, and violence
- Development of health-promoting behaviors (e.g., lifestyle modification).

By teaching and counseling, the nurse plays an important role in each of these areas of health promotion (Figure 14-11). Other developmentally appropriate topics for the nurse to address are vocational counseling and relationship establishment.

Wellness Promotion Decision making by young adults affects their health status. Because young adults tend to take excessive risks, they are at greater risk for violent death from accident, suicide, or homicide (Edelman & Mandle, 1998). Driving recklessly, driving while intoxicated, and engaging in unprotected sex are examples of activities that demonstrate the lack of fear demonstrated by many young adults.

Sexually transmitted disease is a leading cause of infection and resultant reproductive dysfunction among young adults. The information presented about STDs in the discussion of safety considerations for adolescents is also applicable to young adults. Nurses should teach women how to perform a monthly breast self-examination (BSE), and men must learn how to perform a testicular self-examination (TSE). The nurse should also confirm currency of tetanus/diphtheria (Td) immunization.

Safety Considerations Because vehicular accidents are a major cause of health problems among young adults, providing information about driving safety is a must. Another activity that poses a health

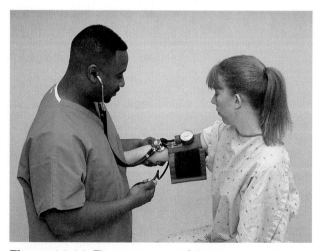

Figure 14-11 The assessment of this young adult's blood pressure is one part of a health-promotion program to help enhance this client's wellness.

risk to many young adults is sunbathing. Exposure to the radiation resulting from direct sunlight or the lighting used in tanning salons is directly linked to skin cancer. According to the American Cancer Society (2000) over 1 million new cases of skin cancer occur every year. Nurses can be influential in decreasing this rate through teaching and modeling safe behaviors.

Middle Adulthood

Middle adulthood (the developmental stage from the ages of 40 to 65 years) is characterized by productivity and responsibility. Many physiological changes occur during middle adulthood. Table 14–16 lists the major changes experienced by the middle-aged person. For most middle-aged adults, the majority of activity

Table 14–16 MIDDLE ADULT: GROWTH AND DEVELOPMENT		
DIMENSION	**CHARACTERISTICS**	**NURSING IMPLICATIONS**
Physiological	*Cardiovascular changes:*	
	Decreased functional aerobic capacity results in decreased cardiac output and a decreased capacity for physical activity.	Instruct cardiac client about necessity of remaining physically active.
	Blood vessels become thicker and lose elasticity.	
	Hypertension (high blood pressure), coronary artery disease, and cerebral vascular accidents ("strokes") may appear.	Teach client about lifestyle modifications related to cardiovascular health:
		• Quitting smoking
		• Avoiding secondary tobacco smoke
		• Practicing good nutrition (low fat, low cholesterol)
		• Engaging in physical activity
	Neurological changes:	
	Changes in cell regulation and repair occur gradually, as does cell atrophy.	Explain age-related changes.
		Provide support and reassurance.
	A gradual loss in efficiency of nerve conduction leads to impaired sensation of heat and cold.	Teach safety precautions regarding:
		• Exposure to sunlight,
		• Sensitivity to heat stroke, and
		• Sensitivity to frostbite.
	Gastrointestinal changes:	
	Slower gastrointestinal motility results in constipation.	Teach client about:
		• Nutrition (increase high-fiber food intake; drink adequate amounts of fluid), and
		• Maintaining physical activity.
	Genitourinary changes:	
	Nephron units diminish in number and size; diminishing blood supply to kidneys.	Teach normal age-related changes.
		Teach signs indicative of dehydration.
	Decreased glomerular filtration rate leads to decrease in urinary output and resultant dehydration.	Inform client of need to maintain adequate fluid intake.
	Integumentary changes:	
	Decreased moisture and turgor of skin and loss of subcutaneous fat leads to development of wrinkles.	Instruct client about effects of sun and of cigarette smoking on the skin.
	Hair thins and turns gray.	Assess client for body image alterations.
		Employ nonjudgmental listening.
	Musculoskeletal changes:	Instruct client about:
	Bone mass and density decreases.	• Need for calcium intake,
	Slight loss of height (from 1 to 4 inches) may occur.	• Importance of decreasing caffeine and alcohol consumption, and
	Intervertebral disks thin.	• Effects of sedentary versus active lifestyle on osteoporosis.
	There is a generalized decrease in muscle tone; appearance becomes "flabby," and agility lessens, leading to an increased risk of injury.	Instruct client of need for proper posture (especially when sitting), exercise, and adequate fluid intake.
		Instruct client on need for adequate physical activity.

continues

Table 14–16 MIDDLE ADULT: GROWTH AND DEVELOPMENT *continued*

DIMENSION	CHARACTERISTICS	NURSING IMPLICATIONS
Physiological (*continued*)	*Endocrine changes:* Decreased metabolism results in reduced production of enzymes and increased hydrochloric acid, leading to acid indigestion and belching.	Instruct client to: • Eat foods that are not spicy or fried, and • Avoid eating within 2 hours before bedtime.
	Reproductive changes: *Women:*	
	Estrogen and progesterone production cease during menopause.	Teach clients about age-related sexual/ reproductive changes.
	Secondary sex characteristics regress (decreased breast size, loss of pubic hair).	Encourage responsible sexual behavior. Teach about prevention of sexually transmitted diseases.
	Vaginal secretions decrease.	
	Note: With no pregnancy risk, some postmenopausal women enjoy sexual activity more.	
	Men:	
	Testosterone level decreases. There is a reduction in the amount of viable sperm. Sexual energy declines, and it takes longer to achieve an erection; however, erection is sustained longer.	
	Adaptation to developing chronic diseases and sexual problems may diminish self-esteem.	
	Grown children leaving home may lead to happiness or depression ("empty nest syndrome").	
Psychosocial	*Erikson:* generativity vs. stagnation stage	
	Adults who have achieved generativity feel good about their lives and comfortable with themselves.	Provide support as the client deals with aging.
	Middle-aged adults become more involved in altruistic acts (e.g., community, volunteer work).	Encourage client to become involved in community activities. Teach leisure skills.
	Family roles usually change (become caregiver to aging parents, become grandparent).	Instruct in the need to care for self while caring for others.
	Havighurst:	
	The middle-aged adult fulfills social and civic responsibilities.	
	Middle-aged adults assist children in becoming independent.	
	The middle-aged adult maintains relationship with partner.	
Cognitive	*Piaget:* will use all stages, depending on the task (e.g., can move between formal operations, concrete operations, and problem-solving as needed).	Encourage middle-aged clients who are anticipating returning to school or engaging in other intellectually stimulating activities.
	The middle-aged adult is able to reflect on the past and anticipate the future.	
	Reaction time diminishes during late middle age.	
	Learning ability remains intact if person is motivated and material is meaningful.	
Moral	*Kohlberg:* postconventional stage	Use nonjudgmental approach when client discusses values.
Spiritual	*Fowler:* conjunctive faith stage	
	The middle-aged adult is able to appreciate others' belief systems.	Encourage use of spiritual support.
	Middle-aged adults are less dogmatic with regard to own beliefs.	Refer to clergy if desired by client.
	Religion is usually a source of comfort.	

Data from Adult Health Nursing (3rd ed.), by P. G. Beare and J. L. Myers, 1998, St. Louis, MO: Mosby–Yearbook. Copyright 1998 by Mosby–Yearbook; Health Promotion throughout the Lifespan (4th ed.), by C. L. Edelman and C. L. Mandle, 1998, St. Louis, MO: Mosby–Yearbook. Copyright 1998 by Mosby–Yearbook; Health Assessment: A Nursing Approach (3rd ed.), by J. Fuller and J. Schaller-Ayers, 2000. Philadelphia: Lippincott. Copyright 2000 by Lippincott Williams & Wilkins; Fundamentals of Nursing: Standards & Practice, by S. DeLaune and P. Ladner, 1998, Albany, NY: Delmar. Copyright 1998 by Delmar.

revolves around work and family, and success and achievement are measured in terms of career accomplishments and family life.

The primary developmental task of the middle-aged adult revolves around the conflict of generativity (a sense that one is making a contribution to society) versus stagnation (a sense of nonmeaning in one's life). When an individual successfully resolves this developmental conflict, acceptance of age-related changes results. Achievement of this developmental task is manifested by the following:

- Demonstrating creativity
- Guiding the next generation
- Establishing lasting relationships
- Evaluating goals in terms of achievement

Evaluation of goals often leads to a midlife crisis, especially if individuals feel they have accomplished little or have not lived up to earlier self-expectations.

Nursing Implications

Middle-aged adults constitute almost half the U.S. population (Edelman & Mandle, 1998). Individuals of the baby-boom generation have entered midlife and will thus require more nursing care to maintain wellness and cope with illness.

Nurses can help middle-aged clients improve their health status (and thus quality of life) by identifying risk factors and providing early intervention. The major risk factors for adults in the middle years can be changed because they are primarily environmental and behavioral. In assisting the middle-aged client to change unhealthy behaviors, the nurse can work on either a one-on-one or group basis.

Wellness Promotion As health educators, nurses can encourage middle-aged adults to assume more responsibility for their own health. The nurse should both encourage clients to obtain influenza and pneumococcal immunizations as recommended by their physicians and confirm currency of Td (tetanus/diphtheria) immunization.

Safety Considerations Automobile accidents, especially those involving the use of alcohol, are a serious health problem among middle-aged adults. Occupational health hazards such as exposure to environmental toxins constitute another significant problem.

Middle adulthood is also the time when a lifelong accumulation of unhealthy lifestyle practices, such as smoking, sedentary habits, and overuse of alcohol, begins to exert adverse effects.

Most middle-aged individuals have more leisure time than in the past, resulting in an increased risk of recreational accidents such as boating accidents, sports-related injuries, and jogging mishaps.

CLIENT TEACHING

Self-Care for Middle-Aged Adults

Self-care topics pertinent to the middle-aged adult include:

- Acceptance of aging,
- Nutrition,
- Exercise and weight control,
- Substance abuse prevention,
- Stress management, and
- Recommendations for health screening (cholesterol screening, prostate examination, mammogram, Pap test).

Older Adulthood

Older adulthood is the developmental stage starting at age 65 and extending to death. Table 14–17 provides an overview of growth and development in the older adult.

Older adults have several psychosocial tasks to accomplish, including:

- Developing a sense of satisfaction with the life that one has lived (finding meaning in one's life),
- Establishing meaningful roles,
- Adjusting to infirmities (if any exist),
- Coping with losses and changes, and
- Preparing for death.

Nursing Implications

Nursing care is important in assisting the aging person to develop a sense of well-being (Eliopoulos, 1997). Nurses who work with elderly clients must be especially sensitive to their own feelings, attitudes, and beliefs about aging and be aware of the potential effects of these responses on their care provided to older clients.

When assessing the older adult for health-related needs, the nurse must learn about the client's background, including family history, work history, hobbies, and achievements (Figure 14-12). Clients should be encouraged to talk about their life experiences. When planning care, it is important to build on the client's lifelong interests. By recognizing each client's unique experiences and assets, the nurse is more likely to individualize care.

When clients express dissatisfaction and regrets about the past, the nurse should listen in a nonjudgmental manner and not try to convince clients that things are really better than remembered or perceived. It is important, though, to help the elderly client put disappointments into perspective by balancing them

Table 14–17 OLDER ADULT: GROWTH AND DEVELOPMENT

DIMENSION	CHARACTERISTICS	NURSING IMPLICATIONS
Physiological	Refer to chapter 28 for a detailed discussion of physiological changes related to aging.	
Psychosocial	*Erikson:* integrity vs. despair stage The older adult accepts own life as it is. A sense of worth is garnered from helping others. *Havighurst:* The older adult adjusts to a decline in physical strength. The older adult fulfills civic responsibilities. Older adults meet social obligations. The older adult develops an affiliation with peers and age group (i.e., sees self as "old"). Retirement from employment affects finances, activities, leisure time, and role identity (positively or negatively). Potential for social isolation increases as significant others and peers die.	Ask the older person for advice. Identify and use the older adult's strengths. Encourage the use of reminiscence. Encourage to express feelings concerning aging. Promote socialization with peers.
Cognitive	*Piaget:* formal operations stage There is no decline in IQ associated with aging. Reaction time is usually slowed. *Memory:* Short-term: Capacity for recall decreases. Long-term: Capacity remains unchanged.	Allow client time to respond to questions or instructions. Be alert for the possibility of medication-induced confusion and resultant impact on memory.
Moral	*Kohlberg:* postconventional stage The older adult makes moral decisions according to own principals and beliefs.	Support decision making. Respect values even when different from own.
Spiritual	*Fowler:* universalizing stage The older adult is generally satisfied with own spiritual beliefs. Older adults tend to act on beliefs.	Listen carefully to determine spiritual needs. Acknowledge losses and encourage appropriate grieving.

Data from Women's Health: Instant Nursing Assessment, *by P. A. Firth and S. J. Watanabe, 1996, Albany, NY: Delmar. Copyright 1996 by Delmar.* Health Promotion throughout the Lifespan *(4th ed.), by C. L. Edelman and C. L. Mandle, 1998, St. Louis, MO: Mosby–Yearbook. Copyright 1998 by Mosby–Yearbook;* Health Assessment & Promotion Strategies through the Life Span *(6th ed.), by R. B. Murray and J. P. Zentner, 1997, East Norwalk, CT: Appleton & Lange. Copyright 1997 by Appleton & Lange.* Fundamentals of Nursing: Standards & Practice, *by S. DeLaune and P. Ladner, 1998, Albany, NY: Delmar. Copyright 1998 by Delmar.*

against accomplishments and achievements. The nurse should encourage family members to engage in a positive life review with the elderly client. Most nursing interventions for elders center around introspection and reflection on their lives. Life review (or reminiscence therapy) promotes a positive self-concept in older people (Heriot, 1999).

Wellness Promotion Health-promotion activities should be implemented with the elderly client to maintain functional independence. Elderly people who are independent are generally healthier. Health-promotion activities are aimed at maximizing the elder's abilities and strengths. Specific topics that are developmentally appropriate for older clients are use of leisure time, increased socialization, regular physical activity, main-

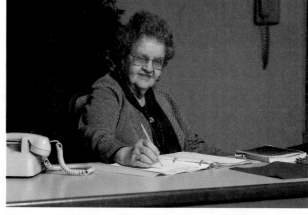

Figure 14-12 This older adult is able to maintain her independence and self-esteem through volunteer work.

taining a positive mental attitude, and developing and maintaining healthy lifestyles. Many older people engage in more health-promoting behaviors than do younger people (Sapp & Bliesmer, 1999). The nurse should both encourage the client to obtain influenza and pneumococcal immunizations as recommended and confirm currency of Td immunization.

Safety Considerations Falls pose a major health threat to elderly persons.

COMMUNITY/HOME HEALTH CARE

Home Safety for Elders

The nurse can encourage the elderly client to create a safe home environment by:

- Ensuring adequate lighting,
- Removing all throw or loose rugs,
- Clearing all walking paths,
- Having a handrail on all stairs, and
- Installing hand-holds in tubs and showers.

CASE STUDY

Mary Jo, age 32, and her two daughters, Sara, age 14, and Katie, age 8, live with Mary Jo's grandmother, age 85. Mary Jo is having difficulty dealing with her daughters and her grandmother.

Consider the following:

1. At what stage of psychosocial development is each member of the household?
2. Compare the cognitive dimensions of these four people.
3. What is the focus of wellness-promotion for each person?
4. What are the safety considerations for each person?

SUMMARY

- Growth is the quantitative changes in physical size of the body and its parts. Development refers to behavioral changes in functional abilities and skills.
- Growth and development of an individual are influenced by a combination of factors including heredity, life experiences, health status, and cultural expectations.
- Maturation is the process of becoming fully grown and developed and involves both physiological and behavioral aspects of an individual.
- During each developmental stage, certain developmental tasks must be achieved for normal development to occur.
- According to Freud, certain developmental tasks must be achieved at each developmental stage; failure to achieve or a delay in achieving the developmental task is the result of a psychosexual fixation in a previous stage.
- Erikson purports that psychosocial development is a series of conflicts that occur during eight stages of life.
- Sullivan theorizes that personality development is strongly influenced by interpersonal relationships.
- Piaget's theory cites four stages of cognitive development: sensorimotor, preoperational, concrete op-

erations, and formal operations. Each stage is characterized by the ways whereby the child interprets and uses the environment.
- Kohlberg's theory describes six stages of moral development through which individuals determine a moral code to guide their behavior.
- Fowler's theory outlines six distinct stages of faith development, and though individuals vary in the age at which they experience each stage, the sequence of stages remains the same.
- Nurses have important roles in promoting the health and safety of individuals at each stage of the life cycle.

Review Questions

1. The fact that development occurs in a proximo-distal manner means that the infant is able to:

   a. crawl before he walks.
   b. raise his head before he is able to sit up.
   c. move his arms before picking up an object with his fingers.
   d. master psychological tasks before establishing a separate identity.

2. The task to be achieved in Erikson's stage of industry versus inferiority is to:
    a. learn self-control.
    b. develop necessary social skills.
    c. develop commitments to others and to a career.
    d. view one's life as meaningful and fulfilling.

3. Piaget's theory relates to a child's:
    a. moral development.
    b. cognitive development.
    c. interpersonal development.
    d. spiritual development.

4. The nurse knows that at birth the neonate's activities are:
    a. reflexive.
    b. adjusting.
    c. purposeful.
    d. continuing.

5. The time for parents to begin teaching (by role modeling) the difference between "right" and "wrong" is during:
    a. infancy.
    b. childhood.
    c. toddler stage.
    d. preschool stage.

6. Immunizations are important during:
    a. infancy.
    b. childhood.
    c. adolescence.
    d. entire life.

7. The nurse working with preadolescent children should:
    a. offer opinions on the child's lifestyle choices.
    b. provide an opportunity for the child to ask questions about health-related concerns.
    c. finish the child's thoughts and sentences to avoid awkward silences.
    d. give a lecture on all the changes to be expected in the next few years; nutrition; and personal hygiene.

8. A great many health problems among adolescents are related to:
    a. nutrition.
    b. sexual behaviors.
    c. activity/exercise.
    d. sleep/rest behaviors.

9. The focus of wellness promotion during middle adulthood should be to:
    a. maintain functional independence.
    b. encourage use of fewer risk-taking behaviors.
    c. encourage client to assume responsibility for own health.
    d. teach about hygiene, nutrition, and substance abuse prevention.

10. The older adult has an increased risk of falls, burns, and other injuries because of:
    a. slower metabolism.
    b. diminished hearing.
    c. decreased ability to see colors.
    d. slower response to environmental changes.

Critical Thinking Questions

1. What is most important in determining a person's behavior: the person's genetic predisposition or the response of other people and socialization?

2. Our society labels certain characteristics as "masculine" or "feminine." How do you think these stereotypes influence the development of young boys and girls in our society?

3. Nurses often encounter clients whose value systems conflict with their own. How will you provide care to sexually active adolescents if you think their behavior is immoral or "wrong"? Is it ethical for you to try to change the adolescent's values so that they become congruent with yours? Should you change your values to be congruent with those of the client?

 WEB FLASH!

- Visit the American Academy of Pediatrics on the web. What information do they offer on such topics as nutrition, safety, discipline, and growth and development?
- What web sites are available for information on elders, adolescents, or middle-age adults?
- What information related to immunizations does the Centers for Disease Control and Prevention (CDC) offer on the Internet?

Health Promotion

Chapter 15
Wellness Concepts

Chapter 16
Stress, Adaptation, and Anxiety

Chapter 17
Loss, Grief, and Death

Chapter 18
Basic Nutrition

Chapter 19
Rest and Sleep

Chapter 20
Safety/Hygiene

WELLNESS CONCEPTS

MAKING THE CONNECTION

Refer to the following chapters to increase your understanding of wellness concepts:

- **Chapter 12, Cultural Diversity and Nursing**
- **Chapter 17, Loss, Grief, and Death**
- **Chapter 28, Nursing Care of the Older Client**

LEARNING OBJECTIVES

Upon completion of this chapter, you should be able to:
- *Define key terms.*
- *Discuss guidelines for healthy living.*
- *Describe the scope of prevention.*
- *Explain the importance of Healthy People 2010.*
- *Make a teaching plan for ways to promote and maintain wellness.*

KEY TERMS

genogram
health
prevention
primary prevention
secondary prevention
tertiary prevention
wellness

INTRODUCTION

The responsibility for maintaining health rests squarely on the shoulders of each individual adult. Parents are responsible for maintaining their children's health and teaching them a healthy lifestyle. Health maintenance involves the whole person and the person's whole life. It includes the prevention of disease and the early detection and treatment of disease. Maintenance of health requires constant effort and a focus on all aspects of a person's life.

Simon (1992) quotes Dr. Wood Hutchinson, who wrote in the *Journal of the American Medical Association* that "our system's philosophy might be condensed in the motto 'millions for health care and not a penny for prevention'." This was written in 1896. Over 100 years have passed and we still spend less than 3 cents of each health dollar on prevention and education.

The United States is the world leader in medical science and education yet is only 16th among nations in life expectancy. We spend more for health care than any other country, yet we rank 24th in infant mortality. In 1991, there were 82,902 positions for residents in specialty areas and only 202 in preventive medicine. Many doctors have not incorporated preventive medicine into their practices (Simon, 1992).

There is no profit in prevention. Insurance premiums buy illness insurance, not health insurance, given that insurance companies often will not pay for preventive testing and treatment. Compensation for clinical care makes illness the priority, not wellness. Diagnosis and treatment of illnesses are what insurance pays for, not health maintenance.

HEALTH

A widely accepted definition of **health** comes from the World Health Organization (WHO), which defines health as a state of complete physical, mental, and social well-being, not merely the absence of disease or infirmity.

Other concepts of health focus on motivation. A eudaemonistic approach to health (from the Greek word *eudaimonia,* meaning "fortunate or happy") views the individual as being motivated by joy and self-fulfillment: Health is the full realization of potential, and illness is an impediment to that realization.

Those who hold the adaptive view of health are motivated by altering the risks in self or the environment through such means as dietary and exercise programs or reducing exposure to environmental hazards. Illness results when the individual is unable to cope with the risks and stresses of daily life.

Some individuals are motivated by being able to meet responsibilities at home, at work, at play, and in the community: Their health focus is role performance. Health is considered achieved when the individual fulfills the obligations and responsibilities to family, job, and community.

Other individuals are motivated by the absence of disease: Theirs is a clinical health focus. As long as no disease is present, the individual considers himself healthy. Personal definition of health influences life choices and personal health decisions.

WELLNESS

Wellness is defined as a state of optimal health wherein an individual moves toward integration of human functioning, maximizes human potential, takes responsibility for health, and has greater self-awareness and self-satisfaction. Floyd, Mimms, and Yelding-Howard (1995), Hafen and Hoeger (1997), and Seiger, Vanderpool, and Barnes (1995) describe the behaviors exhibited by individuals in a state of wellness. These researchers outline seven areas of wellness: emotional, mental, intellectual, vocational, social, spiritual, and physical wellness. Various areas of wellness overlap and none is mutually exclusive.

CLIENT TEACHING

Suppressed Anger in Women
Research has shown that middle-aged women who suppress anger and have hostile attitudes may be at greater risk for developing cardiovascular disease (Matthews, 1998). Nurses can help such women minimize this risk by encouraging them to learn to express negative feelings in a constructive manner, to talk calmly about their feelings, to find other women who may share some of the same concerns and stressors, and to engage in regular exercise routines to relieve stress and tension.

Emotional Wellness

Emotions bridge the gap between mind and body. The person who is emotionally well understands his own feelings and knows when to express them appropriately. This individual accepts his limitations, has the ability to adjust to change, copes with stress in healthy ways, enjoys life, is optimistic and happy, and shows respect and affection to others.

Mental Wellness

The individual who is mentally well is alert, creative, logical, curious, open-minded, clear thinking, and accepting of others. This person also exhibits common sense, a good memory, and a desire for continual learning.

Intellectual Wellness

Intellectual wellness manifests as the ability to think, to process information, and to solve problems. The intellectually well person questions and evaluates information and situations, learns from life experiences, and is flexible, creative, and open to new ideas.

Vocational Wellness

The individual who is satisfied in school and/or job and who works in harmony with others enjoys vocational wellness (Figure 15-1).

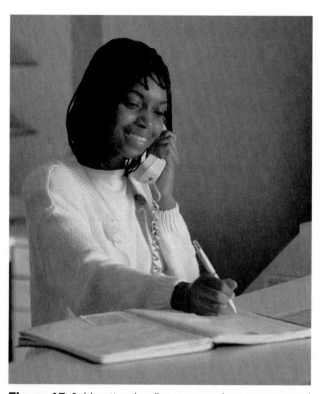

Figure 15-1 Vocational wellness means being content and satisfied with your occupation.

Social Wellness

Social wellness is evident when a person shows concern, fairness, affection, and respect for others; communicates effectively; has satisfying relationships; and interacts well with others. This person has a network of family and friends, is a member of various organizations, and works with a spirit of teamwork. Other behaviors exhibited are honesty, loyalty, confidence, and tolerance.

Spiritual Wellness

Spiritual wellness gives meaning, direction, and purpose to life by way of values, ethics, and morals. The spiritually healthy person has faith, optimism, and high self-esteem.

Physical Wellness

Physical wellness is noted in the person who avoids risky sexual behavior; tries to limit exposure to environmental contaminants; and restricts the intake of alcohol, tobacco, caffeine, and drugs. Regular exercise, a well-balanced diet, and regular physical examinations also enhance physical wellness (Figure 15-2).

HEALTH PROMOTION

Health promotion means more than preventing illness: It means assisting individuals to enhance their health, well-being, and functioning and to maximize their potential. Health promotion focuses on adopting healthy behaviors rather than on avoiding illness. The goal is for individuals to control and improve their health. Health promotion is appropriate for the individual and the population as a whole.

The concept of self-responsibility is important to health promotion, and it must be accepted and acted on in order for wellness to become a reality for an individual. No one else can make a person live a healthy life; self-responsibility is the only way to make changes. An individual can be given information relating to health and wellness, but only that person can change unhealthy or destructive habits. With the exception of small children, each individual must take responsibility

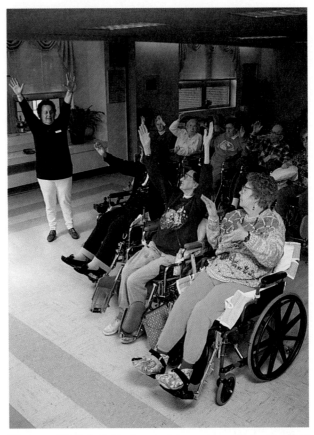

Figure 15-2 Individuals must learn to achieve physical wellness in a manner that accommodates their lifestyle and physical abilities.

for behaviors leading to health and wellness (Figure 15-3). Objectives for healthy living are outlined in the Healthy People 2000 and Healthy People 2010 documents issued by the federal government.

Healthy People 2000

In 1980 and again in 1990, the United States Department of Health and Human Services (USDHHS) released a list of objectives for disease prevention and health promotion in 22 priority areas (USDHHS, 1990). In 1990, more than 10,000 individuals representing 300

PROFESSIONAL TIP

Predictors of Healthy Aging

The most consistent predictors of healthy aging are low serum glucose, normal blood pressure, avoidance of smoking, and maintenance of target weight for height (Reed, 1998). To prevent disease in later years, young adults and even adolescents must keep these four factors in check. Remind clients that it is never too late to modify these four factors to improve health.

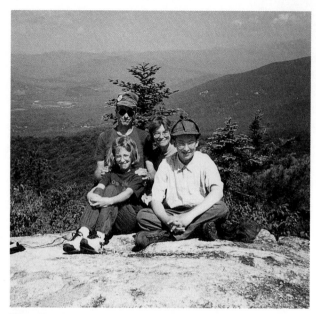

Figure 15-3 Families can engage in activities together to achieve wellness.

national organizations were involved in developing the health objectives for the year 2000. More than 300 health objectives for the nation to achieve by the year 2000 evolved. These objectives were published in a document titled *Healthy People 2000: National Health Promotion and Disease Prevention Objectives,* which addresses three important issues:

- Personal responsibility: Each individual must be health-conscious and must practice responsible, informed health behaviors.
- Health benefits for all people: Everyone must have health benefits in order for the nation to be healthy.
- Health promotion and disease prevention: Health care must change from a treatment focus to a prevention focus to cut costs and to increase the quality of life.

The overall goals include:

- Increasing the span of healthy life for Americans,
- Reducing health disparities among Americans, and
- Achieving access to preventive services for all Americans.

A sample of the objectives is found in Table 15–1. The entire document may be ordered from the United States Department of Health and Human Services, Washington, DC, DHHS Publication No. (PHS) 91–50212.

The USDHHS (2000b) reported on the progress made in meeting the 319 objectives of Healthy People 2000. In 1997, 15% of the goals had been reached or surpassed, and progress had been made in another 44%. Eighteen percent had fallen short of target, 6%

showed mixed results, and 2% showed no change. Eleven percent now have baseline data but no data to evaluate progress, and baselines have not yet been established for 3% of these goals (USDHHS, Healthy People 2000b).

Healthy People 2010

The Healthy People 2000 Consortium met in November 1996 to discuss necessary improvements and modifications to be made for Healthy People 2010 objectives. Over the past 4 years, the consortium worked with a wide range of representatives of national membership organizations, state governments, managed care organizations, and private businesses through focus groups, public meetings, and the Healthy People 2010 website. Several themes that emerged from the meetings and focus groups were earmarked to be addressed in the revised objectives. These include the:

- need to address morbidity and mortality in setting objectives,
- value of packaging the 2010 document into different formats for multiple audiences,
- necessity of linking objectives to community-based health improvement initiatives, and
- importance of using language that is understandable to the general public.

Two goals for the 2010 objectives emerged as a result of these sessions: (1) "Increase Years of Healthy Life," which was retained from the Healthy People 2000 goal, and (2) "Eliminate Health Disparities," a stronger version of the Healthy People 2000 goal "Reduce Health Disparities." These two goals will be supported by four enabling goals concerned with promoting healthy behaviors, protecting health, achieving access to quality health care, and strengthening community prevention. A comparison of select 2000 objectives is presented in Table 15–1, along with baselines, targets, and 2010 objectives.

The 467 objectives for 2010 are grouped into 28 focus areas. New focus areas include disability; people with low income; race and ethnicity; chronic diseases; and public health infrastructure (USDHHS, 2000a).

To expand the ability to track the objectives, new strategies are being developed to improve data collection, especially at the community level, and to improve the ability to measure access and quality of health services.

Healthy People 2010 was released in January 2000.

ILLNESS PREVENTION

Prevention (hindering, obstructing, or thwarting a disease or illness) incorporates both old and new ideas. The taboos, dietary laws, and traditions of various

Table 15–1 SELECTED OBJECTIVES FROM HEALTHY PEOPLE 2000 AND 2010

OBJECTIVE	BASELINE	YEAR 2000 TARGET	REPORT	YEAR 2010 TARGET
Physical Activity and Fitness				
• Increase the proportion of people who engage regularly in light to moderate physical activity for at least 30 minutes per day	22% (1985)	30%	23% (1995) (+)	30%
• Increase the proportion of young people in grades 9 to 12 who participate in daily school physical activity	42% (1991)	50%	27% (1997) (−)	50%
Nutrition				
• Increase the proportion of people aged 2 years and older who meet the Dietary Guidelines average daily goal of no more than 30% of calories from fat	34% (1989–91)	30%	33% (1994–96) (−)	75%
• Reduce the prevalence of BMI at or above 30.0 among people ages 20 years and older	24% males 27% females (1976–80)	20% both groups	34% males 37% females (1988–94) (−)	15%
Tobacco				
• Increase the proportion of cigarette smokers ages 18 years and older who stopped smoking cigarettes for a day	34% (1986)	50%	45.8% (1995) (+)	75%
• Increase the proportion of worksites with a formal smoking policy that prohibits smoking or limits it to separately ventilated areas at the workplace	NA	NA	59% of worksites with 50 or more employees (1992)	100%
Substance Abuse				
• Decrease alcohol-related motor vehicle crash deaths	9.8/100,000 (1987)	5.5/100,000	6.5/100,000 (1997)	3.5/100,000
• Reduce drug-related deaths	3.8/100,000 (1987)	3/100,000	4.7/100,000 (−) (1998)	1.3/100,000
Family Planning				
• Reduce the proportion of individuals ages 15 to 17 who have ever had sexual intercourse	33% of males 27% of females (1988)	15%	27% of males 22% of females (1999)	15%
• Increase the proportion of all females ages 15 to 44 at risk of unintended pregnancy who use contraception	88.2% (1982)	95%	92.5% (1999)	95% (modified to "use effective contraception")
Mental Health and Mental Disorders				
• Reduce suicide rates	11.7/100,000 (1987)	10.5/100,000	11.3/100,000 (1996)	9.6/100,000
Injury/Violence Prevention				
• Reduce firearm-related deaths	14.6/100,000 (1990)	11.6/100,000	13.5/100,000 (1996)	Fewer than 11.6/100,000
• Increase use of bicycle helmets of 9th- to 12th-grade students who ride bicycles		50%	8% (1995)	50%
Maternal, Infant, Child Health				
• Increase the proportion of all pregnant women who begin prenatal care in the first trimester of pregnancy	78.9% (1993)	90%	82.5% (1999)	90%
• Reduce the cesarean delivery rate	24.4/100 (1987)	15/100	21.8/100 (1999)	15/100
Cancer				
• Reduce cancer deaths		130/100,000	130/100,000 (1998) (=)	103/100,000

continues

Table 15–1 SELECTED OBJECTIVES FROM HEALTHY PEOPLE 2000 AND 2010 *continued*

OBJECTIVES	BASELINE	YEAR 2000 TARGET	REPORT	YEAR 2010 TARGET
AIDS/HIV Infection				
• Confine annual incidence of diagnosed AIDS cases among adolescents and adults	29.8/100,000 (1994)		28/100,000 (1998) (+)	12/100,000
• Increase the proportion of those with positive HIV tests who return for counseling	72.5% (1989)	80%	83% (1995) (+)	none
Sexually Transmitted Diseases				
• Reduce prevalence of *Chlamydia trachomatis* infections among 14–24 year olds	12.5% (1996)	5%	10.9% (1998)	3%
• Eliminate sustained domestic transmission of primary and secondary syphillis	84% higher than 1997 (1990)	4/100,000	3.2/100,000 (1998) (+)	0.25/100,000
Immunizatons and Infectious Diseases				
• Reduce indigenous cases of vaccine preventable diseases				
– Diphtheria		0	4 (1997)	0
– Polio		0	0 (1997)	0
– Measles	3,058 (1988)	0	135 (1997)	0
– Rubella	225 (1988)	0	161 (1997)	0
– Mumps	4,866 (1988)	500	612 (1997)	0
– Pertussis	3,450 (1988)	1,000	6,568 (1997) (–)	2,000
• Increase proportion of contacts completing course of preventive therapy for tuberculosis	66.3% (1987)	85%	65.4% (1995) (–)	85%
Environmental Health				
• Reduce exposure of children age 6 and younger who are regularly exposed to tobacco smoke	39% (1986)	20%	27% (1997)	15%

(+) Exceeding target
(–) Receding from target
(=) Met target

Data from U.S. Department of Health & Human Services (USDHHS), Public Health Service (PHS). (2000b). 1998–1999 Progress Review [On-line] Available: http://odphp.osophs.dhhs.gov/pubs/hp2000.

cultural, ethnic, and religious groups were initiated for a reason. If scientific research has not proved these incorrect or harmful, there is no reason not to practice the old ways. New methods of illness prevention emerge as technology expands and health awareness increases.

All stages of life should embody the tenets of preventive health. It must begin before conception with healthy parents and prenatal care and continue through the life span. Scientific advice based on firmly established medical data and reasonable probability should be heeded. Interventions for disease prevention range from lifestyle changes that cost little or nothing to high-tech procedures that are very expensive.

Before the full impact of illness prevention can be discovered, major changes are needed in health care delivery, funding, and insurance coverage. The health care system must insist on more research relating to prevention and must then apply the results of the research to insurance practices. Prevention practices must be supported and funded by the health care system in order for a change from illness treatment to illness prevention to occur. The rewards of such a shift will be enhanced health, longer life expectancy, and a population that feels better, looks better, and functions better.

Illness prevention must be viewed according to the type of prevention and the health care team responsible for its implementation.

Types of Prevention

Prevention extends to all stages of health. There are three types of prevention: primary, secondary, and tertiary. Primary prevention has not historically been supported by our health care system, whereas secondary and tertiary prevention have been, and still are, the main focus. They are also the most expensive.

Primary Prevention

Primary prevention includes all practices designed to keep health problems from developing. Following recommended childhood immunization schedules, not smoking to prevent lung cancer, and eating calcium-rich foods to prevent osteoporosis are all examples of primary prevention. Primary prevention should be the focus for every individual and health care provider. It is usually the least expensive intervention and provides the greatest benefits.

Secondary Prevention

Secondary prevention refers to early detection, diagnosis, screening, and intervention to reduce the consequences of a health problem. That is, disease or illness is identified before the individual has any symptoms or functional impairment. Screening for tuberculosis and performing monthly breast self-examinations are both examples of secondary prevention. When no known methods of primary prevention exist for a specific disease or illness (such as breast cancer), the focus should be on performing self-examinations, and having a regular physical exam, and testing.

Tertiary Prevention

Tertiary prevention refers to caring for a person who already has a health problem; the illness or disease is treated after symptoms have appeared so as to prevent further progression. For example, taking antibiotics for an ear infection should eliminate the infection. Furthermore, potential complications and the disability of hearing impairment are prevented. Rehabilitation is an important aspect of tertiary prevention; this refers to preventing deterioration of a person's condition and minimizing the loss of function. One example is providing range of motion exercises to a client who has had a stroke, to encourage circulation and maintain function in the extremities.

Prevention Health Care Team

The prevention health care team consists of the individual assisted by nurses and the primary physician.

Individual

The individual is the center of the prevention health care team. It is the individual who must incorporate the knowledge related to preventive health care and make the behavioral changes necessary to live a more healthy life.

Individuals should decide those things that they want and expect from health care. Honesty with self, the nurses, and physician is necessary. Clients must be assertive and ask questions of the physicians and nurses and be active, informed health care consumers. The ultimate responsibility for health care belongs with the individual.

Nurses

Nurses, especially nurse practitioners, often do the initial health screening in clinics and physicians' offices. This provides a great opportunity to inquire about lifestyle and the preventive health habits of the client. Nurses can use their excellent listening skills to give clients time to discuss health care habits and ask questions. Nurses are also great teachers of preventive health habits and health promotion activities.

Primary Physicians

Primary physicians generally are family practitioners, pediatricians, or internists: These are the family doctors, the physicians seen on a regular basis. They have the opportunity and obligation to discuss and inquire about preventive health habits. When necessary, they refer clients to specialists for specific problems. After the problem has been resolved, the client returns to the primary physician for further care.

FACTORS AFFECTING HEALTH

A great many factors affect health. They can be categorized into four broad topics:

- Genetics and human biology
- Personal behavior
- Environmental influences
- Health care

Genetics and Human Biology

Inherited traits and the way the human body functions have an impact on an individual's state of health and wellness. An individual's genetic makeup may include inherited disorders, such as sickle-cell anemia, or chromosomal anomalies, such as Down syndrome. Both of these may ultimately affect the individual's quality of life and level of health.

Human biology affects health because normal body functioning prevents some illnesses and makes us more susceptible to others. Production of the female and male hormones, estrogen and testosterone, respectively, are responsible for many of these effects (Hoffman, 1996) (Table 15–2).

Personal Behavior

Personal behavior is the area having the most factors affecting health and wellness, and they are controlled entirely by the individual. It is the individual's decision to use or not to use these factors to promote health and wellness. Factors typically deemed to be under the individual's control include diet, exercise, personal care, sexual relationships, level of stress, tobacco and drug use, alcohol use, and safety.

Table 15–2 EFFECTS OF ESTROGEN AND TESTOSTERONE ON SPECIFIC TISSUES

	HORMONE	
Tissue	**Estrogen (Female)**	**Testosterone (Male)**
Cardiovascular	• Increases arterial dilation • Causes vascular spasms • Improves cardiac function	• Increases size of heart
Liver	• Inhibits production of triglycerides, low-density lipoprotein (LDL) (bad) cholesterol, and free glucose • Decreases drug metabolism, prolonging action	• Produces triglycerides, LDL (bad) cholesterol, and free glucose • Increases drug metabolism, shortening action
Fat	• Encourates fat deposits in breasts, hips, and thighs and suppresses the movement of fat from these areas	• Encourages fat deposits in the abdomen
Gastrointestinal	• Slows motility and favors formation of gallstones	
Respiratory	• Increases respiratory rate and basal body temperature	
Musculoskeletal	• Enhances bone density	• Ensures bone density and strength
Immune	• Enhances antibody production and suppresses T cell-mediated processes (prevents rejection of sperm and fetus)	
Blood	• Suppresses red blood cell (RBC) development • Lowers hemoglobin (Hgb) level • Increases coagulation	• Increases RBC development • Increases Hgb level
Integumentary	• Enhances skin vitality • Increases collagen and water content	• Promotes body hair

Adapted from Our Health, Our Lives, *by E. Hoffman, 1996, New York: Pocket Books. Copyright 1996 by Pocket Books.*

Diet

Healthy eating habits and a proper diet greatly enhance an individual's overall state of health and well-being. Eating both fulfills the basic biological needs of sustenance, nutrition, and hydration and allows individuals to meet social and interpersonal needs (Figure 15-4). All of these factors contribute to overall wellness.

Exercise

Integrating physical activity into daily life is one of the best ways of promoting health. Exercise improves circulation, muscle strength, and emotional well-being; lowers blood pressure; increases endurance; and reduces the chances of heart attack, stroke, and osteoporosis. The individual who exercises regularly looks healthier and feels better.

Many people have joined health clubs in an effort to meet their need for exercise. Health clubs can be a wonderful source of regular exercise, but, also, a source

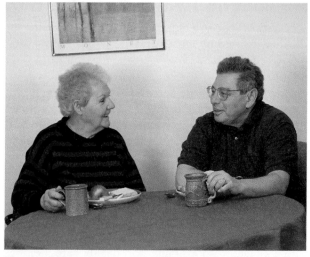

Figure 15-4 Sharing meals together is a wonderful means of meeting both physical and interpersonal needs.

CULTURAL CONSIDERATIONS

Parents' Beliefs about Feeding Children

Many parents:

- Begin feeding cereal and other solid foods earlier than recommended, believing that milk alone will not satisfy their babies' hunger,
- Use food to soothe or console children,
- Believe a heavier child is a healthier child, and
- View having a heavy infant or toddler as evidence of parental competence (Baughcum, 1998).

Nurses can work with these clients by respecting their cultural beliefs while enforcing the notion that a healthy child is a child who is satisfied following a meal and who shows a healthy, normal physical and emotional growth pattern. These factors, not plumpness, are indicators of wellness.

of disease, as reported in *Health-Club Hygiene* (Nov. 6, 1995). For example, perspiration on exercise machines is a prime source of impetigo. Clients should be made aware of such dangers so that they can practice safety precautions, such as wearing thigh-length shorts and always keeping a towel between the body and the exercise equipment.

CLIENT TEACHING

Dietary Guidelines for Americans

Teach clients to develop nutritional wellness by:

Aim for Fitness
- Aim for a healthy weight.
- Be physically active each day.

Build a Healthy Base
- Let the food pyramid guide your meal choices.
- Choose a variety of grains daily, especially whole grains.
- Choose a variety of fruits and vegetables daily.
- Keep food safe to eat.

Choose Sensibly
- Choose a diet that is low in both saturated fat and cholesterol and moderate in total fat.
- Choose beverages and foods to moderate your intake of sugars.
- Choose and prepare foods with less salt.
- If you drink alcoholic beverages, do so in moderation.

From Home and Garden Bulletin No. 232 *(5th ed.), by U.S. Department of Agriculture and U.S. Department of Health and Human Services, 2000.*

CLIENT TEACHING

Preventing Food-Borne Diseases

Share the following tips with clients to educate them in ways to prevent food-borne diseases:

- Allow cooked foods to sit at room temperature for no more than 2 hours.
- Date leftovers, refrigerate, and eat within 5 days.
- Wash dirty dishes in hot (120°F) water, as dirty dishes are an ideal place for bacteria to multiply.
- Keep dishcloths and sponges clean and allow to dry between uses.
- Use a bleach solution to clean cutting boards and countertops.
- Wash all fruits and vegetables in a diluted bleach solution (a bleach to water ratio of 1:100).

Personal Care

The skin protects the body from outside elements. It works with the immune system to defend the body against harmful bacteria, fungi, viruses, and allergens. Regular skin, hair, and nail care will enhance wellness and foster self-esteem. Personal care also includes such wellness habits as proper posture, proper body mechanics, adequate sleep, and dental hygiene.

Sexual Relationships

Establishing intimacy and a sexual relationship with another person is a natural step in growth and development. To maintain health and wellness, the individual will use values, ethics, and morals to guide the development of the relationship. A healthy sexual relationship is based on mutual satisfaction of the parties, a consensual approach to pleasurable activities, and mutual respect for preferences and personal choices.

Level of Stress

Not all stress is harmful. Limited stress makes one more alert and raises one's energy level. The way one responds to or copes with stressors dictates whether the situation is healthy or harmful. For instance, whereas one individual may enjoy the challenge of balancing work and family, another may feel torn by these seemingly conflicting demands and will therefore experience undue stress. Stress results not from an individual's life situation, but from that individual's reaction to and perception of the life situation.

Tobacco and Drug Use

Refraining from tobacco use is a strong step toward health promotion and maintenance. Even when a long-time smoker gives up the habit, the health risks begin to decrease at once, although it will take 10 to 15 years

PROFESSIONAL TIP

Moderate Exercise Reduces Stroke Risk
- Individuals who burn 1,000 to 1,999 calories per week by exercising moderately have a 24% lower risk of suffering a stroke than do those who burn less.
- Individuals who burn 2,000 to 2,999 calories per week by exercising moderately have a 46% lower risk.
- Burning over 2,999 calories a week through moderate exercise lowered the risk of having a stroke by only 20%.
- Moderate exercise includes activities such as brisk walking, dancing, and cycling (Lee & Paffenbarger, 1998).

to eliminate all the effects of smoking from the lungs. The person who smokes exhales secondhand smoke, which presents a health risk to those who do not smoke.

Abuse of both illegal and prescription drugs is a serious medical and social problem in our society. Drugs prescribed by a physician are abused if they are not taken as directed, or if they are taken by anyone other than the client for whom they were prescribed. Many prescribed drugs can be addictive if not taken as directed. Health can be maintained when clients understand the effects, indications, side effects, and interactions of the prescription medications they are taking.

Alcohol Use

The decision to consume alcohol is a personal choice that can influence an individual's state of health. The amount of alcohol consumed will affect sobriety, decision-making ability, and, in many instances, safety. The use of alcohol can play a significant role in drownings, adult fire deaths, traffic fatalities, falling fatalities, and suicides.

Safety

Personal choices concerning safety affect many areas of an individual's life and can be viewed collectively more as a lifestyle choice than individually as separate acts to promote safety. For example, individuals who embrace safety as a fundamental element of health and well-being will ensure safety in their homes by having smoke detectors, fire extinguishers, carbon monoxide detectors, practiced escape plans, locked medicine cabinets, and gates blocking dangerous stairways. These individuals will also most likely buckle their car seat belts, secure their children in child car seats, and obey speed limits when driving. All these elements of safety add up to a healthy lifestyle.

Environmental Influences

Environmental factors that may influence health are numerous, can be natural or man-made, and vary depending on geographic location and living conditions. Exposure to or ingestion of certain natural biological irritants can cause disease, such as results from exposure to poison ivy, and even death, such as results from ingestion of poisonous mushrooms. Exposure to chemicals such as asbestos in older buildings, lead in paint in older houses, and mercury in polluted water sources, can also pose health hazards. Radiation from the sun and certain types of machinery can be harmful in large doses; extreme, prolonged exposure to solar radiation can even result in death. Natural disasters such as hurricanes, floods, volcanic eruptions, droughts, heat waves, blizzards, and other extreme weather conditions pose health risks, as do man-made environmental crises including wars, bombings, pollution, and overpopulation.

Health Care

Most people use the health care system when they are ill, for the treatment of their disease or condition. A more effective use of the health care system, however, is health promotion and disease prevention. Routine physical examinations with minimal testing are invaluable for maintaining health and preventing disease (Figure 15-5). Healthy adults should consider health care services based on factors related to family health history, personal health history, personal habits, or the presence of symptoms that may alter the time frame for suggested health care services.

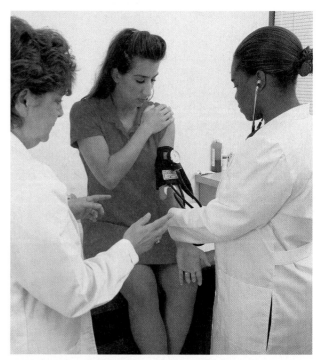

Figure 15-5 Routine physical examinations are essential to maintaining health and preventing disease.

Physical Exam

The physical examination should begin with a review of family health history, personal health history, personal habits (tobacco, alcohol, and drug use, sexual practices), and concerns or questions the client may have. Before visiting the physician, the client should write down questions and concerns so that none will be forgotten. Individuals between the ages of 20 and 39 years should have a complete physical exam every 1 to 3 years; those 40 to 49 years of age, every 1 to 2 years; and those over 50 years of age, every year. Women should have a breast exam with every physical exam obtained before age 40 and yearly thereafter. Men should have a testicular exam with every physical exam and should have a rectal exam to check the prostate at every physical exam obtained after age 40.

Immunizations

Adults who have not had the recommended immunizations as children should discuss this with their primary physicians. Depending on the client's risk factors, the physician may recommend having the immunizations as an adult.

Each adult should have a tetanus booster immunization every 10 years for life. Those at high risk of exposure, such as health care workers and college students; those who have chronic pulmonary, heart, or kidney disease; those who have diabetes; and those 65 years of age and older should have an influenza immunization every year and a pneumococcal pneumonia immunization every 6 years.

Tests

The following tests should be done with every physical exam: complete blood count, blood sugar, cholesterol, urinalysis, stool for blood, and, for women, a Papanicolau (Pap) smear. An electrocardiogram (EKG

PROFESSIONAL TIP

Hepatitis B Vaccine

Health care personnel who may be exposed to blood and body fluids are at risk for contracting the hepatitis B virus. Health care employers are required by law to offer the hepatitis B vaccination without cost to employees who are in direct care positions. Employees have the option of having or refusing this immunization. The vaccine is not contraindicated during pregnancy, and there are no apparent adverse effects to developing fetuses; however, the vaccine may cause shock in individuals who are allergic to baker's yeast.

PROFESSIONAL TIP

Mammograms

The Centers for Disease Control and Prevention (CDC) (2000) reports that 72% of women, age 50 and over, at or above poverty had a mammogram in 1998, but only 53% of women, age 50 and over, living below the poverty threshold had a mammogram in the same year.

or ECG) should be done at ages 20 years and 40 years and every 5 years thereafter (and yearly if the client is at high risk). Women should have a baseline mammogram (Figure 15-6) at age 40 and yearly thereafter. Men should have a testicular exam and rectal exam of the prostate at each physical exam. Each woman should perform a breast self-exam after every menstrual period. Each male should perform a testicular self-exam on a monthly basis.

Dental Exam

A dental exam, prophylaxis, and needed treatment should be performed every 6 to 12 months throughout life.

Eye Exam

An eye exam, including tonometry for glaucoma, should be performed every 2 to 3 years from ages 40 to 49 years and every 1 to 2 years after the age of 50.

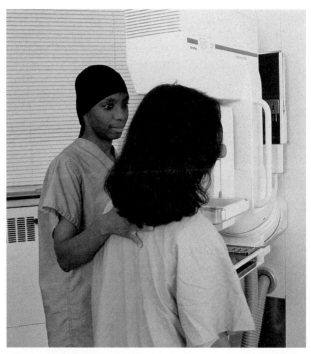

Figure 15-6 Mammograms are a key element to wellness promotion for all women over the age of 40 years.

CLIENT TEACHING

Crucial Health Practices

Simon (1992) states that all the medical progress in the United States from 1900–1990 increased the life span of an average adult by 4 years; but that simple lifestyle changes increased the life span of an average adult by 11 years. He describes 10 crucial health practices:

- Do not use tobacco and drugs.
- Do not consume more than 2 ounces of alcohol per day.
- Eat a diet low in fat, cholesterol, and salt but high in fiber, fruits, vegetables, and fish.
- Exercise regularly—1 hour each week is helpful, 3 is ideal.
- Stay lean.
- Drive cars with air bags and wear seat belts; drive prudently, and never drink before driving.
- Avoid excessive stress.
- Minimize exposure to radiation, ultraviolet rays, chemical pollutants, and other environmental hazards.
- Protect self from sexually transmitted diseases.
- Obtain regular medical care including immunizations and screening tests.

MAKING A GENOGRAM

A **genogram** is a method of visualizing family members, their birth and death dates or ages, and specific health problems. It should include at least four generations: the individual, the children, the parents, and the grandparents. Then it is easy to follow the health problems in the family through the generations. The individual can identify the health problems that may be encountered, take steps to prevent them, and have the appropriate screening tests performed. Figure 15-7 shows a sample genogram.

GUIDELINES FOR HEALTHY LIVING

Because of their education and training, nurses are in a unique position to practice healthy living habits themselves and to promote such habits in their clients. Table 15–3 outlines select causes of death and the controllable lifestyle factors that most contribute to these types of deaths. While it is important to remember that certain health variables such as gender and race cannot be controlled or changed, others such as diet and tobacco use result from individual choice. These lifestyle choices are based on individual preference, and

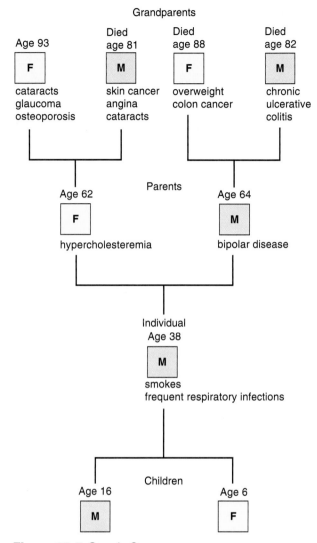

Figure 15-7 Sample Genogram

nurses can help clients make the best choices to promote wellness and optimal functioning. Following is a list of select guidelines, for nurses and their clients, to promote healthy living and wellness in daily life.

Heart Disease:
- Eat a diet low in fat and cholesterol and high in fiber
- Exercise regularly, 30 minutes three to five times a week (walking, swimming, cycling)
- Quit smoking or do not start to smoke
- Handle stress appropriately; use relaxation or meditation
- Do not use caffeine or alcohol excessively
- Maintain appropriate weight for height
- Maintain normal blood pressure
- Have a regular physical exam

Osteoporosis:
- Throughout life, eat calcium-rich foods (milk and milk products) and a balanced diet

Table 15–3 CONTROLLABLE FACTORS FOR TOP 10 CAUSES OF DEATH

CAUSE OF DEATH	CONTROLLABLE FACTORS
Heart disease	Tobacco use, high blood pressure, high cholesterol, lack of exercise, excessive stress, diabetes, obesity
Cancer	Tobacco use, radiation, alcohol abuse, improper diet, environmental exposure
Stroke	Tobacco use, high blood pressure, high cholesterol, lack of exercise
Chronic lung disease	Tobacco use, environmental exposures
Accidents	Alcohol abuse, drug abuse, tobacco use, failure to use seat belts, fatigue, stress, recklessness
Pneumonia and influenza	Chronic lung disease, environmental exposures, tobacco use, alcohol abuse, lack of immunization
Diabetes	Obesity, improper diet, lack of exercise, excessive stress
AIDS	Unsafe sex, neglect to use condom
Suicide	Excessive stress, alcohol abuse, drug abuse
Liver disease	Alcohol abuse, exposure to toxins (ingested and environmental), lack of immunizations

Top 10 Data from National Center for Health Statistics (1997) monthly vital statistics report. 45 (1152) 23, 40–43. [On-line] Available: http://www.youfirst.com/risks.htm

- Get plenty of exercise
- Discuss with the primary care physician the need for a calcium supplement and estrogen replacement therapy (females)
- Do not smoke

Cancer:
- Do not smoke
- Avoid exposure to unnecessary radiation
- Protect skin from ultraviolet rays; use sunscreen
- Avoid exposure to harmful chemicals
- Minimize exposure to pesticides, herbicides, and poisons
- Limit alcohol intake
- Eat a well-balanced diet with adequate fiber
- Exercise
- Practice safe sex
- Have cancer screening tests—mammogram, Pap smear, fecal occult blood test, and rectal exam—with each physical exam

Low-Back Pain:
- Exercise regularly
- Practice good posture
- Use proper body mechanics

Colds and Flu:
- Wash hands frequently
- Use paper tissues and dispose of properly
- Have flu shots yearly
- Follow the Dietary Guidelines for Americans for a balanced diet
- Drink plenty of fluids

Breast Cancer:
- Eat a diet low in fat
- Exercise regularly
- Limit alcohol and caffeine intake
- Perform monthly breast self-examinations
- Have mammograms as recommended by the American Cancer Society

Sexually Transmitted Diseases:
- Practice monogamous sex between noninfected individuals
- Use latex condoms

Tuberculosis (especially for health care workers):
- Mantoux test
- Isoniazid preventive therapy—any newly exposed and infected individual taking a full course of therapy (Reichman & Mangura, 1996)

Urinary Tract Infections:
- Drink plenty of water
- Empty bladder frequently, especially before and after sexual intercourse
- Wear underwear with a cotton crotch
- Wipe from front to back
- Drink cranberry juice
- Avoid bubble bath, douches, and scented or colored toilet paper

Sickle-Cell Anemia and Thalassemia:
- Request genetic screening and counseling if a high-risk group

Cataracts:
- Wear sunglasses and a hat with a brim
- Eat a well-balanced diet
- Do not smoke

Glaucoma:
- Have tonometry performed
- Have an optic nerve exam

Sunburn:
- Always wear sunscreen (with a minimum SPF of 15) when out in the sun

Dental Caries and Periodontal Disease:
- Brush after each meal; floss daily
- Use fluoride toothpaste
- Have a professional cleaning twice a year
- Have a dental exam yearly

Home Safety:
- Lock cupboards containing medicines and cleaning materials
- Maintain working smoke alarms and fire extinguishers
- Use a carbon monoxide alarm in the presence of gas appliances and heaters
- Plan escape routes in case of fire and have fire drills
- Safety proof home against falls
- Know water safety rules

Work Safety:
- Follow workplace safety regulations
- Report unsafe equipment or practices

Travel Safety:
- Wear a seat belt
- Do not drink and drive
- Drive safely and defensively
- Use infant and child seats and restraints
- Wear a helmet when riding a bicycle or motorcycle
- Never swim alone

Weight:
- Follow the Dietary Guidelines for Americans for a balanced diet

CASE STUDY

Use the genogram in Figure 15-8. The individual has a high-level administrative position at a large university. He must attend many luncheon and dinner meetings. Free time is spent reading novels or watching television.

Consider the following:

1. Identify the possible health problems for the individual.
2. List the lifestyle changes the individual must make to lower his risk of health problems.
3. Identify secondary preventive measures the individual should take.
4. Identify the possible health problems for his children.
5. List ways the children can lower their risk for the health problems identified in statement 4.
6. Identify the secondary preventive measures his children should be taking.

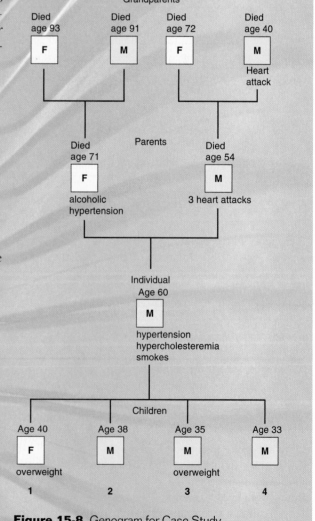

Figure 15-8 Genogram for Case Study

- Exercise 30 minutes daily
- If overweight, eat the least number of servings recommended
- If needed, use raw fruits or vegetables as snacks between meals
- If underweight, eat the largest number of servings recommended
- Eat a nutritious snack between meals

Stress:
- Identify sources of stress
- Establish realistic goals and expectations
- Be flexible
- Express thoughts and feelings
- Do not depend on alcohol or drugs for relaxation
- Exercise
- Practice deep breathing and muscle relaxation
- Get enough sleep
- Have a sense of humor—laugh
- Obtain professional help when needed

SUMMARY

- Wellness includes prevention, early detection, and treatment of health problems.
- The best way to maintain health is to follow the Dietary Guidelines for Americans, exercise regularly, reduce stress, prevent accidents, and receive routine health exams.
- The leading causes of death can be significantly reduced by lifestyle changes.
- Physical, mental, emotional, social, and spiritual aspects play a key role in the ability to resist disease and maintain health and wellness.

Review Questions

1. The person responsible for health maintenance and disease prevention is the:
    a. nurse.
    b. physician.
    c. individual.
    d. nurse practitioner.

2. The Healthy People 2000 objectives:
    a. are related only to physical fitness.
    b. are related only to disease conditions.
    c. address the treatment of disease conditions.
    d. address the issue of personal responsibility for health behaviors.

3. Primary prevention:
    a. begins with the physician.
    b. is curing a disease in a week.
    c. takes place before disease begins.
    d. includes all diseases or conditions.

4. The prevention health care team is composed of the:
    a. dietitian, nurses, and pharmacist.
    b. individual, physician, and nurses.
    c. physician, pharmacist, and laboratory.
    d. radiology, laboratory, and individual.

5. Health is improved by:
    a. not smoking.
    b. drinking alcohol.
    c. eating more sweet foods.
    d. sleeping 3 to 4 hours each night.

6. How often should an individual have a physical exam?
    a. every year.
    b. every two years.
    c. every three years.
    d. it depends on the person's age.

7. A genogram is used for:
    a. building a family tree.
    b. identifying potential health problems.
    c. preventing most diseases and illnesses.
    d. identifying the genes a person inherits.

8. Colds and flu can best be prevented by:
    a. smoking.
    b. staying warm and dry.
    c. washing hands frequently.
    d. having a flu shot every three years.

Critical Thinking Questions

1. How can you assist a client in identifying potential health problems?

2. What kind of preventive health care should be received by a person 20 years old, 42 years old, and 65 years old?

3. How does the nurse's state of health affect client care?

WEB FLASH!

- What information does the Internet provide about Healthy People 2010?
- What information/resources can be found about wellness?

STRESS, ADAPTATION, AND ANXIETY

MAKING THE CONNECTION

Refer to the following chapters to increase your understanding of stress, adaptation, and anxiety:

- **Chapter 1, Holistic Care**
- **Chapter 2, Critical Thinking**
- **Chapter 8, Communication**
- **Chapter 13, Complementary/Alternative Therapies**
- **Chapter 21, Infection Control/Asepsis**
- **Chapter 26, Pain Management**

LEARNING OBJECTIVES

Upon completion of this chapter, you should be able to:
- *Define key terms.*
- *Discuss stress, adaptation, and anxiety as they affect health.*
- *Identify factors contributing to the stress response.*
- *Describe the general adaptation syndrome.*
- *Detail the effects of stress on the whole individual.*
- *Explain stressors inherent in the change process.*
- *Discuss the role of the nurse as a change agent.*
- *Explain nursing interventions that promote positive adaptation to stress.*
- *Develop an individualized stress management plan for use as a nurse.*

KEY TERMS

adaptation	depersonalization
adaptive energy	distress
adaptive measures	endorphin
anxiety	eustress
burnout	fight-or-flight response
catharsis	general adaptation syn-
change	drome (GAS)
change agent	homeostasis
cognitive reframing	local adaptation
conditioning	syndrome (LAS)
crisis	maladaptive measures
crisis intervention	stress
defense mechanisms	stressor

INTRODUCTION

Stress and anxiety are universal experiences that can be either catalysts for positive change or sources of discomfort and pain. Nurses are involved with stress management from a teaching perspective, helping clients learn to cope with the stress imposed by illness, injury, disability, or treatment approaches. Caring for clients who are experiencing a high level of anxiety can also be stress provoking for the nurse. Successful stress management is necessary for the well-being of both clients and nurses. This chapter discusses the major concepts related to stress and anxiety, including strategies for coping with stress.

STRESS

According to Hans Selye (1974), **stress** is a nonspecific response to any demand made on the body. Selye termed such demands **stressors**. Any situation, event, or agent that produces stress is considered a stressor. A stressor is a stimulus that evokes the need to adapt. Stressors can be internal or external. For example, a headache is an internal stressor, whereas a difficult assignment is an external stressor.

Even pleasant events can be stressful in that they evoke the need to adapt. Stressors in themselves are neutral; in other words, a stressor is neither good nor bad. The individual's *perception* of the stressor greatly determines whether the effect on the individual is positive or negative. Any event can be stressful, depending on the person's interpretation of that event.

Response to Stress

Adaptive energy is the term Selye coined to describe the inner force an individual uses to respond or adapt to stress. All persons have adaptive energy; however, the amount of adaptive energy varies from person to person. After an individual has used all of his adaptive energy, the result may be illness, disease, or even death, as he is no longer able to change and adapt to the needs of his environment. Reactions to stress are typically categorized as either general (affecting the entire body) or local (affecting only the involved body part).

General Adaptation Syndrome

Stressors cause structural and chemical changes in the body as the body attempts to maintain **homeostasis**, which is the balance or equilibrium among the physiologic, psychological, sociocultural, intellectual, and spiritual needs of the body. Selye called these responses to stressors the **general adaptation syndrome** (GAS).

Selye divided the GAS into three stages, as illustrated in Figure 16-1. In the first stage, crisis or alarm, the body readies itself to handle the stressors. The physiologic changes may result in symptoms such as cool, pale skin;

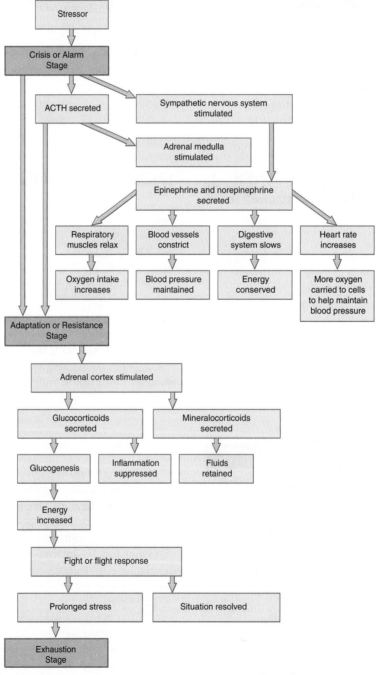

Figure 16-1 Physiological Effects of the General Adaptation Syndrome (GAS) (*Adapted from* Mental Health Concepts, *by C. Waughfield, 1998, Albany, NY: Delmar. Copyright 1998 by Delmar.*)

PROFESSIONAL TIP

Anticipatory Stress

When a person worries about a situation, such as an upcoming exam, the thoughts are stressors that trigger the GAS. The body responds as if the person were *actually* experiencing the events in the present moment, and the individual may feel ill, nauseous, sweaty, or very jittery.

shivering; and sweating of the palms and of the soles of the feet. Severe stress may cause dilated pupils, dry mouth, pounding heart, nausea, and diarrhea.

During the second stage, adaptation or resistance, the body attempts to defend against the stressor through the **fight-or-flight response**. The body becomes physiologically ready to defend itself by either fighting or running away from the danger (stressor).

The third stage, exhaustion, occurs if adaptive energy is inadequate to deal with prolonged or overwhelming stress.

The GAS is the same whether the stressor is actual or imagined, present or potential. In other words, the physiologic reactions of the body are essentially the same regardless of the source of the stress. For example, the mind can imagine a stressor, and the physiologic response (GAS) will be the same as if the body had actually experienced the stressor. According to Selye (1976), all stress reactions involve similar physiologic reactions.

Local Adaptation Syndrome

Selye also described the **local adaptation syndrome** (LAS), which is the physiologic response to a stressor (e.g., trauma, illness) affecting a specific part of the body. For example, if a person experiences a puncture wound on the foot, the LAS is initiated, leading to localized inflammation: The classic symptoms of inflammation (redness, warmth, and swelling) occur at the injured site. The LAS is usually a temporary process that resolves when the traumatized area is restored to its preinjury state. However, if the inflammation does not resolve with the LAS, the individual will then experience the GAS as the entire body becomes diseased.

Manifestations of Stress

The manifestations of stress are numerous and affect every dimension of a person. Common manifestations of stress are outlined in Table 16–1.

Outcomes of Stress

Stress is an experience that provides the individual with two possibilities: (1) an opportunity for personal growth or (2) the risk of disorganization and distress.

Table 16–1 MANIFESTATIONS OF STRESS	
Physiologic	**Cardiovascular/ Respiratory Effects**
	• Increased pulse rate
	• Increased blood pressure
	• Rapid, shallow breathing
	Neurologic Effects
	• Dizziness
	• Headaches
	• Dilated pupils
	Gastrointestinal Effects
	• Nausea
	• Altered appetite
	• Diarrhea or constipation
	Genitourinary Effect
	• Polyuria
	Musculoskeletal Effects
	• Tension
	• Twitching
	Endocrine Effect
	• Increased levels of blood glucose and cortisol
Psychological	• Irritability
	• Increased sensitivity (feelings easily hurt)
	• Sadness, depression
	• Feeling "on edge"
Cognitive	• Impaired memory
	• Confusion
	• Impaired judgment
	• Poor decision making
	• Delayed response time
	• Altered perceptions
	• Inability to concentrate
Behavioral	• Pacing
	• Sweaty palms
	• Rapid speech
	• Insomnia
	• Withdrawal
	• Exaggerated startle reflex
Spiritual	• Alienation
	• Social isolation
	• Feeling of emptiness

From Fundamentals of Nursing: Standards & Practice, *by S. DeLaune and P. Ladner, 1998, Albany, NY: Delmar. Copyright 1998 by Delmar.*

When stressors are responded to appropriately, adaptation is successful, and the body returns to its normal steady state.

The term **eustress** is used to describe a type of stress that results in positive outcomes. Consider for example, students who have an examination scheduled the following week. The stress over the impending test motivates them to study early, and, as a result, they pass the examination. This stress was positive in that it produced motivation to change study habits (an example of growth) and resulted in positive or desired outcomes (high test scores).

When stressors evoke an ineffective response, **distress** is experienced. For example, consider students who have an examination scheduled for the next day. They had plenty of time to study, but because they put it off until the last minute, they take the examination unprepared. As a result of "cramming" all night, they are not alert, do not know the material, and fail the examination; they are experiencing distress.

ADAPTATION

Adaptation is an ongoing process whereby individuals use various responses to adjust to stressors and change. The nurse's goal is to identify and support the client's positive adaptive responses. Adaptation is a holistic response that involves all dimensions of an individual. Individuals, as holistic beings, seek to maintain a steady state in all dimensions of life: physiologic, psychological, cognitive, social, and spiritual. Wellness is an adaptive state; that is, the well person is one who is coping effectively with stressors and thus maintains a high level of well-being. Adaptation may be physiologic, psychological, cognitive, social, or spiritual.

Physiologic adaptation is the way the body responds to stressors affecting the functioning of the body. It may involve the entire body or only a specific area. An individual who lives in the mountains (high elevation) produces more red blood cells to carry enough oxygen to meet the body's needs. The chest also enlarges to allow the lungs to expand to accommodate the needed exchange of oxygen and carbon dioxide.

Psychological adaptation involves the use of defense mechanisms and learning to mentally accept new situations. A person's hardiness includes a sense of commitment, challenge, and control (Kobasa, 1979). A 55-year-old worker who suddenly finds himself unemployed will need to learn to adapt psychologically to the new situation and decide which steps to take next.

Cognitive adaptation involves education, communication, problem-solving ability, and perception of people and the world. A person gains these methods of adaptation as development occurs throughout life. For example, the high-school student will have a different perspective of the world and different problem-solving abilities than will this same individual as a college graduate, due to development and maturity.

Social adaptation involves social relationships with family, friends, and coworkers who may provide support in times of stress. A person unable to cope may withdraw socially. An example of social adaptation

LIFE CYCLE CONSIDERATIONS

Coping Ability
An individual's ability to cope with stressors will depend in part upon age and developmental level.

would be a couple moving to a new town and making new friends and modifying relationships with existing friends.

Spiritual adaptation involves beliefs about a supreme being and a positive sense of life's purpose and meaning. These beliefs are a personal resource for coping with stressors. Following the loss of a loved one, for instance, a family's spirituality and sense of faith may undergo changes.

Coping Measures

Coping measures include all the ways an individual may react to stress. Stress is an automatic response, but individuals can learn to conserve their adaptive energy through conditioning. **Conditioning** occurs when a person is taught a behavior until it becomes an automatic response. Some individuals who are conditioned to do so can handle a great deal of stress, whereas others cannot handle even a small amount of stress. Other factors that affect an individual's ability to cope with stress are the:

- Degree of danger perceived by the individual,
- Immediate needs of the individual,
- Amount of support from others,
- Individual's belief in his own ability to handle the stressful situation,
- Individual's previous successes and failures in coping, and
- Number of concurrent or cumulative stresses being handled by the individual (Waughfield, 1998).

Adaptive Measures

Measures for coping with stress that require a minimal amount of energy are called **adaptive measures** (Figure 16-2). They deal directly with the stressful

CULTURAL CONSIDERATIONS

Adaptive Measures
Nurses must be sensitive to the fact that culture and ethnicity may influence an individual's choice of coping mechanisms. For instance, moaning and chanting may be an expected response to stress in some cultures; the nurse must be careful to view this behavior not as unhealthy, but as a culturally healthy response to a stressful stimulus.

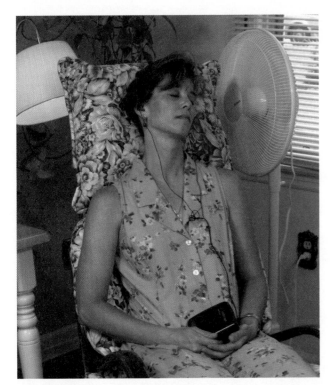

Figure 16-2 Listening to relaxation tapes is a way of coping with stress.

situation or the symptoms thereof. Adaptive measures useful in dealing with stressful situations include the following:

- Use of support people
- Relaxation to relieve tension
- Behavioral change
- Development of more realistic goals
- Problem solving

Defense Mechanisms

Just as the body has physiologic mechanisms (e.g., the immune system, the inflammatory response) to defend against infection and disease, the mind has psychological protective mechanisms. Most of these **defense mechanisms** are unconscious operations that protect the mind from anxiety. Defense mechanisms are employed to achieve and maintain psychological home-

PROFESSIONAL TIP

Defense Mechanisms

The nurse who is unfamiliar with defense mechanisms is likely to be judgmental about clients who do not respond according to the nurse's expectations. If, for example, the nurse tries to break through a client's denial (defense mechanism) too quickly by presenting reality, the client may be overwhelmed by anxiety and will panic.

ostasis, and in many cases, the individual does not consciously decide to use a defense mechanism, but, rather, it will automatically activate.

Defense mechanisms are universal. Their use does not indicate psychosocial imbalance or mental illness. Defense mechanisms are considered to be maladaptive when they become a stereotyped pattern, that is, the only way that an individual responds to a threat. Defense mechanisms are also considered to be maladaptive when they limit the individual's ability to function. Table 16–2 describes and gives examples of various defense mechanisms.

Maladaptive Measures

Measures used to avoid conflict and stress are considered **maladaptive measures**, because they prevent the individual from making progress towards resolving and accepting stress. They may include somatic disorders (transferring stress to an organ, as in an ulcer), rituals, excessive use of alcohol or drugs, excessive eating, or withdrawal from reality.

Crisis

When stressors exceed a person's ability to cope, a crisis occurs. A **crisis** (an acute state of disorganization) occurs when the individual's usual coping mechanisms are no longer effective. Crisis is characterized by extreme anxiety, inability to function, and disorganized behavior. A crisis is time limited; that is, no one can remain in acute disequilibrium for a long period of time because of the degree of discomfort that is experienced. Given the time-limited nature of crisis, a client experiencing a crisis needs immediate intervention to reach a successful resolution. Crisis intervention is discussed later in this chapter.

Crisis can be a negative experience, but it can also present an opportunity for growth and learning. The outcome is unique to each individual's perception and coping abilities. Nurses are challenged to help clients discover the opportunities in their crises, to adapt in positive, healthy manners.

Not every person will experience a crisis as a result of stressful events. Each crisis is unique to the individual; however, some characteristics are common to all crises (Table 16–3). A crisis is *not* a mental illness, even though it is not uncommon for persons experiencing the acute discomfort and anxiety of crisis to fear for their sanity.

ANXIETY

Anxiety is a subjective response that occurs when a person experiences a real or perceived threat to well-being; it is a diverse feeling of dread or apprehension. There is a close relationship between anxiety and stress. Anxiety is the psychological response to a threat, such as the worry that results when an individual oversleeps on a work day. This worry can translate

Table 16–2 DEFENSE MECHANISMS

DEFENSE MECHANISM	DESCRIPTION	EXAMPLE
Denial	Refusal to acknowledge the reality of threatening situations despite factual evidence	A person with heart disease continues to eat fatty foods and fried foods, despite medical advice to the contrary.
Displacement	Transfer of feelings or reactions from one object to another object, usually one that is "safer"	A husband who is angry with his wife yells at the dog instead of dealing with his anger at his wife.
Projection	Attribution of one's own thoughts, feelings, or impulses to others	An adolescent who does not want to go with the crowd states, "My parents won't let me go."
Rationalization	Intellectual explanation or justification of ideas, feelings, or behavior	A student responds after failing a test that "The test had many trick questions on it; I really know the material."
Reaction formation	Expression of a feeling that is the opposite of one's real feeling	A client brings a gift to a nurse with whom he is really angry.
Regression	A return to a previous developmental level	A child who has not sucked her thumb in 2 years starts to do so again when admitted to the hospital.
Repression	The unconscious blocking from awareness of material that is painful or threatening	Adult's claim, despite evidence, that "I never got angry with my parents; we lived in love and harmony."
Suppression	A conscious or unconscious attempt to keep threatening or unpleasant material out of consciousness	Failure to remember a house fire during childhood.
Sublimation	Channeling of socially unacceptable impulses into socially acceptable activities	A young man who deals with aggression by playing football.

Adapted from Psychiatric Mental Health Nursing, *by N. Frisch and L. Frisch, 1998, Albany, NY: Delmar. Copyright 1998 by Delmar.*

into stress, or the person's physiologic response to a stimulus, such as rushing, perspiring, and becoming careless. Anxiety can be both an activator of stress and a response to stress: It is usually activated by stress and may, in and of itself, lead to more stress. Anxiety is a major component of mental health disturbances.

Anxiety is the most common emotional (affective) response to stress. Individuals feel anxious whenever they are threatened, even if the threat is perceived rather than actual. Anxiety occurs on a continuum; some degree of anxiety is necessary, because it serves as a motivator for adaptation. A high level of anxiety, however, can overwhelm a person and impair the ability to think and function. As the severity of anxiety increases, the person is less and less able to function (Figure 16-3). Table 16–4 describes the levels of anxiety.

Table 16–3 CHARACTERISTICS OF CRISIS

- Loss is a component of every crisis. The loss can be actual or perceived and can be related to any significant aspect of the person's life.
- A crisis is experienced as a sudden event.
- A crisis has an identifiable precipitating event.
- The situation is perceived as overwhelming or life threatening.
- Communication becomes impaired.
- The situation cannot be resolved with usual coping skills.
- Intervention is required for equilibrium to be reestablished.

Data from Psychiatric Nursing *(5th ed.), by H. S. Wilson and C. R. Kneisel, 1996, Menlo Park, CA: Addison-Wesley. Copyright 1996 by Addison-Wesley.*

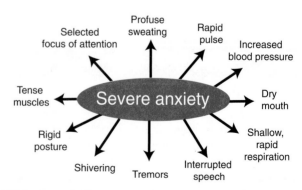

Figure 16-3 Physical and Mental Responses to Severe Anxiety (*From* Mental Health Concepts, *by C. Waughfield, 1998, Albany, NY: Delmar. Copyright 1998 by Delmar.*)

Table 16–4 LEVELS OF ANXIETY

ANXIETY LEVEL	CHARACTERISTICS OF THE ANXIOUS PERSON	NURSING IMPLICATIONS
Mild	• Increased degree of alertness • Increased vigilance • Increased motivation • Readiness for action • Slight increase in vital signs	• This is an optimal time for client teaching, because of heightened awareness and increased perceptual field.
Moderate	• Subjective distress (tension) • Decreased perception and attention • Alert only to specific information • Possible tendency to complain or argue • Possible headache, diarrhea, nausea, or vomiting	• Help the client to determine a cause-and-effect relationship between stressor and anxiety.
Severe	• Increased subjective distress • Feeling of impending danger • Selective attention • Distorted communication • Distorted perception • Feelings of fatigue	• Encourage verbalization. • Encourage motor activity. • Give specific directions.
Panic	• Major perceptual distortion • Immobilization; inability to function • Feelings of terror • Possible harm to self and others	• Provide limits and structure. • Maintain client safety (both physical and psychological).

Data from Interpersonal Relations in Nursing, *by H. E. Peplau, 1952, New York: Putnam. Copyright 1952 by Putnam. And* The Interpersonal Theory of Psychiatry, *by H. S. Sullivan, 1953, New York: Norton. Copyright 1953 by Norton.*

EFFECTS OF ILLNESS

Everyone experiences stress and accompanying anxiety. Anxiety increases during illness and the recovery process. Illness and stress are interwoven to such a degree that it is difficult to determine which precedes the other. When a person's adaptive attempts are unsuccessful, illness occurs. Also, a person who is ill has fewer adaptive resources available to cope with stressors. Even though some stressors may not directly cause illness, stress is a significant component in the onset and progression of many diseases. Table 16–5 lists some disorders commonly associated with stress.

One of the major outcomes of prolonged periods of stress is impairment of the immune system. As the body continues to fight off the actual or perceived threat, steroid production increases. Steroids impair the immune system's ability to function adequately. Thus, the body is less able to protect itself from disease. For example, consider the client recovering from the stress of surgery. Stress affects metabolism and protein synthesis and, thus, can result in inadequate wound healing.

All clients entering the health care system for hospitalization, surgery, or long-term care experience a change in their usual routine. Such changes may evoke anxiety, which can lead to stress.

Being in an unfamiliar environment, losing control over one's schedule, and being dependent on others for care are all issues with which hospitalized or institutionalized clients must cope. Each of these issues is a stressor that requires adaptation on the part of the client in order to maintain a steady state. Most clients

 COMMUNITY/HOME HEALTH CARE

Reducing Stressors

Remember, as a home health or visitng nurse, you are a guest in the client's home. If changes must be made in the home or the way it is kept, provide suggestions that are directly related to the client or the care of the client. Never criticize the home itself or the way it is kept.

Table 16–5 STRESS-RELATED DISORDERS

Respiratory disorders	• Emphysema • Chronic bronchitis • Asthma
Cardiovascular disorders	• Hypertension • Cardiac arrhythmias • Migraine headaches
Endocrine disorders	• Thyroid problems • Amenorrhea, anovulation • Diabetes • Excessive weight gain or weight loss
Musculoskeletal disorders	• Chronic back pain • Arthritis
Genitourinary disorders	• Enuresis • Urinary frequency
Sexual and reproductive disorders	• Low libido • Impotence • Menstrual irregularities
Gastrointestinal disorders	• Colitis • Chronic constipation • Ulcers • Gastritis
Integumentary disorders	• Eczema • Hives • Psoriasis

From Fundamentals of Nursing: Standards & Practice, *by S. DeLaune and P. Ladner, 1998, Albany, NY: Delmar. Copyright 1998 by Delmar.*

do not have the energy to cope with the numerous changes simultaneously with coping with their illnesses. Some cues that a person may be reacting adversely to hospitalization include the following:

• Increased stress response
• Increased level of anxiety
• Increased or impaired use of coping mechanisms
• Inability to function
• Disorganized behavior

Individuals do not have to be hospitalized to experience stressors associated with the client role. Consider for example the person having "minor" surgery at an outpatient center, the employee being treated at the industrial clinic for a work-related injury, or the adolescent being treated by the school nurse. Even clients who are treated through home health agencies experience stressors associated with having a health care provider enter their personal environment.

The greater the threat (or perceived threat), the greater the level of the client's anxiety. The nurse must be sensitive to stress and anxiety stemming from the multiple changes imposed by illness on the client, family, and/or significant others. The nurse's sensitivity to a client's stress reduces the risk of depersonalizing the client.

Depersonalization describes the process whereby an individual is treated as an object instead of a person. Literally, it involves taking away a client's unique aspects by treating him as nonhuman. Nursing interventions should focus on helping the client reduce feelings of unfamiliarity and loss of control.

EFFECTS OF CHANGE

Change, a dynamic process whereby an individual's response to a stressor leads to an alteration in be-

PROFESSIONAL TIP

Promoting Client Control

• *Communicate clearly.* Use terms easily understood by clients and families. Avoid using medical jargon with clients.
• *Answer questions thoroughly.* Validate the client's and family's level of understanding.
• *Teach the use of relaxation techniques,* such as progressive muscle relaxation and guided imagery.
• *Instruct clients in the use of* **cognitive reframing** (a technique whereby the individual changes a negative perception of a situation or event to a more positive, less-threatening perception.)
• *Provide support and reassurance.* The nurse's presence ("being with" the client) can alleviate anxiety. The most therapeutic tool in alleviating client anxiety is the nurse's therapeutic use of self (Figure 16-4).
• *Break down the information shared with clients.* Providing too much information at one time can overwhelm the client, making him less likely to listen. When clients have adequate information, they can make informed decisions and maintain some degree of control over their lives.

From Fundamentals of Nursing: Standards & Practice, *by S. DeLaune and P. Ladner, 1998, Albany, NY: Delmar. Copyright 1998 by Delmar.*

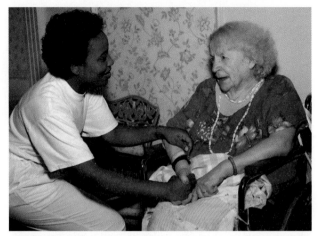

Figure 16-4 Through talking, listening, and touch, the nurse can help relieve the client's feelings of anxiety.

havior, is an inherent part of life; it is the process whereby individuals adapt. Whether it is planned or unplanned, change is both inevitable and constant. Change can be constructive or destructive and is stressful to individuals because it activates the GAS. Characteristics of change are that it:

- Is an inevitable part of life,
- May be eustressful or distressful,
- Can be self-initiated or externally imposed,
- Can occur abruptly or have a gradual onset and insidious progression, and
- Requires energy to effect, as well as to resist.

Nurses, and all health care providers, must be able to initiate and cope with change. Proficiency in critical-thinking and problem-solving skills is necessary for effectively initiating and coping with change.

The pace of change is rapidly increasing in health care agencies, which have been changing and continue to change in response to consumer demands. The following changes have evolved from consumer demands and needs:

- Self-care units
- Abortion clinics
- Sports medicine clinics
- Substance-abuse treatment programs
- Day treatment programs for geriatric and psychiatric clients
- Weight control programs
- Exercise programs

Types of Change

Change is either planned or unplanned. Unplanned change is change that "just happens"; it is unpredictable and may be imposed by others or by uncon-

trollable natural events (e.g., losing one's home in a flood). Conversely, planned change results from a deliberate effort to alter a situation. A marriage is an example of a planned change. In addition to planned change and unplanned change, there are other types of change.

Developmental changes are physical and emotional alterations that occur at different stages of the life cycle. These are generally predictable and occur in a certain progression. For instance, a baby will first learn to roll over, then crawl, then walk. Whereas the exact age for each of these milestones will vary, the sequence generally does not: The majority of infants will crawl before they are able to walk.

Accidental or reactive changes are adaptive responses to external stimuli. These include an individual's efforts to cope with change imposed by others, such as a modification to one's working hours or reaction to a child's baseball game being rescheduled due to the weather.

Covert changes are often subtle and occur without a person's conscious awareness. These might include a gradual shifting of responsibilities as new skills are acquired or developed at work.

Overt changes are obvious and identifiable, and an individual is aware that they are occurring. Although overt changes are usually not under an individual's direct control, such as the restructuring of one's place of employment, the individual must adapt to and accept the new situation in order to continue functioning effectively.

Resistance to Change

Many people tend to resist change because of the energy required to adapt. Conversely, energy is also required to resist change, or to maintain the status quo. Individuals differ in their ability to tolerate (or even thrive on) change.

People tend to resist change for many reasons (Table 16–6). In particular, there are no absolute guarantees that the change will lead to a positive outcome. Uncertainty regarding outcome is a major barrier to change.

It is risky to initiate change, to challenge one's own ideas and those of others. One of the first signs of the need for change is questioning. The nurse who wonders "Why?" "Why not?" or "What if?" is the nurse who will likely take the risk to initiate change activity. The risk taker who is effective is neither reckless nor overly cautious. Successful risk takers "weigh the costs and benefits of their actions. They consider possible outcomes in relationship to the expenditure of available resources" (Talbott, 1993).

Because change is inevitable, nurses must learn ways to deal with change. Resistance manifests as the individual rejecting proposed new ideas without criti-

Table 16–6 BARRIERS TO CHANGE

BARRIER	EXPLANATION
Conformity	Often referred to as "groupthink"; complying with the group's expectations; going along with others to avoid conflict.
Dissimilar beliefs and values	Differences in attitudes and expectations regarding health and illness behaviors; differences between client and nurse that can impede positive change.
Habits	Routine, "set" behaviors are often hard to change.
Satisfaction with status quo	Seeing only advantages to the present system can blind one to the possible need for change. Satisfaction with the way things are now reinforces resistance to change.
Threats to satisfying basic needs	Change may be perceived as a threat to self-esteem, security, or survival.
Fear	Fear of failure and fear of the unknown especially block change.
Unrealistic goals	Set up the individual for failure in change efforts.

From Fundamentals of Nursing: Standards & Practice, *by S. DeLaune and P. Ladner, 1998, Albany, NY: Delmar. Copyright 1998 by Delmar.*

cally thinking about the proposal. Nurses must be willing to take the time to research ideas and make informed decisions as to whether change is worthwhile. Coping with change of any type calls for flexibility, adaptability, and resilience.

The Nurse as Change Agent

Nurses are greatly affected by change. Nurses experience stress daily as a result of changes both within their immediate work environments and in the health care delivery system as a whole. The uncertainty over health care reform is very distressful to some nurses. Others, those with an eustressful outlook, see opportunity for positive change in the future.

In bringing about change to promote positive adaptation, the nurse serves as a **change agent** (a person who intentionally creates and implements change). True change agents constantly seek ways to make improvements. They use critical-thinking skills to develop creative, innovative solutions.

To be most effective, change should be planned and goal directed by people who are proactive. Proactive individuals initiate change rather than respond to change imposed by others. The proactive individual takes action rather than waiting for others to make decisions, solve problems, or become rescuers. On the other hand, a reactive person responds only to externally imposed change. Proactive nurses are change agents who affect the entire health care system as well as individual clients.

Change agents keep the change process moving toward a positive outcome. As an advocate for change, the nurse empowers the client to initiate change in order to adapt more successfully. Client education is a powerful tool for initiating change. Teaching a client about a disease process, a treatment modality, or a lifestyle alteration provides the client with an opportunity to change. Learning results in behavioral changes. The change process is similar to the nursing process, in that change involves assessment, planning, decision making, implementation, and evaluation.

NURSING PROCESS

Nurses can be very instrumental in helping clients both understand their anxiety and learn measures to cope with and control their feelings of stress.

Assessment

When caring for an anxious client, the nurse must first ascertain the client's perception of the situation. This is accomplished by directly asking for the client's input. The nurse must then carefully listen to the client's response. Because the nurse's nonverbal behavior can affect the client's anxiety level, nurses must be aware of their own body language. Because anxiety is a subjective experience, it cannot be directly observed. Therefore, the nurse must look for the signs indicative of anxiety (refer back to Table 16–4).

A thorough assessment of stress and anxiety levels includes eliciting client input to evaluate the following factors:

- Patterns of stressors
- Typical responses to stressful situations
- Cause-and-effect relationships among stressors and thoughts, feelings, and behaviors
- Past history of successful coping mechanisms

Assessing the client's coping abilities can be done in various ways. For example, open-ended questions can be used to determine previously used coping mechanisms. Some sample questions are:

- What is the problem?
- What have you tried before?
- How well did it work?

Identifying the client's coping abilities assists in establishing appropriate nursing diagnoses and developing an effective plan of care. Assessment, which relies heavily on the nurse's observation and listening skills, provides the data necessary for formulating nursing diagnoses.

Nursing Diagnosis

Several nursing diagnoses may apply to clients experiencing anxiety; the most common of these are *anxiety; coping, ineffective individual; denial, ineffective;* and *powerlessness.* Additional North American Nursing Diagnosis Association (NANDA, 2001) diagnoses that may occur in response to stressors include:

- *Impaired Adjustment*
- *Ineffective Role Performance*
- *Disturbed Thought Processes*
- *Defensive Coping*
- *Fear*
- *Post-Trauma Syndrome*
- *Impaired Social Interaction*
- *Spiritual Distress*
- *Hopelessness*
- *Fatigue*
- *Disturbed Sleep Pattern*

Planning/Outcome Identification

Client involvement in planning care is essential because helping clients learn to cope successfully is part of the empowerment process. Planning means exploring with the client self-responsibility issues. A major goal for intervening with an anxious client is to reduce anxiety to a level at which learning and problem solving can occur.

Expected outcomes (goals) appropriate for clients experiencing stress or anxiety may be numerous. A good starting point is to assist the client to:

- Identify situations that increase stress and anxiety levels;
- Verbalize a plan to decrease the effects of common stressors;
- Differentiate positive and negative stressors in the client's life;
- Classify stressors into the following categories: those that can be eliminated, those that can be controlled, and those that cannot be controlled directly by self;
- Demonstrate the accurate use of select stress-management exercises (e.g., progressive muscle relaxation, guided imagery, thought stopping); and
- Verbalize a plan for stress management, including necessary lifestyle modifications.

 Safety: The Client Experiencing Panic
Never leave a panic-stricken client alone. When anxiety has reached the panic level, the client may inflict self-harm. Stay with the highly anxious client or have someone else do so.

Nursing Interventions

Teaching, a major nursing intervention for managing stress, is inherent in holistic nursing practice. Stress management approaches can be taught to clients of every age and developmental stage in all health care settings: acute care (inpatient and outpatient), long-term care, and the home.

Teaching clients to reduce their own levels of stress is a major step in promoting self-care. Client education provides clients with options. Clients who have a thorough understanding of their options can make informed decisions about necessary lifestyle changes (Figure 16-5). Some of the many interventions that can be used with anxious clients follow.

Meeting Basic Needs

There is a close relationship between stress and basic physiologic needs. Anything that interferes with the satisfaction of basic needs evokes the stress response and attendant anxiety. Clients who are cold, hungry, or in pain have higher anxiety levels than do those who are comfortable. When anxiety levels increase, so does the perception of pain. Nurses who empower clients to meet basic needs are laying the foundation for a less stressful, more caring treatment process. By reducing anxiety, the nurse is actually improving the client's potential for recovery.

Minimizing Environmental Stimuli

An individual's immediate environment can influence stress levels. It is important for the nurse to decrease environmental stimuli that may contribute to anxiety. Some specific ways to limit environmental stimuli are to:

- Close the door to the client's room;
- Turn off the television;
- Lower the tone of the telephone ringer or take the phone off the hook, if feasible;
- Turn off the lights or close the blinds; and
- Limit the number of visitors (unless isolation increases the client's anxiety).

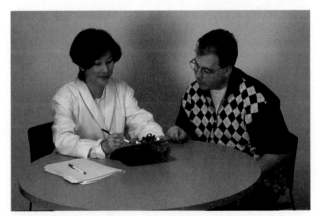

Figure 16-5 ▶ The nurse discusses the options for care and provides the client with the information needed to plan effective lifestyle changes.

Verbalizing Feelings

Encouraging clients to express their feelings is especially valuable in stress reduction. Freud (1959) used the term **catharsis** to describe the process of talking out one's feelings. People instinctively know the value of "getting things off their chest" through verbalization. Verbalization promotes relaxation because: (1) when a feeling is described it becomes real, and after a problem is identified, the person can begin to deal effectively with it; and (2) the actual activity of talking uses energy and, therefore, reduces anxiety.

Involving Family and Significant Others

The client's developmental stage influences the type of intervention for stress management. Children and adolescents have varying coping skills; children of all ages need and rely on their parents or caretakers for security and support (Fennell, 1999). It is important to include the entire family in the care of the client whenever possible (Figure 16-6). Such an approach is useful in decreasing the stress level of everyone involved, because families provide essential support for clients.

Family members who are extremely anxious often have a negative impact on the client's health status. Therefore, nurses must often help family members relax. One way to accomplish this is to provide explanations and information. Thus, it is often necessary for nurses to teach stress-management techniques to the client's family. Researchers concluded that both the client and family benefit from family presence during invasive procedures and resuscitation (Meyers, Eichhorn, Gozzetta, Clark, Klein, Taliaferro, Calvin, 2000).

Using Stress-Management Techniques

A variety of stress-management techniques can easily be taught to clients, families, and significant others.

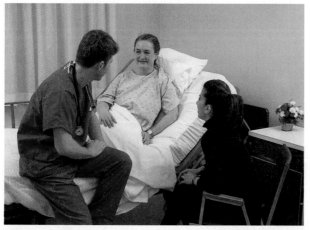

Figure 16-6 The nurse encourages interaction between clients and family members as well as significant others. This involvement helps ease the client's anxiety about issues such as hospitalization and serves as a method to keep the family informed about the client's care.

Some of the most common approaches for managing stress are discussed following.

Exercise   Physical exercise is a powerful way to reduce anxiety. Client teaching should emphasize the need for incorporating exercise into one's lifestyle. Guidelines for establishing an exercise program are:

- Explore the availability of different exercise programs,
- Consult with a health care provider about the safety of a specific exercise program,
- Set realistic goals,
- Plan a routine that allows for warm-up and cool-down periods using stretching exercises, and
- Engage in activities that increase heart rate for a period of time and are followed by a cool-down period.

In other words, if exercise is to reduce anxiety, it must be done on an ongoing and regular basis. The physiologic benefits of regular exercise are listed in Table 16–7. The psychological benefits of exercise include:

- Enhanced feelings of well-being,
- Improved concentration and memory,
- Reduced depression,
- Reduced insomnia,
- Reduced dependence on external stimulants or relaxants,
- Increased self-esteem, and
- Renewed sense of self-control over anxiety.

Relaxation Techniques   Several techniques can help individuals relax (Figure 16-7). Alternative and complementary interventions such as progressive muscle relaxation and guided imagery are useful in helping clients learn specific approaches to achieve relaxation. Meditation and hypnosis can also be very effective in inducing relaxation and relieving stress.

Cognitive Reframing or Thought Stopping
Cognitive reframing is a technique based on a theory

 CLIENT TEACHING

Thought Stopping: A Cognitive Reframing Technique

- Listen to self-talk (thoughts).
- Recognize when the self-talk is negative.
- When a negative thought is detected, do something physical to stop the train of thought. For example, clap your hands or snap a rubber band on your wrist. Tell yourself, "Stop!"
- Replace the negative thought with one that is both positive and realistic.

Like all other relaxation exercises, thought stopping becomes more effective with repetition.

Table 16–7 PHYSIOLOGICAL BENEFITS OF EXERCISE

EFFECT OF EXERCISE	PHYSIOLOGICAL BENEFIT
Promotes metabolism of adrenalin and thyroxine	• Minimizes autonomic arousal and hypervigilance
Reduces musculoskeletal tension	• Reduces feelings of being tense and "uptight"
Improves circulation, resulting in better oxygenation of the bloodstream and the brain	• Increases alertness and concentration, leading to enhanced problem-solving ability
Stimulates **endorphin** (a group of opiate-like substances produced naturally by the brain) production	• Raises the body's pain threshold, produces sedation and euphoria, and promotes a sense of well-being
Decreases cholesterol level	• Reduces the risk of atherosclerosis (a common form of arteriosclerosis characterized by the formation of plaque containing lipids, including cholesterol, on the inner walls of the arteries).
Decreases blood pressure	• Reduces risk of myocardial infarction (heart attack) and cerebral vascular accident (CVA) (stroke)
Increases acidity of blood (lowered pH)	• Improves digestion • Improves energy level • Improves utilization of food for energy (promotes metabolism)
Improves elimination (through lungs, skin, bowels)	• Reduces buildup of toxins in the body.

From "Nutrition, Exercise, and Movement," by L. Keegan, 1999, in B. Dossey, L. Keegan, & C. Guzzetta (Eds.), Holistic Nursing: A Handbook for Practice *(3rd ed.), Gaithersburg, MD: Aspen. Copyright 1999 by Aspen. And "Health Promotion and the Individual," by C. Mandle and R. Gruber-Wood, 1998, in C. Edelmen and C. Mandle (Eds.),* Health Promotion throughout the Lifespan *(4th ed.). St. Louis, MO: Mosby. Copyright 1998 by Mosby.*

proposed by Aaron Beck (1976), who purports that a person's emotional response is determined by the meaning attached to an event. For example, if an event is perceived to be threatening, the client is likely to feel anxious. If the interpretation of the event can be modified, the client will be less anxious. Reframing is a technique used to alter one's perceptions and interpretations by changing one's thoughts.

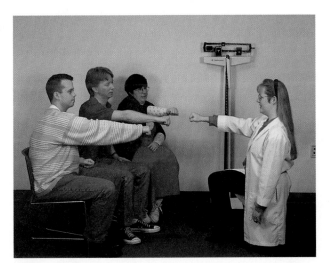

Figure 16-7 The nurse demonstrates the technique of progressive muscle relaxation in a client-education program.

Crisis Intervention

Some clients will be in an acute crisis state and require **crisis intervention**, a specific technique that helps clients regain equilibrium. Crisis intervention is a therapeutic strategy that views individuals as capable of personal growth and as having the ability to influence and control their own lives (Kneisl & Riley, 1996). The five steps of crisis intervention are illustrated in Figure 16-8).

Clients sometimes need more assistance than the nurse is able to provide. Recognition of such situations calls for prompt consultation with and, sometimes, referral to other health care providers, such as:

- Psychiatric clinical nurse specialists,
- Nurse psychotherapists,
- Psychologists,
- Social workers,
- Psychiatrists, or
- Clergy and other counselors.

Evaluation

Evaluating the effectiveness of the client's coping abilities is an ongoing, comprehensive process that must include client input. It is imperative that the nurse evaluate client outcomes as well as the process of delivering nursing care. The family can also be a

Identification of the Problem
It is necessary to be as specific as possible when naming the underlying issue(s). Being specific promotes clarity in planning.

Identification of Alternatives
Client and nurse need to list all the possible options for resolving the crisis. The greater the number of alternatives identified, the greater the likelihood of successful resolution.

Selection of an Alternative
The potential outcomes of each option are examined and one alternative is chosen.

Implementation
The selected alternative is carried out.

Evaluation
The overall effectiveness of the plan is evaluated in terms of process and outcome.

Figure 16-8 Steps of Crisis Intervention (*From* Fundamentals of Nursing: Standards & Practice, *by S. DeLaune and P. Ladner, 1998, Albany, NY: Delmar. Copyright 1998 by Delmar.*)

valuable source of information when evaluating the effectiveness of different stress-reduction approaches.

PERSONAL STRESS-MANAGEMENT APPROACHES FOR THE NURSE

Many stressors are inherent in nursing. Learning to cope successfully with stressors is essential for nurses (Figure 16-9). Two major reasons nurses must cope successfully with stress are to maintain their own wellness and to model health-promoting behaviors to others. In order to help clients learn to manage stress, nurses must first be able to manage their own stress.

High stress levels among nurses are associated with **burnout**, a state of physical and emotional exhaustion that occurs when caregivers deplete their adaptive energy. Nurses who have experienced such an overwhelming degree of stress tend to treat clients in depersonalizing ways. Such nurses also lack feelings

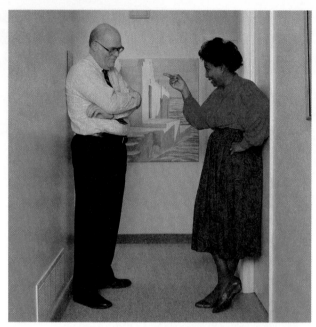

Figure 16-9 Sharing a light and humorous moment with a friend is a wonderful way to relieve stress and regain perspective.

of personal accomplishment. Burnout exacts a high price not only on individual nurses themselves, but also on the profession: Highly qualified professionals leave nursing and, as a result, the quality of care declines.

Several work-related factors can contribute to the development of nursing burnout:

- Job-related stress (for example, the stress evoked by caring for critically ill clients)
- Heavy workload
- Interpersonal conflict in the work environment
- Mandatory overtime and "floating" to other units

Burnout prevention and recovery depend on stress management. A stress-management plan is a continuous process, not the occasional use of a technique or exercise. Development of such a plan begins with self-awareness. The first step to changing nonconstructive or self-defeating practices is to become self-aware. Nurses who care for clients extremely well often fail to take care of themselves. It is essential that nurses learn to care for themselves as well.

Other guidelines that are helpful in changing from a negative to a positive outlook (DeLaune, 1993) include the following:

- Expect to be successful.
- Remember the power of self-fulfilling prophecies and deliberately focus on the positive.
- Let go of the need to be perfect.
- Listen to self-talk.
- Encourage the use of appropriate humor in the workplace.

Nurses can use many strategies to help manage professional and personal stress, as outlined in Table 16–8.

Nurses who cultivate the hardiness factor will likely be resilient to stress. Kobasa (1979) originated the concept of hardiness in the late 1970s. Hardiness consists of a set of attitudes, beliefs, and behaviors that result in individuals being more resilient (or hardy) to the negative effects of stress. There are three components to stress hardiness:

- *Commitment:* becoming involved in what one is doing
- *Challenge:* perceiving change as an opportunity for growth rather than as an obstacle or threat
- *Control:* believing that one is influential in directing what happens to oneself rather than feeling helpless and victimized

According to studies (Kobasa, 1979; Kobasa, Maddi, & Kahn, 1982), individuals who have higher degrees of hardiness are healthier than are individuals with low degrees of hardiness. Such people develop fewer illnesses when they experience multiple stressors.

Many nurses must relearn the value of play and learn when to stop working. Nursing students, who spend many hours a week working and studying, may need to schedule some time for play. By doing so, the student nurse will make a start on managing stress and, thereby, become a more effective care provider.

PROFESSIONAL TIP

Managing Professional Stress

- Develop and maintain active support systems, both at work and away from work. Having friends who are not health care providers helps maintain a sense of balance and separateness between personal and professional domains.
- Develop time-management and decision-making skills. For example, break large tasks down into small, realistic, achievable objectives. This strategy helps you avoid becoming overwhelmed by the seemingly "impossible" task before you.
- Avoid consumption of noxious substances. Practice a substance-free lifestyle to effectively manage stress. Do not depend on unhealthy behaviors such as smoking, overeating, or consuming alcohol or caffeine as avenues to relaxation.
- Nourish your body with a healthy diet and adequate amounts of sleep and rest balanced with activity and exercise. Care for yourself as you would care for your clients.
- Maintain a sense of humor while you work. Humor helps a person maintain a positive outlook; therefore, it can be used to reframe situations so as to reduce distress.

(*Adapted from* Fundamentals of Nursing: Standards & Practice *by S. DeLaune and P. Ladner, 1998, Albany, NY: Delmar. Copyright 1998 by Delmar. Adapted with permission.*)

Table 16–8 STRATEGIES FOR COPING WITH PROFESSIONAL STRESS

STRATEGY	RATIONALE
Using time management methods	When own needs are seen as priorities; you are more likely to schedule time to meet those needs. Time should especially be scheduled to meet highly valued needs.
Focusing on accomplishments instead of the uncompleted tasks	Focusing on unfinished business increases anxiety; paying attention to successes boosts self-esteem.
Practicing slow, focused breathing	Such breathing alleviates muscle tension by increasing the amount of oxygenated blood. Also, consciously thinking about own breathing serves as a diversionary tactic.
Avoiding assumption of responsibility where you have none	You will be less prone to play the role of rescuer who takes on the problems of others.
Knowing your limits	By clarifying your expectations, strengths, and limitations, you will learn to differentiate those things that are really important from the "small stuff" and know when a problem is beyond your control and find ways to accept the problem until you have the resources to deal with it.
Whenever possible, removing yourself from stressors that have a negative impact	Exposure to needless stress and subsequent draining of adaptive resources are minimized.
Identifying and changing the stressors that you can directly influence	Sense of personal power increases, and needless expenditure of energy decreases.
Varying tasks between physical and mental activities	You conserve energy, and the resultant reduction in fatigue helps restore a sense of balance.

Data from "Tips for Managing Stress on the Job," by J. Badger, 1995, AJN, 95(9), 31–33 and "Burnout: Why Do We Blame the Nurse?," by A. Cullen, 1995, AJN, 95(11), 23–27.

SAMPLE NURSING CARE PLAN

THE CLIENT EXPERIENCING ANXIETY

Kathryn is a 38-year-old female who is seeking treatment in the emergency department of a metropolitan hospital. She is tearful, pacing, and wringing her hands. She is complaining of severe chest pain, a pounding headache, and back pain. She is sweating profusely and exhibits fine hand tremors. Her blood pressure and pulse are elevated, and her respirations are rapid and shallow. She says that she hasn't slept well since her husband left her 3 months ago. She states, "I'm afraid I'm losing my mind! My heart is racing and I can't sit still. Help me! I feel like I'm going to die."

Assessment reveals autonomic hyperactivity (rapid pulse, elevated blood pressure), verbalized feelings of apprehension and uneasiness, and restlessness.

Nursing Diagnosis *Anxiety related to threat to self-concept and change in role functioning as evidenced by statement " I'm afraid I'm losing my mind" and the fact that husband left her 3 months ago*

PLANNING/GOALS	NURSING INTERVENTION	RATIONALE	EVALUATION
Kathryn will identify effective coping mechanisms.	Establish a trusting relationship.	Kathryn may perceive the nurse or emergency department as a threat, and, thus, anxiety will increase.	Kathryn is visibly relaxed. Vital signs are within normal limits. Kathryn verbalizes that she is calmer and no longer afraid that she is "losing her mind" or "going to die."
	Have Kathryn identify and describe physical and emotional feelings.	The first step in coping with anxiety is to recognize the anxiety and become aware of feelings in order to link emotions to maladaptive coping responses.	
	Help Kathryn relate cause-and-effect relationships between stressors and anxiety.	Increases Kathryn's sense of control and power over the situation.	
	Encourage Kathryn to use coping mechanisms that have been successful previously.	Increases confidence in own abilities to cope.	
Kathryn will report that anxiety is reduced to a manageable level.	Using therapeutic communication techniques, encourage Kathryn to talk about what has been happening in her life.	Talking about a situation often clarifies it.	

continues

| Kathryn will demonstrate relaxation skills. | Teach Kathryn relaxation techniques (such as imagery and meditation). | The relaxation response is the opposite of the stress response and, therefore, counters the physiologic effects of the stress response. The relaxation response leads to lowered blood pressure, decreased heart rate, and deeper and slower respirations. |

CASE STUDY

Miguel, a 35-year-old lawyer, comes to the emergency medical facility and describes vomiting small amounts of blood for the past several days. He also says that he has been having heartburn and epigastric pain for 3 weeks. The initial interview reveals that his wife asked for a divorce 6 weeks ago because of his long hours at work, which keep him away from the family. He also states that he is working on a very difficult lawsuit.

Vital signs are T 98.6, P 90, R 24, and BP 136/82. A complete blood count and upper GI exam are ordered. He is scheduled to see a clinical specialist to discuss the stressors in his life. At the initial screening, Miguel relates that he has been experiencing frequent headaches and is having difficulty concentrating on his court case, symptoms of moderate to severe anxiety.
(Adapted from Mental Health Concepts, *by C. Waughfield, 1998, Albany, NY: Delmar.)*

The following questions will guide your development of a nursing care plan for the case study.

1. What clinical manifestations indicate that Miguel is experiencing moderate to severe anxiety?
2. What two nursing diagnoses might be appropriate for Miguel?
3. What goal for each nursing diagnosis might be desirable?
4. What nursing interventions would be helpful to Miguel in meeting the goals?
5. How will the evaluation be determined?

SUMMARY

- Stress is an individual's physiologic response to stimuli.
- Individuals who experience prolonged periods of stress are at risk for developing stress-related diseases.
- Anxiety, the psychological response to a threat to the health and well-being of an individual, activates the stress response.
- An individual seeks equilibrium through the process of adaptation. When adaptation is effective, homeostasis (the body's self-regulation of physiologic processes) is maintained.
- Many factors, such as physiologic, psychological, cognitive, or environmental changes, contribute to stress.

- The general adaptation syndrome (GAS), the physiologic response to stress, consists of three stages: alarm, resistance, and exhaustion. The GAS is the same whether the stressor is actual or imagined, present or potential.
- Illness and hospitalization are major stressors for individuals and their families. To alleviate the stress of hospitalization, nursing interventions should reduce the client's feelings of unfamiliarity and loss of control.
- Change can be perceived as stressful because of a fear of failure, a threat to security, or a potential for loss of self-esteem.
- Nursing interventions that promote positive adaptation to stress are to empower clients to meet basic needs; minimize environmental stimuli; encourage verbalization of feelings; include family members

and significant others in client care; and use various stress-management techniques such as progressive muscle relaxation (PMR) and guided imagery.

- Burnout occurs when the nurse is overwhelmed by stress. As a result, the nurse experiences physical, emotional, and behavioral dysfunction, including decreased productivity.

- A stress-management plan for professional nurses involves maintaining support systems; developing time-management and decision-making skills; identifying and changing stressors that can be managed; and knowing personal limits.

Review Questions

1. Physiologic indicators of anxiety include:
   a. warm, dry skin.
   b. constricted pupils.
   c. increased pulse rate.
   d. decreased blood pressure.

2. The body's reaction to any demand made on it (stimulus) is called:
   a. stress.
   b. anxiety.
   c. stressor.
   d. stress response.

3. A major component of mental health disturbances is:
   a. worry.
   b. stress.
   c. anxiety.
   d. adaptation.

4. The general adaptation syndrome (GAS) is the:
   a. behavioral response to stress.
   b. sociocultural response to stress.
   c. psychological response to stress.
   d. physiologic response to stress.

5. The level of anxiety best for client learning is:
   a. no anxiety.
   b. mild anxiety.
   c. severe anxiety.
   d. moderate anxiety.

6. Most defense mechanisms are used unconsciously. The one that is consciously used is:
   a. projection.
   b. regression.
   c. repression.
   d. suppression.

7. The purpose of the first stage of the GAS is to:
   a. alert the individual to danger.
   b. determine the cause of the danger.

   c. mobilize energy needed for adaptation.
   d. prevent the individual from having an unpleasant experience.

8. Symptoms associated with the response to stress are the result of the body's attempt to:
   a. conserve energy.
   b. run from the impending threat.
   c. identify the impending danger.
   d. shield the person from an unpleasant experience.

9. Coping mechanisms to avoid dealing directly with stress are called:
   a. adaptive measures.
   b. maladaptive measures.
   c. nonadaptive measures.
   d. progressive measures.

Critical Thinking Questions

1. Describe the way that you would explain the relationship between stress and illness to a client.

2. A client is exhibiting panic-level anxiety, and you do not want him left alone. You are experiencing severe burnout because of very long work hours and stressful situations that have recently occurred with clients and with other nurses. Your stress level is so high that you feel you cannot even be in the same room with this upset client. If you leave the room to find another nurse to stay with him, he may injure himself; if you stay, you risk your own emotional well-being. How do you deal with this situation?

3. Society often labels people who take care of themselves as selfish. Do you agree? Why or why not? Consider how taking care of yourself can help you be a better care provider to others. What are some specific things you can do now to take better care of yourself?

⚡ WEB FLASH!

- Search the web for information on stress and anxiety. What sites might you recommend to clients and families who are experiencing anxiety and looking for self-help and information sources?
- What resources are listed for caregivers and health care professionals?
- What organizations or professional journals might you search for information on anxiety or stress?

LOSS, GRIEF, AND DEATH

MAKING THE CONNECTION

Refer to the following chapters to increase your understanding of loss, grief, and death:

- **Chapter 6, Legal Responsibilities**
- **Chapter 7, Ethical Responsibilities**
- **Chapter 12, Cultural Diversity and Nursing**
- **Chapter 13, Complementary/Alternative Therapies**
- **Chapter 29, Rehabilitation, Home Health, Long-Term Care, and Hospice**

LEARNING OBJECTIVES

Upon completion of this chapter, you should be able to:
- *Define key terms.*
- *Describe various losses that affect individuals at different stages of the life cycle.*
- *Describe the characteristics of an individual experiencing grief.*
- *Differentiate adaptive grief and pathological grief.*
- *Discuss theoretical perspectives of loss, grief, and death.*
- *Discuss use of the nursing process with a grieving individual.*
- *Discuss the holistic needs of the dying person and his family.*
- *Define the purpose of hospice care.*
- *Develop a plan of care for a dying client.*
- *Discuss nursing responsibilities when a client dies.*
- *Describe ways that nurses can cope with their own grief.*

KEY TERMS

algor mortis	hospice
anticipatory grief	life review
autopsy	liver mortis
bereavement	loss
breakthrough pain	maturational loss
Cheyne-Stokes respirations	mortuary
complicated grief	mourning
death rattle	palliative care
disenfranchised grief	post-mortem care
dysfunctional grief	resuscitation
grief	rigor mortis
grief work	shroud
Health Care Surrogate Law	situational loss
	uncomplicated grief

INTRODUCTION

In contemporary society, individuals constantly experience loss. Frequent episodes of terrorism, natural disaster, and personal crises result in the universal experience of loss. It can be overwhelming to think about real and potential losses. Nurses must be aware of the potential for loss in today's world, as well as the processes whereby individuals react and adapt to losses.

Throughout the life cycle, people are faced with loss, without which growth would not continue. Many people consider loss only in terms of death and dying; however, loss of every type occurs daily.

Every day, nurses encounter clients who are responding to grief associated with losses. Nurses must have an understanding of the major concepts related to loss and grieving. Grief is a response to losses of all types. However, this chapter focuses on grief as a response to death. Nurses also care for dying clients. Thus, this chapter also provides information on meeting the special needs of terminally ill clients and their families.

LOSS

Loss is any situation, either actual, potential, or perceived, wherein a valued object or person is changed or is no longer accessible to the individual. Because change is a major constant in life, everyone experiences losses. Loss can be actual (e.g., a spouse is lost through divorce) or anticipated (a person is diagnosed with a terminal illness and has only a short time to live). A loss can be tangible or intangible. For example, when a person is fired from a job, the tangible loss is income, whereas the loss of self-esteem is intangible.

Losses also occur as a result of moving from one developmental stage to another. An example of such a **maturational loss** is the adolescent who loses the younger child's freedom from responsibility. Other examples of losses associated with growth and development are discussed later in this chapter. A **situational loss** occurs in response to external events usually beyond the individual's control (such as the death of a significant other).

Types of Loss

Not everyone responds to loss in the same way because the significance of the lost object or person is determined by individual perceptions. There are many types of loss, including:

- *Actual loss:* loss of someone or something, such as the death of a loved one or the theft of one's property.
- *Perceived loss:* sense of loss felt by an individual but not tangible to others, such as the perceived loss of self-esteem of a student who was not accepted into a nursing program.
- *Physical loss:* loss of a part or aspect of the body, such as the loss of an extremity in an accident, scarring from burns, or permanent injury.
- *Psychological loss:* emotional loss, such as a woman feeling inadequate after menopause and resultant infertility.

There are four major categories of loss: loss of external objects, loss of familiar environment, loss of aspects of self, and loss of significant other.

Loss of an External Object

When an object that a person highly values is damaged or changed or disappears, loss occurs. The significance of the lost object to the individual determines the type and amount of grieving that occurs. For instance, an individual who loses a family heirloom in a fire may react not only to the lost financial value of the piece, but also to the lost sense of history and heritage that the piece represented.

Loss of Familiar Environment

The loss of a familiar environment occurs when a person moves away from familiar surroundings, for instance to another home or a different community, to a new school, or to a new job. A client who is hospitalized or institutionalized may also experience loss when faced with new surroundings. This type of loss evokes anxiety related to fear of the unknown.

Loss of Aspect of Self

Loss of an aspect of self can be psychological or physiological. Examples of psychological aspects of self that may be lost include ambition, a sense of humor, or enjoyment of life. These feelings of loss may result from life events such as losing a job or failing at a task that the individual deems important. Physiological loss includes loss of physical function or loss resulting from disfigurement or disappearance of a body part, as is the case with amputation or mastectomy. Loss of a physiological aspect of self can result from illness, trauma, or treatment methodologies such as surgery.

Loss of Significant Other

The loss of a loved one is a significant loss. Such a loss can result from separation, divorce, running away, moving to a different area, or death. This chapter focuses on the loss of a significant other as a result of death.

GRIEF

Grief, a series of intense physical and psychological responses that occur following a loss, is a normal, natural, necessary, and adaptive response to a loss. Loss leads to the adaptive process of **mourning**, the period of time during which grief is expressed and resolution and integration of the loss occur. **Bereavement** is the period of grief following the death of a loved one (Figure 17-1).

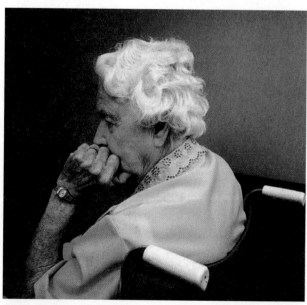

Figure 17-1 Older adults may grieve intensely over the loss of a person or situation that has been a part of their life for many years.

Theories of the Grieving Process

Several theoretical models describe grieving. The theories of Erich Lindemann, George L. Engle, John Bowlby, and J. William Worden are discussed in the following sections.

Lindemann

Following the Coconut Grove fire in Boston in 1944, Lindemann studied survivors and their families. Lindemann coined the phrase **grief work**, which is still used today to describe the process experienced by the bereaved. During grief work, the person experiences freedom from attachment to the deceased, becomes reoriented to the environment where the deceased is no longer present, and establishes new relationships (Lindemann, 1944). Lindemann's classic work is the basis of current crisis and grief resolution theories. Lindemann (1944) and Roach and Nieto (1997) describe Lindemann's theory of a person's reactions to normal grief as:

- *Somatic distress:* The bereaved experience episodic waves of discomfort in durations of 10 to 60 minutes; multiple somatic complaints; fatigue; and extreme physical or emotional pain.
- *Preoccupation with the image of the deceased:* The bereaved experience a sense of unreality, emotional detachment from others, and an overwhelming preoccupation with visualizing the deceased.
- *Guilt:* The bereaved consider the death to be a result of their own negligence or lack of attentiveness; they look for evidence of how they could have contributed to the death.
- *Hostile reactions:* The bereaved's relationships with others become impaired owing to the bereaved's desire to be left alone and the bereaved's feelings of irritability and anger.
- *Loss of patterns of conduct:* The bereaved exhibit generalized restlessness and an inability to sit still; they continually search for something to do.

Engle

Grief is a typical reaction to loss of a valued object. According to Engle, there are three stages of mourning, and progression through each stage is necessary for healing. The grieving process, which may take several years to complete, cannot be accelerated. The goal of the grieving process is for the mourner to accept the loss and let go of the deceased. Engle (1961, 1964) and Roach and Nieto (1997) outline Engle's theory of grief as follows:

- *Stage I: Shock and Disbelief* (can last from minutes to days)
  Disorientation
  Feeling of helplessness

  Denial, which provides protection until the person is able to face reality

- *Stage II: Developing Awareness* (may last from 6 to 12 months)
  Guilt
  Sadness
  Isolation
  Loneliness
  Feelings of helplessness
  Possible anger and hostility toward others
  Increasing emotional pain in response to increasing reality of loss
  Recognition that one is powerless to change the situation

- *Stage III: Restitution and Resolution* (marks the beginning of the healing process; may take up to several years)
  Emergence of bodily symptoms
  Possible idealization of the deceased
  Beginnings of coming to terms with the loss
  Establishment of new social patterns and relationships

Bowlby

According to Bowlby, grief results when an individual experiences a disruption in attachment to a love object. His theory proposes that grief occurs when attachment bonds are severed. The four phases of grieving as cited by Bowlby are:

- Numbness,
- Yearning and searching,
- Disorganization and despair, and
- Reorganization (Bowlby, 1982)

Worden

Worden has identified four tasks that an individual must perform in order to successfully deal with a loss:

- Accept the fact that the loss is real
- Experience the emotional pain of grief
- Adjust to an environment without the deceased
- Reinvest the emotional energy once directed at the deceased into another relationship (Worden, 1991)

Types of Grief

Grief is a universal, normal response to loss. Grief drains people, both emotionally and physically. Because grief requires so much emotional energy, relationships may suffer (Wong, 1996). There are different types of grief, including uncomplicated ("normal"), dysfunctional, anticipatory, and disenfranchised grief.

Nurses play an important role in assisting mourners to develop and understand the normal grieving process and the complex feelings exhibited when grief becomes more complicated. Nurses with a sound knowledge base of both normal grief and dysfunctional grief are better prepared to assist survivors than are nurses who mistakenly believe that all grief is the same.

Uncomplicated Grief

Uncomplicated grief is what many individuals would refer to as *normal grief*. Engle (1961) states that the grief reaction is similar to other physical conditions and draws a parallel between a disease process and the grief process. Both include:

- A common etiologic factor (e.g., loss precipitates grief),
- A predictable symptomatology and course,
- Functional impairment for a period of time, and
- Distress and inability to function normally.

Engle (1961) proposed use of the term **uncomplicated grief** to describe a grief reaction that normally follows a significant loss. Uncomplicated grief runs a fairly predictable course that ends with the relinquishing of the lost object and the resumption of the duties of life. Some of the common reactions experienced by grieving individuals are cited in Table 17–1.

Many grieving people experience feelings of anger or blame; these feelings may be directed toward those perceived to have caused or contributed to the death. Often, the anger associated with grief is directed at one's self, that is, expressed as guilt or depression. Even though the bereaved have done nothing to cause the death, they often believe that somehow they should have been able to prevent it. Some survivors have a strong need to assign blame. If someone else can be blamed, the survivors can rid themselves of any responsibility (Figure 17-2).

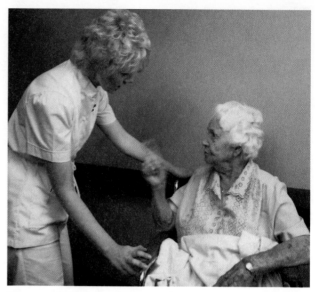

Figure 17-2 Anger is often a response to grief. This nurse is trying to help this client work through the anger she feels following a loss.

Dysfunctional Grief

Dysfunctional grief is a demonstration of a persistent pattern of intense grief that does not result in reconciliation of feelings. Persons experiencing dysfunctional (or pathological) grief do not progress through the stages of overwhelming emotions associated with grief and may fail to demonstrate any behaviors commonly associated with grief. The person experiencing pathological grief continues to have strong emotional reactions, does not return to a normal sleep pattern or work routine, usually remains isolated, and displays altered eating habits. The bereaved may have the need to endlessly tell and retell the story of loss but without subsequent healing. The pathologically

Table 17–1 REACTIONS COMMONLY EXPERIENCED DURING GRIEF (ENGLE)

PHYSICAL REACTIONS	PSYCHOSOCIAL REACTIONS	COGNITIVE REACTIONS	BEHAVIORAL REACTIONS
• Loss of appetite	• Profound sadness	• Inability to concentrate	• Impulsivity
• Insomnia	• Helplessness	• Forgetfulness	• Indecisiveness
• Fatigue	• Hopelessness	• Impaired judgment	• Social withdrawal
• Decreased libido	• Denial	• Decreased problem-solving ability	• Distancing
• Decreased immune functioning (increased susceptibility to illness)	• Anger		
• Multiple somatic complaints (e.g., headache, backache)	• Hostility		
• Restlessness	• Guilt		
	• Nightmares		
	• Ennui (overwhelming sense of emptiness)		
	• Preoccupation with lost object		
	• Loneliness		

PROFESSIONAL TIP

Identifying Dysfunctional Grief

The difference between normal and dysfunctional grief is that the person experiencing dysfunctional grief is unable to adapt to life without the deceased person.

Dysfunctional grief can take several forms, specifically absent grief, distorted grief, or converted grief.

Absent grief is the inability of the person to incorporate the reality of the death into his life. This blocking of reality leads to an incapacity to feel.

Distorted grief blocks the progress of adaptive grieving. The person becomes "stuck" in feelings of guilt and anger, two emotions that are most likely to become distorted. This type of dysfunctional grief usually occurs when the relationship with the deceased was ambivalent or dependent and issues were left unresolved.

Converted grief occurs when the anxiety is expressed as distressing symptoms without the bereaved's being aware of the relationship between the symptom and the loss. The manifestations have no organic basis and can consist of:

- Somatic symptoms: fatigue, headache, tension, sleep changes, weight fluctuations, loss of libido;
- Psychological symptoms: anger, mood instability, diminished coping ability, depression, loss of sense of humor, inability to relax;
- Attitudinal changes: rigid thinking, cynicism, criticism, lack of concern, apathy; and
- Relational differences: irritability, decreased frustration tolerance, distancing.

grieving person is unable to reestablish a routine. Visits to the gravesite or mausoleum may be made often or not at all. A person experiencing dysfunctional grief continues to focus on the deceased, may overvalue objects that belonged to the deceased, and may engage in depressive brooding.

The professional caregiver must be aware of these behaviors and refer the pathologically grieving person to professional counseling.

Anticipatory Grief

Anticipatory grief is the occurrence of grief work before an expected loss actually occurs. Anticipatory grief may be experienced by the terminally ill person as well as the person's family. This phenomenon promotes adaptive grieving and, therefore, frees up the

mourner's emotional energy necessary for problem solving. Although anticipatory grieving may be helpful in adjusting to the loss, it also has some potential disadvantages. For example, in the case of the dying client, anticipatory grieving may lead to family members' distancing themselves and not being available to provide support. Also, if the family members have separated themselves emotionally from the dying client, they may seem cold and distant, and, thus, not meet society's expectations of mourning behavior. This response can, in turn, prevent the mourners from receiving their own much needed support from others (Prichett & Lucas, 1997b).

Disenfranchised Grief

Doka, Rushton, and Thorstenson (1994) describe **disenfranchised grief** as "grief that is not openly acknowledged, socially sanctioned, or publicly shared." Grief can become disenfranchised when an individual either is reluctant to recognize the sense of loss and develops guilt feelings or feels pressured by society to "get on with life." An example of disenfranchised grief is extreme sadness over the loss of a pet when this mourning might be viewed by others as excessive or inappropriate. A mother's sadness over a miscarriage might also be considered disenfranchised grief, as a lengthy period of mourning may not be publicly expected despite the mother's intense feelings of loss and despair.

Factors Affecting Loss and Grief

Studies (Corless, Germino, & Pittman, 1995) conducted to determine factors that influence grieving identify the following variables as possibly affecting the intensity and duration of grieving:

- Developmental stage
- Religious and cultural beliefs
- Relationship with the lost object
- Cause of death

Developmental Stage

Depending on the client's place on the age/development continuum, the grief response to a loss will be experienced differently. Nurses practice in many settings where children, adolescents, and adults, as a result of growth and development, experience changes that result in loss. For example, a pregnant woman will, to some degree, experience loss after delivery of a first child (loss of freedom, independence, and self-focused life), even when the child is normal and healthy. Certain kinds of loss at key developmental points may have a profound effect on a person's ability to both work through the resulting grief and achieve the tasks of the given developmental stage. For example, an adolescent who has lost a parent may have difficulty forming an intimate relationship with members of the opposite sex.

Childhood   Children vary in their reactions to loss and in the ability to comprehend the meaning of death. It is important to understand the way a child's concept of death evolves, because the concept varies with developmental level and may affect mastery of developmental tasks (Table 17–2).

Children who are grieving need explanations about death that are honest and in terms they can comprehend.

Adolescence   Most adolescents value physical attractiveness and athletic abilities. Grief may occur when the adolescent suffers the loss of a body part or function. Because of the strong influence of peer groups, adolescents seek approval of their friends, and they fear being rejected if a loss affects their acceptance by others (e.g., grief after a disfiguring accident is usually intense in adolescents). Even though they have an intellectual understanding of death, adolescents believe themselves to be invulnerable and, thus, immune to death; they reject the possibility of their own mortality.

Early Adulthood   In the young adult, grief is usually precipitated by loss of role or status. For example, unemployment or the breakup of a relationship may

LIFE CYCLE CONSIDERATIONS

Talking with Children about Death

- *Avoid the use of euphemisms.* For example, telling a child that the deceased person has "gone away" may encourage the child to believe that the dead person will return. Also, telling a child that the deceased is "asleep" may lead to the development of sleep phobia in the child.
- *Do not overexplain.* Keep explanations factual and concise; do not offer lengthy explanations of medical conditions.
- *Use simple, concrete terms.* Young children are not able to conceptualize abstract ideas such as "grandma is in a better place now."
- *Show them.* Often, young children do not understand something until they see it. Take them to the funeral home and cemetery.

(*Data from* The 1996 National Directory of Bereavement Support Groups and Services, *by M. M. Wong, 1996, Forest Hills, NY: ADM Publishing.*)

Table 17–2 PERCEPTION OF DEATH BY CHILDREN AND ADOLESCENTS

DEVELOPMENTAL STAGE	PERCEPTION	POTENTIAL DEVELOPMENTAL DISRUPTIONS
Infancy, toddlerhood	• Is not aware of death • Is aware of disruptions in normal routine • Can react to family's expressions of grief	• Death of primary caregiver during the first 2 years of life may have significant long-lasting psychosocial implications.
Preschool	• Views death as temporary separation • Is able to react to the gravity of death in accordance with the reactions of parents or others	• Loss of either parent may have significant psychosocial implications, especially between ages 4 and 6 years (owing to *magical thinking*, wherein children may believe death is their fault). • Problems with development of sexual identity, depending on the gender of the parent lost, the child's identification with that parent, and the child's present state of sexual identity.
School-age	• Appreciates that death is final and inevitable • Fantasizes about and tends to personify death ("the boogie-man")	• Potential nightmares. • Potential death-avoidance behaviors (e.g., hiding under the covers, leaving the lights on, closing closet doors). • Possible intense guilt and a sense of responsibility for the death.
Preadolescence and adolescence	• Recognizes that death is final • Understands that death is inevitable • *Preadolescents:* tend to worry about dying; *adolescents:* tend to deny that death could happen to them	• Loss of a parent may interfere with mastery of the young-adulthood task of forming an intimate relationship with members of the opposite sex

From Fundamentals of Nursing: Standards & Practice, *by S. DeLaune and P. Ladner, 1998, Albany, NY: Delmar. Copyright 1998 by Delmar.*

cause significant grief for the young adult. The concept of death in this age group is primarily a reflection of cultural values and spiritual beliefs.

Middle Adulthood During middle adulthood, the potential for experiencing loss increases. The death of parents often occurs during this developmental phase. As an individual ages, it can be especially threatening when peers die, because these deaths force acknowledgment of one's own mortality.

Late Adulthood During late adulthood, most individuals recognize the inevitability of death. It is challenging for elders to experience the death of age-old friends or to find themselves the last one of their peer group left living. Older adults often turn to their children and grandchildren as sources of comfort and companionship. Cultivating friendships in all age groups helps prevent loneliness and depression.

Religious and Cultural Beliefs

Religious and cultural beliefs can have a significant effect on an individual's grief experience. Every culture has certain religious beliefs about the significance of death, as well as rituals for care of the dying. Beliefs about an afterlife, a supreme being, redemption of the soul, and reincarnation are important aspects that can assist one in grief work.

Relationship with the Lost Person or Object

In general, the more intimate the relationship with the deceased, the more intense the grief experienced by the bereaved. The death of a child poses a particular risk for dysfunctional grieving.

The death of a child is generally thought to be exceptionally painful because it upsets the natural order of things; parents do not expect their children to die before them.

Individuals experiencing parental grief usually have intense reactions and responses (Figure 17-3). The uniqueness of parental grief for a deceased child may lie in the loss of the perceived potential of that child. It is the loss of the hopes of the parents for the child, for "the things that could have been." Table 17-3 suggests some characteristics of parents of infants who have died.

The death of a parent or a sibling can pose a major challenge for children. The child's feelings may often go unrecognized by adults who fail to understand the child's need to mourn. Normal reactions of a child whose sibling has died as an infant, along with nursing responses to these reactions, are given in Table 17-4.

Cause of Death

The intensity of the grief response also varies according to the cause of death, be it unexpected, traumatic, or a suicide.

Table 17-3 CHARACTERISTICS OF PARENTS WHOSE CHILDREN DIE

TYPE OF DEATH	PARENTAL CHARACTERISTICS
Miscarriage and stillbirth	• Parents, especially the mother, may have feelings of intense sadness, anger, or guilt. The death is often inadequately recognized by others, especially if the loss occurs in early weeks of pregnancy. • The death may be considered a personal failure. • Parents may dwell on details, designating blame to themselves or others. • Grief from previous miscarriages may be relived. • Anticipatory grief may occur if the condition of the infant is known early in the pregnancy. • Ambivalence about being pregnant, experienced early in the pregnancy, may increase grief. • Hopes for the future must be modified or changed. • Despair may peak when the parents must leave the hospital or birthplace without the baby.
Neonatal death	• Feelings are similar to those associated with stillbirth. • Parents have had the time to form a bond with the infant, intensifying the grief. • Grief may be intense for both parents.
Sudden infant death syndrome (SIDS)	• Parents are in a state of shock. • Pain is increased by lack of knowledge and misinformation. • Because SIDS usually occurs during the first 6 months of life, parental bonding is complete. • Guilt may be present. • Police may investigate, adding to the guilt. • Grief is acute, because the death is sudden and the parents are not prepared for the loss. • Parents, especially the mother, may be preoccupied with the details of the death.
Abortion	• Shame, secrecy, and guilt may accompany grief. • Highly ambivalent feelings may be present. • Little support or comfort is offered by others. • Feelings of relief are expected, but despair and depression may surface. • No guilt may be felt, especially if the woman did not want a child.

From Healing and the Grief Process, *by S. S. Roach and B. C. Nieto, 1997, Albany, NY: Delmar. Copyright 1997, by Delmar.*

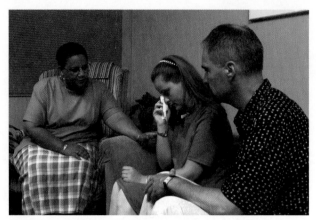

Figure 17-3 This couple discusses grief over the loss of a child.

Table 17–4 REACTION OF SIBLINGS AFTER INFANT DEATH

NORMAL REACTION	NURSING RESPONSE
• Fear of separation from and loss of parents	• Provide reassurance that parents will not abandon them
• Guilt, secondary to feelings of jealousy and anger and to magical thinking in relation to a wish that the infant would go away	• Provide information (at the appropriate level of comprehension) to reassure them that they did not contribute to the cause of death
• Fear about personal needs (that the intensity of parental reactions will interfere with parents' ability to take care of them)	• Continue routine activities to provide assurance that life will go on
• Concern over own health and fear of dying soon	• Encourage parents to avoid overprotectiveness, which reinforces children's fears

Data adapted from "Supporting Families after Sudden Infant Death," by M. McClain and J. Shaefer, 1996, Journal of Psychosocial Nursing and Mental Health Services, 24(4), 30–34.

Unexpected Death The loss occurring as a result of an unexpected death poses particular difficulty for the bereaved in achieving closure. As Roach and Nieto (1997) state, any death, even an anticipated death, is a traumatic experience to the surviving loved ones. Unanticipated death, such as a death from a heart attack, aneurysm, or stroke, leaves survivors shocked and bereaved. Most often, the bereaved are capable of working through the grieving process without complications.

Traumatic Death **Complicated grief** is associated with traumatic death such as death by homicide, violence, or accident. Although traumatic death does not necessarily predispose the survivor to complications in mourning, survivors often suffer emotions of greater intensity than those associated with normal grief.

When loved ones die violently, the bereaved may suffer from traumatic imagery, that is, reliving the terror of the incident or imagining the feelings of horror felt by the victim. Traumatic imagery is a common occurrence in cases of traumatic death. Such thoughts, coupled with intense grief, can lead to post-traumatic stress disorder (PTSD) in the survivors. Nurses must be aware of the possibility of PTSD and be alert for the presence of symptoms, which may include:

• Sleep disturbances, such as recurrent, terror-filled nightmares;
• Psychological distress; and
• Chronic anxiety.

Unless this problem is recognized and the survivors are encouraged to express their intense feelings, they will not be able to progress through the normal, adaptive grieving process.

Suicide The loss of a loved one to suicide is frequently compounded by feelings of guilt among the survivors. They feel guilty for failing to recognize clues that may have enabled the victim to receive help. These feelings of guilt and self-blame can transform into anger at the victim for inflicting such pain, at themselves, and at caregivers. Feelings of shame for having a suicide in the family may also be present. The negative stigma of suicide may prohibit survivors from successfully resolving their grief.

Nursing Care of the Grieving Client

Resolution of a loss is a painful process and must be done by clients in their own way. Nurses can assist by providing support as the client moves through the process of mourning. Rodebaugh, Schwindt, and Valentine (1999) suggest that grief be thought of as a journey through four broad categories titled reeling, feeling, dealing, and healing. Clients are reeling when experiencing shock or disbelief. Feelings may be expressed in various emotions and behaviors. Dealing occurs when they begin to adapt to the loss. Things do not necessarily get better; they just get different. Healing is when the loss becomes part of them, and the acute anguish lessens; it does not mean forgetting. Grief changes people by affecting self-esteem, triggering the development of new ways of coping, and precipitating a new lifestyle without the deceased.

Nurses can play an active role in assisting people to grieve by encouraging clients to do their grief work, that is, to experience their feelings to the fullest in order to work through them. Providing support and

Rituals following Death

- Judaism practices burial of the dead within 24 hours. A 7-day period of mourning, called *Shiva*, begins the day of the funeral.
- In the Muslim faith, men wash the body of a man and women wash the body of a woman after death.
- Buddhists believe that after death, the body should not be disturbed by movement, talking, or crying.
- Hindus pour holy water into the mouth of the dying person. The eldest son arranges for the funeral and cremation within 24 hours of death. Embalming is forbidden.
- Jehovah's Witnesses believe that the soul dies with the body, but 144,000 will be resurrected at the end-time and will be born again as spiritual sons of God.
- Native Americans believe that the spirit lives on after death. Ancestor worship is practiced.

(*From* Health Assessment & Physical Examination (*2nd ed.*), *by M. E. Z. Estes, 2002, Albany, NY: Delmar. Copyright 2002 by Delmar.*)

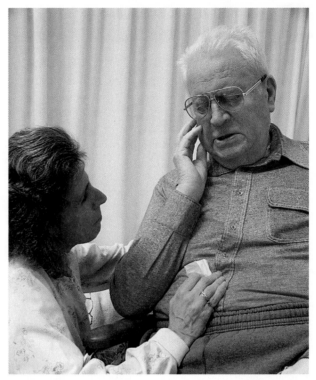

Figure 17-4 The nurse provides support to this client to help him through the grief process.

explaining to the bereaved that it will take time to grieve the loss and to gain some closure to the relationship are both important nursing responsibilities (Figure 17-4).

Assessment

A thorough assessment of the grieving client and family begins with a determination of the personal meaning of the loss. Another key assessment area is deciding the person's progress in terms of the grieving process. The nurse understands that the stages of grieving are not necessarily mastered sequentially, but, instead, that individuals may vacillate in progression through the stages of grief.

Nursing Diagnosis

The North American Nursing Diagnosis Association (NANDA) defines *Dysfunctional Grieving* as "extended, unsuccessful use of intellectual and emotional responses by which individuals, families, communities attempt to work through the process of modifying self-concept based upon the perception of loss" (NANDA, 2001). Another diagnosis that may be applicable is *Anticipatory Grieving*, defined as "intellectual and emotional responses and behaviors by which individuals, families, communities work through the process of modifying self-concept based on the perception of potential loss" (NANDA, 2001).

Planning/Outcome Identification

It is important to clarify the expected outcomes when planning care for the grieving client. Listed below are some expected goals for the person experiencing grief:

- Verbalize feelings of grief
- Share grief with significant others
- Accept the loss
- Renew activities and relationships

Some of these expected outcomes will take a long time to achieve, and some must be achieved before others are mastered. For example, to accept the loss, the person must begin to share grief with others by verbalizing those feelings. Two of the expected outcomes are discussed below.

Acceptance of the Loss Only by going through grief work are individuals able to reach some acceptance and, ultimately, resolution of feelings about the loss. Often, people try to find some meaning in their situations. This search involves introspection, for which spiritual support may be therapeutic.

Renewal of Activities and Relationships The very core of grief work revolves around acceptance of the fact that the needs met by key people in our lives can be met in other ways and by other people. The deceased cannot be replaced; however, enough healing must occur so that new relationships can be initiated.

PROFESSIONAL TIP

Adaptive Grieving

How long does the process of adaptive grieving take? The length of time necessary for grief resolution is as individual as the person experiencing it and depends on the intensity of the grief. Grief is considered to be a "long-term process" (Corless, Germino, & Pittman, 1995). Grief work takes time. There are no definite time frames within which grief should occur. Each person grieves in his own way and at his own pace.

Implementation

Therapeutic nursing care is based on an understanding of the significance of the loss to the client. To understand the client's perspective, the nurse must spend time listening. As the client expresses feelings, the nurse must demonstrate acceptance, even if the client is not responding according to the nurse's expectations or belief system. The nurse's nonjudgmental, accepting attitude is essential during the bereaved's expression of all feelings, including anger and despair. The nurse communicates an understanding of the client's anger and avoids personalizing and using defensive behaviors. The expression of grief is not only appropriate but essential for therapeutic resolution of the loss.

Grieving people need reassurance, counseling, and support. One mechanism of support on a long-term basis is support groups. The nurse must be informed about the availability of such groups within the community in order to make appropriate referrals. When bereaved people join support groups, they will be with others who have experienced similar losses. This sharing decreases the feelings of loneliness and social isolation so common in the grief experience.

Evaluation

People follow their own time schedule for grief work. In general, it takes months or years for grief resolution. Therefore, nurses usually do not have an opportunity to be with the bereaved family when grief work is completed. However, the nurse has a unique opportunity to lay the foundation for adaptive grieving by encouraging the bereaved to share their feelings and to continue to verbalize their experience with significant others. The goals mutually established with client and family are the foundation for evaluation. It is important for nurses to teach grieving individuals that resolution of the loss is generally a process of life-long adjustment.

DEATH

Historically, death has been considered as natural as birth, as simply the last stage of life. The last three decades have brought about significant changes in the cultural perception of death, however. In some cases, dying and death are no longer simple matters but are issues involving ethical concerns and, in some cases, legal intervention by the court system.

Just as each person lives a unique life, each person dies a unique death. Death may be sudden and unexpected, caused by heart attack or accident, for example, or death may be prolonged, coming after a distressing long-term illness. Death may come quietly for the older person who dies during sleep. And some deaths are planned by those who choose to die on their own terms by way of suicide.

Health care workers must understand the legal and ethical issues surrounding dying and death. Understanding the stages of death and dying and the signs of impending death will help prepare the nurse to render sensitive, effective care, both to the client and family and to the client's body after death. Nurses must also come to terms with their own mortality and feelings about death if they are to provide comfort to dying

CULTURAL CONSIDERATIONS

Cultural Influences and Advance Directive Decisions

African American Clients
- Are more likely to select aggressive interventions.
- Are less likely than European American or Hispanic American clients to have documented their end-of-life health care wishes

European American Clients
- Are much more likely to have written advance directives than are members of other cultures.
- Select "no code" more than do Hispanic American or African American clients but less than do Asian American clients

Asian American Clients
- Select "no code" more than do all other groups
- Are less likely to have advance directives

Hispanic American Clients
- Are less likely than are European American or Asian American clients to have written directives
- Are least likely of all groups to select "no code"

(*Data from "Meeting the Challenge of Advance Directives," by P. Haynor, 1998,* American Journal of Nursing, *98(3), 27–32.*)

clients and their families. Health care workers can learn a great deal about life from the dying client.

Legal Considerations

The *Patient Self-Determination Act* (PSDA) was incorporated into the Omnibus Budget Reconciliation Act (OBRA) of 1990. The act was intended to provide a legal means for individuals to determine the circumstances under which life-sustaining treatment should or should not be provided to them. The individual's choices are validated by advance directives. An advance directive is any written instruction, including a living will or durable power of attorney for health care, that is recognized under state law (Taylor, 1995). The act applies to hospitals, long-term care facilities, home health agencies, hospice programs, and certain health maintenance organizations (HMOs). According to the PSDA, all clients entering the health care system through any of these organizations must be given information and the opportunity to complete advance directives if they have not already done so. Clients need to know that in many states, just signing these documents may not be adequate for carrying out their wishes. They may also need to indicate their wishes in regard to artificial feeding, intubation, chemotherapy, surgery, blood transfusions, and transfer to the hospital (for residents in skilled care facilities).

Although the living will and durable power of attorney for health care are legal documents, they do not preclude the need for **resuscitation** (support measures to restore consciousness and life). The medical record must have a written do-not-resuscitate (DNR) order from a physician if this is in agreement with the client's wishes and with the advance directives. In the absence of such an order, resuscitation will be initiated.

PROFESSIONAL TIP

Care of the Dying Client

Dying was once considered to be a normal part of the life cycle. Today, it is often considered to be a medical problem that should be handled by health care providers. Technological advances in medicine have lead to depersonalized and mechanical care of those who are dying.

Our highly technological world calls for application of high-touch interventions with the dying. In other words, appropriate care of the dying is administered by compassionate nurses who are both technically competent and able to demonstrate caring. Huizdos (2000) learned that death is not the enemy— lack of caring is.

Many states also have a **Health Care Surrogate Law** which is implemented in the absence of advance directives. This law varies from state to state. Basically, it provides a legal means for specific individuals to make decisions for the client when the client can no longer do so. The law has developed a hierarchy of individuals who would act in the interests of the client. The spouse is the first person in the hierarchy, followed by children in the event that there is no spouse.

Ethical Considerations

Death is often fraught with ethical dilemmas that occur almost daily in health care settings. Many health care agencies have ethics committees to develop and implement policies to deal with end-of-life issues. Ethics committees are interdisciplinary and may have attorneys and clergy in addition to health care providers as members. Ethical decision making is a complex issue. One of the most difficult dilemmas is determining the difference between killing and allowing someone to die by withholding life-sustaining treatment methods.

The American Nurses Association (ANA) distinguishes relieving pain and mercy killing (euthanasia or assisted suicide). Pain relief is a central value in nursing, whereas euthanasia is viewed as unethical. The ANA's position is that increasing doses of medication to control pain in terminally ill clients is ethically justified, even at the expense of maintaining life (ANA, 1992).

Stages of Dying and Death

In her classic works, Elizabeth Kübler-Ross (1969, 1974) identified five possible stages of dying that are experienced by clients and their families (Table 17–5). Not every client moves sequentially through each stage. These stages are experienced in varying degrees and for varying lengths of time. The client may express anger, and then, a few minutes later, express acceptance of the inevitable, and then express anger again. The value in Kübler-Ross' work is that it helps increase sensitivity to the needs of the dying client.

Denial

In the first stage of dying, the initial shock can be overwhelming. Denial is a useful tool in coping. It is an essential and protective mechanism that may last for only a few minutes or may manifest for months.

In some clients, denial manifests as "doctor shopping" (not to imply that second opinions are not sometimes necessary) or insisting that there must have been a mix-up or mistake in the diagnostic tests. In other clients, denial manifests as simply avoiding the issue. They go about their daily routines as though nothing in their lives has changed. Most people, given the time, will eventually move past the stage of denial.

Table 17–5 KÜBLER-ROSS' STAGES OF DYING AND DEATH	
STAGE	**EXAMPLE**
First Stage: **Denial**	*Verbal:* "This can't be happening to me!" *Behavioral:* Client is diagnosed with terminal lung cancer; client continues to smoke two packs of cigarettes daily.
Second Stage: **Anger**	*Verbal:* "Why me?" *Behavioral:* Client strikes out at caregivers.
Third Stage: **Bargaining**	*Verbal:* Client prays, "Please, God, just let me live long enough to see my grandchild graduate." *Behavioral:* Client tries to "make deals" with caregivers or god.
Fourth Stage: **Depression**	*Verbal:* "Go away. I just want to lie here in bed. What's the use?" *Behavioral:* Client withdraws and isolates self.
Fifth Stage: **Acceptance**	*Verbal:* "I feel ready. At least, I'm more at peace now." *Behavioral:* Client gets financial or legal affairs in order. Client says goodbye to significant others.

Data from On Death and Dying, *by E. Kübler-Ross, 1969, New York: Macmillan. Copyright 1969 by Macmillan.*

LIFE CYCLE CONSIDERATIONS

Reactions to Impending Death
- Persons of all ages generally experience the same feelings and emotions as they progress through a terminal illness.
- Persons of any age who have endured a long illness may view death as a release from their suffering.
- Persons of any age may find it difficult to reach acceptance if they have unfinished business.
- Many people receive satisfaction from **life review** (a form of reminiscence wherein a client attempts to come to terms with conflict or to gain meaning from life and die peacefully).
- Elderly clients may welcome death, especially if they have outlived everyone who was near and dear to them.

Clients may choose to be selective in the use of denial. For example, clients may use denial with certain family members or friends because they are trying to protect those people from the truth. Clients may also use denial from time to time to set aside thoughts of illness and death in order to focus on living.

Anger

The initial stage of denial is often followed by anger. The client's security is being threatened by the unknown. All the normal daily routines have become disrupted. This stage is typically very difficult for family and caregivers because they may feel powerless or useless in terms of helping their loved one through the situation. The client has no control over the situation and, thus, becomes angry in response to this powerlessness. The anger may be directed at self, God, others, the environment, and the health care system. In the client's eyes, whatever is done is not the right thing. Family members may be greeted with silence or with outbursts of anger. Their response, in turn, may be anger, guilt, or despair.

Bargaining

The anticipation of the loss through death may bring about bargaining, through which the client attempts to postpone or reverse the inevitable. The client's bargaining represents an attempt to postpone death and usually has self-imposed limitations. For example, the client will ask to live just long enough to see her first grandchild born in exchange for a promise to perform some service for the church. Most clients bargain in silence or in confidence with their spiritual leader. Caregivers who have cared for terminally ill clients will agree that it is not uncommon for a client to live long enough for some special event (a wedding or birth), only to die shortly afterwards.

Depression

When the realization comes that the loss can no longer be delayed, the client moves to the stage of depression. This depression is different from dysfunctional depression in that it helps the client detach from life and, thus, be able to accept death. Depression in this sense is a therapeutic experience for the dying person. Clients sometimes feel abandoned, as persons who were once friends begin to visit less and less, sometimes severing ties with the client even before death; this may compound the client's feelings of depression and hopelessness.

Acceptance

The final stage, acceptance, may not be reached by every dying client. With acceptance comes growing peace and contentment. The feeling that all that could be done has been done is often expressed during this stage. Reinforcement of the client's feelings and sense of personal worth are important during this stage. Many clients will make an effort to get all of their personal and financial affairs in order.

The client may sleep more, not to avoid reality, but because sleep is needed to fill a physical and emotional need. The client may limit visitors to a few people with whom he feels safe and comfortable. The most significant form of communication at this time is moments of silence.

Nursing Care of the Dying Client

Nursing care of clients who are terminally ill or who are facing and preparing for their own death can be both challenging and rewarding. The death process is typically a very emotional time for clients and their families; compassionate and sensitive nursing care that respects clients' wishes as well as meets their physical needs can help bring peace and dignity to this natural process.

Assessment

Nursing interventions are based on a thorough assessment of the client's holistic needs. Assessment of the dying client includes an ongoing collection of data regarding the strengths and limitations of the dying person and the family.

Nursing Diagnoses

The nurse's assessment of the dying client may lead to any number of diagnoses. One NANDA-approved nursing diagnosis that is applicable for many dying clients is *Powerlessness,* that is, "the perception that one's own action will not significantly affect an outcome; a perceived lack of control over a current situation or immediate happening" (NANDA, 2001). Another response that is often experienced by the dying is described by the diagnosis *Hopelessness,* "a subjective state in which an individual sees limited or no alternatives or personal choices available and is unable to mobilize energy on own behalf" (NANDA, 2001). The

PROFESSIONAL TIP

Information Needed in Assessment of the Dying Client

- Client and family goals and expectations
- Client's awareness of the terminal nature of illness
- Availability of support systems
- Current stage of dying
- History of previous positive coping skills
- Client perception of unfinished business to be completed

(Adapted from Death and Dying, by K. Pritchett and P. Lucas, 1997. In Psychiatric–Mental Health Nursing: Adaptation and Growth *(4th ed., pp. 206–207), by B. S. Johnson (Ed.), 1997, Philadelphia: Lippincott Williams & Wilkins.)*

PROFESSIONAL TIP

Planning Care for the Dying Client

- Schedule time to be available to the client
- Identify areas that are of special concern to the client and make referrals if appropriate (e.g., social worker consult for information on financial assistance)
- Promote and protect individual self-esteem and self-worth
- Balance the client's needs for independence and assistance
- Meet the physiological needs of the client and family
- Respect the client's confidentiality
- Answer all questions and provide factual information to the client and family
- Offer to contact clergy or other spiritual leader

(Adapted from Death and Dying, by K. Pritchett and P. Lucas. In Psychiatric–Mental Health Nursing: Adaptation and Growth *(4th ed., p. 208), by B. S. Johnson (Ed.) (1997) Philadelphia: Lippincott Williams & Wilkins.)*

client may also exhibit *Death Anxiety,* "apprehension, worry, or fear related to death or dying" (NANDA, 2001).

Planning/Outcome Identification

The major goals of nursing care are the physical, emotional, and mental comfort of the client. The goals of nursing care for the dying client are the same as those goals developed for all clients who are unable to meet their own needs. The dying client must be treated as a unique individual worthy of respect, rather than as a diagnosis to be cured. Many dying clients do not fear death but are anxious about a painful death or dying alone.

Promoting optimal quality of life means treating the client and family in a respectful manner and providing a safe environment for the expression of feelings. Planning focuses on meeting the holistic needs of the client and family. These needs are specified in the Dying Person's Bill of Rights (Figure 17-5), which is as relevant today as when it was written in 1975. In planning care, the nurse should make every effort to be sensitive to the dying client's rights.

Implementation

The nurse's first priority is to communicate a caring attitude to the client. A recent study (Czerwiec, 1996) quoted family members of recently deceased hospitalized clients as stating that "the factor that most strongly affects family satisfaction [is] perceiving the staff to have a caring attitude toward the patient and to be acting on his behalf."

The Dying Person's Bill of Rights

- I have the right to be treated as a living human being until I die.
- I have the right to maintain a sense of hopefulness, however changing its focus may be.
- I have the right to be cared for by those who can maintain a sense of hopefulness, however challenging this might be.
- I have the right to express my feelings and emotions about my approaching death in my own way.
- I have the right to participate in decisions concerning my care.
- I have the right to expect continuing medical and nursing attention even though "cure" goals must be changed to "comfort" goals.
- I have the right not to die alone.
- I have the right to be free from pain.
- I have the right to have my questions answered honestly.
- I have the right not to be deceived.
- I have the right to have help from and for my family in accepting death.
- I have the right to die in peace and dignity.
- I have the right to retain my individuality and not be judged for my decisions, which may be contrary to beliefs of others.
- I have the right to expect that the sanctity of the human body will be respected after death.
- I have the right to be cared for by caring, sensitive, knowledgeable people who will attempt to understand my needs and will be able to gain some satisfaction in helping me face my death.

Figure 17-5 The Dying Person's Bill of Rights (*From The Dying Person's Bill of Rghts, by A. J. Barbus, 1975*, American Journal of Nursing, 75(1).

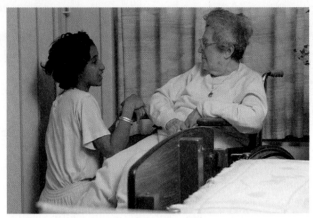

Figure 17-6 Establishing a caring and trusting relationship helps the client come to terms with a terminal illness.

When a client is in denial, it is important for the nurse to approach the client with understanding and the knowledge that moving between the stages of dying is enhanced by a trusting nurse–client relationship. Establishment of rapport facilitates the client's verbalization of feelings (Figure 17-6). The nurse establishes a safe environment wherein the client does not feel embarrassed or chastised for experiencing those feelings. Nurses must understand that clients are not angry with them, but, rather, with the situation they are experiencing.

Terminally ill clients are often given **palliative care**, or care that relieves symptoms, such as pain, but does not alter the course of disease. A primary aim of palliative care is to help the client feel safe and secure.

The nurse can do much to increase the client's feelings of safety by being available when needed. Holding the client's hand and listening are therapeutic measures. Ufema (1995a) suggests asking the client three questions: What do you want? From whom do you want it? and When do you want it? The client needs to know that he has the nurse's support as an advocate for his care and well-being.

Physiological Needs According to Maslow's hierarchy of needs, physiological needs must be met before others, because they are essential for existence. Areas that are often problematic for the terminally ill client are respirations; fluids and nutrition; mouth, eyes, and nose; mobility; skin care; and elimination.

Respirations Oxygen is frequently ordered for the client experiencing labored breathing. Suctioning may be needed to remove secretions that the client is unable to swallow.

Fluids and Nutrition The refusal of food and fluids is almost universal in dying clients. It is believed that the client is not feeling thirst and hunger. Although the issue of permitting dehydration in terminally ill clients is often met with great resistance, the literature supports the concept that forced nutrition has questionable value and may even exacerbate the client's condition (Taylor, 1995). Artificial nutrition often increases the client's agitation, leads to increased use of limb restraints, and increases the risk of aspiration pneumonia (Rhymes, 1993). Hospice nurses have indicated that withholding artificial nutrition is not painful. Regardless, in every situation, the client's own wishes must always take precedence. If the comatose client has not previously made his wishes known, family members must be given accurate and truthful information. For the person in irreversible coma, withholding of artificial nutrition does not cause death; rather, it allows life to take its natural course (Taylor, 1995). Several professional groups have issued statements regarding artificial nutrition and hydration. The American Medical Association, the American Dietetic

Association, and the ANA agree that it is legally, ethically, and professionally acceptable to discontinue nutritional support if the terminally ill client so requests (Taylor, 1995).

Mouth, Eyes, and Nose Oral discomfort is the only documented side effect of dehydration in the terminally ill client (Taylor, 1995). Both the administration of oxygen and mouth breathing increase the need for meticulous oral care. Caregivers can use saliva substitutes and moisturizers to alleviate discomfort. The regular use of toothpaste and a toothbrush may be adequate. The tongue must be given the same attention as is the rest of the mouth, with gentle brushing. Ice chips and sips of favorite beverages should be offered frequently, and petroleum jelly applied to the lips. Oral care must be given every 2 to 3 hours to maintain the client's comfort.

The eyes may become irritated due to dryness. Artificial tears can alleviate this discomfort. A cotton ball should be used to gently wipe the eye from inner to outer canthus (one wipe per cotton ball) to remove any discharge.

The nares may become dry and crusted. Oxygen given by cannula can further irritate the nares. A thin layer of water soluble jelly applied to the nares will help alleviate discomfort. The elastic strap of the oxygen cannula should not be applied too tightly, lest it cause discomfort.

Mobility As the client's condition deteriorates, mobility decreases. The client becomes less able to move about in bed or to get out of bed and requires more assistance. Physical dependence increases the risk of complications related to immobility, such as atrophy and pressure ulcers. Attentive nursing care can prevent the onset of these complications, which increase both client discomfort and the cost of care.

The client should be repositioned at least every 2 hours. It is important to keep in mind that the client may have other disorders that contribute to discomfort related to mobility, such as arthritis or lung disease. The nurse can help the client maintain body alignment with the use of pillows and other supportive equipment and can use positioning techniques to facilitate ease of breathing. Passive range of motion exercises should be performed at least twice a day to prevent stiffness and aching of the joints. The client may prefer to be assisted into a reclining type of chair at intervals throughout the day. Using a wheelchair can also increase the client's environmental space, giving the client more mobility, control, and independence.

Skin Care The prevention of pressure ulcers is a priority. Pressure ulcers are painful, can cause secondary complications such as sepsis, and are costly to treat. Regular repositioning and passive range of motion exercises are two preventive measures. In addition, keeping the skin clean and moisturized will promote healthy tissue. The skin should be inspected once or twice daily, with special attention paid to pressure points and areas where skin surfaces rub together. Gentle massages with soothing lotion are comforting. Bed baths are adequate if the client cannot get into the tub or sit in a shower chair.

Elimination Constipation may occur due to side effects of pain medications and to lack of physical activity. Fluids and foods with high-fiber content can be effective preventive measures for clients with adequate oral intake. Constipation can also be alleviated by maintaining a scheduled time for bowel elimination and administering suppositories, if necessary. A commode with padded arms can be more comfortable than a toilet.

The client may become incontinent of bladder and bowel, so the nurse must check the client frequently, clean the skin with peri-washes, and apply a moisture barrier after each incontinent episode. Incontinent undergarments may increase the client's comfort, especially when the client is out of bed.

Indwelling catheters are never a first choice for bladder management. However, for some clients, the need for frequent cleaning, the discomfort of using a bedpan, or getting out of bed to use the toilet or commode may cause agonizing pain. In these circumstances, the benefits of a catheter greatly outweigh the risks.

Comfort The primary activities directed at promoting physical comfort include pain relief, keeping the client clean and dry, and providing a safe, nonthreatening environment. The nurse who demonstrates a respectful, caring attitude promotes the client's psychological comfort by establishing rapport. The fear of a painful death is almost universal. Pain is a subjective, personal experience, and the client is the best judge of the severity of the pain. Many, though certainly not all, dying clients experience pain. In its position statement on pain relief for the terminally ill, the ANA states that promotion of comfort is the major goal of nursing care (ANA, 1992). Comfort should be maximized by management of pain and other discomforting factors.

The client needs to know that caregivers accept and believe complaints of pain and that they will intervene to prevent and alleviate the pain. The nurse should ask the client to rate the pain on a scale from 0 to 10, with 0 being no pain, and 10 being severe pain. Medication must be given around the clock and not "as needed." A nonnarcotic analgesic may be effective in early stages for mild, intermittent pain. As the pain increases, the client may need to be started on morphine, titrated at increments until adequate pain relief is achieved without severe side effects. Titrating the analgesic dose and interval means finding the lowest dose and the longest interval that will relieve pain. The dosage that should be used is the one that controls the pain to the satisfaction of the client and that causes minimal side effects. For some clients, this may be 10 mg of oral morphine sulfate (MS) every 4 hours. For other clients,

Adjuvant Therapy

Adjuvant therapy may be effective. Nonsteroidal anti-inflammatory agents are beneficial for bone metastases; tricyclic antidepressants and anti-seizure medications for neurogenic pain, and steroids for headaches related to cerebral edema (Rhymes, 1993). Nonpharmacological techniques can be used along with medication. Relaxation techniques, guided imagery, massages, and repositioning may enhance the action of the medications.

it may be 480 mg MS intravenously per hour. The question for the nurse is, what dose can be safely given? No maximum number of milligrams applies to every individual.

The nurse must monitor the client's responses with regard to pain rating and respiratory rate. For example, 10 mg MS given IM may afford pain relief, but if the respiratory rate drops from 12 to 6 per minute, the next dose should be reduced. If the same dose given to another client provides minimal relief, and the client is alert and displays no change in respirations, the next dose should be increased (McCaffery & Pasero, 1999).

The client must be monitored for **breakthrough pain**, or sudden, acute, temporary pain that is usually precipitated by a treatment or procedure or by unusual activity of the client. A supplemental dose of medication is required. If the precipitating factor is known (dressing changes, for example), a dose should be given 30 to 60 minutes before the procedure.

Physical Environment A soothing physical environment can significantly increase the client's comfort. Soft lighting enhances vision without causing the discomfort associated with harsh, glaring light. Complying with the client's request for a night light is also helpful in creating a pleasant and nonthreatening environment. If possible, the client should be offered the opportunity to have the bed or a chair near a window to increase the range of the environment. As the client's circulation becomes more sluggish, body temperature will fall. Lightweight comforters will increase warmth without adding uncomfortable weight. The nurse can help eliminate environmental odors by ensuring adequate ventilation, daily cleaning of the room, removal of leftover food, and frequent linen changes. Noise can be distracting and anxiety provoking, so the nurse and visitors should comply with the client's wishes with regard to the use of radio and television. The telephone can be removed from the room, if the client finds the ringing disturbing.

Psychosocial Needs Death presents a threat to not only one's physical existence, but to one's psychological integrity. The dying person is often tethered to

tubes and electronic gadgetry in an intensive care unit. The client is held captive in a tangle of technology and is kept at a distance from the supportive presence and touch of family and friends.

Technology does not replace touch, concern, compassion, and human companionship. Nurses, through their presence, can humanize the dying person's environment. Families should be encouraged and invited to participate in the client's care, if they desire to do so and the client is willing.

For many clients, maintaining a well-groomed appearance is important. When the client can no longer make requests or give directions for care, caregivers should presume that the client would prefer to maintain the same grooming habits as were previously preferred. Shaving the male client's beard or cleaning and trimming the client's fingernails and toenails, for instance, will help the client maintain a well-groomed appearance and will also promote client dignity. Combing and brushing the hair not only improves appearance, but is also a comforting and relaxing activity for many clients.

Dressing and undressing may become a cumbersome, frustrating, and fatiguing activity. The client who spends time up and about may choose attractive pajamas, housecoats, dusters, or exercise suits. Nurses should advise individuals who may be purchasing clothing for the client to select items that are loose fitting, have few fasteners, and are washable.

COMMUNITY/HOME HEALTH CARE

Equipment To Increase Client Comfort

The following equipment can be rented and may qualify for payment by Medicare or private insurance.

- An electric hospital bed with overhead trapeze, to give the client more control of the environment
- A commode, to extend the client's independence in elimination
- A lifting device, to facilitate getting the dependent client out of bed
- Remote control, for the client who enjoys television
- Portable telephone
- Shower chair and hand-held shower for the bathtub
- Comfort devices such as special mattresses for the bed and cushions for chairs
- Overbed table, for eating or hand activities
- Comfortable chairs close to the bed, to facilitate visits of family and friends

Spiritual Needs Nurses play a major role in promoting the dying client's spiritual comfort. Dying clients are most vulnerable. The moral health and integrity of the broader community can be measured in part by the way we respond to their needs. Dying persons may experience confusion, anger at their god, crises of faith, or other types of spiritual distress.

Dying is a personal and, frequently, lonely process. Table 17–6 provides information on the views of various religions with regard to withdrawal of life support; death; and organ donation. The nurse can serve as a sounding board for the client who expresses values and beliefs related to death. The following are therapeutic nursing interventions that address the spiritual needs of the dying client:

- Communicate empathy
- Play music
- Use touch
- Pray with the client
- Contact clergy, if requested by the client
- Read religious literature aloud, at the client's request

Table 17–6 RELIGIONS AND DYING AND DEATH ISSUES

RELIGION	LIFE SUPPORT WITHDRAWAL	DEATH	ORGAN DONATION
Judaism	Allowed under the right circumstances (when life support is serving only to impede a natural death).	• Suicide is forbidden. • Burial should occur within 24 hours. • Cremation is forbidden.	• Permitted because the procedure saves life. • Rejected by Orthodox Jews. • Autopsy is permitted if it will save future lives.
Islam	Permitted if only serving to prolong death or if client's condition is medically hopeless.	• Suicide is forbidden. • Relatives and friends are present. • Autopsy is permitted to solve a crime or provide further medical knowledge.	• Permitted.
Catholicism/ Orthodoxy	Controversial; permitted if client's condition is hopeless.	• Prayers are offered at time of death. • Burial and cremation are permitted. • Autopsy is permitted.	• Permitted.
Protestantism	Permitted if client's condition is hopeless.	• Prayers are offered at time of death. • Burial and cremation are permitted. • Autopsy is permitted.	• Permitted, although may be rejected by some Baptists or Pentecostals.
Jehovah's Witnesses	Permitted if serving only to prolong death or if quality of life is nonexistent.	• Suicide is not approved. • Autopsy is permitted if legally necessary.	• Individual choice.
Buddhism	Acceptable for those on threshold of death.	• Suicide is criticized. • Cremation is common.	• Controversial.
Hinduism	Supported to allow a natural death.	• Prefer to die at home. • Embalming is forbidden. • Autopsy is discouraged. • Suicide is forbidden.	• Forbidden.
Mormons	A client or family decision.	• Cremation is discouraged. • Autopsy is a family decision.	• A family decision.
Native Americans	Life support is viewed as unnatural and, therefore, unnecessary.	• Complex beliefs about death and treatment of the body.	• Discouraged.

Data from Health Assessment & Physical Examination *(2nd ed.), by M. E. Z. Estes, 2002, Albany, NY: Delmar. Copyright 2002 by Delmar.*

Support for the Family Family members need to be involved in the care of their dying loved one. Guilt may be increased by feelings of powerlessness. Involving family members in the treatment is often a helpful intervention. Families facing the impending death of a loved one require much support from nurses and other caregivers. The nurse's presence, just being there with the family, is extremely important. A recent study showed that "family members indicated that when a loved one is dying, they'd like to know that a nurse will make a special effort to be . . . available" (Czerwiec, 1996).

Each family group has its unwritten rules, its leaders and followers, and its methods for coping with crises. The family's equilibrium is threatened by the impending death. If family members have limited coping skills and inadequate support systems, they need assistance and guidance from the caregivers. Nurses must remember that the rules and coping mechanisms used by the family may not always coincide with the values and beliefs of the staff and that the client's and family's wishes must be respected to the extent possible.

Each family member will grieve the approaching death in her own way. The nurse must be supportive and nonjudgmental. The family needs to know that the staff cares about them as well as the client.

The relationship with the family does not always end with the client's death. Staff members may attend visitations, funerals, or memorial services. If a hospice was involved, the family may participate in a bereavement support program. If the client was a resident in a long-term care facility, family members may return to visit other residents with whom they became acquainted.

Learning Needs Bereaved families need much support and information. The nurse's role is to teach family members what they need to know. For instance, families must be assisted with acquiring the tools that will help them help their loved one. An example might be the need for the family to understand that the dying person needs to conserve energy. Some simple actions on the part of the family could be to schedule activities after a rest period or early in the morning, when the client is strongest. The nurse may need to point out to the family this type of common sense approach, as simple interventions such as these can be overlooked during this highly charged emotional time.

Client and family knowledge deficits can relate to:

- Insufficient information about physical condition,
- Information about the treatment regimen,
- Inability to anticipate medical crises,
- Inexperience with personal threat of death, and
- Unfamiliarity with protocol to follow in case of the need for emergency care outside of the hospital.

CLIENT TEACHING

Guidelines for Teaching a Family Caregiver

- Discuss the nature and extent of the disease process
- Use adult-education principles
- Reinforce material frequently
- Clearly explain the purpose of palliative care while maintaining a sense of realistic hope
- Inform client and family of available community resources; reassure them that they are not alone
- Teach steps for caregiver to follow if an emergency arises at home
- Provide written instructions for caregiver to follow, including important telephone numbers and persons to be contacted
- Inform about the purpose of hospice

Hospice Care **Hospice**, a type of care for the terminally ill, is founded on the concept of allowing individuals to die with dignity and surrounded by those who love them. Clients enter hospice care when aggressive medical treatment is no longer an option or when the client refuses further medical intervention.

Home Care A dying person is often not given the opportunity to be surrounded by family and friends. More than 80% of all reported deaths in the United States occur in health care institutions where people die in unfamiliar, and sometimes intimidating, surroundings (deBlois, 1994).

Impending Death

No one can predict how long a client will be in the terminal stages of illness. A client may exhibit signs of impending death and then rally to live for several more days. It is not uncommon for clients to endure until a member of the family arrives for a last good-bye. The client who has had a long and troublesome illness may be ready to die but needs "permission" to die from a loved one, who says, "It's okay, you can go now." A client may not wish to die when others are present and will wait to take the last breath until everyone has left the room.

Even when death is expected, it is never easy for the family. The family should be thoroughly informed, in simple terms, about what will happen before and after the client's death, including:

- Physical changes that will occur just before and following death
- Pronouncement of death
- Post-mortem care
- Removal of the body

COMMUNITY/HOME HEALTH CARE

An Alternative for the Dying Client

- Family members should be physically and emotionally able to provide care.
- Health care providers should share the responsibility of home care with the family. This sharing could include respite time and frequent visits.

Impending death is signaled by a series of irrevocable events (Durham & Weiss, 1997):

- The lungs become unable to provide adequate gas diffusion.
- The heart and blood vessels become unable to maintain adequate tissue perfusion.
- The brain ceases to regulate vital centers.

Cheyne-Stokes respirations (breathing characterized by periods of apnea alternating with periods of dyspnea) most often herald pulmonary system failure. Secretions accumulate in the larynx and trachea, causing noisy respirations, often called the "**death rattle**."

The heart fails in its pumping function, resulting in poor perfusion, ischemia, and cell death. The skin becomes cool and, possibly, very pale, cyanotic, jaundiced, or mottled. The pulse becomes rapid, irregular, weak, and thready. Death is several hours away if a peripheral pulse is strong and easily palpated. Cold, cyanotic extremities and irregular respirations indicate that death may be expected within an hour or two (Durham & Weiss, 1997).

Inadequate cerebral perfusion hinders the brain's ability to integrate vital functions. The client may be confused and lethargic and may respond only to direct visual, auditory, or tactile stimulation. Pupils no longer react to light and become fixed. The client may "talk" to dead loved ones. A frown or tight facial muscles may indicate pain or discomfort. A client in a coma will move only in response to deep pain. Analgesics should not be withdrawn from a client in a coma.

The care of the client does not cease during this final stage of life. The nursing actions previously described should be continued. The nurse should tell the client in brief, simple terms what is happening as care is rendered. The family should be allowed and encouraged to continue their participation, if that is their wish. The nurse should caution family members that the dying client can hear even in the absence of verbal response, so all comments and conversation should continue to be respectful.

There may be other indications that death is near. The client may report seeing angels (Ufema, 1995b) or hearing beautiful music. These experiences should be

COMMUNITY/HOME HEALTH CARE

When the Client Dies at Home (Expected Death)

The family must:

- Have a list of telephone numbers readily available,
- Have the name and telephone number of the funeral director,
- Know whom to call (physician or hospice nurse or funeral director),
- Know whom not to call (ambulance and emergency services),
- Record the time of death,
- Record the last medications given,
- Record the condition of the client during the last few hours, and
- Record the last time the client was seen by the nurse.

accepted as a natural step in the process of dying. When the final breath is taken, the heart stops beating. Within a few minutes, cerebral death (the point at which brain cells die) occurs, and brain activity ceases.

Care after Death

Caring for the deceased body and meeting the needs of the grieving family are nursing responsibilities. The body of the deceased must be treated in a way that respects the sanctity of the human body (Barbus, 1975). Nursing care includes maintaining privacy and preventing damage to the body. **Post-mortem care** is given immediately after death but before the body is moved to the mortuary.

Several physiological changes occur after death. Body temperature decreases, resulting in a lack of skin elasticity (**algor mortis**). In order to avoid skin breakdown, the nurse must therefore use caution when removing tape from the body. Another physiological change, **liver mortis**, is a bluish-purple discoloration of the skin, usually at pressure points, that is a by-product of red-blood-cell destruction. This discoloration occurs in dependent areas of the body; the nurse should therefore elevate the head to prevent discoloration associated with pooling of blood. Approximately 2 to 4 hours after death, **rigor mortis** occurs: The body stiffens due to contraction of skeletal and smooth muscles. To prevent disfiguring effects of rigor mortis, as soon as possible after death, the nurse should close the client's eyelids, insert dentures (if applicable), close the mouth, and position the body in a natural position.

In preparing the body for family viewing, the nurse strives to make the body look comfortable and natural. This means removing all tubes (if allowed) and preparing and positioning the body as previously described. After the family has viewed the body, identification tags are placed on the body's toe and wrist. The body is then placed in a plastic or fabric **shroud** (a covering for the body after death), and the shroud is tagged. Next, the body is transported to the morgue according to the agency's policy, where it is kept until it can be transported to a **mortuary** (funeral home). In some institutions, the body is kept in the room until the funeral director arrives. The nurse is also responsible for returning the deceased's possessions, such as jewelry, eyeglasses, clothing, and all other personal items, to the family.

Legal Aspects

In most states, the physician is legally responsible for determining the cause of death and signing the death certificate. The nurse may, in certain situations, be the person responsible for certifying the death. It is important for nurses to know their legal responsibilities, which are defined by their respective state boards of nursing.

Autopsy

An **autopsy** (examination of the body after death, by a pathologist to ascertain the cause of death) is mandated in situations where an unusual death has occurred. For example, an unexpected death and a violent death are circumstances that would necessitate an autopsy. Families must give consent for an autopsy to be performed in other situations. The funeral director must know whether an autopsy is to be performed.

Organ Donation

The donation of organs for transplantation is a matter that requires compassion and sensitivity from the caregivers. Health care institutions are required to have policies related to the referral of potential donors to organ procurement agencies. It is important that families of the deceased know the need for and process of organ donation. There is an inadequate supply of organs and tissues to meet the demand for transplants. The following organs and tissues are used for transplantation:

- Kidneys
- Heart
- Lungs
- Liver
- Pancreas
- Skin
- Corneas
- Bones (long bones and middle ear bones)

At the time that the family gives consent for donation, the nurse notifies the donor team that an organ is available for transplant. Time is of the essence, because the organ or tissue must be harvested and transplanted quickly to maintain viability.

Care of the Family

At the time of death, the nurse provides invaluable support to the family of the deceased. Informing the family of the circumstances surrounding the death is extremely important. The nurse provides information about viewing the body, asks the family about donating organs, and offers to contact support people (e.g., other relatives, clergy). Sometimes, the nurse must help the family with decision making regarding a funeral home, transportation, and removal of the deceased's belongings. Sensitive and compassionate interpersonal skills are essential in providing information and support to families.

Nurse's Self-Care

Working with dying clients can evoke both a personal and a professional threat in the nurse. Because many nurses are confronted with death and loss daily, grief is a common experience for nurses. Smith-Stoner and Frost (1998) describe a part of the psyche called the shadow self, where stresses are stored. Unresolved sadness is called shadow grief. Everyone has a shadow self and may have some shadow grief. Nurses often have a great deal of shadow grief, which, if not released, may cause illness and burnout. Frequent exposure to death can interfere with the nurse's effectiveness because of subsequent anxiety and denial.

Whether working in a hospice, a hospital, a long-term care facility, or the home, nurses are at particular risk for experiencing negative effects from caring for the dying. Often, nurses do not want to confront their grief and will use some of the common defenses against grieving: keeping busy, taking care of others, being strong, and suffering in silence. Nurses must avoid pretending that they do not experience grief and subsequent suffering and must instead talk about the intense emotions associated with caregiving. According to Smith-Stoner and Frost (1998), shadow grief may be starting to overwhelm a person if that person experiences the following:

- A loss of energy, spark, joy, and meaning in life
- Detachment from surroundings
- A feeling of being powerless to make a difference
- Increased smoking or drinking
- Unusual forgetfulness
- Constant criticism directed toward others
- Consistent inability to get work done
- Uncontrolled outbursts of anger
- Perception of clients and their families as objects
- Surrender of hobbies or interests

To cope with their own grief, nurses need support, education, and assistance in coping with the death of clients. Staff education should focus on decreasing staff anxiety about working with grieving clients and families; ways to seek support; and ways to provide support to coworkers. Smith-Stoner and Frost (1998) suggest the following ways to cope.

- Take time to cry with and for clients.
- Get physical: run, walk, bicycle, play tennis.
- Ask colleagues to help with tasks; do not try to be "Supernurse."
- Connect to place of worship; pray.

- Look for joy in work. Laughter is a great healer.
- Create a caring circle of friends.
- Listen to music.

Often, the nurse's fears and doubts about death and its meaning surface, causing anxiety related to feelings about mortality. Even though such feelings are normal, caring for the dying client and the client's family can be emotionally draining. Nurses must therefore remember to care for themselves.

PROFESSIONAL TIP

Care for Yourself during Grief

- Do what you do so well: care. By helping the family, you will counter your feelings of helplessness.
- Set aside some time for your own grieving.
- Allow for crying to help ease the pain.
- Know when to ask your coworkers for help.
- Call on someone you can trust, and express your feelings of grief to that person.
- Use support from within your agency—counselors, clergy, support groups.
- Find a way to say goodbye to the deceased client. Rituals bring closure, which is a necessary part of grieving.

(*Adapted from "Please Cry with Me: Six Ways to Grieve," by C. D. Reese, 1996, Nursing96, 26[8], 56.*)

SAMPLE NURSING CARE PLAN

THE CLIENT WITH A TERMINAL ILLNESS/CANCER OF THE LUNG

Mrs. O'Riley, a 78-year-old widow, was diagnosed with cancer of the lung 6 months ago. After a right lower lobectomy, she was discharged to a local skilled-care facility with plans to go home after completing her treatment. Mrs. O'Riley was transported to a cancer center for radiation therapy. After completing the treatments, she resisted the idea of going home, and discharge plans were discontinued. Mrs. O'Riley's condition is deteriorating. She now requires pain medication, is frequently short of breath, has dyspnea, and needs moderate assistance with activities of daily living because of fatigue. She frequently grimaces and says, "Oh, it hurts." Her nutritional intake is marginal because of difficulty swallowing. Mrs. O'Riley is in bed most of the day, getting up only to use the commode. She has two adult children and three grandchildren who live nearby and visit often. They are willing to help their mother get her affairs in order but she resists their efforts. The family very much wants to make their mother's remaining time as comfortable and serene as possible. However, Mrs. O'Riley sometimes defies their attempts to do so.   *continues*

Nursing Diagnosis 1 *Chronic Pain related to disease progression as evidenced by verbal statements, body language, and the need for pain medication*

PLANNING/GOALS	NURSING INTERVENTIONS	RATIONALE	EVALUATION
Mrs. O'Riley will verbalize relief from pain.	Give analgesics as ordered.	Administering regular doses of medication is more effective than waiting until the pain begins.	Mrs. O'Riley's body language and verbal statements indicate freedom from pain.
	Ask client to rate pain on a scale of 0 to 10, with 0 being no pain and 10 being severe pain, to assess the need for beginning morphine. Give morphine as ordered, titrated at increments until adequate pain relief is achieved.	Morphine is the drug of choice for severe pain associated with cancer. The client should begin morphine as soon as it is necessary.	
	Monitor for signs of sudden, acute, temporary pain (breakthrough pain). If the precipitating factor is known, give medication 30 to 60 minutes before the event. For unpredictable breakthrough pain, give the medication as soon as possible.	Breakthrough pain is often precipitated by activity or stress and requires supplemental medication.	
	Assure Mrs. O'Riley that the nurses will help her manage the pain and keep it under control. Give back massages and reposition as necessary for comfort. Assist with progressive relaxation techniques if client agrees.	Clients need reassurance that everything possible will be done to manage the pain.	
	Monitor bowel elimination.	Pain medication may cause constipation.	

continues

Nursing Diagnosis 2 *Ineffective Breathing Pattern related to diminished lung function as evidenced by dyspnea and shortness of breath*

PLANNING/GOALS	NURSING INTERVENTIONS	RATIONALE	EVALUATION
Mrs. O'Riley will be free from moderate or severe dyspnea.	Teach breathing exercises and effective coughing techniques.	Breathing exercises and coughing techniques enhance gas exchange in the alveoli.	Mrs. O'Riley breathes with ease. Dyspnea does not interfere with activities.
	Allow adequate time for physical activities. Postpone activity if dyspnea is present. Provide as much assistance as needed.	Physical exertion increases dyspnea.	
	Administer low-flow oxygen if blood gases indicate need.	Oxygen will ease the effort to breathe but will not be effective unless blood gases indicate the need.	
	Encourage client to drink 8 to 10 glasses of fluid each day.	Adequate fluid intake liquifies respiratory secretions and promotes hydration.	
	Humidify the air with a cold-water vaporizer.	Moisturized air enhances breathing.	
	Assess for signs of respiratory tract infection.	The client is at high risk for respiratory infection.	

Nursing Diagnosis 3 *Ineffective Coping related to terminal illness as evidenced by inability to communicate effectively with family members and to accept their help*

PLANNING/GOALS	NURSING INTERVENTIONS	RATIONALE	EVALUATION
Mrs. O'Riley will express her feelings openly.	Consult Mrs. O'Riley on all aspects of care, giving adequate information. Provide opportunities to express feelings. Acknowledge feelings and let Mrs. O'Riley know that crying and grieving are beneficial.	Mrs. O'Riley needs to be given as much control as she wishes to have. Letting Mrs. O'Riley express her feelings will validate those feelings—she needs to know her feelings are normal and expected.	Mrs. O'Riley is at ease with herself.

continues

| | Listen for clues indicating unfinished business that needs attention. Encourage the process of life review. | There may be something in Mrs. O'Riley's past that needs to be resolved before she can successfully cope with the business of dying. Life review is a process of reflection and pondering of one's past and accepting one's life as having had value and meaning. |
| Mrs. O'Riley will maintain a satisfying relationship with her family. | Encourage family visits. Provide privacy. | Families need privacy in order to feel free to express their emotions. |

CASE STUDY

Mrs. Jason, a 76-year-old with a history of heart failure, has been hospitalized twice within the last year and was critically ill both times. Both times, she was discharged to her home. A home health nurse and a nursing assistant make intermittent visits to monitor her condition and to help with her activities of daily living. Her husband manages the household chores. Mrs. Jason's condition is deteriorating, the shortness of breath becoming more severe. Her energy level is easily depleted, and she is having increasing difficulty getting out of bed. The family is concerned because Mrs. Jason does not have any advance directives. Any attempt to bring up the subject is met with avoidance and a change of subject.

The following questions will guide your development of a nursing care plan for the case study.

1. List the clinical manifestations you would expect Mrs. Jason to experience.
2. Identify four nursing diagnoses to utilize in planning her care.
3. Describe several nursing interventions for implementing palliative care.
4. Describe appropriate interactions with the family to ease their concerns.
5. Cite reasons that Mrs. Jason and her family might benefit from hospice services.

SUMMARY

- Loss is a universal response experienced when someone (or something) of value is no longer available.
- Grief is a psychological response to loss characterized by deep mental anguish and sorrow. Grieving people experience various stages of grief.
- The difference between normal and pathological grief is the inability of the individual to adapt to life without the loved one.
- There are five psychological stages involved in the dying process: denial, anger, bargaining, depression, and acceptance.

- Complicated grief is associated with traumatic death such as by accident, homicide, or suicide.
- Each person dies a unique death.
- Hospice care offers clients an alternative to hospitalization when aggressive medical treatment is no longer an option.
- After death, the nurse focuses on supporting the family and caring for the deceased body.
- Nurses must care for themselves in order to provide quality, compassionate care to the dying person and family.

Review Questions

1. Susan, age 11 years, was left with a distant relative 2 weeks ago. Her parents have not returned or called. Susan is experiencing a:

    a. physical loss.
    b. situational loss.
    c. maturational loss.
    d. anticipational loss.

2. Knowing that a loved one is terminally ill allows family members to begin the grieving process. This is called:

    a. complicated grief.
    b. anticipatory grief.
    c. dysfunctional grief.
    d. disenfranchised grief.

3. A defining characteristic of the NANDA nursing diagnosis *Anticipatory Grieving* is:

    a. prolonged denial or depression.
    b. unsuccessful adaptation to loss.
    c. social isolation or withdrawal from others.
    d. an expression of distress at potential loss.

4. Nursing interventions for a client who has experienced a loss are based on an understanding of:

    a. the degree of the client's depression.
    b. the anger expressed by the client.
    c. the significance of the loss to the client.
    d. the number of support groups available for the loss experienced by the client.

5. The purpose of the Patient Self-Determination Act is to:

    a. serve as an order for "do not resuscitate."
    b. designate a guardian for an incompetent client.
    c. provide a means, instead of a will, to designate what is to be done with a person's property, money, and personal possessions.
    d. provide a legal means for individuals to state those circumstances under which life-sustaining treatment should or should not be provided to them.

6. One of the major goals of hospice care is:

    a. freedom from pain and other symptoms.
    b. free care for all dying clients and their families.
    c. to cure the client using very aggressive medical treatment.
    d. to transfer all dying clients to the hospital when death is imminent.

7. Signs of impending death include:

    a. flushed skin.
    b. slower pulse rate.
    c. increased blood pressure.
    d. Cheyne-Stokes respirations.

8. The nurse must use caution when removing tape from a body because of:

    a. liver mortis.
    b. rigor mortis.
    c. algor mortis.
    d. rimas mortis.

Critical Thinking Questions

1. Find a classmate from a cultural background different from yours. How does your perception of death differ from that of your classmate?

2. Thompson (1994) asks, "Can we afford to leave death in the hands of science, or should we use the benefits of science to provide the dying with a nurturing spiritual environment that feeds the spirit while sustaining the body?" What is your response to this question? What are some ways nurses can promote a "nurturing spiritual environment"?

WEB FLASH!

- What key terms related to loss and death might you search for on the Internet (for instance grief, bereavement)?
- Is there a listing on the Internet of books, videos, or other media on self-care for caregivers to the terminally ill? Are these resources available in your local library?
- What sites can you find that offer information on hospice care?
- Search the web for "Symptoms of terminal illness"; what can you find?

BASIC NUTRITION

MAKING THE CONNECTION

Refer to the following chapters to increase your understanding of nutrition:

- **Chapter 12, Cultural Diversity and Nursing**
- **Chapter 14, The Life Cycle**
- **Chapter 27, Diagnostic Tests**

- **Procedures:** B1, Handwashing; B29, Measuring Intake and Output; I28, Administering Enteral Tube Feedings

LEARNING OBJECTIVES

Upon completion of this chapter, you should be able to:
- *Define key terms.*
- *Describe the role of the nurse in promoting proper nutrition.*
- *Explain the way the body uses nutrients.*
- *Discuss the six types of nutrients.*
- *Describe factors affecting kilocalorie needs.*
- *Explain the food guide pyramid.*
- *Explain the purposes of the Dietary Guidelines for Americans and the recommended dietary allowances (RDAs).*
- *Discuss factors influencing nutrition.*
- *Explain the dietary needs and nutritional assessments for infancy, childhood, adolescence, older adulthood, pregnancy, and lactation.*
- *Explain the relationship between health and nutrition.*
- *Discuss weight management.*
- *Explain the way to determine energy (kcal) needs.*
- *Describe three ways to promote food safety.*
- *Describe the standard hospital diets: regular, soft, liquid, mechanical, and pureed.*
- *Cite the proper procedure for serving a meal tray.*
- *List important points to follow when feeding a client.*

KEY TERMS

absorption
allergy
anabolism
anthropometric
  measurements
atherosclerosis
basal metabolism
body mass index
calorie
catabolism
cholesterol
chyme
complete protein
deglutition
dehydration
diet therapy
dietary prescription/
  order
digestion
empty calories
enriched
enteral nutrition
euglycemia
excretion
extracellular fluid
fat-soluble vitamin
fortified
gluconeogenesis
glycogenesis

glycogenolysis
hyperglycemia
hypoglycemia
incomplete protein
ingestion
insulin
interstitial fluid
intracellular fluid
ketosis
kilocalorie
lipid
mastication
metabolic rate
metabolism
monounsaturated
  fatty acid
nutrition
obesity
oxidation
parenteral nutrition
peristalsis
phospholipid
polyunsaturated
  fatty acid
satiety
triglycerides
villi
vitamin
water-soluble vitamin

INTRODUCTION

Nutrition encompasses all of the processes involved in consuming and utilizing food for energy, maintenance, and growth. These processes are ingestion, digestion, absorption, metabolism, and excretion. Much of the discussion throughout this chapter focuses on ingestion, because this is the process that the individual can control and with which the nurse can be of assistance to the client. This chapter presents basic information regarding proper nutrition and the role of the nurse in assisting clients to meet their nutritional needs. Topics covered include: specific nutrients and their functions in the body; phytochemicals; promoting proper nutrition; factors influencing nutrition; nutritional needs during the life cycle; nutrition and health; weight management; food labeling, quality, and safety; food allergies; and nutrition and the nursing process.

PHYSIOLOGY OF NUTRITION

Five processes are involved in the body's use of nutrients: ingestion, digestion, absorption, metabolism, and excretion.

Ingestion

Nutrition begins with **ingestion**, the taking of food into the digestive tract, generally through the mouth. In special circumstances, ingestion occurs directly into the stomach, through a feeding tube; this situation is discussed later in the chapter.

Digestion

Digestion refers to the mechanical and chemical processes that convert nutrients into a physically absorbable state. Mechanical digestion includes **mastication** (chewing), the breaking of food into fine particles and mixing it with enzymes in saliva; **deglutition** (swallowing of food), the peristaltic waves and mucus secretions that move the food down the esophagus. Chemical digestion is the process whereby enzymes, gastric and intestinal juices, bile, and pancreatic juices change food into the individual nutrients that can be used by the body.

Digestion begins in the stomach (except in the case of some starches, for which digestion begins in the mouth) and is completed in the intestines. **Peristalsis** (coordinated, rhythmic, serial contractions of the smooth muscles of the GI tract) forces **chyme** (an acidic, semifluid paste) through the small and large intestines. Only carbohydrates, proteins, and fats require chemical digestion to make the nutrients available for absorption. Figure 18-1 illustrates the basic elements and functions of the digestive system.

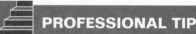

PROFESSIONAL TIP

Role of the LP/VN in Meeting Nutritional Needs

There are several aspects to the role of the licensed practical/vocational nurse (LP/VN) in meeting a client's nutritional needs. These are discussed throughout the chapter and are summarized as follows:

- Teach clients ways to meet their nutritional needs.
- Receive and implement physician's orders.
- Help clients understand their diets.
- Assist clients with eating their meals.
- Report and record observations about nutrient intake and the nutritional status of clients.
- Act as a communication link between the client, the physician, and the dietitian.

Absorption

Absorption is the process whereby the end products of digestion (i.e., individual nutrients) pass through the epithelial membranes in the small and large intestines and into the blood or lymph system. The nutrients are absorbed and taken to the parts of the body that need them. Most nutrients are water soluble and can be absorbed directly through the **villi** (fingerlike projections that line the small intestine) and into the blood. Fats, which are not water soluble, are absorbed first into the lymph system and eventually enter the circulatory system.

Metabolism

The conversion of nutrients into energy by the body is called **metabolism**; this process is the sum total of all the biological and chemical processes in the body as they relate to the use of nutrients in every body cell. Metabolism involves two processes: anabolism and catabolism. **Anabolism** is the constructive process of metabolism, wherein new molecules are synthesized and new tissues are formed, as in growth and repair. This process requires energy. **Catabolism** is the destructive process of metabolism, wherein tissues or substances are broken into their component parts. This process releases energy. During metabolism, energy is also produced by the process of **oxidation**, which is the chemical process of combining nutrients with oxygen. The energy produced by the body is used in a number of ways: electrical energy for brain and nerve activities, chemical energy for metabolism, mechanical energy for muscle contractions, and thermal energy to keep the body warm.

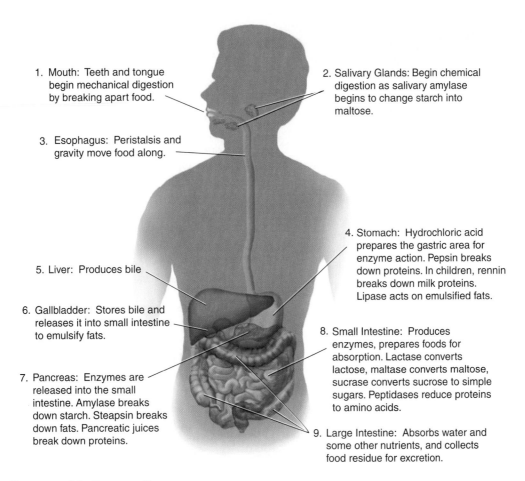

1. Mouth: Teeth and tongue begin mechanical digestion by breaking apart food.

2. Salivary Glands: Begin chemical digestion as salivary amylase begins to change starch into maltose.

3. Esophagus: Peristalsis and gravity move food along.

4. Stomach: Hydrochloric acid prepares the gastric area for enzyme action. Pepsin breaks down proteins. In children, rennin breaks down milk proteins. Lipase acts on emulsified fats.

5. Liver: Produces bile

6. Gallbladder: Stores bile and releases it into small intestine to emulsify fats.

7. Pancreas: Enzymes are released into the small intestine. Amylase breaks down starch. Steapsin breaks down fats. Pancreatic juices break down proteins.

8. Small Intestine: Produces enzymes, prepares foods for absorption. Lactase converts lactose, maltase converts maltose, sucrase converts sucrose to simple sugars. Peptidases reduce proteins to amino acids.

9. Large Intestine: Absorbs water and some other nutrients, and collects food residue for excretion.

Figure 18-1 Functions of the Digestive System

Metabolic rate is the rate of energy utilization in the body; it is expressed in units called calories. One **calorie** is the amount of heat required to raise the temperature of one gram of water by 1° Celsius. Because of the large quantity of energy released during metabolism, the energy is expressed in **kilocalories** (kcal), each of which is equal to 1,000 calories.

Basal metabolism is the amount of energy needed to maintain essential physiologic functions, such as respiration, circulation, and muscle tone, when a person is at *complete* rest, both physically and mentally.

The major factor affecting basal metabolism is body composition. Lean muscle tissue has a higher metabolic rate and thus produces more energy than does fatty tissue. Generally, women have a lower metabolism than men because they have a higher percentage of fat tissue. However, metabolism increases during menstruation, pregnancy, and lactation. Age is also an influence, because growth periods increase metabolism. Glandular activity, especially of the thyroid gland, affects metabolism. The rate of metabolism is governed primarily by the hormones triiodothyronine (T_3) and thyroxine (T_4). Hypothyroid activity, a decrease in the secretion of thyroid hormones, causes a lower rate of metabolism, whereas hyperthyroid activity, an increase in the secretion of thyroid hormones, causes a higher rate of metabolism.

Excretion

Excretion is the process of eliminating or removing waste products from the body. Dietary fiber and other indigestible materials, salts, and other products such as bile and water are formed into feces and excreted from the body as solid waste. Other excretory organs that aid the digestive system in the elimination of wastes includes the kidneys, bladder, sweat glands, skin, and lungs. Most liquid waste is sent through the kidneys and bladder to be excreted as urine. Some liquid waste is removed through the sweat glands of the skin as perspiration. Gaseous waste is eliminated through the lungs.

NUTRIENTS

The body must have six types of nutrients to function efficiently and effectively. These are water, carbohydrates, fats, proteins, vitamins, and minerals. If a person eats a well-balanced diet, all the nutrients the body requires are provided by the food. Table 18–1

Table 18–1 NUTRIENTS, FUEL VALUES, AND DAILY REQUIREMENTS		
NUTRIENT	**FUEL VALUE**	**DAILY REQUIREMENTS**
Water	0	1,000 mL/1,000 kcal eaten
Carbohydrates	1 g = 4 kcal	50% to 60% total kcal per day
Fats	1 g = 9 kcal	25% to 30% total kcal per day
Protein	1 g = 4 kcal	15% to 20% total kcal per day

offers an overview of the first four nutrients in relation to their fuel value (the amount of energy they supply) and their daily requirements.

Nutrients are classified as energy nutrients, organic nutrients, and inorganic nutrients, as shown in Table 18–2.

Energy nutrients release energy for use by the body. Organic nutrients build and maintain body tissues and regulate body processes. Inorganic nutrients provide a medium for the body's chemical reactions, transport materials, maintain body temperature, promote bone formation, and conduct nerve impulses.

The functions of the nutrients are interrelated. Intake changes in one nutrient may lead to functional changes in another. Some examples of interrelated functions are as follows: Iron is better absorbed when vitamin C is present, and calcium absorption depends on the presence of vitamin D.

Water

Water is the most important nutrient. It is more vital to life than is food. Virtually all body functions require water. An individual may live for weeks without food, but for only approximately 10 days without water.

Water is the major constituent in every cell of the body. Approximately 50% to 60% of an adult's weight is due to water, and approximately 70% to 75% of an infant's weight is water. The body's water content decreases with age.

Approximately two-thirds of the water in the body is **intracellular fluid** (ICF), fluid within the cells. The other one-third is **extracellular fluid** (ECF), fluid outside the cells, including plasma fluid, lymph, cerebrospinal fluid, **interstitial fluid** (fluid in tissue spaces around each cell), and GI fluids.

Daily Requirements

The amount of water needed by the body varies based on environmental factors, such as temperature and humidity, and physical factors, such as activity level, metabolic need, functional losses (urine and feces), age, respiratory rate, and state of health. Higher environmental temperatures and vigorous physical activity cause more water loss as perspiration increases. Water lost must be replaced to maintain metabolism. Generally, 1,000 mL of water is needed to process every 1,000 kcal eaten.

A state of relative water balance exists when the body has adequate fluid distributed appropriately as ICF and ECF. A person's daily water intake and output should be equal (Figure 18-2). Excessive intake of fluids is not a problem in a healthy individual; more intake simply causes more output.

Table 18–2 CLASSIFICATION OF NUTRIENTS	
CLASSES	**NUTRIENTS**
Energy nutrients	Carbohydrates
	Fats
	Proteins
Organic nutrients	Carbohydrates
	Fats
	Proteins
	Vitamins
Inorganic nutrients	Water
	Minerals

From Fundamentals of Nursing: Standards & Practice, *by S. DeLaune and P. Ladner, 1998, Albany, NY: Delmar. Copyright 1998 by Delmar.*

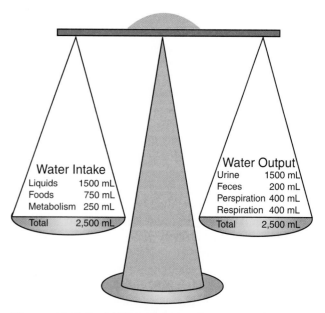

Figure 18-2 Body Water Balance (Approximate figures for a sedentary adult)

Functions

Water has many functions in the body:

- *Solvent:* Water is the liquid in which many substances are dissolved to form solutions.
- *Transporter:* Water carries nutrients, wastes, and other materials throughout the body and to and from each cell via blood, tissue fluids, and body secretions.
- *Regulator of body temperature:* Water is excreted as perspiration when the temperature goes up. Evaporation of perspiration cools the body.
- *Lubricant:* Water is a component of fluid within the joints, called synovial fluid, which provides for smooth movement of the many joints in the body.
- *Component of all cells:* Water gives structure and form to the body.
- *Hydrolysis:* Water breaks apart substances, especially in metabolism.

Classification and Sources

There are three sources of water for the body:

- Liquids consumed, including water, coffee, juice, tea, milk, and soft drinks.
- Foods consumed, especially vegetables and fruits.
- Metabolism, which produces water when oxidization occurs.

Digestion, Absorption, and Storage

Water is not digested but, rather, is absorbed and used by the body as we drink it. It cannot be stored by the body and is excreted daily. Water losses are classified as sensible, that is, the person is aware of the loss, or insensible, that is, the person is not generally aware of the loss. There are four ways the body normally loses water:

- *Urine:* accounts for the greatest amount of water lost from the body (sensible loss)
- *Feces:* contains a small amount of water (insensible loss, except in cases of diarrhea)
- *Perspiration:* varies with temperature, but some fluid is always lost (insensible or sensible loss)
- *Respiration:* releases moisture with every breath (insensible loss)

LIFE CYCLE CONSIDERATIONS

Dehydration

Infants, small children, and elderly persons are more susceptible to dehydration. For them, dehydration occurs more rapidly and is more severe.

PROFESSIONAL TIP

Signs and Symptoms of Dehydration

- Health history reveals inadequate intake of fluids.
- Urine output is decreased.
- Urine specific gravity is > 1.035.
- Weight loss (% body weight) is 3% to 5% for mild, 6% to 9% for moderate, and 10% to 15% for severe dehydration.
- Eyes appear sunken; tongue displays increased furrows and fissures.
- Oral mucous membranes are dry.
- Skin turgor is decreased.
- Venous filling and emptying times are delayed (> 3 to 5 seconds).
- In infants, fontanels are sunken.
- Changes in neurological status may occur with moderate to severe dehydration.

(*From* Health Assessment & Physical Examination (*2nd ed.*), by M. E. Z. Estes, 2002, Albany, NY: Delmar. Copyright 2002 by Delmar.)

Signs of Deficiency and Excess

Abnormal water losses from the body include profuse sweating, vomiting, diarrhea, hemorrhage, wound drainage (burns), fever, and edema. With edema, the water is still in the body, but is not useable.

A deficiency of water is called **dehydration**. Prolonged dehydration results in death.

Some conditions cause an excessive accumulation of fluid in the body. This condition is called *positive water balance.* It occurs when more water is taken in than is used and excreted, and edema results. Hypothyroidism, congestive heart failure, hypoproteinemia (low amounts of protein), some infections and cancers, and some renal conditions can cause such water retention because sodium is not being excreted normally.

Carbohydrates

Carbohydrates are made of the elements carbon, hydrogen, and oxygen. In nutrition, the first letters of these three elements are used as the abbreviation: CHO.

Carbohydrates constitute the chief source of energy for all body functions. They are also the major food source for all people, because they are the least expensive and the most abundant foods.

Daily Requirements

It is recommended that carbohydrates make up 50% to 60% of an individual's kcal intake per day. For example, if an individual's total energy requirement is 2,000 kcal, 50% of this number is 1,000; this number is then divided by 4 (the number of kcal in each gram of carbohydrate, refer to Table 18–1), for an estimated carbohydrate requirement of 250 g/day. It is estimated that current U.S. diets contain only 45% of their kcal from carbohydrates (Townsend & Roth, 2000).

Functions

Carbohydrates constitute the primary source of energy for the body. The body must maintain a constant supply of energy; therefore, it stores approximately one-half a day's supply of carbohydrates in the liver and muscles for use as needed. A sufficient supply of carbohydrates spares proteins from being used for energy, thus allowing proteins to perform their primary function of building and repairing body tissues. Carbohydrates are needed to oxidize fats completely and for the synthesis of fatty acids and amino acids. The central nervous system and erythrocytes rely solely on carbohydrates for energy.

Classification and Sources

Carbohydrates are classified as either simple or complex. Simple carbohydrates are single sugars (monosaccharides) such as glucose, fructose, and galactose found in fruits, honey, and corn syrup. Monosaccharides require no digestion and are quickly absorbed. They are either used immediately for energy or stored as glycogen.

Double sugars (disaccharides), such as sucrose, maltose, and lactose, are two single sugars joined together. They are found in milk, sweeteners, sugar, and molasses. Before they can be absorbed by the body, disaccharides must be separated into monosaccharides through digestion.

Complex carbohydrates (polysaccharides) are composed of many single sugars joined together. Those important in nutrition are starch, glycogen, and dietary fiber (cellulose). The most significant of these polysaccharides in the diet is starch, which is found in grains, grain products, legumes, potatoes, and other vegetables. Complex carbohydrates are digested much more slowly than the simple carbohydrates, and they thus supply the body with energy for a longer period of time.

Glycogen does not come from the foods we eat. Rather, it is a form of carbohydrate made by the liver and stored in the liver and muscles. The body keeps a 12- to 48-hour store of glycogen. This reserve is used between meals and during sleep to maintain **euglycemia** (normal blood glucose level) for body functions. **Glycogenesis** is the process of converting glucose to glycogen. **Glycogenolysis** is the process of changing the glycogen back to glucose when it is needed by the body for energy. **Insulin** is a pancreatic hormone necessary for cells to produce energy and for the liver to produce and store glycogen. Glucose metabolism depends on the availability of insulin.

Dietary fiber has no nutritive value: The human body is unable to digest it. There are two types of dietary fiber: soluble and insoluble. Soluble dietary fiber slows gastric emptying and binds bile acids and cholesterol. This fiber provides **satiety** (a feeling of adequate fullness from food) and lowers the cholesterol level in the blood. Insoluble dietary fiber holds water, which increases fecal bulk and stimulates peristalsis for better elimination. Good sources of both kinds of dietary fiber are whole grains, whole grain products, legumes, and fruits and vegetables with their skins.

Digestion, Absorption, and Storage

Digestion of cooked starches begins in the mouth, when the salivary enzyme ptyalin mixes with the starch in food during chewing. Little digestion takes place in the stomach. Carbohydrate digestion is completed in the small intestine by pancreatic and intestinal enzymes present there. Carbohydrates are used completely, leaving no waste for the kidneys to eliminate.

Glucose and other monosaccharides, the final products of carbohydrate digestion, are absorbed into the blood through the capillaries in the villi of the intestinal mucosa. Fructose and other monosaccharides are converted to glucose in the liver.

Glucose not needed for immediate energy is converted to glycogen by the liver and stored there and in the muscles. Any remaining glucose is then converted to fatty acids and stored as adipose tissue (fat). The body has no way to rid itself of excess carbohydrates; they are either used or stored.

Signs of Deficiency and Excess

A mild deficiency of carbohydrates can result in weight loss and fatigue. A diet seriously deficient in carbohydrates could cause **ketosis**, a condition wherein acids called *ketones* accumulate in the blood and urine, upsetting the acid–base balance. Ketones are produced

PROFESSIONAL TIP

Insulin Levels and the Client Who Is Diabetic

When the secretion of insulin is impaired or absent, the glucose level in the blood becomes excessively high. This condition is called **hyperglycemia** and is usually a symptom of diabetes mellitus. If control by diet is ineffective, insulin injections or an oral hypoglycemic must be used to control blood sugar. When insulin is given, the client's intake of carbohydrates must be carefully controlled to balance the prescribed dosage of insulin. When blood glucose levels are unusually low, **hypoglycemia** results. A mild form of hypoglycemia may occur if one waits too long between meals or if the pancreas secretes too much insulin. Symptoms include fatigue, shaking, sweating, and headache.

PROFESSIONAL TIP

Lactose Intolerance

Many adults are unable to digest lactose and suffer from bloating, abdominal cramps, and diarrhea after drinking milk or consuming milk-based food products such as processed cheese. This reaction is called lactose intolerance. It is caused by insufficient lactase, the enzyme required for digestion of lactose. Special low-lactose milk products can be used instead of regular milk. Lactase-containing products are also available.

when fat oxidation in cells is incomplete. This situation results from an inadequate intake of carbohydrates, which causes an emergency need for energy. Because there are insufficient carbohydrates to fulfill the body's energy needs, an abnormally large amount of fat is metabolized. Ketosis can result from uncontrolled insulin-dependent diabetes mellitus, starvation, or diets extremely low in carbohydrates. It can lead to coma and even death.

Excess carbohydrate consumption is one of the most common causes of obesity. Although some of the surplus carbohydrate is changed to glycogen, the major part of any surplus becomes adipose tissue. Too many carbohydrates may cause tooth decay, irritate the lining of the stomach, or cause flatulence.

Fats

Fats constitute the most concentrated source of energy in the diet. People in developed countries tend to eat diets relatively high in fat. Although fat is an essential nutrient, too much fat is a hazard to good health. The descriptive word for fats of all kinds is *lipids*. **Lipids** are organic compounds that are insoluble in water but soluble in organic solvents, such as ether and alcohol, and include true fats and fatlike compounds such as lipoids and sterols. Fats provide slightly more than twice the calorie content of carbohydrates. Refer back to Table 18–1 for the fuel values and requirements of fats in the diet. Like carbohydrates, fats are composed of carbon, hydrogen, and oxygen, but they have a substantially lower proportion of oxygen.

Daily Requirements

It is recommended that fats make up no more than 25% to 30% of an individual's caloric intake per day. For example, assuming that one's total energy requirement is 2,000 kcal/day, one-quarter (25%) of this would be 500 kcal. Dividing 500 kcal by 9 (the number of kcal in each gram of fat; see Table 18–1) yields an estimated fat requirement of 55.5g/day.

CLIENT TEACHING

Fats

No more than 10% of total kcal should be provided by saturated fats in the diet.

Currently, it is estimated that most American diets obtain 40% to 45% of their kcal from fat.

Functions

Fat has many functions in the body. Fat:

- Provides a concentrated source of energy (more than twice the kcal of carbohydrates);
- Assists in the absorption of fat-soluble vitamins;
- Is a major component of cell membranes and myelin sheaths;
- Improves the flavor of food and delays the stomach's emptying time, providing a feeling of satiety;
- Protects and helps hold organs in place; and
- Insulates the body thus assisting in temperature maintenance.

Classifications and Sources

Fat is formed by one molecule of glycerol being joined to one, two, or three fatty-acid molecules. The most important lipids are as follows:

- **Triglycerides** (true fats), which are composed of one glycerol molecule attached to three fatty-acid molecules. Most dietary fat and body fat are triglycerides.
- **Phospholipids** (lipoids), which are composed of glycerol, fatty acids, and phosphorus. They are structural components of cells, for example myelin (insulating covering of many nerves) and lecithin (a part of cell membranes).
- **Cholesterol** (a sterol), which is not essential in the diet because the liver manufactures approximately 1,000 mg every day. Cholesterol is found in all cell membranes, in brain and nerve tissue, and in blood, and it is excreted in bile. Cholesterol is required for the production of several hormones including estrogen, testosterone, adrenalin, and cortisone. The intake of dietary cholesterol from such sources as animal food products may affect the serum (blood) cholesterol level.

Fats can also be classified by source, visibility, and saturation. The source of fats can be either animal or plant (vegetable). Examples of animal fat are lard, butter, milk, cream, egg yolks, and the fat in meat, poultry, and fish. Examples of plant fat are oils (corn, safflower, olive, cottonseed, peanut, palm, and coconut), nuts, and avocado.

Fats are either visible or invisible. Visible fats are easy to identify, such as butter, oils, margarine, lard, shortening, bacon, salt pork, and the fat around beef. Examples of hidden or invisible fats are those in egg yolks, whole-milk and whole milk products, cheeses, nuts, seeds, olives, avocados, many desserts, and baked goods.

The saturation of a fat refers to its chemical composition. When fatty acids, the main building blocks of fats, contain all of the hydrogen ions possible in the molecule, they are said to be saturated. Saturated fats tend to be solid at room temperature. Generally, animal fats are saturated. Plant fats that are saturated are coconut, palm kernel, and palm oils. Unsaturated fats are missing a hydrogen ion at one or more places in the molecule. They tend to be soft or liquid at room temperature. Plant fats are generally unsaturated, with the exceptions already mentioned. Unsaturated fats are subdivided into monounsaturated and polyunsaturated fats. **Monounsaturated fatty acids** are fatty acids that form glycerol esters with one double or triple bond; foods in this category are nuts, fowl, and olive oil. **Polyunsaturated fatty acids** form glycerol esters that have many carbons unbonded to hydrogen atoms. Foods such as fish, corn, sunflower seeds, soybeans, cottonseeds, and safflower oil contain polyunsaturated fat.

There are three essential fatty acids (linoleic, linolenic, and arachidonic) necessary for growth, cholesterol metabolism, and heart action. They are found primarily in vegetable oils, egg yolks, and poultry.

Digestion, Absorption, and Storage

No chemical breakdown of fats occurs in the mouth, and very little fat digestion takes place in the stomach. When fat reaches the small intestine, digestion begins. The digestive agents for fat are bile, from the gallbladder, and enzymes, from the pancreas and the small intestine. The final products of fat digestion are fatty acids and glycerol. Approximately 95% of dietary fat is absorbed in the small intestine.

Fats not immediately needed by the body are stored as adipose tissue. Approximately 5 g of fat are excreted daily in the feces.

CLIENT TEACHING

Blood Cholesterol
- Blood cholesterol level should not exceed 200 mg of cholesterol/dL of blood.
- To decrease the blood cholesterol level, the client must follow a diet low in saturated fat.
- Weight loss and exercise will also help lower blood cholesterol level.
- A diet high in saturated fat increases the blood cholesterol by 15% to 25%.

LIFE CYCLE CONSIDERATIONS

Children and Cholesterol
If children are not fed high-cholesterol foods on a regular basis, their chance of overusing these foods as adults lessens, as does their risk of heart attack and stroke.

Signs of Deficiency and Excess

Deficiency symptoms occur when fats provide less than 10% of the total daily kcal requirement. Gross deficiency may result in eczema (inflamed and scaly skin condition), retarded growth, and weight loss.

Excess fat in the diet can lead to overweight and heart disease. In addition, studies point to an association between high-fat diets and cancers of the colon, breast, uterus, and prostate.

An elevated level of cholesterol in the blood is thought to be a contributing factor in heart disease, because hypercholesterolemia (high serum cholesterol) is common in clients with atherosclerosis. **Atherosclerosis** is a cardiovascular disease wherein plaque (fatty deposits containing cholesterol and other substances) forms on the inside of artery walls, reducing the space for blood flow.

Protein

Proteins are made of the elements carbon, hydrogen, oxygen, and nitrogen. In nutrition, the first letters of these four elements are used as the abbreviation: CHON.

Protein is the only nutrient that can build, repair, and maintain body tissues. An adequate supply of proteins in the daily diet is essential. All tissues and fluids in the body with the exception of bile and urine, contain some protein. The basic building materials of protein are amino acids. Refer to Table 18–1 for the fuel value and requirements of protein.

Daily Requirements

Daily protein requirement is determined by size, age, gender, and physical and emotional condition. A large person has more body cells to maintain than does a small person. A growing child, a pregnant

LIFE CYCLE CONSIDERATIONS

Proteins
By the age of 4 years, body protein content reaches the adult level of approximately 18% of body weight.

PROFESSIONAL TIP

Daily Allowance of Protein

The National Research Council recommends that protein intake represent no more than 15% to 20% of one's daily kcal intake and not exceed double the amount given in the table of Recommended Dietary Allowances (Appendix C).

woman, or a woman who is breastfeeding needs more protein for each pound of body weight than does the average adult. When digestion is inefficient, fewer amino acids are absorbed by the body; consequently the protein requirement is higher. This is sometimes thought to be the case with elderly clients. Extra proteins are usually required after surgery or severe burns or during infections in order to replace lost tissue and manufacture antibodies. In addition, emotional trauma can cause the body to excrete more nitrogen than it normally does, thus increasing the need for protein-rich foods.

The National Research Council of the National Academy of Sciences considers the average adult's daily requirement to be 0.8 g of protein for each kilogram of body weight. Daily protein requirement is determined by multiplying body weight in kilograms (weight in pounds divided by 2.2) by 0.8. For instance:

$$130 \text{ lb. woman} \div 2.2 \text{ lb/kg} = 59./kg \times 0.8 \text{ g/kg}$$
$$= 47.3 \text{ g protein/day}$$

Recommended dietary allowances of protein are listed in the appendices.

Functions

The primary function of protein in the diet is to provide the amino acids necessary for the synthesis of body proteins, which are used to build, repair, and maintain the body tissues. Protein composes most of the muscles, skin, hair, nails, brain, nerves, and internal organs.

Another function of protein is to assist in regulating fluid balance. Proteins are a vital part of enzymes, hormones, and blood plasma. Many body processes are regulated by enzymes and hormones. Plasma proteins help control water balance between the circulatory system and surrounding tissues. Protein is also used to build antibodies, which help defend the body against disease and foreign substances.

In the event of insufficient stores of carbohydrate and fat (the body's primary and secondary sources of energy), protein, in the form of amino acids, can be converted into glucose and used for energy. This process is called **gluconeogenesis**. However, when pro-

tein is used for energy, it is not available for its primary function. Using protein for energy also results in waste products that are difficult for the kidneys to excrete.

Classification and Sources

Protein is classified by source and completeness. Animal sources include meat, fish, poultry, eggs, milk, and dairy products. Plant sources are grains, legumes, nuts, and seeds.

The completeness of a protein refers to its quality. Of the 22 amino acids, 9 are called essential amino acids, that is, they must be present in the diet because the body cannot synthesize them. **Complete proteins** contain all 9 essential amino acids. All animal proteins, with the exception of gelatin, are complete proteins; the only complete plant protein is soy beans.

Plant proteins (with the exception of soy beans) are **incomplete proteins**; that is one or more of the essential amino acids are missing. Because all plant proteins do not lack the same essential amino acids, they can be combined in various ways to provide all of the essential amino acids. When two plant protein foods are combined to provide the essential amino acids, they are said to be complementary. Some of the common complementary plant proteins are rice and beans (legumes); corn and beans; wheat bread and beans; toast and pea soup; and rice and lentils. Complementary proteins are a very important part of planning a healthy vegetarian diet.

Digestion, Absorption, and Storage

Chemical digestion of protein begins in the stomach, with hydrochloric acid activating the enzyme pepsin. However, most of the digestion takes place in the small intestine through the action of pancreatic and intestinal enzymes. The end products of protein digestion are amino acids. The body can then combine the amino acids to build, repair, and maintain body tissues.

The amino acids are absorbed into the blood by the capillaries in the villi of the intestinal mucosa. Amino acids not used to build proteins are converted to glucose, glycogen, or fat and are stored.

Signs of Deficiency and Excess

When people are unable to obtain an adequate supply of protein for an extended period, muscle wasting occurs, and arms and legs become very thin. At the same time, albumin (protein in blood plasma) deficiency causes edema, resulting in an extremely swollen appearance. The water is excreted when sufficient protein is eaten. People may lose appetite, strength, and weight, and wounds may heal very slowly. Clients suffering from edema become lethargic and depressed. These signs are seen in grossly neglected children or in the elderly poor or incapacitated.

PROFESSIONAL TIP

Vegetarians and Protein

It is essential that clients following vegetarian diets carefully calculate the types and amount of protein in their diets so as to prevent protein deficiency.

LIFE CYCLE CONSIDERATIONS

Vitamins

Vitamin needs vary with the life cycle. Vitamin supplements are generally needed for pregnant or lactating women, infants, and elders.

People suffering from protein energy malnutrition lack both protein and energy-rich foods. Such a condition is not uncommon in developing countries where there are long-term shortages of both protein and energy foods. Children who lack sufficient protein do not grow to their potential size. Infants born to mothers eating insufficient protein during pregnancy can have permanently impaired mental capacities (Townsend & Roth, 2000).

Two deficiency diseases that affect children are caused by a grossly inadequate supply of protein, energy, or both. Marasmus, a condition resulting from severe malnutrition, afflicts very young children who lack both energy and protein foods as well as vitamins and minerals. The infant with marasmus appears emaciated but does not have edema; hair is dull and dry, and the skin is thin and wrinkled. Kwashiorkor results when there is a sudden or recent lack of protein-containing food (such as during a famine). This disease results in edema, painful skin lesions, and changes in the pigmentation of skin and hair (Townsend & Roth, 2000).

It is easy for people living in the developed parts of the world to ingest more protein than the body requires. There are a number of reasons this should be avoided. The saturated fats and cholesterol common to complete protein foods may contribute to heart disease and provide more kcal than are desirable. Some studies seem to indicate a connection between long-term high-protein diets and colon cancer and high calcium excretion, which depletes the bones of calcium and may contribute to osteoporosis. People who eat excessive amounts of protein-rich foods may ignore essential fruits and vegetables, and excess protein intake may put more demands on the kidneys than they can handle (Townsend & Roth, 2000).

Vitamins

Vitamins are organic compounds essential to life and health. They regulate body processes and are needed in very small amounts. They have no fuel value but are required for the metabolism of fats, carbohydrates, and proteins.

Daily Requirements

The Food and Nutrition Board of the National Academy of Sciences—National Research Council has pre-

pared a list of recommended dietary allowances for the 11 vitamins for which it considers current scientific research to be adequate for determining daily recommendations (Appendix C). Vitamin allowances are given by weight in milligrams (mg) or micrograms (μg or mcg).

Vitamins taken in addition to the vitamins received in the diet are called vitamin supplements. Lifestyle choices may affect the need for vitamin supplementation; refer to Table 18–3.

Functions

The functions of vitamins are unique to each individual vitamin. Tables 18–4 and 18–5 list the functions of each type of vitamin.

Classification and Sources

Vitamins are commonly grouped according to solubility. Vitamins A, D, E, and K are fat soluble, and vitamin C and the B-complex vitamins are water soluble; refer to Tables 18–4 and 18–5.

Fat-Soluble Vitamins The **fat-soluble vitamins** (A, D, E, and K) require the presence of fats for their absorption from the GI tract into the lymphatic system and for cellular metabolism. They must attach to protein carriers to be transported through the blood. Excess intake is not excreted but, rather, is stored in the liver and adipose tissue. The body's stored reserve makes daily intake unnecessary. In fact, the reserve can result in toxic levels if large supplemental doses are taken, especially in the case of vitamin A. Deficiencies can occur in conditions that interfere with fat absorption.

Table 18–3 SUPPLEMENTS FOR LIFESTYLE CHOICES	
LIFESTYLE CHOICE	**SUGGESTED SUPPLEMENT**
Restricted diets	B₁₂ (cobalamin)
Extensive exercise program	Riboflavin
Oral contraceptives	Pyridoxine, niacin, vitamin C
Smoking	Vitamin C
Alcohol	Thiamine, folate
Caffeine	B vitamins, vitamin C

Table 18–4 FAT-SOLUBLE VITAMINS

VITAMIN	FUNCTION	SOURCES	DEFICIENCY	TOXIC EFFECTS
A	• Aids in night vision • Promotes growth of bones and teeth • Maintains skin and mucous membranes	• Fish oils • Carrots • Sweet potatoes • Broccoli • Cantaloupe • Green leafy vegetables	• Night blindness • Dry, scaly skin • Diarrhea • Respiratory infections	• From supplementation: anorexia, diarrhea, hair loss, bone pain, liver damage
D	• Stimulates absorption of calcium and phosphorus for good bone mineralization	• Yeast • Fish liver oils • Fortified milk and cereals	• Rickets • Malformed teeth • Bone deformities	• Hypercalcemia • Kidney stones • Cardiovascular damage
E	• Acts as an antioxidant • Maintains cell membrane integrity • Protects red blood cells (RBCs) from hemolysis	• Vegetable oils • Leafy vegetables • Wheat germ	• Increased RBC hemolysis • Rare, except in cases of fat malabsorption	• Depression • Fatigue • Diarrhea • Cramps • Headaches
K	• Responsible for synthesis of prothrombin, needed for normal blood clotting	• Dark-green leafy vegetables • Made by intestinal bacteria	• Rare, except in newborns • Delayed blood clotting	• No toxic effects

Table 18–5 WATER-SOLUBLE VITAMINS

VITAMIN	FUNCTION	SOURCES	DEFICIENCY	TOXIC EFFECTS
C (asorbic acid)	• Builds and maintains strong tissues • Promotes wound healing • Aids in resisting infection • Enhances iron absorption	• Citrus fruits • Green and red peppers • Tomatoes • Melons • Cabbage • Broccoli • Strawberries	• Scurvy • Easy bruising • Delayed wound healing • Swollen, inflamed gums • Secondary infections	• Megadoses: excessive iron absorption • Nausea • Diarrhea
B_1 (thiamine)	• Promotes CHO metabolism • Ensures normal nervous system functioning	• Enriched grains and cereals • Pork • Legumes	• Beriberi • Mental confusion • Anorexia • Fatigue • Muscle weakness	• None known
B_2 (riboflavin)	• Promotes CHO, protein, and fat metabolism • Promotes deoxyribonucleic acid (DNA) synthesis • Aids in protein synthesis	• Milk and milk products • Meat, poultry, fish • Enriched grains and cereals	• Oral lesions • Dermatitis • Cheilosis • Red, swollen tongue • Reddening of cornea	• None known

continues

Table 18–5 WATER-SOLUBLE VITAMINS *continued*

VITAMIN	FUNCTION	SOURCES	DEFICIENCY	TOXIC EFFECTS
Niacin (nicotinic acid)	• Aids in oxidation • Promotes CHO, protein, and fat metabolism • Aids tissue protein building	• Meat, poultry, fish • Legumes • Enriched grains • Peanuts	• Pellegra • Anorexia • Apathy • Weakness • Dermatitis • Diarrhea • Dementia	• Large doses: flushing, itching, hypotension, tachycardia
B_6 (pyridoxine)	• Is necessary for amino acid metabolism • Promotes blood formation • Maintains nervous tissue	• Chicken, fish, pork • Eggs • Whole grains	• Depression • Dermatitis • Abnormal brain wave patterns • Convulsions • Anemia	• Clumsiness • Nerve degeneration
B_{12} (cobolomin)	• Promotes normal function of all cells, especially those of the nervous system • Promotes blood formation • Promotes CHO, protein, and fat metabolism • Aids in synthesis of ribonucleic acid (RNA) and DNA • Is necessary for folate metabolism	• Fresh shrimp, oysters, meats, milk, eggs, and cheese	• Pernicious anemia • Anorexia • Indigestion • Paresthesia of hands and feet • Poor coordination • Depression	• None known
Folate (folic acid)	• Is necessary for synthesis of RNA and DNA • Promotes amino acid metabolism, RBC and white blood cell (WBC) formation • Prevents neural tube defects	• Green leafy vegetables • Milk • Eggs • Yeast	• Glossitis • Diarrhea • Macrocytic anemia	• None known
Pantothenic acid	• Promotes CHO, protein, and fat metabolism	• Animal tissues • Whole-grain cereals • Legumes • Milk	• Not observed in humans	• None known
Biotin	• Promotes CHO and fat metabolism • Is necessary for glycogen formation	• Egg yolk • Yeast • Milk • Soy flours • Cereals • Legumes • Made by intestinal bacteria	• Only induced with long-term total parenteral nutrition (TPN)	• None known

Water-Soluble Vitamins The **water-soluble vitamins** (C and the B-complex vitamins) require daily ingestion in normal quantities because they are not stored in the body. They are absorbed by the capillaries in the intestinal villi directly into the circulatory system. When consumed in excess of the body's need, they are excreted in the urine. Deficiency symptoms develop quickly in response to inadequate intake. Foods should be cooked in the least amount of water possible, because the water-soluble vitamins are released

CLIENT TEACHING

Natural or Synthetic Vitamins

Some people believe that natural vitamins are superior in quality to synthetic vitamins. According to the U.S. Food and Drug Administration (FDA), however, the body cannot distinguish between a vitamin of plant or animal origin and one manufactured in a laboratory. The two types of the same vitamin are chemically identical.

into the cooking water: When the water is discarded, the vitamins are lost.

Digestion, Absorption, and Storage

Vitamins do not require digestion. Fat-soluble vitamins are absorbed into the lymphatic system, whereas water-soluble vitamins are absorbed directly into the circulatory system. Excess amounts of fat-soluble vitamins cannot be excreted but are stored in the liver and adipose tissue. Water-soluble vitamins are excreted through urine, when excess amounts are taken into the body.

Signs of Deficiency or Excess

Vitamin deficiencies can occur and result in disease. Those persons inclined to vitamin deficiencies because they do not eat balanced diets include alcoholics; the poor; incapacitated elders; clients with serious diseases that affect appetite; mentally retarded persons; and young children who receive inadequate care. Deficiencies of fat-soluble vitamins occur in clients with chronic malabsorption diseases such as cystic fibrosis, celiac disease, and Crohn's disease.

Vitamins consumed in excess amounts can be toxic to the body; refer to Tables 18–4 and 18–5.

PROFESSIONAL TIPS

Enriched or Fortified Foods

Foods that have synthetic vitamins added to them during processing are labeled as enriched, or fortified. An example is milk, which frequently has vitamins A and D added to it.

Minerals

Minerals are inorganic elements that help regulate body processes and/or serve as structural components of the body. Like vitamins they have no fuel value (refer to Table 18–1).

Chemical analysis shows that the human body is made up of specific chemical elements. Four of these elements—oxygen, carbon, hydrogen, and nitrogen—make up 96% of body weight. All the remaining elements are minerals, which represent only 4% of body weight. Nevertheless, these minerals are essential for good health.

Daily Requirements

Major minerals are required in amounts greater than 100 mg/day. Trace minerals are those required in amounts less than 100 mg/day.

Functions

The functions of minerals are unique to each individual mineral. Table 18–6 outlines the functions of each mineral.

Classification and Sources

Minerals are generally classified as major minerals and trace elements (Table 18–7). The major minerals occur in large amounts in the body and the required intake is greater than for the trace elements.

Table 18–6 MINERALS

MINERAL	FUNCTION	SOURCES	DEFICIENCY	TOXIC EFFECTS
Calcium (Ca)	• Aids in bone and teeth formation • Promotes muscle contraction and relaxation • Aids blood clotting • Aids in nerve transmission • Promotes normal heart rhythm • Needs vitamin D for absorption	• Milk • Cheese • Sardines • Salmon • Green leafy vegetables • Whole grains	• Rickets • Osteoporosis • Tetany • Poor tooth formation	• Kidney stones • Deposits in joints and soft tissue • May inhibit iron and zinc absorption

continues

Table 18–6 MINERALS *continued*

VITAMIN	FUNCTION	SOURCES	DEFICIENCY	TOXIC EFFECTS
Phosphorus (P)	• Aids in bone and teeth formation • Involved in energy metabolism • Regulates acid–base balance • Ensures structure of cell membranes • Is part of nucleic acids	• Fish, beef, pork, poultry • Cheese • Legumes • Milk • Carbonated beverages	• Rickets • Osteoporosis • Poor tooth formation • Disturbed acid base balance	• Low serum calcium • Kidney stones
Sodium (Na)	• Helps regulate fluid balance and acid–base balance • Regulates cell membrane irritability • Regulates nerve transmission	• Table salt • Milk • Meat • Processed foods • Carrots • Celery	• Hyponatremia • Nausea • Headache • Mental confusion • Hypotension • Anxiety • Muscle spasms	• Hypernatremia • Hypertension • Cardiovascular disturbance • Edema
Potassium (K)	• Maintains fluid balance • Maintains acid–base balance • Regulates muscle activity • Aids in protein synthesis • Aids in CHO metabolism	• Fruits, especially oranges, bananas, and prunes • Red meats • Vegetables • Milk and milk products • Coffee	• Hypokalemia • Fluid and electrolyte imbalances • Tissue breakdown • Cardiac weakness • Muscle cramps	• Hyperkalemia • Muscle weakness • Severe dehydration • Mental confusion • Hypotension • Cardiac arrest
Magnesium (Mg)	• Is necessary for muscle–nerve action • Regulates CHO, CHON, and fat metabolism • Activates enzymes • Aids in bone formation	• Green leafy vegetables • Whole grains • Legumes	• Hypomagnesemia • Tremors • Spasms • Convulsions	• Hypermagnesemia • Central nervous system (CNS) depression • Coma • Hypotension
Chlorine (Cl)	• Helps regulate fluid balance and acid–base balance • Aids digestion as part of hydrochloric acid in stomach	• Table salt • Milk • Meat • Processed foods	• Rare	• Rare
Sulfur (S)	• Serves as component of amino acids • Aids vitamin, enzyme, and hormonal activity • Is part of skin, hair, nails, and soft tissue	• Cheese • Eggs • Poultry • Fish	• None specific	• None specific
Iron (Fe)	• Aids in formation of hemoglobin • Aids in antibody formation	• Meat • Whole grains • Egg yolk • Legumes • Prunes • Raisins • Apricots	• Iron deficiency • Anemia	• Hemochromatosis • GI cramping • Vomiting • Nausea • Shock • Convulsions • Coma

continues

Table 18–6 MINERALS *continued*

VITAMIN	FUNCTION	SOURCES	DEFICIENCY	TOXIC EFFECTS
Iodine (I)	• Is a component of thyroid hormones	• Iodized salt • Seafood (salt water) • Milk	• Cretinism • Goiter	• Hyperthyroidism • Fatal in large amounts
Zinc (Zn)	• Is a component of DNA and RNA • Aids in physical and sexual development • Helps ensure normal taste and smell • Aids in wound healing	• Meats, oysters • Eggs • Milk • Whole grains	• Poor wound healing • Decreased taste and smell • Growth retardation	• Muscle incoordination • Vomiting • Diarrhea • Renal failure
Selenium (Se)	• Acts as an antioxidant • Works with vitamin E	• Seafoods • Meats	• Muscle weakness • Cardiomyopathy	• Selenosis • Nausea • Peripheral neuropathy • Fatigue
Copper (Cu)	• Aids in bone and blood formation • Promotes iron absorption • Is part of myelin sheath	• Seafood • Nuts • Legumes	• Iron-deficiency anemia • Hypocholesterolemia	• None known
Manganese (Mn)	• Aids bone growth • Aids reproduction • Acts as enzyme activator	• Whole-grain cereals • Legumes • Tea	• Unknown	• Unlikely
Flourine (Fl)	• Protects against dental caries • Contributes to bone formation and integrity	• Flouridated water • Tea • Seafood	• Dental caries	• Mottled stains on teeth
Chromium (Cr)	• Associated with glucose metabolism	• Whole grains • Brewers yeast	• Insulin resistance • Impaired glucose tolerance	• Dietary: unlikely
Molybdenum (Mo)	• Helps ensure normal body metabolism	• Milk • Legumes • Whole grains	• Decrease production of uric acid	• Interferes with copper metabolism
Cobolt (Co)	• Is a component of vitamin B_{12} • Aids in RBC formation	• Meat, as B_{12}	• Associated with vitamin B_{12} deficiency	• Unknown

Minerals are found in water and in natural (unprocessed) foods, together with proteins, carbohydrates, fats, and vitamins. Minerals in the soil are absorbed by growing plants. Humans obtain minerals by eating plants grown in mineral-rich soil or by eating animals that have eaten such plants.

Highly processed or refined foods such as sugar and white flour contain almost no minerals. Iron, together with the vitamins thiamin, riboflavin, niacin, and folate is commonly added back to some flour and cereals, which are then labeled enriched.

Most minerals in food occur as salts, which are soluble in water. Therefore, the minerals leave the food and remain in the cooking water when foods are cooked in water. Foods should be cooked in as little water as possible or, preferably, steamed, and any cooking liquid should be saved to be used in soups, gravies, and white sauces. Using this liquid improves the flavor as well as the nutrient content of foods to which it is added.

Supplemental minerals may be required during growth periods and in some clinical situations. Individuals

LIFE CYCLE CONSIDERATIONS

Mineral Supplements

- During adolescence calcium may be needed, if the diet is insufficient.
- Pregnant and lactating women require added calcium, phosphorus, and iron.

with iron deficiency anemia require extra iron. Persons taking potassium-losing diuretics need a potassium supplement. Functions, sources, deficiencies, and toxic effects of minerals are listed in Table 18–7.

Digestion, Absorption, and Storage

Minerals are absorbed in their ionic forms (i.e., carrying a positive or negative electrical charge). The amount of a mineral absorbed by the body is influenced by three factors:

- *Type of food:* Minerals in foods that come from animals are more readily absorbed than those in foods that come from plants.
- *Need of body:* If there is a deficiency of a mineral in the body, more will be absorbed.
- *Health of absorbing tissue:* If absorbing tissue (intestine) is affected by disease, less will be absorbed.

Signs of Deficiency and Excess

Because it is known that minerals are essential to good health, some would-be nutritionists will make claims that "more is better." Ironically, more can be hazardous to one's health when it comes to minerals. In a healthy individual eating a balanced diet, there will be some normal mineral loss through perspiration

Table 18–7   MAJOR MINERALS AND TRACE ELEMENTS

MAJOR MINERALS	TRACE ELEMENTS	
	Essential	**Questionable**
Calcium (Ca)	Iron (Fe)	Arsenic (As)
Phosphorus (P)	Iodine (I)	Boron (B)
Sodium (Na)	Zinc (Zn)	Cadmium Cd)
Potassium (K)	Selenium (Se)	Nickel (Ni)
Magnesium (Mg)	Copper (Cu)	Silicon (Si)
Chlorine (Cl)	Manganese (Mn)	Tin (Sn)
Sulfur (S)	Fluorine (Fl)	Vanadium (V)
	Chromium (Cr)	
	Molybdenum (Mo)	
	Cobalt (Co)	

PROFESSIONAL TIP

Vitamins, Minerals, and Herbs

Since July 1994, the federal Food and Drug Administration has placed limitations on marketing claims for vitamins, minerals, and herbs. The rules are aimed at deterring false or unproven health claims and require that companies selling these products make only claims that are substantiated by broad scientific consensus. Labeling requirements of dietary supplements began in July 1995.

and saliva, and amounts in excess of body needs will be excreted in urine and feces. However, when concentrated forms of minerals are taken on a regular basis and over a period of time, they become more than the body can handle, and toxicity develops. An excessive amount of one mineral can sometimes cause a deficiency of another mineral. In addition, excessive amounts of minerals can cause hair loss and changes in the blood, hormones, bones, muscles, blood vessels, and nearly all tissues. Concentrated forms of minerals should be used only on the advice of a physician. Refer to Table 18–6 for specific signs of deficiency and toxicity of each mineral.

PROMOTING PROPER NUTRITION

Through the years, various ways to promote proper nutrition have been devised. The best known are the four food groups, the food guide pyramid, the *Dietary Guidelines for Americans,* the recommended daily allowances, and the dietary reference intakes.

Four Food Groups (Historical)

For many years, the four food group system constituted a plan to assist people in eating a well-balanced diet. Consuming foods from the four groups—milk, meat, fruit/vegetable, and bread/cereal—provided most nutrients required in a daily diet. The minimum servings given for the four food groups yielded approximately 1,200 kcal. Additional servings were to be added depending on the individual's age and activity level.

Food Guide Pyramid

In 1992, the United States Department of Agriculture introduced the food guide pyramid, which identifies the food groups from which additional servings should be obtained when calorie needs exceed the 1,200 kcal provided for by the minimum servings from the four food groups. The pyramid separates the fruit and vegetable groups and the suggested number of servings from each of these groups. The food guide pyramid also focuses on fat, because most American diets are too high in fat. Figure 18-3 shows the food guide pyramid.

Each food group of the food guide pyramid provides some, but not all, of the nutrients needed each day. Foods in one group cannot replace foods in another group. No one group is more important than another: All are needed.

Bread, Cereal, Rice, and Pasta Group

At the base of the pyramid is the bread, cereal, rice, and pasta group. The nutrients contributed by this group are complex carbohydrates, incomplete protein, the B vitamins, and iron, if the product is whole grain or **enriched** (nutrients that are removed during processing are added back) with iron. Six to eleven servings a day should come from this group. Examples of serving sizes from this group are one slice of bread, one tortilla, 1 ounce (1 cup) dry cereal, and ½ cup cooked cereal, rice, or pasta.

Fruit and Vegetable Groups

On the second level of the pyramid are the foods that come from plants: fruits and vegetables. Most people should eat more of these foods because of the vitamins, minerals, and fiber they supply.

The nutritional contributions of fruits and vegetables are carbohydrates, vitamins, minerals, water, and very small amounts of proteins and fats. Dietary fiber, important for elimination, is found in the skin or pulp of many foods in this group.

Fruits Each person should have two to four servings of fruit every day. Citrus fruits, melons, and berries should be eaten regularly as they are high in vitamin C. Examples of serving sizes from the fruit group are one medium size apple, pear, banana, or orange; ½ cup of cooked, chopped, or canned fruit, or ¾ cup of fruit juice.

Vegetables Three to five servings a day from the vegetable group are suggested. Among the vegetables eaten daily, one should be a dark-green or deep-yellow vegetable to provide vitamin A. Sample serving sizes from the vegetable group include 1 cup of raw leafy vegetables; ½ cup of cooked or chopped raw vegetables; or ¾ cup of vegetable juice.

Milk and Meat Groups

On the third level are the foods that come mostly from animals. These foods have significantly greater amounts of saturated fat or added sugar than do the foods on the first and second levels. Fewer servings should be eaten from this level each day.

Milk The nutritional contributions of the milk group are calcium, protein, riboflavin, fat, carbohydrates, phosphorus, sodium, vitamin B$_{12}$, and vitamin A. If skim milk or skim milk products are used, there is no fat and significantly fewer kcal. All commercial milk

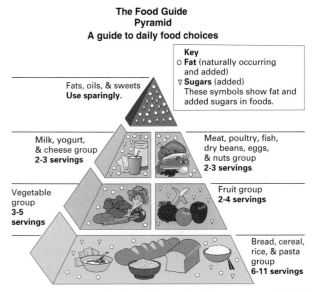

Figure 18-3 Food Guide Pyramid *[Courtesy of the U.S. Department of Agriculture, Center for Nutrition Policy and Promotion, 1996. Food Guide Pyramid (Home and Garden Bulletin, No. 252). Washington, DC: USDA.]*

products are **fortified** (a nutrient not naturally occurring in a food is added to the food) with vitamin D. Vitamin D, not naturally found in milk, is added because the calcium provided by milk is better absorbed when vitamin D is present.

Two to three servings a day are suggested from the milk group. Eight ounces of milk is considered one serving. Other milk products and their serving sizes to provide the equivalent nutrients of 8 ounces of milk are 1½ ounces of cheese, 1 cup of yogurt, 1½ cups of cottage cheese, and 1½ cups of ice cream. The kcal content of these foods varies, with ice cream containing more kcal than the other foods in the milk group.

Meat The meat group contributes protein (especially complete protein), fats, iron, most other minerals, and the B vitamins. Cheese and bacon are not considered part of this group because cheese has too little iron and bacon has too much fat.

The suggested number of servings from the meat group is two to three each day. A serving size is 2 to 3 ounces of meat, fish, or poultry. Other foods that can be substituted for one serving of meat are: two eggs, 4 tablespoons of peanut butter, or 1 cup cooked beans or peas (legumes). Legumes such as dried peas, beans, or lentils can be used instead of meat because of their high protein content. Peanuts as well as many other nuts are high in protein, but they are also typically high in fats and should thus be used sparingly.

Fats, Oils, and Sweets Group

Fats, oils, and sweets are placed at the very top of the pyramid because they do not fit into any of the other food groups. These other food items are considered

empty calories, that is, they generally provide many calories but very few nutrients. Items included are potato chips, cookies, cakes, pies, soft drinks, alcohol, jelly, syrup, fats, oils, salad dressings, pickles, olives, catsup, and mustard. These foods are to be eaten in very small amounts and infrequently, as they have the most fat and added sugar and the least nutritional value of all the foods.

Number of Servings

The number of servings for an individual depends on the number of calories the individual needs. The number of calories needed by a person depends on age, gender, size, and activity. Almost everyone should have the minimum number of servings for each group. Three general calorie levels are suggested, the serving recommendations for which are listed in Table 18–8.

The Vegetarian Diet

There are several vegetarian diets. The common factor among them is that they do not include red meat. Some include eggs, some fish, some milk, and some even poultry. When carefully planned, these diets can be nutritious. They can even contribute to a reduction in obesity, high blood pressure, heart disease, some cancers, and, possibly, diabetes (Townsend & Roth, 2000). They must be carefully planned so that they include all the needed nutrients.

Lacto-ovo vegetarians use dairy products and eggs but no meat, poultry, or fish.

Lacto-vegetarians use dairy products but no meat, poultry, or eggs.

Vegans avoid all animal foods. They use soybeans, chickpeas, meat analogues, and tofu. It is important that their meals be carefully planned to include appropriate combinations of the essential amino acids. For example, beans served with corn or rice, or peanuts eaten with wheat, are complementary proteins. Vegans can show deficiencies of calcium; vitamins A, D, and B_{12}; and, of course, proteins.

Dietary Guidelines

The *Dietary Guidelines* developed by the U.S. Department of Agriculture and the U.S. Department of Health & Human Services were last revised in 1990. They are now stated in positive terms (i.e., "eat . . ."; "consume . . .") instead of negative terms ("avoid . . ."). These guidelines attempt to prevent overnutrition by incorporating some of the concepts of the food guide pyramid (Table 18–9).

Recommended Dietary Allowances

Recommended dietary allowances (RDAs) of essential nutrients are the recommended intake levels judged adequate to meet the known nutrient needs of practically all healthy people. Recommendations are grouped according to infants, children, males, females, and pregnant/lactating women, and are subdivided within those groups according to age. The RDAs are compiled by the Food and Nutrition Board of the National Academy of Sciences and are periodically revised (refer to Appendix C).

Dietary Reference Intakes

The dietary reference intakes (DRIs), according to Barrett (1998), are nutrient-based reference values for use in planning and assessing diets. They are intended to replace the RDAs. The DRIs focus on decreasing the risk of chronic disease through nutrition, rather than on protecting against deficiency diseases, as do the RDAs.

The DRIs encompass four categories:

- Estimated average requirement (EAR) is the amount that meets the estimated nutrient need of 50% of the individuals in a specific group.
- Recommended dietary allowance (RDA) is the amount that meets the nutrient need of almost all (97% to 98%) healthy individuals in a specific age and gender group. It is the EAR plus an increase, based on scientific evidence, to account for variation within the specific group. The RDA should be used to achieve adequate nutrient intake aimed at decreasing the risk of chronic disease.

Table 18–8 SERVINGS FOR THREE CALORIE LEVELS

FOOD GROUP	TOTAL CALORIC INTAKE AND NUMBER OF SERVINGS PER GROUP		
	1,600 calories	**2,200 calories**	**2,800 calories**
Grain	6 servings	9 servings	11 servings
Vegetable	3 servings	4 servings	5 servings
Fruit	2 servings	3 servings	4 servings
Milk	2 to 3 servings	2 to 3 servings	2 to 3 servings
Meat	5 ounces	6 ounces	7 ounces

A 1,600-calorie diet is about right for sedentary women and older adults.

A 2,200 calorie diet is about right for most children, teenage girls, and active women and for many sedentary men. Pregnant and lactating women may need more calories.

A 2,800 calorie diet is about right for teenage boys, many active men, and some very active women.

From U.S. Department of Agriculture, Center for Nutrition Policy and Promotion, 1996. Food Guide Pyramid (Home and Garden Bulletin, No. 252). Washington, DC: USDA

Table 18–9 DIETARY GUIDELINES FOR AMERICANS

AIM FOR FITNESS

- Aim for a healthy weight.
- Be physically active each day.

Following these two guidelines will help keep you and your family healthy and fit. Healthy eating and regular physical activity enable people of all ages to work productively, enjoy life, and feel their best. They also help children grow, develop, and do well in school.

BUILD A HEALTHY BASE

- Use the food guide pyramid to make your food choices.
- Choose a variety of grains daily, especially whole grains.
- Choose a variety of fruits and vegetables daily.
- Keep food safe to eat.

Following these four guidelines builds a base for healthy eating. Let the food guide pyramid guide you so that you get the nutrients your body needs each day. Make grains, fruits, and vegetables the foundation of your meals. This forms a base for good nutrition and good health and may reduce your risk of certain chronic diseases. Be flexible and adventurous, try new choices from these three groups in place of some less nutritious foods or in place of higher calorie foods that you usually eat. Whatever you eat, always take steps to keep your food safe to eat.

CHOOSE SENSIBLY

- Choose a diet that is low in saturated fat and cholesterol and moderate in total fat.
- Choose beverages and foods to moderate your intake of sugars.
- Choose and prepare foods with less salt.
- If you drink alcoholic beverages, do so in moderation.

These four guidelines help you make sensible choices that promote health and reduce the risk of certain chronic diseases. You can enjoy all foods as part of a healthy diet as long as you don't overdo it on fat (especially saturated fat), sugars, salt, and alcohol. Read labels to identify foods that are higher in saturated fats, sugars, and salt (sodium).

From U.S. Department of Agriculture and U.S. Department of Health and Human Services, 2000. Dietary Guidelines for Americans (Home and Garden Bulletin No. 232, 5th ed.). Washington, D.C.: USDA

- Adequate intake (AI) is set when there is insufficient scientific evidence to estimate an average requirement. It is derived through experimental or observational data that show a mean intake that appears to sustain a desired indicator of health, such as calcium retention in bone.
- Tolerable upper intake level (UL) is the maximum intake by an individual that is unlikely to pose risks of adverse health effects in almost all healthy individuals in a specified group. It is not intended to be a recommended level of intake. There is no established benefit for individuals to consume nutrients at levels above the RDA or AI.

FACTORS INFLUENCING NUTRITION

Many factors influence nutrition. Some of the major factors are culture, religion, socioeconomics, fads, and superstitions.

Culture

A person's culture encompasses a total way of life including values, attitudes, and practices. Food practices are a substantial part of a culture. These food habits are based on availability of foods, preparation techniques, methods of serving, and the personal meaning of food (Figure 18-4). American cuisine (cooking style) is a marvelous composite of countless national, regional, cultural, and religious food customs. Consequently, categorizing a client's food habits can be difficult. Nevertheless, it is sometimes helpful to be able to do so to a certain extent. People who are ill commonly have little interest in food, and sometimes foods that were familiar to them during their childhood and youth are more apt to tempt them than other types. The following section briefly discusses some food patterns typical of various cultures, regions, and countries. Of course, there can be and usually are enormous variations within any one classification.

Native American

It is thought that approximately one-half of the edible plants commonly eaten in the United States today originated with the Native Americans. Examples are corn, potatoes, squash, cranberries, pumpkins, peppers, beans, wild rice, and cocoa beans. In addition, wild fruits, game, and fish were used. Foods were commonly prepared as soups and stews or were dried. The original Native American diets were probably more nutritionally adequate than current diets, which frequently consist of an excess of sweet and salty, snack-type, low-nutrient foods. Native American diets today may be deficient in calcium, vitamins A and C, and riboflavin (Townsend & Roth, 2000).

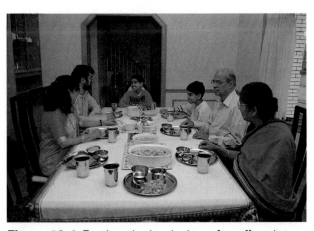

Figure 18-4 Family and cultural values often affect diet.

U.S. Southern

Hot breads such as corn bread and baking powder biscuits are common in the U.S. South because the wheat grown in this area does not make good-quality yeast breads. Grits and rice are also popular carbohydrate foods. Favorite vegetables include sweet potatoes, squash, green beans, and lima beans. Green beans cooked with pork are commonly served. Watermelon, oranges, and peaches are popular fruits. Fried fish is served often, as are barbecued and stewed meats and poultry. These diets have a great deal of carbohydrate and fat and limited amounts of protein in some cases. Iron, calcium, and vitamins A and C may be deficient (Townsend & Roth, 2000).

Mexican

Mexican food is a combination of Spanish and Native American foods. Beans, rice, chili peppers, tomatoes, and corn meal are favorites. Meat is often cooked with a vegetable, as in chili con carne. Corn meal or flour is used to make tortillas, which are served as bread. The combination of beans and corn makes a complete protein. Corn tortillas filled with cheese (called enchiladas) provide some calcium, but the use of milk should be encouraged. Additional green and yellow vegetables and vitamin C-rich foods would also make these diets more well-balanced.

Puerto Rican

Rice is the basic carbohydrate food in Puerto Rican diets. Vegetables commonly used include beans, plantains, tomatoes, and peppers. Bananas, pineapple, mangoes, and papayas are popular fruits. Favorite meats are chicken, beef, and pork. Additional milk is desirable for a more balanced diet (Townsend & Roth, 2000).

Italian

Pastas with various tomato or fish sauces and cheese are popular Italian foods. Fish and highly seasoned foods are common to southern Italian cuisine; whereas meat and root vegetables are common to northern cuisine. The eggs, cheese, tomatoes, green vegetables, and fruits common to Italian diets provide excellent sources of many nutrients, but additional fat-free milk and low-fat meat would make the diet more complete (Townsend & Roth, 2000).

Northern and Western European

Northern and Western European diets are similar to those of the U.S. Midwest, but with a greater use of dark breads, potatoes, and fish, and fewer green-vegetable salads. Beef and pork are popular, as are various cooked vegetables, breads, cakes, and dairy products. The addition of fresh vegetables and fruits would add vitamins, minerals, and fiber to these diets.

Central European

Citizens of Central Europe obtain the greatest portion of their calories from potatoes and grain, especially rye and buckwheat (Townsend & Roth, 2000). Pork is a popular meat. Cabbage cooked in many ways is a popular vegetable, as are carrots, onions, and turnips. Eggs and dairy products are used abundantly. Limiting the number of eggs consumed and using fat-free or low-fat dairy products would reduce the fat content in this diet. Adding fresh vegetables and fruits would increase vitamins, minerals, and fiber.

Middle Eastern

Grains, wheat, and rice provide energy in Middle Eastern diets. Chickpeas in the form of hummus are popular. Lamb and yogurt are commonly used as are cabbage, grape leaves, eggplant, tomatoes, dates, olives, and figs. Black, very sweet coffee is a popular beverage. There may be insufficient protein and calcium in this diet, depending on the amounts of meat and calcium-rich foods eaten. Fresh fruits and vegetables should be added to the diet to increase vitamins, minerals, and fiber.

Chinese

The Chinese diet is varied. Rice is the primary energy food and is used in place of bread. Vegetables are lightly cooked, and the cooking water is saved for future use. Soybeans are used in many ways, and eggs and pork are commonly served. Soy sauce is extensively used, but it is very salty and could present a problem for clients needing low-salt diets. Tea is a common beverage, but milk is not. This diet is typically low in fat (Townsend & Roth, 2000).

Japanese

Japanese diets include rice, soybean paste and curd, vegetables, fruits, and fish. Food is frequently served tempura style, which means fried. Soy sauce (shoyu) and tea are commonly used. Current Japanese diets have been greatly influenced by Western culture. Japanese diets may be deficient in calcium, given the near total lack of milk in the diet (Townsend & Roth, 2000). Although fish is eaten with bones, this may not supply sufficient calcium to meet needs. Japanese diets may contain excessive amounts of salt.

Indian

Many Indians are vegetarians who use eggs and dairy products. Rice, peas, and beans are frequently served. Spices, especially curry, are popular. Indian meals are not typically served in courses as Western meals are. They generally consist of one course with many dishes.

Thai, Vietnamese, Laotian, and Cambodian

Rice, curries, vegetables, and fruit are popular in Thailand, Vietnam, Laos, and Cambodia. Meats and fish are used in small amounts. The wok (a deep, round fry pan) is used for sautéing many foods. A salty sauce made from fermented fish is commonly used. Thai, Vietnamese, Laotian, and Cambodian diets may contain deficient amounts of protein and calcium (Townsend & Roth, 2000).

Religion

Religious beliefs often influence nutrition by placing restrictions on the foods eaten and their preparation. A few examples follow.

Jewish

Interpretations of the Jewish dietary laws vary. Persons who adhere to the Orthodox view consider tradition important and always observe the dietary laws. Foods prepared according to these laws are called *kosher*. Conservative Jews are inclined to observe the rules only at home. Reform Jews consider their dietary laws to be essentially ceremonial and thus minimize their significance. Essentially the laws require the following (Townsend & Roth, 2000):

- Slaughtering must be done by a qualified person and in a prescribed manner. The meat or poultry must be drained of blood, first by severing the jugular vein and carotid artery, then by soaking the meat in brine before cooking.
- Meat and meat products may not be prepared with milk or milk products.
- The dishes used in the preparation and serving of meat products must be kept separate from those used for dairy foods.
- Dairy products and meat may not be eaten together. Six hours must elapse after eating meat before eating dairy products, and at least 30 minutes to 1 hour must elapse after eating dairy products before eating meat.
- The mouth must be rinsed after eating fish and before eating meat.
- The following may not be eaten: animals without cloven (split) hooves or animals that do not chew their cud; hindquarters of any animal; shellfish or fish without scales or fins; birds of prey; creeping things and insects; and leavened (containing ingredients that cause it to rise) bread during Passover.

There are prescribed fast days: Passover Week, Yom Kippur, and Feast of Purim. Chicken and fresh smoked and salted fish are popular, as are noodles, eggs, and flour dishes. These diets can be deficient in fresh vegetables and milk.

Roman Catholic

Although the dietary restrictions of the Roman Catholic religion have been liberalized, meat is not allowed on Ash Wednesday and Fridays during Lent.

Eastern Orthodox

The Eastern Orthodox religion includes Christians from the Middle East, Russia, and Greece. Although interpretations of the dietary laws vary, meat, poultry, fish, and dairy products are restricted on Wednesdays and Fridays and during Lent and Advent.

Seventh Day Adventists

In general, Seventh Day Adventists are lacto-ovo vegetarians, meaning that they use milk products and eggs, but no meat, fish, or poultry. Nuts, legumes, meat analogues (substitutes), and tofu (made from soybeans) may be used. Coffee, tea, and alcohol are considered to be harmful.

Mormon (Latter Day Saints)

The only dietary restriction observed by the Mormons is the prohibition of coffee, tea, and alcoholic beverages.

Islamic

Adherents of Islam are called Muslims. Dietary laws prohibit the use of pork and alcohol, and other meats must be slaughtered according to specific laws. During the month of Ramadan, Muslims do not eat or drink during daylight hours.

Hindu

To the Hindus, all life is sacred, and animals contain the souls of ancestors. Consequently, most Hindus are vegetarians, and do not use eggs in food preparation because eggs represent life.

Socioeconomics

The amount of money available to purchase food certainly influences nutrition. More money, however, does not always mean better nutrition. Often, persons with less money plan their meals and buy food more carefully than do those with higher incomes. Expensive food does not mean better nutrition. Many times, persons with no monetary worries eat what they want, when they want, without paying attention to nutritional value, thereby shortchanging themselves nutritionally.

Fads

Food fads are beliefs that persist for a period of time about certain foods and that generally have no scientific basis. Often, these fads are translated into diets that can be harmful if basic nutrients are missing or are in excess. One of the most popular diets some years ago was the grapefruit and egg diet. One of the more recent fads was the liquid-protein diet. This diet overloaded the body with protein, yet other nutrients were lacking. The excessive amount of protein damaged the kidneys of many people. Indeed, some people died from this fad diet (American Heart Association, 1999).

Superstitions

Superstitions are irrational beliefs about a food that are generally passed down from generation to generation. The nurse should be aware of the beliefs and the facts that contradict them so as to be knowledgeable and respectful. Examples of such superstitions are as follows:

- ***Superstition:*** Toast is less fattening than bread.
  Fact: Only moisture is removed during toasting.
- ***Superstition:*** "Cravings" during pregnancy should be satisfied or the infant will be marked or deformed.
  Fact: Foods eaten or not eaten by the mother do not directly affect the infant; only the nutrients or lack thereof affect the unborn child.

NUTRITIONAL NEEDS DURING THE LIFE CYCLE

As a person grows and develops from birth to old age, nutritional needs change. These changes generally are based on growth needs, energy needs, and utilization of nutrients. A nutritional assessment should be conducted to ascertain the nutritional status of the individual. The following basic assessment should be done for everyone over 1 year old.

- Nutritional status
- Height and weight
- Meal and snack pattern (food record or 24-hour recall)
- Adequacy of intake based on the food guide pyramid
- Food allergies
- Physical activity
- Cultural, ethnic, and family influences
- Use of vitamin/mineral supplements

Infancy

Food and its presentation are extremely important during the baby's first year. Physical and mental development are dependent on the food itself, and psychosocial development is affected by the time and manner whereby the food is offered.

Although babies have been fed according to prescribed time schedules in the past, it is preferable to feed infants on demand. Feeding on demand prevents the frustrations that hunger can bring and helps the child develop trust in people. The newborn may re-

PROFESSIONAL TIP

Nutritional Needs of Infants

It is important to remember that growth rates vary from child to child. Nutritional needs depend largely on a child's growth rate.

quire more frequent feedings, but, normally, the demand schedule averages approximately every 4 hours by the time the baby is 2 or 3 months old (Townsend & Roth, 2000).

Nutritional Requirements

The first year of life is a period of the most rapid growth in one's life. A baby doubles its birth weight by 6 months of age and triples it within the first year. This explains why the infant's energy, vitamin, mineral, and protein requirements are higher per unit of body weight than are those of older children or adults.

During the first year, the normal child needs approximately 100 kcal per kilogram of body weight each day. This is approximately two to three times the adult requirement. Infants who have suffered from low birth weight, malnutrition, or illness require more than the normal number of kcal per kilogram of body weight. The nutritional status of infants is reflected in many of the same characteristics as those of adults.

The American Academy of Pediatrics recommends breast milk for the first 12 months of life, although parents must decide on the method of feeding based on their lifestyle, values, and personal feelings.

Breast Milk Breastfeeding is nature's way of providing a good diet for the baby. It is, in fact, used as the guide by which nutritional requirements of infants are measured.

Mother's milk provides the infant with temporary immunity to many infectious diseases. It is sterile, easy to digest, and usually does not cause GI disturbances or allergic reactions. Breastfed infants grow more rapidly during the first few months of life than do formula-fed

CLIENT TEACHING

Breastfeeding

If the mother works and cannot be available for every feeding, breast milk can be expressed earlier, refrigerated or frozen, and used at the appropriate time, or a bottle of formula can be substituted. Never warm the breast milk in a microwave oven because the antibodies will be destroyed. Instead, warm a cup of water and place the bag of breast milk in the water to heat it.

CLIENT TEACHING

Cow's Milk

Infants under the age of 1 year should not be given regular cow's milk. Because its protein is more difficult and slower to digest than that of human milk, it can cause GI blood loss. The kidneys are challenged by its high protein and mineral content, and dehydration and even damage to the CNS can result. In addition, the fat is less bioavailable, meaning it is not absorbed as efficiently as that in human milk (Townsend & Roth, 2000).

CLIENT TEACHING

Nursing Bottle Syndrome

Infants should not be put to bed with a bottle. Saliva, which normally cleanses the teeth, diminishes as the infant falls asleep. The milk then bathes the upper front teeth, causing tooth decay. Also, the bottle can cause the upper jaw to protrude and the lower to recede. The result is known as the baby bottle mouth, or nursing bottle syndrome. It is preferable to feed the infant the bedtime bottle, cleanse the teeth and gums with some water from another bottle or cup, and then put the infant to bed.

babies, and they typically have fewer infections (especially ear infections). And, because breast milk contains less protein and minerals than infant formula, it reduces the load on the infant's kidneys. Breastfeeding also promotes oral motor development in infants because sucking requires more and different muscles than does bottle-feeding (Townsend & Roth, 2000).

One can be quite confident the infant is getting sufficient nutrients and kcal from breastfeeding if (1) there are six or more wet diapers per day; (2) there is normal growth; (3) there are one or two mustard-colored bowel movements per day; and (4) the breast becomes soft during nursing.

Formula If the baby is to be bottle-fed, the pediatrician will provide information on commercial formulas and feeding instructions. Formulas are usually based on cow's milk, because it is abundant and easily modified to resemble human milk. It must be modified because it has more protein and mineral salts and less milk sugar (lactose) than does human milk. Formulas are developed so that they are similar to human milk in nutrient and kcal values.

When an infant is extremely sensitive or allergic to infant formulas, a synthetic formula may be given. Synthetic milk is commonly made from soybeans. Formulas with predigested proteins are used for infants unable to tolerate all other types of formulas (Townsend & Roth, 2000).

Formulas can be purchased in ready-to-feed, concentrated, or powdered forms. Sterile water must be

mixed with the concentrated and powdered forms. The most convenient type is also the most expensive.

If the type purchased requires the addition of water, it is essential that the amount of water added be correctly measured. Too little water will create too heavy a protein and mineral load for the infant's kidneys; too much water will dilute the nutrient and kcal value such that the infant will not thrive.

Solid Foods The introduction of solid foods before the age of 4 to 6 months is not recommended. The child's GI tract and kidneys are not sufficiently developed to handle solid food before that age. Further, it is thought that the early introduction of solid foods may increase the likelihood of overfeeding and the possibility of the development of food allergies, particularly in children whose parents suffer from food allergies.

An infant's readiness for solid foods will be demonstrated by (1) the physical ability to pull food into the mouth rather than always pushing the tongue and food out of the mouth, (2) a willingness to participate in the process, (3) the ability to sit up with support, (4) having head and neck control, and (5) the need for additional nutrients. If the infant is drinking more than 32 ounces of formula or nursing 8 to 10 times in 24 hours, then solid food should be started.

Solid foods must be introduced gradually and individually. One food is introduced and then no other new food for 4 or 5 days. If there is no allergic reaction, another food can be introduced, a waiting period allowed, then another, and so on. The typical order of introduction begins with cereal, usually iron-fortified rice, then oat, wheat, and mixed cereals. Cooked and pureed vegetables follow, then cooked and pureed fruits, egg yolk, and, finally, finely ground meats. Between 6 and 12 months, toast, zwieback, teething biscuits, custards, puddings, and ice cream can be added.

When the infant learns to drink from a cup, juice can be introduced. Juice should never be given from a bottle because babies will fill up on it and not get

CLIENT TEACHING

Honey

Honey should never be given to an infant because it could be contaminated with *Clostridium botulinum* bacteria.

enough calories from other sources. Pasteurized apple juice is usually given first. It is recommended that only 100% juice products be given because they are nutrient dense (Townsend & Roth, 2000).

By the age of 1 year, most babies are eating foods from all the food guide pyramid's groups and may have most any food that is easily chewed and digested. However, precautions must be taken to avoid offering foods that might cause the child to choke. Examples include hot dogs, nuts, whole peas, grapes, popcorn, small candies, and small pieces of tough meat or raw vegetables. Foods should be selected according to the advice of the pediatrician.

Nutritional assessment for an infant should include the following:

- Height and weight
- Sleeping habits
- Type of feeding (breast- or bottle-fed)
- If breastfeeding, the mother's nutritional status and use of alcohol, tobacco, caffeine, and drugs; infant's feeding schedule (how often fed and for how long)
- If formula feeding, type, frequency, and method of preparation and storage; feeding schedule; amount taken at each feeding
- Use of vitamin/mineral supplements
- If on solid foods, age at introduction, and any reactions or allergies
- Family attitudes about eating, food, and weight

Childhood

Although specific nutritional requirements change as children grow, nutrition always affects physical, mental, and emotional growth and development. Studies indicate that the mental ability and size of an individual are directly influenced by nutrition during the early years.

Eating habits develop during childhood. Once developed, poor eating habits are difficult to change. They can exacerbate emotional and physical problems such as irritability, depression, anxiety, fatigue, and illness. Good eating habits formed in early childhood will generally last a lifetime (Figure 18-5).

Parents should be aware that it is not uncommon for children's appetites to vary. The rate of growth is not constant. As the child ages, the rate of growth actually slows. The approximate weight gain of a child during the second year of life is only 5 pounds. Children between the ages of 1 and 3 years undergo vast changes: Their legs grow longer; they develop muscles; they lose their baby shape; they begin to walk and talk; and they learn to feed and generally assert themselves.

As children continue to grow and develop, their likes and dislikes may change. New foods should be introduced gradually, in small amounts, and as attractively as possible.

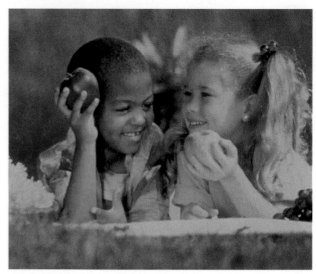

Figure 18-5 Good health radiates from these two children. (*Courtesy of USDA/ARS #K-48191*)

Children should be offered nutrient-dense foods because the amount eaten will be small. Fats should not be limited before the age of 2 years, but meals and snacks should not be fat-laden either. Whole milk is recommended until the age of 2, but low-fat or fat-free should be served from 2 years on. The guideline for fat intake after the age of 2 is 30% or less of total kcal per day, with no more than 10% coming from saturated fats. It is recommended that children not salt their food at the table or have foods prepared with a lot of salt (Townsend & Roth, 2000).

Children are especially sensitive to and reject hot (temperature) foods, but they like crisp textures, mild flavors, and familiar foods. They are wary of foods covered by sauce or gravy. Parents should set realistic goals and expectations as to the amount of food a child needs. A good rule of thumb for preschool children is one tablespoon of new food for each year of age. Table 18–10 details serving sizes according to age. Calorie needs depend on rate of growth, activity level, body size, metabolism, and health.

Nutritional Requirements

The rate of growth diminishes from the age of 1 year until about age 10, thus the kcal requirement per pound of body weight also diminishes during this period. For example, at 6 months, a girl needs approx-

 CLIENT TEACHING

Introducing New Foods

Allowing the child to assist in purchasing and preparing a new food is often a good way of arousing interest in the food and a desire to eat it.

Table 18–10 FOOD PLAN FOR PRESCHOOL AND SCHOOL-AGE CHILDREN BASED ON THE FOOD GUIDE PYRAMID

FOOD GROUP	NUMBER OF SERVINGS	APPROXIMATE SERVING SIZE*			
		AGE 1–2	AGE 3–4	AGE 5–6	AGE 7–12
Milk, yogurt, and cheese	3	½ to ¾ cup or 1 oz	¾ cup or 1½ oz	1 cup or 2 oz	1 cup or 2 oz
Meat, poultry, fish, dry beans, eggs, and nuts	2 or more	1 oz or 1 to 2 tbsp	1½ oz or 3 to 4 tbsp	1½ oz or ½ cup	2 oz or ½ cup
Vegetables	3 or more	1 to 2 tbsp	3 to 4 tbsp	½ cup	½ cup
Fruits	2 or more	1 to 2 tbsp or ½ cup juice	3 to 4 tbsp or ½ cup juice	½ cup or ½ cup juice	½ cup or ½ cup juice
Bread, cereal, rice, and pasta	6 or more	½ slice or ½ cup	1 slice or ½ cup	1 slice or ¾ cup	1 slice or ¾ cup

*Use as a starting point. Increase serving size as energy yields dictate, but maintain variety in the diet by making sure all food groups are still appropriately represented.

Adapted from Food and Nutrition Services, U. S. Department of Agriculture: Meal Plan Requirements and Offer versus Serve Manual, *FNS-265, 1990.*

imately 54 kcal per pound of body weight, but by the age of 10, she will require only 35 kcal per pound of body weight.

Nutrient needs, however, do not diminish. From the age of 6 months to 10 years, nutrient needs actually increase because of the increase in body size. Therefore, it is especially important that young children are given nutritious foods that they will eat.

In general, the young child will need 2 to 3 cups of milk each day, or the equivalent in terms of calcium. However, excessive use of milk should be avoided because it can crowd out other, iron-rich foods and possibly cause iron deficiency. The number of servings of the other food groups is the same as for adults, but the sizes will be smaller. The use of sweets should be minimized because the child is apt to prefer them to nutrient-rich foods. Sweetened fruit juices, especially, should be avoided. Children also need water and fiber in their diets. They need to drink 1 milliliter of water for each kcal. If food valued at 1,200 kcal is eaten, five

8-ounce glasses of water are needed. Fiber needs are calculated according to age. After age 3 years a child's fiber needs are "age + 5g" and no more than "age + 10g." A child who eats more fiber than that might be too full to eat enough other foods to provide all the kcal needed for growth and development. Fiber should be added slowly, if not already in the diet, and fluids must also be increased. Childhood is a good time to develop the lifelong good habit of getting enough dietary fiber to prevent constipation and diseases such as colon cancer and diverticulitis (Townsend & Roth, 2000). In addition to the basic nutritional assessments, dental health should also be assessed.

PROFESSIONAL TIP

Snacks

A child needs a snack every 3 to 4 hours for continued energy. Children often prefer finger foods for snacks. Snacks should be nutrient dense and as nutritious as food served at mealtimes. Cheese, saltines, fruit, milk, and unsweetened cereals make good snacks.

CLIENT TEACHING

Preventing Choking

Instruct parents to:

- Avoid the use of foods that may cause choking in infants and small children (up to 3 years old), such as corn, nuts, raw peas and carrots, celery, small candies, hot dogs, popcorn, and any other small, hard food.
- Offer peanut butter only on bread or a cracker.
- Stress the importance of sitting upright while eating.
- Prohibit running with food or objects in the mouth.

Adolescence

Adolescence is a period of rapid growth that causes major physiologic changes. The growth rate may be as much as 3 inches per year for girls and 4 inches for boys; nutrition plays a role in overall healthy adolescent development. Bones grow and gain density, muscle and fat tissue develop, and blood volume increases (Townsend & Roth, 2000).

Adolescents typically have enormous appetites. When good eating habits have been established during childhood and there is nutritious food available, the teenager's food habits should present no serious problem. However, peer pressure is great at this time, and good eating habits are often forgotten. Many adolescents skip breakfast and/or lunch and then eat at fast-food places (Figure 18-6). Adolescents are concerned with body image and often compare their bodies to those of their peers and of popular media figures. They often restrict food intake, leading to inadequate nutrient intake.

Nutritional Requirements

Because of adolescents' rapid growth, kcal requirements naturally increase. Boys' kcal requirements tend to be greater than girls', because boys are generally bigger, tend to be more physically active, and have more lean muscle mass than girls do (Townsend & Roth, 2000).

Except for vitamin D, nutrient needs increase dramatically at the onset of adolescence. Because of menstruation, girls have a greater need for iron than do boys. The RDAs for vitamin D, vitamin C, vitamin B_{12}, calcium, phosphorus, and iodine are the same for both sexes. The RDAs for the remaining nutrients are higher for boys than they are for girls (Townsend & Roth, 2000).

In addition to the basic nutritional assessments, the following should be assessed for the adolescent client.

PROFESSIONAL TIP

Preventing Eating Disorders

- Encourage healthy dietary habits and adequate exercise.
- Emphasize a healthy lifestyle over physical appearance and weight loss.
- Encourage increased self-esteem and stress a positive self-worth.
- Avoid pressuring children to achieve perfection or perform beyond their abilities.
- Recognize signs and symptoms of eating disorders, and seek professional help when suspected.

(From Health Assessment & Physical Examination *(2nd ed.), by M. E. Z. Estes, 2002, Albany, NY: Delmar. Copyright 2002 by Delmar.)*

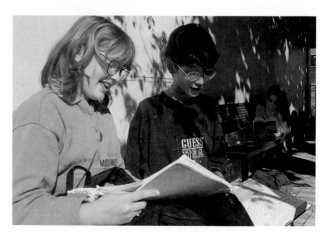

Figure 18-6 Adolescents are vulnerable to peer pressure.

- Use of alcohol, tobacco, caffeine, and drugs
- Use of fad diets
- Family attitude toward thinness and the adolescent's weight

Young and Middle Adulthood

The period of young adulthood ranges from approximately 18 years to 40 years of age. Individuals are alive with plans, desires, and energy as they begin searching for and finding their places in the mainstream of adult life. They appear to have boundless energy for both social and professional activities. They are usually interested in exercise for its own sake and often participate in athletic events as well.

The middle adulthood period ranges from approximately 40 years to 65 years of age. This is a time when the physical activities of young adulthood typically begin to decrease, resulting in lowered kcal requirement for most individuals. During these years, people seldom have young children to supervise, and the strenuous physical labor of some occupations may be delegated to younger people. Middle-age people may tire more easily than they did when they were younger. They may not get as much exercise as they did in earlier years. Because appetite and food intake may not decrease, there is a common tendency toward weight gain during this period (Townsend & Roth, 2000).

Nutritional Requirements

Physical growth is usually complete by the age of 25 years. Consequently, except during pregnancy and lactation, the essential nutrients are needed only to maintain and repair body tissue and to produce energy. During these years, the nutrient requirements of healthy adults change very little.

Despite men's generally larger size, only 11 of the given RDAs are greater for men than for women. Six of the RDAs are the same for both sexes. The iron requirement for women throughout the childbearing years remains higher than that for men. Extra iron is needed to replace blood loss during menstruation and to help build both the infant's and the extra maternal blood needed during pregnancy. After menopause, this requirement for women matches that of men (Townsend & Roth, 2000).

The kcal requirement begins to diminish after the age of 25 years, as basal metabolism is reduced by approximately 2% to 3% per decade. This is a small amount each year, but, after 25 years, a person will gain weight if the total kcal value of the food eaten is not reduced accordingly. An individual's actual need, of course, will be determined primarily by activity and amount of lean muscle mass. Those who are more active will require more kcal than those with a high proportion of fat tissue.

A normal healthy adult should eat a variety of foods as shown on the food guide pyramid. This, along with following the *Dietary Guidelines for Americans,* should provide a healthy diet for the adult. In addition to the basic nutritional assessment, the following should be assessed for the adult client:

- Use of alcohol, tobacco, caffeine, and drugs
- Use of fad diets
- Prescribed restricted diet

Older Adulthood

Physical changes of aging affect nutrition in several ways. The body's functions slow with age, and its ability to replace worn cells likewise diminishes. Metabolic rate slows; bones become less dense; lean muscle mass lessens; eyes do not focus on nearby objects as they once did and some grow cloudy from cataracts; poor dentition is common; the heart and kidneys become less efficient; and hearing, taste, and smell are less acute.

Digestion is affected because the secretion of hydrochloric acid and enzymes diminishes. This, in turn, decreases the intrinsic factor synthesis, which leads to a deficiency of vitamin B_{12}. The tone of the intestines is reduced, possibly resulting in constipation or, in some cases, diarrhea (Townsend & Roth, 2000).

Healthy eating habits throughout life, an exercise program suited to one's age, and enjoyable social activities can prevent or delay physical deterioration and psychological depression during the senior years. The benefits of such pursuits can be said to be circular. The first two contribute largely to one's physical condition, and social activities can prevent or diminish depression, which, if unchecked, can also depress appetite. They give purpose to the day, joy to the heart, and zest to the appetite. Nutrition and lifestyle should be carefully reviewed in any elderly client suspected of having depression.

Food–drug interactions must be monitored closely in the elderly client. Frequently, specific foods will prevent, decrease, or enhance the absorption of a particular drug.

PROFESSIONAL TIP

Food–Drug Interactions

Dairy products should not be consumed within 2 hours of taking the antibiotic tetracycline or the drug will not be absorbed. A person taking a blood clot–reducing drug such as warfarin sodium (Coumadin) must consume vitamin K–rich food in moderation, as this vitamin counteracts blood thinners. Even vitamin supplements can cause interactions. The antioxidant vitamins are not to be taken with blood clot–reducing medications, because they also have a tendency to thin the blood (Townsend & Roth, 2000).

Drug–drug interactions as well as food–drug interactions can contribute to decreased nutritional status. These interactions could affect both appetite and the absorption of nutrients from the food eaten. Careful monitoring is recommended.

Nutritional Requirements

In general, most elderly persons decrease their activity; thus their kcal needs also decrease.

The kcal requirement decreases approximately 2% to 3% per decade, because both metabolism and activity slow. If kcal intake is not reduced, weight will increase. This additional weight increases the work of the heart and puts increased stress on the skeletal system. It is important that the kcal requirement not be exceeded and just as important that the nutrient requirements be fulfilled to maintain good nutritional status. An exercise plan appropriate to one's age and health can be helpful in burning excess kcal and in toning and strengthening the muscles.

Protein needs remain the same or may increase during illness. A well-balanced diet of a variety of foods should supply adequate amounts of vitamins and minerals. An increase in water and dietary fiber is often needed to maintain proper elimination.

In addition to the basic nutritional assessment, the following should be assessed for elderly clients.

- Undesirable change in weight
- Dentition and swallowing
- Appetite
- Vision
- Hand–eye coordination
- Adequacy of daily intake of food
- Ability to self-feed
- Prescribed restricted diet
- Use of alcohol, tobacco, caffeine, and drugs

CLIENT TEACHING

Special Dietary Considerations for Elders

- Give special attention to water needs, regardless of physical activity, because the thirst mechanism is less responsive than in younger people.
- Decrease the kcal requirements in relation to activity: 10% for ages 51–75, and 20% to 25% for ages 75 and older. Bedridden and immobilized persons need a further reduction in kcal. Limit the quantities of empty-kcal foods (sugars, sweets, fats, oils, and alcohol).
- Maintain protein requirements, with 12% to 14% of kcal intake being derived from protein food (meat, eggs, poultry, milk, and cheese).
- Ensure adequate consumption of unsaturated fats, to provide a source of energy, provide the essential fatty acids, utilize the fat-soluble vitamins, and serve as a lubricating agent.
- Select carbohydrates as follows: limit concentrated sweets; use moderate amounts of simple sugars (candy, sugar, jams, jellies, preserves, and syrups); select most sources from complex carbohydrates (fruits, vegetables, cereals, and breads).
- Ensure adequate amounts of vitamin D, calcium, and phosphorus to maintain bone integrity (fortified milk is a good source).
- Consume high-fiber foods (dried fruits, wholegrain cereals, nuts, fresh fruit, and vegetables) to increase satiety and maintain intestinal motility and thereby prevent constipation.
- Maintain a safe, adequate intake of sodium, avoiding canned foods and salted or cured meats high in sodium content for those with cardiac problems and hypertension.
- Include foods from the food guide pyramid in the amounts that meet the RDAs for age 51 and older.

Pregnancy and Lactation

Good nutrition during the 38 to 40 weeks of a normal pregnancy is essential for both mother and child. In addition to her normal nutritional requirements, the pregnant woman must provide nutrients and kcals for the fetus, the amniotic fluid, the placenta, and the increased blood volume and breast, uterine, and fat tissue.

The pregnant woman who follows a nutritionally adequate diet is more apt to feel better, retain her health, and bear a healthy infant than one who chooses her foods thoughtlessly (Townsend & Roth, 2000).

Studies have shown a relationship between the mother's diet and the health of the baby at birth. It is also thought that the woman who consumes a nutritious diet before pregnancy is more apt to bear a healthy infant than one who does not. Malnutrition of the mother is believed to cause growth and mental retardation in the fetus. Infants with low birth weight (less than 5.5 pounds) have a higher mortality (death) rate than those of normal birthweight.

Nutritional Requirements

Despite the saying, the pregnant woman is not "eating for two." No increase in kcal is required during the first 12 weeks of pregnancy. After that time, an extra 300 kcal/day is recommended. This increase can almost be accomplished by drinking two *extra* 8-ounce glasses of 2% milk each day, which supplies 240 kcal. Those two extra glasses of milk also supply the extra calcium, protein, and vitamin D required during pregnancy. The other nutrients that should be increased during pregnancy are folic acid and iron. Folic acid is necessary to prevent neural tube deformities in the fetus. Folic acid has been approved as a supplement for pregnant women. Good sources of folic acid are beef, legumes, wheat germ, and eggs. Good sources of iron are red meat, dried fruit, egg yolk, and wholegrain products. Appendix C lists the RDAs during pregnancy and lactation.

To ensure that the nutritional requirements of pregnancy are met, vitamin supplements may be prescribed in addition to an iron supplement. However, it is *not* advisable for the mother to take any unprescribed nutrient supplement, as an excess of vitamins or minerals can be toxic to mother and infant. Excessive vitamin A, for example, can cause birth defects (Townsend & Roth, 2000).

The mother's kcal requirement increases during lactation. The kcal requirement depends on the amount of milk produced. Approximately 85 kcal are required to produce 100 mL (3⅓ oz) of milk. During the first 6 months, average daily milk production is 750 mL (25 oz), and for this, the mother requires approximately 640 extra kcal a day. During the second 6 months, when the baby begins to eat food in addition to breast milk, average daily milk production slows to 600 mL (20 oz), and the kcal requirement reduces to approximately 510 extra kcal a day.

In addition to the basic nutritional assessment, the following should be assessed for the pregnant client:

- Weight and rate of weight gain
- Diet changes in response to pregnancy
- Cravings for foods or nonfoods (pica)
- Intake of supplemental vitamins/minerals
- Feeding plans (breast or formula)
- Use of alcohol, caffeine, tobacco, or drugs

NUTRITION AND HEALTH

An individual who embraces good nutrition is more likely to have good health than is someone who does not follow good nutritional practices. Of course, all situations of disease or ill health cannot be prevented by good nutrition.

The nutrients in the food we eat may be thought of as the building materials, fuel, and regulators necessary to keep the body functioning. When the body is supplied with nutrients in the proper amounts, it is most likely to function efficiently and effectively. The body is very adaptable and keeps functioning, though less effectively, even when it is not supplied with the proper amounts of nutrients. In this situation, however, the body can become more susceptible to some diseases.

Primary Nutritional Disease

A primary nutritional disease occurs when nutrition is the cause of the disease. Usually, there is an inadequate intake of one or more nutrients. Some examples of such diseases are scurvy, from inadequate intake of vitamin C; rickets, from insufficient intake of vitamin D; and anemia, from a deficiency of iron in the diet.

Excesses of nutrients can also cause illness. These, however, occur when nutrient supplements are taken in excess, rather than from food intake. For instance, excess vitamin D may cause nausea, diarrhea, weight loss, and calcification of the renal tubules, blood vessels, and bronchi. Excess niacin may cause flushing, itching, and hypotension.

Secondary Nutritional Disease

Most nutritional diseases are secondary diseases, that is, they are a complication of another disease or condition. The original disease or condition interferes with digestion or absorption, or there is an increased need for one or more nutrients. For instance, in pregnancy, the body's need for iron increases. Not receiving the increased amount may cause anemia in the mother. In malabsorption disorders, the body is unable to absorb sufficient amounts of certain nutrients. The amount ingested may be adequate, but the body is unable to use it. Rapid excretion from the body, as in diarrhea, does not allow the nutrients to be absorbed and utilized. Uncontrolled, diarrhea can lead to dehydration along with electrolyte and acid–base imbalance.

WEIGHT MANAGEMENT

Maintaining weight at a desired level can be very difficult for some people. Weight management is based on the relationship between the intake and the use of kcal. When these two elements are balanced, weight is maintained at a steady level. A range of 10% over or under the desired weight is considered appropriate.

Determining Caloric Needs

The number of kcal needed to achieve or maintain a desired weight is based on two factors: basal energy needs and total energy requirements.

Basal Energy Need

Basal energy need refers to the number of kcal required to keep an individual alive when at rest. There are two ways to determine basal energy (kcal) needs. One is based on the person's desired weight (Table 18–11), the other on the person's actual weight.

Calculation using desired weight is as follows:

$$\text{Basal energy needs} = \text{desired weight} \times 10$$

Examples
Female: 5 ft 5 in tall
5 ft = 100 lb
5 in =   25 lb
            125 lb desired weight

125 × 10 = 1,250
Basal energy needs = 1,250 kcal

Male: 5 ft 9 in tall
5 ft = 106 lb
9 in =   54 lb
            160 lb desired weight

160 × 10 = 1,600
Basal energy needs = 1,600 kcal

Calculation using actual weight is as follows:

Female weight in kg × 0.9 × 24 = basal kcal
Male weight in kg × 1 × 24 = basal kcal
(Weight in lb ÷ 2.2 = weight in kg)

Examples
Female weighs 130 lb
130 ÷ 2.2 = 59.1 kg
59.1 kg × 0.9 × 24 = 1,276.6
Basal energy needs = 1,276.6 kcal

Table 18–11 DETERMINING DESIRED WEIGHT		
BUILD	**WOMEN**	**MEN**
Medium	100 lb for 5 ft of height, plus 5 lb for each additional inch	106 lb for 5 ft of height, plus 6 lb for each additional inch
Small	Subtract 10%	Subtract 10%
Large	Add 10%	Add 10%

Male weighs 170 lb

170 ÷ 2.2 = 77.3 kg

77.3 kg × 1 × 24 = 1,855.2

Basal energy needs = 1,855.2 kcal

Total Energy Requirements

People do not live their lives at rest. They are active! Kilocalories must be added to the basal metabolic requirements in order to meet the needs of activity. All activity is not equal in kcal needed, however. A person's overall activity level can be divided into sedentary (light, such as watching television), moderate (such as playing a tennis match), or strenuous (such as running a marathon). The following formulas can be used to determine the number of kcal to add given the activity level:

Sedentary: basal kcal × 1.3 = total kcal
Moderate: basal kcal × 1.5 = total kcal
Strenuous: basal kcal × 2.0 = total kcal

Example: The 125-lb woman in the preceding example who is planning on running a marathon would need the following:

1,250 (basal kcal) × 2 = 2,500 kcal

Factors in addition to activity that have an effect on the total kcal need are state of health and climate. A person who is ill needs more kcal to repair tissue. A cold climate requires a person to take in more kcal to provide more thermal energy to maintain body temperature.

Overweight

A person is considered to be overweight when weight is 11% to 19% above the desired weight. **Obesity** is considered present in a person who is 20% or more above the desired weight. Overweight conditions can become serious health hazards by placing increased strain on the heart, lungs, muscles, bones, and joints. Overweight and obese people are more susceptible to diabetes and hypertension and tend to have a shortened life span.

According to the Centers for Disease Control and Prevention (1997), the Third National Health and Nutrition Examination Survey indicated that obesity is rising in the United States. Among children between the ages of 6 and 11 years, 13.7% are overweight; among adolescents ages 12 to 17, 11.5% are overweight. Among adults, 36.4% of men and 33.3% of women are overweight.

Causes

There is no single cause of obesity. Genetic, physiologic, biochemical, and psychological factors may all contribute to overweight conditions. Most often, the cause of being overweight or obese is an energy im-

balance. That is, more kcal are being taken in than are being used. When this occurs, the body stores the excess kcal as adipose tissue. Hypothyroidism is a possible, but rare, cause of obesity. In this condition, basal metabolism is low, thereby reducing the number of kcal needed for energy. Unless corrected, this condition can result in excess weight (Townsend & Roth, 2000).

Treatment

Treatment for an overweight person involves two parts: revised eating habits and exercise. Revised eating habits include reducing daily kcal intake at mealtime, limiting between-meal snacks to fresh fruits or vegetables, and restricting or eliminating empty calories.

One (1) pound of body weight equals 3,500 kcal. Therefore, to lose 1 pound per week, a person must reduce kcal intake by 500 kcal each day. Weight loss should be limited to 1 to 2 pounds per week, unless the client is under strict medical supervision. Diets should be planned according to the minimum servings of the food guide pyramid and should not be reduced to below 1,200 kcal/day in order for the dieter to receive adequate nutrients to sustain health.

Attention should also be given to the preparation of the food. Frying adds many kcal from fat to a food item. Broiling, grilling, baking, roasting, boiling, and poaching are healthy ways to prepare foods. Vegetables should be eaten raw or steamed; the addition of butter, margarine, or sauces should be avoided. Eating habits may be adapted to decrease the amount eaten, and yet provide satisfaction: place food on a smaller plate; cut food into smaller bites; chew each bite at least 12 times; and place the fork on the plate between bites.

Exercise, particularly aerobic exercise, is an excellent adjunct to any weight-loss program. Aerobic exercise uses energy from the body's fat reserves, as it increases the amount of oxygen the body takes in. Examples of aerobic exercise are dancing, jogging, bicycling, skiing, rowing, and power walking. Such exercise helps tone the muscles, burns kcal, increases the basal metabolism so that food is burned faster, and is fun for the participant. Any exercise program must be begun slowly and increased over time so that no physical damage occurs.

Exercise alone can only rarely replace the need to be mindful of diet, however. The dieter should be made aware of the number of kcal burned by specific exercises so as to avoid overeating after the workout.

Underweight

Persons are considered to be underweight when their weight is 10% to 15% below the desired weight. An underweight person is more likely to have nutritional deficiencies because of the decreased intake of food. For women, this can cause complications during pregnancy, when there is an increased need for nutrients. Being underweight may lower a person's resistance to infection. Being severely underweight may even cause death.

Causes

There are several possible causes of being underweight, such as an inadequate intake of food, excessive exercise, poor absorption of nutrients, or severe infection. Occasionally, hyperthyroidism may be the cause. After the adequacy of food intake and the appropriate activity level are ascertained, specific diagnostic tests must be done to determine whether poor absorption, infection, or hyperthyroidism are present.

Treatment

Dietary treatment for an inadequate intake of food is to gradually increase the amount of food eaten. Also, higher-kcal foods can be eaten. Between-meal snacks and a bedtime snack can help increase the intake of food.

If the individual is to gain 1 pound per week, 3,500 kcal in addition to the individual's basic normal weekly kcal requirement are prescribed. This means an extra 500 kcal must be taken in each day. If a weight gain of 2 pounds per week is required, an additional 7,000 kcal each week, or an additional 1,000 kcal per day, are necessary. This diet cannot be immediately accepted at full kcal value. Time will be needed to gradually increase the daily kcal value. In this diet, there is an increased intake of foods rich in carbohydrates, some fats, and protein. Vitamins and minerals are supplied in adequate amounts. If there are deficiencies of some vitamins and minerals, supplements are prescribed (Townsend & Roth, 2000).

FOOD LABELING

In 1990, Congress passed the Nutrition, Labeling and Education Act (NLEA). This was the first legislation on labeling since the 1970s. Prior to this newest legislation, labeling was only required if a nutrient was added or a nutritional claim was made about the product. Now, labeling is required on virtually all retail food products, including bulk foods, fresh produce, and seafood. The nutrition information for fresh produce and seafood is to be displayed or made available at the point of purchase through counter cards, booklets, loose-leaf binders, signs, or tags.

The labels must follow the approved uniform format and use standard serving sizes and household measurements. Information on the label includes calories per serving; calories from fat; total fat, saturated fat, and cholesterol; total sodium; total carbohydrate, dietary fiber, and sugar; amount of protein; and percentages of vitamins A and C, calcium, and iron. A sample food label is shown in Figure 18-7.

Words used to describe nutrient content, such as

Nutrition Facts	
Serving Size ½ cup (114g)	
Servings Per Container 4	

Amount Per Serving	
Calories 90	Calories from Fat 30

	% Daily Value
Total Fat 3g	**5%**
Saturated Fat 0g	**0%**
Cholesterol 0mg	**0%**
Sodium 300mg	**13%**
Total Carbohydrate 13g	**4%**
Dietary Fiber 3g	**12%**
Sugars 3g	
Protein 3g	

Vitamin A	80%	•	Vitamin C	60%
Calcium	4%	•	Iron	4%

• Percent Daily Values are based on a 2,000 calorie diet. Your daily values may be higher or lower depending on your calorie needs:

		Calories	2,000	2,500
Total Fat	Less than		65g	80g
Sat Fat	Less than		20g	25g
Cholesterol	Less than		300mg	300mg
Sodium	Less than		2,400mg	2,400mg
Total Carbohydrate			300g	375g
Fiber			25g	30g

Calories per gram:
Fat 9   •   Carbohydrate 4   •   Protein 4

Figure 18-7 Sample Food Label

low, light, lean, or *reduced,* now have specific, consistent definitions (Table 18–12).

The standardized label and word definitions make it easier for the consumer not only to know the amount of specific nutrients in a food or food product, but also to easily compare foods and food products.

FOOD QUALITY AND SAFETY

When planning an adequate diet, the quality and safety of the food must be considered in addition to the types of foods and serving sizes. To ensure the quality (nutrient content) and safety of food, proper storage, preparation, sanitation, and cooking are necessary; such measures will help prevent or reduce the risk of food-borne illnesses.

Quality of Food

Foods usually begin to lose nutrients when they are harvested, so they are best purchased when fresh in appearance and of bright color. Dates should be checked on all processed foods such as dairy products, lunch and other processed meats, crackers, and breads; all foods should be used prior to their expiration dates. All produce should be cooked until tender and thoroughly done, in the smallest amount of water

Table 18–12 NUTRIENT CONTENT DESCRIPTORS

- **Free, without, no, zero:** The product contains only a tiny or insignificant amount of fat, cholesterol, sodium, sugar, and/or calories. For example, *fat-free* and *sugar-free* contain fewer than 0.5 g per serving. *Calorie-free* has fewer than 5 kcal per serving.

- **Low:** A food described as *low* in fat, saturated fat, cholesterol, sodium, and/or calories could be eaten fairly often without exceeding dietary guidelines. For instance, *low-fat* means no more than 3 g of fat per serving; *low-sodium* means no more than 140 mg of sodium per serving.

- **Lean:** *Lean* means that the product contains fewer than 10 g of fat, 4 g of saturated fat, and 95 mg of cholesterol per serving. *Lean* is not as lean as is *low*.

- **Extra lean:** *Extra lean* means that the product has fewer than 5 g of fat, 2 g of saturated fat, and 95 mg of cholesterol per serving. *Extra lean* is still not as lean as is *low*.

- **Reduced, less, fewer:** Means a diet product contains 25% less of a nutrient or calories. For example, hotdogs might be labeled *25% less fat than our regular hotdogs*.

- **Light/lite:** Means a diet product with ⅓ fewer kcal or ½ the fat of the original. *Light in sodium* means a product with ½ the usual sodium.

- **More:** A food in which one serving has at least 10% more of the daily value of a vitamin, mineral, or fiber than usual.

- **Good source of:** One serving contains 10% to 19% of the daily value for a particular nutrient.

- **High:** One serving contains 20% or more of the daily value for a particular nutrient.

From U.S. Food & Drug Administration (FDA) (1999). The food label [On-line]. Available: http://www.fda.gov/opacom/backgrounders/foodlabel/newlabel.html

COMMUNITY/HOME HEALTH CARE

Resources for Meal Preparation

Ensure that the family has:

- Hot and cold running water;
- A working refrigerator;
- A working oven and range;
- A clean, pest-free kitchen;
- Fresh perishables stored in the refrigerator;
- Adequate food supplies (including canned goods and staples, such as milk and bread), safely stored; and
- Appropriate adaptive equipment, if needed, such as low countertops that facilitate wheelchair access.

From "Home Health Nutrition" by M. Costello, 1996, MedSurg Nursing 5(4), 229–238.

possible to prevent loss of vitamins. Cooking meats via stewing increases mineral loss, so cooking methods that retain the most nutrients should be used instead; these include stir-frying, steaming, microwaving, or pressure cooking.

Safety of Food

There are three aspects to food safety: proper storage, proper sanitation, and proper cooking.

Proper Storage

Foods must be properly stored prior to and after purchase. Packages and jars should be tightly sealed, and cans should not leak or bulge. Any foods that look or smell unusual or show signs of mold or deterioration should be discarded. Hot foods should be kept hot—above 140°F—and cold foods should be kept below 40°F. Foods allowed to stand at temperatures between 40°F and 140°F provide an ideal breeding ground for pathogens. Leftovers must be refrigerated promptly and not allowed to cool before refrigerating.

Proper Sanitation

Proper sanitation means that all cooking utensils, pots, pans, and cutting boards, as well as the cook's hands, have been washed with soap and hot water before preparation begins. To prevent contamination of one food by another, cutting boards, utensils, and the cook's hands should be washed well with soap and hot water between preparation of different foods. A person who is ill should not prepare food. Good hand-washing is a must prior to food preparation and following bathroom use.

Meat, fish, and poultry should be rinsed under cold running water and patted dry with several paper towels before preparing and cooking. A capful of chlorine bleach in a sink one-half full of water can be used to wash fruits and vegetables: leafy vegetables, cauliflower, broccoli, and other fruits and vegetables can be washed in the bleach water for a few minutes, rinsed, and then drained on paper towels.

Proper Cooking

Meats, fish, shellfish, and eggs should be cooked well done to ensure that harmful microorganisms are destroyed (Figure 18-8).

Food-Borne Illnesses

When proper storage, sanitation, or cooking are not maintained, food-borne illnesses often occur. These illnesses range in severity from fairly mild (such as staphylococcal food poisoning) to potentially fatal (such as botulism and *E. coli*). The important thing to remember is that food-borne illness is highly preventable with proper handling, preparation, and storage of food.

It is important to emphasize that nutrition involves the appropriate kinds and amounts of a variety of

Recommended Safe Cooking Temperatures for Home Use

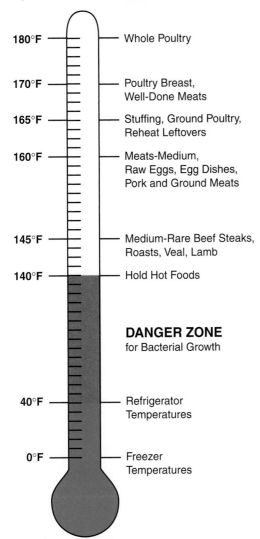

Figure 18-8 Cook foods to a safe temperature. *[From U.S. Department of Agriculture and U.S. Department of Health and Human Services, 2000. Dietary Guidelines for Americans (Home and Garden Bulletin No. 232, 5th ed.). Washington, DC: USDA]*

available foods so that a properly functioning body can digest and use the nutrients in the foods. If the foods are unsafe, they cannot adequately nourish the body.

FOOD ALLERGIES

An **allergy** is an altered reaction of the tissues of some individuals to substances that, in similar amounts, are harmless to other people. The substances causing hypersensitivity are called allergens. A food allergy occurs when the immune system reacts to a food substance, usually a protein. When such a reaction occurs, antibodies form and cause allergic symptoms. An altered reaction to a specific food that does not involve the immune system is called (the specific *food*) *intolerance.*

Allergic Reactions

Allergic reactions are sometimes immediate, or sometimes several hours elapse before signs occur. Allergic individuals seem most prone to allergic reactions during periods of stress. Typical signs of food allergies include hay fever, hives, edema, headache, dermatitis, nausea, dizziness, and asthma (which causes breathing difficulties).

Allergic reactions are uncomfortable and can be detrimental to health. When breathing difficulties are severe, they are life threatening.

Allergic reactions to the same food can differ in two individuals. For example, the fact that someone gets hives from eating strawberries does not mean that an allergic reaction to strawberries will appear as hives in another member of the same family. Allergic reactions can even differ from time to time with the same individual.

Treatment of Allergies

The simplest treatment for allergies is to remove the item that causes the allergic reaction. However, because of the variety of allergic reactions, finding the allergen can be difficult.

When food allergies are suspected, it is wise for the client to keep a food diary for several days and to record all food and drink ingested as well as allergic reactions and the time of their onset. Such records can help pinpoint specific allergens. It is common for other foods in the same class as the allergens to cause allergic reactions as well. Cooking sometimes alters the foods and can eliminate allergic reactions in some people.

Laboratory tests may be used to find the allergen or allergens. The radio allergosorbent test (RAST), for example, may be used to determine which compounds are causing allergic reactions.

 CLIENT TEACHING

Allergies

The client must be taught the food sources of the nutrient or nutrients lacking so that other foods can be substituted that are nutritionally equal to those causing the allergy. It is essential that the client be taught to read the labels on commercially prepared foods and to check the ingredients of restaurant foods carefully. For instance, baked products, mixes, meatloaf, or pancakes may contain egg, milk, or wheat, which may be responsible for the allergic reaction.

After completion of the allergy testing, the client is usually placed on an elimination diet. For 1 or 2 weeks, the client does not eat any of the tested compounds that gave a positive reaction. The client includes in the diet the foods that almost no one reacts to, such as rice, fresh meats and poultry, noncitrus fruits, and vegetables. Sometimes, these diets allow only a limited number of foods and can be nutritionally inadequate. If that is the case, vitamin and mineral supplements may be prescribed.

When relief is found from the allergic symptoms, the client is continued on the diet, and, gradually, other foods are added to the diet at a rate of only one every 4 to 7 days. Those foods most likely to produce allergic reactions are added last until an allergic reaction occurs. The allergy can then be pinpointed, and the offending foods eliminated from the diet. Knowing the cause of the allergy enables the client to lead a healthy, normal life, provided that eliminating these foods does not affect overall nutrition (Townsend & Roth, 2000).

If the elimination of the allergen results in a diet deficient in certain nutrients, suitable substitutes for those nutrients must be found. For example, if a client is allergic to citrus fruits, other foods rich in vitamin C must be found. If the allergy is to milk, soybean milk may be substituted.

NURSING PROCESS

Collection of subjective and objective data regarding the client's nutrition serves as the basis for determining the type of nutritional care the client requires.

Assessment

Proper assessment allows the health care team to determine the degree to which the client's nutritional needs are being met. Assessment must be performed in a logical fashion and should include a nutritional history, physical examination, and the results of laboratory tests.

Subjective Data

Subjective data can be obtained through a nutritional history by asking about food allergies; level of physical activity; cultural, socioeconomic, and religious influences; and the use of alcohol, caffeine, tobacco, drugs, and vitamin or mineral supplements. Several methods can be used in collecting these subjective data: 24-hour recall, food frequency questionnaire, food record, and diet history. Although the history data may indicate adequate nutrition, clients must be reassessed periodically to prevent nutritional problems.

24-Hour Recall The 24-hour recall requires client identification of everything consumed in the previous 24 hours. It is performed easily and quickly by asking pertinent questions. However, clients may be unable

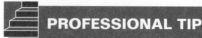

PROFESSIONAL TIP

Nutritional History

Food preferences are an expression of an individual's likes and dislikes. They may be related to the texture of food, how it is prepared, or what was served to the individual during childhood. However, preferences can also be an expression of the person's economic, ecological, ethical, or religious beliefs.

Peer pressures often dictate what teenagers eat. Stress, depression, and alcohol abuse alter the appetite. Medications can alter food absorption and excretion and affect the taste of food. Gastrointestinal disorders can cause anorexia, nausea, vomiting, diarrhea, constipation, discomfort, and pain, all of which may alter eating habits and food preferences.

to accurately recall their intake or anything atypical in the diet. Family members can often assist with these data, if necessary.

Food-Frequency Questionnaire The food-frequency method gathers data relative to the number of times per day, week, or month that the client eats particular foods. The nurse can tailor the questions to particular nutrients, such as cholesterol and saturated fat. This method helps to validate the accuracy of the 24-hour recall and provides a more complete picture of foods consumed.

Food Record The food record provides quantitative information regarding all foods consumed, with portions weighed and measured for three consecutive days. This method requires full client or family member cooperation.

Diet History The diet history elicits detailed information regarding the client's nutritional status, general health pattern, socioeconomic status, and cultural factors. This method incorporates information similar to that collected by the 24-hour recall and food-frequency questionnaire. The history may require more than one interview because of the amount of data to be collected.

Objective Data

A physical examination may elicit findings that suggest nutritional imbalance. Table 18–13 lists physical indicators of nutritional status.

The measurement of a client's intake and output and a daily weight are critical assessments, especially for hospitalized clients. **Anthropometric measurements** (measurement of the size, weight, and proportions of the body) are indicative of the client's calorie–energy expenditure balance, muscle mass, body fat, and protein reserves. The measurements used are body mass index (calculated using weight and height), skinfolds, and limb and girth circumferences.

Table 18–13 PHYSICAL INDICATORS OF NUTRITIONAL STATUS

BODY AREA	GOOD NUTRITION	INADEQUATE NUTRITION
General	Alert, responsive, sleeps well, energetic, seldom ill	Apathetic, easily fatigued, looks tired, often ill
Weight	Appropriate for age, height, body build	Overweight, underweight
Skeleton	Good posture, no malformations	Poor posture
Skin	Good color, no rashes or swelling, smooth, moist, good turgor	Rough, dry, pale, poor turgor
Muscles	Firm, good tone	Flaccid, poor tone
Nails	Pink, firm	Pale, brittle
Eyes	Clear, bright, moist	Dull, pale, dry
Hair	Shiny, smooth	Dull, dry, brittle
Elimination	Regular, soft	Diarrhea or constipation

Body Mass Index Body mass index (BMI) is a measurement used to determine whether a person's weight (in kilograms) is appropriate for height (in meters). It is calculated using a simple formula:

$$BMI = \frac{weight\ (kg)}{[height\ (m)]^2}$$

A BMI of 27 or greater indicates obesity. For example, a person who weighs 65 kilograms and is 1.6 meters tall would have a BMI of 65 kg/(1.6)², or 25.4. Using Table 18–14, find your height and follow the row across to find your weight; then follow the column up to determine your BMI.

Skinfold Measurement Skinfold measurement indicates the amount of body fat. The skinfold is measured by grasping the subcutaneous tissue and taking a reading using a special caliper. Measurements can be taken of the tricep, subscapular, bicep, and suprailiac skinfolds (Figure 18-9).

Table 18–14 BODY MASS INDEX DETERMINATION

How to use this chart:

1. Look down the left column to find your height (*measured in feet and inches*).
2. Look across that row and find the weight nearest your own.
3. Look to the number at the top of the column to identify your BMI.
4. If your number is 27 or greater, you may be at risk.

BMI	25	26	27	28	29	30	31	32	33	34	35	36	37	38	39	40
4'10"	119	124	129	134	138	143	148	153	158	162	167	172	177	181	186	191
4'11"	124	128	133	138	143	148	153	158	163	168	173	178	183	188	193	198
5'	128	133	138	143	148	153	158	164	169	174	179	184	189	194	199	204
5'1"	132	137	143	148	153	158	164	169	174	180	185	190	195	201	206	211
5'2"	136	142	147	153	158	164	169	175	180	186	191	196	202	207	213	218
5'3"	141	146	152	158	163	169	175	180	186	192	197	203	208	214	220	225
5'4"	145	151	157	163	169	174	180	186	192	198	203	209	215	221	227	233
5'5"	150	156	162	168	174	180	186	192	198	204	210	216	222	228	234	240
5'6"	155	161	167	173	179	185	192	198	204	210	216	223	229	235	241	247
5'7"	159	166	172	178	185	191	198	204	210	217	223	229	236	242	248	255
5'8"	164	171	177	184	190	197	203	210	217	223	230	236	243	249	256	263
5'9"	169	176	182	189	196	203	209	216	223	230	237	243	250	257	264	270
5'10"	174	181	188	195	202	209	216	223	230	236	243	250	257	264	271	278
5'11"	179	186	193	200	207	215	222	229	236	243	250	258	265	272	279	286
6'	184	191	199	206	213	221	228	235	243	250	258	265	272	280	287	294
6'1"	189	197	204	212	219	227	234	242	250	257	265	272	280	287	295	303
6'2"	194	202	210	218	225	233	241	249	256	264	272	280	288	295	303	311
6'3"	200	208	216	224	232	240	247	255	263	271	279	287	295	303	311	319
6'4"	205	213	221	230	238	246	254	262	271	279	287	295	303	312	320	328

Used by permission of Knoll Pharmaceutical Company.

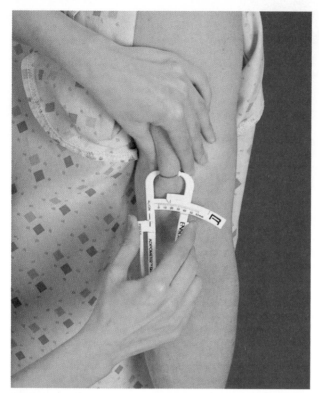

Figure 18-9 Measuring Triceps Skinfold at Midpoint of Upper Arm

Other Measurements Mid–upper-arm circumference serves as an index of skeletal muscle mass and protein reserve. Abdominal-girth measurement serves as an index as to whether the abdomen is increasing, decreasing, or remaining the same. Both of these measurements should be made repeatedly over a span of time, for best assessment.

Laboratory Tests Several laboratory tests provide information about a client's nutritional status. These include the protein indices of serum albumin, pre-albumin, and serum transferrin; hemoglobin; total lymphocyte count; blood urea nitrogen (BUN); and urine creatinine. The serum albumin blood test is used to measure prolonged protein depletion that occurs in chronic malnutrition, liver disease, and nephrosis. The pre-albumin test indicates protein depletion in acute conditions such as trauma and inflammation. Serum transferrin also measures the protein level as indicated

PROFESSIONAL TIP

Creatinine Excretion

Record the client's height and gender on the laboratory request for a creatinine excretion test because the normal values are standardized on the basis of these variables.

by iron stores. Hemoglobin is a measurement of the oxygen- and iron-carrying capacity of the blood. Total lymphocyte count may reflect protein-calorie malnutrition, which inhibits lymphocyte synthesis. Blood urea nitrogen is a nitrogen balance study that indicates the degree to which protein is being depleted or replaced, and urine creatinine excretion indicates the amount of creatinine eliminated by the kidneys.

Nursing Diagnosis

Nursing diagnoses related specifically to nutrition include the following:

Imbalanced Nutrition: Less than Body Requirements
Imbalanced Nutrition: More than Body Requirements
Imbalanced Nutrition: Risk for More than Body Requirements

Other possible nursing diagnoses related to nutritional problems include the following:

Disturbed Body Image
Ineffective Breastfeeding
Impaired Dentition
Deficient Knowledge (specify)
Impaired Oral Mucous Membrane
Pain
Feeding Self-Care Deficit
Chronic Low Self-Esteem
Risk for Impaired Skin Integrity

Planning/Outcome Identification

A plan should be formulated by the nurse and client to achieve mutually agreed-upon goals. The plan is individualized to meet the client's specific needs. These needs may include achieving desired weight, correcting nutritional deficiencies, maintaining a special diet, preventing nutritional disorders secondary to a particular therapy, or improving nutrition to promote health and prevent disease.

Goals for clients with nutritional alterations might be as follows:

Client will maintain intake and output balance.
Client will comply with diet therapy, avoiding high-sodium foods.
Client will gain 2 pounds in 4 weeks.

Implementation

The nurse and client actually carry out the plan through specific actions. Interventions to accomplish the goals may include diet therapy, assistance with meals, weight and intake monitoring, and nutritional support.

Diet Therapy

Diet therapy is the treatment of a disease or disorder with a special diet. A **dietary prescription/order**

is an order written by the physician for food, including liquids. This is similar to a medication prescription written for any medication a client receives. A client must not be given anything to eat or drink without an order. The dietary prescription is written for one or more of the following purposes:

- Provide the client with nutrients needed for maintenance or growth.
- Prepare a client for diagnostic tests.
- Treat the client with a disease or condition.

When the dietary prescription has been received, the dietary department must be notified so that the proper food will be sent to the client.

Many times a client needs some help in understanding changes in the diet and the reasons that the changes are necessary. A basic knowledge of nutrition and diet therapy contributes to the nurse's ability to competently answer the client's questions about nutrition and diet. It is important, however, for the nurse to recognize when to refer questions to the dietitian.

The dietary prescription may be for nothing by mouth, a standard diet, or a special diet.

Nothing by Mouth Nothing by mouth (NPO) status is a type of diet modification as well as a fluid restriction. This intervention is prescribed prior to surgery and certain diagnostic procedures, to rest the GI tract, or when the client's nutritional problem has not been identified.

Standard Diets Each health care agency has standard or house diets. The standard diets include general (sometimes called regular), soft, clear liquid, full liquid, mechanical soft, and pureed.

General, or Regular, Diet The general, or regular, diet is planned in accordance with the food guide pyramid. There are no restrictions of any kind. It is a very adequate diet providing approximately 2,000 kcal a day.

Soft Diet A soft diet provides foods that are easy to chew and swallow, thus promoting mechanical digestion of foods. Foods to be avoided include nuts, seeds (tomatoes and berries with seeds), raw fruits and vegetables, fried foods, and whole grains. The food guide pyramid is the basis for this diet, although fewer kcal, usually approximately 1,800, are provided.

Clear-Liquid Diet The clear-liquid diet, also called the surgical liquid diet, is ordered as preparation for diagnostic tests or as the first meal or two after surgery. It consists mostly of water and carbohydrates, providing approximately 500 kcal/day. This is a very nutritionally inadequate diet but does relieve thirst, aids in hydration, and mildly stimulates peristalsis. Liquids included are water; clear, fat-free broth; tea; coffee; clear and strained fruit juices; jello; popsicles; and carbonated drinks such as lemon-lime soda.

Full-Liquid Diet A full-liquid diet provides approximately 800 to 1,000 kcal per day. It includes all foods that are liquid at room temperature. In addition to the liquids on a clear-liquid diet; milk; milk drinks; cream soups; strained, cooked cereals; ice cream; puddings; all fruit and vegetable juices; and custard are included.

Mechanical Soft or Edentulous Diet A mechanical soft or edentulous diet consists of food fixed especially for a person who has no teeth or has difficulty chewing. The food is either ground or chopped into very small pieces and cooked very soft, to ease the work of chewing.

Pureed Diet A pureed diet provides food that has been blenderized to a smooth consistency. It is prescribed for clients who have difficulty swallowing.

Special Diets The purpose of a special diet is to restore or maintain a client's nutritional status. These diets are variations of the general diet; however, they still must provide all the nutrients of the general diets. Special diets may provide specific amounts of nutrients or may increase or restrict certain foods. Low-residue, high-fiber, liberal bland, fat-controlled, and sodium-restricted are types of special diets.

Low-Residue Diet The low-residue diet of 5 to 10 g of fiber a day is intended to reduce the normal work of the intestines by restricting the amount of dietary fiber and reducing food residue. In some facilities, this diet consists of foods that provide no more than 3 g of fiber a day and do not increase fecal residue. Some low-residue diets limit tough or coarse meats, milk, and milk products. The low-residue diet is prescribed to decrease GI mucosal irritation in clients with diverticulitis, ulcerative colitis, and Crohn's disease. Foods to be avoided include raw fruits (except bananas), vegetables, seeds, plant fiber, and whole grains. Dairy products are limited to two servings per day.

High-Fiber Diet A high-fiber diet contains 25 to 35 g or more of dietary fiber. A high-fiber diet is an integral part of the treatment regimen for diverticulosis because it increases the forward motion of the indigestible wastes through the colon. This diet is believed to help prevent constipation, hemorrhoids, and colon cancer, along with helping in the treatment of diabetes mellitus and atherosclerosis.

The recommended foods for this diet include coarse and whole-grain breads and cereals, bran, all fruits, vegetables (especially raw), and legumes. The diet is

PROFESSIONAL TIP

Opening a Food Tray
Remove the tray cover before moving the overbed table in front of the client. The concentration of odors when the lid is first removed can be nauseating to the client.

nutritionally adequate. High-fiber diets must be introduced gradually to prevent the formation of gas and the discomfort that accompanies it. Eight 8-oz glasses of water also must be consumed along with the increased fiber.

Liberal Bland Diet A liberal bland diet eliminates chemical and mechanical food irritants such as fried foods, alcohol, and caffeine. This diet is prescribed for clients with gastritis and ulcers, because it reduces GI irritation.

Fat-Controlled Diet The fat-controlled diet reduces the total fat ingested by replacing saturated fats with monounsaturated and polyunsaturated fats and restricting cholesterol. This diet is prescribed for clients with atherosclerosis, heart disease, and obesity. Saturated-fat foods to be avoided include animal fats, gravies, sauces, chocolate, and whole-milk products.

Sodium-Restricted Diet Sodium-restricted diets tailor the level of sodium to mild (2 to 3 g); moderate (1,000 mg); strict (500 mg); or severe (250 mg). This diet is prescribed for clients with fluid volume excess, hypertension, heart failure, myocardial infarction, or renal failure.

Assistance with Meals

Assisting with meals consists of preparing the client, preparing the environment, serving the tray, and assisting with eating.

Preparing the Client Before taking a meal tray into a client's room, the nurse must ensure that the client is ready to eat. This means that the client has washed the face and hands, completed oral hygiene, and emptied the bladder, if necessary. The nurse may need to assist with these tasks. The nurse should also help the client into a comfortable eating position; this may be individualized to each client, as not everyone is allowed or able to sit up to eat a meal.

Preparing the Environment The nurse should make every effort to see that the physical environment is as conducive to a pleasant mealtime atmosphere as possible. This may necessitate cleaning and clearing the overbed table so that the tray can be placed on it, tidying the room to remove offensive sights and smells, and brightening the room.

Serving the Tray The nurse should check that the tray contains the diet ordered, that everything on the tray is appropriate for the diet, and that nothing has spilled. For example, if a low-sodium diet tray has a salt packet, the packet should be removed. The nurse should then check the client's ID band against the name on the tray; it is very important that the correct meal is served to each client. The nurse should prepare the food by opening cartons or cutting food, if necessary.

Assisting with Eating The client who needs assistance in eating should be served last. This way, the nurse will have ample time and not have to hurry the client through the meal (Figure 18-10).

Weight and Intake Monitoring

Measuring weight daily or weekly and measuring the amount of food and fluid intake monitors therapy effectiveness.

Recording and Reporting

After the client has finished eating, the tray should be promptly removed. The amount of food eaten should be recorded, usually as the percentage of the meal eaten. When a client with diabetes does not eat all the food on the tray, both the charge nurse and the dietitian must be notified so that a supplemental feeding can be sent later. If the client is on intake and output (I & O), the amount of fluids consumed during the meal must be recorded. Any problems or difficulty in eating as well as likes and dislikes should be reported and documented on the client's medical record.

Nutritional Support

There are two routes for delivery of nutritional support in adult clients: enteral nutrition and parenteral nutrition. **Enteral nutrition** includes both the inges-

PROFESSIONAL TIP

Feeding a Client
- Position yourself at the same level as the client (stand if the bed is high, sit if the bed is low).
- Allow time for prayer, if the client wishes.
- Protect the client's clothing with a napkin.
- Allow time for chewing (do not hurry the client).
- Give bite-size portions.
- Warn about hot foods (do not blow on food to cool).
- Use a separate straw for each liquid.
- Allow the client to choose the order in which the food is eaten.
- Offer pleasant conversation.

PROFESSIONAL TIP

Feeding the Client Who Is Visually Impaired
Clients with impaired vision need established routines that facilitate feeding. For example, foods are usually placed on the plate in a clockwise order: bread at the 12 o'clock position, meat at 3 o'clock, starches at 6 o'clock, and vegetable at 9 o'clock. The plate should have a raised edge so that the food can be scooped to the outside of the plate. Serving liquids in either a glass or a cup with a plastic lid and straw may be helpful in preventing spills.

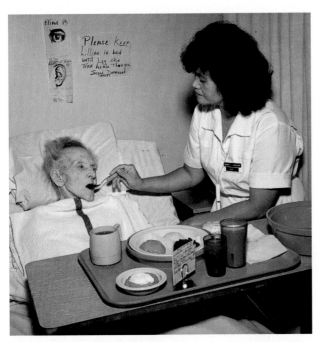

Figure 18-10 Older adults may have health problems that affect their ability to self-feed.

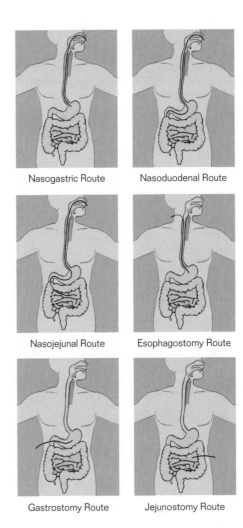

Nasogastric Route   Nasoduodenal Route

Nasojejunal Route   Esophagostomy Route

Gastrostomy Route   Jejunostomy Route

Figure 18-11 Enteral Feeding Routes

tion of food orally and the delivery of nutrients through a GI tube, but is generally used to mean the latter. **Parenteral nutrition** refers to nutrients bypassing the GI system and entering the blood directly.

Enteral Nutrition When clients cannot or will not take food by mouth, but their GI tracts are working, they will be given tube feedings (TF). Sometimes, this may be necessary because of unconsciousness, surgery, stroke, severe malnutrition, or extensive burns. Tube feedings maintain the structural and functional integrity of the GI tract, enhance the utilization of nutrients, and provide a safe economical method of feeding.

Usually, for periods that do not exceed 6 weeks, tube feeding is administered through a nasogastric (NG) tube inserted through the nose and into the stomach or small intestine. When the tube cannot be placed in the nose or when tube feedings will be required for more than 6 weeks, an opening called an ostomy is surgically created into the esophagus (esophagostomy), the stomach (gastrostomy), or the intestine (jejunostomy) (Figure 18-11). The physician selects the route and type of feeding tube. The tubes used for these feedings are soft, flexible, and as small as they can be and still allow the feeding to pass through. Numerous commercial formulas are available, with varying types and amounts of nutrients.

There are three methods for administering tube feedings: intermittent, bolus, and continuous. Usually tube feedings are administered by the continuous infusion method, preferably with a pump. This means the feeding is continuous over a 16- to 24-hour period. Sometimes, the formula is given at half strength at a rate of 30 to 50 mL per hour. This rate may be increased by ap-

proximately 25 mL every 4 hours until tolerance has been established. As soon as the client tolerates the half-strength formula, a full-strength formula is initiated at the appropriate rate. When clients are ready to return to oral feedings, the transfer must be done gradually.

Parenteral Nutrition Parenteral nutrition is the infusion of a solution directly into a vein to meet the client's daily nutritional requirements. It is used if the GI tract is not functional or if normal feeding is not adequate for the client's needs. Formerly called hyperalimentation, it is now frequently referred to as total parenteral nutrition (TPN). The solution used in this intravenous infusion contains dextrose, amino acids, fats, essential fatty acids, vitamins, and minerals. Administration of TPN is generally a function of the registered nurse.

Evaluation

The effectiveness of the plan is evaluated in relation to attaining the desired goals. The nurse must assess whether the goals were met. The plan is continued or modified based on the evaluation.

SAMPLE NURSING CARE PLAN

THE CLIENT WITH ALTERED NUTRITION

Mrs. Vincent, age 58 years, is seen in the clinic for her yearly physical examination. She says, "I hardly have the energy to get up and dressed in the morning. Cleaning the house and doing the laundry make me exhausted." She does not work and is not involved in community activities. Her daily routine involves cooking for her husband, reading, and watching TV for 6 to 8 hours. She loves to bake fresh breads and pastry. She has a history of being overweight and does not exercise. She says, "I eat because I have nothing else to do." Assessment reveals: height, 5'3"; weight, 166 pounds; weight gain, 14 pounds in the past year; sedentary lifestyle; eats in response to having nothing to do.

Nursing Diagnosis *Imbalanced Nutrition: More than Body Requirements, related to excess intake of high-calorie foods, eating in response to boredom, and sedentary lifestyle as evidenced by height–weight relationship and weight gain*

PLANNING/GOALS	NURSING INTERVENTIONS	RATIONALE	EVALUATION
Mrs. Vincent will verbalize factors contributing to excess weight.	Conduct a dietary history, using open-ended statements to assist Mrs. Vincent in exploring factors that may contribute to excess eating.	A nonjudgmental approach to acquiring information will encourage client trust and honesty.	Mrs. Vincent verbalized boredom as the main reason for eating.
Mrs. Vincent will lose 1 to 2 pounds each week while eating well-balanced meals.	Assess Mrs. Vincent's motivation to lose weight.	Having the client's support for the plan will influence success.	Mrs. Vincent is drinking water with meals, chewing her food slowly, and chewing gum while watching TV. She has lost 1.5 pounds in 1 week.
	Suggest methods to adapt eating habits to decrease amount of intake (smaller servings, taking small bites and chewing each bite 12 times, placing the fork on the plate between bites, drinking water with meals, eating only at mealtime, chewing sugar-free gum when watching TV).	Healthy eating habits and tips on recognizing fullness during a meal will help the client eat to satisfy hunger, not boredom.	
	Instruct Mrs. Vincent to maintain a daily dietary intake log: time, food, and amount.	Helps the client recognize her eating patterns and note healthy and unhealthy behaviors.	
	Provide and review the food guide pyramid and *Dietary Guidelines;*	Ensures that the client has information necessary to plan healthy	

continues

	plan with Mrs. Vincent a diet for 1 week, taking into consideration food preferences.	meals within recommended guidelines.	
Mrs. Vincent will engage in 20 to 30 minutes of exercise three times a week.	Review with Mrs. Vincent age-appropriate exercises; emphasize the need for walking.	Changing sedentary lifestyle will increase self-esteem, burn calories, increase energy level, and decrease boredom.	Mrs. Vincent now walks 30 minutes 4 days a week.
Mrs. Vincent will explore outside interests to decrease boredom and increase feelings of self-worth.	Review with Mrs. Vincent community interests outside the home, unrelated to cooking and eating.	Helps the client focus on activities not involving food, thereby decreasing boredom and increasing self-esteem.	Mrs. Vincent will begin volunteering 2 hours three times a week at the church's child care center.

CASE STUDY

Tom, age 27 years, has been HIV positive for 4 years. He is admitted to the hospital complaining of diarrhea and cramping for 3 weeks and a burn wound on his right forearm that will not heal. He states, "I do not have the energy to eat or get dressed. For the past month, I have eaten mainly bread, cereal, milk, and potatoes."

The following questions will guide your development of a nursing care plan for the case study.

1. What subjective and objective data should the nurse gather?
2. Which nursing diagnoses and goals would be appropriate for Tom?
3. List appropriate nursing interventions for helping Tom meet the goals.
4. List teaching Tom will need before leaving the hospital.

SUMMARY

- The LP/VN plays an important role in promoting proper nutrition.
- The six types of nutrients are water, fats, carbohydrates, protein, vitamins, and minerals.
- Water is the most vital nutrient.
- There must always be a balance between water intake and output to maintain health.
- Nutrients build, repair, and maintain body tissue; provide energy; and regulate body processes.
- The food guide pyramid identifies the five food groups for a well-balanced diet along with a range of servings to meet varying kcal needs.
- Nutritional needs vary as an individual moves through the life cycle.
- Nutrition is influenced by culture, religion, socioeconomics, fads, superstitions, age, and health.

- The kcal needs of an individual are based on basal energy needs and activity.
- Weight management is based on the relationship between the intake and the use of kcal.
- Food safety is based on proper storage, proper sanitation, and proper cooking.
- Food-borne illnesses can be fairly mild or fatal.

Review Questions

1. The role of the LP/VN in meeting the nutritional needs of the client includes:
   a. writing the diet order.
   b. preparing food for clients.
   c. preparing a complete diet plan.
   d. answering questions about nutrition.

2. Which of the following would most likely be on a clear liquid diet?

   a. milk shake
   b. tomato soup
   c. orange juice
   d. cranberry juice

3. What is the main function of carbohydrates?

   a. build and repair tissue
   b. provide the body with energy
   c. provide a source of dietary fiber
   d. insulate the body to prevent heat loss

4. What is the fuel value of protein?

   a. 3 kcal/g
   b. 4 kcal/g
   c. 8 kcal/g
   d. 9 kcal/g

5. Which of the following is a complete protein?

   a. milk
   b. gelatin
   c. pinto beans
   d. peanut butter

6. Which of the following is the best source of dietary fiber?

   a. popcorn
   b. chicken
   c. tomato juice
   d. macaroni and cheese

7. Which of the following is true of cholesterol?

   a. It is made in the body.
   b. It has no function in the body.
   c. It is not important in any disease.
   d. It should not be included in the diet.

8. A female client is 5 ft. 5 in. tall and weighs 180 lb. What would be her desired weight?

   a. 115 pounds
   b. 120 pounds
   c. 125 pounds
   d. 130 pounds

9. Why should the nurse advise a client to take an iron supplement with orange juice?

   a. to prevent heartburn
   b. to prevent constipation
   c. to improve absorption of the iron
   d. to improve digestion of the orange juice

10. Where is most of the water in the body found?

    a. inside the cells
    b. in the intestines
    c. in the blood and lymph
    d. in the kidneys and bladder

Critical Thinking Questions

1. What recommendations should be made regarding vitamin supplements?

2. What should the nurse know about nutrition in order to properly care for an obese client?

 WEB FLASH!

- Search the web for information about a vaccine for *E. Coli* O157:H7.
- What resources related to nutrition can be found on the Internet?

REST AND SLEEP

MAKING THE CONNECTION

Refer to the following chapters to increase your understanding of rest and sleep:

- **Chapter 8, Communication**
- **Chapter 9, Nursing Process**
- **Chapter 11, Client Teaching**
- **Chapter 13, Complementary/Alternative Therapies**

- **Chapter 16, Stress, Adaptation, and Anxiety**
- **Chapter 26, Pain Management**

LEARNING OBJECTIVES

Upon completion of this chapter, you should be able to:
- *Define key terms.*
- *Describe the stages of sleep.*
- *Discuss age-related sleep variations.*
- *State the outcomes of sleep deprivation.*
- *Delineate nursing interventions that promote rest and sleep.*

KEY TERMS

biological clock	REM movement
bruxism	disorder
cataplexy	rest
chronobiology	restless leg syndrome
circadian rhythm	sleep
hypersomnia	sleep apnea
insomnia	sleep cycle
jet lag	sleep deprivation
narcolepsy	snoring
parasomnia	somnambulism

INTRODUCTION

The quality of rest and sleep can have a significant impact on a client's health, including physical well-being, mental status, and effectiveness of coping mechanisms. This chapter explores both the importance of rest and sleep and the nursing care that will help clients maintain optimal health when disturbances in rest and sleep patterns threaten to compromise health status.

REST AND SLEEP

Rest and sleep are fundamental components of well-being. All individuals require certain periods of calm and lesser activity so that their bodies can regain energy and rebuild stamina. The need for rest and sleep varies with age, developmental level, health status, activity level, and cultural norms.

Rest refers to a state of relaxation and calmness, both mental and physical. Activity during rest periods can range from lying down to reading a book to taking a quiet walk. When discussing a client's rest patterns, the nurse should try to ascertain those activities and environments that the client defines as restful (Figure 19-1).

Sleep refers to a state of altered consciousness during which an individual experiences fluctuations in level of consciousness; minimal physical activity; and a general slowing of the body's physiologic processes. Sleep generally occurs in a periodic cycle and usually lasts for several hours at a time; disruptions in the usual sleep routine can be distressing to clients and will most likely impair further sleep. As a restorative function, sleep is necessary for physiologic and psychological healing to occur. It is important for clients, their significant others, and health care providers to understand both the normal sleep–wake cycle and the ways sleep affects mood and healing.

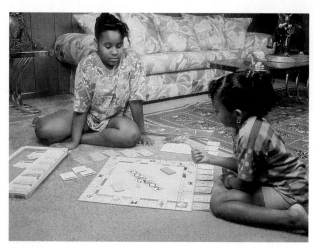

Figure 19-1 Playing a quiet board game can be a relaxing activity for children.

Physiology of Rest and Sleep

The cycles of wakefulness and sleep are controlled by centers in the brain and are influenced by routines and environmental factors. An individual's biological clock also helps determine the specific cycles that will be followed for wakefulness and sleep.

Stages of Sleep

Electroencephalograph (EEG) patterns, eye movements, and muscle activity are used to identify stages of sleep. The stages of sleep are classified in two categories: non-rapid eye movement (NREM) and rapid eye movement (REM) sleep.

NREM Sleep With the onset of sleep, heart rate and respiratory rate slow slightly and remain regular. This first phase of sleep is referred to as non-rapid eye movement, or NREM, sleep. This sleep phase consists of four different stages. As the client enters *stage 1 sleep,* EEG frequency slows overall, but wave spikes occur; the eyes tend to roll slowly from side to side, and muscle tension remains absent except in the facial and neck muscles. In adult clients with normal sleep patterns, stage 1 sleep usually lasts only 10 minutes or so. Stage 1 NREM sleep is of a very light quality, meaning that during this stage, a sleeper can be easily awakened. If awakened, the sleeper often feels as if he has been daydreaming.

Stage 2 sleep is still fairly light sleep; EEG patterns slow further, slow-rolling eye movements stop, and relaxation heightens. Fifty percent of normal adult sleep may be spent in stage 2. After an initial 20 minutes or so of stage 2 sleep, a deep form of sleep, called stage 3 to 4, is entered.

Stage 3 and *stage 4 sleep* are frequently discussed together because of the difficulty in identifying and separating the two. Stage 3 refers to medium-depth sleep, and stage 4 signals the deepest sleep. Each stage lasts 15 to 30 minutes. During these stages, all cortical brain cells appear to be firing at the same time, resulting in large, slow waves on the EEG. Vital signs are significantly lower than during waking hours. When roused from stage 3 to 4 sleep, an adult can take 15 seconds or so to become fully awake. This difficulty in awakening is even more pronounced in children. Stage 3 to 4 sleep is when most sleepwalking, sleeptalking, enuresis, and night terrors occur.

Stage 3 to 4 sleep is felt to have restorative value, necessary for physical recovery. The majority of human growth hormone is secreted at night, peaking during stage 3 to 4 sleep, near the beginning of a sleep period. This growth hormone is required not only for growth but also for normal tissue repair in clients of all ages. Stage 3 to 4 sleep accounts for approximately 25% of sleep in children, declines slightly in young adulthood, gradually declines in middle age, and may be absent in elderly clients.

REM Sleep After the initial 90 minutes or so of NREM sleep in adults, the client enters rapid eye movement, or REM, sleep. The EEG pattern resembles that of the awake state; rapid, conjugate eye movements are present; heart rate and respiratory rate are irregular and often higher than when awake; and muscles, including those of the face and neck, are flaccid, leaving the body immobilized. Dreams occur 80% of the time clients are in REM sleep; these dreams serve as a vehicle for clients to consolidate memories,

---

PROFESSIONAL TIP

Sleep Deprivation

Sleep deprivation can be deadly, and the price tag is staggering. According to the National Sleep Foundation (NSF, 1998), sleep-related accidents cost the U.S. government and businesses $46 billion each year. Drowsy drivers are blamed for 100,000 police-reported crashes each year in the United States, and 31% of commercial truck crashes that are fatal to the driver are caused by drowsiness.

Forty million people in the United States have serious sleep disorders that undermine the quality of their sleep and their health. Many of these sleep disorders are undiagnosed (NSF, 1998). During the past century, the average time asleep for the typical American has been reduced by 20%. The person who is deprived of restful sleep is less alert, less attentive, less able to perform even simple tasks, more irritable, and has poorer concentration and judgment and mood problems that make relationships with family, friends, and coworkers difficult. No matter the cause of sleep deprivation, inadequate sleep reduces the quality of life and is harmful to health.

adapt behaviors, solve problems, and clarify thoughts and emotions. Unlike stage 3 to 4 sleep, which is most abundant during the early portion of a sleep period, REM-sleep periods become longer as the night progresses and the individual becomes more rested.

Sleep Cycle

A **sleep cycle** refers to the sequence of sleep that begins with the four stages of NREM sleep in order, with a return to stage 3 and then stage 2, followed by passage into the first REM stage (Figure 19-2). The duration of a sleep cycle is generally 70 to 90 minutes, and the typical sleeper will pass through four to six sleep cycles during an average sleep period of 7 to 8 hours.

The length of the NREM and REM periods of sleep will change as the overall sleep period progresses and the sleeper becomes more relaxed and re-energized.

There is less need for stage 3 to 4 sleep and more need for REM sleep as the sleep period progresses, and dreams during the REM phases of later sleep may become more vivid and intense. If the sleep cycle is broken at any point, a new sleep cycle will start, beginning again at stage 1 of NREM sleep and progressing through all the stages to REM sleep.

Biological Clock

The **biological clock** is an internal mechanism capable of measuring time in a living organism. It controls the daily fluctuations in hundreds of physiologic processes, including body temperature, respiratory rate, performance, alertness, and a number of hormone levels. According to Coleman (1986), the major characteristics of biological clocks are:

- They are internal physiologic systems that can measure the passage of time;
- They have their own daily cycle length, which is close to, but not exactly, 24 hours;
- When exposed to normal environmental cues, such as the day–night cycle, they can adapt to a 24-hour day; and
- When free of environmental cues, such as the day–night cycle, the organism's internal cycle length determines its behavior.

When external time cues such as day–night, sleep–wake, and mealtimes are inconsistent, a desynchronization, or mismatching, of the circadian biological rhythms occurs. This internal desynchronization disrupts

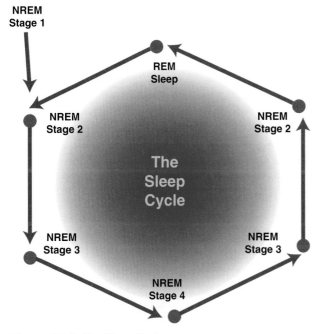

Figure 19-2 The Sleep Cycle

the timing of physiologic and behavioral activity, which, in turn, causes chronic fatigue, disrupted sleep patterns, and decreased performance and coping abilities. An example of desynchronization is that of the newborn, whose biological rhythms are not established until 3 to 4 months of age. At this point, infants will start to develop longer sleep periods at night and become more predictable in their waking and sleeping patterns.

Factors Affecting Rest and Sleep

Several factors can influence the quality and quantity of both rest and sleep. Often, sleep problems result from a combination of many factors.

Degree of Comfort

Comfort is a highly subjective experience. The nurse must assess the degree to which the client's physical

and psychological needs have been met. Whenever basic needs are not satisfied, the person experiences discomfort, which, in turn, leads to physiologic tension and resultant anxiety and, potentially, disturbed sleep and rest. For example, a client experiencing hunger or pain may become restless and irritable and will focus on getting these needs met as opposed to getting restful sleep.

Anxiety

A restless body and mind interfere with the ability to sleep. When trying to go to sleep, many individuals often have intrusive thoughts or muscular tension, which interferes with rest and sleep. Anxiety related to work pressures, family demands, and other stressors does not automatically cease when an individual attempts to go to sleep, and it often results in difficulty falling or staying asleep.

Environment

Environmental factors can either enhance or impair sleep. Lighting, temperature, odors, ventilation, and noise level can all interrupt the sleep process when they differ from the norms of the client's usual sleep environment. The comfort and size of the bed, firmness of the pillow, and habits (snoring or movements) of a sleep partner may all interfere with sleep.

Lifestyle

A fast-paced life filled with multiple stressors can result in a person's inability to relax easily or to fall asleep quickly. Relaxation precedes healthy sleep. Vigorously exercising within an hour of going to bed or performing mentally intense activities just before or after getting into bed often work against getting a good night's sleep.

Another lifestyle factor that interferes with sleep is having a work schedule that does not coincide with an individual's biological clock (e.g., working at times other than the day shift). Approximately 20% of employees in the United States are shift workers (NSF, 2000a). Individuals who frequently change work shifts

PROFESSIONAL TIP

Providing Environmental Comfort
A firm pillow is suggested for side-sleepers, a medium pillow for back-sleepers, and a soft pillow for stomach sleepers (*Pillow Firmness Key,* 1998).

CULTURAL CONSIDERATIONS

Cultural and Societal Expectations Affecting Sleep
Some people perceive sleep as a luxury to be indulged in when they are not too busy with "important" activities. Others view sleep as an absolute necessity. The amount of sleep that a person considers necessary is partially determined by the attitudes of family and culture.

or travel across several times zones face a real challenge in trying to stabilize their biological rhythms and rest comfortably.

Diet

The type of food consumed has an impact on the quality and quantity of sleep. Foods high in caffeine, such as coffee, colas, and chocolate, serve as stimulants and often disrupt the normal sleep cycle. Also, consuming a large, heavy, or spicy meal just before bedtime may cause indigestion, which will likely interfere with sleep. Conversely, going to bed when hungry can also result in sleep problems because the individual may be preoccupied with food and hunger pangs instead of concentrating on sleep.

Drugs and Other Substances

Alcohol and nicotine use can also impair sleep. Small amounts of alcohol may help some people fall asleep; in others, however, alcohol may interfere with REM sleep, causing very restless and nonrefreshing sleep. Nicotine, which is a stimulant, can also impair the sleep cycle by stimulating the body, resulting in difficulty falling and staying asleep. Many medications, both prescription and over the counter, list fatigue, sleepiness, restlessness, agitation, or insomnia as side effects, all of which will have an impact on the quality and quantity of rest and sleep.

Safety: Medications and Sleep
Some medications used to treat high blood pressure, asthma, or depression, may cause sleeping difficulties. For instance, captopril (Capoten) and theophylline (Theomar), used in the treatment of high blood pressure and asthma, respectively, may cause insomnia, whereas trazodone (Desyrel), an antidepressant, can either induce drowsiness or cause insomnia.

Age/Aging

Although sleep and rest patterns are closely tied to lifestyle and other variables, some common variations are based on age.

The neonate (birth–1 month) sleeps in 3- to 4-hour intervals for a total of approximately 16 to 20 hours per day. The newborn usually is very passive, with little

activity occurring during sleep ("sleeping like a baby"), and typically sleeps very soundly. For the first few weeks or even months of life, a baby's biological clock is not attuned to regular day–night patterns, so there is often no difference in sleep patterns between day and night.

The infant averages approximately 12 to 16 hours of sleep per day. As the infant ages, the amount of sleep needed decreases. At approximately 2 months of age, infants can begin to sleep through the night and will typically nap two or three times during the day.

During toddlerhood, the daily average amount of sleep is 12 to 14 hours, which is usually broken down into 10 to 12 hours at night and one or two daytime naps (Figure 19-3). During this stage, bedtime rituals often develop and assume great importance in providing nighttime security. A repeated and predictable nighttime routine such as a bath, brushing teeth, and reading books is helpful in establishing expectations and comfort.

The preschool child sleeps approximately 10 to 12 hours per day. Daytime napping decreases or ceases, unless cultural norms dictate otherwise. Night sleep is often filled with vivid dreams and nightmares, which often awaken children several times during the night.

The school-age child also averages approximately

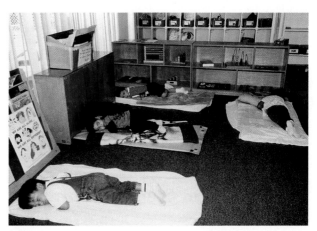
Figure 19-3 Young children require naps and rest periods throughout the day.

10 to 12 hours of sleep daily. Both resistance to bedtime and struggles for independence are hallmarks of the school-age child. During this time, the child may develop fear of the dark and will need reassurance and methods to handle this fear.

Adolescents sleep approximately 8 to 10 hours per day and often decide their own bedtime routines and hours. A high activity level often interferes with regular sleep patterns, and irregular sleeping habits often become the norm at this stage.

The young adult averages approximately 8 hours of sleep per day. During this stage, sleep is often interrupted by young children in the home or by work responsibilities. Lifestyle patterns cause many young adults to experience difficulties falling or staying asleep.

The middle-age adult sleeps approximately 6 to 8 hours per day. Daily stressors may continue to result in insomnia, and use of sleep-inducing medications is common.

Most older adults sleep less at one time than do those who are younger, though overall sleep needs remain constant at 7 to 9 hours (NSF, 2000d). They may go to sleep earlier, wake up more often, get less "deep" sleep, and rise earlier (NSF, 2000a). Often, a daytime nap is taken. The quality of sleep may diminish due to frequent waking, physical pain, and less time spent in stage 3 to 4 sleep. The percentage of REM sleep remains fairly constant.

Physical Factors

The stress imposed by illness often disrupts sleep. Some physical problems can interfere with the ability to fall asleep or stay asleep. Conditions that cause discomfort or pain, such as arthritis, make it difficult to sleep well, as can breathing disorders such as sleep apnea and asthma. Hormonal changes that cause premenstrual syndrome (PMS) or menopause with its hot flashes can disrupt sleep. Even pregnancy, especially during the last few weeks, may make sleeping difficult.

Sleep is especially disrupted when a person is hospitalized. Some factors associated with hospitalization that lead to sleep impairment include:

- Physical or emotional pain,
- Loss of familiar surroundings,
- Loss of routine,
- Fear of the unknown,
- Timing of assessments, procedures, and treatments,
- Intrusive lighting or equipment,
- Noise level (especially unfamiliar noises), and
- Loss of privacy.

Alterations in Sleep Patterns

Sleep disturbances can take many forms and are quite common. Alterations in sleep patterns are generally viewed as either primary sleep disorders (those

wherein the sleep alteration is the fundamental problem) or secondary sleep disorders (those wherein the alteration has a medical or clinical cause that results in or contributes to the sleep alteration). The most common sleep alterations include insomnia, hypersomnia, narcolepsy, sleep apnea/snoring, sleep deprivation, parasomnias, restless leg syndrome, and periodic limb movement disorder.

Insomnia

Insomnia refers to difficulty falling asleep or staying asleep (ASDA, 2000). It affects one in three adults each year in the United States (Cooper, 1998). Insomnia is not a disease, but it may be a manifestation of many illnesses. Causes may include stress, depression, medical problems, caffeine, alcohol, pain, shortness of breath, poor sleep habits, or changes in sleep patterns related to travel or shift work. The person experiencing insomnia often gets caught up in a vicious cycle of not being able to sleep, trying harder to fall asleep, and experiencing increasing anxiety about not sleeping, which, in turn, increases the inability to fall asleep.

Symptoms of insomnia include difficulty falling to sleep, waking frequently during the night, waking very early and not being able to go back to sleep, feeling unrested in the morning and/or tired during the day, and becoming anxious and restless as bedtime arrives. Many who have insomnia actually sleep significantly more than they think they do; thus, there is a discrepancy between perception and reality.

Many times, insomnia may occur only for a night or two. If it continues for more than a few nights or is viewed as very disturbing or disruptive by the individual, a health care provider should be consulted for some relief. Treatment for insomnia is best directed at modifying those factors or behaviors that are causing it.

Hypersomnia

Hypersomnia is an alteration in sleep pattern characterized by excessive sleep, especially in the daytime. Persons suffering from hypersomnia often feel that they cannot get enough sleep at night, and, therefore, they sleep very late into the morning and nap several times throughout the day. Causes of hypersomnia can be physical (such as a disease or use of medications) or psychological (such as a self-imposed short sleep time); treatment depends on addressing the underlying cause.

Narcolepsy

Narcolepsy, another sleep alteration, manifests as sudden, uncontrollable urges to fall asleep during the daytime. Approximately 1 in 2,000 people have narcolepsy (NSF, 2000d). These "sleep attacks" can occur during a conversation or while driving, and they can last from a few seconds to more than 30 minutes. A common characteristic of narcolepsy is **cataplexy**, a sudden loss of muscle control, which may cause the person to fall. The person may also experience vivid dreamlike images as they fall asleep or as they awaken (NSF, 2000d).

Individuals suffering from narcolepsy often achieve adequate sleep at night but are overwhelmed by sleepiness at unexpected and unpredictable periods during the day. There is no cure, but symptoms can be controlled by taking short daytime naps, taking prescribed stimulant medications, or avoiding substances or activities that cause sleepiness.

Sleep Apnea/Snoring

Sleep apnea is characterized by breathing pauses of 30 to 60 seconds during sleep, interspersed between loud **snoring** (noisy breathing during sleep) episodes. The trachea partially closes, and the individual grunts, snorts, and snores. Pulse rate slows and may become irregular. Receptors in the brain, sensing a loss of oxygen, struggle to awaken the sleeper. The unaware sleeper wakes up several hundred times a night for 5 to 10 seconds, takes a deep breath, rolls over, and goes back to sleep, only to start another cycle of apnea. More often than not, sleep apnea victims have no idea that they are not breathing or that they are continually waking up (ASF, 2000f).

The result of sleep apnea is REM-sleep deprivation, which may manifest as daytime sleepiness or chronic fatigue. Persons with sleep apnea have a three to seven times greater risk of falling asleep while driving (NSF, 2000d). Complications can include hypertension and an increased risk of heart attack or stroke. The first line of defense against apnea is treating its cause. Use of a nasal continuous positive airway pressure (CPAP) device, which maintains airflow with a small compressor, may give relief. Dental appliances that reposition the tongue may also help (NSF, 2000d). With some individuals, surgical intervention is required to correct the cause of the apnea.

Sleep Deprivation

Sleep deprivation is a term used to describe prolonged inadequate quality and quantity of sleep, either of the REM or the NREM type. Sleep deprivation can result from age, prolonged hospitalization, drug and substance use, illness, and frequent changes in lifestyle patterns. Sleep and dreaming have a restorative value necessary for mental and emotional recovery, and they appear to enhance the ability to cope with emotional problems. Therefore, sleep deprivation can cause symptoms ranging from irritability, hypersensitivity, and confusion to apathy, sleepiness, and diminished reflexes. Treating or minimizing the factors that cause the sleep deprivation is the most effective intervention.

Parasomnia

Parasomnia refers to a condition wherein a person suffers from profoundly disturbed sleep due to behavioral or physiological events. **Somnambulism** (sleepwalking), sleeptalking, night terrors, REM movement disorder, bed wetting, and **bruxism** (teeth grinding) are the most common parasomnias; the first four are discussed in more detail following. Treatment for parasomnias varies, and care should be focused on helping the client and family understand the given disorder and its potential safety risks.

Somnambulism Sleepwalking, mostly done by children, is typically not remembered by the individual the next morning. The sleepwalker usually moves around furniture very safely, though doors and windows must be kept locked at night to protect the sleepwalker from harm. Sleepwalkers are difficult to rouse during an episode and if awakened are often confused and without any specific recall of events that led to their behavior. Sleepwalking tends to run in families and usually stops at puberty (NSF, 2000d).

Sleeptalking Sleeptalking can occur at any age. It may be a word or two or a long speech, sometimes understandable and sometimes gibberish. The person has no memory of talking, but the sleep partner may have been awakened.

Night Terrors Night terrors, sometimes called sleep terrors, are more common in children and seldom continue into adulthood. Night terrors usually occur during NREM stage 3 to 4 sleep. The child suddenly appears to awaken, thrashes about, sweats, and may even cry. This can last anywhere from 1 minute to approximately 15 minutes. The child remembers nothing in the morning (Brown, 1997). Reassurance by the parents during the episode is the only treatment; the child will eventually outgrow the behavior.

REM Movement Disorder **REM movement disorder** results when the paralysis that normally occurs during REM sleep is absent or incomplete and the sleeper acts out the dream that is occurring. It is most common among older men. Violent behavior and injuries may result. The person *can* remember the dream in the morning. Medication usually is effective in controlling the physical movements.

PROFESSIONAL TIP

Sleep Apnea

Sleep apnea and snoring are more common in obese persons, although the obesity connection is much weaker among older people. Among middle-age people, 4% of men and 2% of women have sleep apnea. After the age of 65, the rate increases to 28% for men and 24% for women (NSF, 2000f).

Restless Leg Syndrome

Restless leg syndrome (RLS) is characterized by the uncomfortable sensations of tingling or crawling in the muscles and by twitching, burning, prickling, or deep aching in the foot, calf or upper leg when at rest (lying down or sitting) (NSF, 2000c). Temporary relief is found by walking, standing, or moving or rubbing the legs (Figure 19-4). The sensations return in seconds or minutes. The legs frequently jump involuntarily if they are not moved. Symptoms worsen at night. If sleep does come, the leg movements awaken the person frequently.

Although the cause is unknown, some cases of RLS have been linked to iron deficiency, dialysis treatment, peripheral neuropathy, pregnancy, excessive caffeine intake, alcohol dependence, smoking, and rheumatoid arthritis (NSF, 2000c). The disorder is more common among women who have passed middle age. Avoiding or reducing both smoking and caffeine and alcohol intake may help. Symptoms may be relieved by the anti-Parkinson drug carbidopa/levodopa (Sinemet).

Periodic Limb Movements in Sleep

Periodic limb movements in sleep (PLMS) is a condition wherein the legs jerk every 20 to 40 seconds throughout the night (NSF, 2000b). It is typically not uncomfortable for the affected person, but may be distressing to the sleep partner. Multiple sleep interruptions occur, leading to daytime sleepiness and nighttime insomnia.

The disorder is quite common in persons over age 65 years. Approximately 45% of elders have at least a mild form of PLMS, which occurs only during sleep and is not as uncomfortable as RLS (NSF, 2000b). Most cases are successfully controlled with carbidopa/levodopa (Sinemet).

NURSING PROCESS

All standardized nursing history tools include questions related to a client's rest and sleep patterns. Care of the client who is diagnosed with a sleep disorder is collaborative, with the nurse participating in an interdisciplinary team providing treatment.

Assessment

Discussion of sleep habits is part of the regular health history. Any client acknowledging a sleep disturbance should be thoroughly assessed to determine sleep routines, sleep alterations, types of disturbance, and impact of sleep problems. Typically, the client is a reliable source for this information, but a spouse or partner who shares sleeping arrangements may be able to add valuable information to the client's report. Ques-

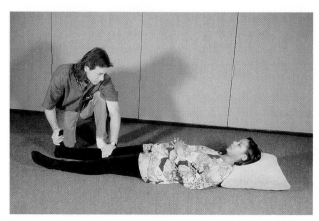

Figure 19-4 Massaging or rubbing the legs often helps relieve the sensations of restless leg syndrome.

tions regarding the client's usual sleep patterns should focus on the following:

- Nature of sleep (restful, uninterrupted)
- Quality of sleep (usual sleep pattern, schedules, hours of sleep, feeling on waking)
- Sleep environment (description of room, temperature, noise level)
- Associated factors (bedtime routines, use of sleep medications or any other sleep inducers)
- Opinion of sleep (adequate, adequate in terms of energy restoration, inadequate, problematic)

Questions regarding altered sleep patterns are intended to discover information such as the following:

- Nature of the problem (inability to fall asleep, difficulty remaining asleep, inability to fall asleep after awakening, restless sleep, daytime sleepiness)
- Quality of the problem (number of hours of sleep versus number of hours spent trying to sleep, number of hours of sleep per night, duration and frequency of naps or other compensatory measures, number of awakenings per sleep period)
- Environmental factors (lighting, bed, noise level, surrounding stimulation, sleep partner)
- Associated factors (relation to meals eaten, activity before retiring, life stressors, work stressors, anxiety level, pain, recent illness or surgery)

 LIFE CYCLE CONSIDERATIONS

Sleep and Aging
- Sleep needs do not decline with age, but stay fairly constant at 7 to 9 hours per day.
- Middle-age and elderly clients are more likely to experience sleep apnea, restless leg syndrome, and periodic limb movement disorder (NSF, 2000e).

Sleep History

To help detect a sleep disorder, ask the client:
- What time do you usually go to bed?
- How long does it take to fall asleep?
- What wakes you up in the morning?
- What time do you wake up in the morning?
- Do you take a nap during the day? When? How long?
- How much food do you eat in the evening?
- Do you drink caffeinated beverages? How much? In the evening?
- Do you drink alcohol? How much? In the evening?
- Do you take medications or herbal supplements to help you sleep?

Communicating with the Client Who Is Sleep-Impaired

- Thoroughly explain procedures before implementation.
- Encourage the client and significant others to verbalize feelings and ask questions.
- Answer questions honestly and completely.
- Identify and support coping mechanisms of the client and family.
- Spend adequate time with the client to facilitate communication.
- Assess and incorporate the client's preferences as much as possible into the plan of care.

- Alleviating factors (mild diet, warm drink before retiring, reading, listening to quiet music, taking a hot bath)
- Effect of problem (fatigue, irritability, confusion)

For clients whose sleep problems do not seem to be well defined, a daily journal of their sleep patterns may prove useful. Other factors such as age, medical diagnosis, occupation, allergies, and psychiatric disorders must also be considered when assessing sleep problems.

Nursing Diagnosis

After information about the sleep impairment has been collected, the data must be analyzed to formulate appropriate nursing diagnoses. Alterations in sleep can manifest as verbal complaints on the part of the client, physical signs such as yawning or dark circles under the eyes, or alterations in mood, such as apathy or irritability. The primary diagnosis for individuals experiencing sleep problems is *Disturbed Sleep Pattern.* According to the North American Nursing Diagnosis Association (NANDA) (2001), *Disturbed Sleep Pattern* is defined as "time-limited disruption of sleep (natural, periodic suspension of consciousness) amount and quality."

Another possible diagnosis related to rest and sleep is *Sleep Deprivation* (NANDA, 2001). This diagnosis is defined as "prolonged periods of time without sustained natural, periodic suspension of relative unconsciousness."

If the client presents with problems in addition to the sleep disturbance, the nurse must be alert to the possibility that the sleep disturbance is the *cause* (not the effect) of another problem. For example, a client may be experiencing *Activity Intolerance related to lack of sleep as evidenced by verbal complaint, extreme fatigue, disorientation, confusion, and lack of energy.*

Planning/Outcome Identification

The plan of care for the client experiencing a sleep-disorder must be individualized. For the nursing care to be effective, client input should be incorporated when developing the plan and goals. It is important to tailor the plan of care and the goals to the true cause related to the sleep disturbance or alteration. For example, if the client is experiencing *Disturbed Sleep Pattern* because of bedwetting, the bedwetting should be targeted for intervention.

Effective planning and goal identification will also take into account that many sleep disturbances require extended periods of time (weeks or months as opposed to days) to correct. Sleep patterns are by nature habitual and intertwined with lifestyle patterns, and these types of disturbances typically require interventions the results of which cannot be seen immediately. When planning care, the nurse should remember to time procedures and treatments in a manner that disturbs sleep time and routines as little as possible.

Nursing Interventions

Several interventions can promote rest and sleep in clients; these are discussed following.

Trusting Nurse–Client Relationship

The quality of the nurse–client relationship can enhance the client's ability to rest and sleep. Knowing that the nurse is a trustworthy individual who genuinely cares about the client's condition allows the client to relax and feel secure. Anxiety can be minimized by the nurse's use of therapeutic communication skills. The therapeutic use of self helps allay client anxiety.

Relaxing Environment

Arranging the immediate surroundings to promote sleep is important for the sleep-impaired client. A place to sleep should be inviting. The nurse should ascertain the type of environment the client finds relaxing, then either provide this environment in the inpatient setting or help the client establish this type of environment in the home setting. For example, the nurse might suggest that the client in the hospital bring the preferred sleeping pillow from home, if doing so will aid in sleeping.

Relaxation Techniques

The client's mood before sleep is of utmost importance. The belief that one can and will sleep affects sleep quality and quantity to a significant extent. The client who is calm and relaxed is likely to fall asleep quickly and stay asleep all night. Relaxation techniques are useful sleep aids (Figure 19-5). Progressive muscle relaxation is especially therapeutic for the person who needs to lessen muscular tension and quiet the mind. A warm bath may be relaxing.

Appropriate Nutrition

Certain foods can actually enhance sleep. Tryptophan, a substance in milk, promotes sleep by stimu-

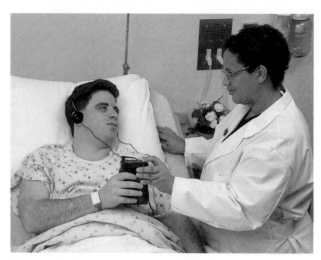

Figure 19-5 To help relieve this client's stress, the nurse is giving him a tape recorder and a relaxation tape.

lating the brain's production of the neurotransmitter serotonin. The old wives' tale that drinking warm milk promotes sleep is supported by scientific data. Other dietary considerations include avoiding large or heavy meals close to bedtime, refraining from eating spicy or other foods that cause gastrointestinal distress, and avoiding caffeine after noon.

Pharmacological Interventions

If unrelieved pain is a factor in the client's sleep disturbance, pain management should be the focus of initial interventions. Many of the nonpharmacological relaxation and imagery interventions can be effective in helping clients with sleep disturbances.

Pharmacological agents that may be therapeutic for clients with sleep disturbances include tricyclic antidepressants, antihistamines, and short-acting hypnotics (McCaffery & Pasero, 1999). The tricyclic antidepressants of choice are amitriptyline (Elavil) or doxepin (Sine-

 CLIENT TEACHING

Managing Sleep Disturbance

To facilitate rest and sleep, the client should be encouraged to:
- Select regular times for going to bed and awakening and try to observe them.
- Avoid "sleeping in" on weekends, vacations, or holidays.
- Limit daytime naps to no more than 30 minutes.
- Take a warm bath before going to bed.
- Avoid stimulating activities, such as strenuous exercise or demanding intellectual activity, during the hour before bedtime and use the time instead to wind down with relaxing activities such as taking a warm bath, reading a book, or sitting by the fire.
- Use bedtime rituals on a consistent basis.
- Practice relaxation techniques, such as neck rolls and muscle relaxation, to release tensions before going to bed.
- Not watch television, study, or talk on the phone while lying in bed and instead accustom the body to using the bed only for sleeping.
- Follow dietary guidelines to avoid caffeine, spicy foods, and heavy meals in the several hours before bedtime

 PROFESSIONAL TIP

Noise Control in Hospitals
- Keep the door to the client's room closed.
- Reduce the volume of paging and telephone systems, especially at night.
- Ensure that unused equipment in the client's room is turned off.
- Turn off or lower the volume on radios and televisions.
- Workers should keep noises to a minimum, especially at night.
- Hold discussions and conferences away from the client's room.

PROFESSIONAL TIP

Variables to Consider in Evaluation

When evaluating the care of the client experiencing a sleep disorder, consider the following questions:

- Were the client's basic needs met?
- Did client education include the family or significant others?
- Was an environment conducive to rest maintained?
- Were therapeutic activities balanced with the client's need for rest and sleep?
- Were the client's bedtime rituals followed as closely as possible?
- Were anxiety-reduction techniques used appropriately?

quan). Amitriptyline (Elavil) improves the client's ability to fall asleep and stay asleep by causing sedation when given 1 to 3 hours before bedtime. Doses of amitriptyline given for sleep disturbances are significantly lower than those given for treatment of depression.

Antihistamines such as hydroxyzine (Vistaril, Atarax) and diphenhydramine (Benadryl) have mild sedative effects that can promote sleep if given at bedtime. If anxiety throughout the day is of concern, low doses of these medications at regular intervals throughout the day may be effective.

The final group of pharmacological agents for sleep disturbances are the short-acting hypnotics. These are *not* recommended for routine or long-term use, as they have been associated with insomnia; however, they may be effective for short-term treatment. When they are used, it is recommended that a hypnotic with a short half-life be chosen.

Client Education

Educating the client about sleep-promoting activities is a good investment of the nurse's time. By providing clients with ways of promoting good sleep habits, the nurse helps them gain a sense of control over their sleep disturbances and boosts their confidence so that they can successfully meet their sleep and rest needs.

Evaluation

The plan of care must be individualized for and negotiated with the client and must be updated on a regular basis and additional interventions initiated as needed. One of the strongest supportive activities the nurse can perform is to ensure that clients understand that there is help for sleep problems and that they are not alone in having difficulty successfully managing their sleep patterns.

SAMPLE NURSING CARE PLAN

THE CLIENT WITH TROUBLE SLEEPING

Six-year-old Jacques Porcheron is brought to your clinic by his father, who states that Jacques has trouble sleeping at night. In the evenings after a dinner of hot dogs, corn or baked beans, and chocolate milk, Jacques reads some books, then watches his favorite superhero video. Afterward, he runs and plays, mimics the actions he sees in the video, and refuses to take a bath or cooperate when getting ready for bed. After being put to bed at 9 P.M., he is up several times for any number of reasons and often is not asleep until midnight. When his father wakes him at 7 A.M. for school, Jacques is disagreeable, tired, and difficult to get moving.

Nursing Diagnosis *Disturbed Sleep Pattern (less than age-normal total sleep time) related to environmental factors (excessive stimulation) and parental lack of knowledge of sleep-promoting behaviors as evidenced by parental complaint, ineffective bedtime rituals, and insufficient hours of sleep for developmental age*

PLANNING/GOALS	NURSING INTERVENTIONS	RATIONALE	EVALUATION
Jacques and his family will determine those sleeping behaviors they would like to achieve.	Explain that the normal sleep requirement for a child of Jacques' age is 10 to 12 hours each day.	Helping the family understand Jacques' sleep requirements will help them be more	Jacques and his family have decided they would like Jacques to *continues*

effective in their management of his bedtime and sleeping habits.

cooperate in getting ready for bed and to be asleep in 30 minutes.

Jacques and his family will develop bedtime rituals to help Jacques wind down from the day.

Teach the family about the effect that certain foods can have on digestion and sleep habits, and identify with them those foods that are good choices for dinner.

Educating the family about the potential adverse effects of certain foods will help them plan meals more appropriately.

Together they have established a bedtime ritual that begins with playing quietly, followed by taking a warm bath, reading two books, brushing teeth, and then going to bed.

Discuss those bedtime activities that can be detrimental to sleep induction.

Understanding those behaviors that can interfere with falling asleep will assist the family in modifying pre-bedtime behaviors

Suggest appropriate bedtime rituals such as taking a bath, brushing the teeth, reading a book, or listening to calming music.

Focusing on quiet activities and having a routine helps the body and mind prepare for bedtime.

Jacques and his family will identify behaviors that are helpful before bedtime.

Explain that overstimulation close to bedtime, such as watching superhero movies and engaging in rowdy play, prevents the body and mind from slowing down and preparing for sleep.

Understanding the psychological and physical implications of overstimulation before bedtime will help the family in choosing more appropriate bedtime activities.

The behaviors identified as helpful include no watching of stimulating videos after 7 P.M. and engaging in quiet play such as reading, arts and crafts, or writing. Some modification to Jacques' diet is planned for the next few weeks.

Emphasize the importance of establishing a calming bedtime routine that is followed every night, especially for the school-age child.

Children Jacques' age are helped by ritual and knowing those things that are expected of them, and they need guidance in practicing routines that are appropriate for bedtime.

Describe an appropriate sleep environment for Jacques, such as a calm room kept at a comfortable temperature and lit only by a night light.

Such an environment promotes sleep and does not interfere with falling back asleep once awake.

CASE STUDY

Mr. Leis, age 74, is hospitalized with deep vein thrombosis. His left thigh hurts when he moves. An intravenous line has been started in his right arm. Mr. Leis reports that it is difficult to fall asleep because of the pain in his leg. Hallway noises and nurses checking on him have awakened him the past 2 nights. He usually goes to bed at 9:30 P.M. but has not been able to fall asleep until 11:30 P.M. He states that he is tired and has been unable to take a nap.

The following questions will guide your development of a nursing care plan for the case study.

1. What other assessments should be done?
2. What nursing diagnosis is appropriate for Mr. Leis?
3. Identify three goals for Mr. Leis.
4. What nursing interventions would be appropriate to meet the goals?

SUMMARY

- Nonpharmacological interventions should be used in promoting rest and sleep.
- The amount of sleep required differs according to developmental stage.
- Pharmacological agents can be therapeutic for clients experiencing sleep pattern disturbances. However, the medications should not be the only interventions used.

Review Questions

1. The first phase of sleep is called:
   a. REM sleep.
   b. deep sleep.
   c. NREM sleep.
   d. light sleep.

2. A new sleep cycle for a client who is awakened during stage 4 NREM sleep will begin in:
   a. REM sleep.
   b. stage 1 sleep.
   c. stage 2 sleep.
   d. stage 3 sleep.

3. Individuals have several rhythms controlled by their biological clocks. The circadian rhythm cycle occurs:
   a. daily.
   b. every year.
   c. every month or so.
   d. several times a day.

4. Irregular sleeping habits often become the norm during:
   a. school-age.
   b. older adulthood.
   c. adolescence.
   d. young adulthood.

5. The older adult:
   a. needs less sleep.
   b. often takes a nap.
   c. experiences less REM sleep.
   d. experiences good-quality sleep.

6. Mitra is waking frequently at night and wakes very early in the morning. She may have:
   a. insomnia.
   b. parasomnia.
   c. narcolepsy.
   d. sleep apnea.

7. Jorge frequently falls asleep while sitting on the couch talking to his wife. He may have the sleep disturbance called:
   a. bruxism.
   b. narcolepsy.
   c. sleep apnea.
   d. hypersomnia.

8. Sleep apnea occurs mostly in:
   a. adolescents.
   b. young adults.
   c. middle-age adults.
   d. elders (those over age 65).

9. REM-sleep deprivation results from:
   a. sleep apnea.
   b. somnambulism.
   c. restless leg syndrome.
   d. periodic limb movements in sleep.

Critical Thinking Questions

1. How are the stages of sleep related to the sleep cycle?

2. What age-related sleep variations should be considered when assessing the sleep habits of neonates, infants, toddlers, adolescents, and elders?

WEB FLASH!

- Search the Internet for the topics sleep and sleep disturbances. What information is available to clients and families?
- Search specific sleep disturbances on the web. How much information can you find?

SAFETY/HYGIENE

MAKING THE CONNECTION

Refer to the following chapters to increase your understanding of safety/hygiene:

- **Chapter 1, Holistic Care**
- **Chapter 6, Legal Responsibilities**
- **Chapter 8, Communication**
- **Chapter 9, Nursing Process**
- **Chapter 12, Cultural Diversity and Nursing**
- **Chapter 13, Complementary/Alternative Therapies**
- **Chapter 15, Wellness Concepts**
- **Chapter 16, Stress, Adaptation, and Anxiety**
- **Chapter 21, Infection Control/Asepsis**

- **Chapter 22, Standard Precautions and Isolation**
- **Chapter 25, Health Assessment**
- **Chapter 27, Diagnostic Tests**
- **Chapter 28, Nursing Care of the Older Client**
- **Procedures:** B1, Handwashing; B16, Bedmaking: Unoccupied Bed; B17, Bedmaking: Occupied Bed; B18, Adult Bath; B19, Perineal Care; B21, Oral Hygiene; B22, Eye Care: Artificial Eye and Contact Lens Removal; B35, Application of Restraints; I27, Assisting a Client with Crutch Walking

LEARNING OBJECTIVES

Upon completion of this chapter, you should be able to:
- *Define key terms.*
- *Describe types of accidents that can occur in health care settings.*
- *Describe the importance of and procedure for correctly identifying clients.*
- *Identify safety factors to be considered before using equipment.*
- *Recount safety measures related to the use of protective restraints.*
- *Detail safety measures related to preventing fire when oxygen is in use.*
- *Discuss factors that influence a client's personal hygiene practices.*
- *Explain the role of assessment in maintaining a safe environment.*

KEY TERMS

body image
chemical restraints
client behavior accident
dental caries
equipment accident
gingivitis
halitosis
hygiene
perineal care

physical restraint
poison
pyorrhea
restraint
self-care deficit
sensory overload
stomatitis
therapeutic procedure accident

- *Describe the modifications that can be used to resolve environmental hazards in institutional and home settings.*
- *Cite nursing interventions that promote a client's personal hygiene.*

INTRODUCTION

Safe care is a basic need of all clients, regardless of setting. Nurses are responsible for providing the client with a safe environment through the delivery of professional, quality nursing care that incorporates safety precautions and hygiene assistance. This chapter describes the nurse's role in these areas.

SAFETY

Safety must be the number one priority in providing client care. The first step in maintaining safety is to raise nurses' awareness regarding risk factors. Prevention is the key to safety. Nurses must be aware of those factors that have the potential to endanger a client's safety. Constant attention to these factors enables the nurse to maintain a safe environment for the client.

A safety committee is required in all health care facilities, with the purpose of maintaining an overall safe facility for clients, employees, and visitors. The committee is composed of representatives from all departments of the facility. Responsibilities range from analyzing environmental safety in the facility to researching illness rates.

Safety is associated with health promotion and illness prevention. A safe environment reduces the risk of accidents and subsequent alterations in health and lifestyle; it also helps contain the cost of health care services (Figure 20-1). Many factors in the environment can threaten safety.

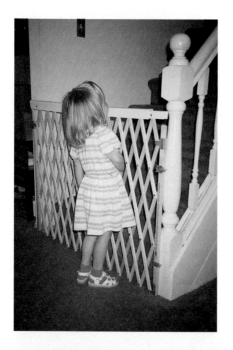
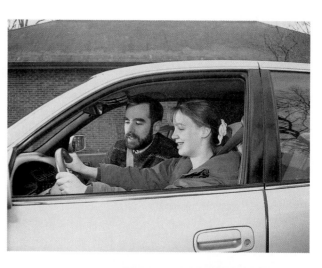
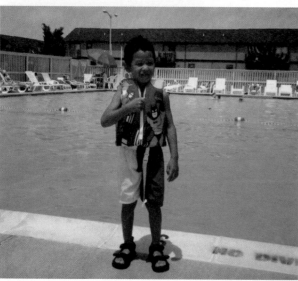
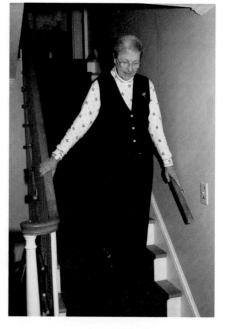

Figure 20-1 Use of stair gates, life vests, seat belts, and handrails minimizes safety risks.

Workplace Safety

Employee Right-to-Know Laws

Under the authority of the Occupational Safety and Health Administration (OSHA) of the Department of Labor and Industry, several states have passed employee right-to-know laws, which state that employees are legally entitled to information regarding hazardous substances or harmful agents in the workplace. Such substances include skin and eye irritants, flammables, poisons, carcinogens, pathogens, and harmful rays (radiation).

Regulations Relating to Hazardous Materials

OSHA also outlines and enforces regulations that all health care facilities must follow with regard to employees' exposure to and handling of potentially infectious materials.

Material Safety Data Sheet

As part of conforming to OSHA regulations, all facilities must have a material safety data sheet (MSDS) for each hazardous substance. The MSDS describes the substance in question, including the associated dangers. Protective equipment, safe handling techniques, and first-aid information are also given. The MSDSs for toxic materials must be kept on site for no fewer than 30 years. All employees must know how to use the MSDS.

FACTORS AFFECTING SAFETY

Client safety and health are influenced by several factors including age, lifestyle/occupation, sensory and perceptual alterations, mobility, and emotional state.

Age

Risk for injury varies with chronological age and developmental stage. Health education about preventive measures can facilitate injury prevention among clients of various age groups.

As infants mature, their potential for injury increases. Infants, toddlers, and preschoolers are explorers of the environment. Most accidents involving individuals in these age groups can be prevented with careful adult supervision to reduce the risk of falls from bed; burns; electrical hazards; choking on small objects; suffocation; and drowning.

As school-age children explore the environment outside the home, their risk for injury increases. Preventive measures during this stage focus on stranger awareness; bicycle, skating, and swimming safety; traffic safety rules; protective equipment for sports; and avoidance of substance abuse.

Adolescents and young adults usually enjoy good physical health; however, their lifestyles put them at risk for injury. Because this age group spends much time away from home, collaborative educational efforts among parents, schools, and community health care providers must focus on environmental safety. High-risk factors for injury and death are automobile accidents, substance abuse, violence, unwanted pregnancies, and sexually transmitted diseases.

Adult risk for injury is generally related to lifestyle, work practices, and behaviors. Preventive measures for adults emphasize nutrition, exercise, and occupational safety. High-risk factors for those in this age group include fatigue, anxiety, sleep pattern disturbances, caregiver role strain, and altered health maintenance.

Because of poor vision and mobility; loss of muscle strength and flexibility; effects of medications and alcohol; chronic diseases such as osteoarthritis, Parkinson's disease, and Alzheimer's disease; and changes in the inner ear that upset the sense of balance, the older adult is prone to falls, especially in the bathroom, bedroom, and kitchen (Walker, 1998). Preventive measures for older adults emphasize slow position changes, good lighting, use of hand rails, application of skid-proof strips in the bathtub or shower, and removal of throw rugs and loose carpets.

Accidents in the Health Care Setting

In the health care setting, accidents are categorized by their causative agent: client behaviors, therapeutic procedures, or equipment:

- **Client behavior accidents** result from the client's behavior or actions. Examples include poisonings, burns, and self-inflicted cuts and bruises.
- **Therapeutic procedure accidents** result from the delivery of medical or nursing interventions. Examples include medication errors, client falls during transfers, contamination of sterile instruments or wounds, and improper performance of nursing activities.
- **Equipment accidents** result from the malfunction or improper use of medical equipment. Examples include electrocution and fire. National and institutional policies establish safety standards with regard to equipment. For example, a facility may attempt to maximize the risk of equipment accidents by requiring that the biomedical engineering department check the equipment inspection label prior to use.

All accidents and incident reports must be fully documented according to institutional protocol.

According to the CDC (2000), one in three adults over age 65 falls each year. Of those who fall, 20% to 30% have mobility and independence permanently reduced and the risk of premature death is increased.

Lifestyle/Occupation

Lifestyle practices, which reflect an individual's personal choices about those activities or habits to pursue, can increase a person's risk for injury and potential for disease. For instance, individuals who operate machinery; experience excessive stress, anxiety, and fatigue; use alcohol and drugs (prescription and nonprescription); and live in high-crime neighborhoods are at increased risk for injury and alterations to health. Risk-taking behaviors such as participating in daredevil activities, driving vehicles at high speeds, and not wearing seat belts are factors that pose a threat to an individual's safety and well-being. Unlike other factors such as age, however, lifestyle/occupation practices are modifiable.

NIOSH (2000) reports that an average of 9,000 U.S. workers sustain disabling injuries each day, costing $145 billion each year. Compare this cost to $33 billion for AIDS and $170.7 billion for cancer.

Sensory and Perceptual Alterations

Sensory functions are essential for accurate perception of environmental safety. Clients who have visual, hearing, taste, smell, communication, or touch perception impairments are at increased risk for injury, as they are often not able to perceive a potential danger.

Mobility

The client whose mobility is impaired is at increased risk for injury, especially from falls. Mobility impairment may result from poor balance or coordination, muscle weakness, or paralysis. Immobility may also precipitate physiologic and emotional complications such as decubitus and depression.

Emotional State

Emotional states such as depression and anger affect a client's perception of environmental hazards and of the degree of risk associated with certain behaviors. These emotional states alter a client's thinking patterns and reaction time. Usual safety precautions may be forgotten during periods of emotional stress.

HYGIENE

Hygiene is the science of health. Care related to hygiene promotes cleanliness, provides for comfort and relaxation, improves self-image, and promotes healthy skin. Client hygiene is an extension of client safety in that proper hygiene protects the client's defense mechanisms against disease. The health of the body's first line of defense, the skin and mucous membranes, is promoted by proper hygiene. Nurses are responsible for ensuring that the client's needs with regard to hygiene are met. The type of care provided depends on the client's ability, needs, and practices.

Factors Influencing Hygiene Practice

Hygiene needs and practices are unique to each client; nurses should provide individualized care based on these needs and practices. Hygiene practices are influenced by several factors including body image, social and cultural practices, personal preferences, socioeconomic status, and knowledge.

Body Image

Body image is the individual's perception of physical self including appearance, function, and ability. Body image is associated with the client's emotions, mood, attitude, and values. A client's body image directly affects the type of personal hygiene practiced, which may change if the client's body image is altered because of illness or surgical procedures. At such times, the nurse should help the client maintain hygiene practices in accordance with the client's pre-illness level of hygiene and personal preferences.

Social and Cultural Practices

Social and cultural practices also directly influence hygiene practices. Clients are socialized to their hygiene practices by family practices in early childhood. As a person ages, hygiene practices are influenced by maturational development and socialization with people outside the family. For example, teenagers are usually concerned with peer acceptance and follow the latest trends in personal hygiene. In later adulthood, hygiene practices may be influenced by coworkers and social networks.

Cultural practices and beliefs are derived from family, religious, and personal values developed during maturation. Clients from diverse cultural backgrounds will have differing hygiene practices. Nurses should maintain a nonjudgmental attitude when assessing or providing hygiene care to clients from different social or cultural backgrounds.

Personal Preferences

Personal preferences influence the timing of bathing; those products that are used for bathing; and the type of bathing performed. For example, some male clients shave before bathing, whereas others prefer to do so after bathing. Some clients prefer to bathe in the morning to facilitate waking, whereas others prefer to bathe before bedtime to encourage relaxation and sleep. Unless the client's health is adversely affected, the nurse should permit the client to practice usual routines and to use hygiene products preferred by the client. Individualized nursing care should incorporate the client's personal hygiene preferences.

Socioeconomic Status

A client's hygiene practices may also be influenced by socioeconomic status. Limited economic resources may affect the type, frequency, and extent of hygiene practiced. Assessment of socioeconomic status provides information about the availability of hygiene supplies. Some clients may not be able to afford deodorants, perfumes, soaps, shampoo, and toothpaste. The nurse can function as an advocate for the client by contacting social services, which can make referrals to community agencies that provide assistance to needy persons, for example, Catholic Charities or a local chapter of the American Association of Retired Persons (AARP).

Knowledge

Knowledge level influences the client's understanding of the relationship between hygiene and health. Thus, knowledge should influence a client's hygiene practices. In order for clients to perform basic hygiene, however, they must have more than such knowledge; they must also be motivated and believe that they are capable of self-care.

Frequently, an illness or surgical procedure results in a knowledge deficit about basic hygiene practices. In such situations, the client may not know the correct procedures or types of hygiene that can be performed. The nurse is responsible for providing the necessary education about hygiene during an illness. Sometimes, the nurse may have to perform all hygiene practices for a client during an illness until the client regains this ability and returns to the former level of independence.

NURSING PROCESS

The nursing process facilitates an understanding of the scope of challenges inherent in providing nursing care to clients at risk for injury or a self-care deficit.

Assessment

Assessment data direct the prioritization of the client's problems and accompanying nursing diagnoses. Clients at risk for injury require frequent reassessment of status, with appropriate changes being made in the plan of care and expected outcomes.

The health history and physical examination data are correlated with the laboratory indicators to identify those clients who are at risk for problems relating to safety, infection, or hygiene. Appropriate risk appraisals may be incorporated into the nursing health history interview.

Subjective Data

The nursing health history interview is the first step in assessment; wherein the client's subjective account of specific health data is elicited. It is important for the nurse to gather complete, pertinent, and relevant information at this point.

Health History Key elements of relevant data regarding the client at risk for injury and infection are obtained in the health history. The client is often asked to complete a health history questionnaire; depending on the client's status, however, the nurse may have to perform an interview to obtain these data. If the client is unable to provide the subjective data, the nurse must designate, either on the questionnaire or in the nursing progress notes, the person who provided the information.

During the nursing health history interview, the client's general health perception and management status should be assessed to ascertain how the client manages self-care. This information will provide data regarding the client's routine self-care and health-promotion needs.

Objective Data

Objective data are gathered through the physical examination and the diagnostic and laboratory findings.

Physical Examination A complete health assessment includes a systematic physical examination, generally conducted from head to toes, in order to obtain objective data relative to the client's health status and presenting problems. When assessing the client to ascertain the level of risk for injury and hygiene deficits, the nurse should focus the physical examination on the following areas and signs:

- Level of consciousness: The Glasgow Coma Scale (GCS) is an objective measurement tool.
- Range of motion: Immobilization of an extremity and/or limited mobility are risk factors for development of joint contractures, skin breakdown, and muscle atrophy.
- Secretions or exudate of the skin or mucous membranes.
- Condition of the skin: Skin condition provides data concerning a client's nutritional and hydration status, continuity of intact skin, hygiene practices, and overall physical abilities.

Risk Factors A comprehensive nursing assessment involves using specifically developed risk assessment tools and appraising the client's environment to detect potential hazards. The client's self-care abilities, used for determining the level of assistance needed in providing hygiene care, are appraised during the health history. The analysis of relevant risk factors alerts the nurse to actual or possible risks. For instance, the risk of impaired skin integrity increases when a person is placed on bed rest. A skin integrity risk appraisal (Table 20–1) should be completed to assist with planning care.

Client in an Inpatient Setting Inpatient clients should be assessed for fall and infection risk factors. The hospitalized or institutionalized client's risk of falling is identified after compiling specific assessment data that are correlated with contributing factors as shown in Table 20–2. Each of these indicators carries a specific weight to determine the client's risk. For example, age over 65 years carries a weight of 3, and diuretic administration carries a weight of 7. The total risk factor for a 65-year-old client receiving a diuretic would thus be 10, placing the client at high risk for falls and requiring the implementation of special fall measures.

The inpatient client should be assessed for falls every shift or as designated by institutional policy. To minimize the chance of falls, the nurse must ensure that the client's environment is safe by keeping the bed in a low position, the side rails up, the nurse call light and personal belongings within easy reach, and

Table 20-1 SKIN INTEGRITY RISK APPRAISAL

AREA OF ASSESSMENT	SCORE
General Physical Condition (Health Problem)	
Good (minor)	0
Fair (major but stable)	1
Poor (chronic/serious, not stable)	2
Mental State/Level of Consciousness (to Commands)	
Alert (responds readily)	0
Lethargic (slow to respond)	1
Semicomatose (responds only to verbal or painful stimuli)	2
Comatose (no response to stimuli)	3
Activity	
Ambulates without assistance/infant	0
Ambulates with assistance	2
Chairfast/out of bed to chair	4
Bedfast/confined to bed	6
Mobility (Extremities)	
Full active range	0
Restricted movement (slightly limited)	2
Moves only with assistance	4
Immobile	6
Incontinence (Bowel and/or Bladder)	
None	0
Occasional (less than twice in 24 hours)	2
Usually (greater than twice in 24 hours)	4
Total (no control)	6
Nutrition (for Age and Size)	
Good (eats/drinks adequately)	0
Fair (eats/drinks inadequately)	1
Poor (unable/refuses to eat/drink)	2
Totally depleted	3

Assess the client's risk status for each indicator on the skin integrity risk appraisal form, then total the numbers from all six indicators. The risk rating is as follows:

   0 to 8: low risk
   9 to 16: moderate risk
   17 to 27: high risk

A rating greater than 8 usually requires implementation of special measures; for example, a protocol to prevent skin breakdown.

Patient Care Admission Sheet courtesy of Tulane University Hospital and Clinic, New Orleans, LA.

Table 20–2 FALL RISK APPRAISAL	
AREA OF ASSESSMENT	**SCORE**
General Factors	1
Restraint (posey, arm, leg)	
Orthostatic changes	
History of falls/crawling out of bed/ syncope (brief loss of consciousness)	
Seizure disorder	
Elimination Function	2
Decreased bladder/bowel tone	
Urgency/frequency	
Incontinence	
Nocturia (excessive urination at night)	
Age	3
Over 65	
Level of Consciousness/Mental Status	4
Lethargy (slow to respond)	
Inability or refusal to follow directions	
Inability or refusal to call for help	
Impaired judgment, memory, awareness	
Confusion, disorientation	
Sensory Deficits	5
Diminished visual acuity, blind, blurred vision	
Slow reaction time	
Mobility/Physical Limitations	6
Decreased mobility in lower extremities	
Ability to rise with assistance	
Amputation/joint difficulties	
Weakness, dizziness, fatigability, vertigo (dizziness), syncope	
Cast, splint	
Use of crutches, cane, walker	
Hemiparesis (one-sided paralysis), paraparesis (loss of function), hemiplegia, paraplegia (loss of function in lower limbs)	
Ataxia (unsteady gait)	
Improperly fitting/smooth soled/no footwear	
Unsteady gait, decreased balance, imbalance	
Medications	7
Sedatives/hypnotics/tranquilizers	
Diuretics/antihypertensives/laxatives	
Narcotics/analgesics/anesthetics	
Antihistamines	
Antiseizures	
Barbiturates/phenothiazines	
Eye drops	
Antipsychotics/antidepressants	

Patient Care Admission Sheet courtesy of Tulane University Hospital and Clinic, New Orleans, LA

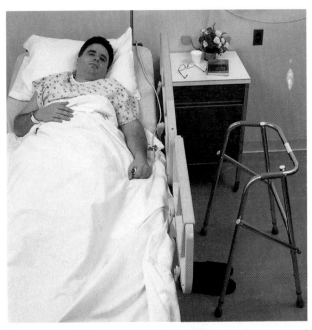

Figure 20-2 This client's risk of falls has been assessed and responded to through the measures shown here.

assistive devices (e.g., a walker) nearby, as shown in Figure 20-2.

Client in the Home An injury risk appraisal provides the nurse with assessment data to determine the client's level of safety knowledge. Injuries in the home primarily result from falls, fires, poisonings, suffocation, and malfunctioning household equipment (Stanhope & Knollnueller, 2000). Home health nurses may use a safety risk appraisal.

The safety risk data assessed in the home environment direct the nurse in planning for the client's and caregiver's education. The home health nurse must prioritize these data when planning the client's care. Assessment, teaching, and outcome evaluation of all safety hazards can take several home visits.

Diagnostic and Laboratory Data Appraising the client's risk for injury also involves evaluating laboratory findings related to an abnormal blood profile (e.g., altered clotting factors, anemic conditions, or leukocytosis). Malnourished clients are at risk for injury.

Nursing Diagnosis

After data collection and analysis, the nurse is able to formulate a nursing diagnosis. The main nursing diagnoses that relate to safety and hygiene deficits are *Risk for Injury* and the *Self-Care Deficit* diagnoses.

Risk for Injury

The primary nursing diagnosis *Risk for Injury* exists when the client is at risk for injury as a result of environmental conditions interacting with the individual's adaptive and defensive resources NANDA, 2001).

COMMUNITY/HOME HEALTH CARE

Home Safety Risk Appraisal

Infants

- Crib side rails stay in the up position while the infant is in the crib.
- Infants are not left unattended, especially on elevated surfaces or in the bath.
- Bath water temperature is 37.8° to 40.6°C (100° to 105°F). Check temperature for comfort with wrist.
- Environment is kept warm and draft free at bath time.
- Bottles are washed with soap and hot water, and formula is refrigerated.
- Toys are soft and have no detachable pieces.
- Car seat has a restraint strap and is used consistently.
- Stroller and carry seat are sturdy and have a restraint strap.
- Fire, police, and poison control numbers are posted by telephones.
- Caregivers know infant cardiopulmonary resuscitation (CPR).

Toddlers/Preschoolers

- Sharp objects are placed out of reach and out of sight.
- Poisons are labeled and placed in a locked cabinet.
- Medications and other toxins have childproof lids and are stored in a locked cabinet.
- Small, hard food objects (peanuts, candy) are kept in locked cabinets.
- Stairs and floor furnaces have gates or barriers.
- Doors and windows have safety locks.
- Electrical outlets are covered.
- Burners on the stove are not left on and unattended.
- Pots with hot liquids are placed on back burners, handles facing toward the back wall.
- Home and yard are free of poisonous plants.
- Play equipment is kept in proper functioning condition; toys have no small parts; crayons are nontoxic.
- Outdoor play is supervised in a fenced area with locks on gates.
- Car seat or seat belt is used consistently.
- Children are supervised when crossing the street.
- Caregivers know child CPR and Heimlich maneuver.

School-Age Children

- Play and sports are supervised.
- Play equipment is kept in proper functioning condition and free of hazards.

- Outdoor play is limited to soft surfaces.
- Bicycle helmet is worn consistently.
- Children are taught not to open the door or speak to strangers while at play.
- Firearms are kept unloaded and in locked cabinets.
- Seat belt is worn at all times.
- Caregivers know child CPR and the Heimlich maneuver.

Adolescents

- Firearm safety is taught.
- Seat belt is worn at all times.
- Teenagers take drivers' education and are cautioned about drinking and driving.
- Caregivers know adult CPR and the Heimlich maneuver.

Adults

- Firearms have safety latches.
- Smoke detectors and fire extinguishers are installed in the home.
- A nondrinking designated driver is chosen.
- Emergency phone numbers are readily available.
- Caregiver knows adult CPR and Heimlich maneuver.

Older Adults

- Stairs have adequate lighting and nonskid surfaces, and rails are in good condition.
- Throw rugs are not present.
- Hallways are uncluttered.
- Carpets are free from frayed ends/pieces.
- Phone cords and other cords are behind furniture.
- Bathtub has rails and a nonslip surface.
- Shower stall has a seat.
- Bathroom is free of drafts.
- Shoes fit properly and have nonskid soles.
- Home is adequately ventilated and heated.
- Home is free of space heaters.
- Pilot lights on gas appliances are functional.
- Electrical appliances are in good working condition.
- Food is properly refrigerated.
- Medications are kept in properly labeled containers with readable print.
- Emergency phone numbers are readily available.
- Fire and police departments are aware that older adult is home alone.
- Caregiver knows adult CPR and Heimlich maneuver.

(From Fundamentals of Nursing: Standards & Practice, *by S. DeLaune and P. Ladner, 1998, Albany, NY: Delmar.)*

Although this diagnostic label does not have defining characteristics as set forth by NANDA, it is categorized as having either internal or external potential hazards. An internal biochemical risk factor for a client with impaired vision would be stated as *Injury, Risk for, related to the risk factor of sensory dysfunction (visual).* In contrast, medications on a nightstand in a home with a toddler present should be identified by a home health nurse as creating an external chemical risk factor for the toddler; the related nursing diagnosis would be stated as *Injury, Risk for, related to the risk factor of medications in the environment.*

Examples of the other risk nursing diagnoses that may be a risk factor for *Risk for Injury* are:

Risk for Aspiration: risk for entry of gastrointestinal secretions, oropharyngeal secretions, or solids or fluids into the tracheobronchial passages

Risk for Falls: increased susceptibility to falling that may cause physical harm

Risk for Latex Allergy Response: at risk for allergic response to natural latex rubber products

Risk for Poisoning: accentuated risk of accidental exposure to or ingestion of drugs or dangerous products in doses sufficient to cause poisoning

Risk for Suffocation: accentuated risk of accidental suffocation

Risk for Suicide: risk for self-inflicted, life threatening injury.

Risk for Trauma: accentuated risk of accidental tissue injury (e.g., wound, burn, fracture)

These seven subcategories of nursing diagnoses provide the nurse with the opportunity to relate specific nursing interventions to the diagnosed problem. For example, the specific nursing diagnosis for the situation of the toddler encountering medications on the nightstand in the home would be *Risk for Poisoning,* related to the risk factor of medications accessible to children. The level of risk would be considered higher if the medications on the client's nightstand were in open containers or if the closed containers did not have childproof caps. This subcategory diagnosis provides for specific nursing interventions directed toward the level of risk for the toddler and toward the need for client teaching.

Self-Care Deficits

A **self-care deficit** exists when an individual is not able to perform one or more activities of daily living (ADL). Three self-care deficits related to hygiene practices are identified by NANDA (2001). These diagnostic labels, together with their defining characteristics and related factors, are presented in Table 20–3.

Table 20–3 SELF-CARE DEFICITS

NURSING DIAGNOSIS AND DEFINITION	DEFINING CHARACTERISTICS	RELATED FACTORS
Bathing/Hygiene Self-Care Deficit: Impaired ability to perform or complete bathing/hygiene activities for oneself	Inability to get bath supplies; inability to wash body or body parts; inability to obtain or get to water source; inability to regulate the temperature or flow of bath water; inability to get in and out of bathroom; inability to dry body	Decreased or lack of motivation; weakness and tiredness; severe anxiety; inadequate to perceive body part or spatial relationship; perceptual or cognitive impairment; pain; neuromuscular impairment; musculoskeletal impairment; environmental barriers
Dressing/Grooming Self-Care Deficit: Impaired ability to perform or complete dressing and grooming activities for oneself	Inability to choose clothing; inability to use assistive devices; inability to use zippers; inability to remove clothes; inability to put on socks; inability to put clothing on upper body; impaired ability to put on or take off necessary items of clothing; impaired ability to obtain or replace articles of clothing; impaired ability to fasten clothing; inability to maintain appearance at a satisfactory level; inability to put clothing on lower body; inability to pick up clothing; inability to put on shoes	Decreased or lack of motivation; intolerance to pain; severe anxiety; perceptual or cognitive impairment; neuromuscular impairment; musculoskeletal impairment; discomfort; environmental barriers; weakness or tiredness
Toileting Self-Care Deficit: Impaired ability to perform or complete own toileting activities	Inability to manipulate clothing; unable to carry out proper toilet hygiene; unable to sit on or rise from toilet or commode; unable to get to toilet or commode; unable to flush toilet or commode	Environmental barriers; weakness or tiredness; decreased or lack of motivation; severe anxiety; impaired mobility status; impaired transfer ability; musculoskeletal impairment; neuromuscular impairment; pain; perceptual or cognitive impairment

From Nursing Diagnoses: Definitions and Classification 2001–2002, by North American Nursing Diagnosis Association, 2001, Philadelphia: Author.

Other Nursing Diagnoses

The client who is at risk for injury or has a self-care deficit may have other associated physiologic or psychological problems. The following nursing diagnoses often accompany diagnostic labels for risk for injury or self-care deficits:

> *Imbalanced Nutrition (specify less than body requirements or more than body requirements)*
>
> *Ineffective Protection*
>
> *Impaired Tissue Integrity*
>
> *Impaired Skin Integrity*
>
> *Social Isolation*
>
> *Risk for Loneliness*
>
> *Individual, Ineffective Coping*
>
> *Impaired Physical Mobility (specify bed, physical, or wheelchair)*
>
> *Hopelessness*
>
> *Powerlessness*
>
> *Deficient Knowledge (specify)*
>
> *Acute Pain*
>
> *Anxiety*
>
> *Fear*

Though not all-inclusive, this list gives an indication of the number of related problems that must be considered when planning care for clients identified as having safety or self-care deficits.

Planning/Outcome Identification

The primary nursing goal is to provide safe care through the identification of actual or potential hazards and the implementation of safety measures. The assessment data are reviewed with the client, and the nurse records the areas where the client indicates a need for change and health teaching, for example, age-related exercise or maintaining a safe environment. These findings are incorporated into the plan of care, reflecting the individualized needs of each client.

During the planning phase, the nurse collaborates with the client and other health care providers to determine the goals, outcomes, and interventions. Identified outcomes provide direction for the nursing care that is implemented to reduce the risk of injury.

Another critical element of the care plan is client/caregiver education related to the identification of potential hazards and health-promotion practices. The nursing care plan should include safety measures to educate the client about preventive actions and modification of an unsafe environment, for example, proper use of a call light or potential hazards related to the side effects of medications.

Table 20–4 outlines the basic components of care planning and outcome measurement for the client who is at risk for injury or has a self-care deficit. Nursing actions are discussed in detail in the following section.

Implementation

Implementation involves continual assessment of client health risks and prioritization of nursing interventions aimed at risk reduction, such as:

- Administration of prescribed medications,
- Provision of balanced nutritional intake,
- Promotion of adequate rest and exercise, and
- Teaching client about health hazards.

Implementation of safety measures may require an alteration in the physical environment as directed by the fall prevention protocol (Table 20–5).

Identify Client

In order to provide safe care, it is essential that nurses correctly match clients with the activity, medication, diet, or treatment ordered for them. The client's well-being can be placed in jeopardy by administration of incorrect care.

The identification (ID) band or bracelet is the primary means of correctly identifying a client. It lists the client's name, room number, bed number, hospital number, and doctor and may include other information such as age, sex, and religion.

This band is placed on the client's wrist upon admission to the hospital. Each time care is given, the band must be checked against the assignment sheet, order sheet, diet card, and medication and treatment sheet or card (Figure 20-3). The client's identity should always be further verified by one other method such as asking the client's name, asking the client to state his name, or obtaining a positive identification from another person. None of these methods is safe when used alone, but when used in conjunction with the ID band, any can help the nurse verify identity.

If a client is discovered without an ID band, care should be withheld until positive identification can be

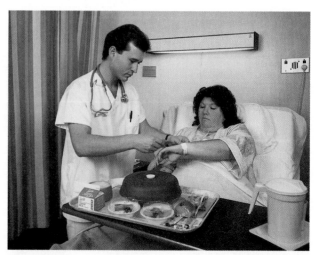

Figure 20-3 Checking the client's ID band ensures that the correct person receives care.

Table 20–4 PLANNING THE CARE OF THE CLIENT WHO IS AT RISK FOR INJURY AND/OR WHO HAS A SELF-CARE DEFICIT

NURSING DIAGNOSIS	GOALS	EXPECTED OUTCOMES	NURSING INTERVENTIONS
Risk for Injury	The client will identify factors that increase the potential for injury.	The client will identify internal and external factors that increase the risk for injury.	Risk identification: analysis of potential risk factors, determination of health risks, and prioritization of risk reduction strategies for an individual
	The client will remain free of bodily injury.	The client will identify and implement safety measures to decrease the risk for injury.	Fall prevention: instituting special precautions with the client at risk for injury
Bathing/Hygiene Self-Care Deficit and Dressing/ Grooming Self-Care Deficit	The client will maintain an optimum functional level of hygiene practices in a safe and effective manner.	The client will participate physically and/or verbally in bathing, dressing, and toileting activities.	Bathing: cleaning of the body for the purpose of relaxation, cleanliness, and healing Perineal care: maintenance of perineal skin integrity and relief from perineal discomfort. Dressing: choosing, putting on, and removing clothes for a person who cannot do same for self.
	The client's skin will remain clean and intact.	The client's skin will remain free of drainage and secretions; intact; and free of redness.	Skin surveillance: collection and analysis of client data to maintain skin and mucous membrane integrity.
Deficient Knowledge related to health hazards	The client will not sustain injuries.	The client will verbalize both feedback of instructions and a willingness to comply.	Teaching, individual: Planning, implementation, and evaluation of a teaching program designed to address a client's particular needs.

Compiled from Nursing Interventions Classification (NIC) *(3rd ed.), by J. C. McCloskey and G. M. Bulecheck (Eds.), 2000, St. Louis, MO: Mosby Yearbook and from* Handbook of Nursing Diagnosis *(8th ed.), by L. Carpenito, 1999, Philadelphia: Lippincott Williams & Wilkins*

made. A new ID band should be placed on the client's wrist as soon as identity is verified.

Most nursing home residents also wear ID bands. Some, however, do not, and other methods of identification, such as photographs, are used. Nurses working in such long-term care facilities must learn to safely use the identification system. Whatever the system, client identification is essential before rendering any care.

Raise Safety Awareness and Knowledge

Nurses in all settings must demonstrate an awareness of safety hazards and must teach clients accordingly. Clients must be made aware of safety precautions in order to prevent injuries. Clients may also need specific safety information regarding the use of oxygen, intravenous equipment, heating devices, and automatic bed controls.

A 1996 Food and Drug Administration (FDA) safety alert addressed entrapment hazards with regard to side rails on hospital beds. The FDA received 102 reports of head and body entrapment incidents that resulted in 68 deaths, 22 injuries, and 12 entrapments without injury (FDA, 1996). These incidents occurred in hospitals, long-term care facilities, and private homes. All reported entrapments occurred in one of the four ways illustrated in Figure 20-4.

Prevent Falls

Most falls occur among clients who are weak, fatigued, uncoordinated, paralyzed, confused, or disoriented. The data obtained from the fall risk appraisal will identify those clients who require special nursing measures to prevent falls. The risk for falls can be reduced by the following:

- Proper supervision
- Orienting the client to the environment and the call system
- Providing ambulatory aids (e.g., a wheelchair or walker)
- Placing personal belongings and the call light within easy reach
- Keeping hospital beds in the lowest position and the side rails up
- Using nonslip mats and rugs
- Illuminating the environment

Specific nursing interventions aimed at preventing falls include wiping up spills; encouraging use of side rails; applying restraints; encouraging use of assistive devices for walking; using proper body mechanics; ensuring adequate lighting; and removing obstacles. These are discussed following.

Table 20–5 ADULT FALL PREVENTION PROTOCOL

Purpose

To direct the nursing management of the client at risk for falls

Supportive Data

Falls account for nearly 90% of injuries reported in hospitalized clients (Whedon & Shedol, 1989). Risk factors for falls include advanced age, dizziness, confusion, use of medications, and physical or mental alterations. Fall prevention is used to increase staff awareness of clients at risk for falls and to provide preventive safety measures.

Content

Assessment

1. Perform client injury risk appraisal and identify fall risks. Update (on nursing care plan) status of fall risks daily or as needed.
2. Assess effects of administered medications that increase the risk of falls.
3. Implement institution's fall prevention program.

Report to Physician

4. Notify physician of previous fall history and identify risk factors for falls.
5. Notify physician of adverse effects of medications that may increase the client's risk of falling.

Client Teaching

6. Orient client to surroundings on admission and as necessary.
7. Instruct client and significant others on safety measures.
8. Instruct client and significant others on correct use of hospital equipment.
9. Instruct client at risk for falls to call for assistance when ambulating or performing ADL.

Environmental Interventions

10. Keep bed in lowest position, brakes locked, and side rails up.
11. Keep call light and frequently used objects within easy reach at the bedside.
12. Keep environment clean and clutter free.
13. Provide adequate lighting at all times.
14. Lock wheels on wheelchair, bed, and stretcher at all times.
15. Provide nonslip footwear, mats, and rugs.
16. Keep hospital furniture in the same place throughout hospital stay.
17. Provide call cord in bathroom.
18. Encourage use of handrails in bathroom and hallways.
19. Provide nonslip mats in the tub or shower.
20. Place high-risk clients in a room near the nurse's station.

Direct Nursing Care

21. Respond promptly to call lights and verbal requests for assistance.
22. Provide assistance with ADL.
23. Maintain close supervision by performing hourly safety assessments.
24. Encourage significant others to stay with high-risk clients.
25. Provide proper equipment for ambulation and elimination needs.
26. Communicate client's injury risk status in shift report.
27. Provide protective devices, such as restraints, for client safety (physician's order necessary).

Evaluation

28. Evaluate client's knowledge of safety measures.
29. Evaluate effectiveness of environmental interventions.
30. Evaluate changes in client's injury risk status.
31. Evaluate effectiveness of direct nursing care.

Documentation

32. Document the following in the client's medical record:
    a. Assessment of client's injury risk status
    b. Nursing care plan
    c. Safety measures implemented
    d. Client education performed
    e. Client outcomes

From "Prediction and Prevention of Patient Falls," by M. B. Whedon and P. Shedol, 1989, Image: Journal of Nursing Scholarship, *21(2), 108–114.*

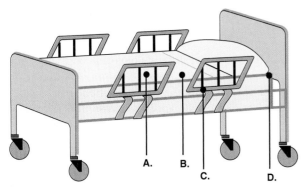

Figure 20-4 Entrapment Hazards Associated with Hospital Bed Side Rails: A. Between the bars of a side rail; B. Between two side rails; C. Between the side rail and mattress; D. Between the headboard or footboard, side rail, and mattress (*Source: Food and Drug Administration, Safety Alert, August 1996*)

Wipe Up Spills Floors must be kept clean and free of spills. Although the housekeeping department usually does the actual washing of floors, it is the nurse's responsibility to either wipe up a spill at the time it occurs or to mark the area as a safety hazard and notify the appropriate person for immediate cleanup (Figure 20-5). Something wet or sticky on the floor can easily cause a weak, unsteady client to slip or trip.

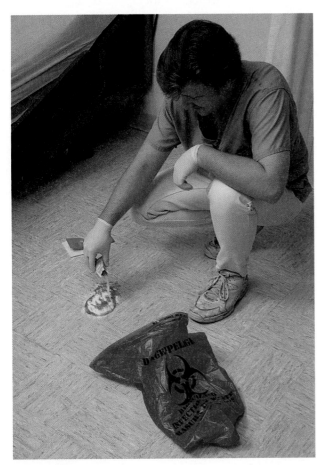

Figure 20-5 Wiping up spills is an important safety measure.

Even those unimpaired by illness, such as visitors and hospital personnel, are at risk.

Encourage the Use of Side Rails Falls from bed are the most common type of accident in hospitals (Easterling, 1990). The reasons are many and varied. Weakness due to illness is a major contributor to such accidents. Confusion and disorientation due to a strange environment, medication, anesthesia, or as a symptom of the client's condition increase the risk of falls.

Side rails are placed on the sides of hospital beds and stretchers to prevent falls. They can be raised and lowered and locked into place. Generally, side rails should be used most of the time (Figure 20-6). For those clients at risk for falls, the side rails should be used all the time.

Many clients resist the use of side rails because of an associated loss of self-esteem: They do not wish to be "treated like children" or to feel dependent. Thorough explanations from the nurse regarding the need for and purpose of side rails, coupled with a positive and respectful attitude will help neutralize resistance. Some facilities allow clients and/or families to sign a release form in the event that side rails are refused. Others may require that a family member or "sitter" provided by the family stay with the client at all times that side rails are not used.

The use of side rails should not give nurses a false sense of security. Beds must still be placed in the lowest position to reduce the height of a fall, should one occur, and clients at risk for falls should still be closely monitored.

Apply Restraints **Restraints** are protective devices used to limit the physical activity of a client or to immobilize a client or extremity. Restraints are used to protect the client from falls, protect a body part, keep the client from interfering with therapies (e.g., pulling out tubes, disconnecting intravenous setups, or removing wound coverings), and reduce the risk of injury to others. Restraints should *never* be used as a substitute

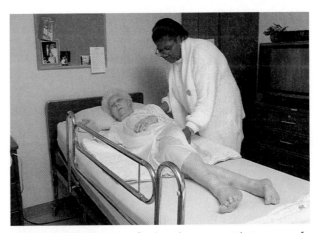

Figure 20-6 The use of side rails can contribute to a safe and secure environment.

PROFESSIONAL TIP

Key Elements of Restraint Documentation

- Reason for the restraint
- Method of restraint
- Explanation given to client and family
- Date and time of and client's response to application
- Duration
- Frequency of observation and client's response
- Safety (release from the restraint along with periodic, routine exercise and assessment for circulation and skin integrity)
- Assessment of the continued need for the restraint
- Client outcome

for close observation and supervision by nursing personnel.

The use of restraints has become very controversial because of client injuries related to these devices. In response, the Omnibus Budget Reconciliation Act (OBRA) of 1987 defines clients' rights and choices and states the following as acceptable reasons for the use of physical restraints:

- Restraints are part of the medical treatment.
- All other interventions have been tried first.
- Other disciplines have been consulted for assistance with the problem.
- Supporting documentation has been provided (Sullivan-Marx, 1994).

The Joint Commission on Accreditation of Healthcare Organizations (JCAHO) has also updated its guidelines on physical restraints. Citing studies, JCAHO stated that the use of restraints may violate clients' rights and cause "physical and psychological harm, loss of dignity . . . and even death" (JCAHO, 2000). Nurses must know the risks they face when physical restraints are or are not used (Richman, 1998).

Once restrained, clients are rendered less able to care for their own basic needs; thus, the nurse's responsibility in meeting these needs increases. Facility policy regarding the use of restraints, the care of the client in restraints, and the method of documentation must be followed precisely.

Restraints used either to limit physical activity or to immobilize a client can be physical or chemical. **Physical restraints** reduce the client's movement through the application of a device. Most states require a physician's order for the application of physical restraints. **Chemical restraints** are medications used to control the client's behavior. Commonly used chemical restraints are anxiolytics and sedatives. The following discussion

is limited to the common types of physical restraints (Figure 20-7):

- Jacket (body restraint): a sleeveless vest with straps that cross in front of the client and are tied to the bed frame or around a chair or wheelchair.
- Belt: straps or belts applied across the client to secure to a wheelchair, stretcher, or bed.
- Mitten or hand: enclosed cloth material applied over the client's hand to prevent injury from scratching.
- Limb or extremity: cloth devices that immobilize one or all limbs by securely tying the restraint to the bed frame or chair.
- Elbow: a combination of fabric and plastic or wooden tongue blades that immobilize the elbow to prevent flexion.
- Mummy: a blanket or sheet that is folded around the child to limit movement and is used when performing procedures on children.

The nursing plan of care should include safety measures to reduce the potential for injury from restraints. Additional safety measures to observe when using restraint devices are as follows:

- Restraints should neither interfere with any treatment (e.g., intravenous therapy) nor aggravate the client's health problem.
- There should be enough slack in the straps to allow the client to move both arms and legs and perform range-of-motion exercises.
- At least once every 2 hours, the nurse must perform circulation and neurological examinations, assessing the color, sensation, temperature, motion, and capillary refill in the area distal to the restraint.
- The client and significant others should be provided psychological support, as needed (Easterling, 1990; Stillwell, 1991).

 Safety: Restraints

- Jacket or belt restraints should not restrict respiratory effort. Placing a restraint too tightly on the diaphragm will inhibit the expansion of the lungs.

- To avoid accidental injury to the extremity in the event that the side rail is released, the restraint strap should be secured to the bed frame, *not* to the side rail.

Encourage the Use of Assistive Devices for Walking Devices used to assist walking include canes, crutches, walkers, and wheelchairs.

Canes Canes are curved walking devices that provide support to one side of the body that is weak. Three common types of canes are the single stick, the tripod (three footed), and the quad (four footed). All types should have a sturdy grip and rubber tips. The tips should be checked frequently for signs of wear.

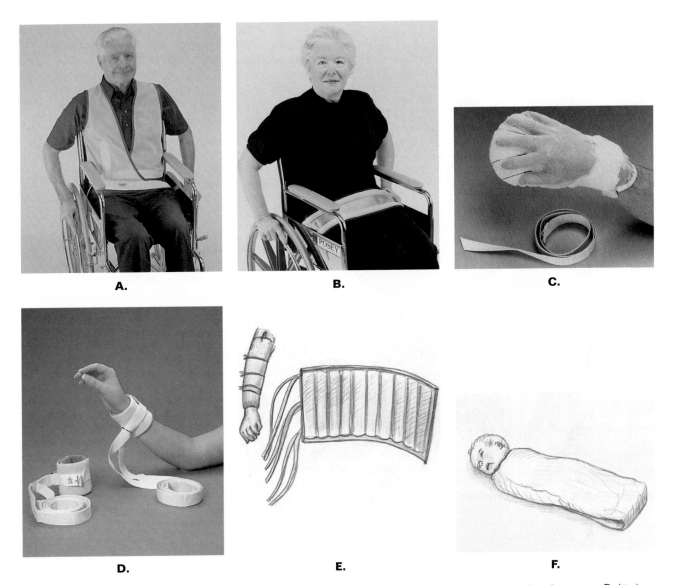

Figure 20-7 Types of Restraints: A. Jacket or vest restraint; B. Belt restraint for chair; C. Mitten or hand restraint; D. Limb or extremity restraint; E. Elbow restraint; F. Mummy restraint. (*Parts A and B courtesy of J.T. Posey Co., Inc.*)

Canes should be held on the strong side of the body (Figure 20-8). The affected side and the cane should move simultaneously while the weight is supported on the strong side. The strong side is moved while the weight is supported on the cane and the weaker side.

Crutches Crutches are wooden or metal staffs used either temporarily or permanently to increase mobility. There are two types of crutches: the axillary crutch and the Lofstrand, or forearm, crutch. The axillary crutch, the type most commonly used, fits under the axilla, with the weight being placed on the handgrips. The Lofstrand crutch has a handgrip and a metal cuff that fits around the arm. This type of crutch is more convenient but not as stable as the axillary crutch.

To prevent slipping, crutches have rubber tips, which must be kept dry. The tips should also be inspected regularly. If tips become loose or worn, they must be replaced immediately. The structure of the crutch must also be inspected regularly. The person's weight will not be properly dispersed if there are cracks or bends in the crutch.

Walkers A walker is a waist-high metal tubular device with a handgrip and four legs. Some walkers have wheels on the front two legs, whereas other walkers have rubber tips on all four legs. Walkers give a sense of security and extra support, as well as independence, to clients. The client first moves the walker forward and then takes a step while balancing the weight on the walker.

Wheelchair A wheelchair is a means of ambulation for clients who are unable to support their weight while standing. The nurse should instruct the client in the safe use of a wheelchair by reminding the client to keep the wheelchair locked when not moving and to lift the footrests out of the way when getting in or out of the wheelchair. The wheelchair should be pushed

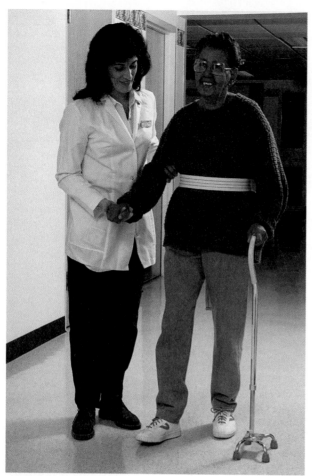

Figure 20-8 A nurse ensures the safety of a client using a quad cane.

slowly from behind and should be backed into doorways and into and out of elevators.

Use Proper Body Mechanics The human body is able to move in many different ways, some more efficient than others. The most effective, safest way of lifting and moving things is through using the principles of body mechanics; including center of gravity, base of support, and body alignment.

Center of Gravity The center of gravity is located in the center of the body, in the pelvic area. Body weight is approximately equal above and below this area. All movement should pivot around this central point. This keeps the weight over the base of support, making it easier to stay balanced. Keeping the back straight and bending at the knees and hips helps to maintain the center of gravity in the pelvic area. If the center of gravity shifts, the body tends to fall.

Base of Support Feet are the base of support. The feet should be kept wide apart when lifting heavy items, as it is easier to stay balanced with a wide base of support. Further, one foot should be kept a little forward of the other to give stability from front to back. Keeping the knees slightly bent allows for quick movement and for jolts to the body to be absorbed.

When turning, the feet rather than the body should be moved, in order to prevent injury to the back.

Body Alignment Proper body alignment requires that the various parts of the body be kept in proper anatomic relationship to each other.

 Safety: Body Mechanics

- Stoop to lift objects from the floor: bend at the hips and the knees, keeping the back straight and base of support wide. The large muscles of the legs can then be used to straighten the body and lift the object.
- Avoid bending from the waist, as doing so strains the lower back muscles.
- To prevent undue stress and strain on the back when caring for clients, adjust the height of the bed to one of comfort and ease.
- Carry objects close to the midline of the body.
- Avoid stretching to reach objects.

Ensure Adequate Lighting Adequate lighting facilitates visualization of environmental hazards. Rooms should be adequately lit so that the client can safely perform ADL and the health care providers can perform procedures. Lighting can be supplemented by lamps and nightlights.

Remove Obstacles Obstacles in heavily traveled areas of health care facilities or homes represent a risk to the client's safety. Older adults or persons who are unfamiliar with the environment are at greatest risk of injury from obstacles. The risk that obstacles pose can be reduced by keeping hallways clear; removing excess furniture from heavily traveled areas; either removing all electrical cords or taping them securely to the floor; removing throw rugs; cleaning up spills immediately; and moving objects that could fall.

Reduce Bathroom Hazards

Bathrooms pose a threat to the client in the home because of the presence of water and the storage of medication. Accidents common to the bathroom are falls, scalds or burns, and poisonings. Such accidents can be reduced with the use of grab bars near the tub, shower, and toilet; nonslip mats in the tub and shower; and a secured bathroom rug near the tub or shower. Other safety measures include checking the temperature of the water before entering the tub or shower; checking the thermostat setting on the water heater; and storing medications in a locked cabinet, out of the reach of children and disoriented or confused adults.

Prevent Fire

Fire is a potential danger to all people in an institutional or home environment. Fire requires the interaction of three elements: sufficient heat to ignite the fire, combustible material (fuel), and oxygen to support the fire.

COMMUNITY/HOME HEALTH CARE

Preventing Fires and Burns

- Turn handles of pots and pans toward the center of the stove to prevent children from pulling them down and burning themselves.
- Keep matches in a metal can and in a place where children cannot reach them.
- Be aware of loose, flowing clothing when cooking, especially over an open flame.
- Avoid using candles for light or heat and never leave a burning candle unattended.
- Install smoke alarms near bedrooms and check batteries twice a year.
- Do not place portable heaters near curtains, which can easily catch on fire.
- Allow only certified electricians to work on wiring in the home.
- Do not place electrical cords under carpeting.
- Do not use multiple plug outlets.
- Do not stick anything into appliances that are plugged in (e.g., a fork in the toaster).
- Teach family members routes of escape from the house, pick a place to meet outside to verify that everyone is safe, and conduct practice fire drills.
- Teach *stop, drop,* and *roll* to extinguish fire on clothing.

Immobilized or incapacitated clients are at increased risk during a fire. Common causes of fire are smoking in bed, discarding of cigarette butts in trash cans, and faulty electrical equipment. Because smoking is a health hazard, many facilities are now smoke free.

Nursing goals are twofold: fire prevention and client protection during a fire. Nursing interventions aimed at preventing or reducing the risk of fire include the following:

- Clearly marking fire exits
- Knowing the locations and operation of fire extinguishers
- Practicing fire evacuation procedures
- Posting emergency phone numbers near all telephones
- Keeping open spaces and hallways clear of clutter
- Checking electrical cords and outlets for exposed or damaged wires
- Educating clients about fire hazards

In the event of a fire, the nurse should follow institutional policy and procedures for fire containment and evacuation (Figure 20-9). Nursing interventions during a fire are directed at protecting the client from injury and containing the fire. If a fire occurs, the nurse should ensure client safety, immediately report the type of fire and its exact location, and evacuate the premises if necessary. Nurses should know the locations and operation of fire extinguishers (Figure 20-10). The four types of fire extinguishers are water, carbon dioxide, regular dry chemical, and multipurpose dry chemical. Each type of fire extinguisher is used for a specific class of fire, as outlined in Table 20–6.

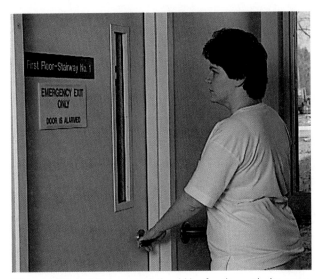

Figure 20-9 All personnel should be familiar with the evacuation plan and emergency exits.

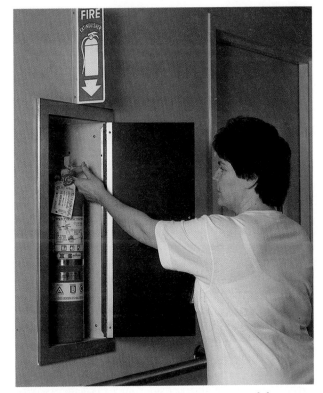

Figure 20-10 Know the location and use of fire extinguishers.

Table 20–6 FIRE EXTINGUISHERS

TYPE	CLASS OF FIRE
Water (type A)	Paper, wood, draperies, upholstery, or rubbish
Carbon dioxide or regular dry chemical (types B and C)	Flammable liquids, flammable gases, or electrical fires
Multipurpose dry chemical (types A, B, and C)	Any type of fire

From Fundamentals of Nursing: Standards & Practice, *by S. Delaune and P. Ladner, 1998, Albany, NY: Delmar. Copyright 1998 by Delmar. Reprinted with permission.*

Ensure the Safety of Equipment

Checking all equipment and supplies carefully before use and refusing to use any damaged goods or equipment can prevent many accidents. A good rule to follow is to never use any piece of equipment that is in any way damaged or not working properly. If a wheel comes off an overbed table, the nurse should not attempt to prop the table up but, rather, should remove it from the room and send it to the appropriate area for repair. The same holds true for smaller supplies given to or used on clients. The safety of clients must always come first.

Glass and Plastic Glass and plastic equipment and supplies should be inspected for cracks and chips before use. The nurse should also check that there are no rough edges that may injure clients.

Disposable Sterile Supplies When using disposable sterile supplies, the nurse should first always check that the package is intact. Any break in or wetness of the wrapper renders it unsterile. Expiration dates should also be verified prior to use.

Electrical Equipment Clients have contact with a variety of electrical equipment in the hospital environment, such as bed controls and intravenous and patient-controlled analgesia (PCA) pumps. Each piece of electrical equipment should have a three-pronged electrical plug that is grounded. A grounded plug transmits any stray electrical current from equipment to ground. To protect the client from electrical injury, the nurse should read the warning labels on all equipment, use only grounded electrical equipment, check for frayed electrical cords, avoid overloading circuits, and report to the biomedical department any shocks received from equipment (Figure 20-11).

Personal electrical appliances that the client is allowed to keep at the bedside, such as shavers, hair dryers, or curling irons, should be safety checked by the biomedical department before being used.

PROFESSIONAL TIP

Oxygen Use

Special precautions must always be taken when oxygen is in use. Because one of the three elements essential to starting a fire is oxygen, the presence of pure oxygen can transform the tiniest spark into a tremendous hazard.

When oxygen is being used, "No Smoking" signs must be posted in the room and on the outside of the door to the room. It is vital that all visitors and other clients understand that the rule applies to everyone in the room, not just to the person receiving the oxygen. Because many critically ill clients use oxygen, it is also necessary for the nurse to caution clergy not to use open flames or candles in any religious rites.

Woolen and nylon blankets should not be used, as they can cause static electricity and thus pose a fire risk in an atmosphere of pure oxygen. Cotton blankets are recommended.

Electrical appliances such as radios and razors are generally not used in the presence of oxygen. Because it is flammable, oil should not be used on oxygen equipment. Hospital policy, as well as equipment itself, must be checked to determine what is safe to be used in a room where oxygen is being used.

Whenever tank oxygen is used, the cylinders must be securely strapped to a holder or cart to prevent the tank from tipping over and knocking off the valve, which could in turn cause a spark that would quickly ignite in the presence of oxygen.

If a client receives an electrical shock, the nurse should turn off the electricity before touching the client. Then, the client's pulse should be checked. If the client has no pulse, CPR should be initiated. If the client has a pulse, the nurse should assess vital signs, mental status, and skin integrity for burns. A physician

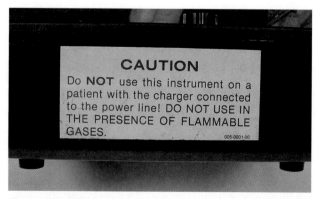

Figure 20-11 Heed warning labels on electrical equipment.

should then be notified of the event, and an incident report should be completed.

Reduce Exposure to Radiation

Clients are exposed to radiation during diagnostic testing and therapeutic interventions. Injury can occur from radiation if overexposure or exposure to untargeted tissues occurs. Exposure to untargeted tissues can result from the dislodgment of radiation implants. General principles of radiation exposure and protection are based on time, distance, and shielding. Protection from radiation therapy involves the following:

- Minimize the time spent in contact with the radiation source (implant or client).
- Maximize the distance from the radiation source (implant or client).
- Use appropriate radiation shields.
- Monitor radiation exposure with a film badge.
- Label all potentially radioactive material.
- Never touch dislodged implants or the body fluids of a client receiving radiation therapy (Eriksson, 1995).

Both the client and the nurse are at risk for radiation injury. The client's risk for injury can be reduced by educating the client about radiation treatment and necessary precautions, placing the client in a private room, and providing a lead apron, when necessary, to protect nontargeted body tissues. The nurse's risk for injury can be reduced by observing all radioactive labels, wearing gloves when handling radioactive body discharges, washing hands, wearing lead aprons, disposing of radioactive substances in special containers, reducing the time of client contact, and wearing badges that measure the amount of radiation exposure.

Prevent Poisoning

A **poison** is any substance that, when taken into the body, interferes with normal physiologic functioning. Poisons may be inhaled, injected, ingested, or absorbed into the body. It is important to realize that many substances can be poisonous if taken in sufficient quantity.

 Safety: Aspirin
Aspirin can be poisonous when taken in sufficient quantity.

Dangerous chemicals may be found in any workplace, but some are specific to the health care industry, such as radioactive isotopes, laboratory dyes, antiseptics, irrigating solutions, disinfectants, and therapeutic drugs. To guard against accidental poisoning in health care facilities, the nurse must be aware of the client's mental and physical condition. The nurse must also ensure that potentially dangerous materials are never left unattended in clients' rooms. Alcohol and other antiseptics or medications used for dressing changes

 LIFE CYCLE CONSIDERATIONS

Vitamins and Minerals

Adult iron preparations are especially poisonous to young children and should be stored in a locked cabinet out of the reach of children.

or other procedures must be removed from the client's room after use.

 Safety: Medications and Cleaning Carts
- Medication trays and cleaning and supply carts should never be left unattended.
- Confused, visually impaired, or very young clients may help themselves to something harmful or something that they may use in a harmful way.
- Medication cupboards and carts must be kept locked when not in use.

On admission, clients are asked whether they have brought any medications to the facility. If so, these medications must be either removed to a safe place or sent home with the client's family. Because family members, in an effort to be helpful, sometimes bring in remedies that the client uses at home, the nurse should check bedside stands periodically to ensure medications or other potentially harmful substances are not being stored there.

The poison control center should be notified when poisoning is suspected. The number can generally be found on the inside cover or first few pages of the telephone book. The person reporting the poisoning should be prepared to state the amount and type of poison ingested, inhaled, or injected and the client's age and symptoms. Clients who have ingested poison should be turned on the side to prevent aspiration while awaiting further treatment. Client education about safety measures can prevent some accidental poisonings (Stanhope & Knollnueller, 2000).

 COMMUNITY/HOME HEALTH CARE

Proper Storage and Use of Medications

Teach clients about:

- Childproofing cupboards where medications are stored,
- The proper use and dosages of medications, and
- The use of special medication containers that are divided into days and times (to help prevent the client from duplicating a medication dose).

CLIENT TEACHING

Measures to Prevent Accidental Poisonings

- Store medications in child-resistant containers (Figure 20-12A).
- Do not take medications in front of children.
- Never call medicine candy.
- Place toxic substances in a locked cabinet out of the reach of children.
- Never remove labels from containers.
- Do not place poisonous substances in food or beverage containers.
- Place poison stickers on toxic substances.
- Keep syrup of ipecac available at all times (Figure 20-12B).
- Display poison control center phone numbers near telephones.

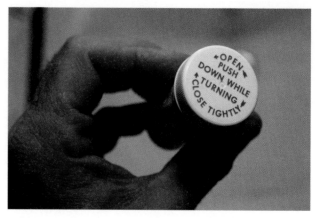

A.

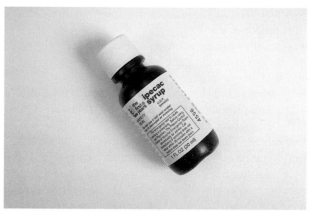

B.

Figure 20-12 Poison Prevention Methods: A. Medications stored in child-resistant containers; B. Syrup of Ipecac

Prevent Choking

To prevent choking on food, special techniques must be used when feeding clients in at-risk categories. Nothing should ever be given by mouth to an unconscious client, because the epiglottis does not function, and choking and suffocation are thus likely. Likewise, to prevent aspiration of vomitus, food and drink are usually withheld before the induction of general anesthesia. After some tests, such as a bronchoscopy, food and drink are withheld until the gag reflex returns.

Prevent Suffocation

Smothering can be prevented by proper nursing observation of at-risk clients such as infants, those who are impaired with regard to ADL, and paralyzed or unconscious clients. Such clients should be repositioned frequently and checked for a patent (open) airway. Soft pillows, mattresses, and comforters, in which they might bury their faces, should not be used. In the presence of oral secretions, the client's head should be turned to the side to prevent choking. Monitors that beep if breathing ceases should be used for at-risk clients.

Prevent Drowning

Infants, young children, and weak or confused clients are most at-risk for drowning. These clients should never be left alone in the bathtub. If the nurse must leave for any reason, either the client must be removed from the tub or another member of the health care team must stay with the client until the nurse returns or the bath is completed.

Clients should be instructed in the use of call systems installed in tub and shower rooms. Clients should also be instructed to first pull the plug in the tub and then call the nurse, should they feel weak or faint.

Reduce Noise Pollution

Noise pollution, or a noise level that is uncomfortable for the client or staff, frequently occurs in the health care setting because of visitor traffic, medical equipment, and personnel. It can result in an unorganized environment, hearing loss, and sensory overload. **Sensory overload** is an increased rate and intensity of auditory and visual stimuli. Sensory overload can alter a client's recovery by inducing or increasing anxiety, paranoia, hallucinations, and depression.

 Safety: Noise Pollution
- Maintain a quiet environment.
- Control traffic.
- Provide earplugs.

Provide for the Client's Bathing Needs

Bathing of clients is an essential component of nursing care. Whether the nurse performs the bath or delegates the activity to another health care provider, the nurse retains the responsibility for ensuring that the hygiene needs of the client are met. The type of bath provided depends on the purpose of the bath and the client's self-care abilities. The two general categories of baths are cleansing and therapeutic.

Cleansing Baths Cleansing baths are provided as routine client care. The purpose of a cleansing bath is personal hygiene. The five types of cleansing baths are shower bath; tub bath; self-help, or assisted, bed bath; complete bed bath; and partial bath.

Shower Bath Most ambulatory clients are capable of taking a shower. Clients with limited physical ability can be accommodated by placing a waterproof chair in the shower. The nurse provides minimal assistance with the shower.

Tub Bath Clients frequently prefer and enjoy a tub bath. Tub baths can also be therapeutic. Clients with limited physical ability should be assisted when entering and exiting the tub.

 Safety: Tub Bath
Check the temperature of the water in the bath tub before allowing the client to enter.

Self-Help Bath A self-help, or assisted, bed bath is used to provide hygiene care for clients who are confined to bed. In the self-help bed bath, the nurse prepares the bath equipment but provides minimal assistance. This assistance is usually limited to washing difficult-to-reach body areas such as the feet, legs, back, and perineal area.

Complete Bed Bath A complete bed bath is provided to clients who are dependent and confined to bed. The nurse washes the client's entire body during a complete bed bath.

Partial Bath In a partial, or abbreviated, bath, only those body areas that would cause discomfort or odor if not washed thoroughly are cleansed. These areas are the face, axillae, hands, and perineal area. The nurse or client may perform a partial bath, depending on the client's self-care abilities. Partial baths may be performed with the client lying in bed or standing at the sink.

Therapeutic Baths Therapeutic baths require a physician's order stating the type of bath, temperature of the water, body surface to be treated, and type of medicated solutions to be used. A therapeutic bath is usually performed in a tub and lasts approximately 20 to 30 minutes. Therapeutic baths are classified as

 PROFESSIONAL TIP

Bathing

- Baths are an excellent time to perform a complete skin assessment.
- The bathing process provides time for the nurse to meet the client's psychosocial needs through assessment and counseling.
- Bathing provides time to educate the client on basic and special hygiene needs.

 PROFESSIONAL TIP

Tub or Shower Bath

- Schedule use of the tub or shower and provide necessary equipment.
- Clean the tub or shower according to agency policy.
- Assist the client with ambulation to and from tub or shower.
- Place bath mat in tub or shower; provide shower chair, if necessary.
- Place "Occupied" sign on door.
- Adjust room temperature and temperature of water.
- Fill tub halfway with water; do not allow the client to soak longer than 20 minutes.
- Assist the client with getting into and out of the tub or shower; provide with a call system.
- Assist with cleansing, as necessary.
- Clean tub or shower after use, according to agency policy.

hot, warm, cool, or tepid; soak or sitz; and oatmeal (Aveeno), cornstarch, or sodium bicarbonate, depending on the prescribed type of bath.

Hot- or warm-water tub baths are used to reduce muscle spasms, soreness, and tension. Hot- or warm-water baths, however, have the potential for causing skin burns. Cool or tepid baths are used to relieve tension or to lower body temperature. The nurse must prevent chilling and rapid temperature fluctuations during a cool or tepid bath by not leaving the client in the tub too long.

A soak can involve the entire body or can be limited to only one body part. In a soak bath, water, with or without a medicated solution, is applied to reduce pain, swelling, or irritation or to soften or remove dead tissue.

Sitz baths cleanse and reduce inflammation in the perineal and anal areas. Sitz baths are commonly used for hemorrhoids or anal fissures and after perineal or rectal surgery. Skin irritations can be soothed with oatmeal (Aveeno), cornstarch, or sodium bicarbonate baths (Shaffer, 1997).

Provide Clean Bed Linen

After a bath, clean linens are placed on the bed to promote comfort. If the client is able to get out of the bed, the nurse can assist the client to a chair and proceed with making the bed.

If the client is unable to get out of the bed, the nurse will need to make an occupied bed. Assistance will be needed if the client is in traction or cannot be turned. Care must be taken to avoid disturbing the traction weights.

Perineal Care

Perineal care may be an embarrassing procedure for both the client and the nurse, especially if the client is of the opposite sex. In this situation, the nurse should provide the client with warm water, a moistened washcloth, soap, a dry towel, and privacy. If the client is unable to perform perineal care, the nurse is responsible for providing this care in a professional and private manner.

Provide Perineal Care

Perineal care is the cleansing of the external genitalia and the perineum and surrounding area. Perineal care is also referred to as *peri-care* or *perineal-genital* care. The purposes of perineal care are to prevent or eliminate infection and odor, promote healing, remove secretions, and provide comfort. Perineal care can be provided separately or as part of the bed bath.

Offer Back Rubs

Back rubs and massages stimulate the client's circulation, relax muscles, and relieve muscle tension as well as provide the nurse with an opportunity to assess the skin. Emollient creams and lotions are used to facilitate the rubbing and lubrication of the skin during a back rub or massage.

The client is positioned either prone or lying on the side. The nurse creates friction and pressure by rubbing the hands on the client's skin. The friction creates heat, which, in turn, dilates the peripheral circulation and increases the blood supply to the skin. The pressure manually stimulates the muscle fibers, which, in turn, relaxes the muscles. Prior to performing a back rub or massage, the nurse must assess for contraindications. Caution should be exercised when massaging limbs; especially the lower limbs, because a thrombus (blood clot) might be dislodged, resulting in an embolus (circulating blood clot). Bony prominences should be massaged lightly to prevent damage to underlying tissue (Shaffer, 1997).

Provide Foot and Toenail Care

Proper foot and toenail care are essential for ambulation and standing. Foot and toenail care are often ignored until problems occur. Common problems with the feet and toenails may be the result of abuse and neglect, such as inadequate foot and toenail hygiene, incorrect nail trimming, poorly fitted shoes, and exposure to harsh chemicals. These problems result in alterations of skin integrity and the potential for infection.

The first sign of foot and toenail problems is usually foot pain or tenderness. These symptoms affect a client's posture and may result in limping and in sub-sequent strain to certain muscle groups. Clients with illnesses such as diabetes mellitus require special foot and toenail care, as these clients experience alterations in circulation that predispose them to foot problems.

The purposes of foot and toenail care are to prevent infection and soft tissue trauma from ingrown or jagged nails and to eliminate odor. Hygiene care of feet and toenails consists of regular trimming of the toenails; cleansing under the toenails; cleansing, rinsing, and drying the feet and toenails; and wearing properly fitted shoes.

If toenails are dirty or thickened, soaking facilitates cleansing. An orangewood stick is used to clean under the toenails, because a metal instrument can roughen the nail and cause it to harbor dirt. The safest instrument for trimming the toenails is the nail clipper; however, some clients feel that cutting the nails makes them brittle. If the client chooses not to cut the nails, they should instead be filed straight across with an emery board. Special attention should be given to drying the areas between the toes. An emollient, such as cold cream, helps to keep toenails and cuticles soft.

Callused areas should never be cut. Repeated soaking usually facilitates the removal of calluses. Lotion should be applied to the feet to maintain moisture and soften callused areas. If the client's feet maintain excessive moisture (sweat), water-absorbent powder should be applied between the toes.

The client should wear clean, properly fitted shoes. Shoes should not be extremely tight, but should be snug enough to provide support to the feet. Each shoe should have an arch support. Shoe size should be large enough so that the shoe is ½ inch longer than the longest toe. Common foot problems can often be alleviated by assessing footwear and providing proper education on footwear and foot and toenail care.

Provide Oral Care

The oral cavity functions in mastication, secretion of mucus to moisten and lubricate the digestive system, and secretion of digestive enzymes. Common problems occurring in the oral cavity include the following:

- Bad breath (**halitosis**)
- Cavities (**dental caries**)
- Plaque
- Periodontal disease (**pyorrhea**)
- Inflammation of the gums (**gingivitis**)
- Inflammation of the oral mucosa (**stomatitis**)

Poor oral hygiene and loss of teeth may affect a client's social interaction and body image as well as nutritional intake. Daily oral care is essential to maintain the integrity of the mucous membranes, teeth, gums, and lips. Through preventive measures, the oral cavity and teeth can be preserved. Preventive oral care consists of rinsing with fluoride; flossing; and brushing.

Fluoride Researchers have determined that fluoride can prevent dental caries. This finding has led to

PROFESSIONAL TIP

Foot and Toenail Care

- Soak feet in warm water and a detergent or in warm oil.
- Use an orangewood stick to clean under the nails and release the cuticle growth from the nail.
- File or cut the nails straight across to prevent ingrown nails.
- Trim the cuticles as necessary.
- Pat all areas dry using a clean towel.
- Apply an emollient.

PROFESSIONAL TIP

Oral Care for the Unconscious Client

Oral care for the unconscious client maintains a clean oral cavity and intact mucous membranes. Special care should be exercised when administering oral care to the unconscious client to prevent both client aspiration and injury to the nurse (from the client biting because of the gag reflex).

- Never use your fingers to hold a client's mouth open; a bite block or padded tongue blade can be used instead.
- Assess for gag reflex.
- Turn the client's head to one side and place a basin under the mouth.
- Use oral suctioning to facilitate removal of secretions; only a small amount of liquids should be used.
- Brush the teeth and tongue in the usual manner. Exercise caution to prevent aspiration.

the fluoridation of water supplies in many communities. Fluoride is a common component of mouthwashes and toothpastes. However, persons with excessively dry or with irritated mucous membranes should avoid commercial mouthwashes because of the alcohol content, which further dries the mucous membranes.

Infants can be given fluoride drops as early as 2 weeks of age to prevent dental caries. Nurses should inform clients that fluoride is an excellent preventive measure against dental caries, but that excessive fluoride usage can affect the color of tooth enamel. To prevent discoloration of the tooth enamel, fluoride should be administered with a dropper directed toward the back of the throat.

Flossing Flossing should be performed daily in conjunction with brushing of the teeth. Flossing prevents the formation of plaque, removes plaque between the teeth, and removes food debris. Dental caries and periodontal disease can be prevented by regular flossing.

Brushing Brushing removes plaque and food debris and promotes blood circulation in the gums. Brushing of the teeth should follow flossing. Teeth should be brushed after each meal. Brushing should be performed using a dentifrice (toothpaste) that contains fluoride to aid in preventing dental caries. An effective homemade dentifrice is the combination of two parts salt and one part baking soda. Dentures should be brushed using the same brushing motion used for brushing the teeth. The oral cavity of a client who wears dentures must also be cleansed.

Provide Hair Care

Hair affects a client's personal appearance and body image. Hair functions to maintain body temperature and as a receptor for the sense of touch. Assessment of hair texture, growth, and distribution provides information on a client's general health status. Common hair problems include dandruff, hair loss, tangled or matted hair, and infestations such as pediculosis and lice. Hair problems can be reduced with daily hair care, which helps to promote hair growth, prevent hair

loss, prevent infections or infestations, promote circulation to the scalp, evenly distribute oils along hair shafts, and maintain the client's physical appearance. Hair care consists of brushing and combing, shampooing, shaving, and mustache and beard care.

Brushing and Combing Hair should be brushed or combed daily in accordance with the client's preferred hairstyle. Brushing and combing stimulate circulation to the scalp, distribute oils along hair shafts, and style the hair. A clean brush or comb should be used. Hair should be brushed from the scalp toward the hair ends. Sensitive scalps should be gently brushed or combed.

Clients who are immobilized may have tangled or matted hair. Care should be taken to prevent pain when combing tangled or matted hair by holding the tangled hair near the scalp while combing. If the client permits, the hair can be braided to prevent tangling or matting, but braiding the hair tightly should be avoided because tight braids may cause pain and hair loss. A nurse must receive written informed consent in order to cut a client's hair.

Shampooing When soiled, the hair should be shampooed according to the client's usual routine. The purposes of shampooing are to stimulate scalp circulation, remove soil from the hair, and facilitate brushing and combing. Hair can be shampooed in the tub, in the shower, at the sink, or in the bed, depending on the client's abilities and preferences.

Clients confined to bed can have their hair shampooed with water or with shampoos that do not require water. Hair is shampooed by thoroughly wetting all hair, applying approximately 1 teaspoon of shampoo, lathering the shampoo, and using the pads of the fingertips to

CULTURAL CONSIDERATIONS

Influences on Hygiene

- All self-care and hygiene practices are influenced by the client's background and cultural values.
- Always ask clients about preferences prior to performing care and demonstrate sensitivity with regard to those practices that may differ from your own.

gently massage the scalp. After shampooing, hair should be rinsed thoroughly, dried with an absorbent towel, combed, and styled as desired by the client.

Shaving Shaving is the removal of hair from the skin surface. Males often shave to remove facial hair, and women may shave to remove leg and/or axillary hair. Operative procedures may also require shaving of an area of the body.

Shaving may be performed before, during, or after the bath. Care should be taken to avoid cutting the skin. Prior to shaving, the area should be washed with soap and warm water to soften the hair. A warm washcloth may be placed over the area for several minutes to facilitate softening of the hair. A shaving cream or mild soap is then applied to the area to ease hair removal. The skin should be pulled taut, and the razor should be held at a 45-degree angle and moved over the skin in short, firm strokes in the direction of hair growth. After the skin is shaved, it should be washed, rinsed, and patted dry.

Safety: Shaving

- Review the client's medical record and the facility's policy regarding the use of razors for shaving.
- Clients prone to bleeding should be instructed to use only electrical razors for shaving.
- The nurse should wear gloves unless using an electric razor.

Mustache and Beard Care Mustaches and beards require daily care. Mustache and beard care consists of keeping the hair clean, trimmed, and combed. Mustaches and beards can be washed with soap or shampoo. Frequently, mustaches and beards require only gentle wiping with a moist washcloth. A mustache or beard should never be shaved off by the nurse without written informed consent from the client.

Provide Eye, Ear, and Nose Care

Eye, ear, and nose care should be included in routine hygiene care.

Eye Care Eyes are continually cleansed by tears and the movement of the eyelids over the eyes. Eyelids should be washed daily with a warm washcloth and from the inner to the outer canthus.

Infection Control: Eye Care

In order to prevent the transfer of pathogens, a new, clean corner of the washcloth should be used for each eye and with each stroke.

Eyelashes function to prevent foreign material from entering the eyes and conjunctival sacs. Eyelashes and eyebrows should be washed as necessary.

Although some artificial eyes (prosthetics) are permanently implanted, others may require daily removal and cleaning: The eye is removed from the eye socket and washed.

Comatose clients have special eye care needs because they lack a blink reflex. These clients require frequent instillations of lubricants or eyedrops to prevent corneal abrasions.

The nursing history should indicate whether the client wears contact lenses, and the routine care and level of assistance required should be recorded on the client's care plan. Clients who can insert, remove, and manage the care of their lenses require minimal assistance from the nurse. If the client is unable to assist with lens care and also has corrective eyeglasses, the nurse can suggest that the client wear eyeglasses during hospitalization. There are two types of contact lenses: hard and soft. Each type requires different cleansing and care. During emergency situations, the nurse should remove the lenses and place them in the appropriate solution.

Ear Care Hearing can be affected by foreign material or wax in the external ear canal. Cleansing of the ears involves cleansing the external ear canal and auricles. Objects should not be inserted into the ear canal. Excess wax or foreign material should be removed by using a warm washcloth to gently wash the external ear and auricles while pulling the ear downward, in the adult client. In children, the ear is pulled up and back. Irrigation of the ear may be necessary to remove dried wax; this will require a physician's order.

PROFESSIONAL TIP

Eye Care for the Comatose Client

- Use a warm washcloth to cleanse eyelids, eyelashes, and eyebrows at least every 4 hours. Clean from the inner to the outer canthus.
- If eyes remain open and the blink reflex is absent, liquid tear solutions should be instilled to prevent corneal drying and ulcerations.
- Eyes can be closed and covered with eye patches or protective shields. Patches or shields should be removed at least every 4 hours to assess the eyes and provide eye care.

Hearing aids amplify sound. The health history should indicate whether the client wears a hearing aid, and the plan of care should discuss the cleaning schedule for the aid. Clients with hearing aids should cleanse the ear mold regularly to ensure proper functioning.

If the hearing aid is not functioning properly, the nurse should check the on–off switch and volume control; the battery (and replace as necessary); the plastic tubing, for cracks and loose connections; and the telephone switch, which should be in the off position unless the client is using the phone. Hearing aids should be handled carefully, because dropping or bumping the hearing aid can damage the delicate mechanisms of the aid. When not in use, the hearing aid should be stored in a container, because dust and dirt can damage the mechanism.

Nose Care The nose provides the sense of smell, prevents entrance of foreign material into the respiratory tract, humidifies inhaled air, and facilitates breathing. Excessive or dried secretions may impair nasal function. Excessive nasal secretions are removed by inserting a cotton-tip applicator moistened with water or saline into the nostrils. The applicator should not be inserted beyond the cotton tip. Excessive nasal secretions in infants may be removed by a suction bulb. The client with a nasogastric tube should receive meticulous skin care to the nose area to prevent skin breakdown.

Evaluation

Evaluation is based on the achievement of goals and expected outcomes, regardless of the setting. Clients with alterations in health-perception–health-management pattern or activity–exercise pattern are at risk for injury and self-care deficits. Keeping the client free from injury requires both frequent reassessment through the use of risk appraisals and timely adjustments to the plan of care in order to facilitate effectiveness of nursing interventions.

It is imperative that the client not only be kept free of injury during hospitalization, but also be helped in developing a true awareness of the internal and external factors that increase the risk for injury. Achievement of this outcome measure is directly related both to the behaviors the client observes while in the hospital and to client teaching. In the home, modifications to ensure a safe environment serve as evidence for the home health nurse that learning has taken place.

The therapeutic value of hygiene is maximized when the client can participate and is kept free from infection and alterations in skin integrity. Evaluation should identify the client's level of functioning in self-care activities. At the time of discharge from the hospital, appropriate referrals should be made to home health care agencies to assist the client in achieving optimal function with regard to safety and hygiene practices.

SAMPLE NURSING CARE PLAN

THE CLIENT AT RISK FOR INJURY

Mr. Simon, age 75 years, presents with coronary heart disease (CHD) upon being admitted to the hospital. He has a family history of CHD. He smokes two packs of cigarettes per day, has diabetes mellitus, and is obese. He has gained 7 pounds in the past month, and exhibits diminished visual acuity, decreased bladder tone, weakness, and syncope. His blood cholesterol is 320 mg/dL, and his high-density lipoprotein (HDL) level is 28 mg/dL. On the GCS, he received a score of 12 (15 is fully oriented; 7 is comatose). His blood pressure is 186/116.

Nursing Diagnosis *Risk for Injury related to failure to adapt to sensory dysfunctions as evidenced by diminished visual acuity and a GCS score of 12*

PLANNING/GOALS	NURSING INTERVENTIONS	RATIONALE	EVALUATION
Mr. Simon will be protected from injury during hospitalization.	Initiate fall-prevention protocol.	Identifies and reduces the risk for injury.	The fall prevention protocol was implemented.
	Place Mr. Simon in a room as close as possible to the nurses' station.	Facilitates faster response time to the client's needs.	When discharged on the third day of hospitalization, Mr. Simon was free of injury.

continues

Place fall-alert signs on Mr. Simon's door and head of bed.	Alerts other health care workers to the client's risk status.
Put the bed alarm on.	Helps monitor client status and facilitates prompt response if the client tries to get out of bed unassisted.
Monitor Mr. Simon and the environment every 2 hours and whenever a caregiver passes by his room.	Provides information on status, progress, and needs of the client; encourages team approach to client care.
Reassess Mr. Simon's injury status every 4 hours.	Identifies changes and, thus, the need to modify the plan of care.
Instruct all caregivers to respond promptly to the call light.	Ensures rapid response to the client's needs.
Teach Mr. Simon to use the call light; reinforce teaching each time before leaving him alone.	Ensures that the client has the means and knowledge to call for assistance if necessary.

CASE STUDY

Manuela, age 30 years, received a broken right arm and a broken right leg in a car accident. The arm and leg are each in a cast.

The following questions will guide your development of a nursing care plan for the case study.

1. What assessment information should be gathered?
2. Identify three nursing diagnoses for Manuela.
3. Formulate possible goals for each nursing diagnosis.
4. Plan nursing interventions for each nursing diagnosis.

SUMMARY

- Maintaining a safe environment for clients must be the highest priority for nurses.
- The best way to ensure safety is to recognize hazards and eliminate them. Prevention is the best safety measure.
- Clients having a high risk factor for injury must be provided extra protection measures.

- Factors influencing client safety are age, lifestyle, sensory and perceptual alterations, mobility, and emotional state.
- The accidents that occur in health care settings relate to client behavior, therapeutic procedures, and equipment.
- Assessment of a safe environment involves performing an injury risk appraisal.

- Nurses can help clients in maintaining a safe environment by resolving or alleviating hazards related to falls, lighting, obstacles, the bathroom, fire, electricity, radiation, poisoning, and noise pollution.
- Safety precautions should be explained thoroughly to clients and/or families.
- Hygiene practices are influenced by body image, social and cultural practices, personal preference, socioeconomic status, and knowledge.
- Basic hygiene practices include bathing, skin care, perineal care, back rubs, foot and nail care, oral care, hair care, and eye, ear, and nose care.

Review Questions

1. Mingo, a 60-year-old diabetic, had his left leg amputated. He is in a semiprivate room with another client who is receiving oxygen. What sign should be posted on the door?

    a. "Amputee"
    b. "No Visitors"
    c. "No Smoking"
    d. "Regular Diet"

2. Felicita, just admitted to the hospital, is overweight, unsteady on her feet, and visually impaired. Her two daughters enter the room as the nurse puts the side rails up on the bed. Felicita begins to cry. The daughters accuse her of being a baby. The best nursing intervention would be to:

    a. tell the daughters to leave until Felicita has calmed down.
    b. explain to the daughters that they are making their mother feel worse.
    c. explain to Felicita that side rails must be used to protect her from falling out of bed.
    d. explain to Felicita and her daughters both the purpose of the side rails and the facility's alternate policy.

3. The priority for nursing care is:

    a. safety.
    b. timeliness.
    c. one-to-one care.
    d. the execution of procedures exactly as written.

4. The use of side rails:

    a. is only needed at night.
    b. is required for all clients.
    c. has caused injury to clients.
    d. relieves the nurse from checking on the client as frequently.

5. Hygiene is considered a safety measure because:

    a. it changes a person's self-image.
    b. the same thing is done for all clients.
    c. it rids the body of all microorganisms.
    d. it promotes the health of the body's first line of defense.

6. The water (type A) fire extinguisher is to be used on:

    a. paper.
    b. flammable gases.
    c. electrical fires.
    d. flammable liquids.

7. If a client receives an electrical shock, the first thing the nurse should do is:

    a. call for help.
    b. unplug the equipment.
    c. check the client's pulse.
    d. move the client out of the room.

Critical Thinking Questions

1. Gloria Hernandez is an 83-year-old widow who fractured her hip when she fell in the bathtub. She had hip replacement surgery yesterday. Tonight she is very confused and is trying to dislodge the bandage and stitches. Mrs. Hernandez is now being restrained for her protection. What other nursing activities could have been implemented prior to the use of restraints? Do you think that restraints will affect Mrs. Hernandez's mental status? If so, in what way(s)? What are some other effects Mrs. Hernandez may experience as a result of being restrained?

2. How is noise a safety factor?

3. How would you approach providing perineal care to someone of the opposite sex or of a similar age?

 WEB FLASH!

- What Internet sources can you locate that relate to safety and hygiene? What types of information are available?
- Which of the resources listed for this chapter have web sites? What kind of information is provided?

Chapter 21
Infection Control/Asepsis

Chapter 22
Standard Precautions
and Isolation

INFECTION CONTROL/ ASEPSIS

MAKING THE CONNECTION

Refer to the following chapters to increase your understanding of infection control/asepsis:

- **Chapter 18, Basic Nutrition**
- **Chapter 20, Safety/Hygiene**
- **Chapter 22, Standard Precautions and Isolation**
- **Chapter 23, Fluid, Electrolyte, and Acid–Base Balance**

- **Procedures:** B1, Handwashing; B2, Use of Personal Protective Equipment; I1, Surgical Asepsis: Preparing and Maintaining a Sterile Field; I2, Performing Open Gloving and Removal of Soiled Gloves; I17, Applying a Dry Sterile Dressing

LEARNING OBJECTIVES

Upon completion of this chapter, you should be able to:
- *Define key terms.*
- *Describe the chain of infection.*
- *Discuss the body's nonspecific and specific immune defenses.*
- *Describe the stages of the inflammatory process.*
- *Discuss the stages of the infectious process.*
- *Identify the signs and symptoms of inflammation and infection.*
- *Explain the principles of medical and surgical asepsis.*
- *Provide client care maintaining the principles of medical and/or surgical asepsis.*

KEY TERMS

acquired immunity
agent
airborne transmission
anthropogenic
antibody
antigen
asepsis
aseptic technique
bactericide
biological agent
carrier
chain of infection
chemical agent
clean object
cleansing
colonization
communicable agent
communicable disease
compromised host
contact transmission
convalescent stage
dirty object
disinfectant
disinfection
edema
erythema
flora
fomite
germicide
handwashing
host
humoral immunity
illness stage
immunization
incubation period
infection
infectious agent
inflammation
localized infection
lymphokine
medical asepsis
mode of transmission
nosocomial infection
pathogen
pathogenicity
physical agent
portal of entry
portal of exit
prodromal stage
purulent exudate
reservoir
resident flora
risk for infection
sebum
spore
sterilization
surgical asepsis
susceptible host
systemic infection
transient flora
vaccination
vectorborne transmission
vehicle transmission
virulence

INTRODUCTION

Nurses are responsible for providing quality care that incorporates infection-control principles. These principles are a major component of a safe environment. This chapter discusses infection-control principles including naturally occurring microorganisms, pathogens, infection and colonization, chain of infection, normal defense mechanisms, stages of the infectious process, and nosocomial infections. Discussion of the nurse's role in controlling infections is also included.

FLORA

Flora are microorganisms that occur or have adapted to live in a specific environment, such as intestinal, skin, vaginal, or oral flora. There are two types of flora: resident and transient. **Resident (normal) flora** are microorganisms that are always present, usually without altering the client's health; an example would be *proprionibacterium* on the skin. Handwashing with soap and water alone is not sufficient to remove resident flora; there must be considerable friction, which is created by rubbing the hands and scrubbing the nails. Resident flora prevent the overgrowth of harmful microorganisms; only when the balance is upset does disease result. **Transient flora** are microorganisms that are episodic (of limited duration); an example would be *staphylococcus aureus*. They attach to the skin for a brief period of time but do not continually live on the skin. Transient flora are usually acquired from direct contact with the microorganisms on environmental surfaces. Handwashing with soap and water is an effective means of removing transient flora (Ellner & Neu, 1992).

PATHOGENICITY AND VIRULENCE

Although most microorganisms found in the environment do not cause disease and infection, there are some that do. Disease-producing microorganisms are called **pathogens**; **pathogenicity** refers to the ability of a microorganism to produce disease. **Virulence** refers to the frequency with which a pathogen causes disease. The factors affecting virulence are the strength of the pathogen to adhere to healthy cells; the ability of a pathogen to damage cells or interfere with the body's normal regulating systems; and the ability of a pathogen to evade the attack of white blood cells (WBCs).

Five types of microorganisms can be pathogenic: bacteria, viruses, fungi, protozoa, and *Rickettsia*.

Bacteria

Bacteria are small, one-celled microorganisms that lack a true nucleus or mechanism to provide metabolism. Therefore, bacteria need an environment that will provide food for survival. Bacteria can be spherical, rodlike, spiral, or curving in shape, usually appearing as single cells, pairs, chains, or groups. Although most bacteria multiply by simple cell division, some forms of bacteria produce **spores**, a resistant stage that withstands unfavorable environments. When proper environmental conditions return, spores germinate and form new cells. Spores are difficult to kill because of their resistance to heat, drying, and disinfectant. The growth rate of bacteria is affected by environmental factors such as changes in temperature and nutrition. The optimal temperature for pathogenic bacteria is 98.6°F.

Bacteria can be found in all environments, yet not all bacteria are harmful or cause disease. Only a small percentage of bacteria are actually pathogenic. Common bacterial infections include diarrhea, pneumonia, sinusitis, urinary tract infections, cellulitis, meningitis, gonorrhea (Figure 21-1), otitis media, and impetigo.

Viruses

Viruses are organisms that can live only inside cells. They cannot get nourishment or reproduce outside cells. Viruses contain a core of deoxyribonucleic acid (DNA) or ribonucleic acid (RNA) surrounded by a protein coating. Some viruses have the ability to create an additional coating called an envelope. This envelope helps protect the cell from attack by the immune system. Viruses damage the cells they inhabit by blocking the normal protein synthesis of the cells and by using the cell's mechanism for metabolism to reproduce.

The same viral infection may cause different symptoms in different individuals, based on the individual's immune response to the invading virus. Some viruses will immediately trigger a disease response whereas others may remain latent for many years. Common viral

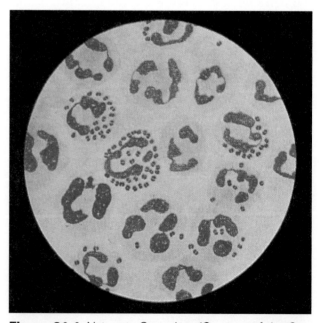

Figure 21-1 Neisseria Gonorrhea (*Courtesy of the Centers for Disease Control and Prevention, Atlanta, GA*)

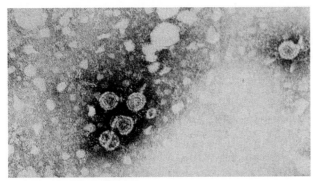

Figure 21-2 Electron Micrograph of Hepatitis B Virus *(Courtesy of the Centers for Disease Control and Prevention, Atlanta, GA)*

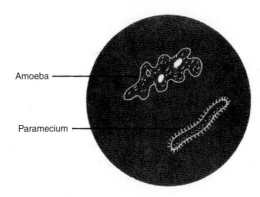

Figure 21-4 Protozoa

infections include influenza, measles, common cold, chickenpox, hepatitis B (Figure 21-2), genital herpes, and HIV.

Fungi

Fungi grow in single cells, as in yeast, or in colonies, as in molds (Figure 21-3). Fungi obtain food from dead organic matter or from living organisms. Most fungi are not pathogenic and make up many of the body's normal flora. Disease from fungi is found mainly in individuals who are immunologically impaired. Fungi can cause infections of the hair, skin, nails, and mucous membranes.

Protozoa

Protozoa are single-celled parasitic organisms with the ability to move (Figure 21-4). Most protozoa obtain their nourishment from dead or decaying organic matter. Infection is spread through ingestion of contaminated food or water or through insect bites. Common protozoan infections include malaria, gastroenteritis, and vaginal infections.

Rickettsia

Rickettsia are intracellular parasites that need to be in living cells to reproduce. Infection from *rickettsia* is

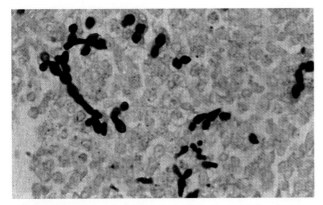

Figure 21-3 Candida Albicans *(Courtesy of the Centers for Disease Control and Prevention, Atlanta, GA)*

spread through fleas, ticks, mites, and lice. Common *rickettsia* infections include typhus, Rocky Mountain spotted fever, and Lyme disease.

INFECTION AND COLONIZATION

Infection and colonization are not synonymous. **Infection** is an invasion and multiplication of pathogenic microorganisms that occurs in body tissue and results in cellular injury; an example is strep throat. These microorganisms are called **infectious agents**. Infectious agents that are capable of being transmitted to a client by direct or indirect contact, through a vehicle (or vector) or airborne route are also called **communicable agents**. Diseases produced by these agents are referred to as **communicable diseases**.

Colonization is the multiplication of microorganisms that occurs on or within a host but does not result in cellular injury; an example of colonization is the normal flora (microorganisms) in the intestines. However, microorganisms that are colonized on a host may be a potential source of infection, especially if host susceptibility increases or the microorganism's virulence increases.

CHAIN OF INFECTION

Neither a susceptible host nor the presence of a pathogen means that an infectious process will occur. The **chain of infection** describes the phenomenon of the development of an infectious process. An interactive process that involves the agent, host, and environment is required. This interactive process must involve several essential elements, or "links in the chain," for transmission of microorganisms to occur. Figure 21-5 identifies the six essential links (elements) in the chain of infection. Without the transmission of microorganisms, an infectious process cannot occur. Therefore, knowledge about the chain of infection facilitates control or elimination of microorganism transmission

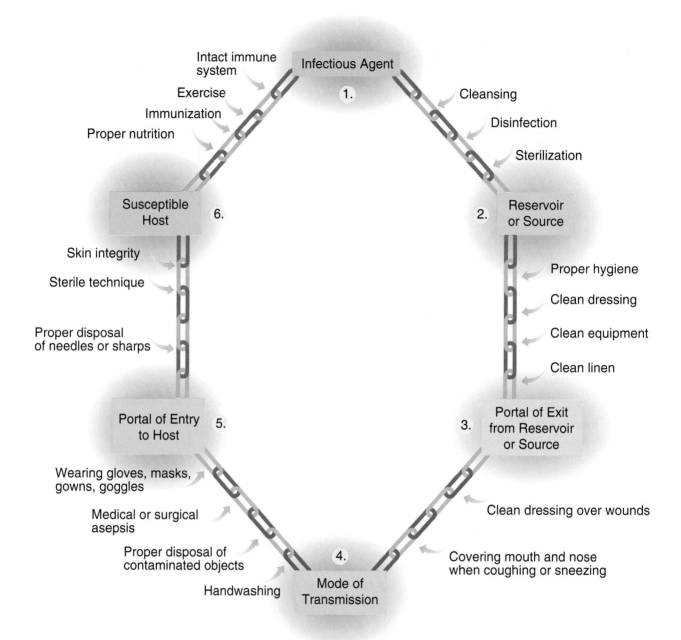

Figure 21-5 The Chain of Infection: Preventive Measures Follow Each Link of the Chain (*Adapted from* Fundamentals of Nursing: Standards & Practice, *by S. DeLaune and P. Ladner, 1998, Albany, NY: Delmar. Copyright 1998 by Delmar.*)

by breaking the links in the chain. Breaking the chain of infection is achieved by altering the interactive process of the agent, host, and environment. Each of the six links in the chain of infection is discussed following.

Agent

An **agent** is an entity that is capable of causing disease. Agents that cause disease may be as follows:

- **Biological agents**: living organisms that invade the host, causing disease, such as bacteria, viruses, fungi, protozoa, and *rickettsia*

- **Chemical agents**: substances that can interact with the body, causing disease, such as pesticides, food additives, medications, and industrial chemicals
- **Physical agents**: factors in the environment that are capable of causing disease, such as heat, light, noise, radiation, and machinery

In the chain of infection, the main concern is biological agents and their effect on the host.

Reservoir

The **reservoir** is a place where the agent can survive. Colonization and reproduction take place while the agent is in the reservoir. A reservoir that promotes growth of pathogens must contain the proper nutrients (such as oxygen and organic matter), maintain proper temperature, contain moisture, maintain a compatible pH level (neither too acidic nor too alkaline), and maintain the proper amount of light exposure. The most common reservoirs are:

- Humans,
- Animals,
- Environment, and
- **Fomites** (objects contaminated with an infectious agent, such as bedpans, urinals, bed linens, instruments, dressings, specimen containers, and other equipment).

Humans and animals can have symptoms of the infectious agents or can be strictly carriers of the agent. **Carriers** have the infectious agent but are symptom free. The agent can be spread to others in both instances.

Portal of Exit

The **portal of exit** is the route by which an infectious agent leaves the reservoir to be transferred to a susceptible host. The agent leaves the reservoir through body secretions including:

- Sputum, from the respiratory tract;
- Semen, vaginal secretions, or urine, from the genitourinary tract;
- Saliva and feces, from the gastrointestinal tract;
- Blood;
- Draining wounds; and
- Tears.

Modes of Transmission

The **mode of transmission** is the process that bridges the gap between the portal of exit of the infectious agent from the reservoir or source and the portal of entry of the susceptible "new" host. Most infectious agents have a primary or usual mode of transmission; however, some microorganisms may be transmitted by more than one mode (Table 21–1). Almost anything in the environment can become a potential means of transmitting infection, depending on the agent.

Contact Transmission

The most important and frequent mode of transmission is **contact transmission**, which involves the physical transfer of an agent from an infected person to a host through direct contact with the infected person, indirect contact with the infected person through a fomite, or close contact with contaminated secretions (Figure 21-6). Sexually transmitted diseases are examples of diseases spread by direct contact. Common viral infections (cold, measles, flu) are spread by close contact with contaminated secretions.

Table 21–1 MODES OF TRANSMISSION

MODE	EXAMPLES
Contact	Direct contact of health care provider with client: • Touching • Bathing • Rubbing • Toileting (urine and feces) • Secretions from client Indirect contact with fomites: • Clothing • Bed linens • Dressings • Health care equipment • Instruments used in treatments • Specimen containers used for laboratory analysis • Personal belongings • Personal care equipment • Diagnostic equipment
Airborne	Inhaling microorganisms carried by moisture or dust particles in air: • Coughing • Talking • Sneezing
Vehicle	Contact with contaminated inanimate objects: • Water • Blood • Drugs • Food • Urine
Vectorborne	Contact with contaminated animate hosts: • Animals • Insects

Airborne Transmission

Airborne transmission occurs when a susceptible host contacts droplet nuclei or dust particles that are suspended in the air. Particle size influences the length of time that the organism can remain airborne. The longer the particle is suspended, the greater the chance it will find an available port of entry to the human host. An example of an organism that relies on airborne transmission is measles. Contaminated droplets containing the measles virus are contained in the spray from sneezing. The droplet can find a portal of entry through the mucous membranes or conjunctiva. Droplets that do not remain airborne or settle out are excluded from this category (Benenson, 1995).

Vehicle Transmission

Vehicle transmission occurs when an agent is transferred to a susceptible host by contaminated inanimate

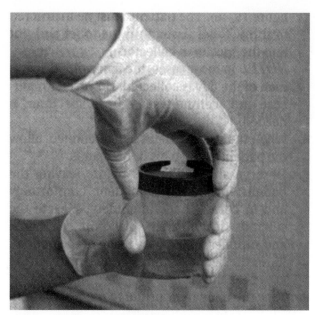

Figure 21-6 Care must be taken in the handling of bodily fluids to prevent the transfer of infectious agents through contact with secretions.

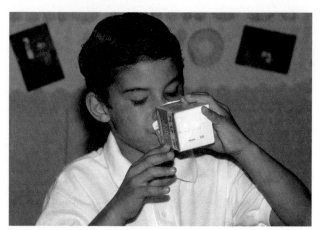

Figure 21-7 Vehicle transmission occurs through contamination of inanimate objects, such as milk.

objects such as water, food, milk (Figure 21-7), drugs, and blood. Cholera, which is transmitted through contaminated drinking water, and salmonellosis, which is transmitted through contaminated meat, are examples of vehicle transmission.

Vectorborne transmission

Vectorborne transmission occurs when an agent is transferred to a susceptible host by animate means such as mosquitoes, fleas, ticks, lice, and other animals (Figure 21-8). Lyme disease and malaria are examples of diseases spread by vectors.

Portal of Entry

A **portal of entry** is the route by which an infectious agent enters the host. Portals of entry include the following:

- Integumentary system, through a break in the integrity of the skin or mucous membranes (for instance, infections of surgical wounds)
- Respiratory tract, by inhaling contaminated droplets (such as cold, influenza, measles)
- Genitourinary tract, through contact with infected vaginal secretions or semen (as in sexually transmitted diseases)
- Gastrointestinal tract, by ingesting contaminated food or water (for example, typhoid, hepatitis A)
- Circulatory system, through the bite of insects (such as mosquito bites resulting in malaria)
- Transplacental, through transfer of microorganisms from mother to fetus via the placenta and umbilical cord (including HIV, hepatitis B)

Host

A **host** is a simple or complex organism that can be affected by an agent. Generally, a human being is considered a host. A **susceptible host** is a person who lacks resistance to an agent and is thus vulnerable to disease. For example, an individual who has not received the measles vaccine is more likely to contract the infection due to the lack of immunity to the infectious agent. A **compromised host** is a person whose normal defense mechanisms are impaired and who is therefore susceptible to infection. For example, a person with a common cold or superficial burns is at greater risk for infection due to the impaired state of the body system mechanisms.

Characteristics of the host influence the susceptibility to and severity of infections. These include:

- Age: As a person ages, immunity declines, thus increasing susceptibility to infection.
- Concurrent diseases: The existence of comorbid diseases indicates an environment susceptible to infection.

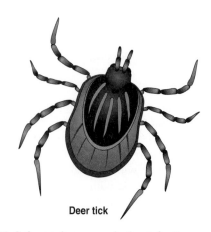

Deer tick

Figure 21-8 Lyme disease and other infections are caused by the bite of a tick.

- Stress: An individual experiencing a compromised emotional state may have altered or decreased immune system response.
- Immunization/vaccination status: Individuals who are not fully immunized are at greater risk for infection.
- Lifestyle: Lifestyle practices such as having multiple sex partners or sharing intravenous drug needles increase an individual's potential for illness.
- Occupation: Forms of employment that involve an increased exposure to pathogens might include dealing with chemical agents (such as asbestos) or handling sharp instruments (such as scalpels).
- Nutritional status: Individuals who maintain targeted weight for height and body frame are less prone to illness.
- Heredity: Some individuals are naturally more susceptible to infection than others (Black & Matassarin-Jacobs, 1997).

Interaction between agent and host occurs in the environment; the environment consists of everything other than the agent and host. Environmental factors that affect the chain of infection are water, food, plants, animals, housing conditions, noise, meteorological conditions, and environmental chemicals. Many of the conditions that promote the transmission of microorganisms are **anthropogenic**, reflecting changes in the relationship between humans and their environments.

BREAKING THE CHAIN OF INFECTION

Nurses focus on breaking the chain of infection by applying proper infection-control practices to interrupt the transmission of microorganisms. Specific strategies can be directed at breaking or blocking the transmission of infection from one link in the chain to the next. A discussion regarding each of the six links follows (refer back to Figure 21-5).

Infection Control: First Line of Defense
Handwashing is the first line of defense against infection and is the single most important practice in preventing the spread of infection.

Between Agent and Reservoir

The first link in the chain of infection is between the agent and the reservoir. The keys to eliminating infection at this point in the chain are cleansing, disinfection, and sterilization. These tactics serve to prevent the formation of a reservoir or environment within which infectious agents can live and multiply.

Cleansing

Cleansing is the removal of soil or organic material from instruments and equipment used in providing client care. Nurses are involved in cleansing instruments after assisting or performing invasive procedures. To reduce the amount of contamination and loosen the material on reusable objects, the objects are cleansed prior to sterilization and disinfection. Cleansing involves the use of water, mechanical action, and, sometimes, a detergent. Contaminated objects are cleansed using a soft-bristled brush to scrub the surface. The steps for proper cleansing are:

1. Rinse the object under *cold* water, because warm water causes proteins in organic material to coagulate and stick.
2. Apply detergent and scrub the object under running water using a soft-bristled brush.
3. Rinse the object under warm water.
4. Dry the object prior to sterilization or disinfection.

Infection Control: Cleansing
Cleansing presents a potential hazard to the nurse in the form of the splashing of contaminated material onto the body. Nurses should wear gloves, masks, and goggles during cleansing.

Disinfection

Disinfection is the elimination of pathogens, except spores, from inanimate objects. **Disinfectants** are chemical solutions used to clean inanimate objects. Bedpans, blood pressure cuffs, linens, stethoscopes,

COMMUNITY/HOME HEALTH CARE

Disinfection

In the home, Lysol and bleach are common disinfectants capable of eliminating several pathogens.

thermometers, and some types of endoscopes are disinfected in the hospital setting. The U.S. Environmental Protection Agency (EPA) licenses (registers) disinfection products and monitors the products to ensure that they work as claimed on the label (Pugliese, 1994). Common disinfectants are alcohol, sodium hypochlorite, quaternary ammonium, phenolic solutions, and glutaraldehyde.

A **germicide** is a chemical that can be applied to both animate (living) and inanimate objects for the purpose of eliminating pathogens. Antiseptic preparations such as alcohol and silver sulfadiazine are germicides.

Sterilization

Sterilization is the total elimination of all microorganisms including spores. Instruments that are used for invasive procedures must be sterilized. Methods of achieving sterilization are moist heat or steam, radiation, chemicals, and ethylene oxide gas. The method of sterilization depends on the type and amount of contamination and the object to be sterilized.

Autoclaving sterilization, which uses moist heat or steam, is the most common sterilization technique used in the hospital setting (Figure 21-9). Boiling water is not an effective sterilization measure, because some viruses and spores can survive boiling water. Objects that have been boiled in water for 15 to 20 minutes at 121°C (249.8°F) are considered clean but not sterile (Department of Labor, 1991).

Between Reservoir and Portal of Exit

Promoting proper hygiene, maintaining clean dressings and linens, and ensuring the use of clean equipment in client care are the methods used to break the chain of infection between the reservoir and the portal

COMMUNITY/HOME HEALTH CARE

Sterilization at Home

Boiling water is still the best and most common sterilization measure used in the home. For example, boiling baby bottles and nipples makes them safe for use.

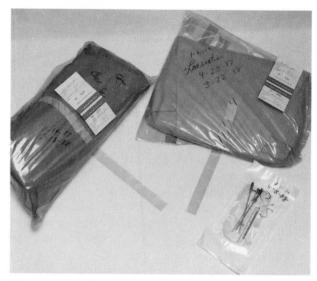

Figure 21-9 Sterilized packages. The strips below each package show the way they looked before sterilization. The strips on the packages have changed color because they have been sterilized.

of exit. The aim at this juncture is to eliminate the reservoir for the microorganism before the pathogen can escape to a susceptible host.

Proper Hygiene

The nurse must teach the client the importance of maintaining the cleanliness and the integrity of the skin and the mucous membranes. Clean skin, hair, and nails will maintain the body's normal flora and eliminate transient flora or infectious agents from the client's system. Bathing and handwashing are important means of eliminating the potential for infection. Clients should be encouraged to practice daily routines of bathing and teeth brushing. The nurse should assist clients who are unable to perform these activities independently.

Clean Dressings

Any open injury or other break in skin integrity represents a potential reservoir for infectious agents or portal of exit for a pathogen to be transferred to another individual. Dressings on open or oozing wounds must be changed and cleaned regularly. To protect both themselves and the client from infection, nurses must follow proper aseptic technique when changing dressings. This technique is discussed in detail later in this chapter.

Clean Linen

Bed linens, dressing gowns, and towels are catchalls for bodily secretions. Infectious agents can be easily transferred from one individual to the next through contact with a client's linens. Linens must be changed regularly, and soiled linens must be properly disposed. When changing linens, the nurse should take care to keep the soiled articles from coming into contact with the nursing uniform. This will prevent the nurse from contracting an infection from the soiled linens or passing the infection on to other clients in her care.

Clean Equipment

All equipment used in the care of a client must be cleansed and disinfected after each use. Although many items such as disposable gowns can be discarded after use, items such as beds and bedpans must be thoroughly cleansed after each use. Clients should be instructed never to share care items. Any nondisposable equipment used in an invasive procedure (such as equipment used in the operating room [OR]) must be sterilized before being used again. To protect themselves, nurses should wear gloves and masks when cleansing equipment to avoid being splashed with contaminated waste products or secretions.

Between Portal of Exit and Mode of Transmission

The goal in breaking the chain of infection between the portal of exit and the mode of transmission is to prevent the exit of the infectious agents. The nurse must maintain clean dressings on all injuries. Clients should be encouraged to cover the mouth and nose when sneezing or coughing, and the nurse must do so as well. Gloves must be worn whenever caring for a client who may have infectious secretions, and care must be taken to properly dispose of any article contaminated with secretions.

Between Mode of Transmission and Portal of Entry

To break the chain of infection between the mode of transmission and the portal of entry, nurses must ensure asepsis and wear barrier protection whenever the care of clients involves contact with body secretions. Gloves, masks, gowns, and goggles are all forms of barrier protection that can be used. Proper handwashing and the proper disposal of contaminated equipment and linens are also keys to preventing the transmission of microorganisms to other clients and health care workers. A thorough discussion of asepsis and disposal of contaminated items is included later in this chapter.

Between Portal of Entry and Host

Maintaining skin integrity and using sterile technique for client contacts are methods of breaking the chain of infection between portal of entry and host. Avoiding needle sticks by properly disposing of sharps also reduces the potential for infection by denying a portal of entry. The goal at this point in the chain is to prevent the transmission of infection to a client or health care worker who has not yet been infected.

Between Host and Agent

Breaking the chain of infection between host and agent means eliminating infection before it begins. There are many ways to reduce the risk of acquiring infection. Proper nutrition, exercise, and immunizations allow an individual to maintain an intact immune system, thus preventing infection.

Proper Nutrition

Proper nutrition assists the body's immune system to function properly. Clients need adequate amounts of protein in their diets to maintain and repair tissue as well as to produce the antibodies needed to fight infection. A balanced diet also allows the body to maintain appropriate acid–base balance.

Exercise

Exercise maintains the body's metabolic rate and, therefore, allows the body to maintain the antibodies and energy necessary to ward off infection.

Immunization

Immunization is the process of creating immunity, or resistance to infection, in an individual. Most immunizations or vaccinations are given in early childhood; examples include vaccinations for measles, mumps, and rubella.

NORMAL DEFENSE MECHANISMS

A host's immune system serves as a normal defense mechanism against the transmission of infectious agents. A unique feature of the immune system is its ability to recognize "self" and "nonself"; that is, the immune system recognizes which agents are not consistent with the genetic composition of the host (self). These agents are usually referred to as antigens (nonself). **Antigens** are foreign proteins that cause the formation of an antibody and react specifically with that antibody. An immune response is mounted against an antigen, which is recognized as nonself, to protect the body from infection. The immune defenses are categorized as nonspecific and specific immune defenses. Nonspecific and specific

CLIENT TEACHING

Inappropriate Use of Antibiotics

- Do not pressure the physician to prescribe antibiotics for every illness. Antibiotics are not always appropriate, for instance, antibiotics are not effective against viruses.
- When antibiotics are prescribed, instruct client to take *all* of the medication as directed.
- Antibiotics taken only until the client feels better allow the microorganisms to become resistant to the antibiotic and the antibiotic will no longer be effective.
- Antibiotics also destroy normal flora microorganisms, and other illnesses may ensue.

immune defenses work in harmony to defend the host from pathogens (Bouman, 1998; Porche, 1998).

Nonspecific Immune Defense

The nonspecific immune defense mounts a response to protect the host from all microorganisms; it is not dependent on prior exposure to the antigen. Nonspecific immune defenses are skin and normal flora; mucous membranes; sneezing, coughing, and tearing reflexes; elimination and acidic environment; and inflammation.

Skin and Normal Flora

The skin is the first line of defense against infection, serving as a physical barrier to infectious agents. Skin cells are shed daily, removing potentially harmful microorganisms. **Sebum** is a substance that is produced by the skin and contains fatty acids that kill some bacteria. The normal flora that reside on the skin and in the body compete with pathogenic flora for food and inhibit the multiplication of pathogens. The balance of normal flora may become disrupted, which allows pathogenic organisms to proliferate and cause infection or superinfection.

Mucous Membranes

Mucous membranes also function as a physical barrier to infectious agents. Mucus produced by these membranes entraps infectious agents and contains substances such as antibodies, lactoferrin, and lysozyme, which inhibit bacterial growth. For example, the cilia of the respiratory tract trap and propel mucus and microorganisms away from the lungs, thereby reducing the potential for infection.

Sneezing, Coughing, and Tearing Reflexes

The sneeze and cough reflexes physically expel mucus and microorganisms from the respiratory tract and oral cavity with force. Tears protect the eyes by continually flushing away microorganisms. Tears also contain **bactericides**, which are bacteria-killing chemicals.

Elimination and Acidic Environment

Elimination patterns and an acidic environment normally prevent microbial growth of pathogenic organisms. Resident flora of the large intestines prevent the growth of pathogens. The mechanical process of defecation evacuates the bowel of feces and microorganisms. Acidity of the urine prevents microbial growth. The flushing action of urination cleanses the bladder neck and urethra of microorganisms and prevents microorganisms from ascending into the urinary tract.

Normal vaginal flora prevent growth of several pathogens. At puberty, lactobacilli ferment and produce sugars in the vagina that lower the pH to an acidic range. The acidic environment of the vagina prevents pathogenic growth.

Inflammation

Inflammation is a nonspecific cellular response to tissue injury. Tissue injury caused by bacteria, trauma, chemicals, heat, or any other phenomenon releases multiple substances that produce dramatic secondary changes in the injured tissue (Figure 21-10). This entire complex of tissue changes and response to injury is referred to as the *inflammatory process* (Table 21–2). The inflammatory process has five stages, which facilitate the localization, neutralization, and resolution of the offending agent within the damaged tissue. The body's response to injury produces the characteristic local and systemic signs of inflammation.

Inflammation is not necessarily the result of invading microorganisms but does have signs and symptoms similar to those of an infection. The primary signs of inflammation and infection are as follows:

- Redness (erythema), the result of increased blood flow to the area
- Heat, the result of increased blood flow and metabolism in the area

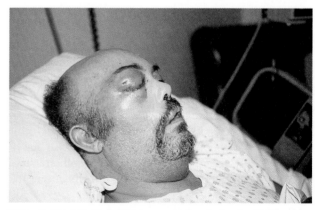

Figure 21-10 Cellulitis, an example of a bacterial infection, is marked by redness, swelling, and pain. *(Courtesy of Dr. Mark Dougherty, Lexington, KY)*

Table 21-2 STAGES OF THE INFLAMMATORY PROCESS

STAGE	DESCRIPTION	RESULT
1	Initial injury precipitates release of chemicals: histamine, bradykinin, serotonin, prostaglandins (reaction products of the complement and blood-clotting systems), and lymphokines (hormonal substances released by sensitized T-cells).	Activates the inflammation process
2	Blood flow increases to the inflamed area (**erythema**).	Produces characteristic signs of redness and increased warmth
3	Increased capillary permeability with leakage of large quantities of plasma out of the capillaries and into the damaged tissue; tissue spaces and lymphatics are blocked by fibrinogen clots.	Initiates the inflammation process; "walls off" infection; results in nonpitting edema
4	Damaged tissue infiltrated by leukocytes, which engulf the bacteria and necrotic tissue. After several days, these leukocytes eventually die and form a cavity of necrotic tissue and dead leukocytes (mainly neutrophils and some macrophages).	Produces purulent exudate (pus)
5	Destroyed tissue cells are replaced by identical or similar structural and functioning cells and/or fibrous tissue.	Promotes tissue healing or the formation of fibrous (scar) tissue, which may reduce the functional capacity of the tissue.

From Fundamentals of Nursing: Standards & Practice, *by S. DeLaune and P. Ladner, 1998, Albany, NY: Delmar. Copyright 1998 by Delmar. Reprinted with permission.*

- Pain, the result of increased pressure on pain sensors in the area
- Swelling (**edema**, a detectable accumulation of increased interstitial fluid), the result of fluid and leukocytes entering the tissues from the circulatory system
- Loss of function, the result of both pain and swelling and the body's way of resting the injured part
- Pus (**purulent exudate**), the result of an infection, a secretion made up of white blood cells, dead cells, bacteria, and other debris

The intensity of the inflammatory process is usually in proportion to the degree of tissue injury. For example, when staphylococci invade the tissues, they release lethal cellular toxins that cause the inflammatory process to develop quickly; the staphylococcal infection is characteristically walled off rapidly before the organism can multiply and spread. Streptococci, on the other hand, do not cause such intense local tissue destruction, and the walling-off process develops slowly, allowing the organism to reproduce and migrate. Therefore, the streptococci have a far greater tendency than do staphylococci to spread throughout the body and cause death, even though staphylococci are far more destructive to the tissue (Guyton & Hall, 1995).

Specific Immune Defense

The specific immune defense mounts an immune response that is specific to the invading antigen. The specific immune defense is activated by the failure of phagocytes to completely destroy the antigen; this causes the production of T lymphocytes (T cells), which regulate the immune response by activating other cells. Stimulated T-cells are referred to as sensitized T cells. These T cells migrate to the area of injury and release chemical substances called **lymphokines**. Lymphokines attract other phagocytes and lymphocytes to the area of injury and assist in antigen destruction.

The T cells also stimulate the production of B cells, which differentiate into plasma cells, producing antibodies specific to the antigen. **Antibodies** are protein substances that counteract and neutralize the effects of antigenic toxins and destroy bacteria and other cells. Antibodies destroy the antigen. The stimulation of B cells and the production of antibodies are collectively referred to as **humoral immunity**.

The B cell activation causes formation of memory B cells. Memory B cells remember the antigen and prepare the host for future antigen invasion. Thus, when the antigen enters the body again, the immune response will occur more rapidly by producing antibodies faster. The formation of these antibodies is referred to as **acquired immunity**, which protects the individual against future invasions of already experienced antigens such as lethal bacteria, viruses, toxins, and even foreign tissues.

The process of **vaccination** (inoculation with a vaccine to produce immunity against specific diseases) provides acquired immunity. There are three ways an individual can be vaccinated:

- By the introduction of dead organisms that are no longer capable of causing disease but still have their

chemical antigens, such as in the cases of typhoid fever, whooping cough, and diphtheria.
- By the introduction of toxins that have been treated with chemicals so that their toxic nature has been destroyed even though their antigens for causing immunity are still intact, such as for tetanus and botulism.
- By the introduction of live organisms that have been attenuated (grown in a special culture media or passed through a series of animals for mutation, rendering the organisms incapable of causing the disease yet still carrying the specific antigen), such as for poliomyelitis, yellow fever, measles, smallpox, and many other viral diseases (Guyton & Hall, 1995).

STAGES OF THE INFECTIOUS PROCESS

Activation of the immune response indicates the occurrence of infection. Infection results from tissue invasion and damage by an infectious agent. There are two types of infectious responses:

- **Localized infections**, which are limited to a defined area or single organ with symptoms that resemble inflammation (redness, tenderness, and swelling), such as a cold sore
- **Systemic infections**, which affect the entire body and involve multiple organs, such as AIDS

Localized and systemic infections progress through four stages: incubation, prodromal, illness, and convalescence.

Incubation Stage

The **incubation period** is the time interval between entry of an infectious agent in the host and the onset of symptoms. During this time period, the infectious agent invades the tissue and begins to multiply to produce an infection; the client is typically infectious to others during the latter part of this stage. For example, the incubation period for varicella (chickenpox) is 2 to 3 weeks; the infected person is contagious from 5 days before any skin eruptions to no more than 6 days after the skin eruptions appear.

 Safety: Incubation Period
Always verify the incubation period of a suspected infection. Keep in mind that, depending on the infectious agent, a client may be able to transmit the infection to another person, even prior to the onset of symptoms.

Prodromal Stage

The **prodromal stage** is the time interval from the onset of nonspecific symptoms until specific symptoms of the infectious process begin to manifest. During this period, the infectious agent continues to

invade and multiply in the host. A client may also be infectious to other persons during this time period. In the client with chickenpox, a slight elevation in temperature will occur during this stage, followed within 24 hours by eruptions of the skin.

Illness Stage

The **illness stage** is the time period when the client is manifesting specific signs and symptoms of an infectious process. The client with chickenpox will experience a further rise in temperature and continued outbreaks of skin eruptions for at least 2 to 3 more days.

Convalescent Stage

The period of time from the beginning of the disappearance of acute symptoms until the client returns to the previous state of health is referred to as the **convalescent stage**. The client with chickenpox will see the skin eruptions and irritation begin to resolve during this stage.

NOSOCOMIAL INFECTIONS

A **nosocomial infection** is an infection that was acquired in a hospital or other health care facility and was not present or incubating at the time of the client's admission. Nosocomial infections are also referred to as *hospital-acquired infections*. These types of infections typically fall into four categories: urinary tract, surgical wounds, pneumonia, and septicemia.

Nosocomial infections also include those infections that become symptomatic after the client is discharged, as well as infections passed among medical personnel. Most nosocomial infections are transmitted by health care personnel who fail to practice proper handwashing procedures or who fail to change gloves between client contacts (Compliance Control Center, 1998).

Hospitalized clients are at risk for nosocomial infections because the environment provides exposure to a variety of virulent organisms to which the client has not typically been exposed in the past; therefore, the

PROFESSIONAL TIP

Nosocomial Infections

Each year more than 2,400,000 nosocomial infections occur in the United States. Annually, nosocomial infections directly cause 30,000 deaths and contribute to 70,000 more deaths. Further, the client's length of stay is increased, costing $2,300 per incident and $4.5 billion annually for the associated extended care and treatment (Compliance Control Center, 1998).

client has not developed any resistance to these organisms. In addition, illness, often the reason for hospital admission, impairs the body's normal defense mechanisms.

Nicolle and Garibaldi (1995) discuss the increased risk of infections in long-term care facilities. The most common endemic infections in this setting affect the urinary tract, upper and lower respiratory tracts, gastrointestinal tract, conjunctiva, and skin. The CDC estimates that 1.5 million cases of nosocomial infection occur annually in long-term care facilities and nursing homes. That is an average of one infection per year per client (Compliance Control Center, 1998).

Clients in long-term care facilities and hospitals often have multiple comorbidities (illnesses), which increases their risk of infection. For example, urologic abnormalities are associated with increased risk for urinary tract infections. Chronic obstructive lung disease and congestive heart failure increase a client's risk of developing pneumonia. Diabetes or vascular insufficiency may lead to more frequent and severe skin infections (pressure ulcers, cellulitis, and vascular ulcers). Because these high-risk clients are housed together, the transmission of pathogens is increased among residents. For instance, organisms may be transmitted through the air (e.g., tuberculosis, influenza), on the hands of staff members (e.g., *Staphylococcus aureus* or uropathogens), and by contaminated items (e.g., *E. coli*).

NURSING PROCESS

Quality nursing care requires the reduction of microorganism transmission in the health care environment. Infection-control practices are directed at controlling or eliminating sources of infection in the health care agency or home. Nurses are responsible for protecting clients and themselves by using infection-control practices.

PROFESSIONAL TIP

Drug-Resistant Organisms

Nosocomial infections are receiving increased attention because of the development of drug-resistant organisms. The common drug-resistant nosocomial infections that occur in acute and long-term care facilities are vancomycin-resistant enterococci (VRE) (Hospital Infection Control Practices Advisory Committee [HICPAC], 1995), methicillin-resistant *S. aureus* (MRSA) (Hartstein, 1995), and multidrug-resistant (MDR) tuberculosis (TB) (Ikeda et al., 1995).

Assessment

The nursing process facilitates an understanding of the scope of challenges inherent in the nursing care of clients at risk for infection. The assessment data guides the prioritization of the client's problem and the appropriate nursing diagnoses. Clients at risk for infection require frequent reassessment of status followed by appropriate changes in the plan of care, goals, and nursing interventions.

The health history and physical examination data are correlated with the laboratory indicators to identify those clients who are at risk for problems related to infection. Appropriate risk appraisals may be incorporated into the nursing health history interview.

Subjective Data

Key elements of relevant data regarding the client at risk for infection are obtained in the health history. During the nursing health history interview, the client's general health perception and management status are assessed to ascertain the ways and degree to which the client manages self-care. This information provides data regarding the client's routine self-care and health-promotion needs. Questions that relate specifically to habits that foster safe, healthy patterns of behavior are appropriate for home health and ambulatory care settings, as well as for inpatient settings.

A comprehensive nursing assessment also involves appraising the client's environment to detect potential hazards and the client's self-care abilities. The analysis of such factors as work environment, immunization status, and other health-related issues alerts the nurse to actual or possible infection risks.

Objective Data

Objective data are gathered through the physical examination and the diagnostic and laboratory findings.

Physical Examination A complete health assessment includes a systematic physical examination, generally conducted from head to toe, in order to obtain objective data relative to the client's health status and presenting problems. When assessing the client to determine the level of risk for infection, the nurse should focus the physical examination on the following areas and signs:

- Range of motion or total immobilization of an extremity. (A client with limited mobility is at risk for developing joint contractures, skin breakdown, and muscle atrophy.)
- Localized infection as manifested by redness, swelling, warmth, tenderness, pain, and loss of movement in a specific body part.
- Systemic infection as manifested by fever with a corresponding increase in pulse and respirations; weakness; anorexia, with possible accompanying findings of nausea, vomiting, and diarrhea; enlarged and/or tender lymph nodes.

- Secretions or exudate of the skin or mucous membranes; crackles or wheezes in the lungs on auscultation.
- Condition of the skin. (Assessment of skin integrity provides data concerning a client's nutritional and hydration status, continuity of intact skin, hygienic practices, and overall physical abilities.)

Diagnostic and Laboratory Data The laboratory indicators for an infection are:

- An elevated leukocyte (white blood cell [WBC]) and WBC differential:

  Neutrophils: increased in acute, severe inflammation

  Lymphocytes: increased in chronic bacterial and viral infections

  Monocytes: increased in some protozoan and rickettsial infections and TB

  Eosinophils and basophils: unaltered in an infectious process

- An elevated erythrocyte sedimentation rate (ESR): increased in the presence of inflammation
- An elevated pH of involved body fluids (gastric, urine, or vaginal secretions): indicative of microorganism presence
- Positive cultures of involved body fluids (blood, sputum, urine, or other drainage): indicative of microorganism growth (Guyton & Hall, 1995).

Nursing Diagnosis

After data collection and analysis, the nurse is able to formulate a nursing diagnosis. The North American Nursing Diagnosis Association (NANDA) identifies one nursing diagnosis related to infection: *Risk for Infection.*

Risk for infection is the state wherein an individual is at increased risk for being invaded by pathogenic organisms (NANDA, 2001). The risk factors that increase a client's susceptibility to infections are as follows:

- Inadequate primary defenses (broken skin, traumatized tissue, decrease in ciliary action, stasis of body fluids, change in pH of secretions, and altered peristalsis)
- Inadequate secondary defenses (decreased hemoglobin, leukopenia, suppressed inflammatory response)
- Inadequate acquired immunity
- Immunosuppression
- Tissue destruction and increased environmental exposure
- Chronic disease
- Malnutrition
- Invasive procedures
- Pharmaceutical agents
- Trauma
- Rupture of amniotic membranes
- Insufficient knowledge to avoid exposure to pathogens (NANDA, 2001)

Clients who are at risk for infection may have other associated physiologic and psychological concerns. The common nursing diagnoses that often accompany *Risk for Infection*:

- *Imbalanced Nutrition: Less than Body Requirements* or *More than Body Requirements*
- *Ineffective Protection*
- *Impaired Tissue Integrity*
- *Impaired Oral Mucous Membrane*
- *Impaired Skin Integrity*
- *Deficient Knowledge* (specify)

This list indicates a number of related problems that must be considered when planning care for the client at risk for infection.

Planning/Outcome Identification

During the planning phase, the nurse collaborates with the client and other health care providers to determine the goals, outcomes, and interventions to reduce the risk of infection. Identified outcomes provide direction for the nursing care that is implemented to reduce the risk of infection. Another critical element of the care plan is client and caregiver education related to the identification of potential hazards and health-promotion practices.

Implementation

Nurses are responsible for providing the client with a safe environment, which includes preventing the transmission of nosocomial infections. Nursing interventions to reduce the risk of infection center around ensuring asepsis and properly disposing of infectious materials to reduce or eliminate infectious agents. **Asepsis** refers to the absence of microorganisms. Providing nursing care using aseptic technique decreases the risk and spread of nosocomial infections. **Aseptic technique** is the infection-control practice used to prevent the transmission of pathogens. There are two types of asepsis: medical and surgical.

Medical Asepsis

The term **medical asepsis** refers to those practices used to reduce the number, growth, and spread of microorganisms. Medical asepsis is also referred to as *clean technique*. Objects are generally referred to as "clean" or "dirty" in medical asepsis. **Clean objects** are considered to have the presence of some microorganisms that are usually not pathogenic. **Dirty** (soiled) **objects** are considered to have a high number of microorganisms, some being potentially pathogenic. Common medical aseptic measures used for clean or dirty objects are handwashing, daily changing of linens, and daily cleansing of floors and hospital furniture.

Handwashing Handwashing is the rubbing together of all surfaces and crevices of the hands using a soap or chemical and water, followed by rinsing in a flowing stream of water. Handwashing is the most basic and effective infection-control measure to prevent and control the transmission of infectious agents. It is the single most important procedure for preventing nosocomial infections (Association for Professionals in Infection Control and Epidemiology [APIC], 1999).

The three essential elements of handwashing are soap or chemical, water, and friction. Soaps that contain antimicrobial agents are frequently used in high-risk areas such as emergency departments and nurseries. Friction physically removes soil and transient flora, and a flowing stream of water rinses it all away.

Infection Control: Handwashing
- Wash hands before and after every client contact.
- The most common cause of nosocomial infections is contaminated hands of health care providers.
- When in doubt, *wash your hands.*

Handwashing should be performed after arriving at work, before leaving work, before and after each client contact, after removing gloves, when hands are visibly soiled, before eating, after excretion of body waste (urination and defecation), after contact with body fluids, before and after performing invasive procedures, and after handling contaminated equipment. A washing time of 10 to 15 seconds is recommended to remove transient flora from the hands. High-risk areas such as nurseries usually require a handwash of approximately 2 minutes duration. Soiled hands usually require more time (APIC, 1999; CDC, 1991; Department of Labor, 1991).

Surgical Asepsis

Surgical asepsis, or sterile technique, consists of those practices that eliminate all microorganisms and spores from an object or area. Surgical asepsis refers to surgical handwashing, establishing and maintaining sterile fields, donning surgical attire (caps, masks, and eyewear), and sterile gloves, gowning, and closed gloving.

Surgical asepsis is practiced by the nurse in the OR, in labor and delivery, and for many diagnostic and therapeutic interventions at the client's bedside. Common nursing procedures that require sterile technique are as follows:

- All invasive procedures, either intentional perforation of the skin (injections, insertion of intravenous needles or catheters) or entry into a bodily orifice (tracheobronchial suctioning, insertion of a urinary catheter)
- Nursing measures for clients with disruption of skin surfaces (changing a surgical wound or intravenous site dressing) or destruction of skin layers (trauma and burns)

Surgical Handwashing Surgical handwashing or scrub is used to remove soil and microorganisms from the skin. Nurses working in the OR perform surgical handwashing to minimize the client's risk for infection. The skin on the nurse's hands and arms should be intact (free of lesions). Agency policy determines the way to perform the scrub with regard to method and timing.

Sterile Field and Equipment The nurse must establish and maintain a sterile field when performing procedures that require sterile technique, such as inserting a urinary catheter or changing wound dressings. Agency policy and supplies vary in different health care settings; the nurse should review the agency's policy and gather all the necessary supplies before preparing the sterile field.

Donning Surgical Attire Surgical nurses are required to wear a surgical mask (Figure 21-11) and a clean cloth or paper cap that covers all of the hair. Protective eyewear (glasses or goggles) is worn during all procedures that pose a threat of body fluids splashing into the eyes. Masks, caps, eyewear, gowns, and gloves are considered barrier precautions because they

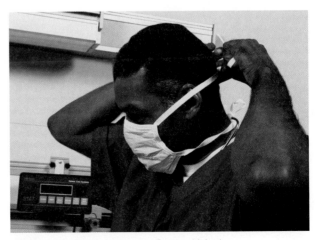

Figure 21-11 Putting on a Surgical Mask

present a physical impediment to the spread of microorganisms.

Donning Sterile Gloves There are two methods of applying sterile gloves: open and closed. The open method is used most frequently when performing procedures that require the sterile technique, such as dressing changes. The closed method is used when the nurse wears a sterile gown.

Gowning and Closed Gloving Nurses in the OR and special procedure areas such as cardiac catheter labs use the closed gloved method when donning a sterile gown. After the surgical scrub, the nurse proceeds to don the sterile gown and gloves using the closed method. The sterile gown serves as a barrier to decrease the risk of wound contamination. The sterile gown also allows the nurse to move freely in the environment with sterile drapes and objects.

Disposal of Infectious Materials All health care facilities must have guidelines for the disposal of infectious-waste materials as required by the OSHA Act of 1991. The types of materials included are:

- Laboratory wastes
- Blood, blood products, and all other body fluids
- Client care items (soiled bed linen and protection pads, urinals, and bedpans)
- Disposable instruments
- Medication and soiled treatment items
- Surgical wastes

All health care workers must be diligent in observing the biological hazard symbol and handling all infectious materials as hazardous.

When disposing of infectious waste, all personnel must be careful to:

- Wear gloves;
- Use the proper containers (red or one labeled with the biological hazard symbol as required by the facility), leakproof plastic bags for waste from client areas (soiled dressings, gloves, linen), and sharps containers for needles, scalpels, and other sharp instruments or devices;

COMMUNITY/HOME HEALTH CARE

Clients at Risk for Infection

Clients at risk for infection should have follow-up visits by the home health nurse to measure the effectiveness of client teaching and to assess resources in the home to prevent the transmission of infections.

- Ensure that all infectious waste is properly labeled;
- Use care when handling plastic bags to avoid punctures and tearing;
- Disinfect carts used to carry infectious waste;
- Dispose of waste in designated areas only; and
- Wash hands after disposing of hazardous materials.

Containers for contaminated sharps should be readily accessible to personnel and maintained in an upright position.

Infection Control: Needle Disposal
- Used needles should not be recapped, bent, or broken.
- Needles should be placed in a puncture-resistant, marked or color-coded container close to the work site.
- Correct disposal decreases the risk of needle punctures to caregivers.

Weltman, Short, and Mendelson (1995) studied disposal-related sharps injuries in a teaching hospital. Of the 361 persons in the study who reported sharps injuries, 72 of the injuries were related to sharps disposal. The majority of exposures to HBV and human immunodeficiency virus (HIV) were due to sharp objects.

Finkelstein and Mendelson (1998) report that results from multicenter studies estimate the transmission rate for HIV as being 0.36% after percutaneous exposure and for hepatitis C virus (HCV) as being 1.8% when injured by hollow-bore needles. Most health care workers acutely infected with HBV will eventually clear the virus, but 5% to 10% percent may develop chronic infection.

Evaluation

Evaluation of the effectiveness of nursing care is based on the achievement of goals and expected outcomes, regardless of the setting. Keeping the client free from infection requires frequent reassessment followed by timely adjustments made in the plan of care in order for nursing interventions to be effective.

It is imperative that the client remain free of infection during hospitalization as well as develop a true awareness of the factors that increase the risk for infection. Adherence to barrier precautions is critical in preventing the spread of infectious agents, especially nosocomial infections to clients, self, and other health care workers. The nurse must correlate the client's diagnostic laboratory results and temperature in evaluating the expected outcome of remaining free of signs and symptoms of infection. If the nurse is caring for a client with an infection, the evaluation should indicate the stage of the inflammatory process.

SAMPLE NURSING CARE PLAN

THE CLIENT AT RISK FOR INFECTION

Mr. Filar, a 38-year-old homeless person, was struck and dragged by a speeding car as he crossed the street. He was taken to the hospital by ambulance. His left leg is broken, and there are lacerations and abrasions on his right side, arm, and leg. The left leg is in a cast and the lacerations have been sutured. Mr. Filar grimaces when he tries to move his legs, but he does not verbalize pain. Mr. Filar is very thin and says that he has not eaten for 2 days.

Nursing Diagnosis 1 *Risk for Infection related to inadequate primary defenses as evidenced by lacerations and abrasions*

PLANNING/GOALS	NURSING INTERVENTIONS	RATIONALE	EVALUATION
Mr. Filar will not have developed an infection in the lacerations and abrasions at discharge.	Thoroughly wash hands using antimicrobial soap before and after caring for Mr. Filar.	Antimicrobial soap is more effective in reducing microorganisms on hands.	Mr. Filar has some redness around one laceration.
	Use sterile technique when caring for lacerations and abrasions.	Prevents introduction of microorganisms into lacerations and abrasions.	
	Apply antibiotic ointment on abrasions, as ordered.	Promotes healing of abrasions.	
	Keep bed linens clean and dry.	Removes any drainage that may harbor microorganisms.	
	Administer oral antibiotics, as ordered.	Prevents or cures infection.	

Nursing Diagnosis 2 *Acute Pain related to physical injury as evidenced by facial grimacing*

PLANNING/GOALS	NURSING INTERVENTIONS	RATIONALE	EVALUATION
Mr. Filar will experience increased comfort and will verbalize that pain is under control within 24 hours.	Use pain scale to determine level of discomfort.	Provides objective measure of pain.	Mr. Filar states that he is experiencing less discomfort by 16 hours but that he still desires pain medication.
	Assist client to a position of comfort and elevate extremities.	Reduces pain and swelling by increasing blood return to the heart.	
	Administer analgesics, as ordered.	Provides comfort.	

continues

Nursing Diagnosis 3 *Imbalanced Nutrition: Less than Body Requirements, related to economic factors as evidenced by extreme thinness and not having eaten for 2 days*

PLANNING/GOALS	NURSING INTERVENTIONS	RATIONALE	EVALUATION
Mr. Filar will eat balanced meals while hospitalized.	Assist Mr. Filar to select foods high in protein, vitamins A and C, calcium, zinc, and copper.	Wound healing depends on the availability of protein, vitamins, and minerals.	Mr. Filar eats everything on his meal trays and the between-meal snacks.
	Provide between-meal snacks, especially milk or milk products.	Snacks will increase overall caloric intake; increased protein will promote wound healing; increased calcium will promote bone healing.	

CASE STUDY

Mrs. Glassel has an open-wound ulcer on her right lower leg.

The following questions will guide your development of a nursing care plan for the case study.

1. What other assessment data should be gathered?
2. What nursing diagnosis is appropriate?
3. Identify two goals for Mrs. Glassel.
4. Identify appropriate nursing interventions.

SUMMARY

- Flora are microorganisms that occur or have adapted to live in a specific environment.
- Pathogens are microorganisms that cause disease; they include bacteria, viruses, fungi, protozoa, and *rickettsia*.
- The elements of the chain of infection include the agent, the reservoir, the portal of exit, the modes of transmission, the portal of entry, and the host.
- The body has two primary defense mechanisms: the nonspecific immune defense, which protects the host from all microorganisms regardless of previous exposure, and the specific immune defense, which is a reaction to a specific antigen that the body has previously experienced.

- Infections progress through four stages: incubation, prodromal, illness, and convalescence.
- Handwashing must be done before and after every client contact and after removing gloves. It is the most important procedure for preventing nosocomial infections.
- Other means of preventing the spread of infection include cleansing equipment, cleansing soiled linen, changing dressings over wounds, practicing barrier precautions, maintaining skin integrity, and receiving all appropriate immunizations.
- The OSHA regulations mandate that sharps be properly disposed of immediately after use.

Review Questions

1. With regard to the chain of infection, the main focus of attention in infection control in a health care facility is the:

    a. portal of exit.
    b. infectious agent.
    c. susceptible host.
    d. mode of transmission.

2. The microorganisms that are always present on a person are called:

    a. resident flora.
    b. colonized flora.
    c. transient flora.
    d. communicable flora.

3. The most important procedure for preventing nosocomial infection is:

    a. sterilizing.
    b. handwashing.
    c. disinfecting.
    d. the use of bactericides.

4. A client with the flu is vulnerable to infection and is called a:

    a. susceptible host.
    b. infectious agent.
    c. compromised host.
    d. anthropogenic agent.

5. Living organisms that invade a host are called:

    a. animated agents.
    b. physical agents.
    c. chemical agents.
    d. biological agents.

6. Fomites are an example of which type of transmission?

    a. contact
    b. vehicle
    c. airborne
    d. vectorborne

7. Lyme disease and malaria are examples of diseases spread by:

    a. contact transmission.
    b. vehicle transmission.
    c. airborne transmission.
    d. vectorborne transmission.

8. The redness noted during the inflammation process is the result of:

    a. fluid entering the tissues.
    b. increased pressure in the area.
    c. increased blood flow to the area.
    d. increased metabolism in the area.

9. Vaccination provides which type of immunity?

    a. humoral
    b. acquired
    c. antibody
    d. lymphokine

10. A client is infectious to other persons during the:

    a. illness stage.
    b. prodromal stage.
    c. incubation period.
    d. convalescent stage.

Critical Thinking Questions

1. How are medical asepsis and surgical asepsis the same? How are they different?

2. How is the chain of infection applicable in everyday life in a person's home?

3. Why are nosocomial infections such a huge problem?

 WEB FLASH!

- What resources can be found on the Internet about infection control and asepsis?
- Visit the web sites of the resources listed for this chapter. What type of information do they provide?

STANDARD PRECAUTIONS AND ISOLATION

MAKING THE CONNECTION

Refer to the following chapter to increase your understanding of Standard Precautions and isolation:

- **Chapter 21, Infection Control/Asepsis**

- **Procedures:** B1, Handwashing; I2, Performing Open Gloving and Removal of Soiled Gloves; A1, Initiating Strict Isolation Precautions

LEARNING OBJECTIVES

Upon completion of this chapter, you should be able to:
- *Define key terms.*
- *Describe each of the eleven aspects of Standard Precautions.*
- *Identify the three transmission-based precautions and when each is to be used.*
- *Apply Standard Precautions in providing appropriate client care.*

INTRODUCTION

For over 120 years, health care facilities and their personnel have struggled to prevent the spread of infections among their clients. This chapter describes some of the historical methods as well as the current methods used to prevent the spread of infections.

HISTORICAL PERSPECTIVE

A hospital handbook published in 1877 recommended placing clients with infectious diseases in a separate facility (Lynch, 1949). These facilities became known as infectious-disease hospitals. Yet, **nosocomial infections** (infections acquired in the hospital that were not present or incubating at the time of the client's admission) continued in these facilities because the infected clients were not separated according to disease, and **aseptic technique** (infection-control practices used to prevent the transmission of pathogens) was seldom, if ever, practiced. To combat the

KEY TERMS

Airborne Precautions
aseptic technique
barrier precautions
Contact Precautions
Droplet Precautions
endemic
epidemic
isolation
nosocomial infection
reverse isolation
Standard Precautions
Transmission-Based Precautions

continuing problem of nosocomial infections in the infectious-disease hospitals, personnel began to set aside a floor or ward for clients with similar diseases (Gage, Landon, & Sider, 1959).

Nursing has always been at the forefront of preventing the spread of infections among clients and personnel. Infectious-disease hospital personnel began practicing aseptic technique as recommended in nursing textbooks published from 1890 to 1900 (Lynch, 1949). Isolation practices and the use of infectious disease hospitals were altered in 1910 when the cubicle system of isolation was introduced in U.S. hospitals (Gage et al., 1959). The cubicle system of **isolation** (separation from other persons, especially those with infectious diseases) placed clients in multiple-bed wards, with hospital personnel using a separate gown when caring for each client, washing their hands in an antiseptic solution after contact with each client, and disinfecting objects contaminated by any client. These nursing procedures were known as *barrier nursing*. Barrier nursing was aimed at preventing transmission of pathogenic organisms to other clients and to health care personnel. The cubicle system of isolation, including the barrier nursing procedures, gave the clients the alternative of receiving care in general hospitals instead of the infectious-disease hospitals (Centers for Disease Control and Prevention [CDC]/Hospital Infection Control Practices Advisory Committee [HICPAC], 1997a).

During the 1950s, infectious-disease hospitals closed, with the exception of the tuberculosis (TB) hospitals, which closed in the 1960s. Thus, by the end of the 1960s, clients with infectious diseases were cared for in general hospitals.

In 1970, the Centers for Disease Control and Prevention (CDC) published *Isolation Technique for Use in Hospitals* (National Communicable Disease Center, 1970), a revised edition of which was released in 1975 (CDC, 1975). This manual introduced and recommended seven categories of isolation: Strict Isolation, Respiratory Isolation, Protective Isolation, Enteric Precautions, Wound and Skin Precautions, Discharge Precautions, and Blood Precautions. By the mid 1970s, 93% of U.S. hospitals had adopted the recommendations of this book (Haley & Schactman, 1980).

By 1980, **endemic** (occuring continuously in a particular population and having low mortality) and **epidemic** (infecting many people at the same time, in the same geographic area) nosocomial infections were surfacing. Some of these infections were caused by multidrug-resistant (MDR) microorganisms, others by newly identified pathogens. Both types required isolation precautions different from those specified in any of the seven isolation categories. As Schaffner (1980) describes, isolation precautions needed to be directed more specifically at nosocomial transmission in special-care units rather than at community-acquired infectious diseases being spread within the hospital.

In 1983, the CDC replaced the 1975 isolation manual with the *Guideline for Isolation Precautions in Hospitals* (Garner & Simmons, 1983). One of the most important changes was the emphasis on decision making by the users as to which guideline was appropriate in a particular situation (Garner, 1984; Haley, Garner, & Simmons, 1985).

Another change was to rename Blood Precautions, primarily used for clients who were chronic carriers of hepatitis B virus (HBV), to Blood and Body Fluid Precautions, which now were to apply to clients with acquired immunodeficiency syndrome (AIDS); body fluids other than blood, such as semen and vaginal secretions; amniotic, cerebrospinal, pericardial, peritoneal, pleural, and synovial fluids; and any other body fluid visibly contaminated with blood. It did not apply to feces, nasal secretions, sputum, sweat, tears, urine, or vomitus unless blood was visible in them.

Until 1985, clients placed in isolation either had a confirmed diagnosis or were suspected of having an infectious disease. Mainly because of the human immunodeficiency virus (HIV) epidemic and those other bloodborne infections often yet unrecognized in a client, it was decided that Blood and Body Fluid Precautions were to be applied universally to all clients, regardless of their presumed infection status (CDC, 1985). Thus, the new name became Universal Precautions.

A new system of isolation called Body Substance Isolation (BSI) was proposed in 1987 as an alternative to the diagnosis-driven isolation system of the 1983 *Guideline for Isolation Precautions in Hospitals*. Body Substance Isolation focused on isolating all moist and potentially infectious body substances (blood, feces, urine, sputum, saliva, wound drainage, and other body fluids) from *all* clients. The use of gloves was the primary method of isolating infectious agents. However, BSI did not contain adequate provisions to prevent droplet transmission, direct or indirect contact transmission, or true airborne transmission of infections. Also, BSI recommended handwashing after removal of gloves only if the hands were soiled (Lynch, Jackson, Cummings, & Stamm, 1987), whereas Universal Precautions recommended handwashing after every removal of gloves (CDC, 1987; CDC, 1988).

In 1991, the Hospital Infection Control Practices Advisory Committee (HICPAC) was established to provide advice and guidance to the Secretary and Assistant Secretary of the U.S. Department of Health and Human Services (USDHHS), the Director of the CDC, and the Director of the National Center for Infectious Diseases (CDC/HICPAC, 1997a). The committee also provides advice to the CDC about updating guidelines and other policy statements related to the prevention of nosocomial infections.

The CDC, with the assistance of HICPAC, revised the *Guideline for Isolation Precautions in Hospitals* in 1996. The new guideline combined the major features of Universal Precautions and Body Substance Isolation into a single set of Standard Precautions, and the specific isolation categories into three Transmission-Based Precautions (CDC/HICPAC, 1997b) (Figure 22-1).

The CDC recommendations are not subject to legal enforcement. However, regulations of the Occupational Safety and Health Administration (OSHA) must be followed by all health care facilities. These regulations, laws enforced through the Department of Labor (OSHA, 1991), ensure that Standard Precautions and Transmission-Based Precautions are followed. According to OSHA regulations, all health care facilities must:

- Determine which employees have occupational exposure.

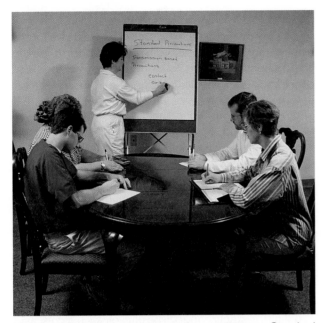

Figure 22-1 Hospital personnel are reviewing Standard Precautions and Transmission-Based precautions.

- Provide hepatitis B vaccine free of charge to all employees with occupational exposure.
- Provide personal protective equipment (e.g., gowns, gloves, masks, goggles) for all employees with occupational exposure.
- Provide adequate handwashing facilities and supplies.
- Provide training regarding these rules to all employees with occupational exposure, both at hire and, then, annually.
- Provide evaluation and follow-up for any employee who experiences an exposure incident.
- Provide appropriate, properly labeled containers for contaminated sharps.
- Provide and prominently display an exposure control plan for staff to follow.

STANDARD PRECAUTIONS

Standard Precautions, listed on the inside back cover of this book, are preventive practices to be used in the care of all clients in hospitals regardless of diagnosis or presumed infection status. These guidelines

PROFESSIONAL TIP

Exposure Incident
- Immediately report all exposure incidents to the proper person in the health care facility.
- The OSHA regulations require initial screening and follow-up care.

CLIENT TEACHING

Standard Precautions
- Assist the client to understand that the techniques and procedures associated with Standard Precautions are designed to prevent the transmission of microorganisms and not to isolate the client.
- Explain why each technique and procedure is used.

are designed to reduce the risk of microorganism transmission from both recognized and unrecognized sources of infection in hospitals (CDC/HICPAC, 1997b).

Standard Precautions apply to:

- Blood
- All body fluids, secretions, and excretions *except* sweat, regardless of whether those fluids contain visible blood
- Nonintact skin
- Mucous membranes

Infection Control: Standard Precautions
- Standard Precautions must be practiced with all clients.
- Standard Precautions represent the most effective means of decreasing the risk of infection among clients and caregivers.

Barrier precautions, used to minimize the risk of exposure to blood and body fluids, involve the use of personal protective equipment, such as masks, gowns, and gloves, to create a barrier between the person and the microorganism and thus prevent transmission of the microorganism. Handwashing, however, is the most basic aspect of Standard Precautions. The other aspects of Standard Precautions are gloves; mask, eye protection, face shield; gown; client-care equipment; environmental control; linen; occupational health and blood-borne pathogens; and client placement.

Handwashing

Hands are to be washed after touching blood, body fluids, secretions, excretions, and contaminated items, regardless of whether gloves were worn. Hands must be washed, immediately after gloves are removed, between client contacts, and any other time when transfer of microorganisms to other clients or environments is possible. To prevent cross-contamination of different body sites on one client, it may be necessary to wash hands between tasks and procedures on that client.

Plain, nonantimicrobial soap is adequate for routine handwashing. An antimicrobial agent or waterless antiseptic agent is needed only for specific circumstances as defined by the facility's infection-control program.

Gloves

Clean, nonsterile gloves are to be worn when touching blood, body fluids, secretions, excretions, and contaminated items. Clean gloves should be put on just before touching mucous membranes and non-intact skin. Gloves must be changed between tasks and procedures being performed on one client if material that may contain microorganisms in high concentrations is touched. Gloves must be removed promptly after use and hands must be washed immediately before touching uncontaminated items or providing care to another client.

Safety: Latex Allergies

- Standard Precautions include the use of gloves when there is a possibility of contact with client body fluids.
- Be alert that health care personnel or the client may be allergic to the latex gloves. Reactions range from an eczematous contact dermatitis to anaphylactic shock.
- Prior to touching clients when wearing latex gloves, ask whether they have a known allergy to latex products. If they do, use non-latex gloves for those clients.

Mask, Eye Protection, Face Shield

A mask and eye protection or a face shield should be worn to protect the mucous membranes of the eyes, nose, and mouth when procedures and client–care activities are likely to generate splashes or sprays of blood, body fluids, secretions, or excretions.

Gown

A clean, nonsterile gown should be worn to protect the skin and prevent soiling of clothing during procedures and client-care activities that are likely to generate splashes or sprays of blood, body fluids, secretions, or excretions. A gown that is appropriate for the activity and potential amount of fluids should be selected. A soiled gown should be removed as promptly as possible, and the hands should be washed to prevent transfer of microorganisms to other clients or environments.

Client-Care Equipment

Client-care equipment soiled with blood, body fluids, secretions, or excretions must be handled in a manner to prevent skin and mucous membrane exposure, clothing contamination, and microorganism transfer to other clients or environments. Reusable equipment must not be used in the care of another client until it has been cleaned and sterilized appropriately. All single-use items must be properly discarded.

Environmental Control

The hospital must have adequate procedures for the routine care, cleaning, and disinfection of environmental surfaces, beds, bed rails, bedside equipment, and other frequently touched surfaces. All personnel must ensure that these procedures are followed.

Linen

Linen that is soiled with blood, body fluids, secretions, or excretions must be handled, transported, and processed in a manner to prevent skin and mucous membrane exposure, clothing contamination, and microorganism transfer to other clients and environments.

Occupational Health and Blood-Borne Pathogens

Care must be taken to prevent injury when using needles, scalpels, and other sharp instruments and when handling, cleaning, and disposing of such items after use. The OSHA regulations state that "contaminated (used) sharps shall be discarded immediately or as soon as feasible in containers that are closable, puncture-resistant, leakproof on the sides and bottom and are labeled or color coded" (OSHA, 1991) (Figure 22-2).

Used needles should never be recapped by using both hands. A one-handed "scoop" method is acceptable. Used needles should never be removed from disposable syringes by hand, nor should they be bent,

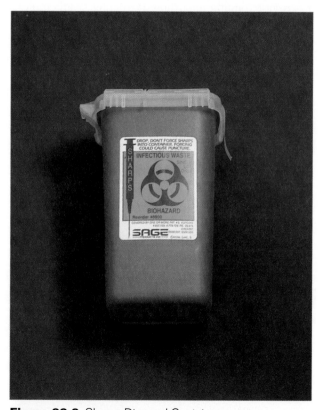

Figure 22-2 Sharps-Disposal Container

broken, or otherwise manipulated by hand. Disposable syringes and needles, scalpel blades, and other sharp items should be placed in designated puncture-resistant containers. Reusable syringes and needles should be placed in a separate puncture-resistant container and transported to the appropriate area for cleaning and sterilizing.

In areas where the need for resuscitation is predictable, mouth pieces, resuscitation bags, or other ventilation devices should be used instead of the direct mouth-to-mouth resuscitation method.

Client Placement

Any client who contaminates the environment or who does not or cannot be expected to assist with maintaining appropriate hygiene or environment control should be placed in a private room. When a private room in unavailable, infection-control professionals must be consulted.

ISOLATION

The 1996 CDC guideline eliminated the previous category-specific isolation precautions and condensed the former disease-specific precautions into three sets of precautions based on the route of transmission: airborne (Figure 22-3), contact (Figure 22-4), or droplet (Figure 22-5). These new, Transmission-Based Precautions are to be used *in addition to* the Standard Precautions. **Transmission-Based Precautions** are practices designed for clients documented as or suspected of being infected with highly transmissible or epidemiologically important pathogens for which additional precautions beyond the Standard Precautions are re-

quired to interrupt transmission in hospitals (CDC/HICPAC, 1997b) (see Table 22–1).

The Transmission-Based Precautions are also to be used in addition to the Standard Precautions in the

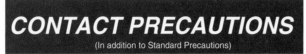

CONTACT PRECAUTIONS
(In addition to Standard Precautions)

VISITORS: Report to nurse before entering

Patient Placement
Private room, if possible. Cohort if private room is not available.

Gloves
Wear gloves when entering patient room.
Change gloves after having contact with infective material that may contain high concentrations of microorganisms (**fecal material** and **wound drainage**).
Remove gloves before leaving patient room.

Wash
Wash hands with an **antimicrobial** agent immediately after glove removal. After glove removal and handwashing, ensure that hands do not touch potentially contaminated environmental surfaces or items in the patient's room to avoid transfer of microorganisms to other patients or environments.

Gown
Wear gown when **entering** patient room if you anticipate that your clothing will have substantial contact with the patient, environmental surfaces, or items in the patient's room, or if the patient is **incontinent**, or has **diarrhea**, an **ileostomy**, a **colostomy**, or **wound drainage** not contained by a dressing. **Remove** gown before leaving the patient's environment and ensure that clothing does not contact potentially contaminated environmental surfaces to avoid transfer of microorganisms to other patients or environments.

Patient Transport
Limit transport of patient to essential purposes only. During transport, ensure that precautions are maintained to minimize the risk of transmission of microorganisms to other patients and contamination of environmental surfaces and equipment.

Patient-Care Equipment
Dedicate the use of noncritical patient-care equipment to a single patient. If common equipment is used, clean and disinfect between patients.

Figure 22-4 Transmission-Based Precautions: Contact Precautions *(From Brevis Corporation, 3310 S. 2700, Salt Lake City, UT 84109. Copyright 1996 by Brevis Corporation. Reprinted with permission.)*

AIRBORNE PRECAUTIONS
(In addition to Standard Precautions)

VISITORS: Report to nurse before entering

Patient Placement
Private room that has:
   Monitored negative air pressure,
   6 to12 air changes per hour,
   Discharge of air outdoors or HEPA filtration if recirculated.
Keep room door closed and patient in room.

Respiratory Protection
Wear an **N95 respirator** when entering the room of a patient with known or suspected infectious pulmonary **tuberculosis**.
Susceptible persons should not enter the room of patients known or suspected to have **measles** (rubeola) or **varicella** (chickenpox) if other immune caregivers are available. If susceptible persons must enter, they should wear an **N95 respirator**.(Respirator or surgical mask not required if immune to measles and varicella.)

Patient Transport
Limit transport of patient from room to essential purposes only.
Use **surgical mask** on patient during transport.

Figure 22-3 Transmission-Based Precautions: Airborne Precautions *(From Brevis Corporation, 3310 S. 2700, Salt Lake City, UT 84109. Copyright 1996 by Brevis Corporation. Reprinted with permission.)*

DROPLET PRECAUTIONS
(In addition to Standard Precautions)

VISITORS: Report to nurse before entering

Patient Placement
Private room, if possible. Cohort or maintain spatial separation of **3 feet** from other patients or visitors if private room is not available.

Mask
Wear mask when working within **3 feet** of patient (or upon entering room).

Patient Transport
Limit transport of patient to essential purposes only.
Use **surgical mask** on patient during transport.

Figure 22-5 Transmission-Based Precautions: Droplet Precautions *(From Brevis Corporation, 3310 S. 2700, Salt Lake City, UT 84109. Copyright 1996 by Brevis Corporation. Reprinted with permission.)*

Table 22–1 PRECAUTIONS RELATED TO TYPE OF DISEASE

PRECAUTION	TYPE OF DISEASE
Standard Precautions	All clients, regardless of disease or condition
Airborne Precautions	In addition to Standard Precautions, used for clients known to have or suspected of having serious illnesses spread by airborne droplet nuclei, including: • Measles • Varicella • Tuberculosis

Contact Precautions	In addition to Standard Precautions, used for clients known to have or suspected of having serious illnesses easily spread by direct client contact or contact with fomites, including:
	• Wound infections
	• Gastrointestinal infections
	• Respiratory infections
	• Skin infections including:
	    Herpes simplex
	    Impetigo
	    Major abscesses, cellulitis, or pressure ulcers
	    Pediculosis
	    Scabies
	    Varicella (Zoster)
	• Viral hemorrhagic infections (Ebola)

Droplet Precautions	In addition to Standard Precautions, used for clients known to have or suspected of having illnesses spread by large particle droplets, including: • Meningitis • Adenovirus • Pneumonia • Influenza • Diphtheria • Mumps • Pertussis • Rubella • Scarlet fever • Parvovirus 19

From Table I Synopsis of Types of Precautions and Patients Requiring Precautions *[On-line], by Centers for Disease Control and Prevention (CDC)/Hospital Infection Control Practices Advisory Committee (HICPAC), 1997, Available: http://www.cdc.gov/ ncidod/hip/isolat/isotab_1.htm*

event of suspicious infections and with clients who are immunosuppressed either from disease or chemotherapy. More than one of the transmission-based precautions is used at the same time for clients with certain infections or conditions.

Isolation precautions are usually ordered by the physician; however, nurses may initiate these precautions whenever a nursing diagnosis related to the infectious process is identified, for example, *Risk for Infection related to decreased resistance of immune system*. Most agencies require nurses to obtain a culture from a draining body area and to initiate isolation precautions when positive cultures are reported. After isolation precautions have been instituted, visitors and all personnel should comply with the agency's policy regarding isolation precautions. Signs should be posted in a prominent location outside the client's room. The signs should indicate the type of isolation precautions and preparation required prior to entering the room (Figure 22-6). The necessary supplies should be readily available.

Clients requiring isolation should be placed in a private room with adequate ventilation and should have their own supplies. Personal belongings should be kept to a minimum, and health care providers

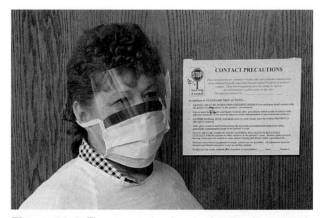

Figure 22-6 The sign on the door to the client's room indicates the type of isolation precaution and preparation needed prior to entering room.

COMMUNITY/HOME HEALTH CARE

Isolation

- Provide the client and family with appropriate written isolation instructions relative to the specific precautions.
- Provide necessary supplies or suggest a list of those things to buy and places to purchase the supplies.

should use disposable supplies and equipment whenever possible. All articles leaving the room, such as soiled linen and collected specimens, should be labeled and either placed in impermeable bags or double bagged.

Reverse isolation, also known as protective isolation, is a barrier protection designed to prevent infection in clients who are severely compromised and highly susceptible to infection. This includes clients who:

- are taking immunosuppressive medications
- are receiving chemotherapy or radiation therapy
- have diseases such as leukemia, which depress resistance to infectious organisms
- have extensive burns, dermatitis, or other skin impairments that prevent adequate coverage with dressings

These clients are at increased risk for infection from their own microorganisms, contact with health care workers whose hands have not been properly washed, and exposure to improperly disinfected and nonsterile items such as air, food, water, and equipment. Nursing responsibilities toward these clients include ensuring that everyone entering the client's room has completed a meticulous handwashing and is properly attired in

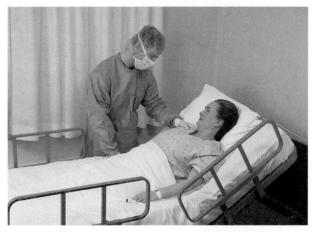

Figure 22-7 Nurse Interacting with Client Requiring Isolation Precautions

gown, gloves, and mask; ensuring that the client's environment is as clear of pathogens as possible; and knowing the institutional policy regarding caring for clients requiring reverse isolation.

CLIENT RESPONSES TO ISOLATION

Isolation precautions are for the client's protection; however, clients who are placed on isolation precautions may experience psychological discomfort (Figure 22-7). Nurses should be alert to symptoms of anxiety, depression, rejection, guilt, or loneliness. Clients should be educated on those isolation precautions that will be practiced and their purposes. Nurses should encourage clients to verbalize their feelings regarding the isolation precautions and should provide the client with intellectual stimulation and diversional activities such as paperback books, crossword puzzles, music, radio, or television. Visitors should be encouraged as a method to alleviate the client's feelings of isolation and loneliness. Wearing appropriate barrier precautions, visitors can safely enter an isolated client's room.

SUMMARY

- Standard Precautions are to be used when caring for *every* client.
- Airborne Precautions are to be used when caring for clients who have or may have serious illnesses spread by airborne droplet nuclei.
- Droplet Precautions are to be used when caring for clients who have or may have serious illnesses spread by large-particle droplets.
- Contact Precautions are to be used when caring for clients who have or may have serious illnesses spread by direct client contact or fomite contact.

PROFESSIONAL TIP

Psychological Interventions for Clients in Isolation

- Explain the pertinent isolation procedures and rationales.
- Discuss the client's feelings about the isolation procedures.
- Convey a sense of empathy and understanding.
- Permit visitors in accordance with isolation precautions.
- Support existing coping mechanisms.
- Visit the client.

CASE STUDY

Joe Spanutius is admitted with a diagnosis of influenza. After 24 hours, the nurses question whether he may also have pediculosis. The physician is out of town for the day.

The following questions will guide your development of a nursing care plan for this case study.

1. On admission, what precautions should be followed for Mr. Spanutius?
2. What additional precautions, if any, should the nurses follow until the physician sees Mr. Spanutius again?
3. What equipment is required and should be available for persons entering Mr. Spanutius' room right after admission?
4. What equipment is required and should be available for persons entering Mr. Spanutius' room after 24 hours?

Review Questions

1. In 1996, the revised *Guideline for Isolation Precautions in Hospitals* combined Universal Precautions and Body Substance Isolation into:
   a. Barrier Precautions.
   b. Contact Precautions.
   c. Standard Precautions.
   d. Transmission-Based Precautions.

2. The use of masks, gowns, and gloves is termed:
   a. Droplet Precautions.
   b. Barrier Precautions.
   c. Contact Precautions.
   d. Standard Precautions.

3. The nursing action most basic to Standard Precautions is:
   a. gloving.
   b. gowning.
   c. handwashing.
   d. wearing a face mask.

4. Airborne Precautions require:
   a. paper masks.
   b. a private room.
   c. the wearing of gloves.
   d. the wearing of a gown.

5. Contact Precautions require:
   a. a private room.
   b. the wearing of a mask.
   c. the wearing of a gown.
   d. the wearing of gloves.

6. Those precautions to be used in the care of all clients in hospitals regardless of diagnosis or presumed infection status are called:
   a. Standard Precautions.
   b. Airborne Precautions.
   c. Universal Precautions.
   d. Body Substance Isolation.

Critical Thinking Questions

1. How are the three Transmission-Based Precautions the same? How are they different?

2. When, where, and why are Standard Precautions to be implemented?

⚡ WEB FLASH!

- What type of information is available on the web about Standard Precautions?
- What web site might you recommend to a client or family for information about Transmission-Based Precautions?

Chapter 23
Fluid, Electrolyte, and
Acid-Base Balance

Chapter 24
Medication Administration

FLUID, ELECTROLYTE, AND ACID–BASE BALANCE

MAKING THE CONNECTION

Refer to the following chapter to increase your understanding of fluid, electrolyte, and acid–base balance:

- **Chapter 25, Assessment**

LEARNING OBJECTIVES

Upon completion of this chapter, you should be able to:
- *Define key terms.*
- *Discuss the importance of pH regulation in the body.*
- *Describe the three buffer systems of the body.*
- *Describe and give examples in the body of diffusion, osmosis, and filtration.*
- *Name the fluid compartments, the fluids contained in them, and the function of those fluids.*
- *Describe the way the kidneys work to maintain fluid and electrolyte balance.*
- *Describe the way the lungs work to maintain pH in the body.*
- *Detail causes, assessment data, nursing interventions, and criteria for evaluating effectiveness of care for clients with a nursing diagnosis of* Deficient Fluid Volume *or* Excess Fluid Volume.
- *Detail causes, assessment data, nursing diagnoses, nursing interventions, and criteria for evaluating the effectiveness of nursing care for clients with sodium, potassium, calcium, and magnesium imbalances.*
- *Relate principles of nursing management for clients receiving fluids and electrolytes via oral supplements, intravenous solutions, enteral feedings, and total parenteral nutrition.*
- *Differentiate the causes, assessment data, and nursing management of metabolic and respiratory acidosis and alkalosis.*
- *Use the nursing process to plan care for a client experiencing a fluid, electrolyte, and/or acid–base imbalance.*

KEY TERMS

acid	hypotonic solution
acidosis	hypoxemia
alkalosis	infiltration
anion	interstitial fluid
arterial blood gases	intracellular fluid
atom	intravascular fluid
base	intravenous therapy
buffer	ion
cation	isotonic solution
compound	isotope
crenation	matter
decomposition	mixture
dehydration	molecule
dialysis	osmolality
diffusion	osmolarity
edema	osmosis
electrolyte	osmotic pressure
element	oxidized
extracellular fluid	permeability
filtration	salt
hemolysis	semipermeable
homeostasis	membrane
hydrostatic pressure	synthesis
hypertonic solution	turgor

INTRODUCTION

The external environment within which we live undergoes continual changes, both small and large. For example, the daily and seasonal temperatures may fluctuate over a wide range. The light intensity may be bright on sunny days and less so on cloudy days. The humidity may be either high or low. These are just a few of the many factors that may change constantly in the external environment. Our bodies must continually adjust to such changes in the external environment. In order for life to continue, however, our internal environment—the one inside our bodies—must remain relatively constant, varying only slightly within narrow ranges. This internal environment consists of the various body fluids such as the fluid inside cells, the blood, tissue fluids that bathe the cells, and other fluids. Constant maintanence of the internal environment within very narrow limits—in equilibrium—is termed **homeostasis**.

HOMEOSTASIS

Homeostasis is an ongoing process; that is, the body simply does not reach a state of equilibrium and remain there. Small changes constantly occur in response to the physiologic processes. As a result, changes occur in the internal environment. The body must therefore continuously make subtle adjustments to maintain the constancy of the internal environment within a range of normal values.

Homeostasis is accomplished by various physiologic processes and the coordinated activities of the organ systems. Some examples are as follows:

- The gastrointestinal (GI) system changes large, complex molecules of ingested food to simpler, less-complex molecules that can be utilized by the cells of the body to produce the energy necessary for life.
- The respiratory system supplies the cells with the constant source of oxygen required to release the energy from the products of digestion.
- The respiratory system also eliminates carbon dioxide, the waste product produced by the cells as a result of energy production.
- The blood acts as a transport mechanism, carrying the products of digestion along with hormones and oxygen to the cells, where these substances are utilized.
- The blood also transports carbon dioxide from the energy-releasing processes of the cells to the lungs, where it will be eliminated.
- All of the activities of the various organ systems are integrated and coordinated through the nervous system and the endocrine system.

When the body loses the ability to maintain homeostasis, and the internal environment changes, the physiologic processes can be interrupted or changed, leading to disease, disorder, or death. In essence, then, maintaining homeostasis is essential to life. Because the processes of homeostasis involve many chemical and physical processes, it is necessary to examine some of these before studying homeostasis in more detail.

CHEMICAL ORGANIZATION

The human body is highly organized. This organization exists in increasing levels of complexity. Most basic is the chemical level. To understand the higher levels of organization, it is necessary to know something about basic chemical and physical principles.

Elements

The cell consists of living matter. **Matter** is anything that occupies space and possesses mass. All matter has certain physical properties such as color, odor, hardness, and density. Matter also has extensive properties such as size, shape, and weight. Matter is composed of basic substances called **elements**. Elements are made of tiny units called atoms. Atoms of each element are alike. Different elements have different kinds of atoms. Presently, 108 elements are recognized. Some examples are iron, gold, carbon, hydrogen, oxygen, nitrogen, and copper. Many of the elements occur in the human body in varying amounts. Some are present in large amounts, and others are found in only trace amounts. The four elements oxygen, carbon, hydrogen, and nitrogen constitute more than 95% of the total body weight of the elements. Some of the elements and their function in the body are presented in Table 23–1.

Atoms

An **atom** is the smallest unit of chemical structure, and no chemical change can alter it. Atoms are made up of three basic particles: protons, neutrons, and electrons. Protons and neutrons are similar in size, but whereas protons have a positive electrical charge, neutrons have no charge. Together, they form the nucleus of the atom. Because the protons have a positive charge and the neutrons are neutral, the nucleus of an atom has a positive charge. The electrons have a negative charge and move in an orbit around the nucleus. There are as many electrons as protons, rendering the overall atom neutral. The number of protons in an atom is called its atomic number. The simplest element is hydrogen. It has an atomic number of 1. One proton with a positive charge forms the nucleus, and one electron moves in an orbit around the nucleus. Hydrogen atoms may or may not have a neutron. A hydrogen atom is illustrated in Figure 23-1.

Depending on the element, other atoms may have more than one proton and one electron shell and may

Table 23–1 ELEMENTS OCCURRING IN THE HUMAN BODY

ELEMENT	APPROXIMATE % OF BODY WEIGHT	FUNCTION
Major Elements		
Oxygen (O)	65.0	Found in both organic and inorganic compounds; as a gas, is necessary in metabolizing glucose and other chemical compounds into energy
Carbon (C)	18.5	Found in all organic compounds such as carbohydrates, protein, lipids, and nucleic acids; necessary for cellular respiration
Hydrogen (H)	9.5	Found in many organic and inorganic compounds; in ionic form, involved in pH; component of water; necessary for life
Nitrogen (N)	3.2	Important in proteins, which are the body's building blocks, an energy source, and a component of hormones
Calcium (Ca)	1.5	Important element in bone and tooth composition; involved in nerve conduction, muscle contraction, and blood clotting
Phosphorus (P)	1.0	Found in bones, teeth, the high-energy carrying compound adenosine triphosphatase (ATP), some proteins, and nucleic acid
Potassium (K)	0.4	Major electrolyte in intracellular fluid; important in muscle contraction and transmission of nerve impulses; activates enzymes; influences cellular osmotic pressure; involved in kidney function and acid–base balance
Sulfur (S)	0.3	Found in some proteins, nucleic acids, and some vitamins and hormones
Sodium (Na)	0.2	Constitutes major electrolyte in extracellular fluid; important in osmoregulation and acid–base balance; necessary for nerve transmission and muscle contraction
Chlorine (Cl)	0.2	Found in extracellular fluid; important in water balance, acid–base balance, and production of hydrochloric acid in the stomach
Magnesium (Mg)	0.1	Important to muscle and nerve function and bone formation and in some coenzymes
Essential Trace Elements		
Present in the human body in minimal amounts, constituting approximately 0.1% of body weight; have known functions		
Cobalt (Co)		Important component of vitamin B_{12}
Copper (Cu)		Necessary for formation of hemoglobin and for bone development
Chromium (Cr)		A cofactor involved with enzymes for fat, cholesterol, and glucose metabolism
Flourine (F)		Gives hardness to teeth and bones
Iodine (I)		Necessary for synthesis of thyroid hormone
Iron (Fe)		Necessary for transportation of oxygen by hemoglobin
Manganese (Mn)		Necessary in activating some enzymes
Selenium (Se)		Acts with vitamin E as an antioxidant; component of teeth
Zinc (Zn)		Found in some enzymes; needed for protein metabolism and carbon dioxide transport
Other Trace Elements		
Have probable, but as yet undetected, functions		

Aluminum (Al)   Nickel (Ni)   Arsenic (As)   Tin (Sn)   Boron (B)   Silicon (Si)   Cadmium (Cd)   Vanadium (V)

have neutrons. The number of protons and neutrons in the nucleus is approximately equal to the atomic weight. Thus, hydrogen has an atomic weight of 1.

Isotopes

The number of protons in the nucleus is the same for all atoms of a given element, but the number of neutrons may vary in atoms of the same element. For instance, all hydrogen atoms have one proton and one electron. However, whereas some hydrogen atoms have one neutron in the nucleus, others have two (Figure 23-2). Atoms of the same element that have differ-

ent atomic weights (i.e., have a different number of neutrons) are called **isotopes**. All of the isotopes of a given element react chemically in the same way.

Some isotopes, called radioactive isotopes, have an unstable nucleus, which decomposes and gives off energy in the form of radiation. This radiation can be in the form of alpha, beta, or gamma rays. All are damaging to cells. Alpha radiation is the least harmful, and gamma radiation is the most harmful. Iodine, oxygen, and cobalt are examples of elements having radioactive isotopes. Some of the radioactive isotopes are useful as biological markers and can be used to track

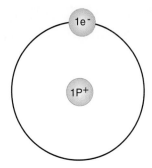

Figure 23-1 Hydrogen Atom Showing Positively Charged Proton in the Nucleus and Negatively Charged Electron in Orbit

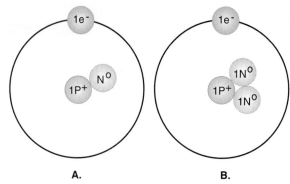

A.   **B.**

Figure 23-2 Isotopes of Hydrogen: A. Deuteridium has one positively charged proton and one neutron in the nucleus and one electron in orbit; B. Tritium has one positively charged proton and two neutrons in the nucleus and one electron in orbit.

metabolic pathways of food. Others such as iodine[131] can be injected in the body and used to track the circulation of blood. Still others such as cobalt[60] are used in cancer treatment.

Molecules and Compounds

Atoms of the same element can unite with each other to form a **molecule**. For example, atoms of hydrogen unite to form a hydrogen molecule. This can be expressed in a chemical equation using the chemical symbol for hydrogen:

$$H + H \rightarrow H_2$$

In this reaction, the atoms on the left are the reactants; the arrow is read as "yield"; and the last symbol is the product—a molecule of hydrogen. A chemical equation uses the chemical symbols of elements and shows the ratios by which they combine. Because atoms of elements always combine in the same ratio under similar conditions, it is possible to predict the nature of a chemical change.

When atoms of two or more different elements combine (react) they form a **compound**. For example, if one atom of sodium (Na) and one atom of chlorine (Cl) react, they form a molecule of the compound called sodium chloride. This is expressed in the following equation:

$$Na + Cl \rightarrow NaCl$$

Compounds can be divided into two groups. Those without carbon are inorganic compounds, and those with carbon are organic compounds. By using chemical equations, chemical changes, called chemical reactions, can be shown. Sometimes, different substances are combined in no specific way, and the components do not have a definite ratio every time. For instance, water, sugar, and table salt mixed without being measured will yield different results depending on the ratio of each substance. Such a combination is called a **mix-**

ture. Its composition may vary each time the components are mixed.

Chemical reactions occur whenever atoms join together or separate. They join together by forming bonds, and they separate by breaking bonds. Either way, new combinations result. When two or more atoms (reactants) bond and form a more complex molecular product, the reaction is called **synthesis**. A sample equation would be as follows:

$$2H \quad + \quad O \quad \rightarrow \quad H_2O$$
hydrogen and oxygen yields water

When the bonding between the atoms in a molecule is broken and simpler products are formed, the reaction is called **decomposition**. If a molecule of sodium chloride is decomposed it forms sodium and chlorine. This can be expressed as follows:

$$NaCl \quad \rightarrow \quad Na \quad + \quad Cl$$
sodium chloride yields sodium and chloride

(decomposition)

It is important to understand that when synthesis occurs, energy is tied up in the bonds formed during the reaction. When decomposition occurs, energy is released. In the cells of the body, these kinds of chemical reactions are repeatedly occurring: Molecules form and decompose. Body cells can utilize these reactions to form energy sources and to free energy to drive the various metabolic processes of the cells.

Ions

When some compounds are placed in water, they decompose, or ionize. The result is an **ion**, an atom bearing an electrical charge. An ion with a positive charge is called a **cation**; an ion with a negative charge is termed an **anion**. For example, sodium chloride in water dissociates to form sodium ions bearing a positive charge and chloride ions bearing a negative charge (Figure 23-3). Because the atoms in this combination are charged, they will conduct electricity. The reaction can be shown as follows:

$$NaCl \rightarrow Na^+ + Cl^-$$
sodium chloride yields sodium and chloride
(cation) (anion)

A compound that dissociates into ions in water is called an **electrolyte**. Many electrolytes are extremely important in body chemistry; some of these are listed in Table 23-2.

WATER

Water constitutes approximately 60% of the total body weight of an adult and is involved in many of the physical and physiological processes of the body. Because water is so integral to the body's processes, fluctuations in the amount of water in the body can have harmful or even fatal consequences.

Water is the major component of blood. Approximately 92% of the body's organic and inorganic compounds dissolve in this water into less-complex molecules and atoms and then are transported throughout the body. Necessary substances such as oxygen and nutrients from the GI system are carried to the cells, where they are utilized. Cellular waste products such as carbon dioxide, urea, and excessive minerals are carried by water to sites of elimination: carbon dioxide to the lungs, urea and minerals to the kidneys.

Water also absorbs heat resulting from muscle contractions and distributes this heat over the body. Water

Table 23–2 **IMPORTANT ELECTROLYTES IN BODY FLUIDS**	
FORMULA	**CHEMICAL NAME**
NaCl	Sodium chloride
Na_2SO_4	Sodium sulfate
Na_2HPO_4	Disodium phosphate
$NaHCO_3$	Sodium bicarbonate
MgCl	Magnesium chloride
$CaCl_2$	Calcium chloride
KCl	Potassium chloride

LIFE CYCLE CONSIDERATIONS

Body Water and Body Size

The amount of body water is inversely proportional to body size. The smaller the body, the higher the water content:

Embryo:	97%
Infant:	77%
Child:	60% to 77%
Adult:	60%
Elders:	45% to 50%

Body water diminishment in elderly persons is related to tissue loss.

in the form of perspiration released from sweat glands in the skin can cool the body by evaporation. Water also can break apart the bonds in large molecules such as starches to form smaller molecules in the digestive process. This type of reaction is called *hydration*.

GASES

Two important gases in the body are oxygen (O_2) and carbon dioxide (CO_2). Because these elements are gases, their molecules are free and can move swiftly in all directions. Oxygen enters the body through the lungs and is transported by the red blood cells throughout the body to the cells. The cells use oxygen in the release of energy from glucose and other molecules. This energy is needed by the cells to carry out their activities. As a result of the energy-releasing processes, carbon dioxide is produced by the cells and transported in the blood to the lungs, where it is eliminated.

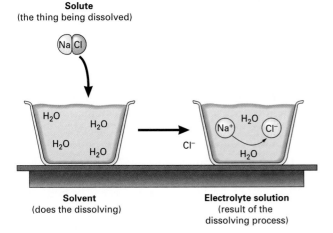

Solute
(the thing being dissolved)

Solvent
(does the dissolving)

Electrolyte solution
(result of the dissolving process)

Figure 23-3 Dissociation of Electrolytes

ACIDS, BASES, SALTS, AND PH

Other chemical substances important for life are acids, bases, and salts; pH is the measure of acid and base strength.

Acids

An **acid** is any substance that in solution yields hydrogen ions bearing a positive charge. As an example, hydrochloric acid (HCl) in water dissociates as shown following:

$$HCl \rightarrow H^+ + Cl^-$$
hydrochloric acid yields hydrogen and chlorine

The hydrogen ion characterizes this as an acid. Important acids in the body are hydrochloric acid, produced in the stomach, and carbonic acid, formed when the carbon dioxide released from cells reacts with some of the water in the extracellular fluid (all body fluids except for those contained within the cells).

Bases

A **base** is a substance that when dissociated produces ions that will combine with hydrogen ions. For example, when sodium hydroxide dissociates in water, it forms a sodium ion bearing a positive charge and a hydroxyl ion bearing a negative charge as shown following:

$$NaOH \rightarrow Na^+ + OH^-$$
sodium hydroxide yields sodium and hydroxyl

The hydroxyl ion is capable of combining with a hydrogen ion to form water. Sodium bicarbonate is an example of a base found in the body.

Salts

A **salt** is formed when an acid and a base react with each other. Salts result from the neutralization of an acid by a base, as illustrated by the following reaction:

$$HCl + NaOH \rightarrow H_2O + NaCl$$
hydrochloric and   sodium   yields water and sodium
acid   hydroxide   chloride

The hydrochloric acid reacts with the sodium hydroxide to form a molecule of water and a molecule of a salt—sodium chloride. When salts are placed in water, they dissociate into a cation and an anion. For instance, in water, the sodium chloride would dissociate into Na^+ and Cl^-. One reason salts are of great biological importance is that many of the compounds that dissociate into ions in living cells are salts. For example, sodium and chlorine ions are present in great amounts in body fluids. Many other salts occur in lesser amounts.

pH

Acid and bases are classified as either strong or weak by the number of hydrogen ions or hydroxyl ions they produce when they dissociate. Strong acids release many hydrogen ions; weak acids release relatively few. The same is true of hydroxyl ions in strong and weak bases. The acidity or alkalinity of a solution is determined by the concentration of hydrogen ions in the solution. Potential hydrogen (pH) indicates the hydrogen ion concentration in a solution, expressed as a number from 0 to 14. A solution with a pH of 7 is neutral, that is, it is neither an acid or a base. A solution with a pH greater than 7 is a base, or alkaline. A solution with a pH below 7 is an acid. The higher above 7 the pH, the more alkaline the solution; the lower below 7 the pH, the more acid the solution. pH is of great biological importance. The human body can tolerate only very slight changes in pH. For example, the pH of human blood ranges from 7.35 to 7.45. Blood pH above or below this range can cause severe or even fatal physiological problems.

Although small amounts of acids may enter the body through food intake, the greatest source of acids—and thus H^+ ions—is cellular metabolism, resulting in products including lactic acid, phosphoric acid, pyruvic acid, and many fatty acids. When blood pH falls below 7.35 as a result of an elevated concentration of H^+ ions, **acidosis** occurs. Rarely does blood pH fall to 7 or become acidic, because death will usually occur first. As acidosis increases, the central nervous system (CNS) becomes involved, and the client may become unconscious. The heartbeat may become weak and irregular, and blood pressure may decrease or even disappear.

When blood pH increases above 7.45, **alkalosis** occurs. Alkalosis is a condition characterized by an excessive loss of hydrogen ions. This happens less often than does acidosis. Symptoms of alkalosis include a heightened state of nervous system activity, resulting in spasmodic muscle contractions, convulsions, and even death.

BUFFERS

Buffers are substances that attempt to maintain pH range, or H^+ ion concentration, in the presence of added acids or bases. Buffers usually occur in pairs in the body fluids. They act to keep the pH of body fluids within normal range. If body fluids become acidic, buffers in the body fluids combine with the excess hydrogen ions and restore normal pH. Likewise, if the body fluids become alkaline, other buffers in the blood combine with the strong bases, converting them to weak bases and restoring normal pH.

Three important buffer systems occur in body fluids: the bicarbonate buffer system, the phosphate buffer system, and the protein buffer system. Because a change in pH of one fluid may bring corresponding changes in the pH of other fluids, an interplay between buffer systems acts to maintain the body's pH. The buffer systems react quickly to prevent excessive changes in the hydrogen ion concentration.

Bicarbonate Buffer System

The bicarbonate buffer system is found in both the extracellular and intracellular fluids and is the body's primary buffer system. It has two components: carbonic acid (H_2CO_3) and sodium bicarbonate ($NaHCO_3$). When a strong acid such as hydrochloric acid is added to this buffer system, the acid will react with the sodium bicarbonate and form a weaker acid (carbonic acid) and a salt (sodium chloride).

HCl	+	NaHCO₃	→	H₂CO₃	+	NaCl
hydrochloric acid	and	sodium bicarbonate	yields	carbonic acid	and	sodium chloride

The strong acid is converted into a weak acid, and the pH is raised toward normal.

If a strong base such as sodium hydroxide is added to this buffer system, the carbonic acid will react with it to form a weak base (sodium bicarbonate) and water.

NaOH	+	H₂CO₃	→	NaHCO₃	+	H₂O
sodium hydroxide	and	carbonic acid	yields	sodium bicarbonate	and	water

The strong base, which initially raised the pH, is converted to a weak base, which will lower the pH toward normal. It is vital to note that hydrochloric acid and sodium hydroxide are substances not normally added to the blood. They are used here only as good examples of the way buffers work. This buffer system normally buffers organic acids found in body fluids.

In the body, bicarbonate helps to stabilize pH by combining reversibly with hydrogen ions. Most of the body's bicarbonate is produced in red blood cells, where the enzyme carbonic anhydrase accelerates the conversion of carbon dioxide to carbonic acid. The production of bicarbonate is illustrated in the following reversible equation:

CO₂	+	H₂O	↔	H₂CO₃	↔	H⁺	+	HCO₃⁻
carbon dioxide		water		carbonic acid		hydrogen		bicarbonate

When the hydrogen ion concentration increases in the extracellular (outside of the cell) space, the reaction shifts toward the left. A decreased concentration of hydrogen ions drives the reaction to the right.

Phosphate Buffer System

The phosphate buffer system is involved in regulating the pH of intracellular fluid and the fluid of the kidney tubules. It has two phosphate compounds: sodium monohydrogen phosphate ($NaHPO_4$) and sodium dihydrogen phosphate (NaH_2PO_4). In the presence of a strong acid such as hydrochloric acid, the sodium monohydrogen phosphate reacts with the acid to form a weak acid (sodium dihydrogen phosphate) and a salt (sodium chloride), thus raising the pH.

HCl	+	NaHPO₄	→	NaH₂PO₄	+	NaCl
hydrochloric acid	and	sodium monohydrogen phosphate	yields	sodium dihydrogen phosphate	and	sodium chloride

When sodium dihydrogen phosphate encounters a strong base such as sodium hydroxide, a weak base (sodium monohydrogen phosphate) and water are formed.

NaOH	+	NaH₂PO₄	→	NaHPO₄	+	H₂O
sodium hydroxide	and	sodium dihydrogen phosphate	yields	sodium monohydrogen phosphate	and	water

Protein Buffers

Proteins are complex substances formed when amino acids bond. Each amino acid contains a carboxyl group (COOH) and an amino group (NH_2). The carboxyl group can ionize and release hydrogen, thus acting as an acid. The amino group can accept hydrogen, thus acting as a base. This ability allows proteins to act as a buffer system. The protein buffer system is found inside cells, especially in the hemoglobin of red blood cells, where the proteins can act to maintain the pH inside the cell. They are also found in the plasma.

SUBSTANCE MOVEMENT

Substances must be able to both enter and leave cells. For example, oxygen and various end products of digestion must enter a cell through the cell membrane for use by the cell. Waste products from cellular processes must be eliminated from the cell. Various ions must also both enter and leave cells. Everything that enters and leaves the cell must pass through the cell membrane. Thus, the cell membrane serves not only as an envelope around the cell, but also as a gatekeeper, regulating which substances can enter and leave the cell. The cell membrane is a very thin and delicate, but complex and living, elastic covering around each cell. It consists of an inner and outer layer of phospholipids in which protein molecules are embedded. Many small channels pass through the membrane. These channels allow some water molecules and some water-soluble substances to pass through the membrane. The ability of a membrane to permit substances to pass through it is called **permeability**. Because a cell membrane allows passage of only certain substances, it is called a selective permeable membrane, or **semipermeable membrane**.

Some substances can pass through the cell membrane without energy expenditure on the part of the cell. This is called passive transport. The passage of other substances requires an expenditure of energy by the cell. This is called active transport.

Passive Transport

There are several types of passive transport: diffusion, osmosis, and filtration.

Diffusion

Diffusion is the tendency of molecules of either gases, liquids, or solids to move from a region of higher molecular concentration to a region of lower molecular concentration until an equilibrium is reached. This movement is due to the kinetic energy in molecules. Kinetic energy causes the molecules to move constantly, colliding with one another and knocking each other about, thus causing them to move farther apart. An example is a drop of black ink placed in a glass of water; over a period of time, the glass of water will turn a uniform black color because of diffusion, as shown in Figure 23-4.

In the body, oxygen moves by diffusion from the lungs to the bloodstream because the oxygen concentration is higher in the lungs and lower in the blood. Carbon dioxide moves by diffusion from the bloodstream, where the concentration of carbon dioxide is higher, to the lungs, for elimination. The size of the channels in the cell membrane can prevent large molecules from passing through the membrane. Some substances, such as glucose molecules, combine with carrier molecules, which carry them into the interior of the cell, where they are released.

The term **dialysis** is used when diffusion is employed to separate molecules out of a solution by passing them through a semipermeable membrane. Dialysis is the process used in the artificial kidney. Blood from a client is circulated through a long, coiled tube. Small, toxic waste molecules such as urea leave the blood and pass through the pores of the tubing by diffusion and out into the fluid surrounding the tubing. The blood, thus cleaned, is then returned to the body.

Osmosis

Osmosis is the diffusion of water through a semipermeable membrane from a region of higher water concentration to a region of lower water concentration. In a solution undergoing osmosis, only the water (solvent) molecules move through the membrane; the dissolved molecules do not (Figure 23-5).

If a cell, having both a membrane that will not allow sodium chloride to pass through and a molecular concentration of 10% sodium chloride, were placed in a container with a 5% sodium chloride solution, the cell would contain 10% sodium chloride and 90% water, and the 5% solution in which it was placed would contain 5% dissolved sodium chloride and 95% water. There would be more water outside than inside the cell; thus, water would pass through the membrane into the cell. Because the cell membrane is elastic, the cell would increase in size as a result of the water accumulation within it facilitated by the process of osmosis. The pressure exerted against the cell membrane by the water inside the cell is called **osmotic pressure**.

A solution that has the same molecular concentration as the cell is called an **isotonic solution**. It neither increases nor decreases the size of the cell. A solution that has a lower molecular concentration than the cell is called a **hypotonic solution**. Placing cells in a hypotonic solution causes them to swell, possibly to the point of eventual rupture. The rupture of red blood cells due to osmosis is called **hemolysis**. As red blood cells swell, the hemoglobin contained within passes to the outside of the cell and into the solution surrounding the cell, rendering the blood cells no longer capable of carrying oxygen. A solution that has a higher molecular concentration than the cell is called a **hypertonic solution**. When placed in such a solution, water leaves the cell, and the cell decreases in size. In the case of red blood cells, they shrivel and become wrinkled. This shrinkage, called **crenation**, leaves the cells incapable of functioning.

In persons who have lost large volumes of blood, it is sometimes necessary to administer additional fluids to maintain blood pressure. Generally, normal saline can be used. This 0.9% sodium chloride solution has approximately the same osmotic concentration as blood. Because it is isotonic, it will not damage the cells. Figure 23-6 shows osmosis in cells with different solution concentrations.

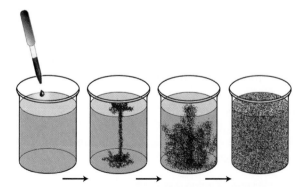

Figure 23-4 Diffusion is the spreading of particles from an area of greater concentration to an area of lesser concentration. Dye put into a beaker of water gradually spreads throughout the water.

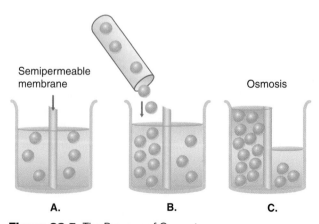

Semipermeable membrane

Osmosis

A.   B.   C.

Figure 23-5 The Process of Osmosis

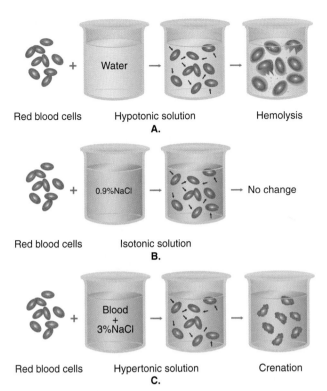

Figure 23-6 Osmosis is the movement of water through a membrane from an area of lower concentration to one of higher concentration. A. In a hypotonic solution, the water moves into the cells, causing them to swell and burst. B. In an isotonic solution, cells are normal in size and shape because the same amount of water is entering and leaving the cells. C. In a hypertonic solution, cells are losing water because water moves from an area of lower concentration (inside the cell) to an area of higher concentration (outside the cell).

Filtration

In **filtration**, fluids and the substances dissolved in them are forced through cell membranes by hydrostatic pressure. **Hydrostatic pressure** is the pressure that the fluid exerts against the membrane. The molecules passing through the membrane are determined by the size of the pores in the membrane. Tissue fluids are formed by filtration. As blood passes through the capillaries, hydrostatic pressure exerted by the pumping action of the heart causes some of the liquid fraction of the blood (but not the cells) to pass out of the capillaries, resulting in the formation of the tissue fluid (Figure 23-7). As the blood circulates through the capillaries of the kidneys, the hydrostatic pressure of the blood causes many materials to leave the blood through the filtration process. These materials pass into the tubules of the kidneys, where the toxic waste products are removed to form urine. The urine is then eliminated from the body.

Active Transport

In the processes discussed thus far, the movement of molecules depends on the concentration of mole-

cules or on pressure. In other words, the cells do not have to expend energy to move the molecules in or out of the cell. In active transport, the cell must use energy to move the molecules. For instance, in the body, sodium ions are in higher concentration in the fluids surrounding the cell than inside the cell. Though some sodium ions can diffuse into the cell, the cell actively transports them through the membrane to the outside. Active transport is accomplished by means of carrier molecules, which can latch onto specific molecules and transport them in or out of the cell. This process requires an expenditure of cellular energy (Figure 23-8). Examples of important ions transported by this process are calcium, sodium, potassium, and magnesium.

FLUID AND ELECTROLYTE BALANCE

Human life is suspended in a saline solution having a salt concentration of 0.9%. This solution, which both surrounds the cells and is contained within them, constitutes the body fluids. The water and electrolytes composing these body fluids come from ingested water and nutrients, and from the water that results from metabolism.

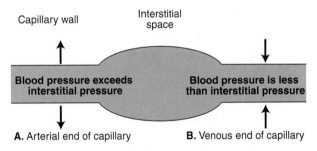

Figure 23-7 Filtration: A. Pressure in the arteriole is greater than interstitial (between the cells) pressure, causing fluid with dissolved substances to move out of capillaries. B. Pressure in venules is less than interstitial fluid pressure, causing fluid and waste products to move back into the capillaries.

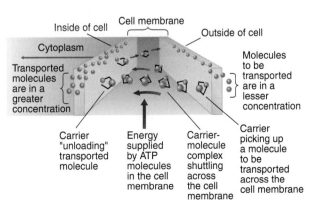

Figure 23-8 Active Transport of Molecules from an Area of Lesser Concentration to an Area of Greater Concentration

For life to continue and the cells to properly function, the body fluids must remain fairly constant with regard to the amount of water and the specific electrolytes of which they are composed. Water is essential because it is the basic component of all the body fluids. Water is involved in many of the metabolic processes in the body and is a by–product of some of these reactions. The various electrolytes all have essential roles in cellular physiological processes. If some of either is lost, it must be replaced, and if either water or an electrolyte is in excess, it must be removed. Maintaining the consistency of this fluid environment is homeostasis.

For cells to survive and carry out their multitude of physiologic functions, they need both a continuing source of water, nutrients, and oxygen and a mechanism to remove cellular wastes. These physiologic processes affect the amount of water, the pH, and the ions both inside and outside the cells. A balance must be maintained between the components of the fluids inside and outside the cell. Because the ions are dissolved in water, these two components are tied together: Anything affecting the amount of water in the body will affect the ion concentration.

Body Fluids

Much of the body weight of an average adult is due to the water in the body fluids surrounding the cells and contained within them. The fluid around the cells cushions them and serves as the medium of exchange. Everything that enters or leaves the cells must pass through this fluid layer.

There are two kinds of body fluids. They can be thought of as being contained within two separate containers, called compartments. The **intracellular fluid** (ICF) compartment contains all of the water and ions inside the cells. By far the largest amount of water in the body, approximately 65%, is found within this compartment.

The extracellular fluid compartment contains the remaining body fluids, called **extracellular fluid** (ECF), or fluid outside the cells. These can be further subdivided into interstitial, intravascular, and other fluids. **Interstitial fluid** is the fluid in the tissue spaces around each cell. The **intravascular fluid** is the plasma in the blood vessels and the lymph in the lymphatic system (Figure 23-9). There are also small amounts of other specialized body fluids such as synovial fluid, cerebrospinal fluid, serous fluid, aqueous and vitreous humor, and the endolymph and perilymph. The proportions of extracellular fluid and intracellular fluid vary with age.

Generally speaking, the major ions in the extracellular fluid are sodium (Na^+), chloride (Cl^-), and bicarbonate (HCO_3^-), although other ions do occur. In the intracellular fluid, the major ions are potassium (K^+), phosphate (PO_4^{--}), and magnesium (Mg^{++}), with lesser

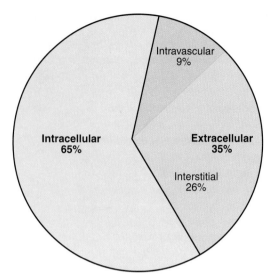

Figure 23-9 Body Fluid Compartments of an Adult

amounts of other ions present. There are also large numbers of protein molecules bearing a negative charge.

Exchange between the Extracellular and Intracellular Fluids

Water and ions moving between the extracellular and intracellular fluids must first pass through the selectively permeable cell membrane. This movement is governed primarily by osmosis. Diffusion and active transport also play a role.

The difference in the ion concentration inside the cell and outside the cell is due primarily to the cell's ability to pump some ions inside and pump others out. If the intracellular fluid becomes hypertonic to the extracellular fluid, water from the extracellular fluid will move by osmosis into the cell to restore the balance, and vice versa.

A fluid balance also occurs between the interstitial fluid and the plasma. This balance is regulated primarily by hydrostatic pressure (blood pressure) and osmotic pressure. When the circulating blood passes from the arterioles into the capillaries, the pressure in the capillaries is higher than that in the interstitial fluid. This forces some of the water from the plasma out of the capillaries and into the interstitial fluid. Due to osmotic pressure, some of the water in the interstitial fluid is forced back into the capillaries in the area where they join the venules. Some water is also returned to the bloodstream through the lymphatic system. If the amount of interstitial fluid returned to the circulatory system lessens and the fluid accumulates in the tissue spaces, the tissues become swollen. This condition is called **edema**. A number of conditions can cause edema, including kidney or liver disease and heart disorders. Many of these conditions can have serious consequences.

When more water is lost from the body than is replaced, **dehydration** occurs. Among the various causes of dehydration are water deprivation, excessive urine production, profuse sweating, diarrhea, and extended periods of vomiting. As water is lost, the amount of water in the interstitial fluid decreases. Water then moves from the cells to the tissue spaces by osmosis, causing an electrolyte imbalance. Circulatory impairment occurs, which in turn affects the kidney's ability to function normally. This condition is corrected by supplying water and the appropriate electrolytes.

Regulators of Fluid and Electrolyte Balance

There must be a balance in the amounts of fluids and electrolytes consumed and lost daily. Under typical conditions, the average adult loses some water through the skin, lungs, and GI tract and loses the largest amount of water through urine production. This can amount to a per-day fluid loss of approximately 2500 mL, depending on conditions.

Skin

In the average adult, an estimated water loss of 300 to 400 mL per day occurs by diffusion through the skin. Because the person is not aware of this water loss, it is called *insensible loss*. Water is also lost through the skin by perspiration. The total amount of water lost through perspiration varies depending on environmental factors and body temperature.

Lungs

In the average adult, an estimated insensible water loss of 300 to 400 mL per day occurs with expired air, which is saturated with water vapor. This amount varies with the rate and depth of respirations.

Gastrointestinal Tract

Although a large amount of fluid—approximately 8,000 mL per day in the average adult—is secreted into the gastrointestinal tract, almost all of this fluid is reabsorbed by the body. In adults, approximately 200 mL of water is lost per day in feces. Severe diarrhea can cause a fluid and electrolyte deficit because the GI fluids contain a large amount of electrolytes.

Kidneys

The kidneys play a major role in maintaining fluid balance by excreting 1,200 to 1,500 mL of water per day in the average adult. The excretion of water by healthy kidneys is proportional to the fluid ingested and the amount of waste or solutes excreted.

When an extracellular fluid volume deficit occurs, hormones play a key role in restoring the extracellular fluid volume. The release of the following hormones into circulation causes the kidneys to conserve water:

- Antidiuretic hormone (ADH): released by the posterior pituitary gland; acts on the distal tubules of the kidneys to reabsorb water
- Aldosterone: produced in the adrenal cortex; causes the reabsoption of sodium from the renal tubules, leading to water retention in the extracellular fluid, thereby increasing its volume
- Renin: released by the juxtaglomerular cells of the kidneys; promotes vasoconstriction and the release of aldosterone

The interaction of these hormones with regard to renal functions serves as the body's compensatory mechanism to maintain homeostasis.

Sodium is the main electrolyte that promotes the retention of water. An intravascular water deficit causes the renal tubules to reabsorb more sodium into circulation. Because water molecules go with the sodium ions, the intravascular water deficit is corrected by this action of the renal tubules.

Fluid and Food Intake

Fluids must be replaced in the amounts lost. The primary source of fluid replacement is water consumption. Approximately 60% may be obtained in this way, with an additional 30% being obtained from foods and 8% to 10% being a product of metabolism (metabolic water) for a total of 2,500 mL. Figure 23-10 illustrates fluid balance.

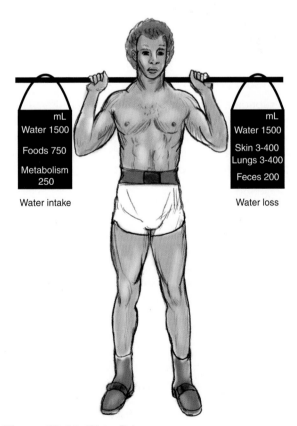

Figure 23-10 Water Balance

Thirst

Water consumption usually occurs in response to the sensation of thirst. This mechanism is poorly understood. It is generally believed to be brought about by the loss of body fluids, which in turn causes a dryness in the mouth and the thirst sensation. Replacing the lost fluids by water consumption causes the sensation to diminish. The thirst mechanism appears to be regulated by the hypothalamus in the brain.

Dehydration is one of the most common and most serious fluid imbalances that can result from poor monitoring of fluid intake. One nursing goal is to ensure that all clients understand both the role that water plays in health and the way to maintain adequate hydration.

DISTURBANCES IN ELECTROLYTE BALANCE

In health, normal homeostatic mechanisms function to maintain electrolyte balance. In illness, one or more of the regulating mechanisms may be affected, or an imbalance may become too great for the body to correct without treatment. Electrolytes are measured by laboratory analysis of a blood sample.

Sodium

Sodium (Na^+) is the major electrolyte in extracellular fluid. It regulates fluid balance through osmotic pressure that results from water following sodium in the body. Sodium stimulates conduction of nerve impulses and helps maintain neuromuscular activity. Excretion occurs primarily via the kidneys. The normal serum sodium for an adult is 136 to 145 mEq/L.

Hyponatremia

A subnormal serum sodium value (< 136 mEq/L) indicates hyponatremia. The cause is either a sodium deficit or a water excess. A hypo-osmotic state exists: The water moves out of the vascular space, into the interstitial space, and then into the intracellular space, causing edema. Hyponatremia may be caused by prolonged vomiting, diarrhea, or gastric or intestinal suctioning.

Hypernatremia

A serum sodium level of > 145 mEq/L indicates hypernatremia. Excess sodium or a loss of water causes a rise in the extracellular osmotic pressure and pulls water out of the cells and into the extracellular space.

Potassium

Potassium (K^+) is the major electrolyte in intracellular fluid. Its concentration inside cells is approximately 150 mEq/L. The normal value range of extracellular (serum) potassium is narrow: 3.5 to 5.0 mEq/L. Consequently, the slightest changes can dramatically affect physiological functions. Potassium maintains normal

PROFESSIONAL TIP

Hypokalemia

Hypokalemia can cause cardiac arrest when:

- The potassium level is < 2.5 mEq/L.
- The client is taking digitalis (a drug that strengthens the contraction of the myocardium and slows down the heart rate). *Hypokalemia enhances the action of digitalis, causing toxicity.*

nerve and muscle activity, especially of the heart, and osmotic pressure within the cells. It also assists in the cellular metabolism of carbohydrates and proteins. The kidneys prefer to retain sodium and excrete potassium, even when both electrolytes are depleted. When potassium is lost from cells, sodium and hydrogen move into the cells. This aids in regulating acid–base balance. Intracellular potassium deficit may coexist with an excess of extracellular potassium.

Hypokalemia

A serum potassium level < 3.5 mEq/L indicates hypokalemia. Excessive loss of gastric fluids and the use of diuretics can place the client at risk for hypokalemia and an acid–base imbalance (metabolic alkalosis). Potassium-wasting diuretics, such as furosemide (Lasix) or chlorothiazide (Diuril) can cause hypokalemia.

 Safety: Potassium Chloride
- Use IV route only when hypokalemia is life threatening or when oral replacement is not feasible.
- Always dilute potassium chloride in a large amount of IV solution.
- Never administer more than 10 mEq/L of IV potassium chloride (KCl) per hour; the normal dose of IV KCl is 20 to 40 mEq/L infused over an 8-hour period.
- Never give KCl intramuscularly (IM) or as an IV bolus; potentially fatal hyperkalemia may result.
- Monitor the IV site frequently for early signs of infiltration, as potassium is caustic to the tissues.

Hyperkalemia

A serum potassium level > 5.0 mEq/L indicates hyperkalemia. Clients with renal disease develop hyperkalemia, because potassium cannot be excreted adequately by the kidneys. Extensive trauma causes potassium to be released from the cells and enter the bloodstream, leading to hyperkalemia. Hyperkalemia inhibits the action of digitalis. This condition is much more critical than is hypokalemia.

Serum Calcium

Approximately 50% of serum calcium is bound to protein. Correlate the serum calcium level with the serum albumin level when evaluating laboratory results. *Any change in serum protein will result in a change in the total serum calcium.*

Calcium and Vitamin D

Vitamin D is necessary for the absorption of calcium from the GI tract. Clients who do not get adequate exposure to the sun or who use sunscreen (which is needed to prevent skin cancer) may not make enough vitamin D to support adequate calcium absorption. Advise these clients to consult their physicians regarding a vitamin D supplement.

Calcium

Calcium (Ca^{++}) plays an essential role in bone and teeth integrity, blood clotting, muscle functioning, and nerve impulse transmission. Vitamin D is required for absorption of calcium from the GI tract. Only 1% of the body's calcium is found in the blood plasma (serum). Normally, 50% of the serum calcium is ionized (physiologically active), with the remaining 50% being bound to protein. Free, ionized calcium is needed for cell membrane permeability. The calcium that is bound to plasma protein cannot pass through the capillary wall and, therefore, cannot leave the intravascular compartment. The normal ionized serum calcium range for an adult is 4.5 to 5.6 mEq/L. Total serum calcium concentration measures both the ionized calcium and the calcium bound to albumin. The normal value range of total serum calcium concentration for an adult is 9.0 to 10.5 mg/dL, with values for the older adult being slightly lower.

Hypocalcemia

Hypocalcemia is indicated by a total serum calcium concentration of < 9.0 mg/dL or an ionized serum calcium level of < 4.5 mEq/L. An ionized serum calcium level of < 3.0 mEq/L is related to tetany. Alkalosis, elevated serum albumin, and the rapid administration of citrated blood increase the activity of calcium binders, thereby decreasing the amount of free calcium.

Hypercalcemia

A total serum calcium level of > 10.5 mg/dL or an ionized serum calcium level of > 5.6 mEq/L indicates

Hypercalcemic Crisis

A rapid increase in the extracellular level of calcium (above 8 to 9 mEq/L) can trigger a hypercalcemic crisis (coma and cardiac arrest). To prevent a hypercalcemic crisis, provide adequate hydration and administer loop diuretics, phosphate, or both, as prescribed by the physician.

hypercalcemia. Generally, three separate evaluations of either total serum calcium or ionized serum calcium are performed before a diagnosis of hypercalcemia is made. Often, hypercalcemia is a symptom of an underlying disease such as metastatic bone tumors, Paget's disease, acromegaly, and hyperparathyroidism, which all increase bone reabsorption and, thereby, foster the release of calcium into circulating blood. Calcium-containing antacids and excess calcium from the diet may also cause hypercalcemia.

Magnesium

Most magnesium (Mg^{++}) is found in intracellular fluid and in combination with calcium and phosphorus in bone, muscle, and soft tissue. Blood serum contains only approximately 1%. Magnesium plays an important role as a coenzyme, in the metabolism of carbohydrates and proteins, and as a mediator, in neuromuscular activity. It is the only cation that is found in higher concentration in cererospinal fluid than in extracellular fluid. When a magnesium deficiency develops, the body conserves magnesium at the expense of excreting potassium. A close relationship exists between magnesium, calcium, and potassium in the intracellular fluid: A low level of one results in low levels of the other two. The normal serum magnesium level for an adult is 1.5 to 2.5 mEq/L.

Hypomagnesemia

A serum magnesium level of < 1.5 mEq/L indicates hypomagnesemia, which most commonly results from chronic alcoholism. Increased renal excretion is associated with prolonged diuretic therapy or use of gentamicin (Garamycin), cyclosporin (Sandimmune), or cisplatin (Platinol).

Hypermagnesemia

A serum magnesium level of > 2.5 mEq/L indicates hypermagnesemia. This condition rarely occurs if kidney function is normal. An increased magnesium level is associated with uncontrolled diabetes (ketoacidosis), renal failure, and ingestion of magnesium antacids (Maalox, Mylanta) or laxatives (milk of magnesia [MOM], magnesium citrate [Citromal]).

PROFESSIONAL TIP

Hyperalimentation

Total parenteral nutrition (TPN) provided continuously (hyperalimentation) and without a magnesium supplement can cause hypomagnesemia.

Safety: Magnesium Level

When the serum magnesium level reaches 10 to 15 mEq/L, respiratory paralysis may occur.

Phosphate

Phosphate (PO_4^{--}) is the main intracellular anion. It appears as phosphorus in the serum, where the normal value range is 1.7 to 2.6 mEq/L. Phosphorus is critical for normal cell functioning. Most phosphorus is found combined with calcium in teeth and bones. Phosphate and calcium exist in an inverse relationship; that is, as one increases the other decreases.

Hypophosphatemia

A client with a serum phosphorus level < 1.7 mEq/L has hypophosphatemia. Rarely does this condition result from decreased dietary intake. More commonly, it stems from respiratory alkalosis. Intense, prolonged hyperventilation can cause severe hypophosphatemia.

Hyperphosphatemia

A client with a serum phosphorus level > 2.6 mEq/L has hyperphosphatemia. This condition most commonly results from renal failure with resultant decreased renal phosphorus excretion. Excessive use of phosphate-containing laxatives or phosphate enemas may cause hyperphosphatemia.

Chloride

Chloride (Cl^-) is the major anion in extracellular fluid. Chloride functions in combination with sodium to maintain osmotic pressure. It also assists in maintaining acid–base balance. When the carbon dioxide level increases, bicarbonate shifts from the intracellular compartment to the extracellular compartment. Chloride, in an effort to maintain homeostasis, then moves

PROFESSIONAL TIP

Hyperphosphatemia

A client with hyperphosphatemia generally remains asymptomatic unless hypocalcemia results, in which case the client may describe both tingling sensations around the mouth and in the fingertips as well as muscle cramps.

into the intracellular compartment. The kidneys selectively excrete chloride or bicarbonate ions depending on the acid–base balance. The normal serum chloride range is 95 to 106 mEq/L.

Hypochloremia

A serum chloride level < 95 mEq/L indicates hypochloremia. Excess losses of chloride may result from prolonged diarrhea or diaphoresis. Loss of hydrochloric acid related to vomiting, gastric suctioning, or gastric surgery may cause hypochloremia.

Hyperchloremia

A serum chloride level > 106 mEq/L indicates hyperchloremia, which usually occurs in conjunction with dehydration, hypernatremia, or metabolic acidosis.

ACID–BASE BALANCE

As described earlier, the body maintains a normal pH within the relatively narrow range of 7.35 to 7.45. Body pH is maintained by the buffer systems, the respiratory system, and the kidneys. A pH below 7.35 is termed acidosis, and a pH above 7.45 is termed alkalosis. Either of these conditions can be brought about by respiratory or metabolic changes.

Regulators of Acid–Base Balance

The body has three main control systems that regulate acid–base balance to counter acidosis or alkalosis: the buffer systems, respirations, and renal control of hydrogen ion concentration. These systems vary in their reaction times in regulating and restoring balance to the hydrogen ion concentration.

Buffer Systems

The buffer systems—bicarbonate, phosphate, and protein—were previously discussed. They react quickly to prevent excessive changes in the hydrogen ion concentration.

Respiratory Regulation of Acid–Base Balance

The respiratory system helps to maintain acid–base balance by controlling the content of carbon dioxide in extracellular fluid. The *rate of metabolism* determines the formation of carbon dioxide. Various intracellular metabolic processes continuously form carbon dioxide in the body. The carbon in foods is **oxidized** (joined with oxygen) to form carbon dioxide.

It takes the respiratory regulatory mechanism several minutes to respond to changes in the carbon dioxide concentration of extracellular fluid. With the increase of carbon dioxide in extracellular fluid, respiration increases in rate and depth so that more carbon dioxide is exhaled. As the respiratory system removes carbon dioxide, less carbon dioxide is present in the blood to combine with water to form carbonic acid. Likewise, if the blood level of carbon dioxide is low, respirations decrease to maintain a normal ratio between carbonic acid and basic bicarbonate.

Renal Control of Hydrogen Ion Concentration

The kidneys control extracellular fluid pH by eliminating either hydrogen ions or bicarbonate ions from body fluids. If the bicarbonate concentration in the extracellular fluid is greater than normal, the kidneys excrete more bicarbonate ions, making the urine more alkaline. Conversely, if more hydrogen ions are excreted in the urine, the urine becomes more acidic. The renal mechanism for regulating acid–base balance cannot readjust the pH within seconds, as can the extracellular fluid buffer system, nor within minutes, as can the respiratory compensatory mechanism; but it can function over a period of several hours or days to correct acid–base imbalance.

Diagnostic and Laboratory Data

The biochemical indicators of acid–base balance are assessed by measuring the **arterial blood gases** (ABGs). The arterial blood gas test measures the levels of oxygen and carbon dioxide in arterial blood. The test assesses pH, partial pressure of oxygen (PO_2 or PaO_2), partial pressure of carbon dioxide (PCO_2 or $PaCO_2$), saturation of oxygen (SaO_2), and bicarbonate (HCO_3). pH has already been discussed.

The PO_2 or PaO_2 expresses the amount of oxygen that can combine with hemoglobin to form oxyhemoglobin, the form in which oxygen is transported through the body. At sea level, the normal range is 80 to 100 millimeters of mercury (mm Hg). The rate at which the oxygen/hemoglobin reaction occurs is influenced by pH. The rate decreases as the pH value decreases.

The PCO_2 or $PaCO_2$ in the blood is a reflection of the efficiency of gaseous exchange in the lungs. At sea level, the normal range is 35 to 45 mm Hg. If the alveoli are obstructed or damaged by disease, carbon dioxide cannot be eliminated and will combine with water to form carbonic acid, which in turn causes acidosis. Conversely, in a person who is hyperventilating, too much carbon dioxide is eliminated, which may trigger alkalosis.

The SaO_2 is the percent of oxygen that combines with hemoglobin in the blood. The normal range is

95% to 100% saturation. This value along with the PO_2 and hemoglobin levels indicates the degree to which the tissues are receiving oxygen. Oxygen saturation can also be measured with a pulse oximeter, a noninvasive technique.

Determining the amount of bicarbonate (HCO_3) in the blood is important because, along with carbonic acid, bicarbonate is a major buffer in the blood. The two substances occur in a ratio of 20 parts bicarbonate to 1 part carbonic acid. Regardless of the carbonic acid and bicarbonate values, the pH of the blood will remain in the normal range as long as the ratio remains 20:1. The normal range for HCO_3 at sea level is 24 to 28 mEq/L. The carbonic acid level is always 3% of the PCO_2 level.

DISTURBANCES IN ACID–BASE BALANCE

The acid–base imbalances are respiratory acidosis and alkalosis and metabolic acidosis and alkalosis. In determining whether the acid–base imbalance is caused by a respiratory or a metabolic alteration, the key indicators are bicarbonate and carbonic acid levels (Figure 23-11). Table 23–3 lists those changes in laboratory values that indicate the various acid–base imbalances.

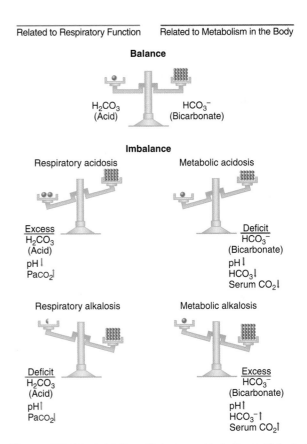

Figure 23-11 Acid–Base Balance and Imbalance (*Adapted from* Fundamentals of Nursing: Standards & Practice, *by* S. DeLaune and P. Ladner, 1998, Albany, NY: Delmar. Copyright 1998 by Delmar. Adapted with permission.)

PROFESSIONAL TIP

Pulse Oximeter Reading

Warming a client's cold hand will provide more accurate results from a pulse oximeter.

Table 23–3 LABORATORY VALUES IN ACID–BASE IMBALANCES

SITUATION	PH	PCO₂	HCO₃
Normal parameters	7.35 to 7.45	35 to 45 mm Hg	24 to 28 mEq/L
Respiratory acidosis			
Acute	< 7.35	> 45 mm Hg	Normal
Chronic	< 7.35	> 45 mm Hg	> 28 mEq/L
Respiratory alkalosis	> 7.45	< 35 mm Hg	Normal
Metabolic acidosis	< 7.35	Normal	< 24 mEq/L
Metabolic alkalosis	> 7.45	Normal	> 28 mEq/L

PROFESSIONAL TIP

Electrolyte Shift

Metabolic acidosis causes an electrolyte shift: Hydrogen and sodium ions move into the cells, and potassium moves into the extracellular fluid. Hyperkalemia may cause ventricular fibrillation and death.

Respiratory Acidosis

When carbon dioxide is not eliminated by the lungs as fast as it is produced by cellular metabolism, the amount of carbon dioxide increases in the blood. It then reacts with water and forms excess hydrogen ions, as shown in the following reaction:

$$CO_2 + H_2O \rightarrow H^+ + HCO_3$$

Respiratory acidosis is characterized by an increased hydrogen ion concentration (a blood pH below 7.35), an increased PCO₂ level (greater than 45 mm Hg), and an excess of carbonic acid. It is caused by hypoventilation or any condition that depresses ventilation. When the respiratory rate and the amount of oxygen supplied to the lungs suddenly lessen, acute respiratory acidosis can occur. This condition can be life threatening, and it must be recognized and corrected quickly. Chronic respiratory acidosis occurs when the respiratory rate is continually depressed.

Clients with respiratory acidosis experience neurological changes resulting from the acidity of the cerebrospinal fluid and brain cells. Hypoventilation causes **hypoxemia** (decreased oxygen in the blood), which in turn causes further neurological impairment. Hyperkalemia may accompany acidosis.

Respiratory Alkalosis

Respiratory alkalosis is characterized by a decreased hydrogen ion concentration (a blood pH above 7.45) and a below normal PCO₂ level (lower than 35 mm Hg). It is caused by hyperventilation (excessive exhalation of carbon dioxide) resulting in hypocapnia (decreased arterial carbon dioxide concentration). As the breathing rate increases, the amount of carbon dioxide in the blood decreases. This in turn increases the pH of the blood.

Hyperventilation can be triggered by anxiety, fear, pain, fever, rapid mechanical ventilation, and hypoxia at high altitudes. This condition is usually self-correcting. As the breathing returns to normal, the carbon dioxide level in the blood increases, and the normal pH is restored. Other causes of hyperventiliation, which involves overstimulation of the respiratory center, include salicylate poisoning, brain tumors, meningitis, encephalitis, and pulmonary embolus.

Metabolic Acidosis

Metabolic acidosis is characterized by an increase in hydrogen ion concentration (blood pH below 7.35) or a decrease in bicarbonate concentration. Such a change may be brought about by kidney disease when the mechanism to excrete excess hydrogen ions is compromised. Diarrhea, diabetes mellitus, and, sometimes, diuretics may also be responsible. The lungs eliminate more carbon dioxide but are usually ineffective in decreasing acids. The kidneys try to increase the pH and the excretion of hydrogen by exchanging sodium ions for hydrogen ions. Metabolic acidosis is most common in individuals with kidney disease or diabetes mellitus.

Metabolic Alkalosis

Metabolic alkalosis is characterized by a loss of acid from the body or a gain in base (increased level of bicarbonate). Blood pH is above 7.45. A gain in base may result from excessive ingestion of antacids and milk. These substances neutralize acids, resulting in alkalosis and hypercalcemia. Excessive oral or parenteral administration of sodium bicarbonate or other alkaline salts (e.g., sodium or potassium acetate, lactate, or citrate) increases the amount of base in extracellular fluid. Loss of gastric fluids from vomiting or suctioning may result in metabolic alkalosis.

The respiratory and renal compensatory mechanisms respond to an increased bicarbonate/carbonic acid ratio. The rate and depth of respirations decreases in an effort to retain carbon dioxide. To counter the pH imbalance of metabolic alkalosis, the arterial carbon dioxide concentration rises, creating respiratory acidosis.

A normal serum potassium level is a prerequisite for renal compensation. In alkalosis, potassium ions enter

PROFESSIONAL TIP

Metabolic Alkalosis

The following clinical conditions can place clients at risk for metabolic alkalosis:

- Vomiting and nasogastric suctioning or lavage cause a loss of hydrochloric acid and chloride. With the loss of the hydrogen and chloride ions, bicarbonate ions are absorbed, unneutralized, into the bloodstream, and the pH of the extracellular fluid rises (alkalosis).
- Diarrhea and steroid or diuretic therapy can cause excessive loss of potassium, chloride, and other electrolytes. The potassium deficit causes the kidneys to exchange hydrogen ions (instead of potassium ions) for sodium ions, which promotes the loss of hydrogen, thereby increasing bicarbonate level.

the cells in exchange for hydrogen ions, causing hypokalemia. Hypokalemia further potentiates metabolic alkalosis because the kidneys conserve hydrogen ions by excreting potassium ions in exchange for sodium ions. When hypokalemia is present, the kidneys cannot function as a compensatory mechanism; they continue to excrete hydrogen, and bicarbonate excess continues.

NURSING PROCESS

The nursing process assists the nurse in planning client care.

Assessment

Assessment data are used to identify clients who have potential or actual alterations in fluid volume. Electrolyte and acid–base imbalances are identified primarily with laboratory data, while fluid balances are identified primarily with the health history and physical examination.

Health History

The nursing history should elicit data in the following areas:

- Lifestyle (sociocultural and economic factors, stress, exercise)
- Dietary intake (recent changes in the amount and types of fluid and food, increased thirst)
- Weight (sudden gain or loss)
- Fluid output (recent changes in the frequency or amount of urine output)
- Gastrointestinal disturbances (prolonged vomiting, diarrhea, anorexia, ulcer, hemmorrhage)
- Fever and diaphoresis
- Burns, trauma, draining wounds

- Disease conditions that can upset homeostasis (renal disease, endocrine disorders, neural malfunction, pulmonary disease)
- Therapeutic programs that can produce imbalances (special diets, medications, chemotherapy, IV fluid or TPN administration, gastric or intestinal suction)

Physical Examination

Because fluid alterations may affect any body system, the nurse performs a complete physical examination and identifies all abnormalities.

Daily Weight Changes in the body's total fluid volume are reflected in body weight. For instance, each liter (1,000 mL) of fluid gained or lost is equivalent to 1 kilogram (2.2 lb) of weight.

Vital Signs Measurement of vital signs provides the nurse with information regarding the client's fluid, electrolyte, and acid–base statuses and the body's compensatory response for maintaining balance. An elevated temperature places the client at risk for dehydration related to an increased loss of body fluid.

Changes in the pulse rate, strength, and rhythm are indicative of fluid alterations. Fluid volume alterations may cause the following pulse changes:

- Fluid volume deficit: increased pulse rate and weak pulse volume
- Fluid volume excess: increased pulse volume and third heart sound

Respiratory changes are assessed by inspecting the movement of the chest wall, counting the respiratory rate, and ascultating the lungs. Changes in the rate and depth may cause respiratory acid–base imbalances or may be indicative of a compensatory response to metabolic acidosis or alkalosis, as previously discussed.

Blood pressure measurements can be used to assess the degree of fluid volume deficit. Fluid volume deficit can lower the blood pressure. A narrow pulse pressure (lower than 20 mm Hg) may indicate fluid volume deficit that occurs with severe hypovolemia.

Intake and Output The client's I&O should be measured and recorded for a 24-hour period to assess for an actual or potential imbalance. A minimum intake of 1,500 mL is essential in balancing urinary output and the body's insensible water loss. Intake includes all liquids taken by mouth (e.g., ice cream, soup, gelatin, juice, and water) and liquids administered through tube feedings (nasogastric or jejunostomy) and parenterally (IV fluids and blood or its components). Output includes urine, diarrhea, vomitus, and drainage from tubes such as gastric suction or surgical drains.

 Safety: Fluid Measurements

To protect both the nurse and the client from transfer of microorganisms, Standard Precautions are always instituted during fluid administration and output measurement.

Thirst The most common indicator of fluid volume deficit is thirst. With a decrease in extracellular fluid volume or an increase in plasma osmolality, the hypothalamus triggers a thirst response.

Food Intake The intake of food also contributes to maintaining extracellular fluid volume. One-third of the body's fluid needs are met with ingested food. Food also provides the body with necessary electrolytes.

Skin Edema and skin turgor are two important indicators related to fluid, electrolyte, and acid–base balances.

Edema Edema is the main symptom of fluid volume excess. Edema may be localized (confined to a specific area) or generalized (occurring throughout the body's tissue). Localized edema is characterized by taut, smooth, shiny, pale skin. The body may retain 5 to 10 pounds of fluid before edema is noticeable (Bulechek & McCloskey, 1999). The dependent body parts—sacrum, back, and legs—should be assessed for peripheral edema. Pitting edema is rated on a four-point scale, as follows:

+0: no pitting

+1, 0 to ¼ inch pitting (mild)

+2: ¼ to ½ inch pitting (moderate)

+3: ½ to 1 inch pitting (severe)

+4: greater than 1 inch pitting (severe)

Turgor Skin **turgor** refers to the normal resiliency of the skin, a reflection of hydration status. When the skin is pinched and released, it springs back to a normal position because of the outward pressure exerted by the cells and interstitial fluid. To measure the client's skin turgor, the nurse uses the thumb and forefinger to grasp and raise and then release a small section of the client's skin. Dehydration is the main cause of decreased skin turgor, which manifests as lax skin that returns slowly to the normal position. Increased skin turgor, which occurs in conjunction with edema, manifests as smooth, taut, shiny skin that cannot be grasped and raised.

Buccal (Oral) Cavity The nurse should inspect the buccal cavity. With fluid volume deficit, saliva decreases, causing sticky, dry mucous membranes and dry, cracked lips. The tongue displays longitudinal furrows.

LIFE CYCLE CONSIDERATIONS

Skin Turgor in Elderly Clients
With aging, the skin loses elasticity, resulting in reduced skin turgor. Assess the tongue for creases or furrows to monitor dehydration in elderly clients (Hogstel, 1994).

Eyes The nurse should inspect the eyes for sunkenness, dry conjunctiva, and decreased or absent tearing, all signs of fluid volume deficit. Puffy eyelids (periorbital edema or papilledema) are characteristic of fluid volume excess. The client may also have a history of blurred vision.

Jugular and Hand Veins Circulatory volume is assessed by measuring venous filling of the jugular and hand veins. The nurse places the client in a low Fowler's position and then:

1. Palpates the jugular (neck) veins. Fluid volume excess causes a distention in the jugular veins (Figure 23-12).
2. Places the client's hand below heart level and palpates the hand veins. Fluid volume deficit causes decreased venous filling (flat hand veins).

Neuromuscular System Fluid and electrolyte imbalances may cause neuromuscular alterations. The muscles lose their tone and become soft and flabby, and reflexes diminish. Calcium and magnesium imbalances cause an increase in neuromuscular irritability. To assess for neuromuscular irritability, the tests for Chvostek's sign and Trousseau's sign are performed. Other neurological signs of fluid, electrolyte, and acid–base imbalances include inability to concentrate, confusion, and emotional lability.

Diagnostic and Laboratory Data

Laboratory tests can reveal imbalances before clinical symptoms are evident in the client. However, unless clients are having the tests for some other reason, symptoms are detected first.

Hemoglobin and Hematocrit Indices Hematocrit (Hct) is affected by changes in plasma volume. For instance, with severe dehydration and hypovolemic shock, hematocrit increases. Conversely, overhydration decreases hematocrit. The hemoglobin (Hgb) level decreases in the event of severe hemorrhage.

Osmolality Osmolality is a measurement of the total concentration of dissolved particles (solutes) per kilogram of water. Osmolality measurements are per-

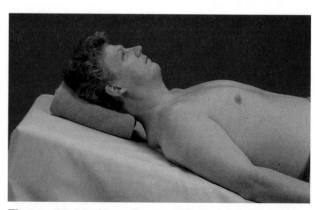

Figure 23-12 Client Position When Assessing Jugular Vein Distention

formed on both serum and urine samples to determine alterations in fluid and electrolyte balance. Osmolality can also be explained in relation to the specific gravity of body fluids. Specific gravity expresses the weight of the solution when compared to an equal volume of distilled water. The osmolality of a solution can be estimated by the specific gravity.

Serum Osmolality Serum osmolality is a measurement of the total concentration of dissolved particles per kilogram of water in serum, recorded in milliosmoles per kilogram (mOsm/kg). The particles measured in serum osmolality include electrolyte ions, such as sodium and potassium, and electrically inactive substances dissolved in serum, such as glucose and urea. Water and sodium are the main entities that control the osmolality of body fluids. Serum sodium is responsible for 85% to 90% of the serum osmolality (McFarland & Grant, 1994). The normal range of serum osmolality is 280 to 295 mOsm/Kg (Noe & Rock, 1994). The value increases with dehydration and decreases with water excess.

In clinical practice, the terms *osmolality* and **osmolarity** (the concentration of solutes per liter of cellular fluid) are often used interchangeably to refer to the concentration of body fluid. However, these terms actually have different meanings, in that *osmolality* refers to the concentration of solutes in the total body water rather than in cellular fluid. The appropriate term to use in conjunction with IV fluid therapy is *osmolarity* (Bulechek & McCloskey, 1999).

Urine Osmolality Urine osmolality is a measurement of the total concentration of dissolved particles per kilogram of water in urine. The particles measured in urine osmolality come from nitrogenous waste (creatinine, urea, and uric acid), with urea being predominant. Urine osmolality varies greatly with diet and fluid intake and reflects the ability of the kidney to adjust the concentration of urine in order to maintain fluid balance. The dehydrated client with normal kidney function will have elevated urine osmolality, whereas the client with shock, hyperglycemia, hemoconcentration, or acidosis will have elevations in both urine and serum osmolalities.

Urine pH The measurement of urine pH reveals the hydrogen ion concentration in the urine, indicating the urine's acidity or alkalinity. When the kidney buffering system is compensating for either metabolic acidosis or alkalosis, the pH of the urine should be within normal range (4.6 to 8.0). This is considered a sign of normal function. However, when the renal compensatory function fails to respond to the blood pH, the urine pH will either increase, with acidosis, or decrease, with alkalosis.

Serum Albumin Albumin is synthesized in the liver from amino acids. Serum albumin plays an important role in fluid and electrolyte balance by maintaining the colloid osmotic pressure of blood, which in turn prevents fluid accumulation (edema) in the tissues. However, serum albumin has a half-life of 21 days and fluctuates according to the level of hydration. Therefore, it is not a good indicator of acute protein depletion. Clinically, this blood test is used to measure prolonged protein depletion, which occurs in chronic malnutrition.

Nursing Diagnosis

NANDA (2001) identifies the primary nursing diagnoses for clients with fluid imbalances as *Excess Fluid Volume, Deficient Fluid Volume, Risk For Deficient Fluid Volume,* and *Risk for Imbalanced Fluid Volume.* Numerous secondary nursing diagnoses may also apply.

Excess Fluid Volume

Excess Fluid Volume exists when the client has edema and increased interstitial and intravascular fluid retention. Fluid volume excess is related to excess fluid in either the tissues of the extremities (peripheral edema) or the lung tissues (pulmonary edema). Factors that put the client at risk for fluid volume excess are:

- Excessive fluid intake (e.g., IV therapy, sodium);
- Excessive loss or decreased intake of protein (chronic diarrhea, burns, kidney disease, malnutrition);
- Compromised regulatory mechanisms (kidney failure);
- Decreased intravascular movement (impaired myocardial contractility);
- Lymphatic obstruction (cancer, surgical removal of lymph nodes, obesity);
- Medications (steroid excess); and
- Allergic reactions.

Assessment findings in the client with fluid volume excess include acute weight gain; decreased serum osmolality (lower than 275 mOsm/Kg), protein and albumin, blood urea nitrogen (BUN), Hgb, Hct; increased central venous pressure (greater than 12 to 15 cm H_2O); and signs and symptoms of edema. The clinical manifestations of edema are relative to the area of involvement, either pulmonary or peripheral (Table 23–4).

PROFESSIONAL TIP

Urine Osmolality

Urine osmolality is a more accurate indicator of hydration than is the specific gravity of urine. Some medications and the presence of protein and glucose solutes in the urine can give a false high specific gravity reading.

Table 23–4 CLINICAL MANIFESTATIONS OF EDEMA	
PULMONARY EDEMA	**PERIPHERAL EDEMA**
Constant cough	Pitting edema in extremities
Dyspnea	Edematous area: tight, smooth
Engorged neck and hand veins	Shiny, pale, cool skin
Moist rales in lungs	Puffy eyelids
Bounding pulse	Weight gain

From Fundamentals of Nursing: Standards & Practice, *by S. DeLaune and P. Ladner, 1998, Albany, NY: Delmar. Copyright 1998 by Delmar. Reprinted with permission.*

Deficient Fluid Volume

Deficient Fluid Volume exists when the client experiences vascular, interstitial, or intracellular dehydration. The degree of dehydration is classified as mild, marked, severe, or fatal on the basis of the percentage of body weight lost. The multiple causes of fluid volume deficit include:

- Excessive fluid loss resulting from diaphoresis, vomiting, diarrhea, hemorrhage, burns, ascites, wound drainage, indwelling tubes, or suction;
- Diabetes insipidus;
- Diabetes mellitus;
- Addison's disease (adrenal insufficiency);
- Gastrointestinal fistula or draining abscess; and
- Intestinal obstruction.

Assessment findings in the client with fluid volume deficit include thirst and weight loss of an amount consistent with the degree of dehydration. Marked dehydration manifests as dry mucous membranes and skin; poor skin turgor; low-grade temperature elevation; tachycardia; respirations of 28 or greater; decreased (10 to 15 mm Hg) systolic blood pressure; slowed venous filling; decreased urine output (fewer than 25 mL/hr); concentrated urine; elevated Hct, Hgb, and BUN; and acidic blood pH (less than 7.4).

Severe dehydration is characterized by the symptoms of marked dehydration plus a flushing of the skin. Systolic blood pressure continues to drop (to 60 mm Hg or below), and behavioral changes (restlessness, irritability, disorientation, and delirium) occur. The signs of fatal dehydration are anuria and coma leading to death.

Risk for Deficient Fluid Volume

Risk for Deficient Fluid Volume exists when the client is at risk of developing vascular, interstitial, or intracellular dehydration resulting from active or regulatory loss of body water in excess of needs. The multiple factors that can place the client at risk for fluid volume deficit were listed previously.

Other Nursing Diagnoses

In clients with a fluid imbalance, the relationship between the primary nursing diagnoses previously discussed and the secondary nursing diagnoses is reciprocal: The primary nursing diagnoses influence and are influenced by the secondary nursing diagnoses. Some commonly identified secondary nursing diagnoses include:

- *Impaired Gas Exchange*
- *Decreased Cardiac Output*
- *Ineffective Breathing Pattern*
- *Anxiety*
- *Disturbed Thought Processes*
- *Risk for Injury*
- *Risk for Infection*
- *Impaired Oral Mucous Membrane*
- *Deficient Knowledge (specify)*

Planning/Outcome Identification

Holistic nursing care for clients experiencing a fluid imbalance requires that the nurse, in collaboration with each client, identify specific goals for each nursing diagnosis. These goals should be individualized to reflect the client's capabilities and limitations and should be appropriate to the diagnosis and the assessment data.

During the planning phase, the nurse also selects and prioritizes nursing interventions to support the client's achievement of expected outcomes based on the goals. For example, if vomiting and diarrhea along with a 5% weight loss and dry mucous membranes led to a nursing diagnosis of *Deficient Fluid Volume,* the goals might include relief from vomiting and diarrhea and achievement of the proper balance of intake and output.

Expected outcomes for the client with a fluid imbalance are not only specific to the primary diagnosis, but also must be relative to the interventions. For example,

PROFESSIONAL TIP

Loss of Gastric Juices

Clients who lose excessive amounts of gastric juices, either through vomiting or suctioning, are prone to not only fluid volume deficit, but also metabolic alkalosis, hypokalemia, and hyponatremia. Gastric juices contain hydrochloric acid, pepsinogen, potassium, and sodium.

an expected outcome for clients receiving IV therapy might be: "IV site remains free of erythema, edema, and purulent drainage" (because these clients are at risk for infection). Achievement of the goals and the client's expected outcomes indicates resolution of the problem.

Implementation

The nurse has a responsibility to collaborate with and advocate for clients to ensure receipt of care that is appropriate, ethical, and based on practice standards. The data obtained from the history serve as the basis for formulating expected outcomes and selecting nursing interventions appropriate to the client's natural patterns as revealed in their history.

The rationale for interventions related to alterations in either fluid, electrolyte, or acid–base balance is based on the goal of maintaining homeostasis and regulating and maintaining essential fluids and nutrients. Clients' adaptive capabilities are kept in mind when selecting interventions based on the clients' perceptions of their support systems, strengths, and options.

Bulechek and McCloskey (1999) address the importance of the nursing interventions relative to fluid therapy by identifying the nurse's responsibilities to:

- Understand the client's metabolic needs and make judgments concerning the outcomes of therapy,
- Perform frequent assessment and monitoring to recognize the adverse effects of fluid and electrolyte therapy and prevent complications, and
- Prevent the rapid depletion of the body's protein and energy reserves.

The nursing activities relative to assessment and implementation often require the same measurements: for example, weight and vital signs. Common interventions that promote attainment of expected outcomes relative to restoring and maintaining homeostasis are discussed following.

Monitor Daily Weight

Daily weight is one of the main indicators of fluid and electrolyte balance. The nurse is responsible for the accurate measurement and recording of the client's daily weight. The physician uses this data along with other clinical findings to determine fluid therapy for the client.

Measure Vital Signs

The frequency with which vital signs are measured depends on the client's acuity level and clinical situation. For example, the vital signs of the typical postoperative client might be taken every 15 minutes until stable, whereas vital signs should be monitored continuously for the client experiencing shock or hemorrhage. Vital sign measurements and other clinical data are used to determine the type and amount of fluid therapy.

PROFESSIONAL TIP

"Strict" I&O

- "Strict" I&O measurement usually involves accounting for incontinent urine, emesis, and diaphoresis and might require weighing soiled bed linens.
- *Gloves should always be worn when handling soiled linen.*

Measure Intake and Output

Intake and output measurements are initiated to monitor the client's fluid status over a 24-hour period. Agency policy relative to I&O may vary with regard to:

- Time frames for charting (e.g., every 8 hours versus every 12 hours),
- Time at which the 24-hour totals are calculated, and
- Definition of "strict" I&O.

 Safety: Removing Gloves Before Charting
To prevent the transfer of microorganisms when the I&O form is removed from the client's room, remove gloves and wash hands before recording the amount of drainage on the form.

The nurse should review the client's 24-hour I&O calculations to evaluate fluid status. Intake should exceed output by 500 mL to offset insensible fluid loss. Intake and output and daily weight are critical components of intervention, because these measurements are also used to evaluate the effectiveness of diuretic or rehydration therapy.

COMMUNITY/HOME HEALTH CARE

Considerations for Measuring I&O
- Elicit client and family member input when selecting household items to be used for intake measurement.
- Provide containers for measuring output, adapting the urinary container to home facilities, and teach client and family about proper washing and storage.
- Teach handwashing technique.
- Provide written instructions on what is to be measured.
- Provide sufficient I&O forms to last between the nurse's visits.
- Identify the parameters for evaluating a discrepancy between the intake and the output and for notifying the nurse or physician.

Securing an accurate I&O requires the full support of the client and family. The client and family members should be taught how to measure and record the I&O.

Provide Oral Hygiene

The nurse is responsible for providing oral hygiene to promote both client comfort and the integrity of the buccal cavity. The frequency of oral hygiene depends on the condition of the client's buccal cavity and the type of fluid imbalance. A client who is dehydrated or permitted no oral fluids for more than 24 hours may have decreased or absent salivation, coated tongue, and furrows on the tongue. Such clients are at risk for developing oral diseases such as stomatitis, oral lesions or ulcers, and gingivitis.

Initiate Oral Fluid Therapy

Oral fluids may be totally restricted—a situation commonly referred to as *nothing by mouth* (NPO, which is from the Latin *non per os*)—or they may be restricted or forced, depending on the client's clinical situation.

Nothing by Mouth Clients are placed on NPO status as prescribed by the physician. On the basis of agency policy and clarification from the physician, the client may be allowed small amounts of ice chips when designated NPO. Common clinical situations that may require NPO status include the need to:

- Avoid aspiration in unconscious, perioperative, and preprocedural clients who will receive anesthesia or conscious sedation;
- Rest and heal the GI tract in clients with severe vomiting or diarrhea or a GI disorder (inflammation or obstruction);
- Prevent the further loss of gastric juices in clients on nasogastric suctioning.

Clients designated NPO should receive oral hygiene every 1 to 2 hours or as needed for comfort and to prevent alterations of the mucous membranes.

Restricted Fluids Fluid intake is commonly restricted in the treatment of fluid volume excess related to heart and renal failure. Intake may be restricted to 200 mL in a 24-hour period. Client and family teaching and collaboration are the main nursing interventions in implementing this measure.

The way fluids are limited should be determined in collaboration with the client. For example:

- Half of the allowed fluid might be divided between breakfast and lunch and
- The remaining half might be divided between the evening meal and before bedtime, unless the client must be awakened during the night for medication.

Forced Fluids "Forcing" or encouraging the intake of oral fluids, mainly water, is sometimes done when treating clients who are at risk for dehydration or who have renal and urinary problems (kidney stones). Compliance is obtained through client education and honoring client preference relative to timing and the type of liquids. A client might, for example, be requested to consume 2,000 mL over a 24-hour period. If the client is intimidated at hearing this amount, which may sound very large, the nurse might explain that the number of glasses to which this volume equates is only eight. This would roughly translate into one glass every 2 hours. The nurse could also tell the client that ice, gelatin, soups, and ice cream all count as liquid.

Maintain Tube Feeding

When the client cannot ingest oral fluids but has a normal GI tract, fluids and nutrients can be administered through a feeding tube as prescribed by a physician.

Monitor Intravenous Therapy

When fluid loss is severe or the client cannot tolerate oral or tube feedings, fluid volume is replaced parenterally through the IV route. **Intravenous** (IV) **therapy** is the administration of fluids, electrolytes, nutrients, or medications by the venous route. The physician prescribes IV therapy to treat or prevent fluid, electrolyte, or nutritional imbalances. The nurse has specific responsibilities relative to IV therapy. Specifically, the nurse must:

- Know why the therapy is prescribed;
- Document client understanding;
- Select the appropriate equipment according to agency policy;
- Obtain the correct solution as prescribed;
- Assess the client for allergies relative to tape, iodine, ointment, or antibiotic preparations to be used for skin preparation of the venipuncture site;
- Administer the fluid at the prescribed rate;
- Observe for signs of **infiltration** (seepage of the fluid into the interstitial tissue as a result of accidental dislodgement of the needle from the vein) and other complications that are fluid specific; and
- Document in the client's medical record the implementation of the prescribed IV therapy.

Evaluation

Evaluation is an ongoing process for clients with fluid, electrolyte, or acid–base imbalances. When evaluating whether the time frames and expected outcomes are realistic (such as whether the intake and output are within 200 to 300 mL of each other), the focus should be on the client's responses. The client's vital signs should be within normal limits. The IV infusion rate should be accurately calculated and reassessed throughout therapy to maintain the client's hydration. The IV site should remain free from erythema, edema, and purulent drainage. The nursing care plan should be modified as necessary to support the client's expected outcomes.

SAMPLE NURSING CARE PLAN

THE CLIENT WITH EXCESS FLUID VOLUME

When brought to the emergency department by his granddaughter, Mr. Gomez, a 68-year-old widower, stated, "I can't breathe." Mr. Gomez has a history of hypertension and heart disease, and he is obese. The practitioner ordered a stat chest x-ray, CBC, and electrolytes, which revealed pulmonary congestion (x-ray), decreased Hct, and decreased Hgb. The physical assessment results were as follows: Wt 162; TPR 97.6, 98, 30 (labored); BP 186/114; shortness of breath, crackles; constant cough; pitting edema (ankles); and engorged neck veins. Mr. Gomez stated, "I thought I could stop taking the heart medication and eat what I wanted when I felt good again."

Nursing Diagnosis 1 *Excess Fluid Volume related to a compromised regulatory mechanism as evidenced by edema, shortness of breath, crackles, decreased Hgb and Hct, and jugular vein distention*

PLANNING/GOALS	NURSING INTERVENTIONS	RATIONALE	EVALUATION
Mr. Gomez will have a balanced I&O for 2 days.	Measure and document hourly I&O; restrict fluids as ordered	Monitors fluid status	Output for the first 3 hours was 2,020 mL; on day two, I&O was indicative of fluid balance.
	Administer diuretics as ordered and document response	Increases excretion of fluids and electrolytes	
Mr. Gomez will identify a specific amount of weight to lose over the next 6 months.	Weigh daily at the same time, with the same scale, and with Mr. Gomez wearing the same clothing	Allows weight to be compared from one day to another	Mr. Gomez identified the need to lose 30 pounds over the next 6 months.
	Discuss with Mr. Gomez the need for weight loss	Allows Mr. Gomez to voice his thoughts about weight loss and provides an avenue to determine number of pounds to be lost	

continues

Mr. Gomez will show normal hydration status prior to discharge.	Measure and document vital signs every hour until shortness of breath subsides, then every 2 hours	Monitors Mr. Gomez's response to therapy	Mr. Gomez demonstrated normal hydration status, as shown by normal levels of Hct and Hgb; BP 156/92; normal breath sounds; and absence of shortness of breath, jugular engorgement, and peripheral edema.
	Hourly assess heart sounds; breath sounds; rate, rhythm, and depth of respirations; and the position Mr. Gomez takes to relieve the shortness of breath	Provides information for use in modifying the plan of care	

Nursing Diagnosis 2 *Deficient Knowledge related to information misinterpretation as evidenced by Mr. Gomez's statement "I thought I could stop taking the heart medication and eat what I wanted when I felt good again."*

PLANNING/GOALS	NURSING INTERVENTIONS	RATIONALE	EVALUATION
Mr. Gomez will demonstrate an understanding of the causes of fluid excess and the role of heart medications, foods, and exercise in assisting with weight reduction.	Assess Mr. Gomez's knowledge of hypertension; decreased cardiac output; digitalis; the effects of a large abdominal girth on breathing; and foods low in sodium, fats, and carbohydrates.	Provides a basis for educating Mr. Gomez about causes, aggravating and alleviating factors, and effects of fluid excess	Mr. Gomez was unable to verbalize understanding of the way that weight, high-sodium diet, and failure to take his heart medications caused the fluid excess. He was referred to home health for client teaching.

SUMMARY

- Homeostasis is the maintenance of the body's internal environment within a narrow range of normal values. It is an ongoing process, with changes constantly occurring in the body.
- Many chemical and physical processes are necessary for homeostasis.
- Ions are electrically charged atoms.
- Compounds that ionize in water are called electrolytes.
- The normal range of blood pH is 7.35 to 7.45. A decrease or increase beyond this range can cause severe or even fatal physiologic problems.
- The bicarbonate buffer system works to regulate pH in both intracellular and extracellular fluids.
- The phosphate buffer system works to regulate the pH of intracellular fluid and fluid in kidney tubules.

- Protein buffers work to regulate pH inside cells, especially red blood cells.
- Substances move in and out of cells by the passive transport methods of diffusion, osmosis, and filtration and by active transport.
- The kidneys regulate fluid and electrolyte balance.
- Sodium is the main electrolyte that promotes the retention of water.
- The slightest decrease or increase in electrolyte levels can cause serious, adverse, or life-threatening effects on physiologic functions.
- Hospitalized clients, especially elderly clients, are at risk for developing dehydration.
- Clients receiving IV therapy require constant monitoring for complications.

CASE STUDY

Mrs. Meisenbach is a 75-year-old woman with diabetes who has been experiencing flu-like symptoms of vomiting and diarrhea for 5 days. She lives alone and does not like to cook. When she got up this morning, she felt weak and dizzy. She called 911 to take her to the clinic. The emergency medical technicians called the practitioner en route, and Mrs. Meisenbach was taken directly to the infusion center, where 1,000 mL of lactated Ringer's solution was started. Later, she was given Gatorade to drink.
Assessment data revealed:

- *Marked thirst*
- *Temperature 99°F*
- *BP 94/74, Resp. 30*
- *Wt 157 lb (loss from 165)*
- *Dry mucous membranes*
- *Apical pulse 108/min*
- *Increased Hct, Hgb, and BUN*

The following questions will guide your development of a nursing care plan for the case study.

1. What other data would you collect?
2. What is the primary nursing diagnosis for Mrs. Meisenbach?
3. What goals would be appropriate for this nursing diagnosis?
4. Identify the nursing interventions and rationale to meet the goals.
5. Ascertain the fluid intake replacement needed. Include the IV and oral fluids.
6. On the basis of the intake, what should have been her output prior to discharge?

Review Questions

1. The basic unit of an element is:
   a. an atom.
   b. the nucleus.
   c. an electron.
   d. small groups of atoms called molecules.

2. The phosphate buffer system is involved in regulating the pH of the:
   a. carbonic acid in the lungs.
   b. carbon dioxide in the lungs.
   c. bicarbonate ions in the lungs.
   d. intracellular fluid and the fluid in the kidney tubules.

3. Diffusion is:
   a. the movement of molecules from a region of high concentration to a region of low concentration.
   b. the movement of molecules from a region of low concentration to a region of high concentration.
   c. the movement of a liquid from a region of high concentration through a membrane to a region of low concentration.
   d. the movement of a liquid from a region of low concentration through a membrane to a region of high concentration.

4. When gas is exchanged in the lungs:
   a. carbon dioxide concentration is equal in the alveoli and lungs.
   b. oxygen concentration is higher in the alveoli than in the blood.
   c. oxygen concentration is higher in the blood than in the alveoli.
   d. carbon dioxide has a higher concentration in the alveoli than in the blood.

5. When blood flows into a capillary bed, the pressure of the blood is:
   a. high in the venule.
   b. low in the arteriole.
   c. high in the arteriole.
   d. low but increases to high.

6. Acidosis and alkalosis are identified by changes in the pH. Which of the following statements is true?

    a. A pH above 7.45 is called acidosis.
    b. A pH above 7.45 is called alkalosis.
    c. A pH increase caused by an increase of bicarbonate in the blood is metabolic acidosis.
    d. A pH decrease caused by an accumulation of carbonic acid results in respiratory alkalosis.

7. The maximum amount of IV potassium chloride that can be infused per hour is:

    a. 5 mEq.
    b. 10 mEq.
    c. 15 mEq.
    d. 20 mEq.

Critical Thinking Questions

1. A client has been vomiting for 3 days and is unable to keep anything down. Besides fluid volume deficit, what other alterations would you expect to find?

2. Because half of serum calcium is bound to another solute in the blood, which other serum level must be considered when monitoring the serum level of calcium?

 WEB FLASH!

- Visit the Intravenous Nurses Society site for standards for IV therapy; certification information; and education.
- Look on the Web for information about IV therapy.

MEDICATION ADMINISTRATION

MAKING THE CONNECTION

Refer to the following chapters to increase your understanding of medication administration:

- **Chapter 6, Legal Responsibilities**
- **Chapter 10, Documentation**
- **Chapter 18, Basic Nutrition**
- **Chapter 21, Infection Control/Asepsis**
- **Chapter 22, Standard Precautions and Isolation**
- **Chapter 27, Diagnostic Tests**
- **Procedures:** B28, Administering a Large Enema/Small (Mini) Enema; B29, Measuring

Intake and Output; I9, Administering an Oral Medication; I10, Withdrawing Medication from an Ampule; I11, Withdrawing Medication from a Vial; I12, Administering an Intradermal Injection; I13, Administering a Subcutaneous Injection; I14, Administering an Intramuscular Injection; I15, Administering an Eye Medication; I16, Instilling an Ear Medication; A6, Administering Medications by IV Piggyback to an Existing IV

LEARNING OBJECTIVES

Upon completion of this chapter, you should be able to:
- *Define key terms.*
- *Describe the influence of drug standards and legislation on medication administration.*
- *Explain the principles of pharmacokinetics, including absorption, distribution, metabolism, and excretion of drugs.*
- *Describe factors that can affect a drug's action.*
- *Explain the different types of medication orders, when each is used, and the nurse's responsibilities for each type.*
- *Discuss principles of safe medication administration.*
- *Discuss potential liabilities for the nurse administering medications.*
- *Develop teaching guidelines for clients regarding medication administration in the home.*
- *Explain procedures for the different methods of medication administration, including the choice of route and site.*

KEY TERMS

absorption	intracath
angiocatheter	intradermal (ID)
aspiration	intramuscular (IM)
bioavailability	intravenous (IV)
butterfly needle	IV push (bolus)
chemical name	metabolism
distribution	onset of action
drug allergy	parenteral
drug incompatibility	patency
drug interaction	peak plasma level
drug tolerance	pharmacokinetics
enteral instillation	phlebitis
excretion	piggyback
flashback	plateau
flow rate	stock supply
generic name	subcutaneous (SC/SQ)
half-life	toxic effect
hypervolemia	trade (brand) name
idiosyncratic reaction	unit dose form
implantable port	vesicant
infiltration	

INTRODUCTION

Medication management requires the collaborative efforts of many health care providers. Medications may be prescribed by a physician, dentist, or other authorized prescriber such as advanced practice registered nurses as determined by individual state licensing bodies. Pharmacists are licensed to prepare and dispense medications. Nurses are responsible for administering medications. Dietitians are often involved in identifying possible food and drug interactions.

Medication administration requires specialized knowledge, judgment, and nursing skills based on the principles of pharmacology. The focus of this chapter is to assist the student in applying knowledge of pharmacology and in acquiring skills in the safe administration of medications. The nursing process is used to direct nursing decisions relative to safe drug administration and to ensure compliance with standards of practice.

DRUG STANDARDS AND LEGISLATION

A drug is a chemical substance intended to elicit a specific effect. An assumption made by nurses before administration of any medication is that the drug will be safe for the client to consume if the dose, frequency, and route are within the therapeutic range for that drug. This assumption is implied in accord with standards that are set to ensure drug uniformity in strength, purity, efficacy, safety, and **bioavailability** (readiness to produce a drug effect).

Standards

Standards have been developed to ensure drug uniformity so that effects are predictable. The *United States Pharmacopeia* and the *National Formulary* (USP and NF) are books of drug standards for use in the United States. The USP and NF list drugs that have been recognized as being in compliance with legal standards of purity, quality, and strength.

The USP has been providing standards for pharmaceutical preparations since its first edition was published in 1851. The NF was first published in 1898 by the American Pharmaceutical Association to provide a listing of drugs that complied with established standards.

Legislation

The Pure Food and Drug Act of 1906 designated the USP and the NF as the official bodies to establish drug standards. It also gave the federal government the authority to enforce these standards. The federal Food, Drug, and Cosmetic Act of 1938 empowered the Food and Drug Administration (FDA) to test all new drugs for toxicity before granting the pharmaceutical com-

pany the approval to market a drug. The federal Food, Drug, and Cosmetic Act of 1938 was amended in 1952 to distinguish prescription (legend) drugs from nonprescription (over-the-counter) drugs and to regulate the dispensing of prescriptions. Testing for drug effectiveness materialized with the Kefauver-Harris Act of 1962 (Lehne, 1998).

The Harrison Narcotic Act of 1914 classified habit-forming drugs as narcotics and began regulating these substances. This law and other drug abuse laws have been replaced with the Comprehensive Drug Abuse Prevention and Control Act (Controlled Substance Act) of 1970. This act defines a *drug-dependent person* in terms of physical and psychological dependence and provides for strict regulation of narcotics and other controlled drugs such as barbiturates through the establishment of five categories of scheduled drugs (see Table 24–1). Any controlled substance must be recorded by the dispensing pharmacist. The Drug Enforcement Agency (DEA) employs pharmacists to inspect all types of records, including prescriptions, to detect the illicit distribution of these substances.

The scheduling of controlled substances must be adhered to by all states as minimum standards; however, an individual state can enact stricter control of these substances. For example, the Controlled Substance Act has codeine in antitussives as a schedule V

Table 24–1 CONTROLLED SUBSTANCES

Schedule (C-I): Includes substances for which there is a high abuse potential and no current approved medical use (e.g., heroin, marijuana, LSD, other hallucinogens, certain opiates and opium derivatives).

Schedule (C-II): Includes drugs that have a high abuse potential and a high ability to produce physical and/or psychological dependence and for which there is a current approved or acceptable medical use.

Schedule (C-III): Includes drugs for which there is less potential for abuse than drugs in Schedule II and for which there is a current approved medical use. Certain drugs in this category are preparations containing limited quantities of codeine. Also, anabolic steroids are classified in Schedule III.

Schedule (C-IV): Includes drugs for which there is a relatively low abuse potential and for which there is a current approved medical use.

Schedule (C-V): Drugs in this category consist mainly of preparations containing limited amounts of certain narcotic drugs for use as antitussives and antidiarrheals. Federal law provides that limited quantities of these drugs (e.g., codeine) may be bought without a prescription by an individual at least 18 years of age. The product must be purchased from a pharmacist, who must keep appropriate records. However, state laws vary, and in many states such products require a prescription.

From PDR Nurse's Handbook 2002 *by G. Spratto & A. Woods, 2002, Albany, NY: Delmar. Copyright 2002 by Delmar.*

drug, but an individual state that identifies abuse of antitussives with codeine may place this drug in the schedule II category, which is more restrictive.

DRUG NOMENCLATURE

A drug may be used as an aid in the diagnosis, treatment, or prevention of disease or under other conditions for the relief of pain or suffering or to improve any physiologic or pathological condition. The terms *drug, medication,* and *medicine* are often used interchangeably by health care providers and laypersons.

Drugs can be identified by their chemical, generic, official, or trade name. The **chemical name** is a precise description of the drug's composition (chemical formula). The *nonproprietary,* or **generic**, **name** in the United States is the name assigned by the U.S. Adopted Names Council to the manufacturer who first develops the drug. When the drug is approved, it is given an *official name,* which may be the same as the nonproprietary name (Lehne, 1998). Drugs with a proven therapeutic value are listed in the USP and NF by their official name. When pharmaceutical companies market the drug, they assign a *proprietary name,* also called a **trade (brand) name**; therefore, one generic drug may have several trade names based on the number of companies marketing the drug. For example, ibuprofen is a generic name; common trade names for this drug are Advil, Excedrin IB, Motrin, and Nuprin. Generic names are not capitalized, but trade names are always capitalized.

DRUG ACTION

Drug action refers to a drug's ability to combine with a cellular drug receptor. Depending on the location of different cellular receptors affected by a given drug, a drug can have a local effect, a systemic effect, or both local and systemic effects. For example, when diphenhydramine hydrochloride (Benadryl) cream is applied to the skin, it elicits only a local effect; however, when this drug is administered in a tablet or injectable form, it causes both systemic and local effects.

Pharmacology

Pharmacology is the study of the effects of drugs on living organisms. This section discusses the pharmacological activities of drug action as it is related to medication management, drug classification, drug preparation, and routes of administration.

Medication Management

The purpose of medication management is to produce the desired drug action by maintaining a constant drug level. Drug action is based on the half-life of a drug. A drug's **half-life** refers to the time it takes the body to eliminate half of the blood concentration level of the original drug dose. For example, if a drug has a half-life of 6 hours, 50% of the drug's original dose is present in the blood 6 hours after administration; in 12 hours after administration, 25% of the drug is present. Because of a drug's half-life, repeated doses are often required to maintain the drug level over a 24-hour interval.

The nurse should understand other terms used to describe drug action: onset, peak plasma level, and plateau. **Onset of action** is the time it takes the body to respond to a drug after administration. A **peak plasma level** is the highest blood concentration of a single drug dose before the elimination rate equals the rate of absorption. Once the peak plasma level is achieved, the blood concentration level will decrease steadily unless another drug dose is given. If a series of scheduled drug doses is administered, the blood concentration level is maintained; maintenance of a certain level is called a **plateau**.

Classification

Drugs are commonly classified by the body system with which they interact (e.g., cardiovascular) or in accord with the drug's approved therapeutic usage (e.g., antihypertensive). Drugs with multiple therapeutic uses are usually classified in accordance with their most common usage.

Preparation and Route

Drugs are available in many forms for administration by a specific route (Table 24–2). The route refers to how the drug is absorbed: oral, buccal, sublingual, rectal, parenteral, topical, and respiratory.

 Safety: Do Not Substitute Drug Forms Drugs prepared for administration by one route should not be substituted by administering the drug prepared for another route. For example, when a client has difficulty swallowing a large tablet or capsule, the nurse should not administer an oral solution or elixir of the same drug without first consulting the physician because a liquid may be more easily and completely absorbed, producing a higher blood level than would a tablet.

Oral Route Most drugs are administered by the oral route because it is the safest, most convenient, and least expensive method. The disadvantage of the oral route is that it acts more slowly than the other routes, such as injectables. Drugs may not be given orally to clients with gastrointestinal intolerance or those on NPO (nothing by mouth) status. Oral administration is also precluded by coma.

Table 24–2 TYPES OF DRUG PREPARATIONS

TYPE	DESCRIPTION
Oral Solids	• Tablets: compressed or molded substances, to be swallowed whole, chewed before swallowing, or placed in the buccal pocket or under the tongue (sublingual)
	• Capsules: substances encased in either a hard or a soft soluble container or gelatin shell that dissolves in the stomach
	• Caplets: gelatin-coated tablets that dissolve in the stomach
	• Powders and granules: finely ground substances
	• Troches, lozenges, and pastilles: preparations designed to dissolve in the mouth
	• Enteric-coated tablets: coated tablets that dissolve in the intestines
	• Time-release capsules: encased substances that are further enclosed in smaller casings that deliver a drug dose over an extended period of time
	• Sustained-release: compounded substances designed to release a drug slowly to maintain a steady blood medication level
Topicals	• Liniments: substances mixed with an alcohol, oil, or soapy emollient that is applied to the skin
	• Ointments: semisolid substances for topical use
	• Pastes: semisolid substances, thicker than ointments, absorbed slowly through the skin
	• Suppositories: gelatin substances designed to dissolve when inserted in the rectum, urethra, or vagina
Inhalants	• Inhalations: drugs or dilutions of drugs administered by the nasal or oral respiratory route for a local or systemic effect
Solutions	• Solutions: contain one or more soluble chemical substances dissolved in water
	• Enemas: aqueous solutions for rectal instillation
	• Douches: aqueous solutions that function as a cleansing or antiseptic agent that may be dispensed in the form of a powder with directions for dissolving in a specific quantity of warm water
	• Suspensions: particles or powder substances that must be mixed with, not dissolved in, a liquid by shaking vigorously before administration
	• Emulsions: two-phase systems in which one liquid is dispersed in the form of small droplets throughout another liquid
	• Syrups: substances dissolved in a sugar liquid
	• Gargles: aqueous solutions
	• Mouthwashes: aqueous solutions that may contain alcohol, glycerin, and synthetic sweeteners and surface-active flavoring and coloring agents
	• Nasal solutions: aqueous solutions in the form of drops or sprays
	• Optic (eye) and otic (ear) solutions: aqueous solutions that are instilled as drops
	• Elixirs: solutions that contain water, varying amounts of alcohol, and sweeteners

From Fundamentals of Nursing: Standards & Practice *by S. DeLaune and P. Ladner, 1998, Albany, NY: Delmar. Copyright 1998 by Delmar. Adapted with permission.*

PROFESSIONAL TIP

Special Considerations Regarding Medication Administration

• Chewable tablets are designed to be chewed before swallowing because chewing enhances gastric absorption.

• Buccal and sublingual medications must be allowed to dissolve completely before the client can drink or eat.

• Suspensions and emulsions should be administered immediately after shaking and pouring from the bottle.

When small amounts of drugs are required, the buccal or sublingual route is used. Drugs administered through these routes act quickly because of the oral mucosa's thin epithelium and large vascular system, which allows the drug to quickly be absorbed by the blood.

Certain oral drugs are prepared for sublingual or buccal administration to prevent their destruction or transformation in the stomach or small intestines. Buccal drugs are designed to be placed in the buccal pocket (superior-posterior aspect of the internal cheek next to the molars) for absorption by the mucous membrane of the mouth. Sublingual medications are designed to dissolve quickly when placed under the tongue. For example nitroglycerin (Nitrostat), an antianginal drug, can be given either sublingually or buccally as prescribed, whereas isoproterenol hydrochloride (Isuprel), a bronchodilator, is given sublingually and methyltesterone (Testred), an androgen, is given only buccally.

Parenteral Route Parenteral drugs are administered with sterile technique by injectable routes. By definition, **parenteral** route refers to any route other than the oral-gastrointestinal tract; however, the medical usage of the term excludes topical administration. There are four routes that nurses routinely use to administer parenteral medications:

- **Intradermal** (ID) is an injection into the dermis.
- **Subcutaneous** (SC or SQ) is an injection into the subcutaneous tissue.
- **Intramuscular** (IM) is an injection into the muscle.
- **Intravenous** (IV) is an injection into a vein.

Other parenteral routes, such as intrathecal or intraspinal, intracardiac, intrapleural, intra-arterial, and intra-articular, are used by physicians and in some cases by advanced practice registered nurses for medication administration.

Topical Route Most topical drugs are given to deliver a drug at, or immediately beneath, the point of application. Although a large number of topical drugs are applied to the skin, other topical drugs include eye, nose and throat, ear, rectal, and vaginal preparations. Drugs directly applied to the skin are absorbed through the epidermal layer into the dermis, where they create local effects or are absorbed into the bloodstream. Drug action varies with the vascularity of the skin, usually requiring several applications over a 24-hour period to cause the desired therapeutic effect.

Transdermal patches, another type of topical preparation, are used to deliver medications such as nitroglycerin (Transdermal-NTG), an antianginal, and certain supplemental hormone replacements for absorption by the blood to produce systemic effects. Some topical drugs, such as eye and nasal drops and vaginal and rectal suppositories, can be applied directly to the mucous membranes. These drugs are absorbed quickly into the bloodstream, and, depending on the drug's dose (strength and quantity), may cause systemic effects.

Inhalants Inhalants such as oxygen and most general anesthetics deliver gaseous or volatile substances that are almost immediately absorbed into the systemic circulation. The inhalants are delivered into the alveoli of the lungs, which promote fast absorption due to:

- Permeability of the alveolar and vascular epithelium
- Abundant blood flow
- Very large surface area for absorption

Oropharyngeal handheld inhalers deliver topical drugs to the respiratory tract to create local and systemic effects. There are three types of inhalers: the metered-dose inhaler, or nebulizer; the turbo-inhaler; and the nasal inhaler. They are explained later in this chapter.

Pharmacokinetics

Pharmacokinetics refers to the study of the absorption, distribution, metabolism, and excretion of drugs to determine the relationship between the dose of a drug and the drug's concentration in biological fluids. Knowledge of pharmacokinetics is used by health care providers in medication management.

The physician, when ordering a drug, is concerned mainly with determining the dose and route that will produce the most therapeutic effects; physicians, pharmacists, and nurses are all involved in identifying appropriate times for drug administration and for avoiding interactions with other substances that could alter the drug's actions. Physicians and nurses monitor the client's response to the drug's action. Drug actions are dependent on four properties: absorption, distribution, metabolism, and excretion.

Absorption

The degree and rate of **absorption**, or passage of a drug from the site of administration into the bloodstream, depend on several factors: the drug's physicochemical effects, its dosage form, its route of administration, its interactions with other substances in the digestive system, and various client characteristics such as age (Springhouse, 2000). Oral preparations, such as tablets and capsules, must first disintegrate into smaller particles for gastric juices to dissolve and prepare the drug for absorption in the small intestines.

Drugs administered intramuscularly are absorbed through the muscle into the bloodstream. Suppositories are absorbed through the mucous membranes into the blood. Intravenous drugs are immediately bioavailable because of their direct injection into the blood.

Distribution

Distribution refers to the movement of drugs from the blood into various body fluids and tissues. The degree of binding between blood proteins and chemical substances can limit the drug's distribution in the body. The actual volume of distribution of any drug can be altered by the client's health condition.

Metabolism

Metabolism refers to the physical and chemical processing of a drug by the body. Most drugs are metabolized in the liver. The rate of metabolism is determined by the presence of enzymes in the liver cells that detoxify the drugs. Certain drugs can also increase the rate of metabolism.

Excretion

Excretion is the elimination of drugs from the body. This occurs mainly through hepatic metabolism and renal excretion. Other organs such as the lungs, exocrine glands, skin, and intestinal tract can eliminate some drugs.

Drug Interaction

Drug interaction refers to the effect one drug can have on another drug. Drug interactions may occur when one drug is administered in combination with a second drug or a short time interval exists between the administration of two different drugs. Drugs can be combined deliberately to produce a positive effect; for example, hydrochlorothiazide (HydroDIURIL), a potassium-depleting diuretic, and spironolactone (Aldactone), a potassium-sparing diuretic, can be combined to maintain a normal blood level of potassium. A positive drug combination can also occur when one drug is deliberately given to potentiate the action of another drug, as in preoperative medications.

Not all drug combinations are therapeutic. Some drug combinations can interfere with the absorption, effect, or excretion of other drugs. For example, calcium products and magnesium-containing antacids can cause inadequate absorption of tetracycline (Tetracyn), an antibiotic, in the digestive tract.

Side Effects and Adverse Reactions

Drug effects other than those that are therapeutically intended and expected are called *adverse reactions*. A nontherapeutic effect may be mild and predictable (side effect) or unexpected and potentially hazardous (adverse effect). There are several types of adverse reactions: drug allergy, drug tolerance, toxic effect, and idiosyncratic reactions.

A **drug allergy** (hypersensitivity to a drug) is an antigen-antibody immune reaction that occurs when an individual who has been previously exposed to a drug has developed antibodies against the drug. The type of reaction may be mild (skin rash, urticaria, headache, nausea, or vomiting) or severe (anaphylaxis). Drug reactions are often manifested in the skin because of its abundant blood supply.

Anaphylaxis is an immediate, life-threatening reaction to a drug, such as penicillin, characterized by respiratory distress, sudden severe bronchospasm, and cardiovascular collapse. If emergency measures are not instituted immediately (administration of epinephrine, bronchodilators, and antihistamines), anaphylaxis can be fatal.

Drug tolerance occurs when the body becomes so accustomed to a specific drug that larger doses are needed to produce the desired therapeutic effect. For example, clients with cancer who experience severe pain may require larger and larger doses of morphine (a narcotic analgesic) to control the pain as the body builds up a tolerance to the morphine.

A **toxic effect** occurs when the body cannot metabolize a drug, causing the drug to accumulate in the blood. Toxic reactions can result after prolonged intake of high doses of medication or after only one dose.

An **idiosyncratic reaction** is a highly unpredictable response that may be manifested by an over-response, an underresponse, or an atypical response. For example, 1 of 40,000 clients will develop aplastic anemia after receiving chloramphenicol (an antibiotic) (Springhouse, 2000).

Food and Drug Interactions

Medication management requires avoidance of possible food and drug interactions. There are three primary types of food and drug interactions:

1. Certain drugs may interfere with the absorption, excretion, or use in the body of one or more nutrients.
2. Certain foods may increase or decrease the absorption of a drug into the body.
3. Other foods may alter the chemical actions of drugs, preventing their therapeutic effect on the body.

Most interaction problems occur with the use of diuretics, oral antibiotics, and anticoagulant and antihypertensive drugs. Clients on sodium-restricted diets should be advised to consult with a pharmacist regarding the sodium content in prescription and over-the-counter drugs. Some drugs can contain almost half the total daily allowance of sodium. Alcohol is also considered a drug. Small amounts of alcohol interact with many drugs, such as antibiotics, antihistamines, anticoagulants, and sleeping pills. Food and drug interactions can vary depending on the dose and the form in which the drug is taken and the client's age, gender, body weight, nutritional status, and specific medical condition.

FACTORS INFLUENCING DRUG ACTION

Individual client characteristics such as genetic factors, age, height and weight, and physical and mental conditions can influence the action of drugs on the body. Sometimes mistaken for drug allergies, genetic factors can interfere with drug metabolism and produce an abnormal sensitivity to certain drugs.

The physician often correlates the client's age, height, and weight when determining the dosage for

LIFE CYCLE CONSIDERATIONS

Age-Related Factors Influence Drug Action and Dosing

- Neonates and infants have underdeveloped gastrointestinal systems, muscle mass, and metabolic enzyme systems and inadequate renal function.
- Elderly clients often experience decreased hepatic or renal function and diminished muscle mass.

---

many drugs. The nurse should make sure that this information is accurately recorded in the client's medical record. The amount of body fat may also alter drug distribution because some drugs such as digoxin (Digoxin), an inotropic drug, are poorly distributed to fatty tissues.

The client's physical condition can also alter the effects of drugs. For example, the drug must be distributed to a larger volume of body fluids in an edematous client than in a nonedematous client; therefore, the edematous client may require a larger drug dose to produce the drug action, whereas a dehydrated client would require a smaller dosage. Diseases that affect liver and renal functions can alter the metabolism and elimination of most drugs.

MEDICATION ORDERS

In health care settings (long-term care facilities and hospitals), medication orders are written on a physician's order form in each client's medical record. When a client is admitted to an inpatient health care facility, the drug order form is stamped with the client's name, room number, age, and weight. The client's weight will be used by the pharmacist in compounding and dispensing drugs.

All orders should be written clearly and legibly, and the drug order should contain seven parts:

1. The name of the client
2. The date and time when the order is written
3. The name of the drug to be administered
4. The dosage
5. The route by which it is to be administered and special directives about its administration
6. The time of administration and frequency
7. The signature of the person writing the order, such as the physician or advanced practice registered nurse

Drug prescriptions written in settings other than acute care facilities may also specify whether the generic or trade name of the drug is to be dispensed, the quantity to be dispensed, and how many times the prescription can be refilled.

The nurse is responsible and held accountable for questioning any medication order if, in the nurse's judgment, the order is in error. The nature of the error may be in any part of the drug order, and the nurse should seek clarification from the physician as necessary. A drug error has serious legal implications if the nurse involved could have been expected, on the basis of knowledge and experience, to have noted the error.

Most agencies have policies relative to medication administration, such as stop dates for certain types of drugs, regularly scheduled times to administer medications as specified in the drug order, and a listing of abbreviations officially accepted for use in the agency. The agency's medical records department maintains the official listing of abbreviations adopted by the medical staff of that agency. Only abbreviations from the official list can be used in any part of the client's medical record at that agency (see appendices).

Types of Orders

Medications are prescribed in different ways, depending on their purpose. Medications can be prescribed as stat, single-dose, scheduled, and prn orders.

Stat Orders

Stat medication orders are those that should be administered immediately, not an hour or two later. Stat drugs are often prescribed in emergency situations to modify a serious physiologic response such as a stat dose of nitroglycerin for a client experiencing chest pain. The nurse should assess and document the client's response to all stat medications.

Single-Dose Orders

Single-dose orders are one-time medications. The nurse should administer single-dose orders either at a time specified by the physician or at the earliest convenient time. These drugs are often prescribed in preparation for a diagnostic or therapeutic procedure; for example, a laxative may be administered in preparation for a lower GI x-ray.

Scheduled Orders

Scheduled orders are administered routinely as specified until the order is canceled by another order. The scheduled orders stay in effect until the physician discontinues or modifies the dosage or frequency with another order or until a prescribed number of days have elapsed as determined by agency policy. The purpose of a scheduled medication order is to maintain the desired blood level of the medication.

Agency policy determines the actual times for administering medications over a 24-hour time interval. For example, t.i.d. drugs may be administered at 0800, 1400, and 2000 or at 0900, 1500, and 2100. Medications ordered qd may have a specified time identified in the order, such as Isophane (NPH) Insulin 10 U SC qd at 0600, or they may be given at the agency's designated time, for example, Lanoxin 0.25 mg po qd would be given at 0900.

When the order specifies the number of days or dosages of the drug the client is to receive, the order has an automatic stop date to discontinue the drug. For example, the order may read tetracycline 250 mg po q6h for 5 days. The nurse should execute this order by administering 250 mg tetracycline orally every 6 hours for 5 days for a total of 20 doses. Day one begins with the administration of the drug and the time the first dose is given.

PRN Orders

A drug may be ordered on a prn (as needed) basis as circumstances indicate. The drug is administered when, in the nurse's judgment, the client's condition requires it. This type of order is commonly written for analgesics, antiemetics, and laxatives. For example, a client may have an order for meperidine (Demerol), a narcotic analgesic, 75 mg IM q3–4h prn. The nurse administers the pain medication on the basis of the assessment of the client's pain and as specified in the order.

SYSTEMS OF WEIGHT AND MEASURE

Medication administration requires the nurse to have a knowledge of weight and volume measurement systems. In the United States there are three different systems of measurement used in medication management: metric, apothecary, and household.

Metric System

The metric system of weights and measures was adopted by the USP in 1890 to the exclusion of all other systems except for equivalent dosages. The Council on Pharmacy and Chemistry of the American Medical Association adopted the metric system exclusively in 1944. Resistance to changing established customs interfered with the exclusive adoption of the metric system. Today, however, the metric system is used in every major country of the world and is used almost exclusively in health care facilities in the United States (*Remington: The Science and Practice of Pharmacology,* 1995).

The metric or decimal system is a simple system of measurement based on units of 10. The basic units can be multiplied or divided by 10 to form secondary units. The decimal point is moved to the right when changing from a larger unit to a smaller unit, and the decimal point is moved to the left when changing from a smaller unit to a larger unit. For example:

5 g	= 5,000 mg		0.5 mg	= 500 mcg
5 mcg	= 0.005 mg		1.25 L	= 1,250 mL
0.25 g	= 250 mg		2.45 kg	= 2,450 g

The basic units of measurement in the metric system are the meter (linear), the liter (volume), and the gram (mass, or weight). Important metric equivalents and abbreviations to remember are:

- Volume (liquid)

  1 milliliter (mL) = 1 cubic centimeter (cc)

  1,000 milliliters = 1 liter (L)

- Weight

  1,000 micrograms (mcg or μg) = 1 milligram (mg)

  1,000 milligrams = 1 gram (g)

  1,000 grams = 1 kilogram (kg)

The metric system uses prefixes derived from Latin to designate subdivisions of the basic units, and prefixes derived from Greek to designate multiples of the basic units (see Table 24–3).

 Safety: Metric System
A zero is *always* placed in front of the decimal for values less than 1 (0.5) to prevent error.

Apothecary System

The apothecary system, which originated in England, is based on the weight of one grain of wheat. Therefore, the basic unit of weight is the grain (gr) and the basic unit of volume is the minim (the approximate volume of water that weighs a grain). Important apothecary equivalents and abbreviations are:

- Volume (liquid)

  60 minums (𝑚) = 1 fluid dram (fl dr, or ʒ)

  8 fluid drams = 1 fluid ounce (fl oz, or ℥)

  16 fluid ounces = 1 pint (pt)

- Weight

  60 grains (gr) = 1 dram (dr, or ʒ)

  8 drams = 1 ounce (oz, or ℥)

  12 ounces = 1 pound (lb)

Table 24–3 METRIC SYSTEM PREFIXES

PREFIX	EXAMPLE
Latin Prefixes— subdivisions of the basic unit	deci (1/10, or 0.1) centi (1/100, or 0.01) milli (1/1,000, or 0.001) micro (1/1,000,000, or 0.000001)
Greek Prefixes— multiples of the basic unit	deka (10) hecto (100) kilo (1,000)

Household System

The household system of measurement is similar to the apothecary system of liquid measures and is the least accurate of the three systems. It is not ordinarily used in dose calculations, but is used as a reference standard to help the client. The units of liquid measure are drop (gtt), teaspoon (tsp), tablespoon (Tbsp), ounce (oz), and cup (Figure 24-1). The 16-ounce pound of the household system *is* used in dose calculations, with 2.2 lb equal to 1 kg.

The USP recognizes the use of the teaspoon as the ordinary practice for household medication administration and states that the teaspoon may be regarded as representing 5 mL (American Hospital Formulary Service, 1996). Household spoons are not appropriate when accurate measurement of a liquid dose is required; therefore, the USP recommends that a calibrated oral syringe or dropper be used for accurate measurement of liquid drug doses.

Household units are often used to inform clients of the size of a liquid dose and are generally used in the calculation of a client's intake and output. Important household equivalents and abbreviations to remember are:

- Volume (liquid)

60 drops (gtt)	=	1 teaspoon (tsp)
3 tsp	=	1 tablespoon (Tbsp)
2 Tbsp	=	1 ounce (oz)
8 oz	=	1 cup (c)
2 cup	=	1 pint (pt)
2 pints	=	1 quart (qt)

- Weight

16 ounces	=	1 pound (lb)

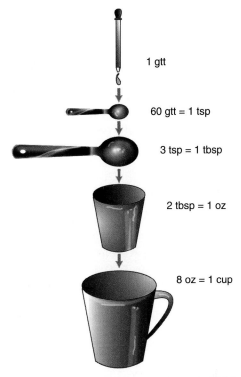

Figure 24-1 Relationship between Household Measures (*From* Medications & Mathematics for the Nurse [8th ed.] by J. Rice, 1998, Albany, NY: Delmar. Copyright 1998 by Delmar. Reprinted with permission.)

APPROXIMATE DOSE EQUIVALENTS

The conversion of metric doses with the apothecary and household systems are *approximate dose equivalents* (Table 24–4). The approximate dose equivalents represent the quantities usually ordered by physicians when using either the metric or apothecary system of

Table 24–4 APPROXIMATE EQUIVALENTS TO THE METRIC SYSTEM

METRIC		APOTHECARY		HOUSEHOLD
Liquid (Volume)				
Liquid	Weight	Liquid	Weight	
0.06 mL	= 60 mg	= 1 ♏	= 1 gr	= 1 gtt
1 mL	= 1 g	= 15–16 ♏	= 15 gr	= 15 gtt
5 mL	= 5 g	= 1 fl dr	= 1 dr	= 1 tsp
15 mL	= 15 g	= 4 fl dr	= 4 dr	= 1 Tbsp
30 mL	= 30 g	= 1 fl oz	= 1 oz	= 1 oz
240 mL	= 240 g	= 8 fl oz	= 8 oz	= 8 oz
380 mL	= 380 g	= 12 fl oz	= 1 lb	= 16 oz
500 mL	= 500 g	= 1 pt	= 16 oz	= 1 pt
1,000 mL	= 1,000 g	= 1 qt	= 32 oz	= 1 qt

Weight	
0.4 mg (400 mcg or μg)	= 1/150 gr
1 mg (1,000 mcg)	= 1/60 gr
4 mg	= 1/15 gr
10 mg	= 1/6 gr
15 mg	= 1/4 gr
30 mg	= 1/2 gr
1000 g (1 kg)	= 2.2 lb

Adapted from Fundamentals of Nursing: Standards & Practice by S. DeLaune and P. Ladner, 1998, Albany, NY: Delmar. Copyright 1998 by Delmar. Adapted with permission.

weights and volumes for drug doses (American Hospital Formulary Service, 1996). If the prepared dosage form is prescribed in the metric system, the pharmacist may dispense the corresponding approximate equivalent in the apothecary system and vice versa. For example, if the physician prescribes morphine gr ¼, the pharmacist may dispense morphine 15 mg. The USP and NF reference *exact equivalents* that must be used to calculate quantities in pharmaceutical formularies and prescription compounding.

Converting Units of Weight and Volume

The nurse has to apply the knowledge of measurement systems and their conversions when the physician prescribes a drug dosage in one system and the pharmacy dispenses the equivalent dose in another. The conversions may be completed with either a proportion or a ratio. For example:

Proportion	Ratio
┌─Means─┐	2 = 6
2 : 4 = 6 : 12	4 12
└──Extremes──┘	

In a proportion, the product (multiplication) of the means equals the product of the extremes. In a ratio, the products of cross-multiplication are equal.

4 × 6 = 24	2 × 12 = 24
2 × 12 = 24	4 × 6 = 24

If one of the terms is unknown, it can be determined by substituting x for the number. The term with the x (unknown) is always put on the left.

2 : x = 6 : 12	2 = 6
	x 12
6x = 24	6x = 24
x = 4	x = 24

Proof that the answer is correct can be determined by substituting the answer for the x and multiplying.

Proportion can be used when converting units of weight and volume, conversions within the metric system, conversions between systems, and in drug dosage calculations. When the physician orders morphine gr ¼ and the pharmacist dispenses morphine 15 mg, the nurse is responsible for ensuring the correct dose. The nurse knows that 1 grain equals 60 milligrams; to convert the ordered dose to milligrams, the nurse should use the following calculation:

$$1 \text{ gr} : 60 \text{ mg} = 1/4 \text{ gr} : x$$

(the grains cancel out)

$$1 x = (60 \text{ mg})(1/4)$$

(divide 60 by 4)

$$x = 15 \text{ mg}$$

Safety: Know What Is Being Calculated
All terms must be labeled (gr, mg, mL, and so on) to avoid errors.

Measurement Conversions within the Metric System

Because the metric system is based on units of 10, dose equivalents within the system are computed by simple arithmetic, either dividing or multiplying. For example, to change milligrams to grams (1,000 mg equals 1 g) or milliliters to liters (1,000 mL equals 1 L), divide the number by 1,000:

$$250 \text{ mg} = x \text{ g}$$

(move the decimal point three places to the left)

$$x = 0.25 \text{ g}$$

or

$$500 \text{ mL} = x \text{ L}$$

(move the decimal point three places to the left)

$$x = 0.5 \text{ L}$$

To convert grams to milligrams or liters to milliliters, the nurse multiplies the number by 1000:

$$0.005 \text{ g} = x \text{ mg}$$

(move the decimal point three places to the right)

$$x = 5 \text{ mg}$$

or

$$0.725 \text{ L} = x \text{ mL}$$

(move the decimal point three places to the right)

$$x = 725 \text{ mL}$$

The nurse may need to convert the volume of liters and milliliters for enemas and irrigating solutions as might be prescribed for bladder and wound irrigations. Intravenous solutions are sterile, prepackaged solutions dispensed in volumes as ordered by the physician, such as 50 mL, 100 mL, 250 mL, 500 mL, or 1,000 mL (1 liter).

Measurement Conversions between Systems

The nurse would have to convert between systems when, for example, the physician orders nitroglycerin (an antianginal drug) gr 1/150 po for chest pain and the dispensed dose is 0.4 mg:

$$1 \text{ gr} : 60 \text{ mg} = 1/150 \text{ gr}: x$$

$$1 \text{ gr } x = (60 \text{ mg})(1/150 \text{ gr})$$

(the grains cancel out)

$$1 x = 60/150 \text{ mg}$$

(divide by 60 by 150)

$$x = 0.4 \text{ mg}$$

The nurse can use proportion when converting pounds to kilograms (2.2 lb = 1 kg). For example, if the client weighs 154 lb, what is the weight in kilograms?

$$2.2 \text{ lb} : 1 \text{ kg} = 154 \text{ lb} : x$$
$$\text{(the pounds cancel out)}$$
$$2.2\, x = 154$$
$$\text{(divide 154 by 2.2)}$$
$$x = 70 \text{ kg}$$

Drug Dose Calculations

Several formulas may be used by the nurse when calculating drug doses. One formula uses ratios based on the *desired dose* and the *dose on hand*. For example, cephalexin hydrochloride (Keftab), an anti-infective cephalosporin, 500 mg po q.i.d. (dose desired) is ordered by the physician; the dose on hand is 250 mg/5 mL. The formula is as follows:

$$\frac{500 \text{ mg (desired dose)}}{250 \text{ mg (dose on hand)}} \times \frac{x \text{ (quantity desired)}}{5\text{mL (quantity on hand)}}$$
$$\text{(cross-multiply)}$$
$$\text{(milligrams cancel out)}$$
$$250\, x = 500 \times 5$$
$$x = \frac{500 \times 5}{250}$$
$$x = 10 \text{ mL}$$

In another example, the physician orders heparin (an anticoagulant) 10,000 units SC; the dose on hand is 40,000 units/mL:

$$\frac{10,000 \text{ units}}{40,000 \text{ units}} \times \frac{x}{1 \text{ mL}}$$
$$\text{(cross-multiply)}$$
$$\text{(units cancel out)}$$
$$40,000\, x = 10,000$$
$$\text{(zeros cancel out)}$$
$$x = \tfrac{1}{4} \text{ mL}$$

Because ¼ mL would be difficult to measure, it is best converted to minums. It is known that 1 mL = 15–16m. It will be best to use 16 so it will come out with a whole number for the answer.

$$1 \text{ mL} : 16m = \tfrac{1}{4} \text{ mL} : x$$
$$\text{(mL cancel out)}$$
$$1\, x = (16)(\tfrac{1}{4})$$
$$x = 4m$$

Pediatric Dosages

"Children are sometimes more susceptible than adults to certain drugs" (*Remington: The Science and Practice of Pharmacology,* 1995, p. 91). Several rules have been devised to calculate infants' and childrens' dosages, such as *Young's Rule, Clark's Rule,* and *Fried's Rule,* but these rules give only approximate dosages. Even when pediatric drug dosages are calculated on body surface area (BSA), they are based on a proportion of the usual adult dose (approximate). Body surface area is considered to be one of the most accurate methods of calculating medication dosages for infants and children up to 12 years of age (Rice, 1998). Regardless of the method used in calculating pediatric drug dosages, the nurse should realize that dosages are approximate and often need adjustment based on the child's response.

Body surface area refers to the square meter surface area method of relating the surface area of individuals to drug dosage. The BSA is based on weight and height and gives an approximate dose by using the following formula:

$$\frac{\text{Body surface area of child}}{\text{Body surface area of adult}} \times \frac{\text{Usual}}{\text{adult}} = \frac{\text{Child's}}{\text{dose}}$$

The BSA of an adult is 1.73 square meters (m²); the 1.73 m² is based on an adult weighing 150 pounds.

A nomogram is used to compute the child's BSA (Figure 24-2). A straight line is drawn from the child's height in the left column to the child's weight in the right column. The point at which this line intersects the body surface area column (designated SA) indicates the child's BSA. For example: A 3-year-old child is 38

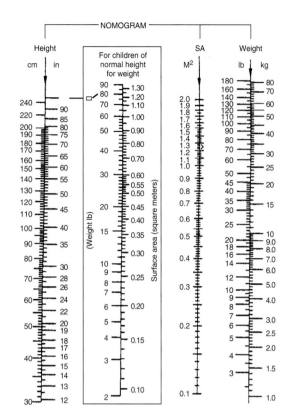

NOMOGRAM

Directions for use: (1) Determine client height. (2) Determine client weight. (3) Draw a straight line to connect the height and weight. Where the line intersects on the SA line is the derived body surface area (M²).

Reprinted with permission from Behrman, R.E., Kliegman, R. and Arvin, A.M., editors. *Nelson Textbook of Pediatrics*, 15th ed. (Philadelphia: W.B. Saunders Company, 1996.)

Figure 24-2 Nomogram for Estimating Body Surface Area (*From* Nelson Textbook of Pediatrics *[15th ed.] by R.E. Behrman, R. Kliegman, & A.M. Arvin, 1996, Philadelphia: Saunders. Copyright 1996 by Saunders. Reprinted with permission.*)

inches tall and weighs 36 pounds. The physician orders meperidine (Demerol) for pain. The average adult dose is 50 mg. How much Demerol should the child receive? From the nomogram the child's BSA is 0.66 m².

$$\frac{0.66 \ (m^2)}{1.73 \ (m^2)} \times 50 \ mg$$

(square meters cancel out)

$$\frac{33}{1.73}$$

(divide 33 by 1.73)

$$= 19.07 \ mg \quad = \quad 19 \ mg$$

Now use the desired dose/dose on hand formula to determine how much to give.

$$\frac{19 \ mg}{50 \ mg} = \frac{x}{1 \ mL}$$

(milligrams cancel out)

(cross-multiply)

$$50x = 19 \ mL$$

$$x = 0.32 \ mL$$

This will have to be given in a tuberculin syringe. Nomograms are used primarily in calculating pediatric drug dosages; however, they are also used when calculating some adult drug dosages such as aminoglycosides and antineoplastic agents.

SAFE DRUG ADMINISTRATION

Nurses must administer numerous drugs daily in a safe and efficient manner. The nurse should administer drugs in accord with nursing standards of practice and agency policy. The safe storage and maintenance of an adequate supply of drugs are other responsibilities of the nurse.

The nurse should document the actual administration of medications on the MAR. The MAR is a medication administration record that contains the drug's name, dose, route, and frequency of administration. Drug data are entered either by the nurse when transcribing the order (hand-written onto the form) or by the pharmacist when dispensing the order (computer-generated form; Figure 24-3).

Guidelines for Medication Administration

To protect the client from medication errors, nurses have traditionally used as a guideline the "five rights" of drug administration as follows:

1. Right drug
2. Right dose
3. Right client
4. Right route
5. Right time

The nurse is legally responsible for knowing the usual dose, the expected action, the side effects, the adverse reactions, and any interactions with other drugs or food of every drug administered. Without this knowledge, the nurse should not administer any medication.

Right Drug

Before administering any medication the nurse compares the medications listed on the MAR or, less frequently, on a medication card against the physician's order. When administering a medication, the nurse should check the label written on the container against the MAR at least three times before giving the drug. The nurse should:

1. Check the label when removing the drug container from the client's medication drawer.
2. Check the drug when removing it from the container.
3. Check the drug before returning it to the client's medication drawer.

PHARMACY MAR

START	STOP	MEDICATION	SCHEDULED TIMES	OK'D BY	0001 HRS. to 1200 HRS.	1201 HRS. to 2400 HRS.
08/31/xx 1800 SCH		PROCAN SR 500 MG TAB-SR · 500 MG · Q6H · PO	0600 1200 1800 2400	JD	0600 LW 1200 LW	1800 MS 2400 JD
09/03/xx 0900 SCH		DIGOXIN (LANOXIN) 0.125 MG TAB · 1 TAB · QOD · PO · ODD DAYS-SEPT.	0900	JD	0900 LW	
09/03/xx 0900 SCH		FUROSEMIDE (LASIX) 40 MG TAB · 1 TAB · QD · PO	0900	JD	0900 LW	
09/03/xx 0845 SCH		REGLAN 10 MG TAB · 10 MG · AC&HS · PO · GIVE ONE NOW!	0730 1130 1630 2100	JD	0730 LW 1130 LW	1630 MS 2100 MS
09/04/xx 0900 SCH		K-LYTE 25 MEQ EFFERVESCENT TAB · 1 EFF.TAB · BID · PO · DISSOLVE AS DIR. START 9-4	0900 1700	JD	0900 LW	1700 GP
09/03/xx 1507 PRN		NITROGLYCERIN 1/50 GR 0.4 MG TAB-SL · 1 TABLET · PRN* · SL · PRN CHEST PAIN		JD		
09/03/xx 1700 PRN		DARVOCET-N 100* 1 TAB · Q4-6H · PO · PRN MILD-MODERATE PAIN		JD		
09/03/xx 2100 PRN		MEPERIDINE*(DEMEROL) INJ · 50 MG · Q4H · IM · PRN SEVERE PAIN W PHENERGAN		JD		2200 (H) MS
09/03/xx 2100 PRN		PROMETHAZINE (PHENERGAN) INJ · 50 MG · Q4H · IM · PRN SEVERE PAIN W DEMEROL		JD		2200 (H) MS

Gluteus	Thigh	Nurse's Signature	Initial		
A. Right	H. Right			Allergies: NKA	Patient: Patient, John D.
B. Left	I. Left	7-3 L. White, R.N.	LW		Patient #: 3-81512-3
Ventro Gluteal					Admitted: 08/31/xx
C. Right	J. Right	3-11 M. Smith, R.N.	MS	Diagnosis: CHF	Physician: J. Physician, MD
D. Left	K. Left				
E. Abdomen	1|2 3|4	11-7 J. Doe, R.N.	JD		Room: PCU-14 PCU

Figure 24-3 Computerized Medication Administration Record (*Adapted from* Fundamentals of Nursing: Standards & Practice *by S. DeLaune and P. Ladner, 1998, Albany, NY: Delmar. Copyright 1998 by Delmar. Adapted with permission.*)

Right Dose

The nurse must know how to reduce the risk of error by correctly calculating doses and having them double-checked before administration. Policy in some agencies, for instance, mandates that two nurses check insulin dosages to ensure accuracy.

To prepare scored or crushed medications the nurse should make sure scored tablets are broken evenly. This practice will prevent overdosage or underdosage of a medication. If the medication has to be crushed with a mortar and pestle, the nurse should thoroughly cleanse the pestle after each use. Cleansing the pestle will avoid mixing different medications and will prevent the client from receiving minute amounts of a medication that may cause serious adverse effects.

Right Client

The nurse should correctly identify the client by asking the client to state his or her full name and by checking the client's identification armband. The nurse should never identify a client solely by calling the person's name because some clients may be confused and will answer to any name.

Right Route

The route of the medication is specified in the written order. The nurse should consult the physician whenever a route is not identified in the prescription, when the route indicated differs from the recommended one, or when the nurse questions the choice of route prescribed. For example, the nurse should not substitute an oral medication for an intramuscular medication simply because the oral medication is available.

Right Time

Medications are generally ordered on a schedule. A drug should not be given more than an hour before or after the scheduled time, or as per agency policy, without first checking with the physician. For the drug's effect to be maintained, the medication has to been given in a timely manner.

Safety: Guidelines for Safe Administration of Medications

- *Never administer medications that are prepared by another nurse.* You are responsible for a medication error if you administer a medication that was inaccurately prepared by another nurse.
- Nurses should listen carefully to the client who questions the addition or deletion of a medication. If a client questions the drug or dose you are preparing to administer, recheck the order.
- If a medication is withheld, indicate the exact reason in the client's record. Legally you are responsible for giving prescribed medications to the client; however, circumstances may prevent you from giving them, and these must be documented.
- Do not leave medications at the client's bedside. The client may forget to take the medication, medications can accumulate, and the client could take two or more of the same medication, causing an overdose.
- Initial the MAR only for those medications you actually have administered. This practice ensures accurate charting by clearly indicating which actions you have performed.
- Advise clients not to take medications belonging to others and not to offer their medications to others. Medications are ordered for each client on the basis of the history, physical examination, and effectiveness of the medication.

In the home health and community care settings, such as a retirement home, the nurse has different responsibilities regarding drug safety (Figure 24-4). The nurse should promote drug safety measures that are appropriate to the environment and inherent risk factors.

Documentation of Drug Administration

A critical element of drug administration is documentation. The standard is *"if it was not documented it was not done."* Many drug errors can be avoided with appropriate documentation. The nurse responsible for

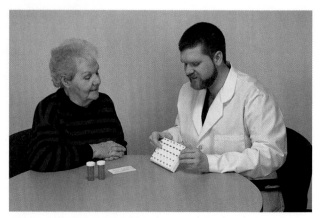

Figure 24-4 Assisting Client at Home with a Pillbox Correlated to the Days of the Month

administering the medication must initial the medication on the MAR for the time the drug was given. Usually there is a space available for a full signature on the record. The nurse should document that a drug has been given *after* the client has received the drug.

If the client refuses to take a medication once it has been prepared, the nurse must indicate that a dose was missed. The nurse should write in the record why the dose was missed and should notify the physician. The client may have refused because the tablet was too large. The medication may be supplied as a liquid so an alternate form of the medication can be given if the physician changes the order to the liquid form. Clients do have the right to refuse medication, but if they understand the actions of a medication, most will be willing to take it. Clients who are scheduled for various diagnostic tests or treatments at the time the medication is to be administered will need to have the medication time rescheduled, and the change will have to be documented.

COMMUNITY/HOME HEALTH CARE

Drug Safety Considerations

- Assist the client in removing outdated prescriptions and over-the-counter drugs from medication cabinets. The chemical composition may change over time, causing a different drug action. Over-the-counter drugs can interact with prescription drugs, either by decreasing or potentiating the effects of the prescription medication.
- Encourage the client or caregivers to maintain drug refills to decrease the risk of missing scheduled medications.
- Use a mechanism such as a paper clock, reminder calendar, or pillbox to help the client or caregiver remember to take or administer prescribed medications as scheduled.

Drug Supply and Storage

Drugs are dispensed by the pharmacy to nursing units through various methods to accommodate the agency's medication system. Once the pharmacy delivers the drugs to a nursing unit, the nurse is responsible for their safe storage.

Scheduled drugs for each client are usually dispensed in a **unit dose form**. Unit dose is a system of packaging and labeling each dose of medication by the pharmacy, often to supply the scheduled drugs for a 24-hour time period. The pharmacy usually delivers the drugs and stores the drugs in the designated area for each client. Unit dose drugs are usually stored in a medication cart that contains individual drawers for each client's medication supply or in the medication room in a separate, organized container for each client. The unit dose system makes it easy for nurses to administer the correct dose, thereby minimizing the number of medication errors.

The nurse, usually at the beginning of each shift, checks the medications in each client's drawer. Some medication carts are locked and the nurse keeps the key. Medication drawers should be removed one at a time from the cart when the nurse is preparing the medication for administration. The client's drawer should never be left unattended on top of the cart. Drugs should not be removed from one client's supply for administration to another client.

Certain drugs may be **stock supplied** (dispensed and labeled in large quantities) and stored in the medication room or other area on the nursing unit. Stock supplies are kept together in a secured area. Certain intravenous fluids and medications must be stored in the medication refrigerator to preserve the integrity of the drug. The Public Health Department and accrediting agencies mandate that only drugs can be stored in the medication refrigerator.

Narcotics and Controlled Substances

Health care agencies have forms to record the supply on hand and the administration of narcotics and controlled substances in accord with federal regulations. These forms usually require the recording of the following information for each drug administered:

- Name of the client receiving the drug
- Amount of the drug used
- Time the drug was administered
- Name of the prescribing physician
- Name of the nurse administering the drug

Nursing practice usually requires that nurses count the narcotics and controlled substances at specified intervals. For example, at the change of shifts, one nurse who is going off duty counts the drugs with a nurse coming on duty. Each drug used must be accounted for on the narcotic record. When the narcotic count does not check, the nurse must report the discrepancy immediately. Narcotics and controlled substances are kept in a double-locked drawer, box, room, or medication-dispensing cart, such as a computer-controlled dispensing system as shown in Figure 24-5. The law requires the use of these safety precautions for narcotics and controlled substances.

MEDICATION COMPLIANCE

Medication compliance can be associated with the client's understanding of why a medication was ordered and how a medication can decrease the likelihood of getting a disease or how it can lessen the effects of an existing disease. When clients do not consistently take their prescribed medications, or when they adjust the scheduling or dose of the medication, they are *noncompliant.*

There are several reasons why clients choose not to take ordered medications. It may be difficult for a hypertensive client who is asymptomatic (without distress) to understand the need to take prescribed medications. If medications are taken, the dose may be altered at the discretion of the client. Medications are costly, and the client may be on a fixed income or unemployed. If the medication does not provide prompt relief, the client may consider the medication useless and discontinue it. The medication may be discontinued if the client experiences undesirable side effects, such as impotence or weight gain.

Compliance can be enhanced if the client is given information on the medication to take home when discharged from the hospital. If the client is elderly, large-type print or illustrations should be used. Caregivers should be included when educating the client. Scheduling the medications around certain activities of daily living may serve as a reminder to the client that the medication must be taken. Providing the client with a telephone number and a name of a nurse to call if questions arise can foster compliance.

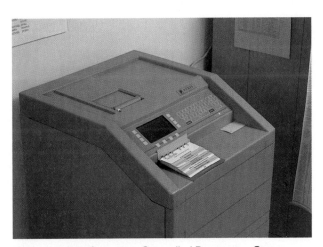

Figure 24-5 Computer-Controlled Dispensing System

The nurse in the community has an opportunity to see how medications are arranged in the client's home. Outdated medications must be discarded. After consulting with the client and caregiver, the nurse can make suggestions that may improve compliance.

Nurses have to remember that many elderly clients take a multitude of drugs. Some drugs actually cancel each other out when taken together, thus eliminating the therapeutic response. A client taking buspirone hydrochloride (BuSpar) and digoxin (Lanoxin) may experience digoxin toxicity. The BuSpar may displace the serum binding of digoxin and increase the toxic levels of that drug (Shannon, Wilson, & Stang, 1999). Nurses must sort through the medications with the client and report back to the physician any drugs taken in addition to those ordered by that physician.

LEGAL ASPECTS OF ADMINISTERING MEDICATIONS

Nurses have learned the "five rights" as a guideline to safe administration of medications. If the nurse gives the wrong medicine to the wrong person, an error has occurred. If the nurse has the right medicine but wrong dose or wrong route, a medication error has occurred. If the nurse gives the medication at the wrong time, an error has occurred. Nurses must inform the physician of the error made. If an antidote must be given, the physician needs accurate information to make appropriate care decisions.

Medication errors must be reported in a timely manner. Knowing the actions and the side effects of drugs will aid the nurse in assessing the client's response and health status. Incident reports are required in some agencies to document medication errors. A report of a medication error must include the name of the medication, dose given, route, time administered, specific error, time the physician was contacted about the error, and what countermeasures were taken.

Sometimes nurses discover errors made by other nurses. These must also be documented and reported.

NURSING PROCESS

The nursing process is vital in planning client care and in ensuring safe and accurate medication administration.

Assessment

Drug administration is based on assessment data obtained from eliciting a drug history, reviewing the client's medical history, performing a physical examination, and obtaining and interpreting relevant laboratory results.

Drug History

A drug history is obtained when a client is admitted to a health care facility. The drug history should contain specific questions about the client's medication background, including allergies, and use of prescription and over-the-counter drugs.

Allergies The nurse should inquire about all food and drug allergies. If the client has had an allergic reaction to a drug, the nurse should have the client describe the details of the reaction: name of the drug; dosage, route, and number of times the drug was taken before the reaction; onset of the reaction; and manifestations of the reaction. The nurse should question the client about possible contributing factors to the allergic reaction, such as concurrent use of stimulants or depressants (tobacco, alcohol, or illegal drugs) or significant changes in nutritional status.

Allergies to foods should also be queried by the nurse because drugs may contain the same elements or nutrients that cause allergic reactions to some foods. For example, clients who are allergic to shellfish may also experience a reaction to drugs that contain iodine. Vaccines are commonly derived from chick embryos and would be contraindicated in clients with allergies to eggs.

Prescription Drugs The nurse should have the client identify all current prescription drugs and describe:

- Why the drug was prescribed and by whom
- The drug's dosage, route, and frequency
- The client's knowledge of the drug's action: side and adverse effects, when to notify the physician, and special administration considerations such as with or without foods

If the client is receiving any drug that requires monitoring before administration, such as insulin (antidiabetic hormone), the nurse needs to make sure the client is checking blood sugar and that the results are within normal limits.

Over-the-Counter Drugs Clients usually have to be questioned separately about nonprescription drugs because they often fail to identify these drugs when asked to list all the medications they take routinely. For example, the nurse must determine if the client takes aspirin, antacids, or laxatives routinely. The client should describe the dosage, route, and frequency of these drugs. Because many drugs are available in topical form, the nurse should also inquire about the use of creams, ointments, patches, or sprays. Clients admitted to inpatient facilities should be asked if they have any over-the-counter drugs with them.

Medical History

The nurse should identify all chronic diseases and disorders and correlate these data with the drugs prescribed by the physician. Preexisting conditions such as liver and kidney dysfunction may require drug alteration because they prolong drug action, thereby increasing the potential for toxicity. The nurse needs to elicit this type of information during the medical history so that these clients can be closely monitored for signs of adverse reactions to drugs.

Biographical Data The client's biographical data, including age, education, occupation, and insurance coverage, may influence the nursing care plan and teaching plan. These data are also used by the nurse when assisting the client in the development of a drug regimen that complements the client's daily routine.

Lifestyle and Beliefs The client's lifestyle and beliefs affect attitudes toward health, use of the health care system, and daily activity patterns. These factors often determine the client's dietary habits and use of illegal drugs or other substances such as tobacco and alcohol.

Sensory and Cognitive Status The nurse should assess for and inquire about sensory deficits such as vision or hearing impairments, weakness or paralysis, or loss of sensation in one or more extremities. These deficits may impair a client's ability to comply with a prescribed drug plan, administer a subcutaneous injection, break a scored tablet, or open a medication container.

The nurse should assess the client's cognitive abilities throughout the drug history interview by noting if the client is alert and oriented and interacts appropriately. Clients who are not able to express their thoughts coherently or who exhibit impaired memory function will require special consideration by the nurse.

Physical Examination

The nurse assesses the client's condition before administering any drug to establish the client's baseline, or normal, health status. For example, the nurse assesses the client's apical pulse before administering digoxin (Lanoxin), an inotropic, so that the heart rate after receiving the drug can be compared with the baseline measurement.

Diagnostic and Laboratory Data

Common laboratory values, such as electrolytes, blood urea nitrogen, creatinine, glucose, complete blood count, and a white blood cell count, are usually monitored over a period of time to identify trends and to measure the body's response to infection.

Nursing Diagnosis

Once the nurse identifies the actual or potential problems, relevant nursing diagnoses can be formulated. The NANDA (2001) nursing diagnoses commonly related to medication administration include:

- *Ineffective Health Maintenance*
- *Deficient Knowledge*
- *Ineffective Therapeutic Regimen Management*
- *Impaired Physical Mobility*
- *Disturbed Sensory Perception*
- *Impaired Swallowing*

Planning/Outcome Identification

The nurse develops the care plan and goals on the basis of the nursing diagnoses. For example, the client with a knowledge deficit related to a newly prescribed drug, insulin, may have the following expected outcomes:

Before discharge the client will:

- Correctly state the actions of insulin in the body.
- Prepare the correct dose of insulin in a syringe three times.
- State the reasons for rotating the injection sites and demonstrate by self-administering insulin to three different sites.
- Correctly identify the onset of action, peak plasma level, and half-life of the insulin preparation prescribed.
- Correctly perform glucometer testing to ensure a normal range of blood sugar before administering the insulin injection.
- Correctly describe the signs of hyperglycemia and hypoglycemia and the appropriate actions to take.

Nursing Interventions

The primary nursing interventions related to medication management are assessment, administration, and teaching. The nurse should use the time spent during medication administration to assess the client's knowledge and response to the drug's action.

The administration of medication requires the implementation of safety guidelines, following the five rights. Medications are administered in accordance with set procedures based on the prescribed route. This section presents procedures and guidelines for medication administration by the following routes: oral, including sublingual and buccal; parenteral; site-specific topical applications; and inhalation.

Drug teaching usually occurs in two phases. The first phase involves a formal teaching session. The nurse explains the drug's action, route, side and adverse effects, and the specific signs of a drug reaction that require physician notification. Clients often need assistance in developing a drug schedule that promotes compliance and complements their lifestyle. Self-administration may require the nurse to teach the client and/or support person specific procedural techniques, such as subcutaneous injection.

CLIENT TEACHING

Written Medication Information

The American Nurses Association and various governing bodies support written medication information for clients that is "scientifically accurate, unbiased in content and tone, sufficiently specific and comprehensive, presented in an understandable and legible format, timely, up to date, and useful." Written medication information should:

- Be appropriate to client literacy level
- Reflect print size appropriate to client's visual abilities
- Give straightforward instructions
- Include generic and trade names
- Prominently display drug warnings
- Outline indications for use, contraindications, and precautions
- List possible adverse reactions and risks, storage, and use

(From American Nurses Association, 1997, American Nurse, 29[2], p. 11.)

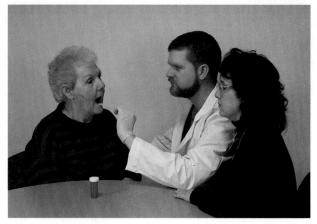

Figure 24-6 Check the client's mouth if unsure that medications have been swallowed.

The second phase of client teaching is ongoing, occurring whenever the nurse administers a drug. The nurse should assess and reinforce the client's knowledge of drugs at each interaction. If the client is being taught self-administration, the drug teaching plan should identify the dates for teaching, and expected outcomes should identify a date for client achievement of targeted goals.

Oral Drugs

Oral administration of drugs is the most common route; however, there are potential risk factors that the nurse must consider. Before administering oral drugs, the nurse should assess the client's ability to take the medication as prescribed. This assessment includes the client's gag reflex, state of consciousness, and presence of nausea and vomiting.

The nurse should protect the client against aspiration when administering any form of oral drugs. **Aspiration** refers to the inhalation of regurgitated gastric contents into the pulmonary system. To prevent aspiration, the nurse checks the client's gag reflex and ability to swallow.

Liquid medications are measured out in a medicine cup that is calibrated, usually in at least two of the three measuring systems. Doses smaller than 1 dr, 1 tsp, or 5 mL are measured in a syringe for acuracy. Solid oral medications are put into a medicine cup or small paper (soufflé) cup, depending on agency policy. Individually wrapped medications should be opened at the bedside.

When administering an oral drug, the nurse should remain with the client until all of the medications have been swallowed. If there is doubt that the client has swallowed a pill, the nurse should don a nonsterile glove and visually inspect the client's mouth with a tongue depressor (Figure 24-6).

Sublingual and Buccal Prior to administering sublingual and buccal drugs, the nurse should assess the integrity of the mucous membranes by inspecting under the client's tongue and in the buccal cavity. If the membranes are excoriated or painful, the nurse should withhold the medication and notify the physician. Some buccal drugs may irritate the mucosa, requiring the nurse to use alternate sides of the mouth to prevent irritation of the mucosa. Drugs given by these

CLIENT TEACHING

Sublingual and Buccal Drug Administration

Sublingual Drugs:

- Keep the medication under the tongue until it dissolves completely to ensure absorption.
- Avoid chewing the tablet or manipulating it with the tongue to prevent accidental swallowing.
- Do not smoke before the drug has completely dissolved because nicotine has a vasoconstriction effect that slows absorption.

Buccal Drugs:

- Keep the medication in place until it dissolves completely to ensure absorption.
- Do not drink liquids for an hour because some tablets take up to an hour to dissolve.
- Do not smoke before the drug has completely dissolved because nicotine has a vasoconstriction effect that slows absorption.

routes are quickly absorbed by the mucosa's thin epithelium and the abundant blood supply.

Enteral Enteral instillation refers to the delivery of drugs through a gastrointestinal tube. Enteral tubes provide a means of direct instillation of medications into the gastrointestinal system of clients who cannot ingest them orally.

There are several types of enteral tubes. A nasogastric tube (NG) is a soft rubber or plastic tube that is inserted through a nostril and into the stomach. The gastrostomy tube is surgically inserted into the stomach through the creation of an artificial fistula. The physician uses an endoscope to insert a percutaneous endoscopic gastrostomy (PEG) tube into the stomach.

The nurse should assess the client for the presence of bowel sounds and check the tube for **patency** and placement before administering a medication. Patency refers to being freely opened. The instillation of drugs is contraindicated when the tube is obstructed or improperly placed, when the client is vomiting, or if bowel sounds are absent.

Safety: Verifying Placement of an Enteral Tube
The usual check for patency and placement of a nasogastric tube is performed as follows:

- Wash hands and don nonsterile gloves.
- Unclamp the tube.
- Create a 20-mL air space in a 50- or 60-mL syringe.
- Attach the syringe to the free end of the tube.
- Place the stethoscope on the left upper quadrant, 3 inches (7.5 cm) below the sternum.
- Gently instill 20 mL of air into the tube while simultaneously listening for a gastric bubble. (The gastric bubble is the "swish" sound heard as the air moves into the stomach.)
- When sound is heard, draw back on the piston of the syringe. (The appearance of gastric contents in the syringe may imply that the tube is in the stomach.) If the nurse fails to hear the swish sound and aspirates gastric contents, the tube may have risen into the client's esophagus. If this occurs, notify the nursing supervisor; do not administer the medication until placement in the stomach is verified. The nursing supervisor may elect to advance the tube into the stomach and check its placement by instilling air and aspirating or by obtaining a physician's order to confirm the tube's placement with an x-ray.

Once the patency and placement of the tube have been determined, the nurse prepares the medication

for instillation as prescribed by the physician. When the physician orders a drug in the tablet or capsule form, the nurse should crush the tablet into minute particles and dissolve the crushed tablet in 15 to 30 mL of warm water before instillation. The instillation of cold solution may cause abdominal cramps. Capsules are prepared for administration by opening the capsule and emptying the contents into a liquid. When the drug has been prepared, the nurse is ready to instill the medication.

PROFESSIONAL TIP

Instilling Drugs into Enteral Tubes
- Wash hands and don nonsterile gloves.
- Place the client in a high or semi-Fowler's position, as the client's condition allows; for an NG tube, unpin the tube from the client's gown to allow manipulation of the tube's free end. Place a linen saver over the bed linens to prevent soilage during administration of the medication.
- Attach the syringe to the free end of the tube, pour 30 ml of medication into the syringe barrel, and open the clamp; for NG tube instillation, hold the NG tube at the client's nose level.
- Hold the syringe barrel at a slight angle and allow the medication to flow at a steady, slow rate; add more medication before the syringe empties to prevent air from entering the stomach. If necessary, adjust the height of the NG tube to achieve a steady flow rate.
- Observe the client while instilling the medication. If the client experiences any discomfort, slow the rate by lowering the height of the syringe.
- When instilling more than one medication, give each separately, with a 5-mL water rinse between medications.
- As the syringe barrel begins to empty with the last of the medication, slowly add 30 to 50 mL of room-temperature water into the syringe to clear the medication from the sides and distal end of the tube to prevent clogging.
- Before the syringe empties of water, clamp the tube, and detach and dispose of the syringe.
- Position the client as appropriate; clients with an NG tube should be placed on the right side with the head of the bed slightly elevated for at least 30 minutes after the instillation.
- Clean area, remove and dispose of gloves in the proper receptacle, and wash hands.
- Document the instillation of the medication on the MAR and record the total amount of fluid instilled on the intake and output sheet.

PROFESSIONAL TIP

Special Considerations for Enteral Tube Management

- When a client is receiving intermittent tube feedings, schedule the medications so as to prevent the two solutions from being given together.
- An adult client should not receive more than 400 mL of liquid at one time. If the administration of feedings and medication coincide, give the medication first to ensure that the client receives the prescribed dosage on time; the feeding may not be given in its entirety.
- When the client is receiving a continuous feeding, stop the feeding and aspirate the gastric contents. If the gastric contents are greater than 150 mL, withhold the medication and notify the physician.
- Never put tablets into tube-feeding bags.
- For clients who have an NG tube for decompression (removal) of gastric contents, turn off the suction for 20 to 30 minutes after the instillation of the medication to allow time for the gastric contents to be emptied into the intestines, where most drugs are absorbed.

Parenteral Drugs

Parenteral medications are given through a route other than the alimentary canal; these routes are intradermal, subcutaneous, intramuscular, or intravenous. The angle of insertion of the syringe or needle and the depth of penetration will indicate the type of injection (Figure 24-7).

Equipment Nurses use special equipment such as syringes, needles, ampules, and vials when administering parenteral medications.

Syringes A syringe has three basic parts: the hub, which connects with the needle; the barrel, or outside part, which contains measurement calibrations; and the plunger, which fits inside the barrel and has a rubber tip (Figure 24-8). The nurse must ensure that the hub, the inside of the barrel, and the shaft and rubber plunger tip are kept sterile. When handling the syringe, the nurse should touch only the outside of the barrel and the plunger's handle.

Most syringes are disposable, made of plastic, and individually packaged for sterility. There are several types of syringes, such as the hypodermic, insulin, and tuberculin (Figure 24-9). When a medication is incompatible with plastic, it is usually prefilled into a single-dose glass syringe. Syringes are often prepackaged with the commonly used needle size and gauge.

The *hypodermic syringe* comes in 2-, 2.5-, and 3-mL sizes. The measurement calibrations (scales) are usu-

ally printed in milliliters and minims. Most syringes are marked in cubic centimeters (cc), and most drugs are ordered in milliters; these are equivalent measurements (1 cc = 1 mL). The hypodermic syringe is used most often when a medication is ordered in milliliters. When the order is written in minims, it is safer to prepare the drug in a tuberculin syringe.

The *insulin syringe* is designed especially for use with the ordered dose of insulin. For example, if the physician writes the order for 30 units of U-100 insulin, the nurse will use an insulin syringe that is calibrated on the 100-unit scale. The nurse should always compare the size of insulin syringe and the dose indicated on the insulin bottle with the physician's order; all three unit doses must be the same.

The *tuberculin syringe* is a narrow syringe, calibrated in tenths and hundredths of a milliliter (up to 1 mL) on one scale and in sixteenths of a minim (up to 1 minim) on the other scale. This syringe is commonly used today to administer small or precise doses, such as pediatric dosages. The tuberculin syringe should be used for doses 0.5 mL or less.

Prefilled single-dose syringes should not be confused with a unit dose. The nurse must be careful to check the prescribed dose against that in the prefilled syringe and discard excess medication. For example, if the physician orders diazepam (Valium) 5 mg IM as a preoperative sedative and the prefilled single-dose contains 10 mg/2 mL, the nurse must calculate dosage

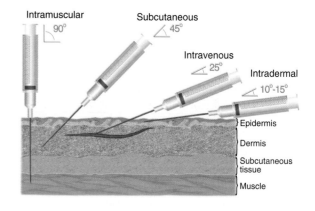

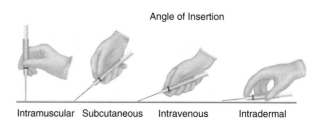

Figure 24-7 Angle of Insertion for Parenteral Injections (*From* Fundamentals of Nursing: Standards & Practice *by* S. DeLaune and P. Ladner, 1998, Albany, NY: Delmar. Copyright 1998 by Delmar. Adapted with permission.)

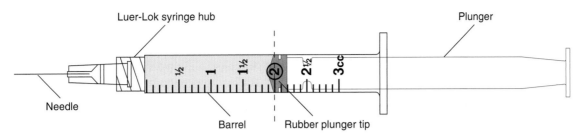

Figure 24-8 The Parts of a Syringe

(5 mg/1 mL) and destroy 1 mL from the syringe before administration.

Needles Most needles today are disposable, made of stainless steel, and individually packaged for sterility. Reusable needles are seldom used today, except in certain areas such as surgery and special procedure rooms; these needles require frequent inspection to ensure that the needle is sharp, and resterilization is necessary between uses.

The needle has three basic parts: the hub, which fits onto the syringe; the cannula, or shaft, which is attached to the hub; and the bevel, which is the slanted part at the tip of the shaft (Figure 24-10). Needles come in various sizes, from ¼ to 5 inches long, and with gauges that range from 28 to 14. The *gauge* of the needle refers to the diameter of the shaft; the larger the gauge number the smaller the diameter of the shaft. Smaller needles (larger gauge) produce less trauma to the body's tissue; however, the nurse has to consider the viscosity of a solution when selecting the gauge.

The *shaft* of the needle indicates its length. The nurse selects the length of the needle on the basis of the client's muscle development and weight and the type of injection, such as intradermal versus intramuscular.

The needle may have a short or a long *bevel*. The length of bevel selected is based on the type of injection. Long bevels are sharp and produce less pain when injected into the subcutaneous or muscle tissues. A short-bevel needle must be used for intradermal and intravenous injections to prevent occlusion of the bevel either by the tissue or by a blood vessel wall.

When the nurse removes a needle from its sterile wrapper, the hub of the needle should be immediately attached to the hub of the syringe to prevent contamination. Likewise, the protective cover should remain on the needle's shaft until the nurse is ready to use the needle.

After an injection, used needles should be disposed of in the proper receptacles, such as a sharps container, to prevent needlesticks. Most agencies have sharps containers in all client care areas. Discussion of the needleless system is found under IV therapy later in this chapter.

Ampules and Vials Drugs for parenteral injections are sterile preparations. Drugs that deteriorate in solution are dispensed as tablets or powders and are dissolved in a solution immediately before injection.

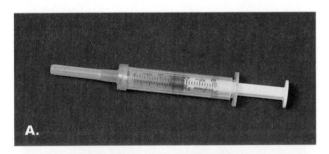

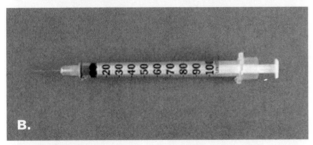

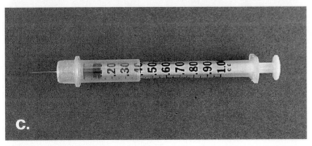

Figure 24-9 Types of Syringes: A. Hypodermic; B. Standard U-100 insulin (*Courtesy of Becton Dickinson Consumer Products*); C. 1-mL tuberculin (*Courtesy of Becton Dickinson and Company*)

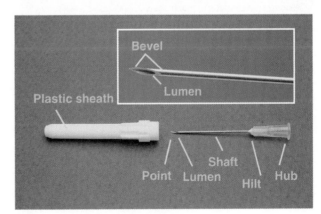

Figure 24-10 Parts of a needle

PROFESSIONAL TIP

Expiration Date

• Manufacturers are required by law to put the expiration date on all drugs.
• Check the expiration date to ensure that the drug is current.
• Return outdated drugs to the pharmacy for proper disposal.

Drugs that remain stable in a solution are dispensed in ampules and vials in an aqueous or an oily solution or suspension.

Ampules are glass containers of single-dose drugs (Figure 24-11). The glass container has a constriction in the stem to facilitate opening the ampule. Because many drugs are irritating to the subcutaneous tissue, the needle on the syringe should be changed after withdrawing a drug from an ampule. The nurse should consider the use of a needle filter when withdrawing medication from an ampule or vial.

Glass, single- or multiple-dose rubber-capped drug containers are called vials (Figure 24-12). The vial is usually covered with a soft metal cap that can be easily removed. The needle on the syringe should be changed after withdrawing a drug from a vial.

Intradermal Injection Intradermal (ID) or intracutaneous injections are typically used to diagnose tuberculosis, identify allergens, and administer local anesthetics. The site below the epidermis is the loca-

tion for administering ID injections; drugs are absorbed slowly from this site. The sites commonly used for ID injection are the inner aspect of the forearm, upper chest, and upper back (Figure 24-13).

The drug's dosage for an ID injection is usually contained in a small quantity of solution (0.01 to 0.1 mL). A 1-mL tuberculin syringe with a short bevel, 25 to 27 gauge, ⅜- to ½-inch needle is used to provide accurate measurement. If repeated doses are ordered, the site should be rotated. Intradermal injections are administered into the epidermis layer by angling the needle 10° to 15° perpendicular to the skin.

Subcutaneous Injection Subcutaneous (SC or SQ) injections are commonly used in the administration of medications such as insulin and heparin because drugs are absorbed slowly, producing a sustained effect. Subcutaneous injections place the medication into the subcutaneous tissue, between the dermis and the muscle. The amount of medication given varies but should not exceed 1.5 mL. If repeated drug doses are to be given, the sites should be rotated.

Common sites for SC injections are the abdomen, the lateral and anterior aspects of upper arm or thigh, the scapular area on the back, and the upper ventrodorsal gluteal area (Figure 24-14). The nurse should

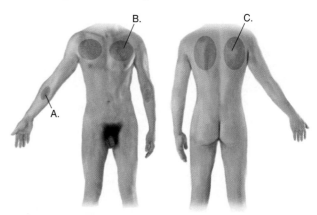

Figure 24-13 Intradermal Injection Sites: A. Inner aspect of the forearm; B. Upper chest; C. Upper back

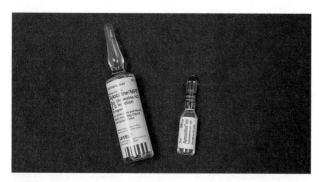

Figure 24-11 Ampules

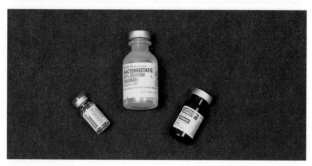

Figure 24-12 Vials

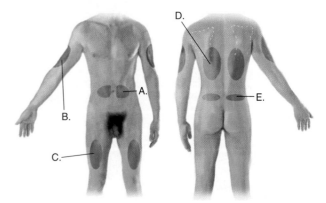

Figure 24-14 Subcutaneous Injection Sites: A. Abdomen; B. Lateral aspect of upper arm; C. Anterior aspect of upper thigh; D. Scapular area on back; E. Upper ventrodorsal gluteal area

select a sterile 0.5- to 3-mL syringe with a 25 to 29 gauge and a ⅜- to ½-inch needle. The medication is administered by angling the needle 45° to 90° perpendicular to the skin.

Intramuscular Injection Intramuscular (IM) injections are used to promote rapid drug absorption and to provide an alternate route when the drug is irri-

tating to subcutaneous tissue. The IM route enhances the absorption rate because there are more blood vessels in the muscles than in subcutaneous tissue. However, the absorption rate may be affected by the client's circulatory status.

There are four common sites for administering IM injections: dorsogluteal and ventrogluteal (gluteus maximus muscle); anterolateral aspect of thigh (vastus lateralis muscle); and upper arm (deltoid muscle). Injection sites are identified by using appropriate anatomic landmarks (Figure 24-15). An IM injection is administered at a 90° angle.

Z-Track Injection The Z-track (zig-zag) technique refers to a method used in administering IM injections, most commonly for administering ventrogluteal and dorsogluteal injections.

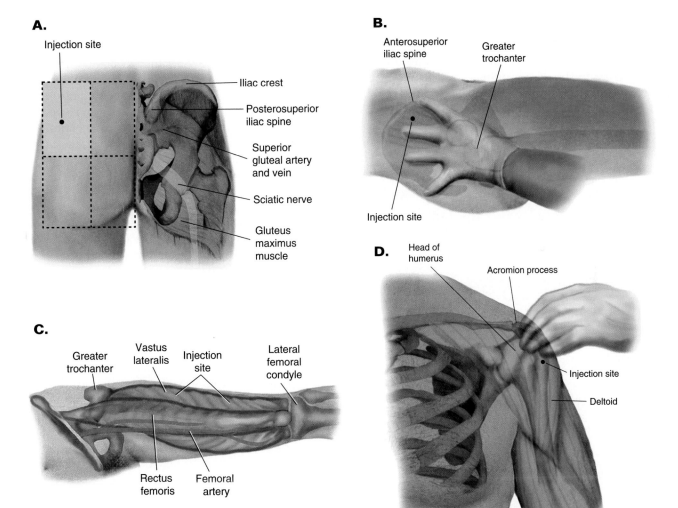

Figure 24-15 Intramuscular Injection Sites: A. Dorsogluteal: Place hand on iliac crest and locate the posterosuperior iliac spine. Draw an imaginary line between the trochanter and the iliac spine; injection site is the outer quadrant. B. Ventrogluteal: Place palm of left hand on right greater trochanter so that the index finger points toward the anteriosuperior iliac spine. Move middle finger to form a V between index and middle fingers; injection site is the middle of the V. C. Vastus lateralis: Identify the greater trochanter. Place hand at the lateral femoral condyle; injection site is middle third and anterior lateral aspect. D. Deltoid: Locate the lateral side of the humerus from two to three fingerwidths below the acromion process in adults or one fingerwidth below the acromion process in children. (*From Fundamentals of Nursing: Standards & Practice by S. DeLaune and P. Ladner, 1998, Albany, NY: Delmar. Copyright 1998 by Delmar. Adapted with permission.*)

LIFE CYCLE CONSIDERATIONS

Primary Site for Administering an IM Injection

- For clients over 7 months old use the ventrogluteal site; the gluteus medius is a well-developed muscle, free of major nerves and large blood vessels.
- The deltoid and dorsogluteal sites should be avoided in infants and children. There is a risk of striking the sciatic nerve when using the dorsogluteal site muscle. The deltoid muscle is not well developed in infants and children.

- For clients under 7 months of age, use the vastus lateralis site.
- Research shows that injuries—including fibrosis, nerve damage, abscess, tissue necrosis, muscle contraction, gangrene, and pain—have been associated with all the common sites (dorsogluteal, deltoid, and vastus lateralis, for example) *except* the ventrogluteal site (Beyea & Nicoll, 1996).

For administration of a Z-track injection, the client is placed in the prone position; the skin is pulled to one side, the needle inserted at a 90° angle and the medication administered (Figure 24-16). The nurse waits 10 seconds, withdraws the needle, and then releases the skin. The site should not be massaged because massaging could cause tissue irritation. Spreading the skin, a common method formerly used for IM injections, in-creases the risk that medication will leak into the needle track and the subcutaneous tissue; this risk is virtually eliminated in the Z-track technique, making it the technique of choice (Beyea & Nicoll, 1996).

Intravenous Therapy Intravenous (IV) therapy requires parenteral fluids (solutions) and special equipment: administration set, IV pole, filter, regulators to control IV flow rate, and an established venous route.

Parenteral Fluids The nurse should confirm the type and amount of IV solution by reading the physician's order in the client's medical record. Intravenous solutions are sterile and are packaged in plastic bags or glass containers. Solutions that are incompatible with plastic are dispensed in glass containers.

Plastic IV solution bags collapse under atmospheric pressure to allow the solution to enter the infusion set. Plastic solution bags are packaged with an outer plastic bag, which should remain intact until the nurse prepares the solution for administration. When the plastic solution bag is removed from its outer wrapper, the solution bag should be dry. If the solution bag is wet, the nurse should not use the solution. The moisture on the bag indicates that the integrity of the bag has been compromised and that the solution cannot be considered sterile. The bag should be returned to the dispensing department that issued the solution. Glass containers are discussed in the section on equipment.

The three types of parenteral fluids are classified based on the tonicity of the fluid relative to normal blood plasma. A solution may be hypotonic, isotonic, or hypertonic. The type of solution is prescribed on the basis of the client's diagnosis and the goal of therapy. The desired effect of the solution is determined as follows:

- Hypotonic fluid: lowers the osmotic pressure and causes fluid to move into the cells. If fluid is infused beyond the client's tolerance, water intoxication may result.
- Isotonic fluid: increases only extracellular fluid volume. If fluid is infused beyond the client's tolerance, cardiac overload may result.

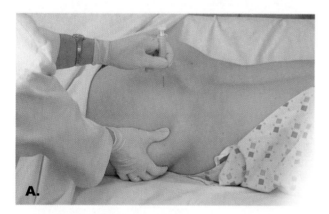

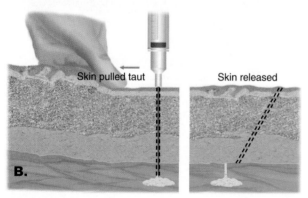

Skin pulled taut   Skin released

Figure 24-16 Z-Track Technique for IM injection: A. With client supine, grasp and pull the muscle laterally before injecting medication. B. Inject medication; keep skin pulled taut for 10 seconds; quickly withdraw the needle and release the skin to seal the site. (*Adapted from* Fundamentals of Nursing: Standards & Practice *by S. DeLaune and P. Ladner, 1998, Albany, NY: Delmar. Copyright 1998 by Delmar. Adapted with permission.*)

- Hypertonic fluid: increases the osmotic pressure of the blood plasma, drawing fluid from the cells. If fluid is infused beyond the client's tolerance, cellular dehydration may result (Bulechek & McCloskey, 2000).

Common intravenous solutions are shown in Table 24–5.

Equipment Intravenous equipment is sterile, disposable, and prepackaged with user instructions. The user instructions are usually placed on the outside of the package and include a schematic that labels the parts, allowing the user to read the package before opening. The syringe tip and port require sterile technique during handling because they are in direct contact with fluids to be infused into the bloodstream.

The administration (infusion) set includes the plastic tubing used to infuse solutions. It contains an insertion spike with a protective cap, a drip chamber, tubing

with a slide clamp and regulating (roller) clamp, a rubber injection port, and a protective cap over the needle adapter (Figure 24-17). The protective caps keep both ends of the infusion set sterile and are removed only just before use. The insertion spike is inserted into the port of the IV solution container.

Infusion sets can be vented or nonvented. The nonvented type is used with plastic bags of IV solutions

LIFE CYCLE CONSIDERATIONS

Choosing IV Equipment

Neonates, infants, and children are at risk for *Excess fluid volume related to rehydration.* Intravenous tubing with a microdrip and special volume control chamber is used to regulate the amount of fluid to be administered over a specific time interval.

Table 24–5 COMMON INTRAVENOUS SOLUTIONS

TONICITY	SOLUTION	CONTENTS (MEQ/L)	CLINICAL IMPLICATIONS
Hypotonic	Sodium chloride 0.45%	77 Na$^+$, 77 Cl$^-$	Daily maintenance of body fluid and establishment of renal function.
Isotonic	Dextrose 2.5% in 0.45% saline	77 Na$^+$, 77 Cl$^-$	Promotes renal function and urine output.
	Dextrose 5% in 0.2% saline	77 Na$^+$, 77 Cl$^-$	Daily maintenance of body fluids when less Na$^+$ and Cl$^-$ are required.
	Dextrose 5% in water (D$_5$W)	38 Na$^+$, 38 Cl$^-$	Promotes rehydration and elimination; may cause urinary Na$^+$ loss; good vehicle for K$^+$.
	Ringer's lactate	130 Na$^+$, 4 K$^+$, Ca^{2+}, 109 Cl$^-$, 28 lactate	Resembles the normal composition of blood serum and plasma; K$^+$ level below body's daily requirement.
	Normal saline (NS), 0.9%	154 Na$^+$, 154 Cl$^-$	Restores sodium chloride deficit and extracellular fluid volume.
	Dextran 40 10% in NS (0.9%) or D$_5$W		A colloidal solution used to increase plasma volume of clients in early shock; *it should not be given to severly dehydrated clients and clients with renal disease, thrombocytopenia, or active hemorrhaging.*
	Dextran 70% in NS		A long-lived (20 hours) plasma volume expander; used to treat shock or impending shock due to hemorrhage, surgery, or burns. *It can prolong bleeding and coats the RBCs (draw type and crossmatch prior to administering).*
Hypertonic	Dextrose 5% in 0.45% saline	77 Na$^+$, 77 Cl$^-$	Daily maintenance of body fluid and nutrition; treatment of FVD.
	Dextrose 5% in saline 0.9%	154 Na$^+$, 154 Cl$^-$	Fluid replacement of sodium, chloride, and calories (170).
	Dextrose 10% in saline 0.9%	154 Na$^+$, 154 Cl$^-$	Fluid replacement of sodium, chloride, and calories (340).
	Dextrose 5% in lactated Ringer's	130 Na$^+$, 4 K$^+$, 3 Ca^{2+}, 109 Cl$^-$, 28 lactate	Resembles the normal composition of blood serum and plasma; K$^+$ level below body's daily requirement; caloric value 180.
	Hyperosmolar saline 3% and 5% NaCl	856 Na$^+$, 865 Cl$^-$	Treatment of hyponatremia; raises the Na osmolarity of the blood, and reduces intracellular fluid excess.
	Ionosol B with dextrose 5%	57 Na$^+$, 25 K$^+$, 49 Cl$^-$, 25 lact., 5 Mg^{2+}, 7 PO$_4^{-}$	Treatment of polyionic parenteral replacement caused by vomiting-induced alkalosis, diabetic acidosis, fluid loss from burns, and postoperative FVD.

From Fluids and Electrolytes With Clinical Applications *(6th ed.), by J. L. Kee & B. J. Paulanka, 1999, Albany, NY: Delmar.*

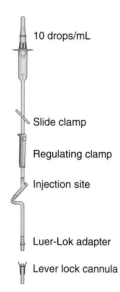

10 drops/mL

Slide clamp

Regulating clamp

Injection site

Luer-Lok adapter

Lever lock cannula

Figure 24-17 Sample Basic Administration Set

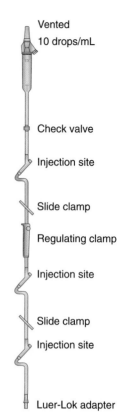

Vented
10 drops/mL

Check valve

Injection site

Slide clamp

Regulating clamp

Injection site

Slide clamp

Injection site

Luer-Lok adapter

Figure 24-18 Sample Vented Administration Set

and vented bottles. The vented set is used for glass containers that are not vented (Figure 24-18).

The drip chamber is calibrated to allow a predictable amount of fluid to be delivered. There are two types of drip chambers: a macrodrip, which delivers 10 to 20 drops per milliliter of solution, and a microdrip, which delivers 60 drops per milliliter. The drip rate, which is indicated on the package, varies with the manufacturer.

The IV tubing has a roller clamp that is used to compress the plastic tubing to control the rate of flow. The end of the IV tubing contains a needle adapter that attaches to the sterile injection device inserted into the client's vein. Extension tubing may be used to lengthen the primary tubing or to provide additional Y-injection ports for the administration of additional solutions.

Intravenous Filters Intravenous filters remove from the solution particulate matter that may cause irritation and **phlebitis** (inflammation of a vein). Intravenous filters come in various sizes; the finer the filter, the greater is the degree of solution filtration. Although studies have shown that IV filters reduce the risk of bacteremia and phlebitis as much as 40%, some agencies do not use IV filters because of cost. Many IV catheters contain an in-line filter. If the catheter has an in-line filter, it is not necessary to add a filter to the tubing.

Needles and Catheters Needles and catheters provide access to the venous system. A variety of devices is available in different sizes to complement the age of the client and the type and duration of the therapy (Figure 24-19). The larger the number, the smaller the lumen of the needle or catheter.

Butterfly (scalp vein or wing-tipped) **needles** are short, beveled needles with plastic flaps attached to the shaft. The flaps (which are flexible) are held tightly together to facilitate ease of insertion and then are flat-

tened against the skin to prevent dislodgment during infusion. These needles are commonly used for short-term or intermittent therapy and for infants and children.

There are several types of catheters used to access peripheral veins. During insertion, some of these catheters are threaded over a needle, and others are threaded inside a needle. **Intracath** is a term used to refer to a plastic tube inserted into a vein. An **angiocatheter** (angiocath, for short) is a type of intracath with a metal stylet to pierce the skin and vein, after which the plastic catheter is threaded into the vein and the metal stylet is removed, leaving only the plastic catheter in the vein.

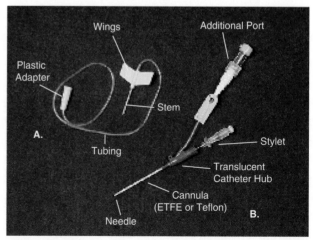

Figure 24-19 Peripheral IV Devices: A. Butterfly; B. Angiocatheter

LIFE CYCLE CONSIDERATIONS

Selecting Needle Gauge

Consider the client's age and body size and the type of solution to be administered when selecting the gauge of the needle or catheter.

- Infants and small children, 24 gauge
- Preschool through preteen, 24 or 22 gauge
- Teenagers and adults, 22 or 20 gauge
- Elderly, 22 or 24 gauge

Peripheral Intravenous and Heparin Locks Peripheral intravenous (PI) and heparin locks are devices that establish a venous route as a precautionary measure for clients whose condition may change rapidly or who may require intermittent infusion therapy. A butterfly needle or peripheral catheter is inserted into a vein and the hub is capped with a lock port, also called a Luer-Lok. The patency of the device is maintained with the injection of either normal saline or heparin (an anticoagulant drug) in accord with the agency's protocol.

Needle-Free System Safety is a concern with IV therapy. Accidental needlestick injuries and puncture wounds with contaminated devices increase the employee's risk for infectious diseases such as AIDS, hepatitis (B and C), and other viral, rickettsial, bacterial, fungal, and parasitic infections. Most health care agencies now use totally needle-free IV systems (Figure 24-20) to decrease the risk of employee injuries.

Vascular Access Devices Vascular access devices (VADs) include various catheters, cannulas, and infusion ports that allow for long-term IV therapy or repeated access to the central venous system. The kind of VAD used depends on the client's diagnosis and the type and length of treatment. Central venous catheters (CVCs) are inserted by a physician.

Another type of VAD is an **implantable port** (a device made of a radiopaque silicone catheter and a plastic or stainless steel injection port with a self-sealing silicone-rubber septum). *Only nurses who have been specially trained are allowed to access an implanted port because of the risk of infiltration into the tissue if needle placement is incorrect.*

Preparing an Intravenous Solution To prepare an IV solution, the nurse should first read the agency's protocol and gather the necessary equipment. Because IV equipment and solutions are sterile, the expiration date on the package should be checked before use. The solution can be prepared at the nurses' work area or in the client's room.

The nurse will prepare and apply a time strip to the IV solution bag to facilitate monitoring of the infusion rate as prescribed by the physician (Figure 24-21). The IV tubing is tagged with the date and time to indicate when the tubing replacement is necessary. Intravenous tubing is changed every 24 to 48 hours according to agency policy. The nurse initials the time strip and the IV tubing tag.

 Safety: Marking an IV Bag
Do not use a felt-tip pen to mark an IV bag. The ink from the pen can leak through the plastic and contaminate the solution.

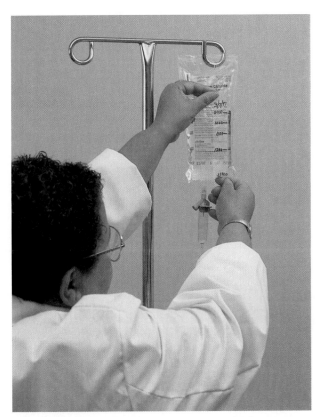

Figure 24-20 Needle-Free System

Luer-Lok injection site
Syringe cannula
Lever lock cannula
T-connector extension set
Three-way stop cock

Figure 24-21 Applying a Time Strip to the IV Container

PROFESSIONAL TIP

Inserting a CVC

When assisting with the insertion of a long-line central catheter, observe the client for symptoms of a pneumothorax: sudden shortness of breath or sharp chest pain; increased anxiety; a weak, rapid pulse; hypotension; pallor or cyanosis. These symptoms indicate accidental puncture of the pleural membrane.

Initiating IV Therapy When initiating IV therapy, the nurse should first consider the type of fluid to be infused and then assess for a venipuncture site. Ellenberger (1999) suggests that the smallest gauge and shortest needle appropriate be selected (22 gauge for maintenance fluids and routine antibiotics, 20 gauge or larger for blood products).

When assessing a client for potential sites, the nurse should consider age, body size, clinical status and impairments, and skin condition. Generally, it is best to begin with the hand and advance up the arm if new sites are needed. Figure 24-22 illustrates common peripheral sites for initiating IV therapy. Venipuncture site contraindications are:

- Signs of infection, infiltration, or thrombosis
- Affected arm of a postmastectomy client
- Arm with a functioning arteriovenous fistula (dialysis)
- Affected arm of a paralyzed client
- Any arm that has circulatory or neurological impairments

Venous blood flows with an upward movement toward the heart, therefore a vein should be selected for puncture at its most distal end to maintain the integrity of the vein. When a vein is punctured with an instrument, such as a needle, fluids can infiltrate (leak from the vein into the tissue at the site of puncture). If IV therapy has to be discontinued for any reason, such as infiltration, it can be restarted above the initial puncture site only.

Locating a Vein With the client's arm extended on a firm surface, place a tourniquet on the arm, tight enough to impede venous flow yet loose enough that

a radial pulse can still be palpated. Next, the index and middle fingers of the nondominant hand are used to palpate a vein. It should feel soft and resilient and not have a pulse. If no vein can be seen or felt, a warm, moist compress may be applied for 10 to 20 minutes, the area may be massaged toward the heart, or the client may open and close the fist (Ellenberger, 1999).

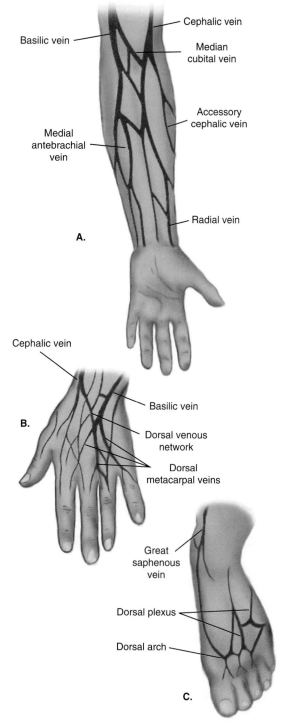

Figure 24-22 Peripheral Veins Used in Intravenous Therapy: A. Forearm; B. Dorsum of the hand; C. Dorsal plexus of the foot

LIFE CYCLE CONSIDERATIONS

Locating a Vein

For clients who are elderly or have fragile veins, eliminate the tourniquet or apply it very loosely if a vein can be palpated.

Safety: Prepping Skin for Venipuncture
When prepping the client's skin for a venipuncture, cleanse the skin with Betadine and wait for it to dry. Do not apply alcohol after the skin has been prepped with Betadine. If these substances are combined, they form a toxic material that may be absorbed through the skin.

Placing the Needle With hands washed and gloved, prepare the selected site according to agency policy. Without touching the prepared site, stabilize the vein by placing your thumb beside the vein and pulling down. Hold the needle at a 10- to 30-degree angle, bevel up to puncture the skin, then lessen the angle to prevent puncturing the back of the vein (Ellenberger, 1999). Secure the needle in place according to agency policy.

Infection Control: Venipuncture
Standard Precautions must be followed when performing a venipuncture.

Administering IV Therapy Once the solution has been prepared for administration, the nurse calculates the rate and explains the procedure to the client. Fluid administration can be continuous, ongoing over a 24-hour period, or intermittent, 1,000 mL ordered once in a 24-hour period. Although fluids may be continuous, the type of fluids can alternate over a 24-hour period. For example, an order might be *add 40 mEq of KCl to first bag of 1,000 mL of normal saline.*

Intravenous medications may be **piggybacked**, connected to an existing IV to infuse concurrently. Intravenous solutions and medications that have been refrigerated should be warmed to room temperature before administration (usually for 30 minutes) to increase the client's comfort.

Regulating IV Solution Flow Rate The flow rate for IV solutions can be regulated by calculating the drops per minute and adjusting the drip rate to that number or by the use of volume controllers and pumps.

Calculating Flow Rate The **flow rate** is the volume of fluid to infuse over a set period of time as prescribed by the physician. The physician will identify the amount to infuse per time period such as: 125 mL per hour or 1,000 mL over an 8-hour period. The hourly infusion rate is calculated as follows:

$$\frac{\text{Total volume}}{\text{Number of hours to infuse}} = \text{mL/hour infusion rate}$$

For example, if 1,000 mL is to be infused over 8 hours:

$$\frac{1,000}{8} = 125 \text{ mL/hour}$$

Calculate the actual infusion rate (drops per minute) as follows:

$$\frac{\text{Total fluid volume}}{\text{Total time (minutes)}} \times \text{Drop factor} = \text{Drops per minute}$$

For example, if 1,000 mL is to be infused over 8 hours with a tubing drop factor of 10 drops per milliliter:

$$\frac{1,000 \text{ mL}}{8 \ (60) \text{ min}} \times 10 \text{ drops/mL} = \frac{10,000 \text{ drops}}{480 \text{ min}} = \begin{array}{l} 20.8, \text{ or } 21, \\ \text{drops/min} \end{array}$$

Another way to calculate the actual infusion rate is to use the hourly infusion rate; for the first example:

$$\frac{125 \text{ mL} \times 10 \text{ drops/mL}}{60 \text{ min}} = 20.8 \text{ or } 21 \text{ drops/min}$$

Volume Controllers and Pumps Controllers are devices that depend on gravity to maintain a preselected flow without adding pressure to IV systems to overcome resistance (for example, Dial-a-Flo or Buretrol). Resistance may develop from the use of a large catheter in a small vein, infusion of a viscous solution, high venous pressure, or a decrease in the height of the container from the IV site. Resistance may cause a decrease in the flow and sound the controller alarm. Volumetric controllers permit flow rates to be set in milliliters per hour.

Pumps are devices that maintain preselected volume delivery by adding pressure to the system when needed. They do not depend on gravity. Pumps may be used for viscous fluids and when large volumes must be delivered in a short period of time. Pumps have maximum pressure limits that, when reached, sound an alarm. Clients are at a greater risk for complications when a drug or solution is administered under high pressure.

Managing IV Therapy Intravenous therapy requires frequent client monitoring by the nurse to ensure an accurate flow rate and other critical nursing actions. These other actions include ensuring client comfort and positioning; checking the IV solution to ensure that the solution, amount, and timing are correct; monitoring expiration dates of the IV system (tubing, venipuncture site, dressing) and changing as necessary; and being aware of safety factors.

PROFESSIONAL TIP

Setting Volume to Be Infused
When setting the volume to be infused (e.g., 1,000 mL), set the volume to be infused slightly lower (e.g., 950 mL) so that the alarm will go off before the fluids are completely gone. This practice will give you time to have the next bag of fluids ready when all 1,000 mL has been absorbed. Having the extra time is especially helpful when dealing with refrigerated fluids that must be warmed to room temperature before being administered. If you will be off duty when the volume will be absorbed and the alarm is set to go off early, tell the oncoming nurse during report.

Catheter Sepsis

If a client complains of chills and fever, check the length of time that the IV solution has been hanging and the needle or catheter has been in place. Assess the client's vital signs, and assess for other symptoms of pyrogenic reactions, such as backache, headache, malaise, nausea, and vomiting. Unexplained fever may be related to catheter sepsis. Pulse rate increases, and temperature is usually above 100°F if IV-related sepsis occurs. Stop the infusion, notify the physician, and obtain blood specimens if ordered.

The nurse must coordinate client care with the maintenance of IV lines. Clients with IV therapy usually require assistance with hygienic measures, including changing the gown. Changing IV tubing when doing site care to decrease the number of times the access device is manipulated will thereby decrease the risk for infiltration and phlebitis. Peripherally inserted devices are changed every 72 hours as directed by the Centers for Disease Control and Prevention (CDC) guidelines.

Hypervolemia **Hypervolemia** (increased circulating fluid volume) may result from rapid IV infusion of solutions. This causes cardiac overload, which may lead to pulmonary edema and cardiac failure. The infusion rate must be monitored hourly to prevent this complication.

If a solution infuses at a rate greater than prescribed, the rate must be decreased to *keep vein open* (KVO) and the physician notified immediately. The nurse must report the amount and type of solution that is infused over the exact time period and the client's response.

Infiltration **Infiltration** (seepage of foreign substances into the interstitial tissue, causing swelling and discomfort at the IV site) may result from inserting the wrong type of device, using the wrong-gauge needle, or dislodgment of the device from the vein. Administration of a drug or solution under high pressure by a pump may also cause infiltration or vein irritation. The client usually complains of discomfort at the IV site. The nurse should inspect the site by palpating for swelling, and feel the temperature of the skin (coolness and paleness of skin are indications of infiltration).

The nurse should also confirm that the needle is still in the vein by pinching the IV tubing. This action should cause **flashback** (blood will rush into the tubing if the needle is still in the vein). If flashback does not occur, the injection port nearest the device should be aspirated. The needle or catheter should be discontinued if it cannot be aspirated and a sterile dressing applied to the puncture site.

After the IV has been removed, the puncture site may ooze or bleed (especially in clients receiving anticoagulants). If oozing or bleeding occurs, pressure is applied and a sterile dressing reapplied until it stops. The degree of edema must be accurately assessed and documented.

Clients may be injured by infiltration. If the IV site becomes grossly infiltrated, the edema in the soft tissue may cause a nerve compression injury with permanent loss of function to the extremity. If a **vesicant** (medication that causes blistering and tissue injury when it escapes into surrounding tissue) infiltrates, it may cause significant tissue loss with permanent disfigurement and loss of function (Hadaway, 1999).

Phlebitis Phlebitis may result from either mechanical or chemical trauma. Mechanical trauma may be caused by inserting a device with too large a gauge, using a vein that is too small or fragile, or leaving the device in place for too long. Chemical trauma may result from infusing too rapidly or from an acidic solution, hypertonic solution, a solution that contains electrolytes (especially potassium and magnesium), or other medications.

Phlebitis may be a precursor of sepsis. Client descriptions of tenderness are usually the first indication of an inflammation. The IV site must be inspected for changes in skin color and temperature (a reddened area or a pink or red stripe along the vein, warmth, and swelling are indications of phlebitis).

If phlebitis is present, the IV infusion must be discontinued. Before removing and discarding the venous device, the nurse should check the agency's protocol to see whether the tip of the device is to be cultured. If so, it must be sent to the laboratory for a culture and sensitivity test. After removing the device, a sterile dressing should be applied to the site and wet, warm compresses to the affected area. Documentation in the nurse's notes must reflect the time, symptoms, and nursing interventions.

Intravenous Dressing Change Intravenous dressing changes require the use of Standard Precautions and aseptic technique. Institutional protocol and the type of intravenous access device and dressing determine the frequency of care. Persistent drainage at the IV site may require dressing changes more frequently or may necessitate changing the IV site.

Intravenous Drug Therapy The intravenous (IV) route is used when a rapid drug effect is desired or when the medication is irritating to tissue. Intravenous administration provides immediate release of medication into the bloodstream; consequently it can be dangerous. Intravenous medications are administered by one of the following methods:

- Intravenous fluid container
- Volume-control administration set
- Intermittent infusion by piggyback or partial fill
- Intravenous push (IVP or bolus)

Adding Drugs to an Intravenous Fluid Container When administering IV medications, regardless of the method used, the nurse should assess the patency of the infusion system and the condition of the injection site for signs of complications such as infiltration and phlebitis. Some IV medications or solutions with high or low pH or high osmolarity are irritating to veins and can cause phlebitis.

Before administering any IV medication, the nurse should note the client's allergies, drug or solution incompatibilities, the amount and type of diluent needed to mix the medication, and the client's general condition to establish a baseline for administering medication. The nurse should check for drug compatibilities of drug additives before injecting a medication into an infusion bag. **Drug incompatibilities** cause an undesired chemical or physical reaction between a drug and a solution, between two drugs, or between a drug and the container or tubing. For example, diazapam (Valium) and chlordiazepoxide hydrochloride (Librium) must not come into contact with a saline solution; insulin should not be added to an infusion bag because the insulin adheres to the inside of the solution bag.

Adding Drugs to a Volume-Control Administration Set A volume-control set is used to administer small volumes of IV solution. These devices have various names as determined by the manufacturer, such as Soluset, Metriset, VoluTrol, or Buretrol. To administer a drug by this method, the nurse should:

- Withdraw the prescribed amount of medication into a syringe that is to be injected into the volume-control set.
- Cleanse the injection port of a partially filled volume-control set with an alcohol swab.
- Inject the prepared medication into the port of the volume-control set.
- Gently mix the solution in the volume-control chamber.

After injecting the medication into the volume-control chamber, the nurse should check the infusion rate and adjust as necessary to the prescribed rate of infusion.

Administering Medications by Intermittent Infusion A common method of administering IV medications is by using a secondary, or partial-fill additive bag, often referred to as an IV piggyback (IVPB). A secondary line is a complete IV set (fluid container and tubing with either a microdrip or a macrodrip system) connected to a Y-port of a primary line. The primary line maintains venous access. The IVPB is used for medication administration (Figure 24-23). When the IVPB medication is incompatible with the primary IV solution, the nurse must flush the primary IV tubing with normal saline before and after administering the medication.

Intermittent Infusion Devices When the client requires only the administration of IV medications

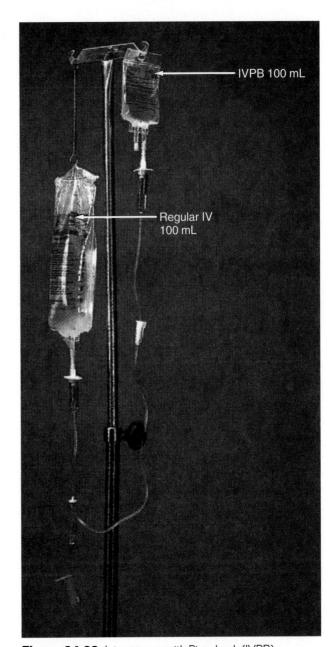

Figure 24-23 Intravenous with Piggyback (IVPB)

without the infusion of solutions, an intermittent infusion device is attached to a peripheral needle or catheter in the client's vein. This device is commonly referred to as a heparin or saline lock (Figure 24-24) depending on the agency's policy regarding the device's maintenance. A lock provides continuous access to venous circulation, eliminating the need for a continuous IV, and it increases the client's mobility.

The device can be used to infuse intermittent IVPB or IV push (also called bolus) medications, or it can be converted to a primary IV. An **IV push (bolus)** is a method of administering a large dose of medication in a relatively short time, usually 1 to 30 minutes. A major consideration for inserting a heparin lock device is that it provides venous access in case of an emergency. Lock devices are routinely used with cardiac clients.

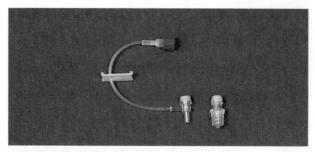

Figure 24-24 Heparin-Locking Device

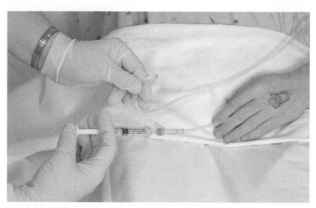

Figure 24-25 Injecting an IV Push (Bolus) Medication into a Peripheral Saline Lock

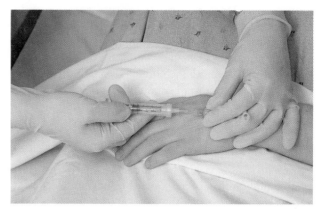

Figure 24-26 Injecting an IV Push (Bolus) Medication into a Primary Infusion Line. The IV tubing must be pinched closed first.

Administering IV Push Medications The method of medication administration by IV push (bolus) injection is determined by the type of IV system. For example, an IV push medication can be injected into a saline or a heparin lock (Figure 24-25) or into a continuous infusion line. When giving an IV push medication into a continuous infusion line, the nurse must stop the fluids in the primary line by pinching the IV tubing closed while injecting the drug (Figure 24-26). This technique is safe and prevents the nurse from having to recalculate the drip rate of the primary infusion line.

Documentation

When IV therapy is begun, the date, time, venipuncture site, number of attempts made, amount and type of fluid, and equipment used are to be documented. Each time the insertion site, venipuncture device, or IV tubing is changed, the reason for the change must be documented (e.g., routine, infiltration). The condition of the insertion site and the fluid type, amount, and flow rate are documented each shift and at intervals specified by agency policy. Any complications are precisely documented along with the nurse's actions.

Blood Transfusion

The purpose of a blood transfusion is to replace blood loss (deficit) with whole blood or blood components. On the basis of the client's unique needs, the physician determines the type of transfusion to administer, either whole blood or a component of whole blood.

COMMUNITY/HOME HEALTH CARE

Blood Temperature

Blood is transported to the client in a container that maintains proper storage temperature for 6 hours. Because the container does not have thermometers and alarms, it is not considered "monitored" storage, and the blood cannot be returned to inventory if the transfusion is canceled (Fitzpatrick & Fitzpatrick, 1997).

Whole Blood and Blood Products Clients with a demonstrated deficiency in either whole blood or a specific component of blood are given a blood transfusion. Whole blood contains red blood cells (RBCs) and plasma components of blood. It is used when the client needs all the components of blood to restore blood volume after severe hemorrhage and to restore the capacity of the blood to carry oxygen.

When the physician prescribes the administration of whole blood or a blood product, the client's blood is typed and crossmatched. Check with the family for donors if time and the client's condition permit. The blood is stored in the blood bank after typing and crossmatching.

Although whole blood has a refrigerated shelf life of 35 days, platelets must be administered within 3 days after they have been extracted from whole blood. If the RBCs and plasma are frozen, their shelf life can be extended up to 3 years (Kee & Paulanka, 1999).

Initial Assessment and Preparation The nurse must perform an initial assessment before administering blood. The nurse should:

• Verify that the client has signed a blood administration consent form and that this consent matches what the physician has prescribed.

LIFE CYCLE CONSIDERATIONS

Initial Assessment

If pediatric, elderly, or malnourished clients are at risk for circulatory overload, notify the blood bank to divide the 500-mL bag of blood into two 250-mL bags or discuss with the physician other alternatives, such as packed RBCs rather than whole blood.

• Verify whether the client has an 18- or a 19-gauge needle or catheter in a vein. The viscosity of whole blood usually requires this gauge needle or catheter to prevent damage to the red blood cells. If blood is to be infused quickly, a 14- or 15-gauge device must be used.
• Ensure patency of the existing IV site.
• Establish baseline data for vital signs, especially temperature, and assess skin for eruptions or rashes.
• Check client's blood type against the label on the whole blood or blood component before administration, to ensure compatibility.
• Assess the client's age and state of nutrition.

Scheduled IV medications should be infused before blood administration. This sequence prevents a reaction to a medication while blood is infusing. If a reaction were to occur, the nurse would not be able to discern whether the medication or the blood was causing the reaction.

Administering Whole Blood or a Blood Component The agency's blood protocol may require that a licensed person sign a form to release the blood from the blood bank and that a blood product be checked by two licensed personnel before infusion. The following information must be on the blood bag label and verified for accuracy: the client's name and identification number, ABO group and Rh factor, donor number, type of product ordered by the practitioner, and expiration date.

Blood should be administered within 30 minutes after it has been received from the bank, to maintain RBC integrity and to decrease the chance of infection. Whole blood should not go unrefrigerated for more than 4 hours. Room temperature will cause RBC lysis, releasing potassium and causing hyperkalemia.

PROFESSIONAL TIP

Transfusion Reaction

The severity of a transfusion reaction is relative to its onset. Severe reactions may occur shortly after the blood starts to infuse. At the first sign of a reaction, stop the blood infusion immediately.

Safety Measures The client should be observed for the initial 15 minutes for a transfusion reaction. Vital signs are usually taken every 15 minutes for the first hour, then every hour while the blood is transfusing.

 Safety: Blood Transfusion Incompatibilities
Only normal saline should be used with a blood product. Blood transfusions are incompatible with dextrose and with Ringer's solution.

There are three basic types of transfusion reactions: allergic, febrile, and hemolytic. Other complications include sepsis, hypervolemia, and hypothermia. An allergic reaction may be mild or severe, depending on the cause. Hemolytic reactions may be immediate or delayed up to 96 hours, depending on the cause of the reaction. The classic symptoms of a reaction and sepsis are fever and chills.

The nursing actions for all types of reactions and complications are given in Table 24–6.

Topical Medications

Topical medications may be administered to the skin, eyes, ears, nose, throat, ear, rectum, and vagina. The medication generally provides a local effect but can also cause systemic effects. Drugs applied directly to the skin to produce a local effect include lotions, pastes, ointments, creams, powders, and aerosol sprays. The rate and degree of the drug's absorption are determined by the vascularity of the area.

Topical drugs are usually given to provide continuous absorption to produce different effects: to relieve pruritus (itching), to protect the skin, to prevent or treat an infection, to provide local anesthesia, or to create a systemic effect. Topical medications are usually ordered two or three times a day to achieve their therapeutic effect.

Table 24–6 NURSING ACTIONS FOR BLOOD REACTIONS

IMMEDIATE NURSING ACTION	OTHER MEASURES
• Stop transfusion. • Keep vein open with normal saline. • Notify the physician.	• Monitor client's vital signs every 15 minutes for 4 hours or until stable. • Monitor I&O. • Send IV tubing and bag of blood back to the blood bank. • Obtain a blood and urine specimen. • Label specimen "Blood Transfusion Reaction." • Process a transfusion reaction report.

Before applying a topical preparation, the nurse should assess the condition of the skin for any open lesions, rashes, or areas of erythema and skin breakdown. The nurse should check with the client and the medical record for any known allergies.

Body oils may interfere with the adhesive properties of the patch, disk, or tape. The skin harbors microorganisms, and lesions can cause encrustation. The nurse should cleanse the area by washing it with soap and warm water, unless contraindicated by a specific order. The skin should be thoroughly dry before applying a topical medication. Open wounds require the nurse to use surgical asepsis.

When the skin is dry, the nurse can apply the medication. When applying a paste, cream, or an ointment, the nurse should follow Standard Precautions and use a sterile tongue depressor to remove the medication from the container; this method prevents cross-contamination. The medication is transferred from the tongue blade to a gloved hand for application. The medication should be applied in long, smooth strokes in the direction of the hair follicles to prevent the medication from entering the hair follicles. A new sterile tongue depressor should be used whenever more medication is removed from the container. Two to 4 hours after the application, the nurse should assess the area for signs of an allergic reaction.

Eye Medications Eye medications refer to drops, ointments, and disks. These drugs are used for diagnostic and therapeutic purposes, to lubricate the eye or socket for a prosthetic eye, and to prevent or treat eye conditions such as glaucoma (elevated pressure within the eye) and infection. Diagnostically, eyedrops can be used to anesthetize the eye, to dilate the pupil, or to stain the cornea to identify abrasions and scars.

 Safety: Prevent Cross-Contamination
- Each client should have his or her own bottle of eyedrops.
- Check the expiration date before administering eyedrops.
- Discard any solution remaining in the dropper after instillation.
- Discard the dropper if the tip is accidentally contaminated, as by touching the bottle or any part of the client's eye.

The nurse should insert medication disks at bedtime because they usually cause blurring of the eyes on insertion. Standard Precautions are used when administering eye care and medications because of the potential contact with bodily secretions.

Ear Medications Solutions ordered to treat the ear are often referred to as *otic* (pertaining to the ear) drops or irrigations. Eardrops may be instilled to soften ear wax, to produce anesthesia, to treat infection or inflammation, or to facilitate removal of a foreign body, such as an insect. External auditory canal irrigations

are usually performed for cleaning purposes and less frequently for applying heat and antiseptic solutions.

Before instilling a solution into the ear, the nurse should inspect the ear for signs of drainage, an indication of a perforated tympanic membrane. Eardrops are usually contraindicated when the tympanic membrane is perforated. If the tympanic membrane is damaged, all procedures must be performed using sterile aseptic technique; otherwise, medical asepsis is used when instilling medications into the ear.

Nasal Instillations Nasal instillations can be performed with different preparations: drops or nebulizers (atomizer or aerosol). Nasal drugs are administered to produce one or more of the following effects: to shrink swollen mucous membranes, to loosen secretions and facilitate drainage, or to treat infections of

 COMMUNITY/HOME HEALTH CARE

Considerations for Use of Nasal Inhalers
- Provide the client with the manufacturer's directions for the specific type of inhaler, such as how to replace a medication cartridge for a nasal aerosol.
- Store inhalers at room temperature.
- Do not puncture or place aerosols in an incinerator because they are prepared under pressure.
- Instruct the client not to allow other people to use the inhaler.
- Caution the client about overuse that could cause a rebound effect, making the condition worse.
- Ensure that the client is knowledgeable about the expected and adverse effects of the drug. Some of these drugs do not produce therapeutic effects for severals days, and some require 2 weeks of continuous use before the drug's effects appear.
- Provide the client with a telephone number to call if assistance is needed.

PROFESSIONAL TIP

Administering Nose Drops

- Gather equipment: MAR; prescribed medication with dropper; emesis basin; and tissues.
- Check the MAR against the written orders and the chart for allergies.
- Wash hands, and follow the five "rights" of drug administration.
- Check the client's identification armband, explain the procedure to the client, and provide for privacy.
- Don nonsterile gloves.
- Instruct the client to blow the nose to facilitate the removal of mucus and secretions.
- Place the client in a supine position and hyperextend the neck. Position the head so that the drops will reach the expected site, as shown in Figure 24-27.
- Squeeze some medication into the dropper.
- Insert the nasal drops about ⅜ inch into the nostril, keeping the tip of the dropper away from the sides of the nares.
- Instill the prescribed dosage of medication and observe the client for any signs of discomfort.
- Instruct the client to remain supine for 5 minutes to prevent the medication from leaking out of the nose.
- Discard any unused medication remaining in the dropper.
- Return the client to a comfortable position and provide the client with the emesis basin and tissues to expectorate any medication that flows into the oropharynx and mouth.
- Remove gloves and wash hands.
- Record on the MAR the drug given, number of drops instilled, and nostril medicated.

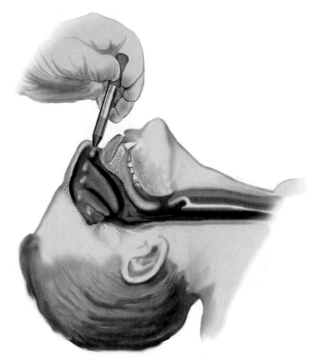

Figure 24-27 Positioning a Client for Nose Drop Instillation

- Instruct the client to clear the nostrils by blowing the nose.
- Client should be in an upright position with head tilted back slightly.

For atomizers:
- Occlude one nostril to prevent air from entering the nasal cavity and to allow the medication to flow freely in the open nostril.
- Insert the atomizer tip into the open nostril and instruct the client to inhale, then squeeze the atomizer once, and instruct the client to exhale.

For aerosols:
- Shake the aerosol well before each use.
- Grasp between thumb and index finger and insert the adapter tip into one nostril while occluding the other nostril with a finger, then press the adapter cartridge firmly to release one measured dose of medication.
- Repeat the above steps as ordered for the other nostril.
- Instruct the client to keep the head tilted backward for 2 to 3 minutes and to breathe through the nose while the medication is being absorbed.

the nasal cavity or sinuses. Because many of these products are nonprescription drugs, clients should be taught their correct usage. For example, nasal decongestants are common over-the-counter drugs used to shrink swollen mucous membranes. However, when these drugs are used in excess, they may have a reverse or rebound effect by increasing nasal congestion.

Although the nose is considered a clean (not sterile) cavity, because of its connection with the sinuses, the nurse uses medical asepsis when performing nasal instillations.

Nebulizers (inhalers) are used to deliver a fine mist containing medication droplets. When the client is discharged with a nasal inhaler, the nurse should teach the client how to store and use the device. The nurse should administer or assist clients with the use of atomizers and aerosols:

Respiratory Inhalants Respiratory inhalants are delivered by devices that produce fine droplets that are inhaled deep into the respiratory tract. These medication droplets are absorbed almost immediately through the alveolar epithelium into the bloodstream. This section addresses only oropharyngeal handheld inhalers.

Oropharyngeal handheld inhalers deliver medications, such as bronchodilators and mucolytics, that produce both local and systemic effects. Bronchodila-

CLIENT TEACHING

Self-Administration with a Metered-Dose Inhaler

- Review with the client the purpose of each prescribed medication. Some clients are ordered several inhalant medications and need to be taught the correct sequencing. For example, fast-acting bronchodilators such as albuterol sulfate (Ventolin) are taken before slower-acting bronchodilators such as salmeterol xinafoate (Serevent).
- Explain that the inhaler must be shaken before each use to mix the medication and the aerosol propellant.
- Remove the mouthpiece and cap from the bottle and insert the metal stem of the bottle into the small hole on the flattened portion of the mouthpiece.
- Instruct the client to exhale, place the mouthpiece into the mouth, and ensure that the lips form a tight seal around the mouthpiece.
- Instruct the client to firmly push the cylinder down against the mouthpiece only once (Figure 24-28) and to inhale slowly until the lungs feel full.
- Ask the client to remove the mouthpiece while holding the breath for several seconds to allow the medication to reach the alveoli, and then to exhale slowly through pursed lips.
- Inform the client that a mouthwash can be used to remove the taste of medication.
- Show the client how to wash the mouthpiece under tepid running water to remove secretions.

tors (drugs that dilate the bronchi) improve airway patency and are used to prevent or treat bronchospasms, asthma, and allergic reactions. Mucolytics are used to liquify tenacious (thick) bronchial secretions.

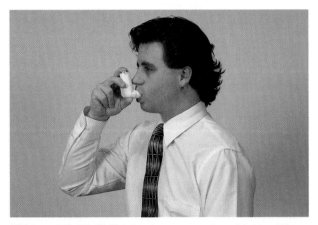

Figure 24-28 Self-Administration with a Metered-Dose Inhaler

Clients must be able to form an airtight seal around the inhaling devices and must be able to assemble the turbo-inhaler. This requirement prevents some clients, such as clients with visual or coordination impairments, from using these devices. Bronchodilators are contraindicated in clients who have a history of tachycardia.

Rectal Instillations Rectal instillations can be in the form of enemas, suppositories, or ointments. Rec-

PROFESSIONAL TIP

Administering a Rectal Suppository

- Gather equipment: MAR; prescribed rectal suppository; water-soluble lubricant, such as K-Y jelly; nonsterile gloves; tissues; bedpan (optional).
- Check the MAR against the written orders and the chart for allergies.
- Wash hands, and follow the five "rights."
- Check the client's identification armband, and explain the procedure to the client.
- Ask the client if he or she needs to void because the client will have to remain in bed after insertion of the suppository. Provide for privacy.
- Don nonsterile gloves.
- Place the client in the Sims', left lateral, position, with the upper leg flexed.
- Fold back the bed linen to expose the rectum.
- Open the package of lubricant and remove the foil wrapper from the suppository. Read the manufacturer's instructions on the wrapper for the recommended time interval the client should retain the suppository after insertion.
- Apply a small amount of lubricant to the smooth rounded end of the suppository to reduce mucosal irritation.
- Lubricate the gloved index finger.
- Instruct the client to breathe through the mouth to relax.
- Insert the suppository into the rectal canal beyond the internal anal sphincter, about 4 inches (10 cm) for an adult and 2 inches (5 cm) for a child to prevent the suppository from slipping out (Figure 24-29). Avoid inserting the suppository into feces.
- Withdraw the finger and wipe the anal area with tissues to provide comfort.
- Instruct the client to remain in the left lateral or supine position for at least 15 minutes until the medication is absorbed and to avoid the urge to defecate for 30 to 40 minutes, or as directed by the manufacturer's instructions.
- Remove gloves, turning them inside out, dispose, and wash hands.
- Record the drug on the MAR: name, dosage, route, and time of administration.

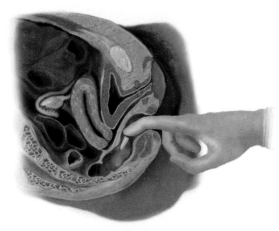

Figure 24-29 Inserting a Rectal Suppository

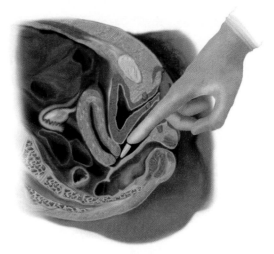

Figure 24-30 Inserting a Vaginal Suppository Along the Posterior Wall of the Vagina

tal ointments are used to treat local conditions and symptoms such as pain, inflammation, and itching caused from hemorrhoids. Rectal suppositories are cone-shaped masses of substances designed to melt at body temperature and to produce the intended effect at a slow and steady rate of absorption.

Suppositories provide a safe and convenient route for administering drugs that interact poorly with digestive enzymes or have a bad taste or odor. They are also used to provide temporary relief for clients who cannot tolerate oral preparations: for example, to relieve nausea and vomiting. Suppositories are also used to relieve pain and local irritation, reduce fever, and stimulate peristalsis and defecation in clients who are constipated.

The nurse should assess the rectum for irritation or bleeding and check sphincter control. Some clients may experience problems in retaining the suppository. The nurse should instruct those clients to remain in the Sims' position for at least 15 minutes or should place the client on the abdomen, if the condition allows, and hold the buttocks closed. The physician should be notified when the client is unable to retain a suppository so that another route can be ordered.

Vaginal Instillations Medications inserted into the vagina are in the form of suppositories, creams, gels, ointments, foams, or douches. These medications may be used to treat inflammation, infections, and discomfort or as a contraceptive measure.

Vaginal creams, gels, or ointments usually come with a disposable tubular applicator with a plunger to insert the drug. Suppositories are usually inserted with the index finger of a gloved hand; however, small suppositories may come with an applicator and the suppository is placed in the applicator's tip. After insertion of these preparations, the client may notice drainage and should be informed that this is expected. The nurse should advise the client to wear a perineal pad to prevent soiling of the underpants.

Sterile technique is usually required by agency policy, especially if there is an open wound when administering a vaginal douche (irrigation). The nurse should ensure that the client does not have an allergy to iodine because many vaginal preparations contain povidone-iodine.

Evaluation

Inherent in safe drug administration is the nursing responsibility to follow the five "rights." Administering medications in accord with these guidelines requires the nurse to verify that safe nursing care was provided to the client. For example, a client receiving a sublingual medication knows not to drink water until the tablet has dissolved completely; the client receiving medications through an NG tube did not aspirate; or

PROFESSIONAL TIP

Contraindications for Rectal Suppositories

- Contraindicated for cardiac clients because insertion may stimulate the vagus nerve, causing cardiac dysrhythmias (abnormal heart patterns).
- Contraindicated for clients recovering from rectal or prostate surgery because suppositories may cause pain on insertion and trauma to the tissues.

CLIENT TEACHING

Tampon Use

Clients should not use tampons after the insertion of vaginal medications because the tampon can absorb the medication and decrease the drug's effect.

PROFESSIONAL TIP

Administering a Vaginal Suppository

- Gather equipment: MAR; prescribed vaginal suppository; disposable applicator if indicated; water-soluble lubricant; nonsterile gloves; tissues.
- Check the MAR against the written orders and the chart for allergies.
- Wash hands, and follow the five "rights" of drug administration.
- Check the client's identification armband, and explain the procedure to the client.
- Ask the client to void because a full bladder may cause discomfort and injury to the vaginal lining when the suppository is inserted. Provide for privacy.
- Don nonsterile glove.
- Place the client in a dorsal recumbent, back-lying position with knees flexed and hips rotated laterally or in a Sims' position if the client cannot maintain the dorsal recumbent position.
- Assess the perineal area, inspect the vaginal orifice, note any odor or discharge from the vagina, and inquire about any problems, such as discomfort or itching.
- If secretion or discharge is present, cleanse the perineal area with soap and warm water to prevent the introduction of microorganisms into the vagina.
- Remove the suppository from the foil wrapper, and if applicable, insert the suppository into the applicator's tip.

- Apply a small amount of lubricant to the smooth rounded end of the suppository to reduce mucosal irritation.
- If not using an applicator, apply a small amount of lubricant to gloved index finger.
- Insert the suppository into the vaginal canal at least 2 inches (5 cm) along the posterior wall of the vagina or as far as it will go to prevent the suppository from slipping out (Figure 24-30). If using an applicator, insert as described above and depress the plunger to release the suppository. Wipe the perineum with clean, dry tissues.
- Instruct the client to remain in bed for 15 minutes until the suppository is absorbed.
- Wash the applicator under cool running water to clean (warm or hot water produces coagulation of protein secretions) and return to appropriate storage in the client's room.
- Remove the gloves, turning them inside out, and dispose of the gloves in the proper receptacle.
- Record on the MAR the drug's name, dosage, route, and date and time of administration; document any evidence of discharge or odor from the vagina.
- Check on the client in 15 minutes to ensure that the suppository did not slip out and to allow the client the opportunity to verbalize any problems or concerns.

the diabetic client can safely self-administer insulin by withdrawing the prescribed dose and administering the injection in the subcutaneous tissues while maintaining sterile technique.

The nurse who identifies a potential medication risk and initiates actions to prevent client injury is performing another form of evaluation. For example, if the client in the home setting cannot remember if the prescribed medications have been taken, providing the client with a daily or weekly pillbox that is filled when the nurse is present prevents the client from taking too much medication or failing to take the dose as ordered.

SAMPLE NURSING CARE PLAN

THE CLIENT WITH DEEP VEIN THROMBOSIS

Mrs. Landry, a 45-year-old, was admitted to your floor with a diagnosis of deep vein thrombosis. She noticed swelling of her left leg about a week ago but decided to treat it at home. Four days later the lower leg was very edematous, warm, and painful to move. After an office visit, Mrs. Landry was admitted to the hospital. This is her first hospitalization. On examination the left leg is warmer than the right. The left thigh circumference is 3 inches larger than the right. The physician ordered a heparin IV drip after a loading dose bolus was given. The drip contained 10,000 units heparin in 500 mL of D_5W at 10 mL/h (200 units/h). The physician anticipates that Mrs. Landry will be weaned off of the heparin drip and started on subcutaneous heparin within 5 days. At the time of discharge she will be given Coumadin.   *continues*

Nursing Diagnosis 1 *Ineffective Tissue Perfusion related to the development of venous thrombi in the deep femoral vein as evidenced by left leg being warmer than right leg and left thigh circumference being 3 inches larger than right thigh circumference.*

PLANNING/GOALS	NURSING INTERVENTIONS	RATIONALE	EVALUATION
Mrs. Landry will: Report an absence of pain.	Maintain on bedrest.	Reduces the possibility of embolus; may decrease the pain and swelling.	Mrs. Landry is able to ambulate without difficulty or pain.
	Apply moist heat to the affected extremity.	Heat provides an analgesic effect; it decreases venospasms and pain.	
Demonstrate an absence of edema.	Elevate the legs above the heart.	Elevation facilitates venous return and decreases the edema.	Mrs. Landry's left thigh is only ½ inch larger than her right thigh.
	Measure the circumference of the left thigh and compare with that of the right thigh.	Measuring the circumference provides a quantitative reference point that can be used to evaluate the swelling.	
Experience the same degree of skin temperature in both legs.	Administer the heparin drip at 200 units/h.	Heparin prevents the conversion of fibrinogen to fibrin and prothrombin to thrombin, thereby limiting the extension of the thrombus.	Mrs. Landry has no temperature difference between her legs.
	Monitor the partial thromboplastin time (PTT).	The partial thromboplastin time is used to monitor heparin therapy because heparin, a short-acting anticoagulant, increases the PTT.	

Nursing Diagnosis 2 *Risk for Injury bleeding related to the administration of an anticoagulant.*

PLANNING/GOALS	NURSING INTERVENTIONS	RATIONALE	EVALUATION
Mrs. Landry will: Not demonstrate evidence of bleeding from gums or nose, in urine or stool, or under the skin.	Advise Mrs. Landry to withhold the medication in the event that bleeding occurs and to notify the physician immediately.	The dose may need to be adjusted.	Mrs. Landry has had no bleeding episodes.
	Encourage the client to discontinue smoking.	Smoking has a tendency to increase the metabolism of the medication, necessitating an increase in the dose.	

continues

Maintain her prothrombin time (PT) or international normalized ratio (INR) within therapeutic range.	Advise the client to watch food intake.	Foods high in fat and foods rich in vitamin K can interfere with the PT.	Mrs. Landry still has many questions about taking the oral anticoagulant on discharge. Discharge followup will be needed to monitor the client's progress on the oral anticoagulant.
	Warn against taking oral contraceptive medication.	There may be a decrease in anticoagulant effect due to the increased production of clotting factors with oral contraceptives.	
	Warn against taking aspirin and other over-the-counter medications.	Aspirin may increase the risk of bleeding; it inhibits platelet formation.	

CASE STUDY

Mrs. Cheng is a 76-year-old client who was discharged from the hospital with cancer of the lungs. Mrs. Cheng elected not to have surgery and was given her first chemotherapy before discharge. She is not accustomed to taking medications. Before the onset of symptoms that necessitated her admission to the hospital, Mrs. Cheng considered herself in good health, only bothered with the discomfort of arthritis in her hands. She is being discharged on the following medications:

- *sulfamethoxazole (Gantanol), a sulfonamide anti-infective, 500 mg/5 mL susp po b.i.d.*
- *granisetron (Kytril), an antiemetic, 1 mg po q12h*
- *morphine sulfate 30 mg po q4h, prn for pain*

The following questions will guide your development of a nursing care plan for the case study.

1. What other assessments would you make about Mrs. Cheng?
2. What two nursing diagnoses with a goal for each might be appropriate for Mrs. Cheng?
3. What nursing interventions might help Mrs. Cheng meet the goals?

SUMMARY

- The *United States Pharmacopeia* and the *National Formulary* outline drug standards for use in the United States.
- The Food and Drug Administration tests all drugs for toxicity before granting a company the right to market a drug.
- Drugs are usually referred to by their generic name, not capitalized, or by their trade name, always capitalized.
- The oral administration route is the safest and least expensive administration route, although it is also the slowest to act.
- Parenteral drugs are injected through intradermal (ID), subcutaneous (SC or SQ), intramuscular (IM), or intravenous (IV) routes and are typically fast-acting.

- The pharmacokinetics of drugs includes absorption, distribution, metabolism, and excretion.
- Safe drug administration is facilitated by following the five "rights": right drug, right dose, right client, right route, and right time.
- Nurses are both morally and legally responsible for correct administration of medications; this includes following institutional policy, considering clients' desires and abilities, fostering compliance, and correctly documenting all actions related to medication administration and medication errors.
- Before administering medications, the nurse must thoroughly assess the client's drug history, medical history, and psychosocial factors that may affect drug acceptance and compliance.
- Oral medications should be poured and measured at eye level to ensure accuracy.

- Although the physician will determine the dose and route of a parenteral drug, the nurse is responsible for choosing the correct gauge and length of the needle to be used.
- The nurse must always carefully monitor client reactions to medications and ensure that clients are appropriately educated as to the actions, side effects, and contraindications of all medications they are receiving.
- Clients receiving intravenous therapy or blood transfusions require constant monitoring for complications.

Review Questions

1. The law that began the regulation of habit-forming drugs is called the:
   a. Kefauver-Harris Act.
   b. Harrison Narcotic Act.
   c. Controlled Substance Act.
   d. Food, Drug, and Cosmetic Act.

2. A client is unable to swallow the pills ordered by the physician. The best action for the nurse is to:
   a. tell the client to chew the pills.
   b. crush the pills and give them to the client.
   c. call the physician for a change in the orders.
   d. ask the pharmacy to send the medications in liquid form.

3. The only household measure used in calculating dosages is the:
   a. drop.
   b. pound.
   c. ounce.
   d. teaspoon.

4. The method considered to be one of the most accurate for calculating medication dosages for infants and children up to 12 years of age is:
   a. Clark's rule.
   b. Young's rule.
   c. weight and height.
   d. body surface area.

5. The client is in the bathroom when the nurse brings the medications. The best action for the nurse is to:
   a. return with the medications when the client is finished in the bathroom.
   b. leave the medications for the client to take when finished in the bathroom.
   c. knock on the bathroom door and give the medications to the client at this time.
   d. ask the nursing assistant to see that the client takes the medications when finished in the bathroom.

6. The best time for the nurse to document medication administration is:
   a. whenever the nurse has time.
   b. before the client receives the medication.
   c. only after the client has received the medication.
   d. toward the end of the shift so all medications can be charted at one time.

7. Sublingual medications are to be:
   a. chewed.
   b. placed under the tongue.
   c. placed between the cheek and teeth.
   d. swallowed with 8 ounces of water.

8. Standard Precautions are required with:
   a. venipuncture.
   b. IM injections.
   c. oral medications.
   d. nasal instillation.

9. An intravenous solution of sodium chloride (0.45%) is:
   a. isotonic.
   b. iso-osmolar.
   c. hypertonic.
   d. hypotonic.

10. A client receiving a blood transfusion tells the nurse, who is taking the first set of 15-minute vital signs, that she is cold (chills) and her chest hurts. The first thing the nurse should do is:
    a. stop the transfusion.
    b. get a warm blanket for the client.
    c. call the blood bank to come and check the blood.
    d. stay with the client and talk quietly to her to help her relax.

Critical Thinking Questions

1. You discover that a similar but incorrect drug (not the drug ordered) is being given IV to a client. What is the first thing you should do? What is your next course of action? How do you feel about the nurse who made the medication error but did not recognize it?

2. How can transfusion reactions be differentiated?

⚡ WEB FLASH!

- Visit the web for sites related to IV therapy, medication administration, and medication errors. What type of information is available?
- Are there any organizations on the web related to medication administration?

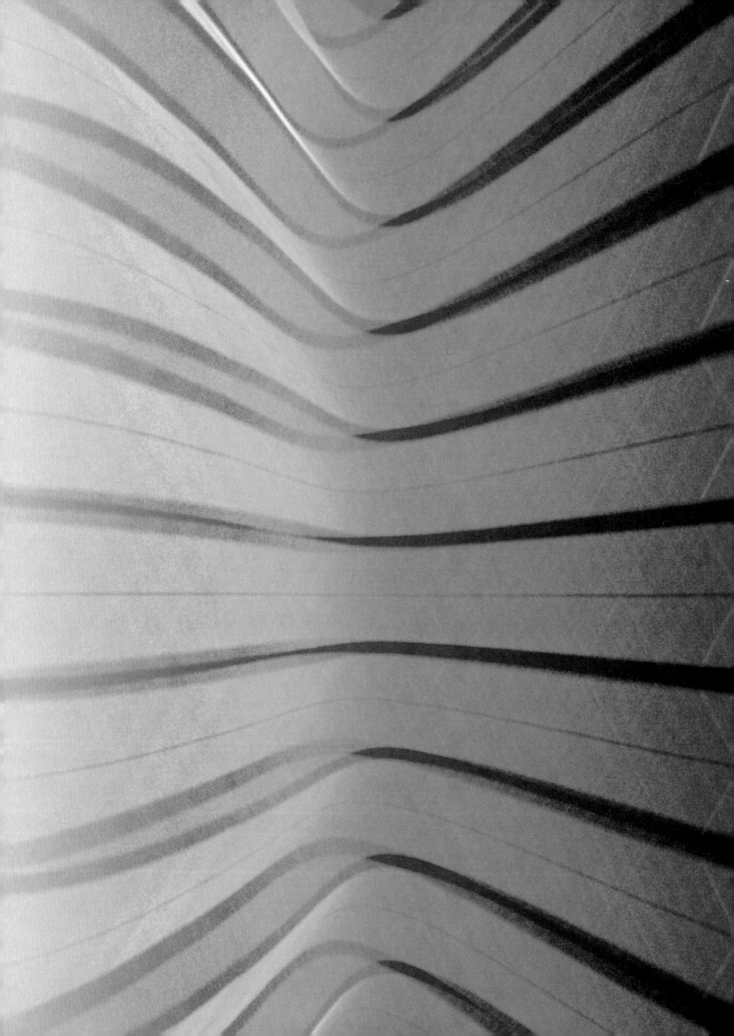

Concepts for Care

Unit 10
Fundamental
Nursing Care

Unit 11
Special Areas of
Nursing care

Unit 12
Leadership/Work
Transition

Chapter 25
Assessment

Chapter 26
Pain Management

Chapter 27
Diagnostic Tests

ASSESSMENT

MAKING THE CONNECTION

Refer to the following chapters to increase your understanding of health assessment:

- **Chapter 8, Communication**
- **Chapter 12, Cultural Diversity and Nursing**
- **Chapter 13, Complementary/Alternative Therapies**
- **Chapter 17, Loss, Grief, and Death**
- **Chapter 23, Fluid, Electrolyte, and Acid-Base Balance**

- **Chapter 26, Pain Management**
- **Chapter 28, Nursing Care of the Older Client**
- **Procedures:** B1, Handwashing; B3, Measuring Body Temperature; B4, Assessing Pulse Rate; B5, Assessing Respirations; B6, Assessing Blood Pressure; B7, Weighing Client, Mobile and Immobile

LEARNING OBJECTIVES

Upon completion of this chapter, you should be able to:
- *Define key terms.*
- *Identify the components of functional health patterns.*
- *Utilize the framework of functional health to facilitate a holistic assessment process.*
- *Analyze the components of the head-to-toe assessment.*
- *Incorporate the four assessment techniques within the head-to-toe assessment.*
- *Utilize the head-to-toe assessment in clinical situations.*

INTRODUCTION

Within the scope of the nursing profession, a complete nursing assessment is necessary to analyze each client's needs in a holistic manner. Nursing assessment includes both physical and psychosocial aspects to evaluate a client's condition. A nurse demonstrates caring, respect, and concern for each client when doing a nursing assessment.

A thorough nursing assessment includes both a health history and a physical examination. To perform

KEY TERMS

adventitious breath
   sound
affect
auscultation
borborygmi
bradycardia
bradypnea
bronchial sound
bronchovesicular
   sound
crackle
cyanosis
dyspnea
eupnea
health history
hyperventilation
hypoventilation
inspection

orthostatic
   hypotension
palpation
percussion
pleural friction rub
pulse amplitude
pulse deficit
pulse rate
pulse rhythm
review of systems
sibilant wheeze
Snellen chart
sonorous wheeze
stridor
tachycardia
tachypnea
vesicular sound

a health history, the nurse interviews the client to identify how the client adjusts to or lives within the environment. This data is subjective data, or information based on client self-report. During the physical examination the nurse collects objective data, which includes observations made by the nurse while utilizing the assessment techniques of inspection, palpation, percussion, and auscultation. Other sources of objective data are laboratory tests, x-rays, and measurements of the client's vital signs, height, and weight.

The health history and the physical examination assist the nurse in focusing on the client as a whole. The initial nursing assessment generally occurs within 8 hours of a client's admission to a health care facility, and continues throughout the stay. In a physician's office or health care clinic, the nursing assessment would be completed immediately. Most institutions have a standard asessment form (Figure 25-1).

Usually a health history is completed prior to the physical examination. However, in emergency situations or when performing care in a health care facility after the initial admitting assessment, it will be necessary to incorporate history-taking within the physical examination. When incorporating a health history within the head-to-toe assessment, the nurse must remember to incorporate questions about the client's habits or usual patterns along with the physical data collected in the head-to-toe assessment. Functional assessment is best done within the framework of the physical assessment since the environment in which each client resides and participates becomes a part of the physical assessment. The functional assessment brings the environment in which the client lives and the physical needs of that client together to establish a holistic picture.

HEALTH HISTORY

A primary focus of the data collection interview is the health history. The **health history** is a review of the client's functional health patterns prior to the current contact with a health care agency. While the medical history concentrates on symptoms and the progression of disease, the nursing health history focuses on the client's functional health patterns, responses to changes in health status, and alterations in lifestyle. The health history is also used in developing the plan of care and formulating nursing interventions.

Demographic Information

Personal data including name, address, date of birth, gender, religion, race/ethnic origin, occupation, and type of health plan/insurance should be included. Factors that are derived from this information may be useful in helping to foster understanding of a client's perspective.

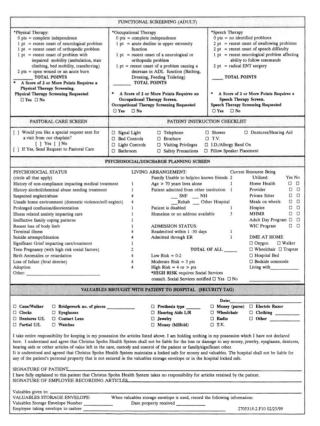

Figure 25-1 Patient Admission Data Base (*Courtesy of Christus Spohn Health System, Corpus Christi, TX*)

continues

Figure 25-1 (*continued*)

Reason for Seeking Health Care

The client's reason for seeking health care should be described in the client's own words. For example, the statement "fell off four-foot ladder and landed on right shoulder; unable to move right arm" is the client's actual report of the event that precipitated his or her need for health care. The client's perspective is important because it explains what is significant about the event from the client's point of view. It is also important to determine the time of the onset of symptoms as well as a complete symptom analysis.

Perception of Health Status

Perception of health status refers to the client's opinion of his or her general health. It may be useful to ask clients to rate their health on a scale of 1 to 10 (with 10 being ideal and 1 being poor), together with the client's rationale for their rating score. For example, the nurse may record a statement such as the following to represent the client's perception of health: "Rates health a 7 on a scale of 1 (poor) to 10 (ideal) because he must take medication regularly in order to maintain mobility, but the medication sometimes upsets his stomach."

Previous Illnesses, Hospitalizations, and Surgeries

The history and timing of any previous experiences with illness, surgery, or hospitalization are helpful in order to assess recurrent conditions and to anticipate responses to illness, since prior experiences often have an impact on current responses.

Client/Family Medical History

The nurse needs to determine any family history of acute and chronic illnesses that tend to be familial. Health history forms will frequently include checklists of various illnesses that the nurse can use as the basis of the questions about this aspect. The client should be instructed that family history refers to blood relatives. It is also helpful to indicate the relative's relationship to the client (e.g., mother, father, sister).

Immunizations/Exposure to Communicable Diseases

Any history of childhood or other communicable diseases should be noted. In addition, a record of current immunizations should be obtained. This is particularly important with children; however, records of immunizations for tetanus, influenza, and hepatitis B can also be important for adults. If the client has traveled out of the country, the time frame should be indicated in order to determine incubation periods for relevant diseases. The client should also be asked about potential exposure to communicable diseases such as tuberculosis or human immunodeficiency virus (HIV).

Allergies

Any drug, food, or environmental allergies should be noted in the health history. In addition to the name of the allergen, the type of reaction to the substance should be noted. For example, a client may report that he or she developed a rash or became short of breath after taking penicillin. This reaction should be recorded. Clients may report an "allergy" to a medication because they developed an upset stomach after ingesting it, which the nurse will recognize as a side effect that would not preclude administration of the drug in the future.

Safety: Assessment for Allergies
It is essential that the nurse explore possible allergies prior to administering any medications. Allergic reactions can be life-threatening and can occur even with very low dosages of medications. A client's sensitivity to a drug can also change over time, resulting in severe reactions even though the client has successfully taken the drug during prior illnesses or experienced only mild reactions to the drug in the past.

Current Medications

All medications currently taken, both prescription and over-the-counter, should be recorded by name, frequency, and dosage. Clients should be reminded that this information should include medications such as birth control pills, laxatives, nonprescription pain relief medications, herbal remedies, and vitamin and mineral supplements.

Developmental Level

Knowledge of developmental level is essential for considering appropriate norms of behavior and for appraising the achievement of relevant developmental tasks. Any recognized theory of growth and development can be applied in order to determine if clients are functioning within the parameters expected for their age group. For example, if the nurse uses Erikson's stages of psychosocial development, validation of an adult client's attainment of the developmental task of generativity versus stagnation can be made by the nurse's statement, such as "client prefers to spend time with his family; very involved in children's school activities."

Psychosocial History

Psychosocial history refers to assessment of dimensions such as self-concept and self-esteem as well as usual sources of stress and the client's ability to cope. Sources of support for clients in crisis, such as family, significant others, religion, or support groups, should be explored.

Sociocultural History

In exploring the client's sociocultural history, it is important to inquire about the home environment, family situation, and client's role in the family. For example, the client could be the parent of three children and the sole provider in a single-parent family. The responsibilities of the client are important data through which the nurse can determine the impact of changes in health status and thus plan the most beneficial care for the client. Patterns related to caffeine and alcohol intake and use of tobacco or recreational drugs should also be explored.

Complementary/Alternative Therapy Use

Lazar and O'Conner (1997) report that 70% of clients using complementary/alternative therapies as well as conventional medicine do not report using these therapies to their healthcare providers. Simple open-ended questions such as "Do you do anything to improve your health?" may provide important information. If a complementary/alternative therapy is mentioned, the nurse might ask if this is something the client would consider using (Hodge & Ullrich, 1999).

Activities of Daily Living

The activities of daily living is a description of the client's lifestyle and capacity for self-care and is useful both as baseline information and as a source of insight into usual health behaviors. This baseline should include information on nutritional intake and eating habits, elimination patterns, rest/sleep patterns, and activity/exercise.

Review of Systems

The **review of systems** (ROS) is a brief account from the client of any recent signs or symptoms associated with any of the body systems. This can most effectively be obtained as the physical examination is being performed. The review of systems relies on subjective information provided by the client rather than on the nurse's own physical examination. When a symptom is encountered, either while eliciting the health history or during the physical examination of the client, the nurse should obtain as much information as possible about the symptom. Relevant data include:

- *Location:* The area of the body in which the symptom (such as pain) is felt.
- *Character:* The quality of the feeling or sensation (e.g., sharp, dull, stabbing).
- *Intensity:* The severity or quantity of the feeling or sensation and its interference with functional abilities. The sensation can be rated on a scale of 1 (very little) to 10 (very intense).
- *Timing:* The onset, duration, frequency, and precipitating factors of the symptom.
- *Aggravating/alleviating factors:* The activities or actions that make the symptom worse or better.

PHYSICAL EXAMINATION

The physical examination is performed in all health care settings (home, outpatient facilities, extended care institutions, and acute care facilities) for all age groups to gather comprehensive, pertinent assessment data. The physical examination provides a complete picture of the client's physiological functioning. When combined with a health and psychosocial assessment, it forms a database to direct decision making. The examination should be performed according to the agency's policy. Policy may vary from one agency to another.

The physical examination is done in a sequential, head-to-toe fashion to ensure a thorough assessment of each system. This method not only prevents the nurse from forgetting to examine an area, it also decreases the number of times the nurse and the client have to change positions.

The nurse performs the physical or the head-to-toe assessment by using specific assessment techniques. These techniques include: inspection, palpation, percussion, and auscultation.

Inspection

Inspection consists of a thorough visual observation of the client. This visual assessment gives the nurse a description of the body's outward response to its internal functioning. Inspection of the skin, for example, can assist the nurse in identifying signs of a fever through the client's flushed facial cheeks. The skin can also be an indicator of a decreased oxygen supply when **cyanosis**, a bluish or dark purple coloration, is noted in the client's lips, skin, or nail beds.

Sharing observations with the client during inspection enhances the holistic data collected. For example, when the nurse mentions the observation of visible scars, the client may discuss previous surgeries or hospitalizations. Instruments such as a penlight and otoscope are often used to enhance visualization.

Effective inspection requires adequate lighting and exposure of the body parts being observed. Beginning nurses often feel self-conscious or embarrassed using the technique of inspection; however, most become comfortable with the technique over time. Nurses must also be sensitive to the client's feelings of embarrassment with the use of inspection and respond to this situation by discussing the technique with the client and using measures such as draping in order to increase the client's comfort level.

Palpation

In **palpation**, the nurse uses the sense of touch to assess texture, temperature, moisture, organ location and size, vibrations, pulsations, swelling, masses, and tenderness. The nurse's finger pads are placed flat against the client's skin, exerting slight pressure for light palpation, as seen in Figure 25-2. Assessment of the kidneys, liver, spleen, bowel, and fundal height may be accomplished through deep palpation, in which more pressure is exerted. Pulses are also palpated. The abdomen is palpated for distention, softness, firmness, rigidity, or tenderness.

Palpation requires a calm, gentle approach and is used systematically, with light palpation preceding deep palpation and palpation of tender areas performed last.

 Safety: Palpation
Deep palpation is a technique requiring significant expertise and should not be employed by beginning nursing students without supervision.

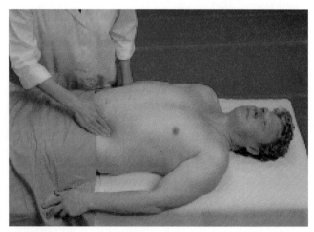

Figure 25-2 Light Palpation

Percussion

Percussion uses short, tapping strokes on the surface of the skin to create vibrations of underlying organs. It is used for assessing the density of structures or determining the location and size of organs in the body. The nurse uses the fingertips to tap the client's body to produce sounds and vibrations. The nurse places the middle finger of the nondominant hand on the client's skin in the area to be percussed, then taps lightly with the middle finger of the dominant hand on the distal phalanx of the middle finger positioned on the body surface (Figure 25-3). The nurse taps twice in one place before moving to a new area. Percussion should not be painful to the client. If it is painful, the percussion should be discontinued and the response documented.

Percussion is a skill that requires much practice to master, and it is important to be familiar with the sounds produced when percussion is used. Table 25–1 describes the various percussion tones.

Auscultation

Auscultation involves listening to sounds in the body that are created by movement of air or fluid. Areas most often auscultated include the lungs, heart, abdomen, and blood vessels. Although direct auscultation is sometimes possible, a stethoscope is usually employed in order to channel the sound (Figure 25-4).

HEAD-TO-TOE ASSESSMENT

Prior to beginning the examination, the nurse should keep in mind some important concepts to be utilized throughout the examination. The client's privacy should be respected by pulling the curtain, closing the door, and providing appropriate draping of the client. When possible, distracting noises such as radio or television and people talking should be eliminated. Assessment should be performed under natural light because fluorescent light can change the color tones of the skin. All procedures should be explained to the client and confidentiality of data acquired during the examination maintained.

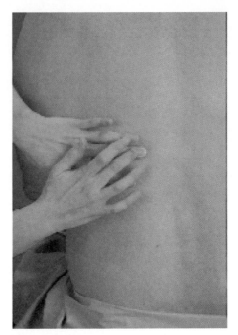
Figure 25-3 Percussion

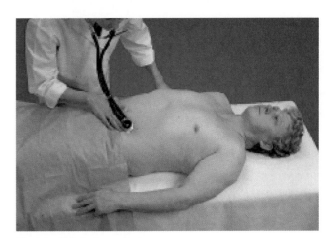
Figure 25-4 Auscultation

 Infection Control: Standard Precautions
Remember to utilize standard precautions when in contact with any body fluids by using gloves, gown, or mask when appropriate.

Table 25–1 DESCRIPTION OF PERCUSSION TONES					
TONE	**INTENSITY**	**PITCH**	**DURATION**	**QUALITY**	**NORMAL LOCATION**
Dullness	Medium	High	Medium	Thudlike	Liver
Flatness	Soft	High	Short	Extreme dullness	Muscle
Hyperresonance	Very loud	Very low	Long	Booming	Child's lung
Resonance	Loud	Low	Long	Hollow	Peripheral lung
Tympany	Loud	High	Medium	Drumlike	Stomach

The nurse should position the client to ensure accessibility to the body part being assessed. Figure 25-5 presents the positions used in conducting a physical examination.

The primary purpose of draping the client is to prevent unnecessary exposure during the examination. Feelings of embarrassment elicit tension and restlessness and will decrease the client's ability to cooperate. The drapes also prevent the client from being chilled.

Sitting

To examine head, neck, back, posterior thorax and lungs, anterior thorax and lungs, breast, axillae, heart, extremities.

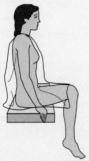

Client can expand lungs; nurse can inspect symmetry. *Institute risk precautions for elderly and debilitated clients.*

Dorsal recumbent

To examine head, neck, anterior thorax and lungs, breast, axillae, heart.

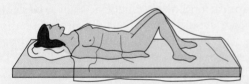

Client comfortable; increases abdominal muscle tension. *Contraindicated in abdominal assessment.*

Prone

To examine posterior thorax and lungs, hip

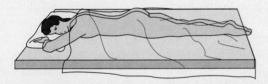

Assessment of hip extension. *Contraindicated in clients with cardiopulmonary alterations.*

Supine

To examine head, neck, anterior thorax and lungs, breasts, axillae, heart, abdomen, extremities.

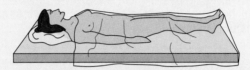

Client relaxed; decreases abdominal muscle tension; nurse can palpate all peripheral pulses. *Contraindicated in clients with cardiopulmonary alterations.*

Sims'

To examine rectum and vagina.

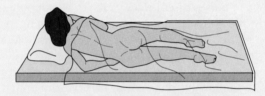

Relaxes rectal muscles. Painful for clients with joint deformities.

Knee-chest

To examine rectum

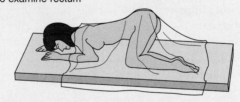

Maximal rectal exposure. *Contraindicated in clients with respiratory alterations.*

Lithotomy

To examine female genitalia, rectum, genital tract.

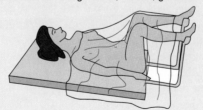

Maximal genitalia exposure; embarrassing and uncomfortable for client. *Contraindicated in clients with joint disorders.*

Figure 25-5 Various Positions for Physical Examination (*Adapted from* Health Assessment and Physical Examination, *(2nd ed.),* by M.E.Z. Estes, 2002, Albany, NY: Delmar. Copyright 2002 by Delmar. Adapted with permission.)

General Survey

The nurse's introduction to the client is an important first step at the start of a complete head-to-toe assessment. It is important for the nurse to identify herself and to express intent for the care of the client and the time frame involved. During this introductory time, it is appropriate for the nurse to utilize inspection to make a general assessment of the client. This overview is the first impression the nurse will have of the client and is the beginning point of the head-to-toe assessment. It includes such aspects as the general state of health and any signs of distress, such as pain or breathing difficulties. It also includes observations regarding the client's awareness of the surroundings, body type and posture, facial expressions, and mood.

The nurse should document the general survey data in an organized fashion to portray a clinical picture of the client. Certain clients such as the elderly, disabled, and abused will require special consideration during the physical examination.

Elderly

When nurses assess elderly clients, it is important to know the normal changes that result from aging. Aging may reduce the body's resistance to illness, tolerance of stress, and the ability to recuperate from illness. The nurse should make sure the client understands and can follow instructions, and allow extra time if the client has difficulty changing positions quickly.

Disabled Clients

When assessing disabled clients, nurses should adapt their interactions to the client's ability; for example, a hearing-impaired client should be given a written questionnaire. An intellectually impaired client might require simple, direct sentences and questions or use of pictures. It is best to determine the client's ability to participate before conducting the examination. To allay

LIFE CYCLE CONSIDERATIONS

The Older Client

- All senses are less acute.
- Endorphin level rises with age, which decreases awareness of painful events.
- Temperature normal range is 96°F to 98.9°F.
- Strength and endurance decline.
- Height decreases.
- Digestive and urinary functions slow down.
- Older clients are prone to constipation and nocturia.
- Respirations are slowed.
- Older clients are prone to fatigue, dizziness, and falls (Andresen, 1998).

CULTURAL CONSIDERATIONS

Cultural Values and Assessment

Cleanliness is highly valued by mainstream American society. However, in some cultures, a daily bath is not perceived as necessary or desirable. In fact, some cultures do not define natural body odors as offensive. It is important to consider the client in the context of cultural beliefs before labeling a client. Think of the terms *dirty, unkempt,* or *foul-smelling.* These value-laden terms can certainly cloud the assessment process and subsequently the care provided to a client.

the disabled client's fears and anxiety, a family member may be allowed to remain with the client during the examination. The nurse should ascertain the client's level of independence and feelings about the disability.

Abused Clients

Nurses must be observant for signs of abuse, especially in the elderly. The symptoms may be psychological as well as physical; for example, refusal to be touched, inability to maintain eye contact, or unwillingness to talk about bruises, burns, or other injuries may indicate abuse. Bruises or lacerations most typically appear on breasts, buttocks, thighs, or genitalia. The nurse should also inspect for healed scarring or burns. The nurse must know state laws and agency policies for reporting possible abuse.

Vital Signs

Once the nurse has established rapport with the client through introductions, measurement of vital signs is the next step in a head-to-toe assessment. Vital signs are the "signs of life" of an individual. They provide a way of connecting the external inspection of each client with the internal functioning of the client's organs. When checking vital signs, the nurse obtains the temperature (T), pulse (P), respirations (R), blood pressure (BP), and pain assessment of the client. See Table 25–2 for normal values and variations. Equipment used for T, P, R, and BP is shown in Figure 25-6.

Temperature

When assessing the client's temperature (T), the nurse can use an electronic, chemical, or mercury thermometer. Body temperature can be taken by 5 routes: oral, rectal, axillary, skin, or tympanic membrane. The route is chosen depending upon the client's age and physical condition. Factors such as age, gender, physical activity, and environment can affect a person's temperature. Consumption of hot or cold food or beverage and smoking 15 to 30 minutes before taking an oral temperature can also affect the result.

Thermometer

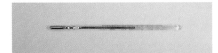

Oral   Slim tip

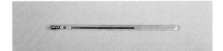

Rectal   Stubby, pear-shaped tip

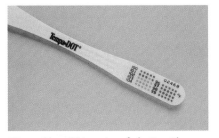

Disposable (chemical), single-use   Thin strips of plastic with chemically impregnated dots that change color to reflect temperature

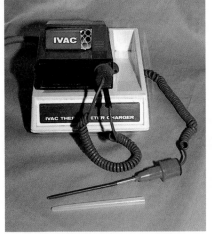

Electronic   Battery-powered display unit with a sensitive probe (blue for oral and red for rectal) covered with a disposable plastic sheath for individual use

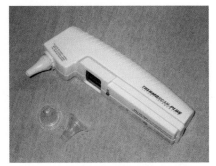

Tympanic   Battery-powered display unit with disposable probe covers.

Stethoscope

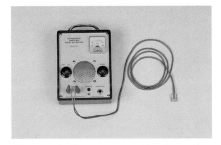

Acoustical   Closed cylinder that prevents dissipation of sound waves and amplifies the sound through a diaphragm. Flat-disc diaphragm transmits high-pitched sounds, and the bell-shaped diaphragm transmits low-pitched sounds.

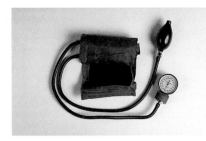

Ultrasound (Doppler)   Battery-operated headset with earpieces attached to a volume-controlled audio unit and ultrasound transducer that detects movement of red blood cells through a vessel.

Sphygmomanometer

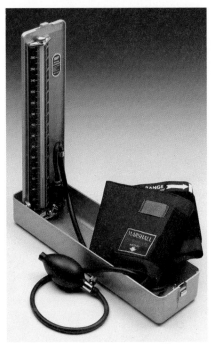

Mercury manometer   Wall or portable unit that contains a mercury-filled glass column, calibrated in millimeters; the mercury rises and falls in response to pressure created when the cuff is inflated. *(Courtesy of Omron Health Care)*

Aneroid manometer   Portable unit with a glass-enclosed gauge containing a needle to register millimeter calibration and a metal bellows within the gauge that expands and collapses in response to pressure variations from the inflated cuff.

Figure 25-6 Equipment Used for Vital Sign Assessment *(From* Fundamentals of Nursing: Standards & Practice, *by S. DeLaune and P. Ladner, 1998, Albany, NY: Delmar. Copyright 1998 by Delmar. Reprinted with permission.)*

Table 25–2 VITAL SIGNS AND VARIATIONS

VITAL SIGN	NORMAL READING		VARIATIONS
Temperature	Axillary	36.5°C or 97.6°F	< 36°C or 96.8°F Hypothermia
	Tympanic	37°C or 98.6°F	> 38°C or 100.4°F Pyrexia
	Oral	37°C or 98.6°F	
	Rectal	37.5°C or 99.6°F	
Pulse	60–100 beats/min.		< 60 Bradycardia
			> 100 Tachycardia
Respirations	16–20 resp./min.		< 16 Bradypnea
			> 20 Tachypnea
Blood Pressure	90/60–140/90		< 90/60 Hypotension
			> 140/90 Hypertension

Pulse

Pulse assessment is the measurement of a pressure pulsation created when the heart contracts and ejects blood into the aorta. Assessment of pulse characteristics provides clinical data regarding the heart's pumping action and the adequacy of peripheral artery blood flow.

There are multiple pulse points (Figure 25-7). The most accessible peripheral pulses are the radial and carotid sites. Because the body shunts blood to the brain whenever a cardiac emergency such as hemorrhage occurs, the carotid site should always be used to assess the pulse in these situations. Pulse point assessments are described in Table 25–3.

Assessment of the client's pulse (P) includes the rate, rhythm, and amplitude.

Pulse rate is an indirect measurement of cardiac output obtained by counting the number of peripheral pulse waves over a pulse point. A normal pulse rate for adults is between 60 and 100 beats per minute. **Bradycardia** is a heart rate less than 60 beats per minute in an adult. **Tachycardia** is a heart rate in excess of 100 beats per minute in an adult.

Pulse rhythm is the regularity of the heartbeat. It describes how evenly the heart is beating: regular (the beats are evenly spaced) or irregular (the beats are not evenly spaced). Dysrhythmia (arrhythmia) is an irregular rhythm caused by an early, late, or missed heartbeat.

Pulse amplitude is a measurement of the strength or force exerted by the ejected blood against the arterial wall with each contraction. It is described as normal (full, easily palpable), weak (thready and usually rapid), or strong (bounding).

Usual assessment of the radial pulse occurs for 30 seconds and the number of beats is doubled for documentation. If the pulse rhythm is irregular, assessment must occur for 60 seconds. In addition, the nurse must assess for a **pulse deficit** (condition in which

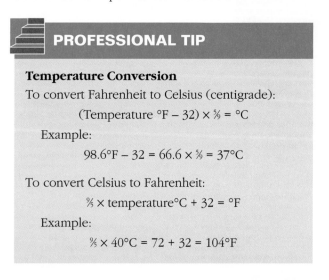

PROFESSIONAL TIP

Temperature Conversion

To convert Fahrenheit to Celsius (centigrade):

$$(\text{Temperature } °F - 32) \times \tfrac{5}{9} = °C$$

Example:

$$98.6°F - 32 = 66.6 \times \tfrac{5}{9} = 37°C$$

To convert Celsius to Fahrenheit:

$$\tfrac{9}{5} \times \text{temperature}°C + 32 = °F$$

Example:

$$\tfrac{9}{5} \times 40°C = 72 + 32 = 104°F$$

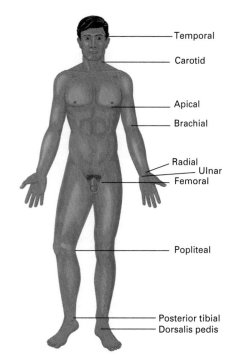

Figure 25-7 Pulse Points

Table 25–3 PULSE POINT ASSESSMENT

PULSE POINT	ASSESSMENT CRITERIA
Temporal: over temporal bone, superior and lateral to eye	Accessible; used routinely for infants and when radial is inaccessible
Carotid: bilateral, under lower jaw in neck along medial edge of sterno-cleidomastoid muscle	Accessible; used routinely for infants and during shock or cardiac arrest when other peripheral pulses are too weak to palpate; also used to assess cranial circulation
Apical: left midclavicular line at fourth to fifth intercostal space	Used to auscultate heart sounds and assess apical-radial deficit
Brachial: inner aspect between groove of biceps and triceps muscles at antecubital fossa	Used in cardiac arrest for infants, to assess lower arm circulation, and to auscultate blood pressure
Radial: inner aspect of forearm on thumb side of wrist	Accessible; used routinely in adults to assess character of peripheral pulse
Ulnar: outer aspect of forearm on finger side of wrist	Used to assess circulation to ulnar side of hand and to perform the Allen's test
Femoral: in groin, below inguinal ligament (midpoint between symphysis pubis and anterosuperior iliac spine)	Used to assess circulation to legs and during cardiac arrest
Popliteal: behind knee, at center in popliteal fossa	Used to assess circulation to legs and to auscultate leg blood pressure
Posterior tibial: inner aspect of ankle between Achilles tendon and tibia (below medial malleolus)	Used to assess circulation to feet
Dorsalis pedis: over instep, midpoint between extension tendons of great and second toe	Used to assess circulation to feet

From Fundamentals of Nursing: Standards & Practice, *by S. DeLaune and P. Ladner, 1998, Albany, NY: Delmar. Copyright 1998 by Delmar. Reprinted with permission.*

the apical pulse rate is greater than the radial pulse rate). A pulse deficit results from the ejection of a volume of blood that is too small to initiate a peripheral pulse wave.

During the pulse assessment, the nurse should integrate questions about endurance, fatigue, and any possible episodes of palpitations, "feeling the heart beating," over the chest area.

Respirations

Respiratory assessment is the measurement of the breathing pattern. Assessment of respirations provides clinical data regarding the pH of arterial blood. Normal

PROFESSIONAL TIP

Carotid Pulse Assessment
When assessing a carotid pulse, apply light pressure to only one carotid artery to avoid disruption of cerebral blood flow. Then assess the other one.

breathing is slightly observable, effortless, quiet, automatic, and regular. It can be assessed by observing chest wall expansion and bilateral symmetrical movement of the thorax. Another method the nurse can use to assess breathing is to place the back of the hand next to the client's nose and mouth to feel the expired air.

Assessment of external respirations (R) should include specific characteristics of respirations as well as the use of any type of oxygen equipment. Each respiration includes one complete inhalation (breathing in) and exhalation (breathing out) by the client. When identifying the characteristics of respirations, the rate, depth, and rhythm of each breath should be determined.

Eupnea refers to easy respirations with a rate of breaths per minute that is age-appropriate. **Bradypnea** is a respiratory rate of 10 or fewer breaths per minute. **Hypoventilation** is characterized by shallow respirations. **Tachypnea** is a respiratory rate greater than 24 breaths per minute. **Hyperventilation** is characterized by deep, rapid respirations. **Dyspnea** refers to difficulty in breathing as observed by labored or forced respirations through the use of accessory muscles in the chest and neck. Dyspneic clients are acutely aware of their respirations and complain of shortness of breath.

It is also important to observe for nasal flaring and the use of accessory muscles for breathing as evidenced by sternal, costal, and subclavicular retractions. The nurse should be aware that children and males typically utilize abdominal muscles to breathe, whereas women use thoracic muscles (Fuller & Schaller-Ayers, 1999). If a client is receiving oxygen, the route and flow rate must be identified.

During the assessment of respirations, the nurse may determine functional ability by asking about any periods of shortness of breath, any difficulty in breath-

PROFESSIONAL TIP

Positioning for Dyspneic Clients
Dyspneic clients should never be placed flat in bed; maintain them in a semi-Fowler's or Fowler's position. To facilitate maximal lung expansion, place the client in a forward-leaning position over a padded, raised overbed table with arms and head resting on the table.

ing with increased exercise, or problems following through with activities of daily living.

Blood Pressure

After checking a client's respirations, the nurse assesses the client's blood pressure (BP). The most common site for indirect blood pressure measurement is the client's arm over the brachial artery.

When pressure measurements in the upper extremities are not accessible, the popliteal artery, located behind the knee, becomes the site of choice. The nurse can also assess the blood pressure in other sites, such as the radial artery in the forearm and the posterior tibial or dorsalis pedis artery in the lower leg. The extremity should be at the level of the heart when blood pressure is measured. Because it is difficult to auscultate sounds over the radial, tibial, and dorsalis pedis arteries, these sites are usually palpated to obtain a systolic reading.

A person's blood pressure is the result of the interaction of cardiac output and peripheral resistance, and will be dependent on the speed with which the arterial blood flows, the volume of blood supplied, and the elasticity of the walls of the artery. The force exerted by the blood against the wall of the artery as the heart contracts and relaxes is called the *arterial pressure*. When the ventricles contract and blood is forced into the aorta and pulmonary arteries, the systolic arterial pressure is measured. This is the first sound heard. When the heart is in the filling or relaxed stage, the force is described as the *diastolic blood pressure*. This is when the last sound is heard. The difference between the systolic and diastolic blood pressures is called the *pulse pressure*. A pulse pressure is usually between 30 and 40 mm Hg.

An accurate reading also requires the correct width of the blood pressure cuff as determined by the circumference of the client's extremity. The bladder cuff must encircle the width and length of the site. According to the American Heart Association (1987), the bladder width should be approximately 40% of the circumference or 20% wider than the diameter of the midpoint

PROFESSIONAL TIP

Contraindications for Brachial Artery Blood Pressure Measurement

When the client has any of the following, *do not* measure blood pressure on the involved side:
- Venous access devices, such as an intravenous infusion or arteriovenous fistula for renal dialysis
- Surgery involving the breast, axilla, shoulder, arm, or hand
- Injury or disease to the shoulder, arm, or hand, such as trauma, burns, or application of a cast or bandage

COMMUNITY/HOME HEALTH CARE

Electronic Sphygmomanometers

Electronic sphygmomanometers are used by clients for self-measurements. A stethoscope is not required because the device electronically inflates and deflates the cuff while simultaneously reading and displaying the systolic and diastolic pressures. The electronic device is useful for clients who must monitor their own pressure at home. However, it must be recalibrated routinely to ensure an accurate reading.

of the extremity. To measure the width of the bladder, the nurse should place the cuff lengthwise on the client's extremity and extend the width to cover 40% of the extremity's circumference (Figure 25-8). Table 25–4 recommends bladder sizes based on different arm circumferences. A falsely elevated reading will result if the bladder is too narrow, and a falsely low reading will result if it is too wide.

This is an appropriate time to ask if the client ever becomes lightheaded or dizzy when moving from a reclining position to a sitting or standing position. This may occur as a result of an abnormally low blood pressure caused by the inability of the peripheral blood vessels to compensate quickly for the change in position and is referred to as **orthostatic hypotension**.

Pain

According to the new Joint Commission on Accreditation of Healthcare Organizations (JCAHO) standards for ambulatory care, behavioral health care, home care, hospital, health care network, long-term care, and long-term care pharmacy, pain is considered the "fifth" vital sign. Pain is to be assessed and recorded along with the client's temperature, pulse, respirations, and blood pressure (JCAHO, 2000a; JCAHO, 2000b). The pain assess-

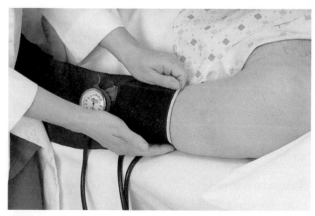

Figure 25-8 Measure width of arm by holding cuff against client's upper arm.

Table 25–4	GUIDELINES FOR SPHYGMOMANOMETER CUFF SELECTION		
MIDPOINT* ARM CIRCUMFERENCE**	**BLADDER CUFF WIDTH****	**LENGTH****
24–32 (average adult)	13	24
32–42 (large adult)	17	32

*Distance between the acromion and olecranon processes.
**Measurement in centimeters (cm).

Adapted from Fundamentals of Nursing: Standards & Practice, *by S. DeLaune and P. Ladner, 1998, Albany, NY: Delmar. Copyright 1998 by Delmar. Adapted with permission.*

ment is to include pain intensity and quality (character, frequency, location, and duration). Regular assessment and followup are according to agency policy. This statement on pain management, "All patients have a right to pain relief," is to be posted in all client care areas (e.g., client rooms, clinic rooms, waiting rooms) (JCAHO, 2000a).

Height and Weight Measurement

Measuring height and weight is as important as assessing the client's vital signs. Routine measurement provides data related to growth and development in infants and children and signals the possible onset of alterations that may indicate illness in all age groups. The client's height and weight are routinely taken on admission to acute care facilities and on visits to physicians' offices, clinics, and in other health care settings.

Height

A scale for measuring height, calibrated in either inches or centimeters, is usually attached to a standing weight scale. This type of scale is used for measuring the height of children and adults. The nurse should ask the client to stand erect on the scale's platform. The metal rod attached to the back of the scale should be extended to gently rest on the top of the client's head, and the measurement should be read at eye level.

Weight

When a client has an order for "daily weight," the weight should be obtained at the same time of day on the same scale, with the client wearing the same type of clothing.

Infection Control: Measuring Weight
When standing on a scale, the client should wear some type of light foot covering, such as socks or disposable operating room slippers, to prevent the transmission of infection and to enhance comfort.

Head and Neck Assessment

The nurse will assess the head and neck and determine the client's mental and neurological status, and the client's overall **affect** (outward expression of mood or emotion).

Hair and Scalp

The hair and scalp of a client should be inspected. The hair distribution, quantity, texture, and color should be noted. The scalp should be smooth and free of any debris or infestations.

Eyes

The eyes should be examined to determine if they are symmetrical. The nurse should look at the eyebrows and eyelids to determine if there is any drooping, which may be a sign of muscle weakness or neurological impairment. The color of the sclera and conjunctiva, as well as the presence of any drainage, should be noted.

The pupils should be assessed to determine their size, shape, and reaction to light. This is accomplished by darkening the room and asking the client to gaze into the distance. The nurse will move a light in from the side and notice if the pupil constricts; this is called the *direct light reflex.* The pupil size in millimeters both before and after the light response (Figure 25-9) is noted. Accommodation is tested by asking the client to focus on an object in the distance; this will dilate the pupils. The client is then asked move his or her gaze to a near object such as a pen or finger held approximately 3 inches from the nose. The pupils should constrict as they focus on the near object and the eyes will converge or move in toward midline. This normal response is documented as PERRLA or Pupils Equal, Round, Reactive to Light and Accommodation.

The nurse should determine if the client utilizes glasses and for what reason, and ask if any eye problems such as blurry vision, diplopia (double vision), or difficulty seeing at night are being experienced.

The assessment of visual acuity is a simple, noninvasive procedure that is performed with the use of a **Snellen chart** (a chart that contains various-sized letters with standardized numbers at the end of each line of letters). The standardized numbers (called the denominator) indicate the degree of visual acuity when the client is able to read that line of letters at a distance of 20 feet.

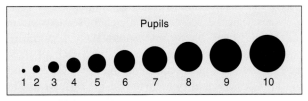

Figure 25-9 Scale Used to Measure Pupil Size, in Millimeters

Nose

The nose should be symmetrical, midline, and in proportion to other features. Any deformity, inflammation, or prior trauma should be noted. The patency of the nostrils can be tested by asking the client to sniff inward while closing off each nostril. The nurse should ask the client if the following are ever experienced: nosebleeds, dryness, or decrease in sense of smell.

Lips and Mouth

The lips and mucous membranes of the mouth are observed for color, symmetry, moisture, or lesions. If the client has dentures or partial plates, the nurse should ask them to be removed for a more thorough inspection of the mouth. Unusual breath odors should be noted. The oral mucosa can be inspected by inserting a tongue depressor between the teeth and the cheek. The mucous membranes and gums should be pink, moist, smooth, and free of lesions. Inspection of the tongue assists in determining the client's hydration. The tongue should be pink with a slightly rough texture. During the examination the nurse can determine if the client is able to enunciate words appropriately and if there have been any voice changes such as hoarseness. Usual dental hygiene practices should be discussed and the client's history of tobacco usage obtained.

Neck

The neck should be assessed to determine if there is full range of motion. The accessory neck muscles should be symmetrical. As the client moves the head, any enlargement of the lymph nodes or thyroid gland should be noted. The nurse should observe for any pulsations in the neck. The carotid pulsation is seen just below the angle of the jaw. Normally there are no other visible pulsations while the client is in the sitting position.

Mental and Neurological Status and Affect

All head-to-toe assessments must incorporate an assessment of the client's mental and neurological status and affect. A client's mental status includes identification of the level of orientation to person, place, and time. Also included within the mental status is the client's responsiveness to the environment. When assessing for responsiveness, the client's ability to follow directions and to respond appropriately to comments and to his or her name when called is observed.

Neurological assessment of the client focuses on the following: level of consciousness (LOC), pupil response, hand grasps, and foot pushes. Each of these assessments will be discussed in the area of the head-to-toe assessment in which it will be observed. The level of consciousness is the client's degree of wakefulness. For example, a client who is alert is fully awake with eyes open and responds to environmental

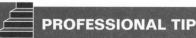

PROFESSIONAL TIP

Common Abnormal Breath Odors

- Acetone breath ("fruity" smell) is common in malnourished or diabetic clients with ketoacidosis.
- Musty smell is caused by the breakdown of nitrogen and presence of liver disease.
- Ammonia smell occurs during the end stage of renal failure from a buildup of urea.

stimuli. The client who is less awake will be drowsy and slow in response to environmental stimuli.

When documenting the client's affect, words such as *pleasant, happy, cooperative, uncooperative, angry, depressed,* or *hostile* should not be used. Instead, the description of affect should focus specifically upon the behaviors exhibited by the client such as facial expression and verbal and nonverbal behaviors. In doing this, the nurse not only maintains the accuracy of the conversation or the behaviors observed, but also maintains the legal appropriateness of the assessment.

Skin Assessment

Assessment of the skin should be performed as each area of the body is assessed. The color of the skin as well as its moisture or dryness should be noted. The nurse should inspect and palpate the client's skin, assessing temperature, turgor, edema, and integrity. Palpation of the skin with the dorsal aspect of the hand on the right and left sides of the body provides a comparison of the client's skin temperature. The client should also be asked if any pain or discomfort in relation to the skin and/or mucous membranes has occurred. Identification of the skin's turgor is best accomplished by pinching the skin of the anterior chest and observing the speed of return of the skin to its previous position. If the skin stays pinched during assessment, it may indicate dehydration, and further assessment should occur.

Palpate dependent areas (sacrum, legs, ankles, feet) for edema. Firmly apply pressure with a finger for 5 seconds. The degree of edema is based on the depth of indentation in centimeters:

1+	equals an indentation of 1 cm or less
2+	equals an indentation of 2 cm
3+	equals an indentation of 3 cm
4+	equals an indentation of 4 cm
5+	equals an indentation of 5 cm or more

The location, size, distribution, and appearance of skin lesions throughout the body should be determined. Documentation of any breaks in or changes in the skin integrity is an important aspect of nursing assessment. Scratches, bruises, skin tears, cuts, and scars from previous injuries or surgeries are examples of

CULTURAL CONSIDERATIONS

Skin Color

- The darker the client's skin, the more difficult it is to assess changes in color.
- Establish a baseline skin color by observing the least pigmented skin surfaces, which include the volar surfaces of the forearms, the palms of the hands, the soles of the feet, the abdomen, and the buttocks. There should be an underlying red tone in these areas. Absence of this red tone may indicate pallor.
- Oral hyperpigmentation often is found in dark-skinned persons. If the hard palate is not hyperpigmented, it has a yellow discoloration in the presence of jaundice.
- The lips may be used to assess jaundice and cyanosis, and the sclera may be used to assess jaundice if a baseline color has been established for each.
- The conjunctiva reflect color changes of cyanosis or pallor.
- Nail beds can be used to note how quickly the color returns after pressure has been released from the free edge of the nail, regardless of the nail bed color.

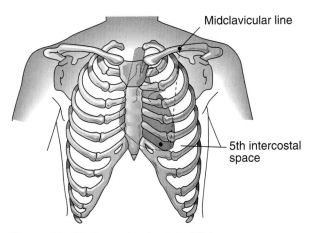

Figure 25-10 Assessing the Apical Pulse

skin characteristics that should be noted. The general hygiene of the skin should be noted, and the client asked about usual skin care routines.

Thoracic Assessment

During thoracic assessment, the nurse will determine the condition of the client's cardiovascular and respiratory systems along with assessment of the breasts.

Cardiovascular Status

Assessment of the client's cardiovascular status by the LP/VN focuses specifically on listening to the apical pulse, identifying heart tones, and checking the nail beds. The apical pulse is determined by using auscultation and palpation. To assess the apical pulse, the nurse must palpate over the apex of the heart at the fourth or fifth left intercostal space at the midclavicular line. A slight, short duration tap against the fingers will be felt, and this is where the apical pulse will be auscultated (Figure 25-10). Listening to the apical pulse is the most accurate assessment of the heart rate, and should occur for 60 seconds. The apical pulse is assessed first with the diaphragm of the stethoscope for the regularity or irregularity of its rhythm. Second, the bell of the stethoscope is used to differentiate the loudness or tones of the heart. Along with the apical pulse, the other pulse points may be assessed now or when the extremities are asessed.

To assess blood perfusion of peripheral vessels and skin, the nurse should note changes in skin temperature, color, and sensation, and changes in the pulses. Feeling the toes for warmth and color provides important information relative to peripheral circulation and tissue perfusion. Because the position of the extremities can affect the skin temperature and appearance, extremities must always be assessed at heart level and at normal room and body temperature. Peripheral pulses should be compared bilaterally, and changes in strength and quality should be noted (Bosley, 1995).

The focus of the functional assessment includes personal habits contributing to or preventing cardiovascular disease. The nurse should determine the client's personal exercise habits and elicit information regarding past chest pain or shortness of breath. The client should describe any pain, its location, duration, precipitating factors, and what is done to alleviate the pain. The nurse should also ask if the client has ever fainted or felt dizzy. Any lower leg swelling and its cause should also be noted.

Respiratory Status

Breath sound assessment is performed after determination of the apical pulse rate. Respiratory auscultation reveals the presence of normal and abnormal breath sounds. During auscultation, the client should be instructed to breathe only through the mouth because mouth breathing decreases air turbulence that could interfere with an accurate assessment.

There are three distinct types of normal breath sounds with their own unique pitch, intensity, quality, location, and relative duration in the inspiratory and expiratory phases of respiration:

- **Bronchial sounds:** loud and high-pitched sounds with a hollow quality heard longer on expiration than inspiration from air moving through the trachea
- **Bronchovesicular sounds:** medium-pitched and blowing sounds heard equally on inspiration and expiration from air moving through the large airways,

posteriorly between the scapula and anteriorly over bronchioles lateral to the sternum at the first and second intercostal spaces
- **Vesicular sounds:** soft, breezy, and low-pitched sounds heard longer on inspiration than expiration that result from air moving through the smaller airways over the lung's periphery, with the exception of the scapular area

Breath sounds that are not normal are described as either abnormal or **adventitious breath sounds**. Adventitious breath sounds include sibilant wheeze (formerly wheeze), sonorous wheeze (formerly rhonchi), fine and coarse crackle (formerly rales), pleural friction rub, and stridor. **Sibilant wheezes** are high-pitched, whistling sounds heard during inhalation and exhalation. A **sonorous wheeze** is a low-pitched snoring sound that is louder on exhalation. Coughing may alter the sound if caused by mucus. **Crackles** are popping sounds heard on inhalation or exhalation, not cleared by coughing. A **pleural friction rub** is a low-pitched grating sound on inhalation and exhalation. **Stridor** is a high-pitched, harsh sound heard on inspiration when the trachea or larynx is obstructed. Breath sounds of the anterior, posterior, and lateral chest wall must be assessed for normal as well as adventitious breath sounds. Adventitious breath sounds must be monitored on a consistent basis. The lungs are assessed from side to side so the two sides can be compared as shown in Figure 25-11.

The functional assessment information to be obtained when assessing the respiratory status of the client includes any difficulty breathing or the presence of a cough. The client should be asked if the cough is nonproductive or productive, and to describe the secretions produced. Terms used to describe secretions expectorated would be *thick, thin, yellow, green.* The client's occupational or home environment may affect breathing patterns; exposure to dust, chemicals, vapors, tobacco, smoke, or paint fumes, and irritants such as asbestos should be noted.

Wounds, Scars, Drains, Tubes, Dressings

When assessing the thorax, the nurse should note any type of wounds, scars, drains, tubes, or dressings the client may have. Assessment of these must include the location, size, and amount of drainage or discharge, and if present, signs of inflammation.

Breasts

Assessment of the breast tissue should be done for both male and female clients. The nurse can begin by inspecting the breasts for size and symmetry. It is common to have a slight difference in size of breasts. Any obvious masses, dimpling (a depression in the surface skin), or inflammation should be noted. The skin nor-

mally is smooth and even in color. The nurse should determine if the nipples and areola are symmetrical in size, shape, and color, and note any discharge from the nipples.

Any abnormal area should be palpated for size, consistency, mobility, tenderness, and location of the lesion. Another area to include in breast assessment is the axillary lymph nodes that drain the breasts. The nurse should palpate the axilla for enlarged or inflamed lymph nodes, ask if there is any tenderness, and also determine if and when the client performs self-breast exams. The nurse can note if the client has had mammography and when the last x-ray was taken.

Abdominal Assessment

During abdominal assessment, the nurse determines the status of the client's gastrointestinal and genitourinary systems. The nurse should also note any type of wounds, scars, drains, tubes, dressings, or ostomies the client may have. Assessment of these must include the location, size, and amount of drainage or discharge, and if present, any signs of inflammation.

Gastrointestinal Status

The abdomen is first inspected for rashes and scars. The nurse should determine if the abdomen is flat, rounded, or distended, and should observe the abdomen for symmetry and visible signs of peristalsis or pulsations. If the abdomen is distended, the client should be asked questions pertaining to bowel movements and urinary status.

Auscultation is the second component of the abdominal assessment of a client's bowel status. A "bubbly-gurgly" sound, caused by peristalsis and movement of the intestinal contents, can be heard by placing the stethoscope on each quadrant of the abdomen and listening for approximately 1 minute. These sounds should be present in all four quadrants of the abdomen, beginning in the right lower quadrant (RLQ) and moving clockwise around the four quadrants as

PROFESSIONAL TIP

Assessment of the Abdomen

Although the usual sequence for implementing assessment techniques is inspection, palpation, percussion, and auscultation, assessment of the abdomen entails a different sequence. Because palpation can affect sounds heard on auscultation, the sequence for abdominal assessment is as follows:

- Inspection
- Auscultation
- Percussion
- Palpation

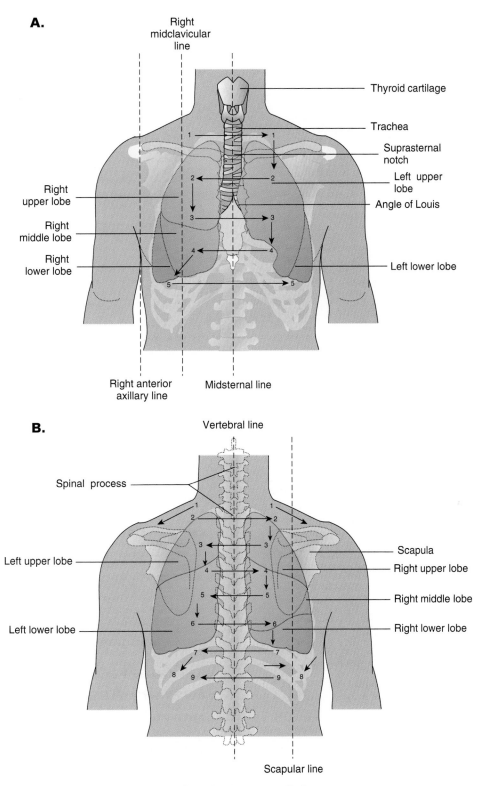

Figure 25-11 Symmetrical Assessment of Breath Sounds: A. Anterior; B. Posterior

shown in Figure 25-12. When approximately 5 to 20 bowel sounds are heard per minute, or 1 at least every 5 to 15 seconds, the bowel sounds are considered active.

The absence of bowel sounds during 1 minute of auscultation in each quadrant is documented as absent bowel sounds. Bowel sounds of less than 5 "bubbly-gurgly" sounds per minute are described as hypoactive, while an excess of 20 or more bowel sounds per minute is defined as hyperactive. High-pitched, loud, rushing sounds heard with or without a stethoscope are termed **borborygmi**. This is caused by the passage of gas through the liquid contents of the intestine.

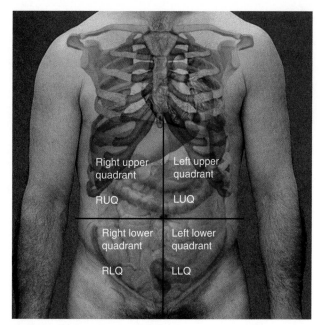

Figure 25-12 The Four Quadrants of the Abdomen (*From Health Assessment and Physical Examination, (2nd ed.), by M.E.Z. Estes, 2002, Albany, NY: Delmar. Copyright 2002 by Delmar. Reprinted with permission.*)

Percussion of the abdomen should occur in all four quadrants. The predominant abdominal percussion sound is tympany caused by percussing over the air-filled stomach and intestines.

Light palpation of the abdomen is done to assess for muscle tone, masses, pulsations, or any signs of tenderness or discomfort. Abdominal muscles may be palpated and should feel relaxed on light palpation, not tightly contracted or spastic. If the client is anxious, muscle contraction may be evident. Palpation of a separation of the rectus abdominous muscle may be felt, especially in clients who are obese or pregnant. The rectus abdominous muscle includes two large, midline muscles that extend from the xiphoid process to the symphysis pubis, and can be palpated midline as the client raises his or her head. Rebound tenderness, indicating possible inflammation of the appendix, may be elicited by depressing the abdomen and quickly withdrawing the fingers. This examination is done at the end of the abdominal assessment because of the possibility of increasing the client's level of pain. If any of the abdominal organs can be felt with light palpation, it is abnormal and should be reported to the nursing supervisor. After assessment of bowel sounds, the nurse should question the client about diet, usual bowel patterns, appetite, weight changes, indigestion, heartburn, nausea, pain, and use of enemas or laxatives.

Genitourinary Status

Assessment of the client's urinary and reproductive status is accomplished mainly by inspection and use of interview skills. Genitourinary assessment includes ex-

CULTURAL CONSIDERATIONS

Genitourinary Assessment
Middle Eastern women often will remain veiled during this assessment.

amination of the abdomen, urinary meatus and genitalia, and assessment of the client's urine.

The abdomen should be inspected for any enlargement or fullness. In the normal adult, the abdomen is smooth, flat, and symmetrical. The urinary meatus should be inspected for any abnormalities such as inflammation and discharge, which may signal a urethral infection.

In females, the appearance of the genitalia (labia, clitoris, vaginal opening) should be observed. Questions to ask the client that focus on the reproductive history include: pregnancies, use of birth control, menstrual cycle history, present sexual activity, use of protection during intercourse, date of the last Pap test, and determination of how any present illness has or will affect sexual activity.

In males, assessment of the genitalia includes inspection of the penis, urethral meatus, foreskin (if uncircumcised), and scrotum. Questions to ask the client that focus on the reproductive history include: present sexual activity, use of protection during intercourse, and also how the present illness has or will affect sexual activity. The nurse should determine if the client performs testicular self-examinations.

Any lesions or ulcerations that may indicate sexually transmitted disease should be noted. The usual voiding pattern and any recent changes should be determined if the client has had any history of urinary tract infections, kidney stones, change in the urinary stream, or painful urination or nocturia.

Musculoskeletal and Extremity Assessment

Symmetry and strength of major muscle groups can be assessed throughout the head-to-toe assessment. Any time during the assessment when the client is repositioned, the range of movement the client utilizes to make that position change can be observed. Asking the client to walk across the room and noting the client's movements and stance when sitting up in bed are observations made to assess gross motor movement and posture. Assessment of the client's handshake gives an estimate of muscle strength. Palpating muscles lightly determines swelling, tone, or any specific changes in the shape of the muscles.

Hand grasps and foot pushes assess the strength and equality of the client's extremities. Upper extremity strength is assessed by having the client grasp the nurse's index and middle fingers of each hand. The grasp should be equal in both hands. Foot pushes assess the lower extremities. The nurse's hands should be placed on the soles of the client's feet. The client is asked to push both feet against the nurse's hands. The push should be equal in both feet. Asking the client to touch the tip of her nose with a finger and then the tip of the nurse's finger as it is moved to different locations tests the client's coordination skills.

Strength and symmetry of some of the major muscle groups can be assessed by watching gait and postural movements. Any aids to ambulation must be noted. Symmetrical examination of muscles should occur in pairs, first one extremity and then the other; equality of size, contour, tone, and strength should be assessed.

The skin of the lower extremities should be carefully assessed to determine color changes, loss of feeling or hair, change in temperature within the extremity and from one extremity to the other, and presence of vari-cose veins, ulcers, and edema. The nurse should determine if the client experiences any leg pain or cramps.

The nurse should ask the client if muscle weakness is experienced or if difficulty or pain when walking or performing routine daily activities occurs. The functional assessment should also include asking the client about routine activities such as cooking, shopping, exercise, yard work, and hobbies. Tolerance limitations can be observed by assessing for stiffness, crepitus, or fatigue during ambulation. Safe and appropriate performance of functions essential for home life and activities of daily living must be determined.

SUMMARY

- Psychosocial needs of clients are identified within the scope of a functional assessment.
- The health history and the physical examination used together present a holistic view of client needs.

CASE STUDY

Tom Turner, age 40, has been admitted to the hospital with pneumonia. He has never been hospitalized before. His wife and three children are at home. Because his wife has just given birth to their third child, Tom's wife cannot drive the other two children to school. Tom provides the sole income for the family, and he has only three more sick days to use at work before he will be off without pay.

Tom's vital signs are BP 120/72, P 100, R 34, T 100.6°F. His breath sounds show sonorous wheezes throughout, cleared by coughing. His cough is frequent and productive of foamy, cloudy, yellow secretions. His apical pulse is 102 and regular, but distant heart tones were noted. The abdomen is firm and distended with hypoactive bowel sounds noted in all four quadrants. He moves all extremities slowly but by himself and with purpose.

Tom is oriented to person, place, and time. His pupils are PERRLA. Hand grips are strong and equal bilaterally, as are foot pushes. He speaks only when spoken to, and his eye contact with staff is minimal. Whenever his wife visits, his voice raises and his heart rate increases about 2–5 beats. At one point, Tom stated, "How much more of this can we take?" Tom's wife mentions that their church would love to help, but Tom refuses to take charity. Tom states, "Any income for this family has to come from me."

Other added information acquired during the assessment includes the fact that Tom has a history of drinking 1 to 2 beers daily, and has not performed testicular self-exams. He eats and drinks what he likes, and he states he really "hates seafood." Usually he bathes daily in the early morning and helps to bathe two of their children each evening. He works 9–5:30 P.M., five days per week, and also some Saturday mornings. Tom pays all of the household bills, and is the sole decision maker of the family.

The following questions will guide your development of a nursing care plan for the case study.

1. List the functional assessment data collected from Mr. Turner that identify psychosocial concerns.
2. What are two possible reasons for identifying the added information about Mr. Turner in the last paragraph?
3. Write two nursing diagnoses that are supported by the health history and physical assessments documented about Mr. Turner.
4. Write goals and nursing interventions for each nursing diagnosis.

- Introduction of the nurse at the beginning of a physical assessment enhances the ability to accomplish the complete assessment.
- Collection of vital signs is the foundation to each head-to-toe assessment and includes: temperature, pulse, respirations, and blood pressure.
- Assessment of a client's mental and neurological status is performed when the nurse obtains information about the client's level of consciousness, pupil response, as well as hand grip and foot push capabilities.
- When describing a client's affect, the nurse must utilize terms that are descriptive of the specific behavior observed, not the nurse's judgment about the behavior.
- Assessing the cardiovascular status of each client includes palpation of specific pulse points.
- Auscultation of lung fields assists in collection of data regarding the breath sounds of the client.
- An abdominal assessment includes use of inspection, auscultation, percussion, and palpation within the four quadrants of the abdomen to establish bowel status and function.
- Through observation of client gait and overall range of movement, the nurse is able to obtain some knowledge of the symmetry and strength of muscles.
- During the assessment of wounds, drains, dressings, and other external devices, the nurse must maintain accurate documentation of the amount of drainage, color, or other changes.

Review Questions

1. Jim's apical pulse is 102. He states to the nurse that he can feel his heart pounding. Which of the following charting terms would accurately describe Jim's statement of concern regarding his heart rate?

    a. bradycardia
    b. changing of rhythm
    c. palpitation
    d. tachycardia

2. Mrs. Jones is 54 years old. While performing the assessment overview, Mrs. Jones states, "I just get so lightheaded when I first get up in the morning." Mrs. Jones most likely has:

    a. cyanosis.
    b. hypertension.
    c. orthostatic hypertension.
    d. orthostatic hypotension.

3. During the physical head-to-toe assessment of the client, the nurse checks the pulse and blood pressure. Which of the four assessment techniques did the nurse utilize?

    a. auscultation, palpation, and inspection
    b. auscultation, percussion, and inspection
    c. auscultation and palpation
    d. palpation and inspection

4. Upon admission to your unit, the client verbalizes an increased pain in her left leg. What would be the pertinent assessment information to collect about this client?

    a. Listen to the client's bowel sounds.
    b. Check circulation in the right leg.
    c. Assess both of the client's legs.
    d. Ask the client about her current diet.

5. Which of the pulses should be palpated when assessing circulation to the lower extremities?

    a. dorsalis pedis
    b. femoral
    c. temporal
    d. popliteal

6. How often a nurse assesses a client's vital signs depends upon the:

    a. availability of personnel.
    b. doctor's orders.
    c. nurse's discretion.
    d. client's condition.

7. The nurse checks the radial pulse for 30 seconds and multiplies by 2. She notices an irregularity in the beat. What is the next action the nurse should take?

    a. Check the radial pulse for 60 seconds.
    b. Listen to the apical pulse for 60 seconds.
    c. Listen to the apical for 30 seconds and multiply by 2.
    d. Continue with the rest of the assessment.

Critical Thinking Questions

1. How do you feel about performing a complete physical assessment on a client?

2. How do you feel when you receive a complete physical assessment?

 WEB FLASH!

- Search the Internet for information regarding physical examination (assessment). What type of information is available?
- Are there any organizations on the Internet that focus on physical examination (assessment)? Are they specific by age group (children, elderly)?

PAIN MANAGEMENT

MAKING THE CONNECTION

Refer to the following chapters to increase your understanding of pain management:

- **Chapter 8, Communication**
- **Chapter 12, Cultural Diversity and Nursing**
- **Chapter 13, Complementary/Alternative Therapies**
- **Chapter 17, Loss, Grief, and Death**

- **Procedures:** I9, Administering an Oral Medication; I10, Withdrawing Medication from an Ampule, I11, Withdrawing Medication from a Vial; I12, Administering an Intradermal Injection; I13, Administering a Subcutaneous Injection; I14, Administering an Intramuscular Injection

LEARNING OBJECTIVES

Upon completion of this chapter, you should be able to:
- *Define key terms.*
- *Identify the four components of pain conduction.*
- *Discuss the gate control theory of pain.*
- *Describe the types of pain.*
- *List three guidelines that should be included in a thorough pain assessment.*
- *Identify three general principles of pain management.*
- *List the nurse's responsibilities in administration of analgesics.*
- *Identify site of action of both nonopioid and opioid analgesics.*
- *Describe three examples of nonpharmacological measures for pain relief.*
- *Discuss nursing interventions that promote comfort.*

INTRODUCTION

Pain is a phenomenon that crosses all specialties of nursing. No matter the setting a nurse practices in, including neonatal intensive care, intraoperative, home care, or clinics, the nurse will be exposed to challenges in pain management. While other health care team members address pain management with clients, it is the nurse who spends the most time with the client experiencing pain. For example, in an acute care setting,

KEY TERMS

acupuncture
acute pain
adjuvant medication
afferent pain pathway
analgesia
analgesic
ceiling effect
chronic acute pain
chronic nonmalignant
  pain
chronic pain
colic
cryotherapy
cutaneous pain
distraction
efferent pain pathway
endorphin
epidural analgesia
gate control pain
  theory
hypnosis
intrathecal analgesia
ischemic pain
mixed agonist-
  antagonist
modulation

myofascial pain
  syndromes
neuralgia
nociceptor
noxious stimulus
pain
pain threshold
pain tolerance
patient-controlled-
  analgesia
perception
phantom limb pain
progressive muscle
  relaxation
recurrent acute pain
referred pain
reframing
relaxation technique
somatic pain
tolerance
transcutaneous
  electrical nerve
  stimulation
transduction
transmission
visceral pain

the physician orders the **analgesics** (substances that relieve pain) for the client, but may only spend 10 to 15 minutes each day with that client. The nurses are the ones who are present 24 hours a day, administer the medications, assess the client's response, and report the response to the physician. It is for this reason the nurse is often called the "backbone" or "cornerstone" of pain management. The nurse's role can be pivotal in relieving the client's pain.

Studies have documented undertreatment of pain of all types and in all age groups (Liebeskind & Melzack, 1987). In one such study, the researchers interviewed medical and surgical clients, finding that 58% had experienced excruciating pain in the previous 72 hours. Fifty-five percent of these clients could not recall a nurse asking about their pain (Donovan, Dillon, & McGuire, 1987). Another study examined pain management in metastatic cancer clients in an outpatient setting. Forty-two percent of the clients with pain were not given adequate analgesic therapy (Cleeland, Conin, Hatfield, Edmonson, Blum, Stewart, & Pandya, 1994).

It is generally thought that this undertreatment of pain is partially due to the lack of knowledge in both physicians and nurses. It is, therefore, important for the nurse to understand not only the psychological and physiological components that add up to the pain experience, but also the wide range of interventions available to provide relief. Another reason for undertreatment may be the health care workers' own biases regarding pain. Consequently, nurses should also recognize their own responses to pain and how they respond to others' expressions of pain.

The experience of pain is a factor that can have a significant impact on a client's health. It is a personal experience that can affect all other aspects of an individual's health, including physical well-being, mental status, and effectiveness of coping mechanisms. This chapter provides an overview of the complex phenomenon of pain, including: pain definitions, pain physiology, and pain assessment. Strategies to control pain will also be discussed, including pharmacological, noninvasive, and invasive techniques.

DEFINITIONS OF PAIN

The phenomenon of pain is evidenced in ancient history with references being made as far back as the Babylonian clay tablets. Aristotle (4th century B.C.) described pain as an emotion, being the opposite of pleasure. While emotions certainly play an important role in pain perception, we now know there is much more to the experience than the feelings involved.

In the Middle Ages, pain was viewed with religious connotations. Pain was seen as God's punishment for sins, or as evidence that an individual was possessed by demons. This definition of pain is still embraced by some clients, who might tell the nurse that the suffering is their "cross to bear." Pain relief may not be the goal for those individuals who believe in this definition of pain. Spiritual counseling may need to be implemented before this person is willing to work toward relief.

Currently, the most widely accepted definition of **pain** is that developed by the International Association for the Study of Pain (IASP). This organization defines pain as "an unpleasant sensory and emotional experience associated with actual or potential tissue damage or described in terms of such damage" (Merskey & Bogduk, 1994). This definition incorporates both the sensory and emotional components of pain. It also acknowledges that evidence of actual tissue damage is not required in order for the pain to be considered real.

Many pain experts emphasize the subjective nature of pain. Unlike a blood pressure or a blood glucose measurement, the intensity of discomfort the client is feeling cannot be measured with an instrument. McCaffery and Pasero (1999) say it best by defining pain as "whatever the person experiencing it says it is, existing whenever [he or she] says it does." This philosophy is emphasized in professional pain management guidelines. For example, the 1994 Agency for Health Care Policy and Research (AHCPR)—now called Agency for Healthcare Research and Quality (AHRQ)—from the guideline for cancer pain states, "Health professionals should ask about pain, and the patient's self-report should be the primary source of assessment." Guidelines are still published under the old name. The American Pain Society (APS) also stresses the importance of self-report: "Pain is always subjective. . . . The clinician must accept the patient's report of pain" (1999).

Though pain has had many definitions throughout humankind's history, research in pain physiology has shown that pain is a complex phenomenon. Pain is often difficult for clients to describe and nurses to understand; yet it is among the most common complaints that cause individuals to seek health care. Until recently, pain was viewed as a symptom that required diagnosis and treatment of the underlying cause. It is now clear that pain itself can be detrimental to the health and healing of clients. McCaffery and Pasero (1999) write that pain control, not just relief from pain once it occurs, must be recognized as a priority in the care of clients in all settings.

NATURE OF PAIN

A major function of the pain experience is to signal ongoing or potential tissue damage (Schecter, Berde, & Yaster, 1993), as is seen in the pain of cancer and chronic illness. Pain can also be a protective mechanism to prevent further injury, as is seen in clients who guard or protect an injured body part. The sensation of pain as the warning of potential tissue damage may be absent in people with hereditary sensory neuropathies, congenital nerve or spinal cord abnormalities, diabetic neuropathy, multiple sclerosis, leprosy, alcoholism, and nerve or spinal cord injury (Brand & Yancey, 1993).

COMMON MYTHS ABOUT PAIN

Because pain is subjective (dependent on the client's perception) and cannot be objectively measured by another individual through a laboratory test or diagnostic data, pain is often misunderstood and misjudged. A client's report of level of pain will vary on the basis of cultural and experiential backgrounds, and the nurse's interpretations of a client's pain will be filtered through the nurse's own biases and expectations. Misalignment of the nurse's view and the client's perception of pain can often lead to undermedication and unnecessary suffering on the client's part. Some common myths related to pain are discussed in Table 26–1.

TYPES OF PAIN

Pain can be qualified or described in two basic ways: by its cause or origin and by its description or nature. Pain categorized by its origin is either cutaneous, somatic, or visceral. Pain categorized by its nature is either acute or chronic.

Pain Categorized by Origin

Cutaneous pain is caused by stimulation of the cutaneous nerve endings in the skin and results in a well-localized "burning" or "prickling" sensation; getting a knot in the hair that is pulled out during combing may cause cutaneous pain. **Somatic pain** is nonlocalized and originates in support structures such as tendons, ligaments, and nerves; jamming a knee or finger will result in somatic pain. **Visceral pain** is discomfort in the internal organs and is less localized and more slowly transmitted than cutaneous pain. Visceral pain is often difficult to assess because the location may not be directly related to the cause. Pain originating from the abdominal organs is often called **referred pain** because the sensation of pain is not felt in the organ itself but instead is perceived at the spot where the organs were located during fetal development (Figure 26-1).

Pain Categorized by Nature

It is important to understand the difference between acute and chronic pain, as they each present a different clinical picture.

Acute Pain

Acute pain is most frequently identified by its sudden onset and relatively short duration, mild to severe intensity, and a steady decrease in intensity over a period of days to weeks. Some forms of acute pain may have a slower onset. Once the **noxious stimulus** (underlying pathology) is resolved, the unpleasant sensation usually disappears (Table 26–2). It can usually be associated with a specific injury, condition, or disease that has caused tissue damage. Acute pain should diminish as healing occurs. Everyone has experienced acute pain, for example: headaches, toothaches, needle

Table 26–1 COMMON MYTHS ABOUT PAIN	
MYTH	**FACT**
• The nurse is the best judge of a client's pain.	• Pain is a subjective experience; only the client can judge the level and severity of pain.
• If pain is ignored, it will go away.	• Pain is a real experience that is appropriately treated with nursing and medical intervention.
• Clients should not take any measures to relieve their pain until the pain is unbearable.	• Pain control and relief measures are effective in lowering the pain level, which will help clients function more normally and comfortably.
• Most complaints of pain are purely psychological (e.g., "it's all in your head"); only "real" pain manifests in obvious physical signs such as moaning or grimacing.	• Most clients report honestly on their perception of pain, both physical and emotional, and need effective intervention and teaching; physical responses to pain vary greatly depending on experience and cultural norms, and visible expressions of pain are not always reliable indicators of its severity.
• Clients taking pain medications will become addicted to the drug.	• Addiction is unlikely when analgesics are carefully administered and closely monitored.
• Clients with severe tissue damage will experience significant pain; those with lesser damage will feel less pain.	• Individuals' perceptions of pain are subjective; the extent of tissue damage is not necessarily proportional to the extent of pain experienced.
• Clients ask for pain medication when they need it.	• Many clients do not ask for medication because they are afraid of side effects, do not want to bother the nurse, have cultural norms and beliefs against it, or believe pain is inevitable and untreatable.

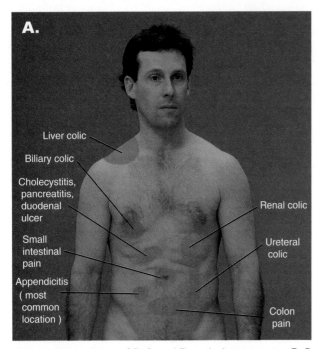
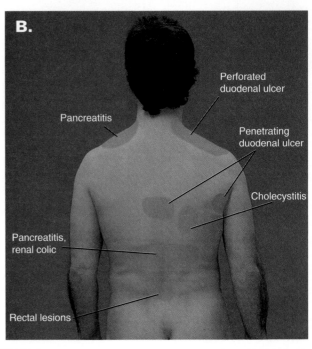

A.

Liver colic

Biliary colic

Cholecystitis,
pancreatitis,
duodenal
ulcer

Small
intestinal
pain

Appendicitis
(most
common
location)

Renal colic

Ureteral
colic

Colon
pain

B.

Perforated
duodenal ulcer

Pancreatitis

Penetrating
duodenal ulcer

Cholecystitis

Pancreatitis,
renal colic

Rectal lesions

Figure 26-1 Areas of Referred Pain: A. Anterior view; B. Posterior view

Table 26–2	ACUTE VERSUS CHRONIC PAIN	
	ACUTE	**CHRONIC**
Time Span	Less than 6 months	More than 6 months
Location	Localized, associated with a specific injury, condition, or disease	Difficult to pinpoint
Characteristics	Often described as sharp, diminishes as healing occurs	Often described as dull, diffuse, and aching
Physiologic Signs	• Elevated heart rate • Elevated BP • Elevated respirations • May be diaphoretic • Dilated pupils	• Normal vital signs • Normal pupils • No diaphoresis • May have loss of weight
Behavioral Signs	• Crying and moaning • Rubbing site • Guarding • Frowning • Grimacing • Complains of pain	• Physical immobility • Hopelessness • Listlessness • Loss of libido • Exhaustion and fatigue • Complains of pain only when asked

sticks, burns, skinned knees, muscle pain, childbirth, postoperative pain, fractures, and a sprained ankle. The client will describe the pain as highly localized and is usually able to pinpoint the hurt. Acute pain is often described as sharp, although if the pain is deep, it may be described as dull and aching. Accompanying signs will be those of the activation of the sympathetic nervous system, that is, the fight-or-flight response. Therefore, the client will exhibit elevated heart rate, respiratory rate, and blood pressure. The client may become diaphoretic and have dilated pupils. These signs resemble those of anxiety, which often accompanies acute pain. Behaviors may include crying and moaning, rubbing the site of pain, guarding, frowning, and grimacing. The client will often verbally complain of the discomfort.

Recurrent acute pain is identified by repetitive painful episodes that may recur over a prolonged period or throughout the client's lifetime. These painful episodes alternate with pain-free intervals. Examples of recurrent pain often seen in children include recurrent abdominal, chest, or limb pain that occurs in 5% to 10% of school-age children; headaches; and sickle cell pain crises with vaso-occlusion that leads to ischemia or infarction (Schecter et al., 1993). Examples of recurrent pain experienced by adults include migraine headaches, sickle cell pain crises, and the pain of angina pectoris due to hypoxia of the myocardium.

Chronic Pain

Chronic pain is generally identified as long-term (lasting 6 months or longer), persistent, nearly constant, or recurrent pain that produces significant negative changes in the client's life. Unlike acute pain, chronic pain may last long after the pathology is resolved. Although severe chronic persistent pain is experienced by some infants, children, and adolescents, it is much more common in the adult population (Schecter et al., 1993). More than 30% of all persons in the United States experience chronic pain, with the most common chronic pain in adults being back pain (Vasudevan, 1993).

Chronic acute pain occurs almost daily over a long period, has the potential for lasting months or years, and has a high probability of ending. Severe burn injuries and cancer are examples of pathophysiology that leads to chronic acute pain, which may last for long periods before the condition is cured or controlled. In some cases, the pain ends only with the death of the client, as in the case of those terminally ill with cancer (McCaffery & Pasero, 1999). This type of pain is also known as *progressive pain.*

Chronic nonmalignant pain, also called *chronic benign pain,* occurs almost daily and lasts for at least 6 months, with intensity ranging from mild to severe. McCaffery and Pasero (1999) identify three critical characteristics of chronic nonmalignant pain in that it:

- is due to non–life-threatening causes.
- is not responsive to currently available methods of pain relief.
- may continue for the remainder of the client's life.

Examples of pathophysiology leading to chronic nonmalignant pain include:

- Many forms of **neuralgia** (paroxysmal pain that extends along the course of one or more nerves)
- Low back pain
- Rheumatoid arthritis
- Ankylosing spondylitis
- **Phantom limb pain** (a form of neuropathic pain that occurs after amputation with pain sensations referred to an area in the missing portion of the limb)
- **Myofascial pain syndromes** (a group of muscle disorders characterized by pain, muscle spasm, tenderness, stiffness, and limited motion)

When chronic nonmalignant pain is severe enough to disable the client, it is identified as *chronic intractable nonmalignant pain syndrome.*

The signs and symptoms of chronic pain can look very different from those of acute pain. The body cannot tolerate the sympathetic nervous system signs for such a long period of time and, therefore, adapts. The vital signs will often be normal, with no accompanying pupil dilatation or perspiration. Lack of these signs may prompt some health care workers to question the client's description of pain.

The signs and symptoms of chronic pain, such as hopelessness, listlessness, and loss of libido and weight, are similar to those of depression. The client will often complain of exhaustion and fatigue. Behaviors include no complaints of pain unless asked and physical inactivity or immobility that can lead to functional disability. The crying, moaning, guarding, and grimacing that most clinicians associate with pain are absent. Treatment of chronic pain is more complex than that of acute pain. Chronic pain is viewed by pain experts as a disease state, rather than a symptom (Bonica, 1990). Management includes identifying the cause of pain, recognizing emotional and environmental factors that may be contributing to the pain, and rehabilitation to improve the client's functional abilities.

PURPOSE OF PAIN

Pain serves an important purpose as a protective mechanism. For example, if a person touches a hot stove, the pain signal will cause the person to pull the hand away immediately. The skin would be seriously burned if this did not happen. Pain not only protects, but it prompts clients to seek out medical care.

Pain is also useful as a diagnostic tool. Characteristics of the pain, such as the quality and duration, can give important clues in determining a client's medical diagnosis. For example, in acute appendicitis, the clinician looks for rebound tenderness (the pain increases when pressure is released) when palpating the abdomen. This particular type of pain helps to confirm the diagnosis of appendicitis rather than other gastrointestinal disorders.

PHYSIOLOGY OF PAIN

There are two known endogenous (developing within) analgesia systems in humans: the opioid system and the nonopioid system. The opioid system is best known and is mediated by a family of chemicals known as **endorphins** (endogenous neuropeptides that have morphinelike effects). The nonopioid system is mediated by monoamine substances such as norepinephrine and serotonin.

When pain occurs, sensory input from injured tissue causes peripheral **nociceptors** (receptive neurons for painful sensations) and central nervous system (CNS) pain pathways to enhance subsequent responses to pain stimuli. Thus, long-lasting changes in cells within the spinal cord **afferent** (ascending) and **efferent** (descending) **pain pathways** may occur after a brief noxious stimulus.

Physiological responses (such as elevated blood pressure, pulse rate, and respiratory rate; dilated pupils; pallor; and perspiration) to even a brief acute pain episode will begin showing adaptation within a short period, possibly minutes to a few hours. Physiologically, the body cannot sustain the extreme stress response for other than short periods of time. The body conserves its resources by physiological adaptation: returning to normal or near normal blood pressure, pulse rate, and respiratory rate; normal pupil size, and dry skin with little evidence of poor perfusion, *even in the face of continuing pain of the same intensity.*

Stimulation of Pain

The specific action of pain varies depending on the type of pain. In cutaneous pain, cutaneous nerve transmissions travel through a reflex arc from the nerve ending (point of pain) to the brain at a speed of approximately 300 feet per second, with a reflex response causing an almost immediate reaction. This explains why, when a hot stove is touched, the person's hand jerks back *before* there is conscious awareness that damage is occurring (Figure 26-2). After a hot stove is touched, a sensory nerve ending in the skin of the finger initiates nerve transmission that travels through the dorsal root ganglion to the dorsal horn in the gray matter of the spinal cord. From there, the impulse travels though an interneuron that synapses with a motor

neuron, which exits the spinal cord at the same level. This motor neuron, and the stimulation of the muscle it innervates, is responsible for the swift movement of the hand away from the hot stove.

In the case of the hot stove, the sensory neuron synapses not only with an interneuron but also with an afferent sensory neuron. The impulse travels up the spinal cord to the thalamus, where a final synapse conducts the impulse to the cortex of the brain. Once the signal reaches the cortex and is interpreted by the brain, the information is available on a conscious level. It is then that the person becomes aware of the intensity, location, and quality of pain. This information is interpreted in light of previous experience, adding the affective component to the pain experience. Efferent or descending motor neuron response is conducted from the brain through the spinal cord, where it synapses with a motor neuron that exits the spinal cord and innervates the muscle.

In visceral pain, transmission of pain impulses is slower and less localized than in cutaneous pain. The internal organs (including the gastrointestinal tract) have a minimal number of nociceptors, which explains why visceral pain is poorly localized and is felt as a dull aching or throbbing sensation. However, internal

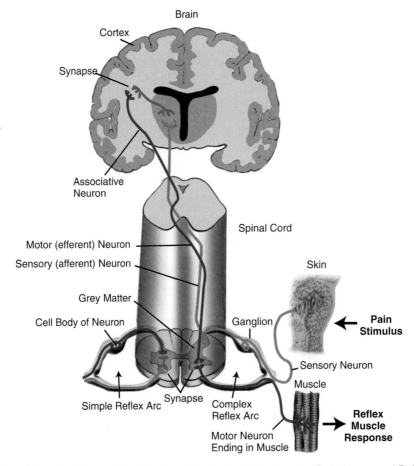

Figure 26-2 Reflex Arcs *(From* Fundamentals of Nursing: Standards & Practice, *by S. DeLaune and P. Ladner, 1998, Albany, NY: Delmar. Copyright 1998 by Delmar. Reprinted with permission.)*

PROFESSIONAL TIP

Sensation of Pain

It takes 0.2 grams of pressure per square millimeter for the cornea of the eye to feel pain, as opposed to 20 grams on the forearm, 200 grams on the sole of the foot, and 300 grams on the fingertips (Brand & Yancey, 1993).

organs have extreme sensitivity to distension. The cramping pain of **colic** (acute abdominal pain), for example, results when:

- Flatus or constipation causes distension of the stomach or intestines
- There is hyperperistalsis, as in gastroenteritis
- Something tries to pass through an opening that is too small

The physiology of **ischemic pain**, or pain occurring when the blood supply of an area is restricted or cut off completely, also differs from that of cutaneous pain. The restriction of blood flow causes inadequate oxygenation of the tissue supplied by those vessels, as well as inadequate metabolic waste product removal. Ischemic pain has the most rapid onset in an active muscle and a much slower onset in a passive muscle. Examples of ischemic pain are muscle cramps, sickle cell pain crisis, angina pectoris, and myocardial infarction. When ischemic pain occurs in a muscle that continues to work, a muscle spasm (cramp) is the outcome. If the blood supply to the heart is severely restricted or completely cut off and is not restored quickly, a myocardial infarction will occur.

Safety: Ischemic Pain

Supplemental oxygen and pain medication must be administered quickly to clients with ischemic pain to minimize oxygen deprivation and prevent infarction (tissue death).

In acute pain episodes, substances released from injured tissue lead to stress hormone responses in the client. This causes an increased metabolic rate, enhanced breakdown of body tissue, impaired immune function, increased blood clotting, and water retention. It triggers the fight-or-flight reaction leading to tachycardia and negative emotions.

The Gate Control Theory

Theories of pain transmission and interpretation attempt to describe and explain the pain experience. Early pain theorists focused on the neuroanatomical and neurophysiological mechanisms while failing to consider the psychological, social, cultural, and developmental factors involved (Stevens, 1994).

In 1965, Melzack and Wall proposed the **gate control pain theory**, which was the first to recognize that the psychological aspects of pain are as important as the physiological aspects. The gate control theory combines cognitive, sensory, and emotional components—in addition to the physiological aspects—and proposes that they can act on a gate control system to block the individual's perception of pain. The basic premise of this theory is that transmission of potentially painful nerve impulses to the cortex is modulated by a gating mechanism in the spinal cord and by CNS activity. As a result, the level of conscious awareness of painful sensation is altered.

The theory suggests that nerve fibers that contribute to pain transmission converge at a site in the dorsal horn of the spinal cord. This site is thought to act as a gating mechanism that determines which impulses will be blocked and which will be transmitted to the thalamus. The image of a gate can be useful in teaching clients and their families about pain relief measures. If the "gate" is closed, the signal is stopped before it reaches the brain, where **perception** (being aware of) of pain occurs. If the gate is open, the signal will continue on through the spinothalamic tract to the cortex, and the client will feel the pain. Whether the gate is opened or closed is influenced by the impulses from peripheral nerves (the sensory components) and nerve signals that descend from the brain (motivational-affective and cognitive components). For example, stimulation of some types of peripheral nerves by cutaneous stimulation such as massage can close the gate, whereas stimulation of the nociceptors will open the gate.

If a person is anxious, the gate can be opened by signals sent from the brain down to the mechanism in the dorsal horn of the spinal cord. On the other hand, if the person has had positive experiences with pain control in the past, the cognitive influence can send signals down to the gating mechanism and close it. The gate theory offered a great benefit by suggesting new approaches to relieving both acute and chronic pain. Pain could be relieved by blocking the transmission of pain impulses to the brain by both physical modalities and by altering the individual's thought processes, emotions, or other behaviors.

Conduction of Pain Impulses

Conduction of pain impulses refers to the physiologic processes that occur from the initiation of the pain signal to the realization of pain by the individual. There are four processes involved in the conduction of this signal. The first of these, **transduction**, is the step where a noxious stimulus triggers electrical activity in the endings of afferent nerve fibers (nociceptors). Once the signal is triggered, **transmission** occurs. The impulse travels from the receiving nociceptors to the spinal cord. Projection neurons then carry the message to the thalamus, and the message continues to the somatosensory cortex. This is where the third step, perception of pain, occurs. It is here that neural messages are converted into the subjective experience. The fourth process, **modulation**, is a central nervous system pathway that selectively inhibits pain transmission by sending blocking signals back down to the dorsal horn of the spinal cord.

FACTORS AFFECTING THE PAIN EXPERIENCE

McCaffery and Pasero (1999) point out that *the client is the only authority about the existence and nature of his or her pain*. Many factors account for the differences in clients' individual responses to pain, including age, previous experience with pain, drug abuse, and cultural norms.

Age

Age can greatly influence a client's perception of the pain experience. Clients may continue pain behaviors they learned as children and may also be reluctant to admit pain or seek medical care because of fear of the unknown or fear of the impact that treatment may have on their lifestyle. Older adults may often ignore their pain, viewing it as an unavoidable consequence of aging; family and health care members may inadvertently support this stereotype and be less than responsive to an older client's complaints of pain.

Previous Experience with Pain

Clients' previous exposures to pain will often influence their reactions. Coping mechanisms that were used in the past may affect clients' judgments about how the pain will affect their lives and what measures are within their control to successfully manage the pain on their own. Client teaching about pain expectations and management methods can often allay client fears and lead to more successful pain management, especially in those clients who do not have previous pain experience or who have memories of a previous devastating pain experience that they do not wish to repeat.

LIFE CYCLE CONSIDERATIONS

Elders and Pain
Older clients often are resigned to living with pain believing that nothing can be done. Pain often is not reported by older clients for fear of being labeled a "bother" or "complainer." The nurse should convey empathy and encourage the client to request pain relief as needed.

Drug Abuse

According to Compton (1999), a drug abuser is likely to be *less* tolerant of pain than someone who does not use drugs. Drug abuse may cause changes in the central nervous system that result in an exaggerated neurophysiologic response to painful stimuli. To keep a drug abuser comfortable, withdrawal must be prevented.

Cultural Norms

Cultural diversity in pain responses can easily lead to problems in pain management. Laboratory studies on subjects of various cultures found no significant difference among the groups in the level of intensity at which pain becomes appreciable or perceptible. However, the same studies showed that the subjects differed significantly in the level of intensity or duration of pain the client was willing to endure. Expression of pain is also governed by cultural values. In some cultures, tolerance to pain, and therefore "suffering in silence," is expected; in others, full expression of pain may include animated physical and emotional responses. The nurse must be careful not to equate the level of expression of pain with the level of actual pain experienced, but to instead consider cultural and other influences that affect the expression of pain.

JCAHO STANDARDS

New pain management standards were included in the 2000–2001 standards of the Joint Commission on Accreditation of Healthcare Organizations (JCAHO). They will first be scored for compliance in 2001.

The health care organizations will be expected to:

- Recognize the right of patients to appropriate assessment and management of pain;
- Assess the existence and, if so, the nature and intensity of pain in all patients;
- Record the results of the assessment in a way that facilitates regular reassessment and follow-up;
- Determine and assure staff competency in pain assessment and management and address pain assessment and management in the orientation of all new staff;
- Establish policies and procedures that support the appropriate prescription or ordering of effective pain medications;
- Educate patients and their families about effective pain management; and
- Address patient needs for symptom management in the discharge planning process (JCAHO, 1999).

NURSING PROCESS

The nursing process will provide the correct framework for managing a client's pain.

Assessment

Assessment of the client's pain is a crucial function of the nurse. During the assessment process, nurses need to be aware of their own values and expectations about pain behaviors. Just as the client's experience and cultural background help determine how pain is demonstrated, nurses' cultures and experiences help determine which pain behaviors are viewed as acceptable. Nurses need to be aware of these values and avoid biases when assessing client pain and planning client care. Once a self-assessment about pain has been conducted, the nurse is ready to assess the client.

Pain assessment tools are the single most effective method of identifying the presence and intensity of pain in clients. *These tools must be used, and the results must be believed.* Figure 26-3 shows the Initial Pain Assessment Tool developed by McCaffery and Beebe and found in AHCPR's acute pain management guideline (AHCPR, 1992). This tool is particularly effective when clients have complex pain problems because it assesses location, intensity, quality, precipitating and alleviating factors, and how the pain affects function and quality of life. Once this tool is completed, another less detailed tool can be used for ongoing monitoring of the client's pain level.

The JCAHO (2000a) now considers pain as the "fifth" vital sign. It is to be assessed and recorded along with the client's temperature, pulse, respiration, and blood pressure.

Subjective Data

Gathering subjective information regarding the client's pain is the first step in pain assessment. The nurse should determine a client's pain threshold and pain tolerance level. **Pain threshold** is the level of intensity at which a person feels pain. It will vary with each individual and with each different type of pain. **Pain tolerance** is the level of intensity or duration of pain the client is willing or able to endure.

The client's description of the pain should cover several qualifiers, including its location, onset and duration, quality, intensity, aggravating factors (variables

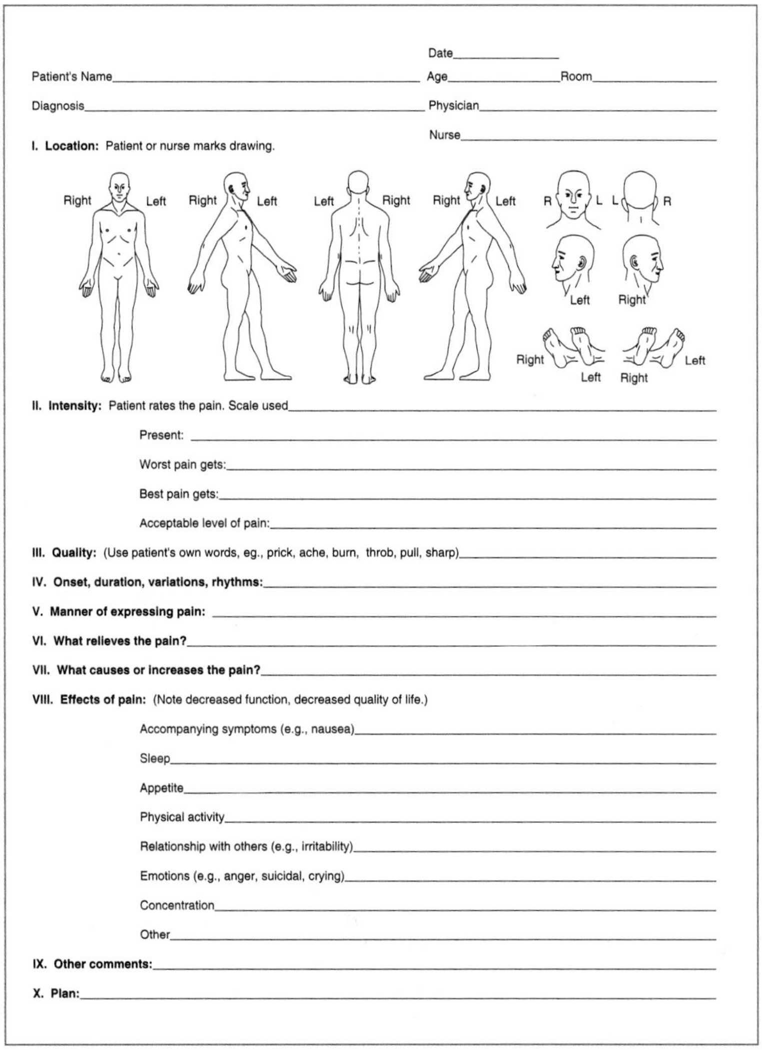
Date______
Patient's Name______ Age______ Room______
Diagnosis______ Physician______
Nurse______

I. Location: Patient or nurse marks drawing.

II. Intensity: Patient rates the pain. Scale used______

Present: ______

Worst pain gets: ______

Best pain gets: ______

Acceptable level of pain: ______

III. Quality: (Use patient's own words, eg., prick, ache, burn, throb, pull, sharp)______

IV. Onset, duration, variations, rhythms:______

V. Manner of expressing pain: ______

VI. What relieves the pain?______

VII. What causes or increases the pain?______

VIII. Effects of pain: (Note decreased function, decreased quality of life.)

Accompanying symptoms (e.g., nausea)______

Sleep______

Appetite______

Physical activity______

Relationship with others (e.g., irritability)______

Emotions (e.g., anger, suicidal, crying)______

Concentration______

Other______

IX. Other comments:______

X. Plan:______

Figure 26-3 Initial Pain Assessment Tool *(From* Pain: Clinical Manual for Nursing Practice *[2nd ed.], by M. McCaffery and A. Beebe, 1999, St. Louis, MO: Mosby. Copyright 1999 by Mosby. Reprinted with permission.)*

PROFESSIONAL TIP

Location of Pain

During intershift report on a postoperative client recovering from abdominal surgery, the nurse reported that the client had stated she had pain and had been medicated with IM Demerol. When greeting her client, the nurse asked the client about the pain she had experienced during the night. The client replied, "Oh, it is fine now, I only had a headache." The night nurse had assumed the client's pain was in her surgical site and chose the medication accordingly. The headache probably could have been relieved with a milder medication. All reports of pain must be thoroughly asessed prior to any interventions being implemented.

CLIENT TEACHING

Pain at Night

- It is common for pain to be worse at night when there are fewer distractions. Knowing that this is normal can be reassuring because the client may attribute the increased pain to complications.

that worsen the pain, such as exercise, certain foods, or stress), alleviating factors (measures the client can take that lessen the effect of the pain, such as lying down, avoiding certain foods, or taking medication), associated manifestations (factors that often accompany the pain, such as nausea, constipation, or dizziness), and what pain means to the client.

Whenever subjective and objective data conflict, the subjective reports of pain are to be considered the primary source.

Location The client can point to the location of the pain on the client's own body or locate it on a body diagram on a pain assessment tool. The client should be asked if there is more than one site of pain; if the pain radiates, and if so to where; and ask if the pain is deep or superficial.

Onset and Duration The nurse should ask the client how long the pain has existed; what, if anything, triggers its onset; and if there are any patterns to the pain; for example, whether it is worse at certain times of the day or night.

Quality The nurse should ask the client what the pain feels like, and record the words used to describe the pain. Clients may use sensory-type words, such as "pricking," "radiating," "burning," or "throbbing." However, some clients use words that have an affective connotation, such as "fearful," "sickening," or "punishing." Other words used may be evaluative, such as "miserable" or "unbearable." The quality of pain provides information that may be useful in diagnosing the cause of the pain. For example, pain described as "burning" or "freezing" is usually neuropathic in origin.

Intensity The client may have difficulty in judging the intensity of pain. However, it is important to obtain an estimate of the severity of the pain. This information allows the clinician to evaluate the effectiveness of pain relief measures tried by comparing intensity before and after the interventions.

Pain intensity scales are an effective method for clients to rate the intensity of their pain (Figure 26-4). The simple descriptive pain-intensity scale and the visual analog scale (VAS) are best used by showing the scale to the client and asking the client to point to the spot on the scale that corresponds to the present pain. The pain scale most frequently used with adolescent and adult clients is the verbal 0 to 10 scale. No equipment or supplies are needed, and it requires only enough time to ask one question: "On a scale of 0 to 10, with 0 being no pain at all and 10 being the worst pain you could ever have, how much do you hurt right now?" If there are multiple painful areas, this question can be asked regarding each area.

Although developed for use with children, the FACES Pain Rating Scale (Figure 26-5) can be used effectively with clients when a language barrier exists. A translator should be used initially to explain what the faces represent.

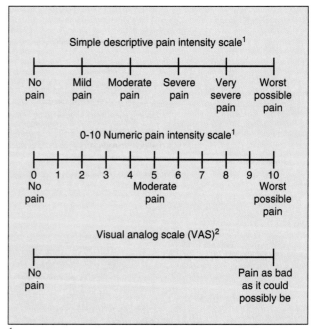

[1] If used as a graphic rating scale, a 10-cm baseline is recommended.
[2] A 10-cm baseline is recommended for VAS scales.

Figure 26-4 Pain Intensity Scales: Three Commonly Used Self-Report Intensity Scales *(Courtesy of Agency for Health Care Policy and Research, 1992.)*

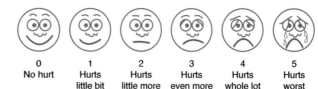

0	1	2	3	4	5
No hurt	Hurts little bit	Hurts little more	Hurts even more	Hurts whole lot	Hurts worst

Figure 26-5 Wong/Baker FACES Pain Rating Scale *(From Wong, D. L., Hockenberry-Eaton, M., Wilson, D., Winkelstein, M. L., Ahmann, E., DiVito-Thomas, P. A.: Whaley and Wong's Nursing Care of Infants and Children, ed. 6, St. Louis, 1999. Mosby, p. 1153. Copyrighted by Mosby-Year Book, Inc. Reprinted by permission.)*

LIFE CYCLE CONSIDERATIONS

Children and Pain Assessment

Children provide a special challenge in pain assessment. Two useful tools for assessing pain in children are the Wong/Baker FACES Pain Rating Scale, the Oucher scale.

- The Wong/Baker FACES Pain Rating Scale can be used with children as young as 3 years. It helps children express their level of pain by pointing to a cartoon face that most closely resembles how they are feeling (Figure 26-5).
- The Oucher pediatric pain intensity scale (Figure 26-6) consists of two scales: a 0 to 100 numeric scale and a 6-point facial scale. If the child can count from 1 to 100 by ones or by tens, the numeric scale can be used; if not, the facial scale can be used. The facial scale has been successfully used in children as young as 3 to 4 years.

A new pain assessment tool is the "Painometer" developed by Dr. Gaston-Johansson (Mattson, 2000). The client positions a pointer between "no pain" and "worst possible pain." Quantifying numbers are on the back. The client also indicates the quality of pain by selecting sensory and affective descriptors from a list.

Aggravating and Alleviating Factors The nurse should question the client about what makes the pain worse and what makes the pain better, including behaviors or activities that influence the pain. This information provides input into developing the plan of care for the client in pain. If there are specific activities that relieve the pain, the nurse can incorporate them into the care plan. Being aware of activities that increase the pain can allow for interventions that may prevent the pain. For example, if physical therapy exercises trigger an increase in pain, the nurse can administer an analgesic as ordered prior to treatment.

Associated Manifestations The initial pain assessment should include the impact of pain on the activities of daily living. Pain may cause changes in sleep

CULTURAL CONSIDERATIONS

Language Barrier and Pain

The Faces Pain Rating Scale can be used effectively with clients when a language barrier exists. A translator should be used initially to explain what the faces represent.

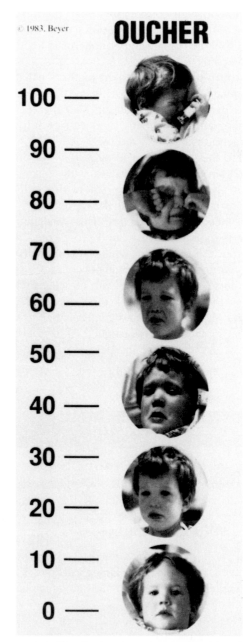

Figure 26-6 The Oucher Pain Assessment Tool: For Use with Children 3–12 Years of Age. Caucasian, Hispanic, and African American versions are available. *(The Caucasian version of the Oucher, developed and copyrighted by Judith E. Beyer, RN, PhD, 1983.)*

patterns or the ability to work and carry out the many roles in a client's life. Pain may affect appetite, mood, sexual functioning, or the ability to participate in recreational activities. If pain is interfering with daily life, the client's quality of life can be greatly affected.

Pain is fatiguing. It requires a significant amount of energy to deal with pain. The longer a person suffers from pain, the greater the level of fatigue. Although there is no conscious awareness of pain during sleep, there may be a dream-state awareness (McCaffery & Pasero, 1999). The stress response (which can be seen even in clients under general anesthesia) continues, and the body physiologically pays the price. Clients also wake up with considerably more pain than they had going to sleep, thereby requiring even more intervention (pharmacologic and nonpharmacologic) to reduce the pain.

Meaning of Pain Due to the motivational-affective components of the pain experience, the meaning of pain can have a great impact on how the client perceives the pain. A frequently cited classic study on this phenomenon was conducted by Beecher (1956), who compared the pain perceived by soldiers wounded in battle to pain perceived by civilians with similar surgical wounds. He found that only 32% of the soldiers required narcotics for pain relief, whereas 85% of the civilians needed the narcotics. This was interpreted that for the soldiers, the wound represented a ticket away from the battlefield, while for the civilians, the surgical wound was a depressing event.

The nurse should explore with the client what implications the pain may have for the individual. Does it mean that the client's cancer is metastasizing? Or that the client's condition is worsening? All of these interpretations may influence the pain experience for the client.

Objective Data

As discussed when addressing acute versus chronic pain, the objective data often presents a different picture depending on the type of pain the client is experiencing.

Physiologic Acute pain activates the sympathetic nervous system, and the client may exhibit the following: elevated heart rate, elevated respiratory rate, elevated blood pressure, diaphoresis, pallor, muscle tension, and dilated pupils. These signs resemble those of anxiety, which often accompanies acute pain. The signs and symptoms of chronic pain show adaption, and, therefore, are different from those of acute pain, with vital signs being normal and no accompanying pupil dilation or perspiration.

Behavioral Acute pain behaviors may include crying and moaning, rubbing the site of pain, restlessness, a distorted posture, clenched fists, guarding the painful area, frowning, and grimacing. The client usually speaks of the discomfort and may be restless or afraid to move.

The client in chronic pain may demonstrate behaviors similar to those of depression such as hopelessness, listlessness, and loss of libido and weight. Chronic pain also often leads to physical inactivity or immobility, which can lead to functional disability.

Clients' behavioral adaptation may yield no report of pain unless questioned specifically. **Distraction** (focusing attention on stimuli other than pain) may also be used by clients. McCaffery and Pasero (1999) recognize that clients often minimize the pain behaviors they are able to control for a number of reasons including:

- To be a "good" client and avoid making demands
- To maintain a positive self-image by not becoming a "sissy"

PROFESSIONAL TIP

Assessing the Effect of Pain on Sleep

Questioning clients about the effect pain has on their sleep habits will help clarify the intensity of the pain and its effect on the clients' patterns of daily living. The nurse should ask the client whether the pain:

- Prevents the client from falling asleep
- Makes finding a comfortable sleeping position difficult
- Wakes the client from a sound sleep
- Keeps the client from falling back asleep once awakened
- Leaves the client feeling tired and unrefreshed after a sleeping session

---

CULTURAL CONSIDERATIONS

Perception of Pain

Culture determines the way persons derive meaning from their lives and also determines appropriate behaviors. One's cultural upbringing teaches behaviors, including those that are exhibited when in pain. People from different cultures use different types of words to describe pain (for example, in sensory or emotional terms). These differences should not be ignored, but the nurse also needs to be careful not to prejudge a client based on cultural background or ethnicity. Due to the unique experience of pain, the person will exhibit individualized behaviors even though they are influenced by cultural upbringing.

- By using distraction as a method of making pain more bearable (young children are particularly adept at this)
- Exhaustion

Occasionally, there is a discrepancy between pain behaviors observed by the nurse (objective data) and the client's self-report of pain. Client pain behaviors (AHCPR, 1992) include splinting of the painful area, distorted posture, impaired mobility, insomnia, anxiety, attention seeking, and depression. Discrepancies between behaviors and the client's self-report can be due to good coping skills (e.g., relaxation techniques or distraction), stoicism, anxiety, or cultural differences in expected pain behaviors. Whenever these discrepancies occur, they should be addressed with the client, and the pain management plan must be renegotiated accordingly.

Ongoing Assessment

The initial assessment obtains a baseline of information regarding the client's pain. Subsequent assessments provide information regarding the effectiveness of the interventions. Physiologic and behavioral signs, and most important, the client's subjective pain ratings of the intensity will all help the health care team determine whether the interventions should be continued or changed. Pain assessments should be performed to coincide with when the intervention should be providing the most relief. For example, the onset of intravenous morphine is rapid, peaking approximately 20 minutes after administration. If the client has not ob-

tained relief by 20 minutes, the intravenous morphine was ineffective, and the plan of care would need to be changed.

Recording Pain Assessment Findings

No matter which pain assessment tool is chosen, it will be of little effect unless the pain rating and related information are recorded in a manner easily understood by the health care team. Figure 26-7 is a flow sheet (McCaffery & Beebe, 1989) that is an excellent record in an acute care setting. It provides one place to document the majority of information used to make pain management decisions, including pain rating, vital signs, analgesic administered, and level of arousal.

Nursing Diagnoses

The two primary nursing diagnoses used to describe pain are *Acute Pain* and *Chronic Pain*. According to the North American Nursing Diagnosis Association (NANDA, 2001), *Acute Pain* is defined as "an unpleasant sensory and emotional experience arising from actual or potential tissue damage or described in terms of such damage . . . [with] sudden or slow onset of any intensity from mild to severe, with an anticipated or predictable end and a duration of less than 6 months" (p. 129). *Chronic Pain* is defined the same as *Acute Pain,* with the last phrase replaced by "constant or recurring without an anticipated or predictable end and a duration of greater than 6 months" (p. 130).

Pain may be the etiology (cause) of other problems, for example: *Impaired Physical Mobility,* related to

Patient _____ Date _____
Pain rating scale used* _____
Purpose: To evaluate the safety and effectiveness of the analgesic(s)
Analgesic(s) prescribed: _____

Time	Pain rating	Analgesic	R	P	BP	Level of arousal	Other**	Plan and comments

May be duplicated for use in clinical practice.
*Pain rating: A number of different scales may be used. Indicate which scale is used and use the same scale each time.
**Possibilities for other columns: bowel function, activities, nausea and vomiting, and other pain relief measures. Identify the side effects of greatest concern to patient, family, physician, and nurse.

Figure 26-7 Flow Sheet for Pain Management Documentation *(From* Pain: Clinical Manual for Nursing Practice, *[2nd ed.], by M. McCaffery and A. Beebe, 1999, St. Louis, MO: Mosby. Copyright 1999 by Mosby. Reprinted with permission.)*

arthritic hip pain. Whether the pain is addressed in the problem statement or the etiology will be determined by the client's primary problem. There are many diagnoses that can be related to the client in pain depending on the effects of the pain:

- *Activity Intolerance*
- *Anxiety*
- *Constipation*
- *Deficient Knowledge (specify)*
- *Disturbed Body Image*
- *Disturbed Sleep Pattern*
- *Disturbed Thought Processes*
- *Fatigue*
- *Fear*
- *Hopelessness*
- *Impaired Physical Mobility*
- *Impaired Social Interaction*
- *Ineffective Breathing Pattern*
- *Ineffective Individual Coping*
- *Ineffective Role Performance*
- *Ineffective Therapeutic Regimen Management*
- *Powerlessness*

Planning/Outcome Identification

When planning care for the client experiencing pain, mutual goal setting is of utmost importance. After assessing the client's perception of the problem, the nurse and client can work together in developing realistic outcomes. Both nonpharmacologic and pharmacologic interventions should be considered in planning strategies to return clients to control or to maintain them at desired levels of functioning and pain.

When asking about the client's goal for pain relief, the nurse often has to state, "We can't usually get rid of all your pain, but if we could get it down to a place that it didn't bother you so much, what would that be?" That way the client, the family, and health care professionals involved will all be aware of the goal for pain relief and can adjust the plan of care accordingly.

Often several approaches must be combined for adequate relief to be obtained. No matter which type of intervention is being utilized, there are general principles that apply: individualization, prevention, and utilization of a multidisciplinary approach.

Individualize the Approach

A variety of pain relief measures can be tried in many combinations until the goal of pain relief is reached. This often means some trial-and-error of interventions until the right combination is found. It is important to include measures that the client believes will be effective. The cognitive component of pain perception can have a powerful influence on the effectiveness of interventions. This may mean including folk remedies or nonscientific relief measures. It is important to keep an open

mind. This comes with the caution that the nurse needs to avoid those remedies that may harm the client.

Use a Preventive Approach

Pain is much easier to control if it is treated before it gets severe. Interventions should be implemented when pain is mild, or when it is anticipated. For example, medicate a client prior to a painful dressing change or treatment rather than waiting for the pain to occur.

Use a Multidisciplinary Approach

Pain relief is a complex phenomenon requiring input from various members of the health care team. The nurse's role is pivotal in managing a client's pain. The physician also plays a key role, diagnosing and treating the medical cause of the pain, which includes prescribing appropriate medications. In complex cases, other professionals, such as physical therapists, psychologists, social workers, or chaplains may be needed. The multidisciplinary team approach is the most successful way to manage chronic pain and improve the quality of a client's life.

Nursing Interventions

Pharmacologic and nonpharmacologic interventions can both be effective in caring for clients with pain. In some cases of mild pain, nonpharmacologic techniques may be the primary intervention, with medication available as "backup." In cases of moderate to severe pain, nonpharmacologic techniques can be an effective adjunctive, or complementary, treatment.

There are three categories of pain control interventions: (1) pharmacological, (2) noninvasive, and (3) invasive. Each category will be discussed separately, but these methods are often used in combination.

Pharmacological Interventions

Drug therapy is the mainstay of treatment for pain control. The American Pain Society (1999) and AHCPR (1992, 1994) have published guidelines that provide specific recommendations for the use of drug therapy in pain control. These guidelines were developed by panels of experts who analyzed current research available on pain control and represent concise information that can help nurses, physicians, and other health care workers to effectively administer medications for pain relief.

The World Health Organization (WHO) has made worldwide relief of cancer pain one of their primary goals (1990). In order to help meet this goal, it developed an analgesic ladder to help the clinician determine which analgesic to prescribe (Figure 26-8). Combining analgesics and the use of adjuvant medication provides effective pharmacologic intervention for clients with pain. **Adjuvant medications** are those drugs used to enhance the analgesic efficacy of opioids, to treat con-

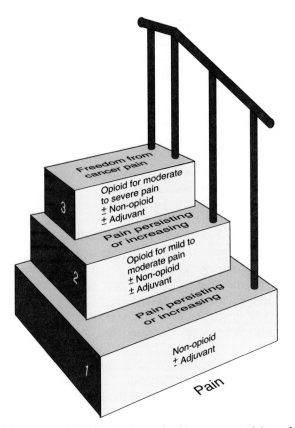

Figure 26-8 WHO Analgesic Ladder gives guidelines for choosing analgesic therapy for cancer pain based on the level of pain the client is experiencing. (*Courtesy of World Health Organization, 1990. Used with permission.*)

current symptoms that exacerbate pain, and to provide independent analgesia for specific types of pain. The ladder recommends that the analgesic, plus or minus an adjuvant, is chosen based on the level of pain the client is experiencing. For mild pain, the ladder recommends a nonopioid. If the pain persists or if the client has moderate pain to begin with, WHO recommends a weak opioid, plus or minus the nonopioid, plus or minus an adjuvant. If pain persists, a strong opioid is used. The *nonopioid should be continued,* and an adjuvant medication should be considered (AHCPR, 1994). This ladder gives health care workers guidelines in determining if the drug regimen is appropriate for the client with cancer pain.

Nurses' Role in Administration of Analgesics The nurse is the health care professional who spends the most time with the client in pain and is the team member who is most often able to assess the effectiveness of pain control interventions. When analgesics are prescribed, the nurse is often given choices of drug, route, and interval. For example, the postop client may have the following orders:

- Morphine 10–15 mg IM or IV q2–4h prn severe pain
- Vicodin i–ii tabs q3–4h prn moderate pain

When this client complains of pain, which analgesic should the nurse administer? Which route? Which dose? How frequently? The nurse in this situation carries a large responsibility in making these decisions. The nurse also has autonomy in making these decisions. The client may not be aware of all the available choices. Each nurse may make a different decision, often based on the nurse's own biases.

These choices and autonomy require responsibility on the part of the nurse. McCaffery and Pasero (1999) identify the following as the responsibilities of the nurse in administering analgesics. The nurse must:

- Determine whether or not to give the analgesic, and if more than one is ordered, which one
- Assess the client's response to the analgesic, including assessing the effectiveness in pain relief and occurrence of any side effects
- Report to the physician when a change is needed, including making suggestions for changes based on the nurse's knowledge of the client and pharmacology
- Teach the client and family regarding the use of analgesics

Principles of Administering Analgesics "How an analgesic is used is probably more important than which one is used" (McCaffery & Pasero, 1999). There are principles that should be applied in the administration of analgesics, no matter which one is given.

Establishing and maintaining a therapeutic serum level is important. Figure 26-9 illustrates the peaks and valleys that often occur when analgesics are administered in the traditional prn (as needed) manner. When the dose is administered on an intermittent schedule, a larger dose is often required, causing the client to have a peak serum drug level in the sedation range. The client must wait for the return of pain before requesting the next dose of analgesic. Depending on the length of time it takes to obtain the medication and,

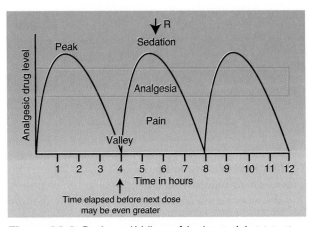

Figure 26-9 Peaks and Valleys of Analgesic Administration. (*From Pain: Clinical Manual for Nursing Practice [2nd ed.], by M. McCaffery and A. Beebe, 1999, St. Louis, MO: Mosby. Copyright 1999 by Mosby. Reprinted with permission.*)

CLIENT TEACHING

Pain Management

Clients and their families must be educated regarding:
- The importance of taking or requesting pain medication before the pain becomes severe and more difficult to control
- The numerous nonpharmacologic approaches that clients can use to augment their pharmacologic pain management
- The individualization of pain management (The client may be taking different medications or different dosages than other individuals.)

once taken, to reestablish an adequate blood level, there could be a period of up to an hour or so with inadequate pain control.

Preventive Approach Pain is much easier to control if treated when it is anticipated or at a mild intensity. Once pain becomes severe, the analgesics ordered may not be effective enough to relieve it. Many clinicians still teach their clients to wait to take medication until they are sure they really need it. This practice leads to uncontrolled pain. There are two ways the preventive approach may be implemented:

- ATC (around the clock)—When pain is predictable, for example, the first few days following surgery or with chronic cancer pain, the medication is administered on a scheduled basis. This prevents the peaks and valleys of serum drug level that can lead to oversedation or toxicity and recurrence of pain, respectively. If the analgesics are ordered by the physician to be given PRN, it can still be a nursing measure to administer the drugs ATC, as long as they are given within the time constraints of the order.
- PRN (Latin for *pro re nata,* which means "as required")—Pain cannot always be predictable, therefore PRN dosing may be required. For some clients this may be used in addition to scheduled dosing for "breakthrough" pain (pain that surpasses the level of **analgesia**, or pain relief, that the steady level of analgesics is providing). Examples of this include a cancer client on prolonged-release morphine who needs extra analgesics to participate in activities such as shopping or receiving visitors. Another example would be the orthopedic client who is receiving regularly scheduled analgesics for postop pain who needs additional pain relief for therapy sessions. In order to implement the preventive approach with PRN dosing, the medications should be given as soon as the pain appears, or when it is anticipated to begin.

Titrate to Effect Due to the unique nature of the pain experience, the analgesic regimen needs to be titrated until the desired effect is achieved. This involves adjusting the following:

- *Dosage*—Some clients may require more or less than the standard dose. There are many factors that may influence the pharmacokinetics in an individual client. The individual's response is assessed and the dosage of the analgesic is regulated accordingly. In clients with chronic cancer pain, opioid analgesics are recommended to be increased until pain relief is obtained or unacceptable side effects occur. This may be done due to the lack of a **ceiling effect** (the dosage beyond which no further analgesia occurs) in pure opioids. The lack of a ceiling effect means there is no limit to the dose that can be given. For example, cancer clients have been known to receive over 1 gram per hour intravenously. Because the dosage is gradually increased, the client develops a **tolerance** (requiring larger and larger doses of an analgesic to achieve the same level of pain relief) to the side effects of the opioid.
- *Interval*—Some clients metabolize the analgesics faster than others. For example, young adults tend to metabolize opioids faster, therefore they may need more frequent doses. Older clients tend to metabolize them slower, therefore they will require a longer interval between doses.
- *Route*—The appropriate route is chosen depending on how rapidly pain relief is required, the client's ability to take medications orally, the client's diagnosis, and assessment of the client's response to the current route. Intravenous administration provides the most rapid onset of pain relief. All other routes require a lag time for absorption of the analgesic into the circulation. In postoperative pain, IV is the preferred route for opioids when the oral route is not appropriate. If IV access is not available, sublingual, rectal, or transdermal routes should be considered (AHCPR, 1992).

  With cancer pain, the oral route is preferred. If these clients are unable to take oral medications, rectal and transdermal routes are preferred since they are less invasive than other routes (AHCPR, 1994). In addition, tolerance develops at a slower rate with the oral route compared to the more invasive routes.
- *Choice of drug*—If one drug is not providing relief or has unacceptable side effects, another analgesic may be tried.

The key to administering an analgesic is to monitor the client's response to it. This includes assessing the effectiveness of pain relief and the occurrence of side effects.

Classes of Analgesics There are three classes of drugs used for pain relief: (1) nonopioid analgesics; (2) opioid analgesics; and (3) analgesic adjuvants already discussed (WHO, 1986). Nonopioid and opioid analgesics will be addressed separately, as indications and side effects are different for each one.

Nonopioids The medications in this category are useful for a variety of painful conditions, including surgery, trauma, and cancer (American Pain Society, 1999). The indications include mild to moderate pain, and they are used in conjunction with opioids. These drugs differ from opioids in several ways in that they:

- Are subject to the ceiling effect
- Do not produce the effect of tolerance or physical dependence
- Are antipyretic and should not be given in cases where they may mask an infection

Ketorolac is the only NSAID available in parenteral form and has proven useful in clients on NPO status who would benefit from a NSAID. Even when administered intramuscularly or intravenously, ketorolac produces significant gastric irritation and the potential for gastric bleeding. The most frequent use of ketorolac is orally or intramuscularly in adults, but some pediatric centers have used it intravenously under strict supervision for a limited course (less than 5 days) in children and adolescents with great success.

Action Action of these drugs is thought to inhibit prostaglandin formation. If prostaglandins are inhibited, the sensory neurons are less likely to receive the pain signal. Thus, this class of analgesics works in the peripheral nervous system.

Opioids The opioid analgesics fall into three classes: pure opioid agonists, partial agonists, and **mixed agonist-antagonists** (a compound that blocks opioid effects on one receptor type while producing opioid effects on a second receptor type). Pure agonists are those that produce a maximal response from cells when they bind to the cells' opioid receptor sites. Morphine (the gold standard against which all other opioids are measured), fentanyl (Duragesic), methadone (Dolophine), hydromorphone hydrochloride (Dilaudid), and codeine are pure agonists. Meperidine (Demerol), although classified as a pure agonist, is not recommended except in clients with a true allergy to all other narcotics, because of its neurotoxicity. Meperidine produces clinical analgesia for only 2.5 to 3.5 hours when given intramuscularly in adults.

PROFESSIONAL TIP

Ketorolac

Ketorolac should not be used in a client with any history of renal dysfunction, gastric irritation, bleeding problems, low platelet count, or allergy to aspirin or other NSAIDs.

Unlike the NSAIDs, pure agonist opioids are not subject to the ceiling effect. As the dosage is increased, there is increasing pain relief.

Action Opioids act in the central nervous system by binding to opiate receptor sites on afferent neurons. The pain signal is stopped at the spinal cord level, and does not reach the cortex where pain is perceived.

Side Effects The only limiting factor in the use of pure agonist opioids is the degree of side effects, particularly respiratory depression and constipation. Other side effects include pruritus and nausea, but the degree to which they are present from each medication varies among individuals. Clients must be instructed regarding these normal responses to opioids and informed that it does not mean that they are allergic to them. A true allergy to opioids would be indicated by a rash or hives that starts after receiving the opioid, a local histamine release at the site of infusion, or anaphylaxis. Clients also need to know that the pruritus and nausea generally subside after 4 to 5 days of opioid therapy. In the meantime, an antihistamine such as diphenhydramine hydrochloride (Benadryl) or hydroxyzine hydrochloride (Atarax, Vistaril) may be used for pruritus, and an antiemetic such as metoclopromide hydrochloride (Clopra) or trimethobenzamide hydrochloride (Tigan) can be used to treat the nausea.

Almost all medications used to treat side effects have their own side effect of sedation. Thus, there is the possibility of a cumulative effect of severe sedation. These medications must be used with caution

PROFESSIONAL TIP

Types of Nonopioid Drugs

- *Salicylates*—These include aspirin and other salicylate salts. Common side effects of aspirin include gastric disturbances and bleeding due to the antiplatelet effect. Some of the salicylate salts, such as choline magnesium trisalicylate (Trilisate) and salsalate (Salgesic) have fewer gastrointestinal and bleeding effects than aspirin.
- *Acetaminophen*—This is a nonsalicylate that is similar to aspirin in its analgesic action, but has no anti-inflammatory effect. Its mechanism of action for pain relief is not known.
- *NSAIDs*—The effectiveness of these drugs varies, with some being close to the effectiveness of aspirin and acetaminophen, while others are much stronger. Clients tend to vary in response, so once the maximum recommended dose has been tried with ineffective results, it would be worth trying another NSAID. The drugs in this group inhibit platelet aggregation, and are contraindicated in clients with coagulation disorders or on anticoagulation therapy.

LIFE CYCLE CONSIDERATIONS

Effects of meperidine (Demerol)

- In the elderly, most of whom show decreased glomerular filtration rates, there is generally a higher peak and longer duration of action as it takes longer to excrete the opioid as well as its toxic metabolite, normeperidine.
- In pediatric clients receiving intravenous meperidine, analgesia may last for only 1.5 to 2.0 hours.

and appropriate monitoring until the client's response is determined. Ondansetron hydrochloride (Zofran) is one antiemetic on the market with little, if any, sedative effect. It has recently received Food and Drug Administration (FDA) approval for use with postoperative nausea and has been effective in clients with refractory nausea and vomiting unresponsive to other antiemetics. The current cost per dose, close to $100 in many hospitals, limits its use to the extreme nausea associated with cancer chemotherapy or to clients with refractory nausea and vomiting.

Mixed agonist-antagonist opioids are believed to be subject to the ceiling effect for pain relief, as well as a ceiling effect for respiratory depression. Mixed agonist-antagonist opioids activate one opioid receptor type while simultaneously blocking another type. Butorphanol tartrate (Stadol), pentazocine hydrochloride (Talwin), and nalbuphine hydrochloride (Nubain) are the most frequently used in pain management.

Opioid antagonists include naloxone (Narcan) and naltrexone (Trexal), with the most commonly used being naloxone (Narcan). They work by blocking opioid stimulation of receptor sites. Naloxone effectively reverses opioid side effects of sedation, respiratory depression, and nausea *while it completely reverses any pain control.*

PROFESSIONAL TIP

Constipation and Opioids

Clients who are expected to require opioid analgesics for more than 1 or 2 days should be administered a stool softener as soon as they are taking fluids orally. While they are still NPO, a glycerin or bisacodyl (Dulcolax) suppository should be administered if the client has not had a bowel movement in 1 or 2 days.

Alternative Delivery Systems Opioids are administered in more than just the traditional oral, subcutaneous, intramuscular, intravenous, and rectal routes.

Patient-Controlled Analgesia Patient-controlled analgesia (PCA) is most often delivered by a device that allows the client to control the delivery of intravenous, epidural, or subcutaneous pain medication in a safe, effective manner through a programmable pump (Figure 26-10). This system helps to eliminate the time required for the nurse to draw up the medication, and allows the client to feel some control over the pain. The pump has the safety feature of locking out once a maximum dose has been reached. This prevents the client from overdosing. Requirements for the use of PCA are the cognitive ability to understand how to use the pump and the physical ability to push the button. The PCA has been successfully used with many types of pain and in many settings, including pediatrics and home health.

Oral PCA is relatively new in hospitals and, according to Pasero (2000), is becoming increasingly popular. Client teaching is the key for success. The client must understand how pain, pain medication, and pain relief are related and how to maintain a pain-relief diary. A Velcro®-sealed wrist pouch is applied to the client with one or two doses of the prescribed oral analgesic, even controlled substances, in the pouch. The client notifies the nurse when a dose is taken, so it can be replaced. If the client does not comply with the oral PCA policy, it is discontinued.

Epidural/Intrathecal Analgesia Epidural analgesia refers to administering the opioid via a catheter that terminates in the epidural space, the space outside the dura mater that protects the spinal cord. **Intrathecal analgesia** refers to administering the drug directly into the subarachnoid space. These may be administered as a one-time injection by the anesthesiologist, or via a catheter that has been placed. Both of these

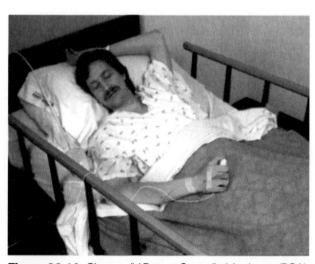

Figure 26-10 Client on IV Patient-Controlled Analgesia (PCA)

CLIENT TEACHING

Timed-Release Tables

Teach clients and families the difference between extended-release and immediate-release tablets. Emphasize that the extended-release tablets become immediate-release if crushed (e.g., for a client who has difficulty swallowing the tablet).

LIFE CYCLE CONSIDERATIONS

Injections and Children

Because children lack the cognitive ability to weigh the pain of injection against the pain relief from the medication, oral and rectal routes are preferred over injections.

routes are occasionally referred to as *intraspinal anesthesia.* Because the opioid is delivered close to the site of action, these routes require much lower doses of opioid (usually morphine [Duramorph] or fentanyl [Sublimaze] are used) for pain relief. The incidence of systemic side effects is also much lower with these routes. Duration is longer than systemic routes, for example, the duration of one dose of intrathecal morphine can last 24 hours.

Transdermal Analgesia Another route of opioid administration is the transdermal patch. The only opioid drug currently available via this route is fentanyl (Duragesic). This medication is on an adhesive patch that attaches to the skin. It is available in 25, 50, 75, and 100 mcg/hour dosages. The fentanyl transdermal patch allows slow infusion of the drug through the skin. The fentanyl patch is indicated for continuous pain with high dosage requirements. The advantage of this route is that it is simple to apply and it is effective for 72 hours. The disadvantage is that dosage adjustments are difficult to make due to the slow infusion rate. In addition, side effects may not be reversed as rapidly as when opiates are administered via the oral route.

LIFE CYCLE CONSIDERATIONS

Opioid Analgesia in the Elderly

- Cheyne-Stokes respiratory patterns are not unusual during sleep in the elderly and should not be used as a reason to restrict appropriate opioid pain relief unless accompanied by unacceptable degrees of arterial desaturation (less than 85%).
- The elderly experience a higher peak and longer duration of effect of opioid medications and are more sensitive to sedation and respiratory depressant effects.
- Opioid dose titration must be based on analgesic effects and degree of side effects such as sedation, urinary retention, constipation, respiratory depression, or exacerbation of Parkinson's disease (AHCPR, 1992).

Local Anesthesia Local anesthetics are effective for pain management in a variety of settings. Topical anesthetics are available for teething, sore throats, denture pain, laceration repair, and intravenous catheter insertions. One topical anesthetic, EMLA cream, is a mixture of local anesthetics, combining prilocaine and lidocaine (Xylocaine). It produces complete anesthesia for at least 60 minutes when topically applied on intact skin. Another topical anesthetic, TAC, is available for anesthesia during closure of lacerations. It is a combination of tetracaine hydrochloride (Pontocaine) 0.5%, adrenaline (epinephrine) 1:2000, and cocaine 11.8% in a normal saline solution that can be applied directly to the open wound surface in place of local anesthetic infiltration with a needle. This allows pain-free cleansing of the laceration as well as suturing. Because both adrenaline (epinephrine) and cocaine cause vasoconstriction, TAC cannot be used in areas supplied by end-arteriolar blood supply such as digits, the ear, or the nose. It also is contraindicated on burned or abraded skin because this could lead to increased systemic absorption of cocaine and tetracaine, thus placing the client at risk for seizures.

Noninvasive Interventions

Noninvasive relief measures consist of cognitive-behavioral strategies and physical modalities that use cutaneous stimulation. These treatments can be used to supplement pharmacological therapy and other modalities to control pain. Clients and their families can also be instructed to utilize these treatments at home and in inpatient settings.

Cognitive-Behavioral Interventions The cognitive-behavioral interventions influence the cognitive and the motivational-affective components of pain perception. These methods can not only help influence the level of pain, but also help the client gain a sense of self-control.

Trusting Nurse–Client Relationship Establishment of a therapeutic relationship is the foundation for effective nursing care of the client experiencing pain. Clients who trust their nurses to be there, to listen, and to act are the clients who are most likely to be comfortable.

Relaxation **Relaxation techniques** (a variety of methods used to decrease anxiety and muscle tension) result in decreased heart rate and respiratory rate, and decreased muscle tension. These signs and symptoms are opposite of the effects of sympathetic nervous system activation that occurs with acute pain. The body's response to pain is almost "tricked" into reversing itself when relaxation exercises are implemented.

Relaxation exercises help reduce pain by decreasing anxiety and decreasing reflex muscular contraction. There are a wide variety of relaxation techniques, including focused breathing, progressive muscle relaxation, and meditation. Simple techniques should be used during episodes of brief pain (for example, during procedures) or when pain is so severe that the client is unable to concentrate on complicated instructions.

To teach simple relaxation techniques, the nurse can instruct the client to: (1) take a deep breath and hold it; (2) exhale slowly and concentrate on going limp; and (3) start yawning (McCaffery & Pasero, 1999). The yawning triggers a conditioned response in the client, that is, the body associates yawning with relaxation and will relax when the client yawns. The technique can be enhanced if the nurse starts yawning. It is so contagious that even the client compromised by severe pain will usually start yawning with the nurse.

A more complex technique is **progressive muscle relaxation**, a strategy in which muscles are alternately tensed and relaxed. This type of technique is especially useful for clients who do not know what muscle relaxation feels like. By purposely contracting and releasing the muscle groups, the client is able to compare the difference and identify feelings of relaxation. Meditative relaxation techniques are also available, including audiotapes sold in most bookstores.

Relaxation is a learned response. The more frequently the client practices these techniques, the more skilled the body will be in learning to relax. Ideally, the best time to teach the client these methods is when pain is controlled, or before the pain occurs (for example, in the preoperative period).

Reframing **Reframing** is a technique that teaches clients to monitor their negative thoughts and replace them with ones that are more positive. Teaching a client to view pain by replacing an expression such as, "I can't stand this pain, it's never going away," with one such as, "I've had similar pain before, and it's gotten better," is an example of effective reframing.

Distraction Distraction focuses one's attention on something other than the pain, therefore placing pain on the periphery of awareness (McCaffery & Pasero, 1999). Successful use of distraction does not eliminate the pain; it makes it less troublesome to the client. The main disadvantage of distraction is that as soon as the distractive stimuli stop, the pain returns in full force. For this reason, the most appropriate use of distraction techniques is for the relief of brief, episodic pain. For example, it can be effective for procedural pain or the period of time between administration of an analgesic and the onset of the drug. Examples of distraction include:

- Active listening to recorded music (have the client tap fingers in rhythm to the beat)
- Reciting a poem or rhyme (children do this well)
- Describe a plot of a novel or movie
- Describe a series of pictures

Guided Imagery Guided imagery is using one's imagination to provide a pleasant substitute for the pain. This modality incorporates features of both relaxation and distraction. The client imagines a pleasant experience, such as going to the beach or the mountains. The experience should include use of all five senses in order to fully involve the client in the image.

The images chosen need to be ones that are pleasant for the client. Describing an ocean cruise would not be appropriate for a person who becomes seasick.

Humor The old saying, "Laughter is the best medicine," carries some truth to it. While there is nothing very funny about pain, laughing has been shown to provide pain relief. The act of laughing can cause distraction from the pain, induce relaxation by taking deep breaths and releasing tension, release endorphins, and provide a pleasant substitute for pain. Norman Cousins (1991) relates obtaining 2 hours of pain relief from watching episodes of the Candid Camera television show and Marx Brothers films. The nurse can implement this technique by encouraging the client to watch humorous movies, read funny books, or listen to comedy routines. Because different people see humor in different types of situations, the nurse needs to be sensitive to what the client views as funny.

PROFESSIONAL TIP

Cognitive–Behavioral Interventions
Cognitive–behavioral interventions should be introduced as early as possible so that clients can learn and practice the techniques before experiencing intense pain, which impairs learning.

PROFESSIONAL TIP

Using Distraction
Distraction should never be used as the *only* pain management intervention, but it can be extremely helpful while waiting for other techniques to take effect.

Biofeedback Biofeedback training is another method that may be helpful for the client in pain, especially one who has difficulty relaxing muscle tension. Biofeedback is a process through which individuals learn to influence their physiological responses to stimuli. Through the use of biofeedback, clients can alter their pain experience.

Cutaneous Stimulation The technique of cutaneous stimulation involves stimulating the skin to control pain. It is theorized that this technique provides relief by stimulating nerve fibers that send signals to the dorsal horn of the spinal cord to "close the gate." The main advantage of these therapies is that many techniques are easy for the nurse to implement, and easy to teach the client and family to perform. They are not usually meant to replace analgesic therapy, but to complement it.

The site chosen on which to apply the skin stimulation will depend on the client's diagnosis, treatments or procedures being performed, and client preference. There are several options to choose from:

- *Site of pain*—Apply stimulation directly to the site.
- *Around the pain*—Apply stimulation in circular motion around the site.
- *Proximal*—Apply between site of pain and the center of the body (McCaffery and Pasero refer to this as "between pain and the brain").
- *Contralateral*—Apply stimulation to the opposite side of the body. (This is effective due to the crossing over of the nerves in the spinal cord.)
- *Acupuncture points*—Stimulation is applied to specific sites defined by Oriental medicine that is based on a system of meridians.
- *Trigger points*—Apply stimulation to areas that cause referred pain, pain felt in a point other than the point of origin.

Heat and Cold Application In addition to stimulating nerves that can block pain transmission, superficial heat application serves to increase the circulation to the area, which can promote oxygenation and nutrient delivery to the injured tissues. It can also decrease joint and muscle stiffness. Heat is contraindicated in cases of acute injury because it can increase the initial response of edema. It is also contraindicated in rheumatoid arthritis flare-ups, and over topical applications of mentholated ointments. Heat treatments should be limited to 20- to 30-minute intervals because maximum vasodilatation occurs in that time.

Cryotherapy (cold applications) induces local vasoconstriction and numbness, therefore altering the pain sensations. It is contraindicated in any condition where vasoconstriction might increase symptoms, for example, peripheral vascular disease. For best results, cold therapy should be limited to 20- to 30-minute intervals. Either heat or cold can be used as cutaneous

CLIENT TEACHING

Hot or Cold Applications

Teach the client or family that hot or cold applications:

- Must have at least one layer of towel between the heating or cooling device and the skin
- Should be placed on the skin only for short periods of time
- Should not be applied to tissue that has been exposed to radiation therapy (AHCPR, 1994)

stimulation unless one is specifically contraindicated. Cold often provides faster relief (McCaffery & Pasero, 1999). If the client has used heat or cold before, the nurse should incorporate the modality that the client believes will be the most effective. Combining the two might provide better relief. An example of this would be to apply a hot pack for 4 minutes, followed by an ice pack for 2 minutes, repeated 4 times. In a hospital setting, a physician order is required for this therapy.

Acupressure and Massage One of the first responses to pain is to rub the painful part. Instinctively people seem to understand the pain-relieving aspects of this intervention. In addition to blocking the pain transmission through nerve stimulation, massage can also promote relaxation. Acupressure is a type of massage that consists of continuous pressure on or the rubbing of acupuncture points. It is based on the same principles as acupuncture, but needles are not used. Massage also provides a form of nonverbal communication that can be therapeutic on its own.

Mentholated Rubs Ointments or lotions containing menthol are thought to provide relief by providing a counterirritation to the skin. The menthol gives the client the perception that the temperature of the skin has changed (becoming either warmer or cooler). This alters the sensation of pain or provides a distraction from the pain. Client response varies to mentholated rubs; some gain effective relief, while others have poor results. Their use is contraindicated on broken skin, on mucous membranes, or if pain increases.

Transcutaneous Electrical Nerve Stimulation **Transcutaneous electrical nerve stimulation** (TENS) is the process of applying a low-voltage electrical current to the skin through cutaneous electrodes. This modality modulates the pain transmission as do other cutaneous stimulation methods but also distracts the client from pain. Research supports the effectiveness of using TENS for the relief of postoperative pain (AHCPR, 1992). It has also been used successfully in many pain syndromes, for example: chronic low back pain, menstrual cramps, temporomandibular joint (TMJ) syndrome, phantom limb pain, and others. It is administered by health professionals especially trained in its use, usually a physical therapist. Other modalities of pain management should *not* be abandoned while a trial of TENS occurs.

 Safety: TENS Contraindications
- No electrodes should be placed in the area over or surrounding demand cardiac pacemakers.
- No electrodes can be placed over the uterus of a pregnant woman.

Exercise Exercise is an important treatment for chronic pain because it strengthens weak muscles, helps mobilize joints, and helps restore balance and coordination. Passive range of motion should not be used if it increases pain or discomfort. Immobilization is frequently used for clients with episodes of acute pain or to stabilize fractures; however, prolonged immobilization should be avoided whenever possible because it can lead to muscle atrophy and cardiovascular deconditioning.

Psychotherapy Psychotherapy may be beneficial to many clients, particularly those:

- In whom the pain is difficult to control
- Who are clinically depressed
- Who have a history of psychiatric problems

Some psychotherapists use **hypnosis** (a state of heightened awareness and focused concentration) to help clients alter their perception of pain. Hypnosis can be effective in modifying the pain response, but it should be used only by specially trained professionals.

Positioning The final noninvasive technique is proper positioning and body alignment. Moving the client with the least possible stress on joints and skin will minimize exposure to painful stimuli. This includes supporting joints appropriately and maintaining wrinkle-free sheets.

Invasive Interventions

Invasive interventions are meant to complement behavioral, physical, and pharmacological therapies in those clients who do not obtain relief from those measures alone (AHCPR, 1994). Invasive measures are indicated primarily for chronic cancer pain and in some cases of chronic benign pain. These procedures are usually tried only when noninvasive measures have been attempted first with poor results.

Nerve Block Neural blockade is the process of injecting a local anesthetic or neurolytic agent into the nerve. An anesthetic agent may be injected to act as a diagnostic tool in order to identify the nerves involved in a pain syndrome. A neurolytic agent is a chemical agent that causes destruction of the nerve and, therefore, creates an interruption in the pain signal.

Neurosurgery Neurosurgical measures for pain control include neurostimulation procedures and destructive or ablative procedures. Neurostimulation procedures involve the implantation of electrical stimulation devices that send impulses to different parts of the nervous system. Some of these devices stimulate areas of the brain; others stimulate the spinal cord. Relief is thought to be provided by blocking the afferent fiber input at the spinal cord level, or by stimulating release of endorphins using the body's ability to modulate pain.

Destructive or ablative procedures are used to destroy part of the nervous system that conducts pain. By interrupting the pain signal, it is prevented from reaching the cortex where realization of pain occurs. These procedures are reserved for clients with terminal illness.

Radiation Therapy Radiation can be used as a palliative measure for pain relief in clients with cancer. It can relieve both metastatic pain and pain caused by tumors at the primary cancer site. It enhances other pain management strategies such as analgesic therapy because it is aimed specifically at the cause of the client's pain. When administered for pain relief, the smallest dose of radiation is utilized to minimize the side effects that accompany radiation therapy.

Acupuncture **Acupuncture** is the insertion of small needles into the skin at selected (or hoku) sites. The specific sites will be chosen after the practitioner takes a detailed history and uses traditional Oriental diagnostic techniques. The needles used for acupuncture have rounded ends that enter the skin without cutting the tissue. The practitioner may twirl or vibrate the needles manually or electrically. It is important that the nurse keep an open mind when the client chooses this therapy, or the client may be reluctant to discuss its use.

The advantages and disadvantages of selected pain therapies are outlined in Table 26–3.

Evaluation

Evaluating the efficacy of the pain management interventions is ongoing, with client input throughout the process. Evaluation focuses primarily on the client's subjective reports. Objective data used to evaluate pain management efficacy include:

- Client's facial expression and posture
- Presence (or absence) of restlessness
- Vital sign monitoring
- Ongoing use of pain assessment tools

Table 26–3 ADVANTAGES AND DISADVANTAGES OF SELECTED PAIN THERAPIES

INTERVENTION	ADVANTAGES	DISADVANTAGES
Relaxation, Imagery, Biofeedback, Distraction, and Reframing	• May decrease pain and anxiety without drug-related side effects. • Can be used as adjuvant therapy with most other modalities. • Can increase client's sense of control. • Most are inexpensive, require no special equipment, and are easily administered.	• Patient must be motivated to use self-management strategies. • Requires professional time to teach interventions.
Psychotherapy, Structured Support, and Hypnosis	• May decrease pain and anxiety for clients who have pain that is difficult to manage. • May increase client's coping skills.	• Requires skilled therapist.
Cutaneous Stimulation (Superficial Heat, Cold, Massage)	• May reduce pain, inflammation, or muscle spasm. • Can be used as adjuvant therapy with most other modalities. • Relatively easy to use. • Can be administered by clients or families. • Relatively low cost.	• Heat may increase bleeding and edema after acute injury. • Cold is contraindicated for use over ischemic tissues.
Transcutaneous Electrical Nerve Stimulation (TENS)	• May provide pain relief without drug-related side effects. • Can be used as adjuvant therapy with most other modalities. • Gives patient sense of control over pain.	• Requires skilled therapist to initiate therapy. • Potential risk of infection, bleeding.
Acupuncture	• May provide pain relief. • Can be used as adjuvant therapy with most other therapies.	• Requires skilled therapist.

Adapted from Agency for Health Care Policy and Research, Clinical Practice Guideline. Acute Pain Management: Operative or Medical Procedures and Trauma, *1992 [AHCPR Publication No. 92-0032], Rockville, MD: Author.*

SAMPLE NURSING CARE PLAN

THE CLIENT WITH CHRONIC PAIN

Sally Jeffries, a 48-year-old woman, injured her back 3 years ago while lifting some boxes of paper at work. Since that time, she has had 4 epidural steroidal injections for the pain associated with 2 ruptured discs. Her pain has been intermittent with some alleviation from the epidural injections. Her last epidural was 3 months ago. She arrives at the clinic stating, "I just don't know how I can go on like this. The pain has been tolerable until last night. I'm hurting so bad!" She is tearful and pacing, saying, "It hurts too much when I sit down." Verbalizes pain is "9" on a 1 to 10 pain intensity scale. Blood pressure is 148/90. Pulse is strong and regular at 92. She has guarded movements.

Nursing Diagnosis 1 *Chronic Pain, related to muscle spasm and ruptured discs as evidenced by back injury 3 years ago and client statement "I just don't know how I can go on like this. The pain has been tolerable until last night. I'm hurting so bad!"*

PLANNING/GOALS	NURSING INTERVENTIONS	RATIONALE	EVALUATION
Ms. Jeffries will verbalize a decrease in pain.	Assess Ms. Jeffries's level of pain, determining the intensity at its best and worst.	Determines a baseline for future assessment.	After practicing relaxation techniques,

continues

PLANNING/GOALS	NURSING INTERVENTIONS	RATIONALE	EVALUATION
	Listen to Ms. Jeffries while she discusses the pain; acknowledge the presence of pain.	Acknowledging Ms. Jeffries's pain decreases anxiety by communicating acceptance and validating her perceptions.	Ms. Jeffries rates her pain as a 2 to 3 on the pain intensity scale.
	Discuss reasons why pain may be increased or decreased.	Helps Ms. Jeffries determine a cause-and-effect relationship between pain and specific activities.	
Ms. Jeffries will practice selected noninvasive pain relief measures.	Teach relaxation techniques such as deep breathing, progressive muscle relaxation, and imagery.	Reduces skeletal muscle tension and anxiety, which potentiates the perception of pain.	Ms. Jeffries demonstrates the use of deep breathing and progressive muscle relaxation.
	Teach Ms. Jeffries and her family about treatment approaches (biofeedback, hypnosis, massage therapy, physical therapy, acupuncture, and exercise).	Makes Ms. Jeffries and her family aware of the availability of treatment options.	
	Teach Ms. Jeffries about the use of medication for pain relief. Provide accurate information to reduce fear of addiction.	Lack of knowledge and fear may prohibit Ms. Jeffries from taking analgesic medications as prescribed.	
	Encourage Ms. Jeffries to rest at intervals during the day.	Fatigue increases the perception of pain.	

Nursing Diagnosis 2 *Anxiety related to chronic pain as evidenced by pacing and tears*

PLANNING/GOALS	NURSING INTERVENTIONS	RATIONALE	EVALUATION
Ms. Jeffries will verbalize an increase in psychological and physiological comfort level.	Assess Ms. Jeffries's level of anxiety.	To collect baseline data to be used in measuring a decrease or increase in anxiety level.	After practicing relaxation techniques, Ms. Jeffries rates her pain as a 2 to 3 on the pain intensity scale. She voices concern that the pain will soon come back.
	Encourage Ms. Jeffries to verbalize angry feeling.	Anger is often a component of chronic conditions because of the prolonged sense of powerlessness.	
Ms. Jeffries will demonstrate ability to cope with anxiety as evidenced by normal vital signs and a verbalized reduction in pain intensity.	Speak slowly and calmly.	Avoids escalating Ms. Jeffries's anxiety level and increases the likelihood of her comprehension.	After a relaxation session, her vital signs returned to normal limits. Ms. Jeffries denies feeling angry.

CASE STUDY

Johnny Prince, a 27-year-old male, is admitted to the medical unit diagnosed with hemophilia and septic arthritis in his left ankle. He has a history of epilepsy, arthritis, artificial knee joints (bilateral), and two hip surgeries. Medications taken at home include: factor VIII, phenobarbital 100 mg hs, and Naprosyn 5 mg tid. His chief complaint is swelling and severe pain in his left ankle.

Current RX: *Colace, Milk of Magnesia, ceftriaxone sodium (Rocephin) IV piggy-back, phenobarbital 100 mg qhs, FeSO₄, multivitamins, vitamin C, oxacillin (Bactocill), factor VIII 20,000 IVP q12h, hydromorphone HCl (Dilaudid) 8 mg po q8h (hold SBP < 90, resp. < 12), MS 4 mg IVP q4h prn, flurazepam HCl (Dalmane) 30 mg po qhs prn.*

The following questions will guide your development of a nursing care plan for the case study.

1. What will you include in assessing Mr. Prince's pain?

2. What factors in his history will influence his pain perception?

Your pain assessment gives you the following information:
- Location—through center of ankle.
- Intensity—pain at time of assessment is 5 (medicated 30 minutes prior to interview) on scale of 0 to 10; worst is 25, best is 3.
- Quality—describes pain as throbbing at times, a jabbing pain. It hurts worse between 9 and 10 A.M., and 9 and 12 at night. Mainly worse when medicine wears off.
- Effects of pain—only gets 2 or 3 hours of sleep, often dreaming about it. Pain makes him avoid activity, get grumpy and snappy. Concentration turns totally to pain.
- Behaviors—he yells at times, but does not like to. He would prefer to "sweat it out." Also grimaces, grips hands, and tries repositioning.

3. Why did the physician order the analgesics on that schedule?

4. Mr. Prince requests a dose of morphine. The narcotic drawer has the following available in prefilled syringe cartridges: 2 mg per cc, and 8 mg per cc. Which cartridge(s) should the nurse select?

5. Why is the morphine ordered IVP, not IM?

6. Why did the physician order colace and Milk of Magnesia?

7. What are some noninvasive relief measures that might be tried with Mr. Prince?

8. Write two individualized nursing diagnoses and goals for Mr. Prince.

9. What teaching will Mr. Prince need before discharge?

SUMMARY

- *Pain* may be defined as "an unpleasant sensory and emotional experience associated with actual or potential tissue damage," and "whatever the client says it is, existing whenever the client says it does."

- The gate control theory proposes that several processes (sensory, motivational-affective, and cognitive) combine to determine how a person perceives pain.

- Assessment of pain helps establish a baseline of data, and helps to evaluate the effectiveness of interventions.

- Several factors influence the perception of pain, including age, previous experience with pain, and cultural norms.

- The subjective data to gather include: location of pain, onset and duration, quality, intensity (on a scale of 0 to 10), aggravating and relieving factors, and how pain affects the activities of daily living.

- The three general principles to follow with pain relief measures are: (1) individualize the approach; (2) use a preventive approach; and (3) use a multidisciplinary approach.

- The nurse carries a great deal of autonomy in administering analgesics, which leads to specific responsibilities for which the nurse is accountable.

- Pharmacologic agents can be therapeutic for clients experiencing pain. However, the medications should not be the only interventions used.

- Noninvasive treatments for pain relief are measures that can supplement pharmacological and invasive treatments for pain relief.
- Invasive techniques are interventions used when the noninvasive and pharmacological measures do not provide adequate relief. Methods include nerve blocks, neurosurgery, radiation therapy, and acupuncture.

Review Questions

1. According to McCaffery and Pasero, pain may be defined as:

   a. discomfort resulting from identifiable physiologic or iatrogenic sources.
   b. a syndrome of behavioral and physical manifestations that can be objectively identified by the nurse.
   c. whatever the patient says it is, existing whenever and wherever the patient says it does.
   d. a sensory response to noxious stimuli.

2. Which of the following is a useful tool for assessing the intensity of pain that is easy to use?

   a. the gate control scale
   b. acute pain monitor
   c. numeric pain scale
   d. pressure pain monitor

3. Mr. Levy, 45, has experienced chronic low back pain since a fall 8 years ago. He describes his pain as "a gnawing, constant dull pain" that makes him feel tired. The nurse caring for him recognizes that one of the differences between acute and chronic pain characteristics is:

   a. acute pain is more severe.
   b. chronic pain is often described as dull and is difficult to localize.
   c. chronic back pain is often not real.
   d. acute pain is more diffuse and difficult to describe.

4. Nancy Johnson, 84 years old, is recuperating from a total hip replacement. Morphine, 8 mg IV q4h prn, is prescribed for Ms. Johnson. Her respiratory rate is 18, her pulse rate is 96 beats per minute, and her blood pressure is elevated slightly above her normal level. She is complaining of severe pain, 8 on a scale of 0 to 10. The most appropriate initial nursing intervention is:

   a. question the physician regarding the dosage amount for a client this age.

   b. turn her and then reevaluate her need for opioid analgesia.
   c. administer the medication as ordered.
   d. advise Ms. Johnson to cough and breathe deeply since you are unable to give her anything for pain until her respiratory rate is 20.

5. Ms. Redgrave, 55 years old, is hospitalized with an exacerbation of rheumatoid arthritis. She has a favorite television show she watches every afternoon. She reports feeling comfortable during this show and seldom requests pain medication when she is watching it. The nurse's assessment of this phenomenon is that:

   a. the assessment of pain that prompted hospitalization is inaccurate.
   b. Ms. Redgrave is bored and the boredom usually makes her pain seem worse.
   c. inactivity is the best approach to Ms. Redgrave's pain.
   d. distraction is an effective modifier of the pain experience for Ms. Redgrave.

6. One of the general principles of pain management is:

   a. anticipated or mild pain is easier to relieve than severe pain.
   b. the more experience a person has with pain, the better that person will be able to tolerate it.
   c. no pain, no gain.
   d. the cause of pain must be identified in order to relieve it.

Critical Thinking Questions

1. What are the differences between somatic, cutaneous, visceral, referred, ischemic, acute, and chronic pain?

2. How would you decide which noninvasive technique to use with a client?

 WEB FLASH!

- Search the Internet for the organizations listed in the Resources for this chapter at the end of the book. What kind of information is available for clients, families, and health care professionals?
- Search the word *pain* on the Internet. What information is available?

CHAPTER 27

DIAGNOSTIC TESTS

MAKING THE CONNECTION

Refer to the following chapters to increase your understanding of diagnostic tests:

- **Chapter 13, Complementary/Alternative Therapies**
- **Chapter 25, Assessment**
- **Procedures:** B30, Urine Collection: Closed Drainage System; B31, Urine Collection: Clean Catch Female, Male; I3, Performing Urinary Catheterization: Male Client; I4, Performing Urinary Catheterization: Female client; I26, Skin Puncture; A3, Venipuncture

LEARNING OBJECTIVES

Upon completion of this chapter, you should be able to:
- *Define key terms.*
- *Discuss the relevant client teaching guidelines for the care of the client before, during, and after diagnostic testing.*
- *Describe the common specimen collection methods.*
- *Describe common invasive and noninvasive diagnostic procedures.*
- *Discuss nursing responsibilities for the common diagnostic procedures.*

KEY TERMS

agglutination	aspiration
agglutinin	bacteremia
agglutinogen	barium
analyte	biopsy
aneurysm	cation
angiography	central line
anion	computed
antibody	tomography
antigen	conscious sedation
arteriography	contrast medium
ascites	culture

cytology	Papanicolaou test
electrocardiogram	paracentesis
electroencephalogram	phlebotomist
electrolyte	pneumothorax
endoscopy	port-a-cath
enzyme	radiography
fluoroscopy	sensitivity
hematuria	stable
invasive	stress test
ketone	thoracentesis
lipoprotein	transducer
lumbar puncture	trocar
magnetic resonance	type and cross-
imaging	match
necrosis	ultrasound
noninvasive	urobilinogen
occult blood	venipuncture
oliguria	void

INTRODUCTION

Health care providers use the findings from a thorough history and physical examination to determine the need for diagnostic testing. The client's history and presenting symptoms determine those diagnostic procedures that are necessary to formulate a medical diagnosis and course of treatment. The challenge of cost-effective health care pushes practitioners to rely on basic assessment and to be selective with regard to expensive diagnostic tests. To reflect the emphasis on cost containment, the nurse's role has changed from doing for the client to teaching clients to do for themselves. The role of the nurse is to teach the client, family, and significant others about the procedures involved in diagnostic testing, the steps to be taken in preparation for the specific test(s) in question, and the care that will follow the procedure. Although the primary focus is on teaching, the nurse may assist in performing various noninvasive and invasive procedures. Nurses must be aware of the implications of diagnostic testing so as to deliver appropriate nursing care to the client.

To understand the nature of diagnostic tests, nurses must review anatomy and physiology. Knowing the anatomic and physiologic functions of the body will assist nurses in relating certain diagnostic tests to specific disease processes and in understanding the meaning of test results.

This chapter discusses common diagnostic tests. The terms *test* and *procedure* are used interchangeably throughout the chapter. The term *practitioner* is used in this chapter to refer to either the physician or an advanced practice registered nurse. Most state boards of nursing allow advanced practice registered nurses to order and perform certain diagnostic tests.

DIAGNOSTIC TESTING

Diagnostic tests are either noninvasive or invasive. **Noninvasive** means that the body is not entered with any type of instrument; the skin and other body tissues, organs, and cavities remain intact. **Invasive** means that the body's tissues, organs, or cavities are accessed through some type of procedure making use of instruments.

Nursing Care of the Client

Diagnostic testing is a critical element of assessment. In collaboration with feedback from the client, assessment data are used to formulate nursing diagnoses, a plan of care, and outcome measures. Ongoing client assessment and evaluation of the client's expected outcomes require the incorporation of diagnostic findings.

 Safety: Diagnostic Testing
To protect your health and safety, as well as that of other health care providers and the client, use Standard Precautions whenever performing invasive or noninvasive procedures.

Preparing the Client for Diagnostic Testing

The nurse plays a key role in scheduling and preparing the client for diagnostic testing. When tests are not scheduled correctly, not only is the client inconve-

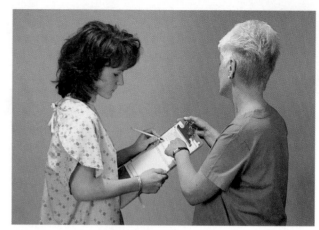

Figure 27-1 Preparing a Client for Diagnostic Testing

nienced, but interventions may be delayed, which may place the client's health at risk. The institution is also at risk to lose money. Table 27–1 outlines a sample protocol of the nursing care to prepare a client for diagnostic testing.

During the assessment of the client, the nurse must ensure that the client is wearing an identification band and understands those things to be done. It is also the nurse's responsibility to see that needed consent forms have been signed (Figure 27-1).

Other key nursing measures in ensuring client safety are to establish baseline vital signs, identify known allergies, and assess the effectiveness of teaching. In ambulatory and outpatient centers, the nurse might have only one opportunity to assess and record vital signs. It is important for the nurse to confirm that the vital signs are normal values *for the client*. To accurately assess the client's response to anesthetic agents and the procedure performed, the nurse must compare the vital signs taken during and after the procedure to those obtained before as baseline data.

The client must be made aware of those things to expect during the procedure. Such teaching can both increase the level of cooperation and decrease the degree of anxiety. The client's family should also be informed of what will happen during the procedure and approximately how long the procedure should last. Nurses must also know the institution's specific protocols and procedures, because these are not standardized in all practice settings.

Care of the Client during Diagnostic Testing

Although client care must be individualized according to the specific procedure, general guidelines for client care during a procedure are outlined in Table 27–2. Protocols are used to assist the nurse with client care.

Standard Precautions are initiated when exposure to body fluids presents a threat to the safety of the caregiver or client. Protective barriers, such as gloves and a gown, should be used during invasive procedures.

Table 27–1 PROTOCOL: PREPARING THE CLIENT FOR DIAGNOSTIC TESTING

Purpose	To increase the reliability of the test by providing client teaching on the reason the test is being performed, those things the client can expect during the test, and the outcomes and side effects of the test
	To decrease the client's anxiety about the test and the associated risks
Supportive Data	Increase the client's knowledge, thereby promoting cooperation and enhancing the quality of the testing
	Decrease the time required to perform the tests, thereby increasing cost effectiveness
	Prevent delays by ensuring proper physical preparation
Assessment	Ensure that the client is wearing an identification band
	Review the medical record for allergies and previous adverse reactions to dyes and other contrast media; a signed consent form; and the recorded findings of diagnostic tests relative to the procedure
	Assess for the presence, location, and characteristics of physical and communicative limitations or pre-existing conditions
	Monitor the client's knowledge of both the reasons for the test and those things to expect during and after testing
	Monitor vital signs, including pain, of the client who is scheduled for invasive testing, to establish baseline data
	Assess client outcome measures relative to the practitioner's preferences for preprocedure preparations
	Monitor level of hydration and weakness for clients who are designated nothing by mouth (NPO)
Report to Practitioner	Notify practitioner of allergy, previous adverse reaction, or suspected adverse reaction following the administration of drugs
	Notify practitioner of any client or family concerns not alleviated by discussions with nurse
Interventions	Clarify with practitioner whether regularly scheduled medications are to be administered
	Implement NPO status, as determined by the type of test
	Administer cathartics or laxatives as denoted by the test's protocol; instruct clients who are weak to call for assistance to the bathroom
	Teach relaxation techniques, such as deep breathing and imagery
	Establish intravenous (IV) access if necessary for the procedure
Evaluation	Evaluate the client's knowledge of those things to expect
	Evaluate the client's anxiety level
	Evaluate the client's level of safety and comfort
Client Teaching	Discuss the following with the client and family, as appropriate to the specific test:
	• The reason for the test and those things to expect
	• An estimation of how long the test will take
	• Specifics of NPO status, including amount of water to drink if oral medication is to be taken
	• Cathartics or laxative: amount, frequency
	• Sputum: cough deeply, do not clear throat
	• Urine: voided, clean-catch specimen; timing of collection
	• Removal of objects (e.g., jewelry or hair clips) that will obscure x-ray film
	• Contrast medium:
	Barium: taste, consistency, after effects (lightly colored stools for 24 to 72 hours; possibly, obstruction/impaction)
	Iodine: metallic taste, delayed allergic reaction (itching, rashes, hives, wheezing and breathing difficulties)
	• Positioning during the test
	• Positioning posttest (e.g., immobilize limb after angiography)
	• Posttest (encourage fluid intake if not contraindicated)
Documentation	Record in the client's medical record:
	• Practitioner notification of allergies or suspected adverse reaction to contrast media
	• Presence, location, and characteristics of symptoms
	• Teaching and the client's response to teaching
	• Responses to interventions (client outcomes)

Table 27-2 PROTOCOL: CARE OF THE CLIENT DURING DIAGNOSTIC TESTING

Purpose	To increase cooperation and participation by allaying the client's anxiety To provide the maximum level of safety and comfort during a procedure
Supportive Data	Encourage relaxation of the muscles and thus facilitation of instrumentation by increasing the client's participation and comfort Ensure both efficient use of time during the test and reliable results from the test with proper preparation of the client
Assessment	Check the client's identification band to ensure the correct client Review the medical record for allergies Assess the client's reaction to the preprocedure sedatives administered prior to the induction of anesthesia during the procedure Assess airway maintenance and gag reflex, if a local anesthetic is sprayed into the client's throat Assess vital signs, including pain, throughout the procedure and compare to baseline data Assess the client's ability to maintain and tolerate the prescribed position Assess the client's comfort level (pain) to ensure the effectiveness of the anesthetic agent Assess for related symptoms indicating complications specific to the procedure (e.g., accidental perforation of an organ)
Report to Practitioner	Notify the practitioner of any client concerns or questions not answered in discussions with the nurse Notify the practitioner of any family members present and their location during the procedure Notify the practitioner when the client is positioned properly and the anesthetic agent has been administered to the client
Interventions	Institute Standard Precautions or appropriate aseptic technique for the specific test Report to all personnel involved in the test any known client allergies Place the client in the correct position, drape, and monitor to ensure that breathing is not compromised Remain with the client during induction and maintenance of anesthesia If the procedure requires the administration of a dye, ensure that the client is not allergic to the dye; if the client has not received the dye before, perform the skin allergy test according to the manufacturer's instructions that accompany the medication Maintain the client's airway and keep resuscitative equipment available Assist the client to relax during insertion of the instrument by telling the client to breathe through the mouth and to concentrate on relaxing the involved muscles Explain what the practitioner is doing so that the client knows what to expect Label and handle the specimen according to the type of materials obtained and the testing to be done Report to the practitioner any symptoms of complications Secure client transport from the diagnostic area Posttest in the diagnostic area: • Assist the client to a comfortable, safe position • Provide oral hygiene and water to clients who were designated NPO for the test, if they are alert and able to swallow • Remain with the client awaiting transport to another area
Evaluation	Evaluate the client's ventilatory status and tolerance to the procedure Evaluate the client's need for assistance Evaluate the client's understanding of what was performed during the procedure Evaluate the client's understanding of findings identified during the procedure Evaluate the client's knowledge of what to expect after the procedure
Client Teaching	Discuss the following with the client and family, as appropriate to the specific test: • Those things that occurred during the procedure • Questions and concerns of the client or family member • Those things to expect during the immediate recovery phase • Those things to report to the nurse during the immediate recovery phase
Documentation	Record in the client's medical record: • Person who performed the procedure • Reason for the procedure • Type of anesthesic, dye, or other medications administered • Type of specimen obtained and where it was delivered • Vital signs and other assessment data such as client's tolerance of the procedure or pain/discomfort level • Any symptoms of complications • Person who transported the client to another area (designate the names of persons who provided transport and the destination)

The nurse is responsible for labeling any specimen with the client's name and room number (for hospitalized clients), and the date, time, and source of the specimen. Some specimens may need to be taken immediately to the laboratory or placed on ice (e.g., arterial blood gases [ABGs]).

Ongoing assessment of the client's status is required during the procedure. The patency of the client's airway should be continuously assessed, as it may be compromised by the client's position, by anesthesia, or by the procedure itself. During an invasive procedure, the nurse also must monitor for signs and symptoms of accidental perforation of an organ (e.g., sudden changes in vital signs).

The nurse has the following additional responsibilities:

- Preparing the procedure room (e.g., ensuring adequate lighting)
- Gathering and charging for supplies to be used during the procedure
- Testing the equipment to ensure it is functional and safe
- Securing proper containers for specimen collection

Practitioners usually have preference cards within the diagnostic testing area that specify the type of equipment to be used, the position in which to place the client, and the type of sedative or anesthesic agent to be used.

Some diagnostic tests are performed with the registered nurse administering IV sedation, also called conscious sedation. **Conscious sedation** is a minimally depressed level of consciousness during which the client retains the ability to maintain a continuously patent airway and respond appropriately to physical stimulation or verbal commands (Somerson, Husted, & Sicilia, 1995). The nurse managing conscious sedation is usually functioning in an expanded role that requires additional education and demonstrated ability beyond that afforded by basic education.

Care of the Client after Diagnostic Testing

Postprocedure nursing care is directed toward restoring the client's prediagnostic level of functioning (Table 27–3). Nursing assessment and interventions are based mainly on the nature of the test and whether the client received anesthesia.

The client is monitored closely for signs of respiratory distress and bleeding. Some diagnostic procedures require that vital signs be measured every 15 minutes for the first hour, and then at gradually longer intervals until the client is **stable** (alert and with vital signs within the client's normal range).

Some diagnostic tests require the use of medications that are excreted through the kidneys. The client's in-take and output (I&O) is monitored by the nurses for 24 hours. The client is taught to monitor I&O and to report **hematuria** (presence of blood in the urine).

 Safety: Radioactive Iodine and Urine Collection
Clients receiving radioactive iodine must have their urine collected and properly discarded in a special container, according to agency policy for handling radioactive medical wastes.

When clients are discharged after diagnostic testing, they should receive written instructions. Most agencies have discharge forms on which the nurse documents teaching regarding medications, dietary and activity restrictions, and signs and symptoms to be reported immediately to the practitioner. Clients may also need to have follow-up appointments made for them.

LABORATORY TESTS

Common laboratory studies are usually simple measurements to determine the amount or number of **analytes** (i.e., measured substances) present in a specimen. Laboratory tests are ordered by the practitioner to:

- Detect and quantify the risk of future disease,
- Establish or exclude diagnoses,
- Assess the severity of the disease process and formulate a prognosis,
- Guide the selection of interventions,
- Monitor the progress of the disorder, or
- Monitor the effectiveness of the treatment.

Specimen Collection

The scheduling and sequencing of laboratory tests are important functions of the nurse. All tests requiring **venipuncture** (the use of a needle to puncture a vein to aspirate blood) are grouped together so that the client is subjected to only one venipuncture. Fasting laboratory and radiological studies are scheduled on the same day so that the client is required to fast for only 1 day. Appropriate scheduling increases the client's comfort level and satisfaction.

 PROFESSIONAL TIP

Documentation of Specimen-Collection Difficulties
Document on the laboratory requisition slip and in the nurses' notes any difficulty experienced during collection of a specimen. Such problems may indicate adverse effects related to the nature of the test and thus must be reported and treated immediately.

Table 27–3 PROTOCOL: CARE OF THE CLIENT AFTER DIAGNOSTIC TESTING

Purpose	To restore the client's prediagnostic level of functioning by providing care and teaching relative to both those things the client can expect after a test and the outcomes or side effects of the test
Supportive Data	Decrease client anxiety by increasing the client's participation and knowledge of expected outcome measures after a diagnostic test Through proper postprocedure care and client teaching, alert the client to those signs and symptoms that must to be reported to the practitioner
Assessment	Check the identification band and call the client by name Assess the client closely for signs of airway distress, adverse reactions to anesthesic or other medications, and other signs that may indicate accidental perforation of an organ Assess for bleeding those areas where a biopsy was performed Assess the client's vital signs, including pain Assess vascular access lines or other invasive monitoring devices Assess the client's ability to expel air, if air was instilled during a gastrointestinal test Assess the client's knowledge of those things to expect during the recovery phase
Report to Practitioner	Notify the practitioner of any signs of respiratory distress, bleeding, or changes in vital signs; adverse reactions to anesthetic, sedative, or dye; and other signs of complications Notify the practitioner of any client or family concerns or questions not answered in discussions with the nurse Notify the practitioner when any results are obtained from the diagnostic test Notify the practitioner when the client is fully alert and recovered (for an order to discharge)
Interventions	Implement the practitioner's orders regarding the postprocedure care of the client Institute Standard Precautions or surgical asepsis as appropriate to the client's care needs Position the client for comfort and accessibility so as to facilitate performance of nursing measures Monitor vital signs according to the frequency required for the specific test Observe the insertion site for hematoma or blood loss; replace pressure dressing, as needed Monitor the client's urinary output and drainage from other devices Enforce activity restrictions appropriate to the test Schedule client appointments as directed by the practitioner
Evaluation	Evaluate the client's respiratory status, especially if an anesthetic agent was used Evaluate the client's tolerance of oral liquids Evaluate the client's understanding of the procedural findings of when the practitioner expects to receive written results Evaluate the client's knowledge of those things to expect after discharge
Client Teaching	Based on client assessment and evaluation of knowledge, teach the client or family about the following: • Dietary or activity restrictions • Signs and symptoms that should be reported immediately to the practitioner • Medications
Documentation	Record in the client's medical record on the appropriate forms: • Assessment data, nursing interventions, and achievement of expected outcomes • Client or family teaching and demonstrated level of understanding • Written instructions given to the client or family members

Accuracy in laboratory testing requires that:

- The practitioner's order be transcribed onto the correct requisition form,
- All requested information be written on the form (e.g., the client's full name and medical number),
- Pertinent data that could influence the test's results, such as medications taken, be included,
- Collection of the specimen from the correct client be confirmed by checking the identification band, and
- Laboratory results be placed in the correct medical record.

Venipuncture

Venipuncture can be performed by various members of the health care team. Although laboratories employ **phlebotomists** (individuals who perform venipuncture) to collect blood specimens, the nurse must know how to perform venipuncture, because nurses routinely perform venipuncture in the home, long-term care settings, and hospital critical care units.

Venipuncture can be performed by using either a sterile needle and syringe or a vacuum tube holder with a sterile two-ended needle. Test tubes are used to collect blood specimens. Test tubes have different colored stoppers to indicate the type of additive in the test tube. Collection tubes are universally color coded as follows:

- Red: no additive
- Lavender: ethylenediaminotetraacetic acid (EDTA)
- Light blue: sodium citrate
- Green: sodium heparin
- Gray: potassium oxalate
- Black: sodium oxalate

Arterial Puncture

Assessment of ABGs reveals the ability of the lungs to exchange gases by measuring the partial pressures of oxygen (PaO_2) and carbon dioxide ($PaCO_2$) and evaluates the potential of hydrogen (pH) of arterial blood. Blood gases are ordered to evaluate:

- Oxygenation,
- Ventilation and the effectiveness of respiratory therapy, and
- Acid–base balance in the blood.

Arterial blood samples are drawn from a peripheral artery (e.g., radial or femoral) or from an arterial line. The arterial blood sample is collected in a 5-mL heparinized syringe. To prevent clotting, the syringe is then rotated to mix the blood with the heparin. The blood sample is then placed on ice to reduce the rate of oxygen metabolism.

In some agencies, it is within the scope of nursing practice to perform radial artery puncture; however, femoral artery puncture is usually performed only by an advanced practitioner, because of the associated increased risk of hemorrhage. Although it is not common practice for student nurses to draw ABG samples, students often assist with the procedure and care for the client after the procedure.

Regardless of who performs the arterial puncture, the nurse is responsible for assessing the client for symptoms of postpuncture bleeding or occlusion. Direct pressure must be applied to the puncture site until all bleeding has stopped (for a minimum of 5 minutes). Symptoms of impaired circulation include the following:

PROFESSIONAL TIP

Arterial Blood Gases

To ensure an accurate determination of the client's actual blood gases, ABGs should not be drawn within 30 minutes after any respiratory treatment.

CLIENT TEACHING

Postarterial Puncture

The client should *immediately* notify the nurse if any pain or numbness occurs in the arm or leg after an arterial puncture. These symptoms indicate impaired circulation.

- Numbness and tingling
- Bluish color
- Absence of a peripheral pulse

Capillary Puncture

Skin punctures are performed when small quantities of capillary blood are needed for analysis or when the client has poor veins. Capillary puncture is also commonly performed for blood glucose analysis. Figure 27-2 illustrates a capillary puncture of a fingertip.

Central Lines

Blood samples can also be collected from central lines. A **central line** refers to a venous catheter inserted into the superior vena cava through the subclavian or internal or external jugular vein. Central lines are used in the treatment of alterations in fluid or electrolyte balance, such as severe dehydration due to vomiting. Insertion is necessary when a peripheral route cannot be obtained. Central lines can be used for treatment and to withdraw blood for analysis.

The first sample of blood drawn from the central line cannot be used for diagnostic testing; it must be discarded, with the volume of discard being directly related to the dead space (catheter size) (Laxson & Titler, 1994). The agency's protocol should indicate the volume to discard relative to the type and size of catheter.

The care of central lines requires strict sterile technique. The practitioner must write an order to allow a blood sample to be obtained from a central line.

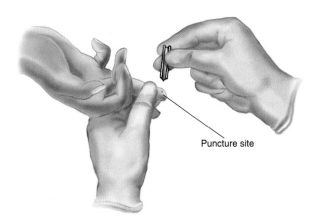

Puncture site

Figure 27-2 Capillary Puncture of Fingertip

Implanted Port

Some clients have a **port-a-cath** (a port that has been implanted under the skin) over the third or fourth rib. The port has a catheter that is inserted into the superior vena cava or right atrium through the subclavian or internal jugular vein. The implanted port is used for the same purpose as is a central line. Blood can be withdrawn for sampling by accessing the port while using strict sterile technique. Accessing a port should be performed only by a nurse who has the education to be able to properly do so. Students are not usually taught how to access an implanted port.

Urine Collection

Urine can be collected for various studies. The type of testing determines the method of collection. The different methods of urine collection are as follows:

- Random collection (routine analysis)
- Timed collection (24-hour urine)
- Collection from a closed urinary drainage system
- Sterile specimen (catheterized)
- Clean-voided specimen

Client teaching depends on the client's age and the method of collection. The method of collection should be written on the laboratory requisition.

Safety: Standard Precautions and Urine Collection
All urine collection requires the use of Standard Precautions to prevent the transmission of microorganisms among nurses, clients, and other health care providers. All specimen containers should be sealed in a biohazard bag prior to transport to the laboratory.

Random Collection The practitioner usually writes the order for a UA (routine urine analysis), which is also called a random collection. The specimen can be collected at any time using a clean cup. The container does not have to be sterile. The specimen should be taken immediately to the laboratory to prevent both bacteria growth and changes in the urine's analytes.

Timed Collection Timed collection is done over a 24-hour period. The urine is collected in a plastic gallon container that contains preservative(s), some of which are caustic.

For a timed collection, the client is told to **void** (eliminate urine) and discard the specimen at the beginning of the collection. Timing for a 24-hour urine collection begins after the first voiding has been discarded. For example, if the client voids at 1000 hours (24-hour [military] time), that urine should be discarded, but all other urine specimens until 1000 hours the following day saved. The client can void throughout the test into a clean container, then pour the urine into the collection bottle. Toilet tissue should not be dropped into the container used to catch the urine. The collection container should be refrigerated or kept on ice throughout the 24 hours to retard bacterial growth and stabilize the analytes.

Collection from a Closed-Drainage System A sterile specimen can be collected from a client with an indwelling Foley catheter and closed drainage system. A sterile specimen is used for urine culture. The urine specimen should *not* be obtained from the drainage bag, because the analytes in the urine drainage bag change, leading to inaccurate results, and bacteria grows quickly in the drainage bag. The catheter's closed drainage tubing has an aspiration port that is used for sterile specimen collection.

Sterile Specimen Sometimes a sterile urine specimen is required when the client does not have an indwelling catheter and closed drainage system. In such cases, the client is catheterized. A small amount of urine is allowed to run out of the catheter into a basin, then the urine is allowed to run into a sterile specimen bottle.

Clean-Voided Specimen Clean-voided (clean-catch, or midstream) specimen collection is done to secure a specimen uncontaminated by skin flora. Different aseptic techniques are used for women and men. The female client is instructed to cleanse from the front to the back and then void into the specimen bottle; the male client is instructed to cleanse from the tip of the penis downward and then void into the specimen bottle.

Stool Collection

The nurse should first explain to the client the reason for collection of the stool specimen. The client can then be instructed to defecate into a clean bed pan or container, discarding used tissue in the toilet. Stools can be collected for a one-time defecation or over 24, 48, or 72 hours. If stools are to be collected over a prolonged period of time, all must be placed into a container and refrigerated. Once all stools have been collected, the container should be labeled with the client's name, the date and time, and the test to be performed on the specimen. All stool specimens are placed in a biohazard bag before being transported to the laboratory.

Safety: Collecting Stool from a Client with Hepatitis

When collecting a stool specimen from a client with hepatitis, write on the requisition form that the client has hepatitis. Doing so alerts laboratory personnel to be especially careful when handling the specimen.

Specific Tests

Many tests can be performed on the blood. Tests specific to the hematological system are described in Table 27–4.

Type and Crossmatch

A **type and crossmatch** is a laboratory test that identifies the client's blood type and determines the compatibility of blood between a potential donor and recipient (client). There are four basic blood types: A, B, AB, and O. The blood types are determined by the presence or absence of A or B antigens. **Antigens** are substances, usually proteins, that cause the formation of and react specifically with antibodies. **Antibodies** are immunoglobulins produced by the body in response to bacteria, viruses, or other antigenic substances. Type A and type B are antigens that are classified as **agglutinogens**, or substances that cause **agglutination** (clumping of RBCs). **Agglutinins** are specific kinds of antibodies whose interaction with antigens manifests as agglutination.

Blood types are also designated as either positive or negative, depending on the presence or absence of the Rh factor. The Rh factor is an antigen that may be found on the RBC. The designation *Rh positive* means the antigen is present; *Rh negative* means the antigen is absent. An individual's blood type and Rh are determined genetically.

Crossmatch determines the compatibility of the donor's blood with that of the recipient. In the laboratory, a sample of the recipient's blood is mixed with the blood of a possible donor. If the blood sample is compatible, the mixed sample does not agglutinate.

Blood Chemistry

Blood chemistry tests are often grouped together into profiles, or panels, requiring one requisition and a single venous specimen. Tests performed include glucose, electrolytes, enzymes, lipids, creatinine, and protein values. Other tests that may be performed on a blood specimen are listed in Table 27–5.

Blood Glucose Blood for glucose measurement is obtained by either skin puncture or venipuncture; glucose is measured as either fasting (FBS) or nonfasting (usually 2 hours postprandial) blood sugar. This test is used to screen for diabetes mellitus. If the results are abnormal, the practitioner may order a glucose tolerance test, the most accurate test for diagnosing hypoglycemia and hyperglycemia (diabetes mellitus).

Serum Electrolytes An **electrolyte** is a substance that, when in solution, separates into ions and conducts electricity. Some electrolytes act on the cell membrane, allowing for the transmission of electrochemical impulses in nerve and muscle fibers. Other electrolytes determine the activity of different enzymatically catalyzed reactions necessary for cellular metabolism (Guyton & Hall, 2000).

Cations are ions that have a positive charge, such as sodium (Na^+), potassium (K^+), calcium (Ca^{++}), and magnesium (Mg^{++}). **Anions** are ions that have a negative charge, including chloride (Cl^-), bicarbonate (HCO_3^-), and phosphate (HPO_4^{--}).

Blood Enzymes **Enzymes** are globular proteins produced in the body that catalyze chemical reactions within the cells by promoting the oxidative reactions and synthesis of various chemicals, such as lipids, glycogen, and adenosine triphosphate (ATP). Enzyme tests play a key role in diagnosing the degree of tissue damage, mainly to the myocardium and, to a lesser degree, to the brain.

Elevations in plasma levels of intracellular enzymes occur in the presence of myocardial **necrosis** (tissue death as the result of disease or injury). Enzymes are released into the bloodstream in proportion to the degree of cellular damage. The enzymes are not used as single diagnostic values in determining a diagnosis but, rather, are reviewed in relation to other diagnostic studies.

Blood Lipids An elevated serum lipid level is one of the controllable contributing risk factors to CHD. **Lipoproteins** (blood lipids bound to protein) are measured along with cholesterol.

Table 27–4 TESTS SPECIFIC TO THE HEMATOLOGIC SYSTEM

TEST	EXPLANATION/NORMAL VALUES	NURSING RESPONSIBILITIES

Red blood cells (RBCs)	Number of RBCs per mm^3 of blood. May be low in clients with rheumatoid arthritis. Clients living in high altitudes may have an elevated RBC level.
	Normal:
	    Male: 4.6–5.9 million/mm^3
	    Female: 4.2–5.4 million/mm^3
		The client is not required to fast for the test.

White blood cells (WBCs)	Number of WBCs per mm^3 of blood. Elevation is associated with infectious processes. Normal: 4300–10,800 mm^3	The client is not required to fast for the test. Exercise, stress, last month of pregnancy, labor, previous splenectomy, and eating may increase level and alter differential values. Note medications taken that may affect test; aspirin, heparin, and steroids may increase WBC level, whereas antibiotics and diuretics may decrease WBC level.

Differential count
Neutrophils
 	
  Segs (mature neutrophils)
  Bands (immature
    neutrophils)
	Percentage of types of WBCs in 1 mm of blood.
	Increase in bacterial infections and trauma.
	Normal:
	  Segs: 50%–65%
	  Bands: 0%–5%
		The client is not required to fast for the test.

Eosinophils	Increased in allergic reactions or parasitic infestation. Normal: 1%–3%	Corticosteroid therapy causes a decreased level.
Basophils	Increased in allergic reactions and during healing periods. Normal: 0.4%–1.0%	Steroids cause a decreased level.
Lymphocytes	Increased in viral infections and other diseases, such as pertussis and tuberculosis (TB). Decreased in acquired immunodeficiency syndrome (AIDS). Normal: 25%–35%	Steroids cause a decreased level.
Monocytes	Increased in chronic diseases, such as malaria, TB, Rocky Mountain spotted fever. May be low in clients with rheumatoid arthritis. Normal: 4%–6%	

Hemoglobin (Hgb)	Measures the oxygen-carrying capacity of the blood.
	Normal:
	    Male: 14–18 g/dL
	    Female: 12–16 g/dL
	Critical value: < 5 g/dL
		The client is not required to fast for the test.
		Sample may be drawn from a finger of a child or the heel of an infant.

Hemoglobin electrophoresis	Detects abnormal forms of hemoglobin. Performed after positive sickle cell test. If the hemoglobin electrophoresis is negative, the client has the sickle cell trait. If the hemoglobin electrophoresis is positive, the client has sickle cell anemia.
	Normal:
	    Hgb S: 0%
	    Hgb F: < 2%
	    Hgb Ca: 0%
		If the client has had a blood transfusion within the last 12 weeks, the results of the test may be altered.

Hematocrit (Hct)	Measures the percentage of blood cells in a volume of blood. Clients living in high altitudes may have an increased level.
	Normal:
	    Male: 42%–52%
	    Female: 37%–47%
	Critical value: < 15%
		The client is not required to fast for the test.

continues

Table 27–4 TESTS SPECIFIC TO THE HEMATOLOGIC SYSTEM *continued*

TEST	EXPLANATION/NORMAL VALUES	NURSING RESPONSIBILITIES
Platelet count	Measures the number of platelets per cubic milliliter of blood. Normal: 150,000–400,000/mm^3 Critical level: < 50,000 and > 1 million/mm^3	Instruct the client that strenuous exercise and oral contraceptives increase platelet level. Instruct the client that aspirin, acetaminophen, and sulfonamides decrease platelet level. If the client has a low platelet count, maintain digital pressure to the puncture site.
Bleeding time	Measures the length of time for a platelet plug to occlude a small puncture wound. Normal: 1–9 minutes (Ivy method) Critical value: > 12 minutes	Notify the laboratory if the client is taking aspirin, anticoagulants, or other medications that may affect the clotting process.
Prothrombin time (PT, protime)	Measures the effectiveness of several blood-clotting factors. Normal: 11–12.5 seconds INR: 2.0–3.0 In the presence of anticoagulant therapy, the values should be 1½–2 times the normal value. Critical value: > 20 seconds In the presence of anticoagulant therapy, the critical value should be > 3 times the normal critical value.	Ensure that the blood specimen is drawn before the daily dose of warfarin (Coumadin) is administered. Instruct the client that alcohol intake may increase PT and that a diet high in fat may decrease PT. Note those medications taken that may affect results; salicylates, sulfonamides, and methyldopa (Aldomet), as these may increase PT, whereas digitalis and oral contraceptives decrease the level. Instruct the client not to take any medication without notifying the physician, as medications may affect the PT level.
International normalized ratio (INR)	Normal: 2–3 (2.5–3.5 for the client with a mechanical prosthetic heart valve). The INR is more accurate than PT in monitoring warfarin (Coumadin) therapy.	The daily warfarin (Coumadin) dose should be given after blood has been drawn for the INR.

Partial thromboplastin time (PTT), also called activated partial thromboplastin time (APTT)	Normal:
	  PTT: 60–70 sec
	  APTT: 30–40 sec
	In the presence of anticoagulant therapy, the normal value is 1.5–2.5 times the control value.
	Critical value:
	  APTT: > 70 seconds
	  PTT: > 100 seconds
		If the client is receiving intermittent heparin doses, schedule the APTT to be drawn 30–60 minutes before the next heparin dose.
		If heparin is given continuously, the blood specimen can be drawn at any time.
		If APTT is greater than 100 seconds, the client is at risk for bleeding, and the physician is notified.
		The antidote for heparin is protamine sulfate.
		Note whether the client is taking antihistamines, vitamin C, or salicylates, as these prolong PTT time.

D dimer test (fragment D dimer, fibrin degradation fragment)	Measures a fibrin split product that is released when a clot breaks. Confirms the diagnosis of disseminated intravascular coagulation (DIC). Normal: negative for D-dimer fragments	Note whether the client is on thrombolytic therapy, as the results of this test would be increased from negative to positive.

Table 27–5 ADDITIONAL TESTS PERFORMED ON BLOOD SPECIMEN

TEST	EXPLANATION/NORMAL VALUES	NURSING RESPONSIBILITIES
Acid phosphatase	Acid phosphatase is an enzyme found in highest concentrations in the prostate gland. An elevated level is seen in clients with prostatic cancer that has metastasized to other body parts. If tumors are treated successfully, the level will decrease. A rising level may indicate a poor prognosis. Normal: 0.11–0.60 U/L	Tell the client that no food or drink restrictions are associated with this test. Apply pressure to the venipuncture site. Observe the site for bleeding.

continues

Table 27–5 ADDITIONAL TESTS PERFORMED ON BLOOD SPECIMEN *continued*

TEST	EXPLANATION/NORMAL VALUES	NURSING RESPONSIBILITIES
Adrenocorticotropic hormone (ACTH), corticotropin	Determines the function of the anterior pituitary. Because of diurnal variation, specimens should be drawn in both morning and evening. Normal: A.M.: 15–100 pg/mL, or 10–80 ng/L P.M.: < 50 pg/mL, or < 50 ng/L	Emotional or physical stress or recent radio-isotope scans can interfere with test results. Drugs that may increase ACTH level include corticosteroids, estrogens, ethanol, and spironolactone. Explain the procedure to the client. This is especially important to decrease the client's stress level. Evaluate the client for increased stress level. Initiate NPO status after midnight. The blood specimen must be drawn with a heparinized syringe, chilled by placing the specimen on ice, and immediately transported to the lab.
ACTH stimulation test, cortisol stimulation test, cosyntropin test	Monitors plasma cortisol level to indicate adrenal gland response to ACTH. Normal: Rapid: ↑ 7 µg/dL above baseline 24 hours: > 40 µg/dL 3 days: > 40 µg/dL	Note those medications taken that may affect results: cortisone, estrogens, hydrocortisone, and spironolactone may increase plasma cortisol level. Explain the procedure to the client. Initiate NPO status after midnight. For all tests, obtain baseline serum cortisol level. Rapid test: Administer IV injection of cosyntropin over 2 minutes. Draw blood specimen at 30 and 60 minutes after injection. 24-hour test: Start an IV infusion of cosyntropin in 1 liter normal saline and run at 2 U/h for 24 hours. Draw plasma cortisol level after 24 hours. 3-day test: Administer 25 units cosyntropin IV over 8 hours for 2 or 3 days. At the end of 3 days, draw plasma cortisol level.
Alanine aminotransferase (ALT, formerly serum glutamic pyruvic transiminase [SGPT])	ALT is an enzyme released in response to liver injury. Normal: 5–35 U/L	Note those medications taken that affect results: many medications may increase level, including antibiotics, narcotics, oral contraceptives, and many others.
Albumin	Albumin, a protein formed by the liver, is responsible for maintaining colloidal osmotic pressure. Indicates how well the liver is functioning. Normal: 3.5–5.0 g/dL	Note those medications taken that may affect results; steroids and hormones such as insulin, and growth hormones may increase level, whereas oral contraceptives and liver toxic drugs may decrease level.
Alkaline phosphatase	Alkaline phosphatase is an enzyme found in many tissues. The highest concentrations are found in the liver, biliary tract, and bone. Detection is important for determining possible liver and bone cancers. Normal: 30–85 ImU/mL	Fasting may be required. Apply pressure to the venipuncture site. Observe the site for bleeding.
Alpha-fetoprotein (AFP)	Test for tumor marker; elevated in nonsemi-nomatous testicular cancer. Performed between 16 and 18 weeks of pregnancy. A high level is suggestive of neural tube defects, whereas a low level may suggest Down syndrome. Normal: 0.9 ng/mL	Apply pressure to site and watch for bleeding or hematoma. First sample must be drawn between 15–20 weeks of gestation.
Amylase	Amylase is an enzyme secreted by the pancreas. Elevation indicates pancreatitis. Normal: 56–190 IU/L	Note those medications taken that affect test results; steroids, aspirin, alcohol, some narcotics, some diuretics, and other drugs may increase level, whereas citrate, glucose, and oxalates may decrease level.
Antidiuretic hormone (ADH), vasopressin	Determines the production of ADH by the posterior pituitary. Normal: 1–5 pg/mL, or < 1.5 ng/L	Explain the procedure to the client. The blood specimen should be collected in a plastic, not glass, container.

continues

Table 27-5 ADDITIONAL TESTS PERFORMED ON BLOOD SPECIMEN *continued*

TEST	EXPLANATION/NORMAL VALUES	NURSING RESPONSIBILITIES
Antidiuretic hormone (ADH), vasopressin (*continued*)		Note those medications taken that may interfere with test results. Drugs that elevate ADH level include acetaminophen, barbiturates, cholinergic agents, estrogen, nicotine, oral hypoglycemic agents, some diuretics such as thiazides, and tricyclic antidepressants. Drugs that decrease ADH level include alcohol, beta-adrenergic agents, morphine antagonists, and phenytoin (Dilantin). Client should fast for 12 hours before the test. Evaluate the client for high level of physical or emotional stress.
Antinuclear antibodies (ANAs)	ANA attack cell nuclei. The result is positive in 95% of clients with systemic lupus erythematosis. Levels are low in clients with mononucleosis, rheumatic fever, and liver diseases. Normal: negative	Fasting is not required. Hydralazine (Apresoline) and procainamide (Pronestyl) may increase level. A radioactive scan in the past week may alter results; inform the lab, if applicable.
Antistreptolysin O (ASO)	High titer indicates presence of *beta-hemolytic streptococcus*, which may cause rheumatic fever or acute glomerulonephritis. Upper limit of normal varies with age, season, and geographic area. Normal: 　Adult: < 1 : 100 　12–19 years: < 1 : 200 　2–5 years: < 1 : 100	There are no food or fluid restrictions. Antibiotics decrease ASO level. Check urine output if ASO is elevated. Urine output of less than 600 mL/24 h is associated with acute glomerulonephritis.
Antithyroid microsomal antibody, antimicrosomal antibody, microsomal antibody, thyroid autoantibody, thyroid antimicrosomal antibody	Used to detect thyroid microsomal antibodies found in clients with Hashimoto's thyroiditis. Normal: titer < 1 : 100	Explain the procedure to the client.
Aspartate aminotransferase (AST, formerly serum glutamic oxaloacetic transiminase [SGOT])	AST is an enzyme that indicates inflammation of heart, liver, skeletal muscle, pancreas, or kidneys. Normal: 　Male: 7–21 U/L 　Female: 6–18 U/L	Avoid intramuscular (IM) injections; record date and time of any injections. Avoid hemolysis. Withhold medications that affect results, for 12 hours if possible; several medications, such as antihypertensives, cholinergic agents, anticoagulants, digitalis, and others, may increase level, as may exercise.
Arterial blood gases (ABGs)	Direct measurement of the pH, PaO_2, and $PaCO_2$, and calculated measurement of HCO_3^- and SaO_2 from samples of arterial blood. pH = expresses the acidity or alkalinity of the blood. PaO_2 = partial pressure of oxygen in the blood. $PaCO_2$ = partial pressure of carbon dioxide in the blood. SaO_2 = arterial oxygen saturation. HCO_3^- = bicarbonate ion concentration in the blood. The oxygen content of the blood expressed as a percentage of the oxygen carrying capacity of the blood. Normal: 　pH: 7.35–7.45 　PaO_2: 80–100 mm Hg 　$PaCO_2$: 35–45 mm Hg 　HCO_3^-: 22–26 mEq 　SaO_2: > 95% (at sea level)	Explain that an arterial sample of blood is required. Arterial punctures cause more discomfort than venous. Instruct the client not to move. Assess the adequacy of collateral circulation. The blood sample is drawn in a syringe containing heparin. After the specimen has been obtained, rotate the syringe to mix the blood and heparin. The blood sample is placed on ice and taken immediately to the lab. Apply pressure to the arterial site for 3 to 5 minutes or 15 minutes if client is on an anticoagulant. Assess site for bleeding.

continues

Table 27–5 ADDITIONAL TESTS PERFORMED ON BLOOD SPECIMEN *continued*

TEST	EXPLANATION/NORMAL VALUES	NURSING RESPONSIBILITIES
Bilirubin	Measures bilirubin in the blood. Indicates how well the liver is functioning. Normal: 0.1–1.0 mg/dL	Note those medications taken that affect results; steroids, antibiotics, oral hypoglycemics, narcotics, as well as others may cause increased level, whereas barbiturates, caffeine, penicillins, and salicylates may cause decreased level. Fasting may be required. Do not shake the tube; protect the tube from light.
Blood glucose, fasting blood sugar, (FBS)	Measures blood level of glucose (serum values). Results depend on method used by laboratory. Normal: 70–115 mg/dL Diabetic: ≥ 126 mg/dL Critical values: 　> 400 mg/dL 　< 50 mg/dL	Client must fast (except for water) for 6–8 hours before test. Withhold insulin or oral antidiabetic medications until blood is drawn. Be certain client receives medications and meal after fasting specimen drawn. Cortisone, thiazide, and loop diuretics cause increase.
2 hour post prandial glucose (2h PPG) or 2 hour post prandial blood sugar (2h PPBS)	Measures blood glucose 2 hours after a meal. Normal: 70–140 mg/dL Diabetic: > 140 mg/dL	Instruct the client to eat entire meal and then to not eat anything else until blood is drawn. Notify the laboratory of the time meal was completed.
Blood urea nitrogen (BUN)	Measures urea, end product of protein metabolism. Normal: 5–25 mg/dL	Initiate NPO status 8 hours prior to test, if possible. Note the client's hydration status. Note those medications taken that may affect results, including phenothiazines, nephrotoxic drugs, diuretics (hydrochlorthiazide [Hydro-Diuril], ethacrynic acid [Edecrin], furosemide [Lasix]); antibiotics (bacitracin, gentamicin, kanamycin, methicillin, neomycin); antihypertensives (methyldopa [Aldomet], guanethidine [Ismelin]), sulfonamides, propranolol, morphine, lithium, carbonate, salicylates.
CA-15-3	CA-15-3 (cancer antigen) is a tumor marker for monitoring breast cancer. Because benign breast or ovarian disease can also cause elevations, it has limited use in diagnosis. Normal: < 22 U/mL	Fasting is not required. Apply pressure to the venipuncture site. Observe the site for bleeding.
CA-19-9	CA-19-9 (cancer antigen) is a tumor marker used primarily in the diagnosis of pancreatic carcinoma. Normal: < 37 U/mL	Fasting is not required. Apply pressure to the venipuncture site. Observe the site for bleeding.
CA-125	CA-125 (cancer antigen) is a tumor marker especially helpful in making the diagnosis of ovarian cancer. Normal: 0–35 U/mL	Fasting is not required. Apply pressure to the venipuncture site. Observe the site for bleeding.
Calcitonin, HCT, thyrocalcitonin	Determines thyroid and parathyroid activity. Also used as a tumor marker to detect thyroid cancer and several other cancers. Normal: basal 　Male: ≤ 19 pg/mL, or ≤ 19 ng/L 　Female: ≤ 14 pg/mL, or ≤ 14 ng/L	Note those medications taken that may increase calcitonin level, including calcium, cholecystokinin, epinephrine, glucagon, pentagastrin, and oral contraceptives. Explain the procedure to the client. The client should fast overnight but may have water.
Carcinoembryonic antigen (CEA, carcinoembryonic antigen)	CEA was thought to be a specific indicator of the presence of colorectal cancer, but has been found in clients with a variety of carcinomas. It is especially useful in monitoring treatment response in breast and gastrointestinal cancers and is occasionally the first sign of tumor recurrence. Normal: < 5 ng/mL	Fasting is not required. Apply pressure to the venipuncture site. Observe the site for bleeding. Note whether the client smokes or has a disease that will alter results, such as hepatitis, cirrhosis, or colitis.

continues

Table 27–5 ADDITIONAL TESTS PERFORMED ON BLOOD SPECIMEN *continued*

TEST	EXPLANATION/NORMAL VALUES	NURSING RESPONSIBILITIES
Cardiac enzymes	Indicates possible tissue damage if elevated.	Neither fasting nor NPO status is necessary.

Serum AST	Normal:
	  Male: 7–21 U/L
	  Female: 6–18 U/L
		Pattern of elevated levels of AST, CPK, and LDH is indicative of myocardial infarction (MI).

Creatine kinase CPK (CK)	Normal:
	  Male: 55–170 U/L
	  Female: 30–135 U/L
		CPK is the first enzyme elevated after MI, and peaks within the first 24 hours.

CK isoenzymes	Present in skeletal muscle, brain, lungs, and heart muscle. Normal:	Elevation of an isoenzyme indicates damage to tissue in a specific organ; CK-MB is specific for myocardial cells.

CK-MM (muscle)
    CK-BB (brain)
    CK-MB (heart)
	95%–100%
	0%–1%
	< 3%–4% (> 5% in MI)	

Lactic dehydrogenase (LDH) LDH isoenzymes	Normal: 70–180 mg/dL, or 95–200 U/L	LDH_1 value greater than LDH_2 value is indicative of an acute MI. LDH_5 is elevated with congestive heart failure (CHF).

LDH_1 (heart and erythrocytes)
    LDH_2 (reticuloendothelial system)
    LDH_3 (lungs and other tissues)
    LDH_4 (kidney, placenta, pancreas)
    LDH_5 (liver and striated muscles)
	*17.5%–28.3%
	*30.4%–36.4%
	*18.8%–26.0%
	*9.2%–16.5%
	*5.3%–13.4%	

Cardiac troponin I and T	Proteins found in cardiac muscle. Protein is released when the muscle is injured or dead. Troponin I elevated level in 4–6 hours Normal: <1.5 ng/mL Troponin T elevated level in 3–4 hours Normal: <0.1 ng/mL	Explain to client that blood sample is needed. Text very expensive. Often used in the ED.
CD4 T-cell count	Predictor of HIV progression; baseline taken after positive HIV test. Normal: 500–1000/mm^3 Critical value: < 200/mm^3	Explain the meaning of the test. Provide follow-up explanation of test results.
Cholesterol (lipid profile)	Lipid necessary for steroid, bile, and cell membrane production. Normal: < 200 mg/dL (total)	Have client fast 12 to 14 hours prior to test. No alcohol 24 hours prior to test. Diet intake 2 weeks prior to test will affect results. Note those medications taken that may affect results; steroids, phenytoin, diuretics, and others may elevate level, whereas MAO inhibitors, some antibiotics, lovastatin, and others may decrease level. If elevated, increased risk of coronary artery disease (CAD), hypertension, and MI.
High density lipoprotein (HDL)	Normal: 30–70 mg/dL	
Low density lipoprotein (LDL)	Normal: 60–160 mg/dL	
Very low density lipoprotein (VLDL)	Normal: 25%–50%	
Triglycerides	Normal: 40–150 mg/dL	Elevated level in CAD; level increases when LDL level increases.

Complement assay (total complement, C3 and C4)	Decreased levels in autoimmune diseases due to depletion of complement by antibody–antigen complexes.
	Normal:
	  C3: Male: 80–180 mg/dL
	      Female: 76–120 mg/dL
	  C4: 15–45 mg/dL
		Fasting is not required.

Coombs' test (direct antiglobulin test)	Detects whether immunoglobulins are attached to RBCs. Normal: negative	Note whether the client is taking ampicillin (Unasyn), captopril (Capoten), indomethacin (Indocin), or insulin, as these cause false-positive results.

*% of total LDH

continues

Table 27–5 ADDITIONAL TESTS PERFORMED ON BLOOD SPECIMEN *continued*

TEST	EXPLANATION/NORMAL VALUES	NURSING RESPONSIBILITIES

Cortisol, hydrocortisone	Determines adrenal cortex function. There is normally a diurnal variation, with higher level around 6 to 8 A.M. and lowest levels around midnight.
	Normal:
	  8 A.M.: 6–28 µg/dL, or 170–625 nmol/L
	  4 P.M.: 2–12 µg/dL, or 80–413 nmol/L
		Note whether the client has been under physical or emotional stress as either can artificially elevate plasma cortisol level.
		Likewise, recent use of radioisotopes can interfere with test results.
		Note those medications taken that may affect results. Drugs that may increase plasma cortisol level include estrogen, oral contraceptives, and spironolactone (Aldactone). Drugs that may decrease plasma cortisol level include androgens and phenytoin (Dilantin)
		Explain the procedure to the client. Two specimens are drawn—one at 8 A.M. and another at 4 P.M. Assess the client for physical or emotional stress and report to the physician.
		Indicate times of collection on laboratory requisitions.

C-reactive protein test (CRP)	An abnormal protein appears in the blood of clients with an acute inflammatory process. Used to monitor the progress of clients with autoimmune disorders such as rheumatoid arthritis. Negative except in pregnancy. More sensitive than erythrocyte sedimentation rate (ESR).	Some labs may require clients to fast, except for water, for 4 to 12 hours prior. Note those medications that may affect results: nonsteroidal anti-inflammatory drugs (NSAIDs), steroids, and salicylates may decrease level, whereas oral contraceptives and intrauterine devices (IUDs) may increase level. Inform laboratory, if applicable.
Culture	Identifies pathogens in blood. Normal: None	There are no food or fluid restrictions.
Dexamethasone suppression test (DST), prolonged/rapid DST, cortisol suppression test (ACTH suppression test)	Monitors plasma cortisol level to measure adrenal gland function. Normal: nearly 0 cortisol level	Stress can interfere with test results. Note those medications taken that may affect results, including barbiturates, estrogens, oral contraceptives, phenytoin (Dilantin) spironolactone, steroids, and tetracyclines. Explain the procedure to the client. Weigh the client for baseline weight. Rapid test: Administer dexamethasone 1 mg orally at 11 P.M. with milk or antacid. Administer sedative, if ordered. At 8 A.M. before client rises, draw plasma cortisol level. Overnight 8-mg dexamethasone suppression test: If no cortisol suppression occurs, repeat test using 8 mg dexamethasone. If there is still no cortisol suppression, a prolonged test over 6 days involving six 24-hour urine collections should be done.
Electrolytes	Determines blood electrolyte levels. First four are the most commonly measured.	Sodium and potassium are necessary for cardiac electrical conduction.
Sodium (Na⁺)	Measures level of serum sodium. Function in the body: Major electrolyte in extracellular fluid, regulates fluid balance, stimulates conduction of nerve impulses, helps maintain neuromuscular activity. Normal: 135–145 mEq/L	There are no food or fluid restrictions.
Potassium (K⁺)	Measures level of serum potassium. Function in the body: Major electrolyte in intracellular fluid, maintains normal nerve and muscle activity, assists in cellular metabolism of carbohydrates and proteins Normal: 3.5–5.0 mEq/L	There are no food or fluid restrictions. If the client has hypokalemia or hyperkalemia, evaluate the client for cardiac dysrhythmias.
Chloride (Cl⁻)	Measures level of serum chloride Function in the body: Major electrolyte in extracellular fluid, functions in combination with sodium to maintain osmotic pressure, assists in maintaining acid–base balance Normal: 100–110 mEq/L	There are no food or fluid restrictions.

continues

Table 27–5 ADDITIONAL TESTS PERFORMED ON BLOOD SPECIMEN *continued*

TEST	EXPLANATION/NORMAL VALUES	NURSING RESPONSIBILITIES
Electrolytes (*continued*)		

Calcium, total/ionized Ca^{++}	Indicates parathyroid gland function and calcium metabolism. Because ionized calcium is un-affected by serum albumin, it can give more accurate results; however, most laboratories do not have the equipment to perform the test.
	
	Normal:
	  Total: 9.0–10.5 mg/dL, or 2.25–2.75 nmol/L
	  Ionized: 4.5–5.6 ng/dL, or 1.05–1.30 nmol/L
		Note those medications taken that may affect results. Drugs that may increase serum calcium level include calcium salts, hydralazine, lithium, thiazide diuretics, parathyroid hormone (PTH), thyroid hormone, and vitamin D.
		
		Drugs that may decrease serum calcium level include acetazolamide, anticonvulsants, aspara-ginase, aspirin, calcitonin, cisplatin, cortico-steroids, heparin, laxatives, loop diuretics, magnesium salts, and oral contraceptives. Vitamin D and excessive milk ingestion can also interfere with test results.
		
		Explain the procedure to the client.
		
		Fasting is not required for serum calcium, but might be required if other blood chemistry tests are to be drawn.

Magnesium (Mg^{++})	Measures level of serum magnesium Function in the body: Combines with calcium and phosphorous in intracellular bone tissue, essential for neuro-muscular contraction, synthesis of protein, and body temperature regulation Normal: 1.5–2.5 mEq/L	There are no food or fluid restrictions.
Phosphate (PO$_4$$^{--}$)	Measures level of serum phosphate Function in the body: An essential intracellular electrolyte, exists in an inverse relationship with calcium Normal: 1.8–2.6 mEq/L	Initiate NPO status after midnight. Intravenous fluids containing glucose are sometimes discontinued several hours before the test.
Bicarbonate (HCO$_3$$^{-}$) (total carbon dioxide content or carbon dioxide capacity)	Always in a 20 : 1 ratio with carbonic acid. Normal: 24–30 mEq/L	There are no food or fluid restrictions. Loss of gastric contents is the most common reason for increased level.
ELISA	Screening test used to indicate the presence of HIV Normal: negative	Inform the client that if the first ELISA test is positive, a second ELISA will be drawn before confirmation is done with Western blot. Provide pretest counseling. Obtain informed consent. Provide or arrange for post-test counseling.

Erythrocyte sedimentation rate (ESR or sed rate test)	Measures, in mm, RBC descent in a normal saline solution after 1 hour. Level is increased in inflammatory, infectious, necrotic, or cancerous conditions, due to increased protein content in plasma. Used to monitor the course of therapy for clients with autoimmune diseases, such as rheumatoid arthritis.
	
	Normal:
	  Male: 1–13 mm/h
	  Female: 1–20 mm/h
		The test should be performed within 3 hours after the blood is drawn. Menstruation or pregnancy may increase level. Ethanbutal, quinine, aspirin, cortisone, and prednisone may alter results.

Folic acid (Folate level)	Measures folic acid level in the blood. Normal: 5–20 ug/mL, or 14–34 mmol/L	Fasting is not required. Instruct the client not to drink any alcoholic beverages before the test. The test is drawn before folic acid medications are administered. Note whether the client is taking phenytoin (Dilantin), primidone (Mysoline), methotrexate, antimalarial agents, or oral contraceptives, as these cause decreased level.

continues

Table 27–5 ADDITIONAL TESTS PERFORMED ON BLOOD SPECIMEN *continued*

TEST	EXPLANATION/NORMAL VALUES	NURSING RESPONSIBILITIES

Follicle-stimulating hormone (FSH)	Determines anterior pituitary function. Usually measured with luteinizing hormone level.
	
	Normal: varies with phase of menstrual cycle
	  Follicular: 5–20 mU/mL
	  Midcycle peak: 15–30 mU/mL
	  Luteal: 5–15 mU/mL
	  Postmenopause: 50–100 mU/mL
	  Male: 5–20 mU/mL
		Note whether client is taking estrogen or progesterone, as these may decrease FSH level. Recent use of radioisotopes can also interfere with test results.
		
		Explain the procedure to the client.
		
		Indicate on the laboratory requisition the date of the last menstrual period (LMP) or that the client is postmenopausal. Indicate use of estrogen or progesterone on laboratory requisition.
		
		The client should be relaxed and recumbent for 30 minutes before the test.

Gamma-glutamyl transpeptidase (GGT or GGTP)	Enzyme that detects liver cell dysfunction.
	Normal:
	  Female, < 45 years: 5–27 U/L
	  Female, > 45 years; male: 8–38 U/L
		The client must fast for 8 hours prior to test.
		
		Note those medications taken that interfere with results; alcohol, dilantin, and phenobarbital may elevate results, whereas oral contraceptives and clofibrate may decrease results.

Globulin	Key for antibody production. Indicates how well the liver is functioning. Normal: 2.3–3.3 g/dL	Note those medications taken that affect results (see albumin).
Glucose tolerance test (GTT)	Evaluates blood and urine glucose 30 minutes before, and 1, 2, 3, and 4 hours after a standard glucose load. Normal: blood glucose ≤ 140 mg/dL within 2 h. urine negative for glucose Diabetic: blood glucose 200 mg/dL or greater, 2 hr after a load of 75 g anhydrous glucose	The client must fast (except for water) for 6–8 hours prior to the test. Withhold drugs that interfere with results. After administration of glucose load, withhold all food. The client should drink water, however. Collect urine specimens at hourly periods. Administer meal and medications after test is completed.

Glycosylated hemoglobin (GHb)	Measures glycohemoglobin, evaluating average blood glucose level over 120 days.
	Normal: 4%–8%
	  Good control: 7.5% or less
	  Fair control: 7.6%–8.9%
	  Poor control: ≥ 9% or more
		Fasting is not required.
		
		Blood can be drawn at any time.

Growth hormone (GH), human growth hormone (HGH), somatotropin hormone (SH)	Determines the function of the anterior pituitary, although other tests such as the growth stimulation test are more accurate.
	Normal:
	  Males: < 5 ng/mL, or < 5 µg/L
	  Female: < 10 ng/mL, or < 10 µg/L
		The client should fast but may have water.
		
		Random measurement of growth hormone is not adequate because the hormone is not secreted constantly.
		
		A radioactive scan within the week; stress; exercise; or decreased blood glucose level can interfere with test results.
		
		Drugs that may increase GH level include amphetamines, arginine, dopamine, estrogens, glucagon, histamine, insulin, levodopa, methyldopa, and nicotinic acid.
		
		Drugs that may decrease GH levels include corticosteroids and phenothiazines.
		
		Explain the procedure to the client.
		
		The client should be well rested and not emotionally or physically stressed.
		
		Additional blood specimens should be obtained during sleeping hours.
		
		Additional information for the laboratory requisition includes fasting time, time of specimen collection, and the client's recent activity.
		
		Because GH half-life is only 20–25 minutes, the specimen should be taken to the laboratory immediately.

continues

Table 27–5 ADDITIONAL TESTS PERFORMED ON BLOOD SPECIMEN *continued*

TEST	EXPLANATION/NORMAL VALUES	NURSING RESPONSIBILITIES
GH stimulation test, GH provocation test, insulin tolerance test (ITT), arginine test	Indicates growth hormone deficiency Normal: > 10 ng/mL, or 10 µg/L	This test is not to be done on a client with epilepsy, cerebrovascular disease, MI, or decreased basal plasma cortisol levels. Explain the procedure to the client and parents. Initiate NPO status after midnight, except for water. To prevent multiple puncture, a heparin lock should be inserted. Baseline GH, cortisol, and glucose levels are done. An injection of insulin or arginine is given. Blood specimens for growth hormone are drawn at 0, 60, and 90 minutes after injection. Blood glucose level is monitored every 15 to 30 minutes. Blood glucose must drop to 40 mg/dL for effectiveness. Monitor client for signs and symptoms of hypoglycemia. This test takes approximately 2 hours. Although the test can be performed by a nurse, a physician should be readily available. If vigorous exercise is used instead of medication, the client should run or stair-climb for 20 minutes. Blood specimens are drawn at 0, 20, and 40 minutes. At the conclusion of the test, the client is given cookies and punch or IV glucose. Blood specimens should be taken to the laboratory immediately after being drawn.
Hepatitis B surface antigen (HB$_s$AG)	A positive result indicates presence of hepatitis or that the person is a carrier. Normal: negative	
Human chorionic gonado-tropin (hCG)	Test for tumor marker; elevated in germ cell testicular cancer. Normal: Male: 0 Female, pregnant: < 5.0 mIU/mL Female, abnormal pregnancy or chorio-carcinoma: > 25 mIU/mL	Apply pressure to the site and observe for bleeding or hematoma.
Human leukocyte antigen DW4 (HLA-DW4)	Positive (present in 50% of clients with rheumatoid arthritis. Normal: negative	Fasting is not required.
Lupus erythematosus test (LE prep)	Positive in 70%–80% of clients with systemic lupus erythematosus. May be positive in clients with rheumatoid arthritis. Used to diagnose and monitor the course of treatment for clients with systemic lupus erythematosus. Normal: negative	Fasting is not required. May be ordered daily for 3 days. Note whether the client is taking Apresoline, Pronestyl, oral contraceptives, quinidine, penicillin, Aldomet, tetracycline, isoniazid, or reserpine, as these may cause false-positive results.
Luteinizing hormone (LH) assay	Determines anterior pituitary function. It can be used to determine whether ovulation has occurred. Can also determine whether gonadal insufficiency is primary or secondary. Normal: Males: 7–24 mU/mL Females: 6–30 mU/mL	Note whether the client is taking estrogen or progesterone, as these may decrease LH level. Recent use of radioisotopes can also interfere with test results. Explain the procedure to the client. Indicate on the laboratory requisition the date of the LMP or that the client is postmenopausal.
Parathyroid hormone (PTH), parathormone	Measures the quantity of PTH to determine hyperparathyroidism or whether hypercalcemia is caused by parathyroid glands. Normal: < 2,000 pg/mL	Recent use of radioisotope can interfere with test results. Explain the procedure to the client. Initiate NPO status after midnight, except for water. Obtain morning blood specimen and indicate time of collection.

continues

Table 27–5 ADDITIONAL TESTS PERFORMED ON BLOOD SPECIMEN *continued*

TEST	EXPLANATION/NORMAL VALUES	NURSING RESPONSIBILITIES
Phosphorus	Determines the level of phosphorus in the blood. Normal: 3.0–4.5 ng/dL, or 0.97–1.45 nmol/L	Laxatives or enemas containing sodium phosphate can increase serum phosphorus level. Note those medications taken that may affect results. Drugs that may increase serum phosphorus level include methicillin and excessive vitamin D. Recent carbohydrate ingestion including IV administration causes decreased serum phosphorus level, as do antacids and mannitol. Explain the procedure to the client. Initiate NPO status after midnight. Discontinue IV fluids containing glucose for several hours before test, if possible.
Plasma renin assay, plasma renin activity (PRA)	Measures the amount of renin and is used as a screening procedure to detect essential or renal hypertension. When combined with plasma aldosterone level, determines adrenal cortex activity. Normal: 　Upright position, sodium depleted or restricted diet: 　　20–39 years: 2.9–24 ng/mL/h 　　> 40 years: 2.9–10.8 ng/mL/h 　Upright position, sodium repleted or normal diet: 　　20–39 years: 0.1–4.3 ng/mL/h 　　> 40 years: 0.1–3.0 ng/mL/h	Pregnancy, salt intake, or licorice ingestion can interfere with test results. Time of day (early in the day), a low-salt diet, or an upright position increases renin value. Note those medications taken that may interfere with test results, including antihypertensives, diuretics, estrogens, oral contraceptives, and vasodilators. Explain the procedure to the client. The client should maintain a normal diet with sodium restricted to 3 grams per day for 3 days before the test. Drugs and licorice should be discontinued for 2 to 4 weeks before the test. The client should stand or sit upright for 2 hours before blood is drawn. Client position, dietary status, time of day, and drugs should be recorded on the laboratory requisition. Blood specimen should be placed in ice and taken immediately to the laboratory. After blood specimen is obtained, the client may resume a normal diet and restart medications.
Polymerase chain reaction (PCR)	Detects HIV-specific DNA (virus). Normal: negative	Explain the meaning of the test. Provide follow-up explanation of test results.
Progesterone assay	Determines ovulation and function of corpus luteum. Adrenal tumors can elevate level. Normal, midcycle: 300–2,400 ng/dL	Recent use of radioisotopes or hemolysis resulting from rough handling of blood specimen can interfere with test results. Note those medications taken that may interfere with test results, including estrogen and progesterone. Explain the procedure to the client. Indicate the date of LMP on the laboratory requisition.
Prolactin level (PRL)	Determines anterior pituitary secretion. Among the problems indicated by an elevated level are pituitary tumors or primary hypothyroidism. Normal: 　Female, or male: 0–20 ng/mL 　Pregnant: 20–400 ng/mL	Note those medications taken that may affect results. Drugs that may increase prolactin level include phenothiazines, oral contraceptives, reserpine, opiates, verapamil, histamine antagonists, monoamine oxidase (MAO) inhibitors, and antihistamines. Drugs that may decrease prolactin level include ergot alkaloid derivatives, clonidine, levodopa, and dopamine. Explain the procedure to the client. The blood specimen should be obtained in the morning and placed on ice if not taken immediately to the laboratory
Prostate-specific antigen (PSA)	PSA is an antigen detected in all males; level increases with prostatic cancer. It is more sensitive and specific than the acid phosphatase. Normal: < 4 ng/mL	Fasting is not required. Apply pressure to the venipuncture site. Observe the site for bleeding.

continues

Table 27–5 ADDITIONAL TESTS PERFORMED ON BLOOD SPECIMEN *continued*

TEST	EXPLANATION/NORMAL VALUES	NURSING RESPONSIBILITIES
Rheumatoid factor (RF)	Abnormal protein in serum of approximately 80% of clients with rheumatoid arthritis. Formed as a result of the reaction of IgM to an abnormal IgG. Also elevated in clients with other autoimmune diseases such as systemic lupus erythematosus. Normal: < 60 IU/mL	Fasting is preferred.
Schilling test	Determines vitamin B_{12} absorption by the intestine. Differentiates between pernicious anemia and gastrointestinal malabsorption problems. Normal: 8%–40% of the radioactive vitamin B_{12} is excreted in the urine within 24 hours.	Collect the urine for a 24- to 48-hour period. Laxatives are not given during the test, as they decrease the absorption of vitamin B_{12}.
Serum acid phosphatase (prostatic)	Serum measurement of prostatic acid phosphatase, elevated in malignancy; because it detects cancer in the later stages, no longer commonly used. Normal: 0.0–0.8 U/L	Apply pressure to the site. Observe the site for bleeding or hematoma.
Serum alkaline phosphatase	Serum measurement of alkaline phosphates, elevated in malignancy. Normal: 30–120 U/L	Apply pressure to the site. Observe the site for bleeding or hematoma.

Serum creatinine	Specific indicator of renal disease.
	Normal:
	  Male: 0.6–1.5 mg/dL
	  Female: 0.6–1.1 mg/dL
		Note those medications taken that may affect results, including amphotericin B, cephalosporins (cepfazolin [Ancef], cephalothin [Keflin]), methicillin, ascorbic acid, barbiturates, lithium carbonate, methyldopa (Aldomet), triamterene (Dyrenium).

Sickledex (sickle-cell test)	Screening test to determine the presence of Hgb S. Normal: no Hgb S If results are positive, a hemoglobin electrophoresis test is done.	There are no food or fluid restrictions. Note on the laboratory requisition whether the client had a blood transfusion in the past 3 to 4 months.
Thyroid-stimulating hormone (TSH), thyrotropin	Determines thyroid function as well as monitors exogenous thyroid replacement. Normal: 2–10 μU/mL, or 2–10 mU/L	Recent use of radioisotopes may affect test results. Severe illness may decrease TSH level. Note those medications taken that may affect results. Drugs that may increase TSH level include antithyroid drugs, lithium, potassium iodide, and TSH injection. Drugs that may decrease TSH level include aspirin, dopamine, heparin, steroids, and T_3. Explain the procedure to the client. The client should be relaxed and recumbent for 30 minutes before the test.
TSH stimulation test	Differentiates between primary and secondary hypothyroidism. Normal: none given	Explain the procedure to the client. Obtain baseline level of radioactive iodine intake or serum T_4. Administer 5–10 units of TSH intramuscularly for 3 days. Repeat radioactive iodine intake or T_4 as indicated for comparison studies.
Thyrotropin-releasing hormone (TRH) test, thyrotropin-releasing factor (TRF) test	Assesses the responsiveness of the anterior pituitary by its secretion of TSH in response to an IV injection of TRH. Also tests the function of the thyroid gland. Normal: undetectable to 15 μU/mL	Pregnancy may increase TSH response to TRH. Note those medications taken that may modify TSH response, including antithyroid drugs, aspirin, corticosteroids, estrogens, levodopa, and T_4. Explain the procedure to the client. Any thyroid preparations should be discontinued for 3–4 weeks before the test.

continues

Table 27–5 ADDITIONAL TESTS PERFORMED ON BLOOD SPECIMEN *continued*

TEST	EXPLANATION/NORMAL VALUES	NURSING RESPONSIBILITIES
Triiodothyronine (T_3) radio-immunoassay (T_3 by RIA)	Determines thyroid gland function Normal: 110–230 ng/dL, or 1.2–1.5 nmol/L	Radioisotope administration may interfere with test results. Pregnancy increases T_3 results. Note those medications taken that may affect results. Drugs that may increase T_3 level include: estrogen, methadone, and oral contraceptives. Drugs that may decrease T_4 level include anabolic steroids, androgens, phenytoin (Dilantin), propranolol (Inderal), reserpine, and salicylates (high dose). Explain the procedure to the client. Determine whether exogenous T_3 is being taken. With physician's approval, withhold those drugs that would interfere with test results.
Triiodothyronine (T_3) serum free	Measures the amount of free T_3 that actually enters the cells and is active in metabolism. A true indicator of thyroid activity. Can be used to diagnose thyroid status in pregnant females or clients on drugs that can interfere with results of other tests. Normal: 0.2–0.6 ng/dL	Explain the procedure to the client. Blood specimens for T_3 and T_4 uptake must be obtained to calculate T_3.
Thyroxine (T_4) Screen	Directly measures the amount of T_4 present. Normal: radioimmunoassay: 5–12 μg/dL, or 65–155 nmol/L	X-ray iodinated contrast studies may increase T_4 levels. Pregnancy will increase T_4 level. Note those medications taken that may affect results. Drugs that may increase T_4 level include clofibrate, estrogens, heroin, methadone, and oral contraceptives. Drugs that may decrease T_4 level include anabolic steroids, androgens, antithyroid drugs, lithium, phenytoin (Dilantin), and propranolol (Inderal). Explain the procedure to the client. Evaluate the client's drug history. If needed, instruct the client to stop exogenous T_4 medications for 1 month prior to test.
Thyroxine index free, FTI, FT_4 Index	Measures the amount of free T_4 that actually enters the cells and is active in metabolism. A true indicator of thyroid activity. Can be used to diagnose thyroid status in pregnant females or clients on drugs that can interfere with results of other tests. Normal: 0.8–2.4 ng/dL, or 10–31 pmol/L	Recent radionuclear scans can interfere with test results. Explain the procedure to the client. Blood specimens for T_4 and T_3 uptake must be obtained to calculate T_4.
Total iron-binding capacity (TIBC)	Determines the ability of iron to bind to a protein called transferrin. Normal: 250–420 ug/dL, or 45–73 umol/L	If possible, initiate NPO status 8 hours prior to the test. A recent blood transfusion or a diet high in iron may affect test results. Note whether the client is taking oral contraceptives, as these increase TIBC level.

Triglycerides	Form of fat produced in the liver.
	Normal:
	    Male: 40–160 mg/dL
	    Female: 35–135 mg/dL
		Instruct the client to fast for 12–14 hours prior to the test, and to have no alcohol for 24 hours before. Dietary intake for 2 weeks prior to the test affects results.

Total protein	Total measure of albumin and globulin. Normal: 6.4–8.3 g/dL	Note medications taken that affect results (see Albumin, this table). Instruct the client to avoid eating foods high in fat for 24 hours before the test.

Uric acid (serum, urine)	Elevated in gout.
	Normal, serum:
	    Male: 2.1–8.5 mg/dL
	    Female: 2.0–6.6 mg/dL
		There are no food or drink restrictions. Note those medications and other substances taken that may affect results, including ascorbic acid, diuretics, levadopa, allopurinol, and Coumadin.

continues

Table 27–5 ADDITIONAL TESTS PERFORMED ON BLOOD SPECIMEN *continued*

TEST	EXPLANATION/NORMAL VALUES	NURSING RESPONSIBILITIES
Uric acid (serum, urine) (*continued*)	Normal, urine: 250–750 mg/24 h	Label container with client's name and date/times of collection. Note those medications and other substances taken that may affect results, including corticosteroids and cytotoxic agents.
VDRL (Venereal Disease Research Laboratories), RPR (rapid plasma reagin), FTA-ABS (fluorescent treponemal antibody-absorption test), Reiter test, fluorescent antibody Treponema pallidum immobilization (TPI) test (performed only at Centers for Disease Control [CDC] in Atlanta)	Blood tests for presence of syphilis. Normal: negative or nonreactive	Explain the test to the client, including amount of blood to be drawn.
Western blot	Confirmatory test for the presence of antibodies to HIV. Normal: negative	Provide pretest counseling. Obtain informed consent. Provide or arrange post-test counseling.

Urine Tests

Urinalysis is performed to assist in the diagnosis of various conditions. Urine specimens are obtained to measure substances such as amylase, catecholamines, chloride, and certain hormones. Substances not normally found in the urine include RBCs, white blood cells (WBCs), protein, glucose, ketones, and casts. Tests often performed on a urine specimen are found in Table 27–6.

Urine pH

The pH is governed by the hydrogen ion concentration in the urine. Disorders such as diabetes mellitus, dehydration, diarrhea, emphysema, and starvation make the urine acidic. Chronic renal failure, renal tubular acidosis, urinary tract infections, and salicylate poisoning cause the urine to be alkaline.

Specific Gravity

Specific gravity measures the number of solutes in a solution. Urea and uric acid (the by–products of nitrogen metabolism) have the greatest influence on the specific gravity of urine. A urinometer and cylinder are used to measure specific gravity (Figure 27-3). The urinometer has a specific gravity scale and a weighted mercury bulb. A fresh urine specimen is poured into the cylinder, then the urinometer is twirled into the cylinder. When the urinometer stops spinning, the urinometer is read at eye level.

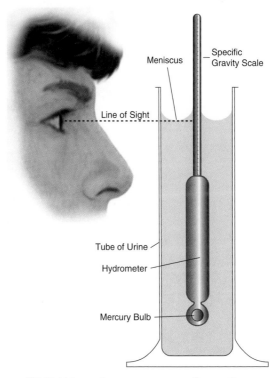

Figure 27-3 Urinometer measures specific gravity.

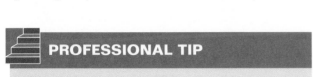

PROFESSIONAL TIP

Drugs and Laboratory Tests

Note drugs the client is taking when those drugs may influence the results of laboratory tests.

PROFESSIONAL TIP

Testing for Blood Lipid Level

To allow for the proper balance between the vascular and extravascular compartment and ensure valid test results, the blood should always be drawn after the client has been sitting quietly for 5 minutes.

Specific gravity increases with conditions that increase fluid loss from the body. Decreases in specific gravity result from renal disease. When the amount of urine increases and the specific gravity decreases, there is an absence of the antidiuretic hormone (ADH), usually triggered by diabetes insipidus (a disorder of the posterior pituitary gland).

Urine Glucose

When the blood level of glucose exceeds the renal threshold (180 mg/dL), glucose spills into the urine. Many agents are available for measuring the glucose content of urine, although these agents are not as accurate as is measuring the blood glucose level.

Urine Ketones

Ketones, products of incomplete fat metabolism, are completely metabolized by the liver under normal conditions. The most common cause of ketonuria (excessive ketones in the urine) is diabetes.

Urine Cells and Casts

Normally, the urine is free of blood cells and casts. When the renal system is impaired, as in cases of renal damage or failure, nephritis, and urinary stones or infections, the following can occur:

Table 27–6 TESTS PERFORMED ON URINE

TEST	EXPLANATION/NORMAL VALUES	NURSING RESPONSIBILITIES
Urinalysis		Explain the procedure and purpose to the client and assist with specimen collection, if needed.
Color	Clear amber	Ensure that specimen is taken to the laboratory in a timely manner.
Odor	Pleasantly aromatic until left standing; offensive and unpleasant in kidney infection.	
pH	4.6–8.0	
Specific gravity	1.005–1.030	
Glucose	Negative	
Acetone (ketone)	Negative	
Casts	Rare	
Albumin (protein)	Negative	
RBCs	2–3/HPF	
WBCs	4–5/HPF	
Bilirubin	Negative	
Bacteria	Negative	

Aldosterone Assay	A blood test or 24-hour urine collection to evaluate the adrenal cortex, especially for tumors. The 24-hour urine is more reliable, but the blood specimen is more convenient.
	
	Normal, blood:
	    Supine: 3–10 ng/dL, or 0.08–0.30 nmol/L
	    Upright:
	        Male: 6–22 ng/dL, or 0.17–0.61 nmol/L
	        Female: 5–30 ng/dL, or 0.14–0.80 nmol/L
	Normal, urine: 2–80 μg/24 h, or 5.5–72.0 nmol/24 h
		Strenuous exercise and stress can increase aldosterone level.
		
		Excessive licorice ingestion can decrease aldosterone level.
		
		Posture, dietary sodium, and pregnancy can interfere with test results.
		
		Note those medications taken that may affect results. Drugs that may increase aldosterone level include diazoxide, hydralazine, and nitroprusside. Drugs that may decrease aldosterone level include fludrocortisone and propranolol (Inderal).
		
		Explain the procedure to the client. The client should follow a normal diet with 3 grams of sodium/day and no licorice for at least 2 weeks before the test. Medications should be stopped for at least 2 weeks before the test, if possible.
		
		Blood: Blood should be drawn before the client gets out of bed. A second blood specimen might be obtained 4 hours later. Indicate on laboratory requisition time and client position. Transport blood specimen on ice to the laboratory.

continues

Table 27–6 TESTS PERFORMED ON URINE *continued*

TEST	EXPLANATION/NORMAL VALUES	NURSING RESPONSIBILITIES
Aldosterone Assay (*continued*)		24-hour urine: Initiate 24-hour urine collection after discarding first specimen. Post signs with times of collection. Each voiding does not have to be measured. Instruct the client not to contaminate urine with feces or toilet tissue. Force fluids unless medically contraindicated. Collection must be preserved and refrigerated. Indicate times of collection and any drugs that might interfere with results on laboratory requisition. Send collection to laboratory immediately upon conclusion.
Bence Jones Protein	Bence Jones proteins are immunoglobulins typically found in the urine of clients with multiple myeloma. They may also be associated with tumor metastases to the bone and chronic lymphocytic leukemia. Normal: no Bence Jones proteins present in urine.	Instruct the client to collect an early morning urine specimen of at least 50 mL. Instruct the client not to contaminate specimen with toilet paper or stool.
Creatinine clearance	Normal: Male: 95–135 mL/min Female: 85–125 mL/min Minimum: 10 mL/min to maintain life	Instruct the client about the 24-hour urine test. Encourage hourly water intake. Keep urine on ice or in special refrigerator. Drugs that affect results include phenacetin, anabolic steroids, thiazides, ascorbic acid, levodopa, methyldopa (Aldomet), phenolsulfonphthalein (PSP) (test).
17-hydroxycorticosteroids (17-OHCS)	24-hour urine test that measures adrenal cortex function. Normal: Male: 4.5–10.0 mg/24 h Female: 2.5–10.0 mg/24 h	Emotional or physical stress or licorice ingestion may increase adrenal activity. Note those medications taken that may affect results. Drugs that may increase 17-OHCS level include acetazolamide, chloral hydrate, chlorpromazine, colchicine, erythromycin, meprobamate, paraldehyde, quinidine, quinine, and spironolactone. Drugs that may decrease 17-OHCS level include estrogens, oral contraceptives, phenothiazines, and reserpine. Explain the procedure to the client. Initiate 24-hour urine collection after discarding first specimen. Post signs with times of collection. Each voiding does not have to be measured. Instruct the client not to contaminate urine with feces or toilet tissue. Force fluids unless medically contraindicated. Collection must be refrigerated. Indicate on laboratory requisition times of collection and any drugs that might interfere with results. Send collection to laboratory immediately upon conclusion.
17-ketosteroids (17-KS)	24-hour urine test that measures adrenal cortex function. Normal: Male: 7–25 mg/24 h, or 24–88 μmol/24 h Female: 4–15 mg/24 h, or 14–52 μmol/24 h	Stress may increase adrenal activity. Note medications taken that may affect results. Drugs that increase 17-KS level include antibiotics, chloramphenicol, chlorpromazine, dexamethasone, meprobamate, phenothiazines, quinidine, secobarbital, and spironolactone. Drugs that may decrease 17-KS level include estrogen, oral contraceptives, probenecid, promazine, reserpine, salicylates (prolonged use), and thiazide diuretics. Explain the procedure to the client. With physician's approval, withhold all drugs for several days before test. Monitor client for stress and report to physician. Initiate 24-hour urine collection after discarding first specimen. Post signs with times of collection. Each voiding does not have to be measured. Instruct the client not to contaminate urine with feces or toilet tissue. Force fluids

continues

Table 27–6 TESTS PERFORMED ON URINE *continued*

TEST	EXPLANATION/NORMAL VALUES	NURSING RESPONSIBILITIES
17-ketosteroids (17-KS) (*continued*)		unless medically contraindicated. Collection must be preserved and refrigerated. Indicate on laboratory requisition times of collection and any drugs that might interfere with results. Send collection to laboratory immediately upon conclusion.
Urine cortisol, hydrocortisone	24-hour urine test that measures adrenal cortex function. Normal: 10–100 μg/24 h, or 27–276 nmol/24 h	Pregnancy or stress increases cortisol level. Recent radioisotope scans can interfere with test result. Note medications taken that may interfere with test result, including oral contraceptives and spironolactone. Explain the procedure to the client. Assess for stress and report to physician. Initiate 24-hour urine collection after discarding first specimen. Post signs with times of collection. Each voiding does not have to be measured. Instruct the client not to contaminate urine with feces or toilet tissue. Force fluids unless medically contraindicated. Collection must be preserved and refrigerated. Indicate on laboratory requisition times of collection and any drugs that might interfere with results. Send collection to laboratory immediately upon conclusion.

Vanillylmandelic acid (VMA) and catecholamines (epinephrine, norepinephrine, metanephrine, normetanephrine, dopamine)	24-hour urine test that diagnoses pheochromocytoma and other adrenal tumors.
	Normal:
	  VMA: 2–7 mg/24 h, or 10–35 μmol/24 h
	  Epinephrine: 0.5–20.0 μg/24 h, or < 275 nmol/24 h
	  Norepinephrine: 15–80 μg/24 h
	  Metanephrine: 24–96 μg/24 h
	  Normetanephrine: 75–375 μg/24 h
	  Dopamine: 65–400 μg/24 h
		Certain foods (e.g., tea, coffee, cocoa, vanilla, chocolate), vigorous exercise, stress, or starvation may increase VMA level.
		Uremia, alkaline urine, or iodinated contrast dyes may falsely decrease VMA level.
		Note those medications taken that may affect results. Drugs that may increase VMA level include caffeine, epinephrine, levodopa, lithium, and nitroglycerine. Drugs that may decrease VMA level include clonidine, disulfiram (Antabuse), guanethidine, imipramine, MAO inhibitors, phenothiazines, and reserpine. Drugs that may increase catecholamine level include ethyl alcohol, aminophylline, caffeine, chloral hydrate, clonidine (chronic therapy), contrast media (iodine containing), disulfiram (Antabuse), epinephrine, erythromycin, insulin, methenamine, methyldopa, nicotinic acid (large doses), nitroglycerin, quinidine, riboflavin, and tetracyclines. Drugs that may decrease catecholamine level include guanethidine, reserpine, and salicylates.
		Explain the procedure to the client. The client should be on a VMA-restricted diet for 2–3 days before the test. Items restricted include coffee, tea, bananas, chocolate, cocoa, licorice, citrus fruit, anything with vanilla, and aspirin. Client should not take antihypertensive drugs before the test.
		Initiate 24-hour urine collection after discarding first specimen. Post signs with times of collection. Each voiding does not have to be measured. Instruct the client not to contaminate urine with feces or toilet tissue. Collection may need to be preserved (consult laboratory) and is to be refrigerated. Indicate times of collection and any drugs that might interfere with results.

- Bleeding, resulting in RBCs in the urine
- Accumulation of epithelial cells accompanied by cast formation
- WBCs in the urine, which indicate infection

Stool Tests

Stool specimens are collected for examination of both normal substances (such as urobilinogen) and blood, bacteria, and parasites (Table 27–7).

Urobilinogen

Urobilinogen is a colorless derivative of bilirubin formed by the normal bacterial action of intestinal flora on bilirubin. It increases in the presence of severe hemolysis and decreases in the presence of most biliary obstructions.

Occult Blood

Occult blood is invisible on inspection; it is blood in the stool that can be detected only with a microscope or by chemical means. In the gastrointestinal tract, the digestive process acts on blood, making it occult. Random sampling for occult blood is done to diagnose gastrointestinal bleeding, ulcers, and malignant tumors.

To decrease the possibility of a false-positive result when occult blood is to be used to confirm suspicions of a gastrointestinal disorder, the client is placed on a 3-day diet free of meat, poultry, and fish. Common drugs that can cause a false-positive test for occult blood are salicylate, steroids, and indomethacin.

Parasites

The gastrointestinal tract can harbor parasites and their eggs (ova). Whereas some of these parasites are harmless, others cause clinical symptoms. With the exception of pinworms (which can enter the body through both the oral and anal routes), most common parasites enter the body through the mouth when contaminated water or food is ingested.

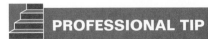

PROFESSIONAL TIP

Cultures

All culture tests should be performed before initiating antibiotic therapy so as to identify the type of pathogen and its sensitivity to specific antibiotics.

Culture and Sensitivity Tests

Culture refers to the growing of microorganisms to identify the pathogen. Culture and **sensitivity** (C&S) tests are performed to identify both the nature of the invading organism and its susceptibility to commonly used antibiotics. Sensitivity allows the practitioner to select the appropriate antibiotic therapy. All C&S specimens should be taken immediately to the laboratory.

Blood Culture

Bacteremia is bacteria in the blood. The blood culture should be obtained while the client is experiencing chills and fever. A series of three venipuncture collections are performed using strict sterile technique. The needle should be changed after the specimen is collected and before injecting the blood sample into the test tube.

Throat (Swab) Culture

The throat normally hosts many organisms. Throat cultures serve to isolate and identify such pathogens as beta-hemolytic streptococci, *Staphylococcus aureus,* meningococci, gonococci, *Bordetella pertussis,* and *Corynebacterium diphtheria*. A throat swab is commonly done to identify streptococcal infections, which, if left untreated, can cause rheumatic fever or glomerulonephritis.

To obtain a throat swab, the nurse uses a wooden blade to depress the tongue and swabs the white patches, exudate, or ulcerations of the throat using a

Table 27–7 TESTS PERFORMED ON STOOL

TEST	EXPLANATION/NORMAL VALUES	NURSING RESPONSIBILITIES
Stool occult blood (guaiac) Fecal occult blood test (FOBT) Hemocult	Fecal occult blood screening studies may be utilized as possible indicators of colorectal cancer. Normal: negative for blood	Place a smear of stool on a card. Medications such as anticoagulants, aspirin, iron preparations, NSAIDs, and steroids may cause a false-positive result, whereas vitamin C may cause a false negative. Red meat should not be ingested for 3 days prior to the test. For premenopausal women, wait at least 4 days after menstrual period. Wear gloves when obtaining and handling the specimen.
Stool O & P (ova & parasite)	A positive result indicates infection. Normal: negative	Place the stool specimen in a container and take warm to the laboratory.

sterile applicator. The applicator should not touch any other parts of the mouth. Once the swab is obtained, the applicator should be placed in a sterile container.

Sputum Culture

Sputum tests performed include culture, smear, and cytology. Sputum is created by the mucous glands and goblet cells of the tracheobronchial tree and is raised by coughing. Sputum is sterile until it reaches the throat and mouth, where it comes in contact with normal flora. To yield a more accurate identification of pulmonary organisms, sputum can be obtained by tracheobronchial suctioning and transtracheal aspiration.

In addition to the same organism(s) found in a culture, a sputum smear identifies eosinophils, epithelial cells, and other substances. Smears are helpful in diagnosing asthma (eosinophils) and fungal infections. The specimen must be refrigerated if it cannot be taken immediately to the laboratory.

Sputum **cytology** (the study of cells) is performed to diagnose cancer of the lungs. The specimen should be collected early in the morning and after a deep cough.

Urine Culture

Urinary C&S tests are performed whenever a urinary tract infection is suspected.

Stool Culture

Stool C&S is performed to identify bacterial infections. If the client has diarrhea, a rectal swab can be taken and used as a specimen. Fecal material must be visible on the swab in order for the laboratory to perform the test.

Papanicolaou Test

The **Papanicolaou test** (a smear method of examining stained exfoliative cells), commonly called a Pap smear, is performed to evaluate the cellular maturity, metabolic activity, and morphological variations of cervical tissue. Papanicolaou testing can also be done on specimens from other organs, such as bronchial aspirations and gastric secretions.

RADIOLOGICAL STUDIES

Radiography (the study of film exposed to x-rays or gamma rays through the action of ionizing radiation) is used by the practitioner to study internal organ structure. When used in conjunction with a **contrast medium** (a radiopaque substance that facilitates roentgen imaging of the body's internal structures), **fluoroscopy** (immediate, serial images of the body's structure and function) reveals the motion of organs. X-rays are valuable to the practitioner in either formu-

CLIENT TEACHING

Pap Smear

Advise female clients to prepare for a Pap smear by:

- Avoiding intercourse, douches, and vaginal creams for 24 hours before the test and
- Informing the practitioners if they are menstruating, as the test will need to be delayed.

Cervical Pap smear testing is recommended every 2 to 3 years after the onset of sexual activity. Annual testing is indicated for those women who:

- Are over 40 years of age,
- Have a family history of cervical cancer, and/or
- Previously had a positive Pap smear.

lating a diagnosis or helping to determine the necessity for other studies (e.g., a lung lesion requiring biopsy to differentiate between a benign or malignant tumor).

Certain radiological tests require a contrast medium that might interfere with other diagnostic studies. Barium and iodine are commonly used contrast media. Laboratory blood samples measuring thyroid function should be drawn before initiating an intravenous pyelogram (IVP), where radioactive iodine dye is administered. If the client needs both an IVP and a barium enema, the IVP is performed first because the barium is likely to decrease visualization of the kidneys. Commonly performed radiological studies are described in Table 27–8.

Safety: X-rays
- Prior to scheduling x-rays, question the client about the possibility of pregnancy, asthma, and allergic reactions to contrast media (iodine) as well as to other foods and drugs.
- If the client has not previously received iodine, note this on the requisition to indicate that allergic status is unknown.

PROFESSIONAL TIP

Contrast Media

Carefully monitor those clients who are scheduled for dye injection studies and have a history of allergies to any foods or drugs (particularly fish or iodine), because such allergies may predispose these clients to allergic reactions to contrast media.

Table 27–8 RADIOLOGIC STUDIES

TEST	EXPLANATION/NORMAL VALUES	NURSING RESPONSIBILITIES
Radiograph (x-ray)	Most common diagnostic study. Identifies traumatic disorders, i.e., fractures, dislocations, tumors, bone disorders, joint deformities, bone density, and changes in bone relationships. Performed by a technician.	Explain the procedure to the client. Prepare the client as ordered. No specific post procedure care is required. Administer an analgesic, especially for the arthritic client.
Abdominal x-rays	Determines diaphragm position and gas and fluid distribution in the abdomen.	No preparation is required.
Adrenal angiography, Adrenal arteriogram	Study of adrenal glands and arterial system after injection of radiopaque dye to detect benign or malignant tumors or hyperplasia of the adrenal glands. Normal: no growth or enlargement	Assess for allergy to shellfish or iodine; arteriosclerosis; pregnancy; or blood disorders, as they preclude the test. Explain the procedure to the client. Assess for allergies. Informed and written consent must be obtained before the procedure. Note whether client has been taking anticoagulants. Initiate NPO status after midnight. Mark peripheral pulses with a pen before the procedure. Inform the client that a warm flush may be felt when the dye is injected. Observe the puncture site. Monitor vital signs. Monitor peripheral pulses, color, and temperature of extremities. Institute bed rest for 12–24 hours. Apply cold compresses to puncture site, if needed. Force fluids to prevent possible dehydration from the dye.
Adrenal venography	Involves insertion of a catheter through the femoral vein and into the adrenal vein to withdraw a blood specimen to detect the function of each adrenal gland. A contrast dye is injected to visualize size and position of the adrenal glands. Normal: no growth or enlargement	Explain the procedure to the client. Assess for allergies. Obtain informed and written consent. Inform the client that a burning sensation may be experienced when the dye is injected. Although this study involves the venous system, monitor vital signs and injection site as well as pulses, temperature, and color of extremities.
Arthrogram (-graphy)	Visualization of a joint. Radiopaque dye or air is injected into the joint cavity to outline soft tissue, usually on knee/shoulder joints. Local anesthetic and sterile technique are used. Performed by a physician; takes approximately 30 minutes.	Explain the procedure to the client. Obtain informed consent. Client wears an elastic bandage for several days; check for edema. Administer a mild analgesic for pain. Monitor for increased pain. Neither fasting nor sedation is required.
Barium enema	An enema of barium is given while x-rays are taken of the large intestine.	Initiate NPO status the night before. Administer the ordered medication to clean the bowel. Observe the results of the laxatives, and inform the x-ray department if there have been no results. After the test, force oral fluids and administer a cleansing enema, as ordered. Document status of abdomen and stools.
Barium swallow	The client drinks a glass of barium while x-rays are taken of the esophagus and cardiac sphincter.	Initiate NPO status the evening before. Explain the procedure and the time frame for results. Encourage the client to drink fluids and eat fiber after the test. A laxative is sometimes given after the test. The client should be instructed that bowel movements will be white for 1–2 days. During the test, the client will be tilted on the x-ray table in various positions. There may be repeated pictures taken at ½-hour intervals as the barium moves through the bowel. Document the client's tolerance of the procedure and passage of the barium. Because the procedure can be lengthy, encourage the client to take reading material.
Cardiac catheterization (cardiac angiogram, coronary arteriogram)	A catheter is passed into the right and/or left side of the heart to determine oxygen level, cardiac output, and pressure within the heart chambers.	Assess the client for allergy to iodine or shellfish. The client is to fast for 6 hours prior to the test, but medications can be taken with sips of water. Inform the client of the possibility of feeling warm or flushed during the test.

continues

Table 27–8 RADIOLOGIC STUDIES *continued*

TEST	EXPLANATION/NORMAL VALUES	NURSING RESPONSIBILITIES
Cardiac catheterization (*continued*)		After the procedure, assess the peripheral pulses every 15 minutes for 2–4 hours, or according to physician's orders. Assess color, temperature, and pulse in the extremity below the catheter insertion site. Instruct the client to keep the involved extremity straight for 6–8 hours.
Chest x-ray	Provides a two-dimensional image of the lungs without using contrast media. Used to detect the presence of fluid within the interstitial lung tissue or the alveoli; tumors or foreign bodies; and the presence and size of a pneumothorax. The size of the heart can also be determined by chest x-ray.	Explain the test to the client. If appropriate, inquire whether the client may be pregnant, to prevent exposure of the fetus to x-ray. The client is generally required to stand for various views; if the client is unable to stand, views may be obtained with the client in a sitting position, or a portable x-ray may be obtained. Instruct the client to inspire deeply and hold the breath. Instruct the client to remove all metal objects from the chest and neck area and to don a hospital gown that does not have snap closures.
Conduitogram	Radiopaque dye is injected through a catheter into either the conduit or a piece of ileum to assess by means of x-ray the length and emptying ability of the conduit as well as the presence of stricture or obstruction.	A conduit is a connection between the bladder or pouch and the outside of the body. Explain the procedure to the client. Assess the client for allergies to iodine-based dye.
Fistula gram	Radiopaque dye or barium is given to drink, and x-rays are taken as the dye or barium passes through the gastrointestinal tract. The dye shows the location of the fistula and how it is connected to the gastrointestinal tract.	Initiate NPO status as ordered. Explain the procedure and the time frame for the results and identify the person who will give the client the results.
Fluoresce in angiography	Following IV injection of sodium fluorescein, rapid-sequence photographs of the fundus are taken with a special camera. Visualization of microvascular structures of the retina and choroid are enhanced, allowing evaluation of the entire retinal vascular bed.	Instill eye drops to dilate the pupils. Start an IV so the sodium fluorescein can be injected. Remove the IV following completion of the test. Inform the client that skin and urine may be yellow for 24–48 hours.
Gallbladder series	X-ray visualization of the gallbladder.	Administer dye tablets the evening before the test. Provide a low-fat or fat-free meal the evening before. Initiate NPO status except for water after taking the dye.
Hysterosalpingogram	Radiopaque dye is instilled through the cervix. Used to diagnose uterine cavity and tubal abnormalities. Performed as a part of an infertility workup.	Explain the procedure and prepare the client in the lithotomy position. The test is done in the radiology department. Inquire about allergies to iodine or other dyes. Assist the physician.
Intravenous pyelogram (IVP)	Infusion of radiopaque dye into a vein, allowing visualization of the urinary system. The renal pelvis, ureters, and bladder can be seen.	Explain the procedure to the client. Explain that client will experience a warm feeling during dye injection. Ask the client about allergy to iodine or shellfish. Serve a light supper, then initiate NPO status overnight. Administer a laxative or enema. Schedule test before barium studies. Post-test, observe for untoward reaction to dye. Encourage fluids for 24 hours to eliminate dye.
Kidney-ureter-bladder x-ray (KUB)	Shows abnormalities such as calculi, tumors, or changes in anatomic position.	Explain the procedure to the client. No preparation is required.
Long bone x-rays	Serial x-rays of the long bones to determine bone growth.	Explain the procedure to the client. Instruct the client to keep extremities still while the x-ray is being taken. Shield ovaries, testes, or pregnant uterus. Remove all metallic objects from area being x-rayed.

continues

Table 27–8 RADIOLOGIC STUDIES *continued*

TEST	EXPLANATION/NORMAL VALUES	NURSING RESPONSIBILITIES
Lymphangiogram	A contrast dye is injected into the lymph vessels in the hands or feet to examine the lymph vessels and nodes. Used to stage lymphomas and evaluate the effectiveness of chemotherapy and radiation therapy. Normal: Normal-sized lymph nodes with no malignant cells	The dye remains in the lymph nodes for 6 months to 1 year, so disease progress can be evaluated with an x-ray. Obtain informed consent. Inform the client that if a blue-colored dye is used, the skin and urine may have a bluish discoloration. Assess the client's breath sounds after the procedure, as lipoid pneumonia is a possible complication if the dye gets into the thoracic duct.
Mammography	Used to diagnose benign and malignant disorders of the breast.	Explain the procedure to the client. The breast will be compressed, possibly causing discomfort for several seconds. Explain that it is important to have a baseline mammogram done between the ages of 35 and 40 and a breast examination done by a physician or nurse practitioner every 3–4 years. For women ages 40–49, a mammogram should be performed every 1–2 years; for those over 50, an annual mammogram is recommended along with an annual breast examination by physician or nurse practitioner.
Myelogram	X-ray of spinal subarachnoid space following injection of an opaque medium.	Follow nursing responsibilities for lumbar puncture in Table 27-14. Inform the client that the table may be tilted during the procedure. Obtain informed consent according to facility guidelines. Withhold the meal prior to procedure. Administer a light sedative, if ordered. Postprocedure care is determined by the type of medium used; follow physician's orders for activity and fluids.
Pouchogram	Installation of radiopaque dye into the Kock or Indiana pouch. Done with the continent ostomies to determine the state of healing and size of the pouch created.	Assess the client for allergy to iodine. Explain the procedure to the client.
Pulmonary angiography	Assesses the arterial circulation of the lungs. Most often used to detect pulmonary emboli.	Explain the procedure to the client. Assess for allergy to iodine or shellfish. Inform the client that an arterial puncture is required, usually of the femoral artery, and that injection of the dye may cause a flushing or warm sensation due to vasodilation. After the study, assess the arterial puncture site frequently for evidence of bleeding. Assess vital signs and respiratory status. The client may be required to lie flat for up to 6 hours if the femoral artery is used for access. Obtain informed consent per facility policy.
Renal angiography	A catheter is inserted into the femoral artery and threaded into the renal artery. Dye is injected to show blood vessels in the kidney.	Initiate NPO status; administer enema. Assess client for allergy to iodine or shellfish. Check vital signs and peripheral pulses. Institute post-test bedrest, with leg straight. Monitor vital signs, peripheral pulses, urine output, and puncture site.
Voiding cystourethrography	The bladder is filled with dye, and x-rays are taken to observe bladder filling and emptying. Detects structural abnormalities of the bladder and urethra and reflux into the ureters.	Administer enema. Insert a Foley catheter and inject dye into bladder while x-rays are taken. Remove catheter and ask the client to void while more x-rays are taken. Allow the client to express feelings, as this test may be embarrassing.

continues

Table 27–8 RADIOLOGIC STUDIES *continued*

TEST	EXPLANATION/NORMAL VALUES	NURSING RESPONSIBILITIES
Computed tomography (CT) scan	Provides a three-dimensional cross sectional view of tissues. Computer-constructed picture interprets densities of various tissues. Most useful for viewing tumors in the chest, abdominal cavity, and brain.	Explain the procedure to the client. Obtain informed consent. Remove wigs and hairpins and clips for head CT. Initiate NPO status 8 hours prior to scan. Assess for iodine allergy. Observe for signs of anaphylaxis, if dye is used. Check for claustrophobia. Inform the client that the test will take approximately 45 minutes to 1 hour. The client must lie still on a hard, flat table and will be put through a large machine. Because barium will interfere with the test, schedule tests using barium either after or 4 or more days before the scan.
Cardiac positron emission tomography (PET) scan	Radioactive tracers are injected intravenously prior to the test. Nuclear imaging is used to confirm tissue that has adequate blood supply and tissue that has become impaired due to a lack of blood.	Instruct the client not to have caffeine for 18 hours and not to smoke for 4 hours prior to the test. Initiate NPO status from 10 P.M. the evening before the test, except for medications and water. Obtain informed written consent. Encourage the client to drink fluids after the procedure to facilitate faster excretion of the radioactive material.
Orbital CT scan	Allows visualization of abnormalities not readily seen on standard x-rays, delineating size, position, and relationship to adjoining structures. The orbital CT is a series of images reconstructed by a computer and displayed as anatomic slices on an oscilloscope. It identifies space-occupying lesions earlier and more accurately than do other x-ray techniques. It also provides three-dimensional images of orbital structures, especially the ocular muscles and optic nerve. Enhancement with a contrast agent may help define ocular tissue and circulation abnormalities.	Explain the test and the procedure to the client: that the client is positioned on an x-ray table; that the head of the table is moved into the scanner; that the scanner rotates during the test and may make loud, crackling sounds; that if an IV contrast agent is required, the client may feel flushed and warm or experience a transient headache; and that salty taste, nausea, and vomiting may occur following injection of the IV contrast dye. Reassure the client that the reaction is common and she may signal the technician if she is unable to tolerate the test.

Chest X-Ray

The most common radiological study is the noninvasive, noncontrasted chest x-ray. Radiographic projections of chest x-ray films are taken from various views (Figure 27-4), because the practitioner needs multiple views of the chest to assess the entire lung field. To prepare for a chest x-ray, the client should remove all clothing from the waist up and don a gown. The client should also remove all metal objects (jewelry), as metal will appear on the x-ray film, thereby obscuring visualization of parts of the chest. Pregnant women are advised against x-rays; however if x-ray is absolutely necessary, the woman should be draped with a lead apron to protect the fetus.

Computed Tomography

Computed tomography (CT) is the radiological scanning of the body. X-ray beams and radiation detectors transmit data to a computer that transcribes the data into quantitative measurement and multidimensional images of the internal structures. Figure 27-5 illustrates the sagittal, transverse, and coronal planes used in CT scanning.

The procedure requires the client's informed consent. Because the client will be positioned on the scanning table and told to remain motionless, the client's cooperation is essential during the CT scanning. The nurse should prepare the client by providing an explanation and pictures of what to expect.

Safety: Contrast Media
If a contrast medium is used, observe the client for indicators of allergic reaction to the dye, such as respiratory distress, urticaria, hives, nausea, vomiting, decreased production of urine (**oliguria**), and decreased blood pressure.

PROFESSIONAL TIP

Computed Tomography
Assess the client's ability to relax, and review imagery relaxation. Sedation can be administered with an order from the practitioner.

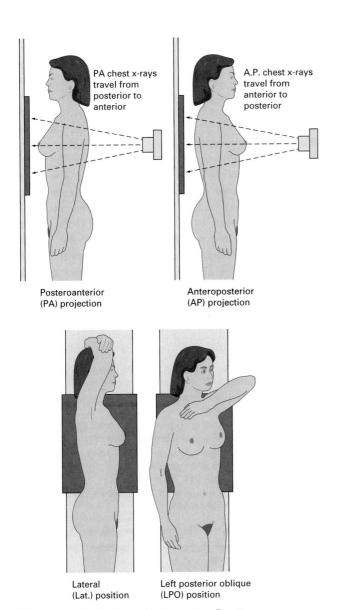

Figure 27-4 Radiographic Projection Positions

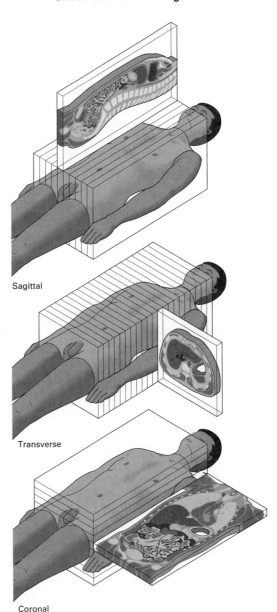

Figure 27-5 Computed Tomography

Barium Studies

Barium (a chalky white contrast medium) is a preparation that permits roentgenographic visualization of the internal structures of the digestive tract. The results of barium studies can reveal congenital abnormalities, lesions, spasm, reflux, stricture, obstruction, inflammation, ulceration, varices, and fistula.

Angiography

Angiography allows visualization of the vascular structures through the use of fluoroscopy in conjunction with a contrast medium. The test reveals the blood flow to the heart, lungs, brain, kidneys, and lower extremities. It is also useful in diagnosing an **aneurysm** (weakness in the wall of a blood vessel).

Arteriography

Arteriography is the radiographic study of the vascular system following injection of a radiopaque dye through a catheter. The practitioner uses fluoroscopy to thread the catheter through a peripheral artery and into the area to be studied, such as the aorta or the cerebral, coronary, pulmonary, renal, iliac, femoral, or popliteal artery. The client is placed on a cardiac monitor. Dye is injected through the vascular catheter, and a rapid sequence of films is taken to visualize the vasculature.

Dye Injection Studies

Iodine is a common dye used in radiographic studies. Iodine injection might cause the client to experience the following temporary symptoms: shortness of breath; nausea; and a warm to hot flushed sensation. Most dye injections studies are invasive and thus require written consent.

ULTRASONOGRAPHY

An **ultrasound,** also called an echogram or sonogram, is a noninvasive procedure that uses high-frequency sound waves to visualize deep body structures. To ensure accuracy, this procedure should be scheduled before any studies requiring the use of a contrast medium or air, because the contrast medium would reflect the sound waves differently than body structures do. The client is instructed to lie still during the procedure.

Ultrasound is used to evaluate the brain, thyroid gland, heart, vascular structures, abdominal aorta, spleen, liver, gallbladder, pancreas, and pelvis. An ultrasound is commonly done during pregnancy to evaluate the size of the fetus and placenta. A full bladder is needed to ensure visualization.

To increase the contact between the skin and the **transducer** (instrument that converts electrical energy to sound waves), a coupling agent (lubricant) is placed on the surface of the body area to be studied. The transducer emits waves that travel through the body tissue and are reflected back to the transducer and recorded. The varying density of body tissues deflects the waves into a differentiated pattern on an oscilloscope. Photographs can be taken of the sound wave pattern on the oscilloscope. Table 27–9 describes some ultrasound tests.

Table 27–9 ULTRASOUND TESTS

TEST	EXPLANATION/NORMAL VALUES	NURSING RESPONSIBILITIES
Ultrasound	High-frequency ultrasound waves are sent into the body, and echoes are recorded as they strike tissues of different densities, producing an image or photograph. Useful in distinguishing between cystic and solid masses. Most often used to assess the pelvis, heart, and abdomen. Diagnostic for cysts, tumors, pregnancy, fetal gestational age, and multiple gestation.	Explain the procedure to the client. Most ultrasound tests require no special preparation: Pelvic sonogram: Instruct the client to have a full bladder. Abdominal sonogram: Initiate NPO status at bedtime; prepare bowel as directed. Gallbladder sonogram: Initiate NPO status for 12 hours and institute a fat-free diet the evening before the test. Vaginal sonogram: Client does not need to have a full bladder.
Doppler ultrasound	Determines patency of veins and arteries in conditions such as arterial occlusive disease, arteriosclerotic disease, or Raynaud's disease. Normal: audible "swishing" sound of the Doppler when placed over vessel A Doppler unit with blood pressure cuffs can measure the pulse volume of arteries and veins. An AB index is obtained by dividing the blood pressure reading in the ankle by the blood pressure reading in the arm (brachial artery). This is known as the ankle-to-brachial arterial blood pressure. There should be a less than 20 mm Hg difference between the pressure in the lower extremity as compared to the pressure in the upper extremity. Normal, AB index: 0.85 or greater	Inform the client that the procedure is painless. Remove clothing from the extremity being evaluated. Instruct the client not to smoke for 30 minutes prior to the test, because nicotine causes vasoconstriction of the vessels. Remove conductive or acoustic gel from the skin after the test is completed.
Echocardiogram	An ultrasound of the heart to determine hypertrophies, cardiomyopathies, or congenital defects. Very helpful in diagnosing valve abnormalities and pericardial effusion.	Explain the procedure to the client and assure the client that there is no discomfort during the procedure, although some pressure may be felt on the chest wall from the transducer.
Thyroid ultrasound	Detects the size, shape, and position of the thyroid gland.	Explain the procedure to the client: that the client will lie supine, with the neck hyperextended; that breathing or swallowing will not be affected by the sound transducer; that a liberal amount of lubricating gel will be placed on the neck for the transducer; and that a series of photos will be taken over a 15-minute period. Assist the client in removing the lubricant.
Transrectal bladder ultrasound	Produces an image of the prostate or bladder and surrounding tissue.	Explain the procedure to the client.

Table 27–10 MAGNETIC RESONANCE IMAGING

TEST	EXPLANATION/NORMAL VALUES	NURSING RESPONSIBILITIES
Magnetic resonance imaging (MRI)	Uses magnetic field and radio waves to detect edema, hemorrhage, blood flow, infarcts, tumors, infections, aneurysms, demyelinating disease, muscular disease, skeletal abnormalities, intervertebral disk problems, and causes of spinal cord compression. Provides greater tissue discrimination than do chest x-ray or CT scans. Performed by qualified technologist. Takes approximately 1 hour.	Assess the client for the presence of metal objects within the body (i.e., shrapnel, cochlear implants, pacemakers). Explain the procedure to the client: that the client will be required to lie still for up to 20 minutes at a time; that the client will be placed within a scanning tunnel; that sedation may be required if the client has claustrophobic tendencies; that the magnet will make a loud thumping noise as images are obtained (provide earplugs as necessary). As the test may require up to 2 hours to perform, have the client void prior to entering the scanning tunnel. Obtain informed written consent, per facility policy.

MAGNETIC RESONANCE IMAGING

Magnetic resonance imaging (MRI) uses radiowaves and a strong magnetic field to make continuous cross-sectional images of the body. A noniodine IV paramagnetic contrast agent may be used during the study. The study reveals lesions and changes in the body's organs, tissues, and vascular and skeletal structures (Table 27–10).

RADIOACTIVE STUDIES

Radionuclide imaging (nuclear scanning) uses radionuclides (or radiopharmaceuticals) to image the morphological and functional changes in the body's structure. A scintigraphic scanner is placed over the area of study to detect emitted radiation and produce a visual image of the structure on film. Radiopharmaceutical agents are administered by various routes, with consideration given to time delays of absorption. The results reveal congenital abnormalities, lesions, skeletal changes, infections, and glandular and organ enlargement (Table 27–11).

Table 27–11 RADIOACTIVE STUDIES

TEST	EXPLANATION/NORMAL VALUES	NURSING RESPONSIBILITIES
Scan (radioisotope test)	A radioactive substance or isotope is taken up by the part of the body being examined. Organ sites most frequently studied are the liver, spleen, lungs, heart, urinary tract, thyroid, and brain. The radioactive substance is given orally or intravenously by nuclear medicine personnel.	Explain the procedure to the client: that the client must lie still for 30–60 minutes and that the machine makes clicking noise at times. For liver, spleen, lung, thyroid, and brain scans, no special preparation is required. For a heart scan, initiate NPO status the evening before. For a kidney scan, hydrate as ordered.
Brain scan	A radioactive agent is injected into a vein and allowed to circulate to the brain; the brain is then scanned in successive layers and a picture composite of the structures developed. Useful in identifying structural lesions, whether vascular or tumors.	No food or fluid restrictions. The test takes approximately 2 hours. Obtain informed consent according to facility guidelines. Explain that the client may experience a hot feeling when dye is injected. Assess for allergies, especially to iodine or shellfish. Administer a light sedative, if ordered.

Radioactive iodine uptake, (RAIU), iodine uptake test, ^{131}I uptake	Uses oral radioactive iodine to determine thyroid function by the thyroid's ability to trap and retain iodine.
	Normal:
	  2 hours: 4%–12% absorbed
	  6 hours: 6%–15% absorbed
	  24 hours: 8%–30% absorbed
		The client who is allergic to iodine or shellfish or is pregnant should not have the test.
		
		Exogenous iodine preparations or recent x-ray studies using iodinated contrast material will decrease thyroid gland uptake.
		
		continues

Table 27–11 RADIOACTIVE STUDIES *continued*

TEST	EXPLANATION/NORMAL VALUES	NURSING RESPONSIBILITIES
Radioactive iodine uptake, (*continued*)		Note those medications taken that may affect results. Drugs that may increase RAIU level include barbiturates, estrogen, lithium, phenothiazines, and TSH. Drugs that may decrease RAIU level include ACTH, antihistamines, saturated solution of potassium iodine, thyroid drugs, antithyroid drugs, and tolbutamide.
Radionuclide angiography (multiplegated radioisotope scan, multigated acquisition scanning, MUGA)	A radioisotope is injected to evaluate the function of the left ventricle. The ejection fraction (a comparison of the volume of blood pumped by the left ventricle to the total volume of blood left in the ventricle) is measured.	Obtain informed written consent per agency policy.
Renal scan	Uses radioactive material (gallium 67) to show blood flow in the kidneys.	Check policy on disposal of client's urine for first 24 hours. Pregnant nurses should not care for clients undergoing this test because of the associated radiation.
Technetium pyrophosphate scanning	Important in diagnosing acute MIs, with the best accuracy obtained at 48 hours after the client experiences symptoms suggestive of an infarct. A tracer or radioisotope, which is injected intravenously, accumulates in the damaged or infarcted tissue areas, called hot spots.	Instruct the client not to smoke or consume caffeine or alcohol for 3 hours before the test. Inform the client that the test will take 45–60 minutes.
Thyroid scan, thyroid scintiscan	Uses a radioactive substance to visualize the size, shape, position, and function of the thyroid gland. Normal: no growth or enlargement	Assess for allergy to iodine or shellfish and for pregnant. Recent exposure to iodine-containing foods or x-ray iodinated contrast agents can interfere with test results. Drugs that can interfere with test results include cough medicines, multiple vitamins, some oral contraceptives, and thyroid drugs. Explain the procedure to the client. Certain drugs may have to be restricted for weeks before the test. Obtain a history concerning previous contrast x-ray studies, nuclear scans, or intake of thyroid-suppressive or antithyroid drugs. Fasting is usually not required. The scan may be taken 2 hours or 24 hours after oral ingestion of the radioactive substance. The client should be instructed to remove all jewelry, metal objects, and dentures before the scan. The scan takes approximately 30 minutes. Neither isolation nor specific urine precautions are necessary.
Ventilation-perfusion scan	Assesses ventilation and perfusion of the lungs. Most often used to detect the presence of pulmonary emboli.	Assess for allergy to iodine and shellfish. Explain the procedure to the client: that a radioactive contrast media will be introduced via an IV access and inhalation of radioactive gas and that the client will be required to hold the breath for short periods as images are obtained. Obtain informed written consent per facility policy.

ELECTRODIAGNOSTIC STUDIES

Electrodiagnostic tests use devices to measure the electrical activity of the heart, brain, and skeletal muscles. Electrical sensors (electrodes) are placed at certain anatomic points to measure the tone, velocity, and direction of the impulses. The impulses are then transmitted to an oscilloscope or printed on graphic paper. Table 27–12 describes the various electrodiagnostic studies.

Electrocardiography

An **electrocardiogram** (ECG or EKG) is a graphic recording of the heart's electrical activity. The client may be asked not to smoke or drink caffeinated beverages

Table 27–12 ELECTRODIAGNOSTIC STUDIES

TEST	EXPLANATION/NORMAL VALUES	NURSING RESPONSIBILITIES
Electrocardiogram (ECG or EKG)	Electrodes are placed on the skin to record wave patterns of the electrical conduction of the heart. Detects myocardial damage, rhythmic disturbances, and hyperkalemia.	Explain the procedure to the client. Inform the client that the test is painless.
Electroencephalogram (EEG)	Record of electrical activity generated in the brain and obtained through electrodes applied to the scalp or microelectrodes placed in brain tissue during surgery.	Withhold caffeine due to stimulant effect. Serve meal so that blood sugar will not be altered. Explain the procedure to the client: that the test takes approximately 45 minutes to 2 hours; that electrical shock will not occur; that the procedure is painless and that there are no after effects; that the client may be asked to open and close the eyes during the test and that there may be flashing lights or small electrical stimulations.
Electromyography (EMG)	Detects primary muscular disorders. A needle electrode is inserted into the muscle being examined. Measures electrical activity of skeletal muscle at rest and during voluntary muscle contraction.	Explain the procedure to the client. Obtain informed written consent. Instruct the client to refrain from consuming caffeine and smoking for 3 hours before the test. Assure client that the needle will not cause electrocution. Inform the client that there will be temporary discomfort when the needle electrode is inserted. Observe the site for hematoma or inflammation after the test. The procedure takes approximately 1 hour.
Electroretinogram (ERG)	A record of the changes in the retina's electric potential following stimulation by light. Clinically useful in some clients with retinal disease. Performed by placing a contact lens electrode on the anesthetized cornea. The electrical potential recorded on the cornea is identical to the response that would be obtained if the electrodes were placed directly on the surface of the retina.	Explain the test and procedure to the client.
Esophageal motility studies (manometry)	Evaluates muscle contractions and coordination by using a tube with transducers. Used as a diagnostic tool for disorders of the esophagus and lower esophageal sphincter (LES).	Initiate NPO status 6–8 hours prior to the test.
Holter monitor	A portable EKG monitors and records the electrical conduction of the heart for a period of 24 hours. The heart rhythm is compared to client activities.	Instruct the client to engage in normal daily activities and to keep a journal of symptoms experienced in performing these activities.
Stress test	An EKG taken as the client exercises. Evaluates the effects of exercise on the heart. Often, the client is asked to walk on a treadmill, the incline of which is elevated at various times throughout the test. Used frequently on clients who have CAD.	Explain the procedure to the client. Encourage the client to wear good walking shoes during the test.
Thallium test (myocardial perfusion scan)	A radioactive tracer (Thallium^{201}) is injected and accumulates in myocardial tissue that is well perfused. Accumulation is lessened in areas of myocardial tissue that are not well perfused, areas called "cold spots." The client may be asked to perform exercise, such as riding a bike, during the test to evaluate the perfusion of myocardial tissue during exercise.	Instruct the client to refrain from eating and drinking for 3 hours prior to the test.

for 24 hours before the test, as nicotine and caffeine can affect heart rate.

Electrodes are applied to the chest wall and extremities. A lubricating gel applied to the electrodes increases the conduction of electrical activity between the skin and electrodes. The client is instructed to lie still during the pain-free test. The test can reveal abnormal transmission of impulses and electrical position of the heart's axis.

A portable cardiac monitor (Holter monitor) is a device that records the heart's electrical activity. It produces a continuous recording over a specified time (e.g., 24 hours). The portable unit allows the client to ambulate and perform regular activities. Clients are instructed to maintain a log of those activities that result in the heart beating faster or irregularly. The practitioner reviews the ECG tracing in relation to the client's log to determine whether certain activities, such as walking, are associated with abnormal transmission of impulses.

Stress Test

A **stress test** measures the client's cardiovascular fitness. It demonstrates the ability of the myocardium to respond to increased oxygen requirements (the result of exercise) by increasing the blood flow to the coronary arteries.

The client is connected to an ECG machine and asked to walk on a treadmill. Continuous ECG recordings are made of the client's heart response (rate, electrical activity, and cardiac recovery time) to frequent changes in the treadmill's speed and slope. The test is stopped immediately if the client experiences any symptoms of decreased cardiac output (chest pain, dyspnea, fatigue, or ischemic changes revealed by the ECG monitor).

Thallium Test

Thallium[201] is a radioactive isotope that emits gamma rays and closely resembles potassium. Although a radioactive study, the thallium test is discussed here because it is often performed in conjunction with an ECG. Thallium is rapidly absorbed by normal myocardial tissue but is slowly absorbed by areas with poor blood flow and damaged cells. During the test, thallium is administered intravenously and the scanner detects the radiation and makes a visual image. The light areas on the image represent heavy isotope uptake (normal myocardial tissue), whereas the dark areas represent poor isotope uptake (poor blood flow and damaged cells).

There are two types of thallium test: resting imaging and stress imaging. Resting imaging can detect a myocardial infarction within its first few hours. Stress imaging (thallium stress test) is performed while the client is on a treadmill and being monitored with an ECG. At peak stress, the IV thallium is injected. Scan-

ning is performed 3 to 5 minutes postinjection and again in 2 to 3 hours. The test is stopped immediately if the client becomes symptomatic for ischemia.

Electroencephalography

An **electroencephalogram** (EEG) is the graphic recording of the brain's electrical activity. During the procedure, electrodes are placed on the client's scalp. The electrodes transmit impulses from the brain to an EEG machine. The machine amplifies the brain's impulses and makes a recording of the waves on strips of paper. An EEG can reveal not only the presence of a seizure disorder or intracranial lesion, but also the type. The absence of the brain's electrical activity is used to confirm death.

ENDOSCOPY

Endoscopy is the visualization of a body organ or cavity through a scope. An endoscope (a metal or fiberoptic tube) is inserted directly into the body structure to be studied (Figure 27-6). A light and, in some studies, a camera at the end of the scope allow the practitioner to assess, via direct visualization or television picture, for lesions and structural problems. The endoscope has an opening at the distant tip that allows the practitioner to administer an anesthetic agent and to lavage, suction, and biopsy tissue. Common endoscopic procedures are listed in Table 27–13.

After the procedure, the nurse must monitor vital signs, observe for bleeding, and assess for procedural risks (e.g., return of the gag and swallowing reflexes following a bronchoscopy performed under local anesthesia).

ASPIRATION/BIOPSY

Aspiration is performed to withdraw fluid that has abnormally collected or to obtain a specimen. To min-

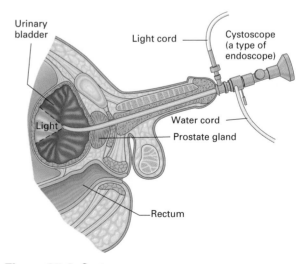

Figure 27-6 Cystoscope

Table 27-13 ENDOSCOPIC PROCEDURES

TEST	EXPLANATION/NORMAL VALUES	NURSING RESPONSIBILITIES
Endoscopy	Permits visual examination of internal structures of the body using specially designed instruments. The observation may be done through a natural body opening or through a small incision. A biopsy of suspicious areas may then be done for further study.	Explain the procedure to the client. Initiate NPO status 8–10 hours before test, except for sigmoidoscopy, before which a liquid diet should be followed for several days prior to the examination. Administer a laxative and then a cleansing enema.
Arthroscopy	Endoscopic procedure for direct visualization of a joint. Done in an operating room under sterile conditions and local or general anesthesia.	Perform frequent neurovascular checks. Elevate the client's leg. Apply compression dressing. Administer analgesic for discomfort.
Bronchoscopy	Direct visual examination of the bronchi through a fiber optic scope. Used to remove foreign bodies, for aggressive pulmonary cleansing, and to obtain sputum and tissue specimens.	Explain the procedure to the client: that the client must be NPO for at least 6 hours prior to the test; that, if ordered, preprocedure sedation is administered; that an IV access will be obtained and sedation given during the procedure via this route. Following the procedure, frequently assess vital signs and respiratory status. Assess the client for unusual amounts of bleeding. Inform the client that sputum may be blood tinged initially following the procedure. Maintain the client in a side-lying position until the gag reflex returns. Withhold all food and fluids until the client is fully awake and has a gag reflex. Obtain written informed consent per facility policy.
Colonoscopy	Examination of the rectum, colon, cecum, and ileocecal valve.	Initiate sedation. Cleanse the bowel. Offer only clear liquids after cleansing. Initiate NPO status for 6–8 hours prior to the test. Inform the client that flatulence and cramping will be experienced after the test.
Cystoscopy	A cystoscope is passed through the urethra and into the bladder to examine the interior of the bladder for inflammation, stones, tumors, or congenital abnormalities. A biopsy may be performed, and small stones may be removed. Ureteral catheters may be inserted to obtain urine from each kidney. May require topical, spinal or general anaesthesia.	Explain the procedure to the client. Obtain informed written consent. Check vital signs. Instruct in deep breathing, if general anesthesia is to be used. Allow a full liquid diet if topical anesthetic is to be used. Monitor I&O.
Endoscopic retrograde cholangiopancreatogram (ERCP)	Examination of the common bile duct (CBD) and biliary and pancreatic systems following injection of dye. Sphincterotomy, stone crushing, and stone removal can be done.	Initiate sedation. X-ray is used in conjunction. Initiate NPO status 6–8 hours prior to examination. Schedule PT, PTT, and bleeding time tests prior to this examination. Inform the client that the test can last up to 2 hours.
Esophagogastro-duodenoscopy (EGD)	Examination of the esophagus, stomach, and duodenum. Biopsies can be taken, and dilations done.	Initiate sedation. Initiate NPO status 6–8 hours prior to the examination.
Flexible sigmoidoscopy	Examination of the sigmoid colon and rectum.	Sedation is optional. Administer enemas prior to examination. Inform the client to expect some flatulence and cramping after the examination.
Laparoscopy	Examination of the internal pelvic structures by direct visualization with a laparoscope. Usually performed under general anesthesia. Diagnostic for pelvic disorders and infertility problems.	Explain the procedure to the client. Prepare the client, conduct pre- and postoperative assessment, and institute interventions. Provide discharge instructions on activity and follow-up.

imize client discomfort when the skin is pierced by the needle, a local anesthetic is administered in the area to be studied.

A stylet with an outer, hollow-bore needle is used to pierce the skin. Once the needle is in place, the stylet is withdrawn, leaving only the outer needle to aspirate the fluid. A **biopsy** (excision of a small amount of tissue) can be obtained during aspiration or in conjunction with other diagnostic tests (e.g., bronchoscopy). Table 27–14 outlines various aspiration/biopsy procedures.

Table 27–14 ASPIRATION/BIOPSY PROCEDURES

TEST	EXPLANATION/NORMAL VALUES	NURSING RESPONSIBILITIES
Aspiration Procedures		
Arthrocentesis	Procedure to obtain fluid from a joint using strict sterile technique. The knee is anesthetized, the sterile needle is inserted into joint space, and synovial fluid is aspirated. Used to diagnose infections, crystal-induced arthritis, and synovitis, and to inject anti-inflammatory medications. Performed by physician. Takes approximately 10 minutes.	Explain the procedure to the client. Obtain informed consent. Assess site for edema, pain. The client should fast if possible. Apply pressure dressing and ice.
Bone marrow aspiration	Evaluates how well the bone marrow is producing RBCs, WBCs, and platelets. Normal: adequate numbers of RBCs, WBCs, and platelets.	Inform the client that pressure will be felt when the physician aspirates the bone marrow. Assess the site for bleeding after the procedure is completed. Institute bed rest for at least 30 minutes after the test.

Gastric analysis, tube and tubeless test	Determines the amount of hydrochloric (HCl) acid in the stomach. If no HCl acid is present, that indicates parietal cells are malfunctioning. Parietal cells secrete the intrinsic factor that is essential for vitamin B_{12} absorption. Used to diagnose pernicious anemia.
	 Normal tube test:
	     Basal acid output: 2–5 mEq/h
	     Maximal acid output 10–20 mEq/h
	 Normal, tubeless test: presence of dye in urine (usually blue or blue-green in color)
		If the client is having the tube test, initiate NPO status after midnight and instruct the client not to smoke prior to the test. Inform the client that a nasogastric tube is inserted prior to the test so that gastric contents can be aspirated after the administration of pentagastrin.
		 If the client is having the tubeless test, inform the client of the possibility of a blue or blue-green discoloration of urine.
		 Note any medications taken that affect results; antacids, anticholinergics, and cimetidine (Tagamet) decrease HCl level, whereas adrenergic-blocking agents, cholinergics, steroids, and alcohol elevate HCl level.

Lumbar puncture (LP)	A needle is inserted into the subarachnoid space to measure CSF pressure and/or to obtain a specimen. Normal pressure: 60–180 mm water pressure Normal specific gravity: 1.007 Normal glucose: 60–80 mg/100 mL Normal complete blood count (CBC): 0 Normal WBC: 0–5 cells/mm^3	Obtain informed written consent. Have the client empty the bowel and bladder prior to procedure. Position the client in the dorsal recumbent position on the side of bed of physician's choice. Place the hips at the edge of the bed, client's back to the physician. Assist in setting up a sterile field and pouring solutions, if not included in the tray. Assist the client to maintain the position. Postprocedure, deliver the specimen to the lab for testing, keep the client flat in bed for 3–24 hours or as ordered by physician; encourage fluid intake to replace fluids lost; and monitor vital and neurological signs.
Peritoneal aspiration	Fluid is withdrawn from the abdominal cavity by inserting a needle into the abdomen. The specimen in analyzed for infection or bleeding.	Have the client empty the bladder prior to the procedure. Prepare the abdomen by scrubbing it with a surgical prep solution and draping it with a sterile drape. Post procedure, dress the site with a sterile dressing and monitor the site for further drainage. Assess vital signs one time post procedure.
Pericardiocentesis	Fluid is removed from the pericardial sac for analysis or to relieve pressure.	Inform the client that the procedure will be done under a local anesthetic and that pressure may be felt when the needle is inserted. Position the client in the semi-Fowler's position during the procedure and attach to an EKG monitor. Postprocedure, take vital signs every 15 minutes and monitor EKG rhythm.
Thoracentesis	Removal of fluid for diagnostic purposes. May also obtain biopsy, instill medications, and remove fluid for client comfort and safety.	Explain the procedure to the client. Obtain informed consent. Position the client in an upright sitting position, leaning forward. *continues*

Table 27–14 ASPIRATION/BIOPSY PROCEDURES *continued*

TEST	EXPLANATION/NORMAL VALUES	NURSING RESPONSIBILITIES
Thoracentesis (*continued*)		Have client rest the arms on an overbed table to facilitate this position. Explain to the client that the area will be anesthetized prior to the procedure. Instruct the client to hold as still as possible during the insertion of the thoracentesis needle. Assist the physician during the procedure. Deliver the specimen to the laboratory as soon as possible. Observe the thoracentesis site for bleeding following the procedure. Assess breath sounds before and after the procedure. Report absent breath sounds immediately.
Biopsy procedures	Removal of sample tissue for microscopic study. Tissue may be quickly frozen or placed in formalin before it is chemically stained and thinly sliced for analysis. Frozen section analysis takes only a few minutes and is often completed while a client is still in surgery. The full biopsy analysis takes 24–48 hours to complete but is the most accurate means of establishing a cancer diagnosis. Tissue biopsy is essential to confirming the type of cancer, the amount of lymph node involvement, and whether the cancer was successfully removed.	Explain the procedure to the client. Follow the physician's orders and/or agency protocol for client preparation. Obtain informed written consent.
Breast biopsy	Performed with or without local or general anesthesia and by aspiration, needle biopsy, excision, or incision. Tissue or fluid is obtained and sent to pathology for examination and identification of abnormal cells. New method of obtaining breast biopsies may be done with the stereotactic mammography studies.	Explain the procedure to the client. Have the client undress down to the waist. Cleanse the biopsy region and shave the area, if needed. Drape the breast and adjacent skin. Provide emotional support prior to, during, and following the procedure. Monitor vital signs. Apply a sterile dressing or bandage. Instruct the client in post-biopsy wound care.
Cardiac biopsy	Done during a cardiac catheterization. The tissue sample is taken from the apex or septum to determine toxicity related to drugs; inflammation; or rejection of a transplanted heart.	Preparation is the same as for Cardiac Catheterization (refer back to Table 27-8). After the procedure, observe the client for symptoms of a perforation, such as chest pain, decreased blood pressure, or dyspnea.
Endometrial biopsy	Obtained with special biopsy instruments and used to diagnose endometrial tissue abnormalities.	Explain the procedure to the client. Prepare the tissue preservation agent and label and send the sample to pathology. Assist the client in relaxing during the procedure, to offset the discomfort/cramping she may experience.
Liver biopsy	Obtained by inserting a needle into the liver. May be done with ultrasound or CT scan to guide needle placement. Evaluates cirrhosis, cancer, and hepatitis.	Schedule H&H, PT, PTT, and platelet tests prior to the procedure. Instruct the client to refrain from using NSAIDs including aspirin for 1 week prior to the procedure. Prepare the site by scrubbing it with a surgical prep solution and draping with a sterile towel. Monitor for signs of hemorrhage post procedure by frequently monitoring vital signs and pain. Have the client lie on the right side. Support the biopsy site with a towel or bath blanket for 2 hours. Monitor the site for ecchymosis.
Prostatic biopsy	Removal of a small piece of tissue for microscopic examination.	Monitor for and educate the client about signs and symptoms of hemorrhage, infection, and post-procedure pain.
Testicular biopsy	Determines presence of sperm and rules out vas deferens obstruction.	Monitor for and educate the client about signs and symptoms of infection or hemorrhage.
Thyroid biopsy	Excision of thyroid tissue for histological examination after noninvasive tests prove abnormal or inconclusive. Can be obtained through needle biopsy or open surgical biopsy under general anesthesia.	Explain the procedure to the client. Obtain informed written consent. Assess for allergies. Have coagulation blood studies done. Assess for bleeding and respiratory and swallowing difficulties after the test. To prevent undue strain on the biopsy site, instruct the client to put both hands behind the neck when sitting up. Warn the client that a sore throat is possible after the biopsy.

Bone Marrow Aspiration/Biopsy

The sternum and iliac crest are common sites for bone marrow puncture. During a bone marrow puncture, a fluid specimen (aspiration) or a core of marrow cells (biopsy) can be obtained. Both tests are commonly done concurrently to obtain the best possible marrow specimen. The test can reveal anemias; cancers such as leukemia, multiple myeloma, or Hodgkin's disease; or the client's response to chemotherapy.

Client positioning is determined by the site to be used, supine for the sternum and side lying for the iliac crest. The site is prepped to decrease the skin's normal flora in the area to be punctured. The nurse should explain to the client that pressure may be experienced as the specimen is withdrawn. The client should not move when the specimen is being withdrawn, as a sudden movement may dislodge the needle.

After the procedure, the client should be kept on bedrest for 1 hour. The nurse should monitor vital signs to assess for bleeding (rapid pulse rate, low blood pressure), and the client instructed to report to the practitioner any bleeding or signs of inflammation.

Paracentesis

Paracentesis is the aspiration of fluid from the abdominal cavity. This test can be diagnostic, therapeutic, or both. With end-stage liver or renal disease, for instance, **ascites** (an accumulation of fluid in the abdomen) occurs. Pressure caused by the ascites can interfere with breathing and gastrointestinal functioning. Aspiration in this instance is therapeutic. If a culture specimen is taken, it is also diagnostic.

The client should be instructed to void and the nurse should weigh the client before the procedure. The client should be placed in a high-Fowler's position in a chair or sitting on the side of the bed. The skin is prepped, anesthetized, and punctured with a **trocar** (a sharply pointed surgical instrument contained in a cannula). The trocar is held perpendicular to the abdominal wall and advanced into the peritoneal cavity. When fluid appears, the trocar is removed, leaving the inner catheter in place to drain the fluid. The client's vital signs are observed for changes resulting from the rapid removal of fluid.

After the procedure, a sterile dressing is applied to the puncture site, and the client monitored for changes in vital signs and electrolytes. The nurse should instruct the client to record the color, amount, and consistency of drainage on the dressing after discharge.

Thoracentesis

Thoracentesis is the aspiration of fluids from the pleural cavity. The pleural cavity normally contains a small amount of fluid to lubricate the lining between the lungs and pleura. Infection, inflammation, and trauma may cause an increased production of fluid, which can impair ventilation.

To facilitate access to the rib cage, the client should be positioned with the arms crossed and resting on a bedside table (Figure 27-7). The nurse should instruct the client not to cough during insertion of the trocar. The practitioner selects, preps, and anesthetizes the puncture site. The trocar is usually inserted into the intercostal space at the location of maximum dullness to percussion. The site should be above the ninth rib posteriorly and above the seventh rib laterally.

During the procedure the client must be carefully monitored for symptoms of a **pneumothorax** (collection of air or gas in the pleural space, causing the lungs to collapse), such as dyspnea, pallor, tachycardia, vertigo, and chest pain. After the procedure, the nurse assesses for signs of cardiopulmonary changes and a mediastinum shift, as indicated by bloody sputum and changes in vital signs.

Cerebrospinal Fluid Aspiration

Lumbar puncture (LP, "spinal tap") is the aspiration of cerebrospinal fluid (CSF) from the subarachnoid space. The specimen is examined for organisms, blood, and tumor cells. A spinal tap is also performed:

- To obtain a pressure measurement when blockage is suspected,
- During a myelogram, or

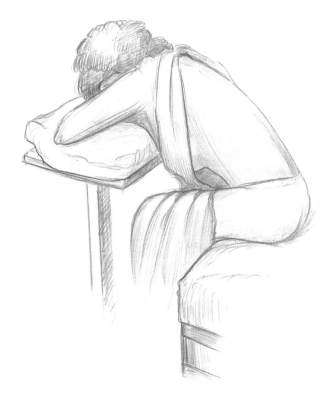

Figure 27-7 Client Position for Thoracentesis

- To instill medications (anesthetics, antibiotics, or chemotherapeutic agents).

The client assumes a lateral recumbent position, with the craniospinal axis parallel to the floor, the flat of the back perpendicular to the procedure table. The client should assume a flexed knee–chest position to bow the back, thereby separating the vertebrae. Most clients require assistance in maintaining this position throughout the procedure. To do so, the nurse stands facing the client and places one hand across the client's shoulder blades and the other hand over the client's buttocks.

The practitioner selects, preps, and anesthetizes the puncture site (usually interspace L3–L4, L4–L5, or L5–S1). The needle and stylet are inserted into the mid-sagittal space and advanced through the longitudinal subarachnoid space (Figure 27-8).

Once in the subarachnoid space, the stylet is removed, leaving the needle in place. An initial CSF pressure reading is taken. If the pressure reading is greater than 200 mm H_2O or falls quickly, only 1 or 2 mL of CSF is withdrawn for analysis. If the pressure is less than 200 mm H_2O, an adequate specimen is withdrawn slowly.

After the pressure reading is taken, the stopcock is turned to allow the CSF to slowly flow into a sterile test tube. A sterile cap is placed on the test tube, and the sample is taken to the laboratory for analysis. Rapid withdrawal of CSF can cause a transient postural headache. The client's cardiorespiratory status is monitored throughout the procedure.

OTHER TESTS

Other diagnostic tests are described in Table 27–15.

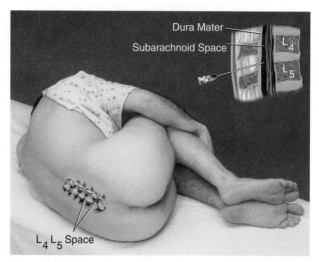

Figure 27-8 Lumbar puncture: Position of client and insertion of the needle into the subarachnoid space are shown.

 PROFESSIONAL TIP

CSF Pressure

The client should remain relaxed and quiet during the initial pressure reading, because straining increases CSF pressure.

After the procedure, pressure is applied to the puncture site, followed by a sterile bandage to prevent leakage of CSF. The client's neurological and cardiorespiratory statuses are then assessed. A postural headache is the most common complication of a lumbar puncture.

Table 27–15 OTHER TESTS

TEST	EXPLANATION/NORMAL VALUES	NURSING RESPONSIBILITIES
Arterial plethysmography (pulse volume recorder)	Determines arteriosclerotic disease in the upper extremities and occlusive disease in the lower extremities. Done by applying three blood pressure cuffs to an extremity. The cuffs are connected to a pulse volume recorder, which records the amplitude of each pulse wave. If there is a decrease in the amplitude of the pulse wave, an occlusion is in the artery proximal to the cuff. A decrease of 20 mm Hg of pressure indicates arterial occlusion. The test is not as reliable as arteriography but also does not have the risks associated with an arteriogram. Normal: normal arterial pulse waves	Explain to the client that the test is painless. Instruct the client to lie still during the test. Instruct the client not to smoke for 30 minutes prior to the test. Instruct the client to remove clothing from the extremity on which the test is to be done.

continues

Table 27–15 OTHER TESTS *continued*

TEST	EXPLANATION/NORMAL VALUES	NURSING RESPONSIBILITIES
Audiometric testing	Evaluates both bone and air conduction and determines the degree of hearing loss. The client wears headphones, through which a series of tones is delivered at different frequencies. The client signals to the audiologist when the tones are audible. The results are recorded on an audiogram. The client is kept in a sound proof booth during the test.	Explain the procedure and its purpose to the client. Ensure that the client is not claustrophobic.
Brainstem auditory-evoked response (ErA and BAER)	Detects hearing dysfunctions of the central nervous system and cochlear nerve (cranial nerve VII). Valuable for testing comatose clients, clients with neurological damage, and children. An altered appearance of the brainstem waveforms or a delay or loss of a waveform indicates an abnormality including a possible cochlear lesion or acoustic neuroma.	Explain the procedure and its purpose to the client particularly that the client will be in a darkened room and will have both electrodes attached to the head and earphones in place.
Caloric test	Assesses alteration in vestibular function. The client is placed in a supine or Fowler's position and each ear is irrigated with cold and then warm water. A decreased response or failure to respond within 3 minutes indicates that an abnormality may be present. Most commonly done on comatose clients. A punctured eardrum or Meniere's disease may contraindicate the test. Normal: vertigo, nystagmus, nausea, vomiting, and unsteady gait.	Explain the procedure and its purpose to the client. Tell the client that nystagmus, vertigo, nausea, vomiting, and an unsteady gait represent a normal response. Stay with the client and have an emesis basin and tissues available.
Color vision tests	Most common color vision tests use pseudoisochromatic (seemingly the same color) plates comprising patterns of dots of the primary colors superimposed on backgrounds of randomly mixed colors. A client with normal vision can identify the patterns; a client with a color deficiency cannot distinguish between pattern and background.	Explain the test and procedure to the client.
Colposcopy	Direct visualization of the vagina and cervix through a high-powered microscope. Acetic acid or other solution is applied to the tissue to dehydrate the cells for improved visualization. Used to diagnose cervical dysplasia or carcinoma in situ of the cervix. Biopsies may be obtained as needed.	Explain the procedure and prepare the client in the dorsal lithotomy position. Assist with the procedure. Prepare biopsy specimens for pathological examination.
Culture and sensitivity (C&S)	Determines presence of microorganism and identifies the antibiotic that will kill or inhibit growth of microorganism. Drainage from infected lesions is obtained with a sterile swab and is incubated in order to identify the causative organism and to determine antibiotic sensitivity. Normal: negative for microorganism growth.	Ensure that the specimen has been obtained before initiating antibiotic therapy. Specimens should be taken to the laboratory within 30 minutes of being obtained.
Cytology	The study of cells and fluids obtained from various organs by scrapings, brushings, or needle aspiration. Cytologic smears, such as the Pap smear, are routinely done to study cells from the female genital tract. A cytological smear showing evidence of malignancy is followed by a biopsy to facilitate a more comprehensive diagnosis.	Explain the procedure to be used for obtaining cells and fluids for study. Follow agency protocol for client preparation.
Dark field examination of wart scrapings	Microscopic examination to differentiate genital warts from syphilis condylomata.	Take a careful client history. Examine the genital area carefully and provide scalpel and slide, if specimen is to be obtained. Explain the procedure thoroughly to the client.
Dilatation and curettage (D&C)	Surgical scraping of the endometrial lining, performed under general, epidural, or paracervical anesthesia and on an outpatient basis. Diagnostic or therapeutic for uterine bleeding disorders.	Explain the procedure to the client. Perform pre- and postoperative assessment and provide care. Provide discharge instructions related to activities and follow-up appointments.

continues

Table 27–15 OTHER TESTS *continued*

TEST	EXPLANATION/NORMAL VALUES	NURSING RESPONSIBILITIES
Dynamic infusion cavernosometry and cavernosography (DICC)	Group of diagnostic tests that measure neuro-vascular events of penile erection.	Perform baseline assessment, monitor during the procedure, and assess for postoperative complications; advise the client of possible discomfort related to the injection. Explain the procedure to the client. Assess for allergies. If preferred by the laboratory, initiate NPO status after midnight. Restrict iodine and thyroid preparations a week before test. Inform the client that radioactive iodine may be given orally or intravenously. Withhold food for 45 to 60 minutes after the iodine is given. Provide the client with a list of times to report to radiology. Tell the client that he will lie supine for test, which takes about 30 minutes, and that neither isolation nor specific urine precautions are necessary.
Huhner test (post-coital test)	Performed in the office. The couple has intercourse 2 hours before the appointment. A sample of secretions is removed from the vagina and placed on a microscopic slide. The sperm are observed for number and motility in the cervical mucous. Normal: a minimum of 20 sperm per field that demonstrate good motility	Explain the procedure to the client and schedule it near client's normal ovulation. Prepare the client in the lithotomy position. Assist the physician or nurse practitioner with the procedure. Perform microscopic observations as directed.
Nocturnal tumescence penile monitoring	Various devices are attached to the penis at night to monitor swelling (tumescence).	Explain to the client that the test will require application of a device to the penis and that the device is to be worn while sleeping. Show the client the device and explain how to apply it.
Ophthalmoscopic examination	Examination of the fundus (posterior eye) using an ophthalmoscope. Magnifies vascular and nerve tissue of the fundus, including the optic disk, retinal vessels, macula, and retina. Used to diagnose diseases of the eye and aberrations in the refractive mechanism.	Explain the test and procedure to the client.
Otoscopic examination	Visual examination of the ear canal using an otoscope. The examiner looks for signs of inflammation, discharge, or foreign bodies. The tympanic membrane is normally pearly gray. The position and color of the membrane are noted as is any unusual appearance.	Explain the procedure and its purpose to the client. The ear should be clear of cerumen. Tilt the head away from the examiner and pull the earlobe up, back, and out to straighten the auditory canal. In children, pull the earlobe down and out to straighten the canal.
Papanicolaou (Pap) smear	Cells are obtained from the external and internal cervical canal. Used to diagnose cervical dysplasia or cancer.	Explain the procedure. Have client empty bladder and undress. Position client in dorsal lithotomy position. Help client relax during procedure. Prepare microscopic slides for pathology. Instruct the client on the importance of having an annual Pap smear.
Past-point testing	Measures the ability or inability to accurately place a finger on some part of the body, usually the client's or examiner's face and fingers. For example, the examiner will instruct the client to close her eyes and touch her nose, then, with eyes open, touch the examiner's nose or the examiner's index finger.	Explain the test and procedure to the client. Explain that it is painless and represents a helpful measure of vestibular function (coordination).
Patch testing	Allergens within occlusive patches are applied to normal skin (usually the upper back) for 48 hours. If the client is allergic to a specific allergen, an erythematous skin reaction will occur.	Clean and dry the skin where the patches are to be applied. Tell the client that the patches must be left in place for the full 48 hours.
Pelvic examination (recommended annually for women over 18 through menopause)	Performed by a physician or nurse practitioner. The external and internal pelvic structures are visualized, the pelvic organs are palpated via bi-manual examination, and the cervix is examined via a speculum. A Pap smear and rectovaginal exam are also performed, and cultures and wet smears may be obtained.	Explain the procedures to the client; prepare the client by having her void and undress; position the client on the examination table in a dorsal lithotomy position; help the client to relax during the examination, prepare slides and culture medium; obtain other supplies; and assist with the procedure.

continues

Table 27–15 OTHER TESTS *continued*

TEST	EXPLANATION/NORMAL VALUES	NURSING RESPONSIBILITIES
Prostatic smears	Microscopic examination of prostatic secretions obtained via rectal massage performed by a physician.	Explain to the client that to obtain the specimen, the prostate must be massaged via the rectum and that this will cause some discomfort.
Pulmonary function tests (PFTs)	A group of studies used to evaluate ventilatory function. Measurements are obtained directly via spirometer or calculated from the results of spirometer measurements. Bronchodilators may be used during the study. Measurements included are: Tidal volume: the amount of air inhaled and exhaled during a normal respiration. Inspiratory reserve volume: the amount of air inspired at the end of a normal inspiration. Expiratory reserve volume: the amount of air expired following a normal expiration. Residual volume: the amount of air left in lungs after maximal expiration. Vital capacity: the total volume of air that can be expired after maximal inspiration. Total lung capacity: the total volume of air in the lungs when maximally inflated. Inspiratory capacity: the maximum amount of air that can be inspired after normal expiration. Forced vital capacity: the capacity of air exhaled forcefully and rapidly following maximal inspiration. Minute volume: the amount of air breathed per minute.	Explain the procedure to the client, PFTs should not be done within 1–2 hours after a meal. After the test, monitor respiratory status. Advise the client to avoid activity and to rest following the test, as fatigue may result.
Pulse oximetry	A noninvasive procedure. A transdermal clip is placed on a finger or earlobe to detect the arterial oxygen saturation (SaO_2). Normal: > 95% (at sea level)	Explain the procedure to the client. Assess peripheral circulation, as this may alter results. Place the sensor on the earlobe, fingertip, or pinna of the ear. Keep the sensor intact until a consistent reading is obtained. Observe and record readings. Report to the physician measurements below 95%.
Rinne test (tuning fork)	Detects loss of hearing in one or both ears. Tuning fork is struck and placed against the mastoid bone to measure the sound conduction through the bone. The tuning fork is then placed beside and parallel to the ear to test conduction through the air. If the sound is louder when the tines are placed beside the ear, hearing is normal or the hearing loss is sensorineural. If the sound is louder when conducted through the bone, the hearing loss is conductive.	Explain the procedure and its purpose to the client.
Romberg test	Assesses vestibular (balance) function. The client stands with the eyes closed, arms extended in front, and feet together. Normal: slight swaying.	Explain the procedure and its purpose to the client. Stand close and reassure the client that someone will catch him if he begins to fall.
Schiller test	Performed during colposcopy. An iodine solution is applied to the cells of the cervix. Abnormal cells turn white or yellow. Aids in visualization of abnormal tissue and indicates areas for biopsy. Normal: cells turn brown	Explain the reason for the application of the solution. Assist with the biopsy procedure as necessary. Label tissue specimens and send to histology.
Segmented bacteriologic localization cultures	The first 5–10 mL of urine is collected, the next 200 mL is discarded, then 5–10 mL is collected midstream. The prostate is then massaged until prostatic secretions can be collected. Finally, 5–10 mL urine is collected before the bladder is emptied. Four samples are needed in sterile culture tubes.	Ensure that the client is well hydrated and has a full bladder.
Semen analysis	Determines the presence, number, and motility of sperm.	Teach the client about proper collection of sperm.

continues

Table 27–15 OTHER TESTS *continued*

TEST	EXPLANATION/NORMAL VALUES	NURSING RESPONSIBILITIES
Skin scrapings	A lesion is scraped with an oiled scalpel blade. The cells are then examined under a microscope. Used to diagnose fungal lesions.	Explain the procedure and its purpose to the client.
Slit-lamp examination	The cornea is examined with the aid of a slit lamp. A slit-like beam facilitates visualization of the layers of the cornea and lens, facilitating evaluation of the thickness of these structures and the location of disease processes. Useful in detecting and evaluating abnormalities of anterior segment tissues and structures. May reveal disorders such as iritis, corneal abrasions, conjunctivitis, and lens opacities (cataracts).	Explain the procedure and its purpose to the client.
Speech audiometry (Spondee threshold)	Evaluates ability to hear and understand the spoken word. A series of two-syllable words commonly recognized by their vowel sounds (like *toothbrush* and *baseball*) are delivered through earphones. When the client correctly repeats the word, the sound intensity is recorded in decibels. The test is normally conducted in a soundproof booth.	Explain the procedure and its purpose to the client. Ensure that the client is not claustrophobic.
Sputum analysis	Sputum samples are examined for the presence of bacteria, fungi, molds, yeasts, and malignant cells. Appropriate antibiotic therapy is determined via C&S studies.	Explain the procedure and its purpose to the client. Obtain specimens early in the morning to prevent contamination via ingested food or fluids. Instruct the client to breathe deeply and cough, so as to facilitate collection of a specimen originating from the lower respiratory tract. If necessary, pulmonary suctioning may be used to induce such a specimen. Instruct the client to expectorate sputum into the appropriate container. Deliver specimens to the laboratory as soon as possible.
Tonometry	Used to measure intraocular pressure and to aid in the diagnosis and follow-up evaluation of glaucoma. Two types of tonometric devices are used for assessment: applanation and indentation. An applanation tonometer is the most accurate and commonly used device and measures the force (delineated by the reading on the tension dial on the tonometer) required to flatten a small, standard area of the cornea. An indentation tonometer measures the deformation of the globe in response to a standard weight placed on the cornea. Before use of either apparatus, the eyes are anesthetized with a local ophthalmic solution, such as benoxinate with fluorescein or tetracaine, so that the pressure from the tonometer will not be felt. Normal: 12–22 mm Hg	Explain the procedure and its purpose to the client. Explain to the client that this test measures the pressure within the eyes and that although the test requires the client's eyes to be anesthetized, the anesthesia will wear off shortly after the examination is complete. Reassure the client that the procedure is painless.
Typanometry	Measures the movement of the eardrum in response to air pressure in the ear canal. Evaluates the presence of fluid in the middle ear and is commonly used to evaluate otitis media in children or adults.	Explain the procedure and its purpose to the client. Inform the client a small burst of air is introduced through the otoscope, which may produce an uncomfortable sensation.
Tzanck smear	Fluid from the base of a vesicle is applied to a glass slide, stained, and examined under a microscope. Used to diagnose herpes zoster, herpes simplex, varicella, or pemphigus. Normal: negative	Describe to the client how the laboratory technician will obtain the specimen and that although the procedure will likely not be painful, the client must remain still to prevent injury. Provide scalpel blade, glass slide, and stain for collection.
Urethra pressure profile (UPP)	Assesses functional urethral length and general competency of the urethra and sphincter, either at rest or during coughing, straining, or voiding. Functional profile length is the length from bladder outlet to the point in the urethra where urethral	Explain the procedure and its purpose to the client: that it is often performed when the bladder is empty and the client is at rest; that it may be performed simultaneously with CMG; and that the client may be asked to cough or

continues

Table 13–15 OTHER TESTS *continued*

TEST	EXPLANATION/NORMAL VALUES	NURSING RESPONSIBILITIES

Urethra pressure profile (UPP) *(continued)*	pressure equals intravesical pressure. Used to diagnose stress or overflow incontinence or urethral obstruction.
	
	Normal:
	  Male: bladder outlet through membranous urethra
	  Female: bladder outlet through mid-urethra
		void. Provide privacy, as the test can be embarrassing.

Uroflowmetry	Noninvasive assessment of urination. An electronic device connected to a funneled commode calculates the rate of urine flow, volume voided, and time taken to void.	Explain the procedure and its purpose to the client. Instruct the client to void as usual, leaving client alone to do so, if possible.
Venous plethysmography (cuff pressure test)	Assists in determining patency of veins. Two blood pressure cuffs are placed on the extremity, one proximally (occlusion cuff) and one distally (recording cuff). The cuffs are attached to pulse volume recorders. The occlusion cuff is inflated to 50 mm Hg pressure to occlude the venous flow of blood; the recording cuff is inflated to 10 mm Hg pressure. The pulse volumes are recorded and then the occlusion cuff is rapidly deflated. The pulse volume of the extremity should return to the preocclusion volume within 1 second if there is no occlusion in the venous system. A delay in the return of volume pressure is indicative of a thrombus. Normal: return of volume pressure to preocclusion value within 1 second after deflation of occlusion cuff The test is often done in conjunction with a doppler ultrasound. The test is not as reliable as a venogram.	Nursing responsibilities are the same as for Arterial Plethysmography (see beginning of table).
Visual acuity	Used to test distant and near visual acuity and to identify refractive errors in vision. Distant visual acuity is measured with a standardized visual acuity chart, e.g., a Snellen chart. Near visual acuity is measured with a Jaeger card (a card with print in graded sizes). Visual acuity is recorded as a fraction, with the numerator representing the distance to the chart and the denominator representing the distance at which a normal eye can read the line. Thus, the larger the denominator, the poorer the client's visual acuity. For example, if the client's vision is normal, results are expressed as 20/20, which means that the smallest symbol one can identify at 20 feet is the same symbol the normal eye can identify from the same distance.	Explain the procedure and its purpose to the client. Have the client stand the specified distance from the eye chart, usually 10 feet. Instruct the client to first cover one eye and then the other. If the client wears glasses, perform the test first with the client's glasses on and then with the client's glasses off.
Weber test (tuning fork)	Detects loss of hearing in one or both ears. Tuning fork is struck and the handle is placed in the middle of the forehead. Clients with normal hearing or bilateral deafness will hear or not hear the sound equally in both ears. Clients with unilateral hearing loss will hear the sound only in the unaffected ear.	Explain the procedure and its purpose to the client.
Wood's light examination	Skin and hair are examined under ultraviolet light (black light) in a darkened room. Used to diagnose fungal infections (tinea) of hair and skin.	Explain the procedure and its purpose to the client. Reassure the client that the rays are not harmful.

SUMMARY

- Most invasive procedures require that the client give informed consent.
- Nurses prepare clients for diagnostic testing by ensuring client understanding and compliance with preprocedural requirements.
- Clients, families, and significant others must be involved in the testing process. The nurse must advise them of the estimated time required to perform the procedure.
- To help offset the discomfort and anxiety experienced during procedures, the nurse teaches the client how to perform relaxation techniques such as imagery.
- After a diagnostic test, the nurse provides care and teaches the client those things to expect, including the outcomes or side effects of the test.
- The role of the nurse in diagnostic testing is to facilitate the scheduling of diagnostic tests, perform client teaching, perform or assist with procedures, and assess clients for adverse responses to procedures.
- Nurses should schedule diagnostic procedures to promote both client comfort and cost containment.
- Standard Precautions are used when obtaining a specimen for diagnostic examination or when assisting with an invasive procedure.
- Before the procedure, the nurse is responsible for obtaining baseline vital signs and assessing the client's preparation for testing.
- After the procedure, the nurse assesses the client for secondary procedural complications and performs any necessary nursing interventions.

Review Questions

1. Scheduling and sequencing of laboratory tests are important functions of the:

    a. nurse.
    b. physician.
    c. phlebotomist.
    d. laboratory supervisor.

2. The most commonly used site for capillary puncture in neonates and infants is the:

    a. heel.
    b. toetip.
    c. earlobe.
    d. fingertip.

3. When collecting a 24-hour urine specimen, the nurse knows:

    a. to put a large bottle at the client's bedside.
    b. the collection begins at the time of the first discarded voiding.

    c. that the client must urinate at a specific start time.
    d. to teach the client how to void in the large collection bottle.

4. The nurse knows that glucose spills into the urine when the blood glucose level exceeds the renal threshold of:

    a. 120 mg/mL.
    b. 140 mg/mL.
    c. 160 mg/mL.
    d. 180 mg/mL.

5. Occult blood may be found in which type of specimen?

    a. blood
    b. stool
    c. urine
    d. sputum

6. When scheduling a series of tests, the nurse knows to schedule:

    a. a barium enema before an upper GI.
    b. an ultrasound after all other tests.
    c. an upper GI before a gallbladder x-ray.
    d. a gallbladder x-ray before any barium studies.

7. A test that combines a radioactive scan with an electrodiagnostic study is a:

    a. MUGA.
    b. brain scan.
    c. thallium stress test.
    d. radioactive iodine uptake test.

Critical Thinking Questions

1. If a client's blood type is AB positive, what are the possible blood types of the client's parents? Can the client receive Rh-negative blood? Explain your answer.

2. The physician orders gallbladder x-rays, a barium swallow, an upper GI, and a barium enema. In which order should these tests be scheduled? Why?

 WEB FLASH!

- Search the web for "diagnostic tests." How many sites can you find? What type of information is available?
- Search the web for the specific diagnostic tests discussed in this chapter. How many tests have sites devoted to them? Is the information for health professionals or the general public?

UNIT
11
Special Areas of Nursing Care

Chapter 28
Nursing Care of the Older Client

Chapter 29
Rehabilitation, Home Health,
Long-term Care, and Hospice

NURSING CARE OF THE OLDER CLIENT

MAKING THE CONNECTION

Refer to the following chapters to increase your understanding of the older adult:

- **Chapter 8, Communication**
- **Chapter 23, Fluid, Electrolyte, and Acid–Base Balance**
- **Chapter 11, Client Teaching**

- **Chapter 14, The Life Cycle**
- **Chapter 15, Wellness Concepts**
- **Chapter 18, Basic Nutrition**
- **Chapter 20, Safety/Hygiene**

LEARNING OBJECTIVES

Upon completion of this chapter, you should be able to:
- *Define key terms.*
- *Describe stereotypes associated with older adults.*
- *Discuss the biological and psychosocial theories of aging.*
- *Cite the normal physiologic changes that occur with aging.*
- *List the normal functional changes that occur with aging.*
- *Describe key factors of optimal health maintenance in the aging adult.*
- *Identify funding and policy changes that have influenced elder care.*
- *Identify common disorders related to aging.*
- *Detail nursing interventions for each disorder.*
- *Discuss areas wherein the nurse can advocate for older adults on the individual, community, state, and national levels.*

KEY TERMS

activities of daily living
Balanced Budget Act
delirium
dementia
gerontological nursing
gerontologist

gerontology
Health Care Financing Administration
Omnibus Budget Reconciliation Act
polypharmacy

INTRODUCTION

Gerontology is the study of the effects of normal aging and age-related diseases on human beings. It is a general term used by all health care and social services disciplines. Aging (senescence) is a complex phenomenon that occurs on the continuum of human life, beginning with birth and continuing throughout the lifespan, and on into the end stages of life and death.

The phrase *older adult* is very subjective and has historically meant persons who are 65 years of age and older. However, there is a great deal of debate among **gerontologists** (gerontological specialists in advanced practice nursing, geriatric psychiatry, medicine, and social services) as to whether this specific age delineation should continue to be used. The practice of using 65 years of age as a dividing line for social welfare benefits began in the 1880s when Otto von Bismark randomly selected that age for benefits in Germany. It should be noted that there was no standardized clinical basis for establishing this age as the dividing line between young and old. Longer average life-expectancy rates (76.5 years for both genders, 73.6 years for men, and 79.4 years for women) (National Council on Aging [NCOA], 2000) along with a decline in the average number of children per family since the late 1960s have changed U.S. demographics. As a result, there is a great need to support and strengthen independence among older adults, and to value and utilize their life experiences in the areas of career, family, and community.

Retirement age is now less consistently determined by a mandatory age limit. Rather, retirement frequently is offered when the employee meets a formula of combined age and years of service. Since the 1990s, benefit penalties have been imposed on Social Security beneficiaries up to 70 years of age and who continue to earn incomes over a minimum amount. This was changed in April 2000 when the Senior Citizens' Freedom to Work Act of 2000 was signed into law by the president. This eliminates the Social Security retirement earnings test in and after the month in which a person is 65 years of age (the current full retirement age) (Social Security Administration [SSA], 2000).

Currently, the clinical delineation of an older adult is still someone who is 65 years of age or older; older-old adults are defined as those individuals 85 years of age or older. In 1900, there were a total of 3.1 million individuals over the age of 65 in the United States; by 1996, there were 33.2 million, 3.8 million of whom were over the age of 85 years (AARP, 1998). It is projected that by the year 2030, the number of older individuals in the United States will reach 69.4 million (Figure 28-1) including 8 million over the age of 85 (Administration on Aging [AoA], 2000). The most rapid increase is expected to occur in the years 2010–2030, when the "baby-boomers" reach age 65.

The aging of the United States and the world is a phenomenon that will impact all areas of society. The age range of 65 to 100+ years potentially comprises three generations: parents, grandparents, and great-grandparents. No other age group has the potential for as much diversity in both strengths and needs, both psychosocial and physical. Burggraf and Barry (2001) suggest ways these facts may affect gerontology, such as:

- More nurses will be needed for home health care and parish or neighborhood nursing.
- There will be more opportunities for gerontologic nurse-consultants.
- Nurse-researchers will be needed to study trends in aging.
- Preventing elder abuse.

The future will also place demands on those who were born from the late 1950s to the late 1960s. Many in this age group chose to focus first on career, delaying marriage and childrearing until in their thirties.

They have thus been labeled "the sandwich generation" to denote the challenges they will face in meeting social and financial responsibilities later in life as they work to provide for children entering college and for aging parents and, sometimes, grandparents and, in a few instances, great-grandparents.

This chapter presents an overview of influences on the older client, including the social impacts of aging. Also examined are theories of aging; myths and realities of aging; health promotion and aging; physiologic and functional changes that normally occur with aging; and some common disorders of aging along with nursing interventions to assist clients to achieve optimal outcomes related to those disorders.

As caregivers for older adults, nurses and other members of the client's health care team must also understand the budgetary and policy decisions that can affect the care they will provide to their clients. Thus, this chapter concludes with a short discussion on health care financing for elder care in the 21st century.

GERONTOLOGICAL NURSING

The acceptance of **gerontological nursing** as a separate nursing specialty that addresses and advocates for the special care needs of older adults has not been realized without a struggle. In 1961, gerontological nursing attained national recognition with the creation of its own division of nursing within the American Nurses Association (ANA). Nurses in the United States who were aware of the trends toward an aging population realized the importance of taking such a step. The charter members of the Division of Gerontological Nursing deserve a great deal of credit for their vision and commitment to developing gerontology education and recognizing the special nursing care needs of older adults. The major topics addressed in the over-

Number of persons 65+: 1900 to 2030

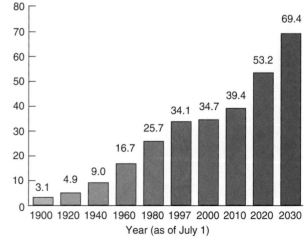

Figure 28-1 Number of Persons Over Age 65: 1900–2030 *(From* A Profile of Older Americans, *by The Administration on Aging and the AARP, 1998)*

view of the expanding scope of practice for gerontological nursing included (Bahr, 1994):

- The historical evolution of gerontological nursing practice based on population statistics;
- The way that ageism in U.S. society has affected the profession of nursing, the health care delivery system, and the care of older adults;
- Nursing education and care of older adults with a perspective derived from studies of the attitudes and interests of nursing personnel and nursing students;
- The delineation of various aspects of nursing care of older adults, including clinical practice based on the ANA Standards of Nursing Practice; select theories of nursing applied to the care of older adults; and the expanding scope of gerontological nursing, in general, and the roles of clinical nurse specialists and geriatric nurse practitioners, in particular; and
- Trends in gerontological nursing and long-term care.

The battle continues against the stereotyping of older adults, both in the health professions and in the community at large. There are many stereotypes or preconceived notions associated with aging and being old. Stereotypes are usually generated in an attempt to categorize people or to set standards that can be applied to large groups of people. They are often based on an individual's experience with persons in that group. Stereotypes may be true of some individuals, but not of a collective group.

Health professionals, in particular, must be diligent in avoiding age prejudice, as believing stereotypes can influence interactions between older adults and caregivers. The caregiver may treat the older adult as a child in an old body. This approach is demeaning to elders and strips individuals of their self-esteem and dignity. Clients with cognitive or expressive deficits cannot always process questions or comments quickly or follow through with responses. Nurses and caregivers must never make the mistake of believing that clients do not understand verbal and, especially, nonverbal messages. Elders are a diverse group; they deserve respect and, through their memories and life examples, can teach a great deal to younger persons about life and survival and coping skills. Learning from clients and their families and assisting clients to find activities that enhance the quality of life (regardless of state of health) make caring for older adults a rewarding and satisfying experience.

Aging is universal, progressive, and irreversible and eventually leads to death. The aging process itself, however, is very individualized and is independent of chronological age. The way whereby an individual ages is influenced by genetics; lifestyle; availability and quality of health services; cultural beliefs; and socioeconomic status. Certain physiologic changes are expected with aging (Figure 28-2), although there exists considerable variation in the time of onset, rate, and degree of these changes. In order to render effective

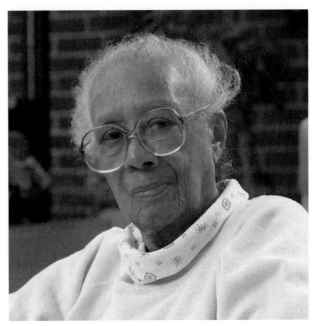

Figure 28-2 The aging process is a normal and natural part of growth and development.

and compassionate care to elderly clients, nurses working in gerontology must be familiar with the normal processes as well as the common disorders of aging.

THEORIES OF AGING

At this time, no single theory of aging has been universally accepted by practitioners in gerontology. Aging is a complex issue that must take into account the psychosocial, cultural, and experiential aspects of living. Several biological theories of aging have been proposed to explain the physiologic and functional changes that are observed in older adults. Psychosocial theories of aging strive to explain the behaviors and social interactions of older adults. These theories are summarized in Table 28–1. It should be noted, however, that each generation is unique and that biological and psychosocial theories of aging are thus unlikely to be universal. Also, as more knowledge is garnered from scientific studies (e.g., the study of the impact on cells of auto-oxidization by free radicals and the study of dietary chemical exposure) and gene sequencing efforts (e.g., the human genome project), it is likely that the biological theories of aging will change as well.

MYTHS AND REALITIES OF AGING

Myths are fictitious ideas. Myths about elders are abundant and do not reflect the reality of the aging population. Following are some common myths associated with aging, based (in part) on data from the United States Bureau of Census and *A Profile of Older Americans* developed by the American Association of Retired Persons (AARP) in 1998.

Table 28–1 THEORIES OF AGING

BIOLOGICAL THEORIES

Title	Major Premise
Somatic mutation theory	Radiation or miscoding of enzymes causes changes in the DNA. Changes associated with aging are the result of decreased function and efficiency of the cells and organs.
Programmed aging theory	The life span is programmed within the cells. This genetic clock determines the speed at which the person ages and eventually dies.
Cross-linkage, or collagen, theory	Collagen is the principal component of connective tissue and is also found in the skin, bones, muscles, lungs, and heart. Chemical reactions between collagen and cross-linking molecules cause loss of flexibility, resulting in diminished functional mobility.
Immunity theory	The thymus becomes smaller with age. The ability to produce T-cell differentiation decreases. This impairs immunologic functions and results in increased incidence of infections, neoplasms, and autoimmune disorders.
Stress theory	Stress throughout the lifetime causes structural and chemical changes in the body. These changes eventually cause irreversible tissue damage.

PSYCHOSOCIAL THEORIES

Title	Major Premise
Activity theory	Roles and responsibilities change throughout the lifetime. Life satisfaction depends on maintaining an involvement with life by developing new interests, hobbies, roles, and relationships.
Disengagement theory	There is decreased interaction between the older person and others in his social system. The disengagement is inevitable, mutual, and acceptable to both the individual and society.
Continuity theory	Successful methods used throughout life for adjusting and adapting to life events are repeated. Characteristic traits, habits, values, associations, and goals remain stable throughout the lifetime, regardless of life changes.

Myth: Senility is an expected result of aging.

Reality: Senility is an outdated term once used to refer to any form of dementia that occurred in older people. Dementia is a result of disease, can affect adults of all ages, and is not a natural consequence of aging. Although some slight declines are noted in short-term memory from the age of 40 on, most people adjust through the use of memory aids such as lists and calendars. Long-term memory can actually become clearer with age. Even for a client with dementia, long-term memory can remain somewhat intact long into the disease process. Thus, nurses

CULTURAL CONSIDERATIONS

Aging

At the same time that diversity continues to broaden in the United States, it remains important to understand the individual needs of clients. As with all clients, it is important to assess the older client's religious beliefs, traditions, and culture and to evaluate the ways that these may influence the client's health beliefs and health practices. Not only can caregivers make the mistake of not fully assessing the client's beliefs about health in elders, they can also be misled themselves by myths about aging that exist in U.S. society.

and caregivers find that interventions such as reminiscence, memory photo books, and activities that draw on the client's long-practiced skills provide positive client outcomes (Figure 28-3).

Myth: Incontinence is an expected result of aging.

Reality: Incontinence is not an expected outcome of aging and, in most cases, can be reversed through assessment and treatment. The challenge is that many people are embarrassed to discuss this problem with family or primary providers. Also, in long-term care settings, both the belief in this myth and the historically low staffing levels have served to dissuade clinical efforts at providing the needed nursing interventions (prompted voiding; consistent, nonhurried, timed voiding) to reverse urinary incontinence. In settings where care is provided to older adults, lack of funding, lack of policy support and education, and inconsistent enforcement of adequate staffing levels have often had a negative impact on client health outcomes. By developing urinary incontinence treatment programs, care facil-

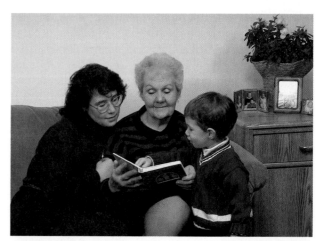

Figure 28-3 Sharing memories and photographs with younger family members is valuable for all generations.

ities could improve clinical outcomes for clients and also reduce health care costs.

Myth: Older adults are no longer interested in sexuality or sexual activity.

Reality: Sexuality is a lifelong need. Elders can be and are sexually active, regardless of age. Although sexual function may be affected by changes in the reproductive systems, persons of both genders are capable of orgasm into old age. Despite interest and desire, physiologic or psychological problems and medication side effects may present barriers to intercourse. In such situations, sexuality without coitus can provide elders with love and intimacy. It is important to remember that human beings are social beings. Just as small babies can fail to thrive without human touch (hugs, nurturing, companionship, valuing of the individual), so can older adults fail to thrive without these same human interactions and support (Figure 28-4).

A national survey by NCOA in 1998 revealed that half of those age 60 and older were sexually active. Approximately 72% of those were as satisfied or more satisfied with their sex lives compared to when they were in their forties (NCOA, 2000).

The medication sildenafil citrate (Viagra) has proven beneficial to many older couples as they work to meet their sexual health needs. The debate over the acceptance and funding of this medication for erectile dysfunction sheds light on just how far U.S. society still has to go in debunking this myth and replacing it with the truth that normal human sexuality needs continue throughout the life span.

Myth: Most people spend the last years of their lives in nursing homes.

Reality: According to NCOA (2000), in 1996 only 4.2% of those over age 65 lived in nursing homes. The percentage rises steeply with age, however (1% of those 65 to 74 years of age, 4% of those 75 to 84

years of age, and 20% of those over 85 years of age). For many, that stay will involve rehabilitation following surgery, a fracture, or stroke before returning home after a short hospital stay. The late 1990s have seen a growing interest in the use of alternative care options for elders (retirement communities, assisted living centers, group homes, respite care, and partial hospitalization/adult day programs). However, the majority of older adults continue to live in communities with varying levels of assistive services or support as they age. The projected trends in long-term care needs are for continued use of alternate settings that will support interventions to meet residents' physical, psychosocial, cultural, spiritual, cognitive, and mental health needs.

Traditionally, elders in long-term care facilities have been taken from home environments where they have likely experienced the highest level of independence they have had in their lifetimes (to choose when to get up, eat, go to bed, and the like), and have been placed in settings where very few, if any, choices, including care decisions, are made based on their preferences. Gerontological nurses have an ongoing responsibility to help recreate the way care is provided to elderly clients and to advocate for individual choices for older clients in long-term care facilities. Nurse leaders must learn to think in new ways about long-practiced trends in elder care in the United States and to work with older clients and their families to envision and create better trends.

Myth: All elderly persons are financially impoverished.

Reality: Income range varies among those over 65 years of age, just as it does among those in younger groups. However, the high costs of medications does disproportionately affect those over age 65, who are more likely to have one or more chronic conditions that require management with medication. In the past, lack of reimbursement for preventive assessment, treatments, and medications led many elders to go without medications or to delay care until they were too ill to wait any longer. This resulted in increased use of acute care services in hospitals.

In 1996, families headed by persons over 65 years of age had a median income of $28,983, despite the fact that the median net worth of older households (assets over expenses) is $86,300 (AARP, 1998). The challenge for most elders below the median (especially older women, who often have lower retirement incomes) is that most of their assets are tied up in the family home or in other nonliquid holdings. Thus, when an acute illness strikes, there is little financial reserve to help cover costs.

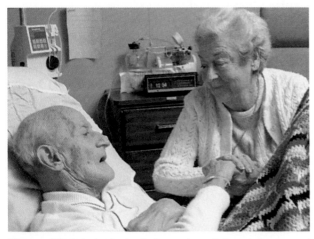

Figure 28-4 Individuals of all ages benefit from intimacy and companionship.

HEALTH AND AGING

Like all age groups, elders can do much to adopt a healthy lifestyle that will enhance their remaining years.

Activities of Daily Living

Being well groomed enhances the self-esteem of all older adults. Adaptive devices and techniques are available for those who need assistance with the **activities of daily living** (ADLs), basic care activities that include mobility, bathing, hygiene, grooming, dressing, eating, and toileting.

Mobility

Many assistive devices are available to help the older client maintain mobility and independence. Handrails can decrease the risk of falls while the person is walking (Figure 28-5); they are also useful in the tub and, when used in conjunction with a plastic riser, can help the older adult get on and off the toilet safely.

Bathing

Skin dryness increases with aging; thus, it may be preferable for older adults to bathe or shower only two to three times per week and to take sponge baths in between. A gentle soap should be used sparingly for the bath, after which a moisturizing lotion should be applied. The individual or caregiver should be instructed to inspect the skin during bathing for any indication of skin breakdown, lumps, or changes in moles.

With aging oil secretion decreases in the scalp, and hair can thus become dry. Shampooing one or two times per week is usually adequate for most elders, and a simplified hairstyle may be helpful to those with limited mobility in the arms. The use of mild shampoos and conditioners can also enhance hair texture.

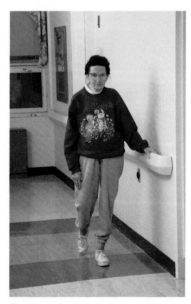

Figure 28-5 Handrails allow clients more independence when ambulating.

Hygiene

Fingernails may become more brittle with aging. Keeping the client's fingernails clean and short can prevent accidental injury or scratches to fragile older skin. Impaired circulation is common among older adults, and special attention should thus be given to care of the feet and lower extremities. Because toenails frequently become thick and tougher with aging, soaking the feet prior to trimming the toenails may ease the task. For clients with circulation or skin integrity problems of the feet and toes or for clients with diabetes, a referral to a podiatrist should be made for nail trimming. During bathing, the client's feet should be monitored for discomfort; inflammation; broken skin; color changes such as redness, pallor, or cyanosis (blue or purple discoloration resulting from lack of circulation); heat or coldness; cracking between toes; and corns or calluses.

The need for adequate oral care does not diminish with aging. Dental problems can result in poor eating habits and inadequate nutrition. Inadequate brushing and dental check-ups can lead to gingivitis (bleeding and edematous gums), which, if left untreated, can progress to periodontal disease that can destroy connective tissue, alveolar bone, and periodontal ligaments. The nurse must therefore monitor clients for proper oral care. For those clients with dentures, the nurse must inspect the dentures for cleanliness and proper fit. Clients with dentures must brush the dentures and the gums regularly with a soft brush and a mild cleanser. It is helpful to label dentures with the client's name to facilitate identification of the dentures in the event that the client is admitted to a hospital or an assistive care setting.

Grooming

Good grooming is important in promoting the older client's self-esteem and confidence. Keeping the hair neat and tidy, choosing attractive clothing and jewelry, and making decisions about makeup and other personal care practices will all contribute to the older client's sense of well-being and independence (Figure 28-6).

Male clients may feel much better with a clean shaven face. Infection-control principles demand that each razor (either electric or blade) be used for only one individual, and that that razor be marked with the client's name. Women may also require attention to facial hair, as estrogen levels decrease after menopause. It is not uncommon for older women to notice hairs on the chin or upper lip that were not there in younger days. Also, both men and women are likely to notice graying and diminished hair on legs, underarms, and pubic areas as they age.

Dressing

Dressing may be difficult for clients who have restricted joint movement, paralysis, or limited endurance

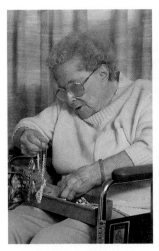
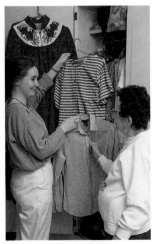

Figure 28-6 Good grooming for the older client includes choosing personal items such as jewelry and clothing.

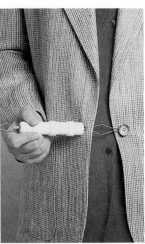
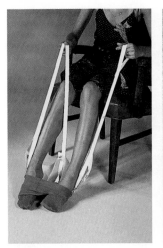

Figure 28-7 Assistive devices such as these for pantyhose and buttons are available to help clients dress independently. *(Courtesy of Maddak, Inc.)*

due to health problems. Many choices are available to ease dressing, such as elastic waists, velcro fasteners, and assistive reaching and dressing devices (Figure 28-7).

Eating

Many older adults are able to maintain the ability to self-feed, thereby promoting independence and self-esteem. Neurological and musculoskeletal alterations may, however, affect ability to self-feed. Dysphagia, or difficulty swallowing, may place the older client at increased risk of choking, and diminished taste sensation may affect the desire to eat.

Toileting

Toileting habits also change with aging. Bowel elimination problems can often be prevented as clients age by:

- Ensuring adequate fiber intake,
- Ensuring adequate fluid intake,
- Ensuring regular daily exercise, and
- Developing regular elimination habits.

For the client in the hospital or a long-term care facility, it is helpful to:

- Maintain previously effective habits such as reading on the toilet or drinking warm liquids upon arising, and
- Assist the client to the toilet approximately 30 minutes after eating, to take advantage of the gastrocolic reflex.

As a result of the physical changes that occur with aging, increased frequency of urination may be noted in elders of both genders. It is not uncommon for older adults to self-limit fluid intake due to a fear of incontinence. This habit is unhealthy and should thus be discouraged. Cases of incontinence should be assessed to determine the cause and type, so that appropriate interventions and treatment can be implemented. Timing

the use of prescribed diuretics in the morning rather than the evening can prevent the increased need for urination at night, which is especially helpful to older clients who are being treated for congestive heart failure (CHF).

Exercise

What was once accepted as the normal deterioration of old age is now considered the result of disuse through sitting and bed rest. Research indicates that high-intensity, progressive resistance training can improve muscle strength and muscle size in frail elderly clients. Walking and all other maneuvers required for ADLs are also beneficial. Exercise programs should be individually planned and should take into consideration the older person's:

- General health status (Figure 28-8),
- Physiologic disorders (if present),
- Preference for solidarity or group activity,
- Physical environment, and
- Financial status.

PROFESSIONAL TIP

Bowel Patterns in Elderly Clients

It is extremely important that caregivers of older adults monitor bowel patterns. Long periods of constipation (> than 2 to 3 days) should alert caregivers to the need for interventions to minimize the likelihood of bowel impaction, which can ultimately be life threatening if left untreated. Evacuation aids such as laxatives, lubricants, stool softeners, and enemas all have side effects and should thus be avoided if at all possible. Dietary changes or an exercise regimen should be introduced first.

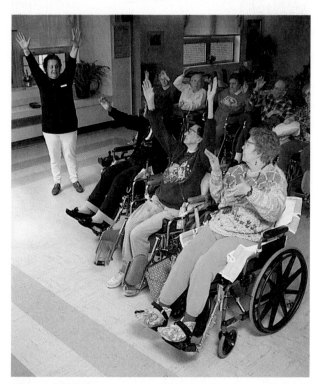

Figure 28-8 Exercise is important to all clients and should be tailored to interests and ability levels.

Nutrition

For many older adults, cultural heritage, religious rites, ethnic practices, and family traditions are linked to food. The physiologic, psychological, sociological, and economic changes of aging may compromise nutritional status. Elders must follow a balanced diet, often with lowered intakes of sugar, caffeine, and sodium. There are no universally accepted dietary guidelines specific to older adults. A dietitian can determine the needed food intake for a specific individual by taking into account the individual's height, ideal weight, activity level, and disease processes.

The National Institutes of Health (NIH) recommends 1,000 mg of calcium per day for both men and women over the age of 25. Postmenopausal women 50 to 65 years of age who are not receiving estrogen therapy have been reported to need 1,500 mg of calcium per day (Yen, 1995). It is important to note that calcium supplements should also contain vitamin D to provide for optimal metabolism by the body. The need for additional supplements depends on the older individual's nutritional status and ability to maintain an adequate diet. Growing discussion supports the needs for adequate protein intake, to maintain both skin integrity and bone density; moderate carbohydrates intake due to the metabolism of carbohydrates to sugars; and, whenever possible, the acquisition of needed calcium from dietary intake of unprocessed natural cheeses (Peskin, 1999).

It is important that nurses be knowledgeable about community services designed to help older clients meet their nutritional needs. Such services include grocery transportation and delivery services, homebound meals (e.g., Meals on Wheels), group meals at senior food sites, and the Food Stamp program. Nurses and caregivers should also realize that socialization and companionship are necessary components of adequate dietary intake, and should thus ensure that these areas are addressed as part of any food-assistance intervention.

Psychosocial Considerations

Older adults, like all individuals, have psychosocial and cognitive needs for lifelong learning. Many colleges have developed education program options for elder students (often at no tuition), and employers are beginning to recruit older workers for part-time positions (recognizing their historically good work ethic and experience). Many elders continue to volunteer countless hours each year, offering to help meet the social service needs of their communities. These efforts can result in feelings of productivity and self-worth for the older adult. Mental activity and emotional involvement are as necessary to the overall well-being as is physical activity. Older clients can benefit from building on their long-practiced skills to develop interesting and stimulating activities or hobbies. Such activities may be of an individual or group nature. Socialization with people of all age groups can help not only the older participants, but also the young and middle-age participants, by illustrating that aging is not a disease but, rather, a rich and natural part of the life process.

Strengths

Older adults generally have suffered many losses over the years. Some losses are slight and require only minor adaptation, whereas others may significantly affect the person. Physiologic changes or disease processes may result in losses, causing impairments in:

- Communication,
- Vision and learning,
- Mobility,
- Cognition, or
- Psychosocial skills.

If the impairment is severe, the individual could lose some degree of independence, and adaptations may be required. Furthermore, losses can cascade for the older client, as one loss contributes to another. For example, if an elderly person with diabetes were to lose her driver's license due to impaired vision related to diabetic retinopathy, socialization might be restricted, which in turn might increase her feelings of loneliness and diminished self-esteem. If, however, her spouse provides caregiving and transportation, these adaptations might allow her to remain active socially while still living in her home. If her spouse later dies, and her health continues to decline, a move to an assisted living facility may become necessary, if other community adaptations are unavailable. She would then be faced with adapting to the loss of both her home and her spouse.

Health care professionals should remember that persons who have lived for many years are survivors and can adapt to life changes better if they are allowed to utilize their existing strengths. They are often much stronger and more ingenious and enterprising than they are given credit for. The strengths of each individual (including past coping skills) must be identified and utilized when planning care and assisting the older client to find new ways to adapt and maintain optimal independence in a new setting.

Health Promotion and Disease Prevention

Older adults must be alerted to means of preventing disease and reducing risks. Being knowledgeable about self-care and participating in screening tests are important components of health maintenance. For older men, annual prostate examinations and a regular prostate specific antigen (PSA) level lab test, which can detect prostate cancer in the early stages, are recommended every 1 to 2 years. For older women, annual mammograms and Pap smears, and monthly breast self-examinations represent means of detecting breast and gynecological cancers in the early stages. Nurses can teach their clients habits for healthy living and inform them of signs and symptoms that require medical investigation. Older clients who have been exposed to environmental chemicals, tobacco, or extensive alcohol use over many years often experience serious health consequences as they reach older age. Older clients of any age can benefit from healthy lifestyles and from disease-prevention interventions such as being inoculated yearly against influenza and every 6 years against pneumonia; assessment of tuberculosis (TB) status; and adequate safe food and clean water intake.

In many cases, by the time a person reaches 65 to 70 years of age, that person has been prescribed medication to address at least one ongoing (chronic)

PROFESSIONAL TIP

Identifying Strengths of Older Adults as Part of Assessment

Assessment should include the identification of strengths as well as problems. Strengths are utilized to achieve or maintain optimal physical, mental, and emotional function. All of the following can be considered strengths:

- Cognitive health
- Freedom from or successful adaptation to deficits or impairments
- A history of healthy lifestyle with regard to diet, sleep, stress management, exercise, and chemical abuse (none)
- Adequate functional ability to carry out ADL
- Freedom from incapacitating physical discomfort and pain
- A physically safe living environment
- Feelings of security in present environment
- Realistic knowledge about capabilities
- Pattern of avoiding dangerous situations and unnecessary risks
- Compliance with health care regimen
- Capability with regard to managing own environment
- An intact support system
- Satisfying relationships with others
- Opportunities for sexual expression
- Access to transportation
- Adequate functional mobility
- Successful adaptation to life changes and crises
- History of relinquishing roles as phases of life require and replacing them with satisfying new roles
- A pattern of successful mourning for losses

- Participation in groups: religious, community, hobbies
- Membership in family whose members respect each other and are willing to give and receive help when necessary
- Successful problem-solving skills
- Willingness to seek information to improve situation
- Evidence of initiative and self-confidence in abilities and judgment
- Participation in self-care by making decisions and accepting responsibility for decisions
- A well-defined value system
- Acceptance of that which cannot be changed
- Successful use of assertive skills
- Strong spiritual beliefs and ability to find comfort and strength in spiritual and religious practices
- Enthusiastic appreciation for aging, with demonstrative embrace of the positive aspects and adaptation to the negative aspects
- Participation in healthy reminiscing; evidence of few regrets about life past
- Joyful appreciation for nature, art, music, hobbies, and activities
- A well-developed sense of humor

medical problem (e.g., hypertension, heart disease, diabetes, allergies, gastrointestinal disorders). The challenge many elders face is that side effects from one medication are often treated with another prescription medication. If the client then goes to different doctors, these doctors may prescribe even more medications to address the same or other health concerns. This is called **polypharmacy**, or the problem of clients taking numerous prescription and over-the-counter medications for the same or various disease processes, with unknown consequences from the resulting combinations of chemical compounds and cumulative side effects. In many settings, primary care providers, nurses, clinical pharmacists, and social workers collaborate on interdisciplinary teams to assist the older client and the family to oversee the client's medication management, as well as other health needs.

Among the biggest challenges facing older clients are shorter hospitalization stays and reduced time with physicians in the physician's offices. There is less time to ensure that the follow-up services the client will need are understood and in place and less time to educate client and family about medication regimens, including timing and possible interactions with other prescription and over-the-counter drugs or herbal remedies that the client may also be taking. The nurse, as part of the interdisciplinary team, plays a vital role as client advocate when ensuring that older clients have the teaching, services, and follow-up care they need.

PHYSIOLOGIC CHANGES ASSOCIATED WITH AGING

Although the aging process brings with it many physiologic changes, it should be remembered that aging and disease are not synonymous. Whereas the physiologic changes of aging described following are normal for most people, the medical disorders described are not considered normal.

Respiratory System

Review the anatomy and physiology of the respiratory system. The following respiratory changes result from the aging process:

- The muscles of respiration become less flexible, causing decreased vital capacity of the lungs.
- Decrease in functional capacity results in dyspnea on exertion or stress; usual activity does not affect breathing.
- Effectiveness of the cough mechanism lessens, increasing the risk of lung infection.
- The alveoli thicken and decrease in number and size, causing less effective gas exchange and, in individuals who also have chronic lung disease, intensifying respiratory deficits.

- Structural changes in the skeleton, such as kyphosis (seen in clients with osteoporosis as an often asymetrical convex curve of the spine) can decrease diaphragmatic expansion. Kyphosis in older clients can lead to a need for small, more frequent meals to balance nutritional requirements and respiratory function due to the restriction of adequate space for expansion and contraction of the diaphragm. It can also create skin integrity risks, as the bony prominences of the client's back press against the backs of chairs.

Common respiratory disorders related to aging include the following:

- Respiratory tract infection (RTI)
- Chronic obstructive pulmonary disease (COPD)
- Pulmonary tuberculosis (TB)

Nursing Interventions: Respiratory Tract Infections

1. Advise discussing the pneumovaccine with the primary care provider.
2. Advise obtaining annual influenza vaccine.
3. Assist the client to assume a position of comfort and assist with medications and respiratory treatments, as ordered.
4. Avoid distention of bowel, bladder, or stomach, any of which can increase breathing discomfort.
5. Allow adequate time for nursing care.
6. Administer humidified oxygen therapy, as prescribed.
7. Administer analgesics and antipyretics, as prescribed.

PROFESSIONAL TIP

TB in the Elderly Client

Elders can be vulnerable to TB because of:

- An ineffective cough reflex and the resulting inability to clear the lungs.
- An altered immune system and a reduced response to extrinsic antigens. Not only are elders at increased risk of infection via a new contagion, but older clients who contracted TB years ago and have been in remission since can experience reexacerbation. The risk of reexacerbation increases in cases where the initial infection was remote and healed (encapsulated) such that the immune system's memory of the T cells has been lost. Facilities where health care is provided to older clients and to immune compromised clients thus must regularly assess the TB status of both their clients and their employees.

8. Assess for signs of dehydration and ensure that fluids are accessible to the client, unless contraindicated.
9. Review diagnostic data and monitor lung sounds and intake and output every 8 hours or as needed given changes in the client's condition. Weigh the client daily, assessing for fluid retention.
10. Monitor for any signs of respiratory distress (cyanosis of lips, mucous membranes, or nailbeds) and obtain pulse-oximetry readings, as needed.

Nursing Interventions: Chronic Obstructive Pulmonary Disease

1. Assist the client to a position of comfort.
2. Teach the client to use pursed-lip breathing to avoid hyperventilation when short of breath.
3. Teach the client diaphragmatic breathing for use when active.
4. Teach proper use of inhalers. Steroid inhalers should be used first, with a full 60-second wait between puffs; after waiting 3 minutes, any bronchodilator inhalers that are prescribed should then be used, also with a 60 second wait between puffs.
5. Teach the client to cough and clear the airway.
6. Adminster chest physiotherapy (e.g., percussion, postural drainage), if prescribed.
7. Establish a schedule for ambulation, gradually increasing the distance ambulated.
8. Assist with active assistive range of motion exercises.
9. Monitor for signs and symptoms of infections (e.g., fever, blood-tinged or thick, greenish colored sputum, and diminished lung sounds) and immediately report same to the registered nurse and the primary care provider.
10. Monitor breathing and pulse rate and administer oxygen, if necessary, during periods of increased activity.

PROFESSIONAL TIP

COPD

Remember that in the client with COPD, breathing may not be triggered by a higher level of carbon dioxide as it would in clients without COPD, because the client with COPD always has a consistently high CO_2 level. The breathing impulse is instead triggered by a low level of oxygen. Increasing the oxygen level by more than 1 to 2 L/h in the client with COPD can shut shut down the trigger to breathe, and can drive the client into respiratory failure.

11. Suggest smoking cessation programs, if the client is a smoker.

 Safety: Oxygen and Smoking
Ensure that no smoking is allowed around clients on oxygen therapy.

Nursing Interventions: Pulmonary Tuberculosis

1. Monitor clients for TB status and for symptoms including fever, night sweats, weight loss, and cough producing blood-tinged sputum.
2. Inform the client, family, and caregivers of the need for adequate isolation techniques.

 Infection Control: TB
Remember that TB is spread through droplets when a client sneezes or coughs (direct and indirect contact). Consult the infection-control nurse on the client's interdisciplinary team and work to protect the client and others from transmission of *Mycrobacterium tuberculosis* and other infections.

3. Evaluate the client's risk for infection with the human immunodeficiency virus (HIV) and related pneumocystic pneumonia.
4. Monitor that the client's psychosocial needs are being adequately met while the disease is being pharmacologically addressed with medications like isoniazid (Laniazid). Tell the client and family that the entire course of medication must be completed.
5. Monitor the client's nutrition intake and provide supplements as necessary to maintain adequate body weight.
6. Provide for rest periods throughout the day. Encourage the older client with TB to monitor activity level and length of visits by family so as not to become overtired.

Cardiovascular System

Review the anatomy and physiology of the cardiovascular system. The following cardiovascular changes result from the aging process:

• Cardiac output and recovery time decline. The heart requires more time to return to a normal rate after a rate increase in response to activity.
• The heart rate slows.
• Blood flow to all organs decreases. The brain and coronary arteries continue to receive a larger volume than do other organs.
• Arterial elasticity decreases, causing increased peripheral resistance and, in turn, a rise in systolic blood pressure and a slight rise in diastolic blood pressure.
• Veins dilate, and superficial vessels become more prominent.

Common cardiovascular disorders related to aging include the following:

- Peripheral vascular disease (PVD)
- Hypertension
- Chronic congestive heart failure (CHF)

Nursing Interventions: Peripheral Vascular Disease

1. Assess the lower extremeties, including the peripheral pulses, for signs of arterial or venous insufficiency.
2. Evaluate lifestyle factors that may aggravate or advance atherosclerosis, such as a high-carbohydrate, high-fat diet and little exercise.
3. Teach the client about the disease, including treatment, medication actions and side effects, and signs of thrombosis.
4. Educate the client and caregivers about the care and inspection of the lower extremeties.
5. Provide instructions on interventions specific to the client's type of PVD (arterial or venous).

Nursing Interventions: Hypertension

1. Evaluate food intake patterns, especially of cholesterol, fats, sodium, and carbohydrates. Make recommendations based on findings.
2. Evaluate for fluid retention.
3. Recommend a smoking cessation program, if necessary.
4. Advise the client to avoid alcohol use.
5. Recommend and facilitate a consistent and appropriate exercise program.
6. Discuss the relationship of stress to hypertension and provide resources from which the client can learn relaxation techniques.
7. Provide information on medications and the importance of taking daily blood pressure medications as prescribed, regardless of health status on any given day.
8. Arrange for and encourage regular blood pressure checks and teach the client or significant others proper use of blood pressure equipment, if applicable.

Nursing Interventions: Chronic Congestive Heart Failure

1. Frequently monitor serum digitalis level and monitor for any signs of digoxin toxicity, for which older clients are at increased risk due to the decreased rate of renal clearance of the drug. Withhold the digoxin and immediately contact the registered nurse and the physician if abnormal serum level or signs and symptoms of toxicity are present.

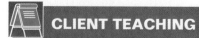

CLIENT TEACHING

Digoxin Toxicity

Possible signs and symptoms of digoxin toxicity include the following:
- Disturbances in cardiac rhythms
- Fatigue
- Listlessness
- Anorexia
- Nausea
- Visual disturbances (halos around lights)
- Shaking
- Unsteady gait
- Confusion

2. Take the apical pulse for a full 1 minute before administering digoxin. Withhold the medication if the apical pulse is below 60, and consult the registered nurse and the physician if this or any other significant changes in vital signs are noted.
3. Monitor the client's blood pressure and lung sounds.
4. Monitor electrolyte levels, blood urea nitrogen (BUN), and creatinine level to observe system changes including decreased kidney efficiency.
5. Monitor for signs of fluid retention such as intake and output (output too small), weight gain, shortness of breath, or coughing.
6. Encourage alternating periods of activity with periods of rest.
7. Encourage the client to maintain a level of exercise/physical activity appropriate to physical condition.
8. Teach the client and family about the safe use of the prescribed medications.
9. For clients on diuretics, which deplete potassium, monitor fluid intake and level of potassium, ensuring adequacy of each. Encourage administration of diuretics early in the day, unless contraindicated, to prevent increased urination at night.

Gastrointestinal System

Review the anatomy and physiology of the gastrointestinal system. The following gastrointestinal changes result from the aging process:

- Tooth enamel thins.
- Periodontal disease rate increases.
- Taste buds decrease in number, and saliva production diminishes.
- Effectiveness of the gag reflex lessens, resulting in an increased risk of choking.

- Esophageal peristalsis slows, and the effectiveness of the esophageal sphincter lessens, causing delayed entry of food into the stomach and increasing the risk of aspiration.
- Hiatal hernia may occur.
- Gastric emptying slows. Food remains in the stomach longer, decreasing the capacity of the stomach.
- Peristalsis and nerve sensation of the large intestine decreases, contributing to constipation.
- The incidence of diverticulosis increases with age.
- Liver size decreases after age 70.
- Liver enzymes decrease, slowing drug metabolism and the detoxification process.
- Emptying of the gallbladder lessens in efficiency, resulting in thickened bile, increased cholesterol content, and increased incidence of gallstones.

PROFESSIONAL TIP

Determining Alterations in Nutrition

- Height and weight: Record actual body weight, usual body weight, and ideal body weight. If usual weight has varied significantly from the ideal for several years, the use of height/weight tables may be meaningless. Compare actual body weight to usual body weight to determine present status.
- Review laboratory values: hematocrit, hemoglobin, total iron-binding capacity, total protein, BUN.
- Determine whether client is on a weight-loss diet.
- Determine whether client was edematous when initially weighed and has lost weight with treatment.
- Evaluate cognitive status. Cognitively impaired clients may be unaware of hunger or be unable to attend to the task of eating.
- In clients with central nervous system damage, evaluate the presence of sensory–perceptual deficits that interfere with eating.
- Evaluate ability to pick up utensils and glasses and to get items from table to mouth.
- Evaluate dental/oral status: status of teeth/dentures, gums, presence of oral dryness (xerostomia).
- Determine presence of impaired swallowing.
- Determine whether client has distaste for certain food groups.
- Assess knowledge in regard to nutrition and food purchase and preparation.
- Determine whether client is taking medications that interfere with taste or food absorption.
- Determine whether financial status interferes with food purchasing.
- Evaluate for history of compulsive eating.

Common gastrointestinal disorders related to aging include the following:

- Over-/undernutrition
- Constipation
- Dehydration
- Dental disorders

Nursing Interventions: Over-/ Undernutrition

1. Assess nutritional status.
2. Provide nutritional instruction based on assessment findings.
3. Advise on community nutrition programs (e.g., Meals-on-Wheels, senior center food sites, food pantries, and Food Stamp program).

Nursing Interventions: Constipation

1. Assess food and fluid intake.
2. Make recommendations based on assessment findings (e.g., increase fiber intake, increase fluid intake).

COMMUNITY/HOME HEALTH CARE

Nutritional Status

Evaluate the following when assessing a client's nutritional status in the home:

- Ability to shop for and prepare meals (Figure 28-9)
- Mealtime environment, for unpleasant odors, noises, and visual stimuli
- Table setting, for appealing table cover, centerpiece, colorful dishes
- Appropriateness of food storage system (cabinets, refrigerator, freezer)

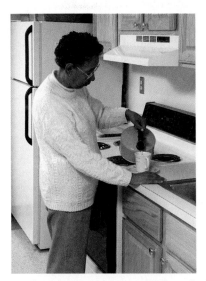

Figure 28-9 Cooking and preparing foods in the home are important skills to maintaining a nutritionally healthy lifestyle.

3. Discuss the relationship of exercise to bowel activity.
4. Discuss the importance of routine for regular bowel elimination.
5. Advise avoiding the overuse of laxatives.
6. Monitor adequate bowel elimination and provide interventions (e.g., prune juice, senna bars, milk of magnesia, as ordered) to assist the client in returning to a normal bowel elimination routine.

Nursing Interventions: Dehydration

1. Identify the reason for dehydration (i.e., inadequate fluid intake or excessive fluid output).
2. Identify the reason and corresponding interventions for inadequate fluid intake:
   • Fluids are inaccessible due to the client's physical limitations: offer fluids on a regular basis throughout the day.
   • The client dislikes water or other available fluids: identify fluid choices.
   • The client restricts fluids due to a fear of incontinence: explain the relationship of decreased fluid intake to bladder infections and arrange for assistance, as needed, for toileting.
3. Identify the reasons for any excessive fluid output and treat accordingly.

Nursing Interventions: Dental Disorders

1. Teach the oral hygiene procedures of brushing and flossing and facilitate and encourage brushing of the teeth and gums and flossing of the teeth, as tolerated.
2. Inspect the mouth regularly for signs of dental disorders.
3. Advise regular dental checkups.

Reproductive System: Female

Review the anatomy and physiology of the female reproductive system. The following reproductive changes result from the aging process:

• Estrogen production decreases with the onset of menopause.
• Ovaries, uterus, and cervix decrease in size.
• The vagina shortens, narrows, and becomes less elastic, and the vaginal lining thins. Secretions decrease and become more alkaline, resulting in increased incidence of atrophic vaginitis. These changes may result in discomfort during coitus, which can often be rectified with the use of a water-based lubricant. As at any age, protected intercourse (safe sex) through the use of a latex condom should be advised with new partners.
• Supporting musculature of the reproductive organs weakens, increasing the risk of uterine prolapse.
• Breast tissue diminishes, and nipple erection lessens during sexual arousal.

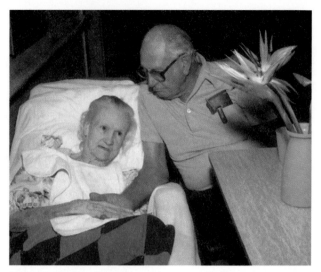

Figure 28-10 Sexuality and companionship remain important throughout the life span.

• Libido and the need for intimacy and companionship in older women remain unchanged (Figure 28-10).

Common female reproductive system disorders related to aging include the following:

• Breast cancer (the risk of which increases with age)
• Altered sexuality patterns related to physiologic changes, medications, changes in body image, or psychosocial changes such as the loss of significant other or a move to a setting that provides some level of assistive care (i.e., group home, assisted living center, or care facility)

Nursing Interventions: Female Reproductive System Disorders

1. Teach and encourage monthly breast self-exams and yearly mammograms for early detection and treatment of disorders.
2. Establish rapport and encourage the client to verbalize feelings and concerns related to sexuality, body image, and self-esteem.
3. Complete a sexual history and recommend interventions based on findings. Support the client's needs for companionship and intimacy throughout the life span.
4. Recommend that a bone density scan be discussed with the client's primary care provider to allow for early detection and treatment of osteoporosis.
5. Encourage annual gynecological examinations with the client's primary care provider.

Reproductive System: Male

Review the anatomy and physiology of the male reproductive system. The following reproductive changes result from the aging process:

- Testosterone production decreases, resulting in decreased size of the testicles.
- Sperm count and viscosity of seminal fluid decrease.
- Although more time is required to obtain erection, the older man often finds that he and his partner can enjoy longer periods of lovemaking (greater control) prior to ejaculation. As at any age, protected intercourse (safe sex) through the use of a latex condom should be advised with new partners.
- The prostate gland may enlarge.
- Impotency may occur. Medications and other medical interventions have been successful in reversing impotency problems in many older males. A thorough evaluation by the primary care provider and a urologist can provide clients with available options given health status and current medication regimen.
- Libido and the need for intimacy and companionship remain unchanged in older males.

Common male reproductive disorders related to aging include the following:

- Altered sexuality patterns related to physiologic changes, medications, changes in body image, or psychosocial changes such as the loss of significant other or a move to a setting that provides some level of assistive care (i.e., group home, assisted living center, or care facility)
- Benign prostatic hypertrophy (BPH)

Nursing Interventions: Male Reproductive System Disorders

1. Establish rapport and encourage the client to verbalize feelings and concerns related to sexuality, body image, and self-esteem.
2. Complete a sexual history and recommend interventions based on findings. Support the client's needs for companionship and intimacy throughout the life span.
3. Provide client and family education regarding the signs and symptoms of prostate disorders (e.g., difficulty in starting the urine stream, a smaller urine stream, frequent urination, frequent nighttime awakening for the purpose of urinating, or, in severe cases, the failure or inability to urinate).
4. Teach and encourage monthly testicular self-exam and yearly digital rectal examinations of the prostate gland by a primary care provider. The benefits of a PSA lab test performed every 1 to 2 years to facilitate early detection and treatment of prostate cancer are currently under research and debate.

Endocrine System

Review the anatomy and physiology of the endocrine system. The following endocrine changes result from the aging process:

- Alterations occur in both the reception and the production of hormones.
- Release of insulin by the beta cells of the pancreas slows, causing an increase in blood sugar.
- Thyroid changes may lower the basal metabolic rate.

The most common endocrine disorder related to aging is diabetes mellitus type 2.

Nursing Interventions: Diabetes Mellitus Type 2

1. Arrange for a consultation with a dietitian to assess nutritional status and to provide food-management instruction.
2. Teach the client, family members, or caregivers (as appropriate) the procedure for blood glucose monitoring specific to the equipment the client will be using.
3. Develop a personal exercise program with the client based on the client's physical condition, mental status, resources, and interests.
4. Provide information on prescribed oral hypoglycemic medications.
5. Teach the causes, signs, and treatment of hypoglycemia and hyperglycemia.
6. Advise on self-care and on careful monitoring of the extremities and of sores on the skin, to minimize threats to skin integrity.
7. Encourage the client to wear shoes and to have nails trimmed by a podiatrist, if unable to safely perform self-care.

Musculoskeletal System

Review the anatomy and physiology of the musculoskeletal system. The following musculoskeletal changes result from the aging process:

- Muscle mass and elasticity diminish, resulting in decreased strength, endurance, coordination, and increased reaction time.
- Bone demineralization occurs, causing skeletal instability and shrinkage of intervertebral disks. The flexibility of the spine lessens, and spinal curvature often occurs.
- Joints undergo degenerative changes, resulting in pain, stiffness, and loss of range of motion.

Common musculoskeletal system disorders related to aging include the following:

- Osteoporosis
- Degenerative arthritis
- Fractured hip

Nursing Interventions: Osteoporosis

1. Make dietary recommendations to ensure adequate intake of calcium, protein, and vitamin D.

2. Recommend a smoking cessation program, if necessary.
3. Advise the client to avoid alcohol.
4. Encourage the client to take a calcium supplement in conjunction with vitamin D, as ordered by the client's primary care provider.
5. Recommend consultation with the primary care provider regarding either estrogen replacement therapy (ERT) options for females, or the use of medications like alendronate sodium (Fosamax) to address bone density loss associated with osteoporosis.
6. Teach the client, family, and caregivers about measures to reduce the risk of falling and sustaining fractures.
7. Recommend evaluation (via x-ray) for the presence of stress, or compression, fractures of the spine in cases of severe back pain that occurs with or without a fall. In clients with osteoporosis, these fractures can occur more easily because the vertebrae are compacted by shrinkage of the intervertebral spaces as a consequence of aging.
8. Provide adequate pain control for back pain or other musculoskeletal discomfort.
9. Monitor for adequate dietary intake of calories and fluids and for effective elimination patterns.
10. Teach, encourage, and assist clients to establish exercise programs appropriate to their capabilities. Especially promote exercise programs that include walking or other weight-bearing activities, as tolerated (Figure 28-11).

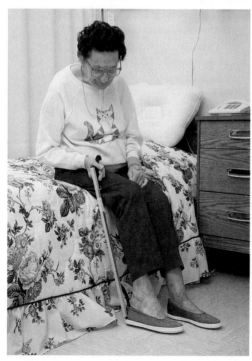

Figure 28-11 This elderly client is able to ambulate and remain active with the help of an assistive device.

Nursing Interventions: Degenerative Arthritis

1. Suggest a schedule for alternating periods of activity and rest.
2. Advise a weight reduction plan, if necessary, to eliminate extra strain on affected joints.
3. Teach, assist, and encourage the client to establish an exercise program that emphasizes gentle stretching and movement of all joints. For those clients who are more independent, exercise programs in warm water can have positive outcomes.
4. Provide adequate pain control. Teach clients and caregivers to monitor for gastrointestinal distress related to arthritis medications such as nonsteroidal anti-inflammatory drugs (NSAIDs) and to be aware that enteric coated medications cannot be crushed, as they are designed to protect the stomach by dissolving in the duodenum.
5. Encourage the client to seek ongoing evaluation by the physician, as new arthritis medications such as celecoxib (Celebrex) are continually being developed and trialed.

Nursing Interventions: Fractured Hip

NOTE: Nursing interventions may vary depending on whether the older client has an open reduction/internal fixation fracture (ORIF) or total hip arthoplasty (THA).

1. Maintain postoperative positioning as appropriate to the client's form of treatment.
2. Provide adequate pain control prior to physical therapy and on an ongoing basis through the recovery process.
3. Prevent complications, including skin breakdown, RTIs, infections at the surgical site, and dislocation of the prosthesis or internal fixation device.
4. Facilitate and monitor with the registered nurse the client's consistent use of antiembolism stockings as ordered and the administration of anticoagulant medications and the related monitoring of lab values, to decrease the risk of pulmonary embolism (which can be a significant risk to older clients after hip fracture and/or hip replacement).
5. Teach the client about fall prevention. Evaluate the client's environment (home, room, bathroom) for safety with regard to mobility and make recommendations for rectifying any threats to safety.

Integumentary System

Review the anatomy and physiology of the integumentary system. The following integumentary changes result from the normal aging process:

- Subcutaneous tissue and elastin fibers diminish, causing the skin to become thinner and less elastic.

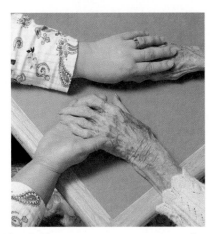

Figure 28-12 Hyperpigmentation is a normal result of the aging process.

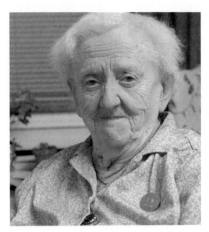

Figure 28-13 Gray hair results from a reduction in melanin production.

- Ability of melanocytes to produce even pigmentation diminishes, resulting in hyperpigmentation or liver spots, typically on the hands and wrists (Figure 28-12).
- Eccrine, apocrine, and sebaceous glands decrease in size, number, and function, resulting in diminished secretions and moisturization and, thus, pruritis.
- Body temperature regulation diminishes due to decreased perspiration and, many times, decreased circulation.
- Capillary blood flow decreases, resulting in slower wound healing.
- Blood flow decreases, especially to lower extremities.
- Vascular fragility causes senile purpura.
- Cutaneous sensitivity to pressure and temperature diminishes.
- Melanin production decreases, causing gray-white hair (Figure 28-13).
- Scalp, pubic, and axillary hair thin, and women display increased facial hair on the upper lip and chin.
- Nail growth slows, nails become more brittle, and longitudinal nail ridges form.

Common integumentary disorders related to aging include the following:

- Pressure ulcers (alteration in skin integrity)
- Herpes zoster (shingles)
- Skin cancer (included because the risk of skin cancer increases with age)

Nursing Interventions: Alteration in Skin Integrity

1. Perform a pressure ulcer risk assessment upon the client's admission to the health care setting (Figure 28-14).
2. Implement pressure ulcer prevention protocol for clients at risk for pressure ulcer formation. It is important to consider and document pressure relieving interventions for all surfaces that the client will sit or lay on during the course of the day (Table 28–2).
3. Encourage adequate intake of protein and fluids to help ensure good skin integrity.

 Infection Control: Skin Integrity
It is the nurse's responsibility to educate caregivers (including other staff members, as necessary) about the need to thoroughly wash and dry the client's perineal area, and to keep linens and clothing clean and dry, especially when incontinence is a problem. Such education may also include instruction on maintaining client privacy; properly retracting, cleansing, and repositioning the foreskin of an uncircumcised older male client; and proper cleansing of the skin folds of an older female client's perineal area. Clients and caregivers should also be instructed to cleanse front to back only and to not rinse and reuse washcloths again or use them on other body areas. These simple hygiene and infection-control guidelines can help maintain the client's skin integrity and can also prevent unnecessary infections.

Nursing Interventions: Herpes Zoster

1. Treat the pain.
2. Treat the ulcer with medications (e.g., acyclovir [Zovirax] topical cream), as ordered, to reduce the length of time of the outbreak.
3. Develop a plan to ensure continuity in meeting the client's psychosocial needs, and allow the client time to share concerns.

 Infection Control: Herpes Zoster
Prevent cross-infection from drainage from the vesicular eruptions by practicing proper handwashing and implementing appropriate isolation procedures, especially if the client is in the hospital or another health care facility.

Date of assessment: _____   Nurse: _____

Pressure ulcer present on admission: No _____ Yes _____ Stage _____

A score of 11 or more places a client at risk for pressure ulcer formation. Preventive protocol should be established.

Activity		Total	Level of Consciousness		Total
Ambulant without assistance	0		Alert	0	
Ambulant with assistance	2		Slow verbal response	1	
Chairfast	4		Responds to verbal or painful stimuli	2	
Bedfast	6	_____	Absence of response to stimuli	3	_____
Mobility—Range of Motion			**Nutritional Status**		
Full range of motion	0		Good (eats 75% or more of required intake)	0	
Moves with minimal assistance	2		Fair (eats less than 75% of required intake)	1	
Moves with moderate assistance	4		Poor (minimal intake, consistent weight loss)	2	
Immobile	6	_____	Unable/refuses to eat/drink, emaciated	3	_____
Skin Condition			**Incontinence—Bladder**		
Hydrated and intact	0		None	0	
Rashes or abrasions	2		Occasional (fewer than 2/24 hours)	1	
Decreased turgor, dry	4		Usually (more than 2/24 hours)	2	
Edema, erythema, pressure ulcers	6	_____	Total (no control)	3	_____
Predisposing Disease Process			**Incontinence—Bowel**		
No involvement	0		None	0	
Chronic, stable	1		Occasional (formed stool)	1	
Acute or chronic, unstable	2		Usually (semi-formed stool)	2	
Terminal	3	_____	Total (no control, loose stool)	3	_____

Figure 28-14 Pressure Ulcer Risk Assessment

Table 28–2 PROTOCOL FOR CLIENTS AT RISK FOR PRESSURE ULCERS

OBJECTIVE	INTERVENTIONS	OBJECTIVE	INTERVENTIONS
Relieve pressure	• Establish positioning schedule. • Place pressure relieving mattress on bed, cushions on chair. • Teach client wheelchair exercises. • Stand and/or ambulate client in chair frequently. • Use wheelchair for transporting only. • Allow client to sit on bedpan, commode, or toilet for only brief periods. • Check areas of pressure under casts, braces, splints, slings, prostheses.	Prevent spasticity and contractures	• Avoid quick, rough movements. • Do range of motion exercises at least twice daily. • Assess for synergy patterns when positioning. • Administer oral antispasmodics if ordered.
Relieve friction and shearing	• Use turning sheet for positioning in bed and chair. • Keep head of bed lower than 30 degrees unless contraindicated. • Use supportive devices to prevent sliding in chairs. • Use appropriate transfer techniques. • Do not use powder on skin. • Place bed cradle under top covers.	Maintain hydration/ nutritional status	• Assess nutritional status. • Investigate causes of anorexia. • Correct underlying nutritional deficits. • Encourage additional fluids, unless contraindicated. • Give high protein supplement, if necessary. • Monitor weight weekly.
Prevent moisture/ maceration	• Implement scheduled toileting or bladder retraining program. • Use absorbent incontinent briefs or pads. • Check incontinent clients frequently. Wash and rinse thoroughly. Apply moisture barrier. • Avoid use of plastic/rubber sheets, protectors.		Continue with routine skin care. Do skin checks with each position change.

Nursing Interventions: Skin Cancer

1. Teach clients and caregivers both cancer prevention methods and skin self-examination to detect lesions early. Early detection and treatment of skin cancers are essential to optimal client outcomes.
2. Provide information in both verbal and written form and in collaboration with the client's multidisciplinary team, regarding treatment (surgery, chemotherapy, radiation, and other options).
3. Monitor for signs of infection at the lesion site.
4. Ensure that the client's psychological, psychosocial, spiritual, and dietary needs are also addressed.

Neurological System

Review the anatomy and physiology of the neurological system. The following neurological changes result from the aging process:

- Neurons in the brain decrease in number, resulting in decreased production of neurotransmitters and, thus, reduced synaptic transmission.
- Cerebral blood flow and oxygen utilization decrease.
- Time required to carry out motor and sensory tasks requiring speed, coordination, balance, and fine-motor hand movements increases.
- Short-term memory may somewhat diminish without much change in long-term memory.
- Night sleep disturbances occur due to more frequent and longer wakeful periods.
- Deep-tendon reflexes decrease, although reflexes at the knees remain fairly intact.

Many disorders that affect the neurological system are not unique to elders. However, the risk of acquiring one of these disorders increases with age. One of the most common diagnoses among elders in long-term care facilities is dementia, particularly one form of dementia called Alzheimer's disease (AD). **Dementia** is an organic brain pathology characterized by losses in intellectual functioning. The clinical manifestations associated with dementia are never considered normal aging changes.

It is important for care providers to assess the length of onset of confusion or cognitive changes in the client. Generally, dementia describes declines that have a slow onset of greater than 6 months, whereas **delirium** (or acute confusion) describes cognitive changes that have a shorter onset of 6 months or less. Acute confusion can occur independently or as an exacerbation of a current dementia-related disorder in the client. Acute confusion can result from many stresses such as infections, medication side effects, drug interactions, metabolic imbalances, dehydration, or injuries from falls (e.g., subdural hematomas). Elimination of the causative factor can often turn the acute confusion around in a relatively short period of time to the pre-exacerbation level of functioning, unless further pathology to the brain has occurred.

Mental Health in the Elderly

Mood disorders including depression, bipolar disorder, anxiety disorders, late onset psychosis, sleep disorders, substance abuse, schizophrenia (chronic and late onset), and other psychiatric diseases certainly occur among older clients and often go unaddressed or are ineffectively treated. Appropriate assessment, treatment, and clinical management of these clients require effective interdisciplinary teams comprising a geriatric psychiatrist; a neurologist; a clinical nurse specialist specializing in gerontology and mental health; a licensed social worker; a clinical pharmacist; other multidisciplinary team members (including direct care nurses and staff and activity therapists); and the client's family and, whenever possible, the client.

Nursing Interventions: Alzheimer's Disease

1. Before diagnosis, encourage a medical and psychological diagnostic workup including a mental status examination.
2. Facilitate orientation in the early stages of the disease with calendars, lists, and consistent schedules.
3. Arrange an environment that is therapeutic, consistent, calm, and safe and that alternates rest with activities that require the use of long-practiced skills.
4. Encourage and facilitate access for the client and family to support groups where they can independently share their feelings and concerns and have questions addressed.
5. When assistance is needed with ADLs, implement consistent routines with consistent caregivers but allow for delay of care if needed due to client stress or irritability. Encourage independence of the client while assisting with ADLs (e.g., offer a warm washcloth for client to wash the face and assist with those ADLs that the client cannot complete without assistance).
6. Monitor general health status. Treat any underlying medical problems. Provide adequate pain control, as needed, and monitor for lack of sleep to minimize the risk of violent behavior (Andersen, 1999). Observe for the client's better times of the day, and plan activities or interventions accordingly.

PROFESSIONAL TIP

Neurological System in the Elderly Client

In the absence of pathology, intellect and capacity for learning remain unchanged with aging.

7. Build a trusting relationship with the client. Use clear, simple directions and treat clients with respect and as individuals, building on their strengths and their unique interests and histories. Doing so demonstrates appreciation for the individual and can help build the client's self-esteem.

8. Be aware that as much is communicated to the AD client through the caregiver's nonverbal behavior and tone and volume of voice as is communicated through actual words. A calm attitude allows the client time to process and retrieve information when spoken to or asked a question.

9. Support the client's mobility within a safe environment, recognizing that as the disease progresses, baseline wandering often increases as a coping skill, whereas verbal communication often decreases (Fetters, 1994). Bean bag chairs, low mattresses, bed and chair alarms, positional (anti-sliding) wedges for chairs, merry walkers that support independent mobility, and assisted-ambulation programs to build leg strength are all therapeutic interventions for AD clients as the disease progresses and represent preferable alternatives to the use of restraints.

10. Monitor for changes in baseline behaviors and for intensity of wandering (both pacing or lethargy), as either often indicates underlying infections, metabolic imbalances, or stress. Encourage clients to alternate periods of activity and rest.

Nursing Interventions: Depression

1. Assess for signs of a physical basis for any fatigue (e.g., infection, pain, altered nutritional status, or shortness of breath upon exertion).

2. Administer treatment for underlying physiologic problems, if applicable.

3. If symptoms persist, encourage the client to have a medical diagnostic workup with a geriatric psychiatrist, if such a workup has not yet been done.

4. Monitor for verbal or nonverbal signs of suicidal thoughts/intent. Determine whether the client has a plan.

5. Provide one-on-one supervision of the client as needed and assure the client that the caregiver will keep him safe. If appropriate for the client, seek an agreement that he will not try to harm himself.

6. Administer antidepressant medication as ordered. Provide client and family education regarding medication, including length of time before therapeutic results should occur, and potential side effects. Report immediately to the registered nurse and primary care provider any extrapyramidal side effects (e.g., tremors, drooling, pin rolling of the fingers, shuffling gait) that are observed.

7. If the client is not assessed as being at risk for suicide but is isolating in his room, establish small goals with the client (e.g., coming out of the room and sitting safely in the hallway with the nurse for 5 minutes two times per day and for meals). Advance to more challenging goals as the client demonstrates increased tolerance for social interaction.

8. Facilitate the client's reintegration into a healthy support system and provide small community group time for the client to share his views.

Nursing Interventions: Transient Ischemic Attack

1. Assess for risk factors for stroke and for the existence of any previous carotid vascular tests for potential blockage (stenosis).

2. Provide client and family education explaining the relationship between risk factors and transient ischemic attack (TIA) and stroke.

3. Provide teaching to assist in reducing risk factors.

4. Monitor orthostatic blood pressure and encourage clients to change positions slowly to decrease the risk of falling.

Urinary System

Review the anatomy and physiology of the urinary system. The following urinary changes result from the aging process:

- Nephrons in the kidneys decrease in number and function, resulting in decreased filtration and gradual decrease in excretory and reabsorbtive functions of the renal tubules.
- Glomerular filtration rate decreases, resulting in decreased renal clearance of drugs.
- Blood urea nitrogen increases. The creatinine clearance test is a better indicator than is BUN of renal function in elders.
- Sodium-conserving ability diminishes.
- Bladder capacity decreases, causing increased frequency of urination, including nocturia.
- Renal function increases when the older client lies down, sometimes causing a need to void shortly after going to bed.
- Bladder and perineal muscles weaken, resulting in the inability to empty the bladder and predisposing the elderly client to cystitis.
- Incidence of stress incontinence increases in older females.
- The prostate may enlarge in older males, causing urinary frequency or dribbling.

Common urinary disorders related to aging include the following:

- Incontinence
- Urinary tract infections (UTIs)

Nursing Interventions: Incontinence

1. Complete an assessment for bladder management (Figure 28-15).
2. Identify the type of incontinence present (Table 28–3).
3. Implement an appropriate bladder management program (Table 28–4).
4. Frequently monitor for skin impairment.
5. Offer absorbent incontinent pads or briefs that draw the moisture away from the skin.
6. Teach all caregivers, the client, and the family the importance both of adequate cleansing of the genital area (proper retraction and cleansing of the foreskin in the older uncircumcised male and proper cleansing of the skin folds of the older female), legs, and back and of the use of clean linens, to ensure that the client's skin is kept clean and dry. Apply a moisture barrier cream as needed to prevent skin maceration from excessive exposure to moisture.
7. Teach and employ effective infection-control techniques (e.g., wipe and clean [from front to back only] after toileting and when bathing).
8. Encourage referral to discuss medical options (in addition to nursing interventions) for treatment of incontinence.
9. Allow the client to voice concerns over incontinence and assist to overcome any adverse effects on psychosocial functioning.

Nursing Interventions: Urinary Tract Infections

NOTE: Elderly persons frequently do not present with the usual signs and symptoms of UTIs. Falling or signs of acute confusion (more than usual) may often be the major clinical manifestations.

1. Monitor fluid intake and output. Increase intake unless contraindicated. Offer cranberry juice frequently, per ordered diet.
2. Teach and encourage client to empty the bladder every 3 to 4 hours.
3. Encourage the client to take all medication as prescribed.

Table 28–3 TYPES OF URINARY INCONTINENCE

TYPE	CHARACTERISTICS
Functional	Bladder emptying is unpredictable but complete. Incontinence is related to impairment of cognitive, physical, or psychological functioning or to environmental barriers.
Urge	Incontinence occurs immediately after the sensation to void is perceived.
Reflex	Incontinence is related to neurogenic bladder and central nervous system or spinal cord injury. Bladder fills, and uninhibited bladder contractions cause loss of urine.
Stress	Increased abdominal pressure is higher than urethral resistance. Stress associated with coughing or laughing causes incontinence.
Total	Unpredictable, unvoluntary, continuous loss of urine.

To be completed and reviewed every 90 days or as frequently as needed based on outcome and response.

CLIENT_____ Adm No. _____ Date_____ Diagnoses_____ Birthdate_____

Bladder function: History of infection or other urinary problem._____ Urinalysis: Date_____

Protein___ Glucose__ Ketones__ RBC__ WBC__ Bacteria__ Crystals__ Sp.Gr.__ Culture: Date_____ Result_____

Treatment_____

BUN___ Ser.Creatinine___ Tot.Pro.___ FBS___ To be completed after 2-week assessment period

Frequency of voiding_____ Average amount_____ Is client aware of need to void?____ Urgency?_____ Dribbling?____

Incontinence preceded by laughing, sneezing_____

Medications affecting bladder function/continence_____

Mental status: Short-term memory_____ Orientation_____ Able to express self_____

   Able to follow directions_____ Reaction to incontinence_____

Hydration baseline: Daily average fluid intake: Days_____ Eve._____ Night_____

Mobility/self-care skills: Ambulatory/self_____ Cane_____ Walker_____ Requires assist of one or two_____

   Weight-bearing_____ Propels self by w/c_____ Transfers self_____ Requires assistance_____

   Can manage clothing_____ Cleanses self after toileting_____ Washes hands_____

Figure 28-15 Assessment for Bladder Management

Table 28–4 BLADDER MANAGEMENT TECHNIQUES

PROGRAM	DESCRIPTION
Kegel exercises	Used for stress incontinence in cognitively alert persons. Exercises strengthen pelvic floor musculature.
Scheduled toileting	Client is on a fixed schedule of toileting—usually every 2 hours. Technique can be used to facilitate voiding and emptying of the bladder.
Habit training	Client is toileted according to individual pattern of voiding. Several days must be spent assessing pattern.
Bladder retraining	Restores normal pattern of voiding/continence. Requires accurate assessment before establishing schedule with progressive shortening or lengthening of toileting intervals. Client must be cognitively alert.
Prompted voiding	Client is prompted to toilet at regular intervals and is given social reinforcement for appropriate toileting behavior.

4. Use proper infection-control techniques to minimize the risk of infection, including maintaining sterile technique for any urinary catheterization procedure (for urinalysis, assessment for bladder retention, or insertion of indwelling catheter), to prevent unnecessary introduction of bacteria into the bladder.

5. Teach female clients to wipe from front to back only; cleanse thoroughly after bowel movements; avoid bubble baths, colored toilet paper, douches, and vaginal sprays; and wear underwear made from cotton rather than synthetic fibers.

6. Teach the client and caregivers that hematuria (blood in the urine) and fever indicate the need for immediate assessment and intervention, as these signs and symptoms can signify a potentially serious infection or condition. Any signs and symptoms of bladder infection should be immediately reported to the registered nurse and the physician.

Sensory Changes

Review the anatomy and physiology of the sensory system. The following sensory changes result from the aging process:

Vision

- With aging, the lens becomes less pliable and less able to increase its curvature in order to focus on near objects, causing presbyopia (trouble seeing objects up close) and decreased accomodation. The lens also yellows, causing distorted color perceptions, with greens and blues washing out and warm colors such as reds and oranges becoming more distinct. The incidence of cataracts also increases.

- Accommodation of pupil size decreases, resulting in both decreased adjustment to changes in lighting and decreased ability to tolerate glare. For instance, high-gloss tile floors in hallways can appear like hills and valleys to older clients, especially those with perceptual deficits; this may increase anxiety and safety risks.

- Vitreous humor changes in consistency, causing blurred vision. Changes in the anterior chamber may increase the pressure of the aqueous humor, resulting in glaucoma.

- Lacrimal glands secrete less fluids, causing dryness and itching. Entropion or ectropion (turning of the eyelids inward or outward) occasionally occurs in older clients. These conditions can not only impact vision, but can increase the risk of infection due to dryness and ineffective blinking. In these conditions, obtaining an order for artificial tears, lacrilube, and eye drop treatments for dryness or infection may be necessary.

Infection Control: Eye Care
To decrease infection risks, remind all caregivers to wash from the center outward when washing clients' eyes.

Common vision disorders related to aging include the following:

- Presbyopia
- Cataract
- Glaucoma
- Age-related macular degeneration

Nursing Interventions: Visual Impairment

1. Teach visually impaired clients adaptive techniques for ADL, such as extra lighting.

2. Advise regular examination by an ophthalmologist.

3. Provide preoperative and postoperative care and teaching to clients undergoing cataract surgery, including lifting and bending restrictions as well as measures to prevent infection.

4. Teach proper eye drop administration techniques to all clients who are prescribed eye drops, including holding the drop in the eye with the lid closed for 30 seconds after administration.

5. Ensure that older clients have their glasses on when needed to decrease perceptual and spatial deficits.

Hearing

- As aging occurs, the pinna becomes less flexible, the hair cells in the inner ear stiffen and atrophy, and cerumen (earwax) increases.
- The number of neurons in the cochlea decrease, and the blood supply lessens, causing the cochlea and the ossicles to degenerate.
- Presbycusis, the impairment of hearing in older adults, is often accompanied by a loss of tone discrimination. High-frequency tones are lost first; thus, keeping the voice low and calm and decreasing any background noise can improve the client's comprehension of the caregiver's message.

Nursing Interventions: Hearing Impairment

1. Assess for ear pain; drainage; inflammation; abnormalities; surgeries; perforations; or impacted cerumen.
2. Evaluate medication regimen and assess for ototoxicity, if medication history reveals such a risk.
3. Advise hearing testing by an audiologist, if the previous assessments are negative.
4. Monitor the care and use of a hearing aid by the older client with unilateral or bilateral aids (Figure 28-16). Provide teaching and assistance as needed for cleaning the hearing aid(s) and replacing batteries.
5. Instruct caregivers and family about the communication and socialization needs of the client. For some older clients, either the use of a small erasable board to augment verbal questions or communication with written text represents a therapeutic intervention for hearing impairment. If writing dexterity or ability is also impaired, a story board that has pictures indicating the client's needs (e.g., bathroom, food, rest) can assist the client to independently communicate needs to caregivers.

ELDER ABUSE

One million older persons (60 years or over) may be abused each year (Wolfe, 1998). It is suspected that many cases are not reported. Some signs of abuse are similar to the normal process of aging (e.g., recurrent fractures and osteoporosis, malnourishment and poor appetite). The possibility for abuse should be considered when caring for older clients. They are vulnerable because of physical or cognitive impairment, social isolation, and dependence.

Forms of Abuse

- *Physical*—deliberate harm, inappropriate use of drugs or physical restraints

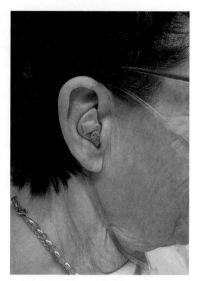

Figure 28-16 Hearing aids help compensate for hearing loss that results from aging.

- *Psychological*—threats, intimidation, humiliation, insults, verbal harassment, isolation
- *Sexual*—any sexual activity without consent or when the client is incapable of giving consent
- *Neglect*—failure of the caregiver to meet physical, emotional, or social needs of the older client
- *Financial*—misuse of or taking possessions or money assets
- *Abandonment*—desertion by the caregiver

Legal Requirements of Reporting

Most states require health care providers, including nurses, to report cases when elder abuse is suspected. States not requiring reporting, encourage it. A "reasonable belief" is the standard for reporting that a vulnerable older person has been or is likely to be abused, neglected, or exploited (Stiegel, 1995). Failure to report could result in a misdemeanor charge against the health care provider and, in some states, disciplinary action by the licensing agency (Morris, 1998).

PROFESSIONAL TIP

Reporting Elder Abuse
- Check state statute and employer's policy for reporting abuse.
- If suspected abuser is a health care provider, many states require reporting to the licensing agency.

SAMPLE NURSING CARE PLAN

THE CLIENT WITH ALZHEIMER'S DISEASE (AD)

Mrs. Jane Rodriguez, 64 years old, was admitted to the Alzheimer's unit of a long-term care facility. Last month, Mrs. Rodriguez was visiting her daughter in another state and wandered away from the daughter's home. Mrs. Rodriguez was found 60 miles away, unharmed but completely disoriented and agitated. Mrs. Rodriguez had worked as a nursing assistant before she retired. She is a widow and has two children in the same community where the nursing home is located, in addition to the daughter she was visiting in another state. Unless reminded, Mrs. Rodriguez does not shower or change clothes. She awakens at least once each night and asks for breakfast.

Nursing Diagnosis 1 *Disturbed Thought Processes related to progressive dementia as evidenced by disorientation to time and place, loss of short-term memory, inability to concentrate, and periods of agitation*

PLANNING/GOALS	NURSING INTERVENTIONS	RATIONALE	EVALUATION
Mrs. Rodriguez will remain calm and will not experience agitation and anxiety as a result of her disorientation and memory loss.	Provide Mrs. Rodriguez with clues for orientation: "Good morning, Mrs. Rodriguez. My name is Jean, and I will help you today." Avoid putting her on the spot by asking questions she may not answer, such as "Do you know what day this is?"	People in the early stages of Alzheimer's disease may become agitated because their world is always unfamiliar to them. The issue is not whether individuals with a dementia are oriented, but whether they can cope with their environment.	Mrs. Rodriguez remained calm and showed no signs of agitation or anxiety.
	Place a large sign on Mrs. Rodriguez's door with her name printed in large letters to help her find her room.	Short-term memory loss makes it impossible for Mrs. Rodriguez to remember where her room is or where the bathroom is. If she still recognizes her name, posting it on the door will help her find her way.	
	Have family bring in snapshots and photos to stimulate reminiscence.	Reminiscing can be a satisfying activity. It is especially helpful if the photos are from an earlier, happier time such as when her children were young. Long-term memory may still be intact, allowing her to recall these happier times.	

continues

Avoid changing Mrs. Rodriguez's room. Put items back in the same place all the time.

Consult with activities staff in planning self-expressive, non-fail activities that require little concentration (e.g., painting with nontoxic paints, modeling with nontoxic clay).

If Mrs. Rodriguez is resistant to care, provide clear, simple, non-threatening instructions and delay care as needed until she is calmer.

Consistency in the environment (as well as in routine and staff) reduces frustration.

Appropriate activities prevent boredom, which can lead to irritation. It is important to plan non-stressful, noncompetitive, failure-proof activities in order to prevent frustration.

Persons with cognitive deficits often vary between combativeness and cooperation. Often, delaying care for even 10 to 15 minutes when resistance is encountered improves client outcomes. Also, exploring and understanding the antecedents to a client's combative behavior allows caregivers to intervene early and to change the environment or the approach to better ensure positive client outcomes (Andersen, 1999).

Nursing Diagnosis 2 *Risk for Injury related to risk factors of mode of transportation and cognitive and affective factors as evidenced by wandering behavior, impaired judgment, and disorientation*

PLANNING/GOALS	NURSING INTERVENTIONS	RATIONALE	EVALUATION
Mrs. Rodriguez will remain free of injury while retaining as much independence and freedom as possible.	Lock up tools, medicines, and chemicals. Keep only nonpoisonous plants on the unit. Arrange furniture so that walkways are open. Pad sharp corners of tables and chests. Cover electrical outlets and hot radiators. Place electrical cords and telephone wires out of reach.	Persons with Alzheimer's disease do not recognize unsafe acts or conditions due to loss of impulse control and loss of judgment. They do not comprehend cause and effect.	Mrs. Rodriguez has experienced no injury.
	Provide assurance during fire drills.	Unusual activity of any sort increases agitation, especially when noise level is increased.	

continues

Nursing Diagnosis 3 *Bathing/Hygiene Self-Care Deficit and Dressing/Grooming Self-Care Deficit related to perceptual or cognitive impairment (memory loss and sensory–perceptual deficits) as evidenced by needing a reminder to shower and change clothes*

PLANNING/GOALS	NURSING INTERVENTIONS	RATIONALE	EVALUATION
Mrs. Rodriguez will complete ADL with minimal assistance now and with increasing assistance as the disease progresses.	Use verbal cues and hand-over-hand assistance with ADL. Instruct staff to avoid doing tasks that Mrs. Rodriguez can do by herself. Watch for signs of frustration and irritation and intervene when appropriate.	Using these simple techniques can minimize the need for assistance, thereby increasing feelings of self-esteem.	Mrs. Rodriguez participates in ADL.
	Ask family to bring in clothing that is easy to manipulate. Set clothing out in the order it is to be put on.	Dressing is one of the more difficult tasks to accomplish. Appropriate clothing can simplify the activity.	
	Consider tub baths rather than showers. Provide privacy, check the temperature of the bathroom, and do not leave the client alone.	Showers are frequently threatening or confusing to persons with Alzheimer's disease. Tub baths are also more relaxing.	

Nursing Diagnosis 4 *Disturbed Sleep Pattern related to disorientation as evidenced by wakefulness at night*

PLANNING/GOALS	NURSING INTERVENTIONS	RATIONALE	EVALUATION
Mrs. Rodriguez will experience fewer periods of wakefulness during the night. If she awakens, she will remain calm and free of agitation.	Avoid stimulating activities prior to bedtime. Establish a consistent bedtime routine. Take Mrs. Rodriguez to the bathroom and allow sufficient time for complete bladder emptying.	Overstimulation prior to bedtime may increase anxiety, preventing sleep. Having the client participate in relaxation activities and repeating the client's long-practiced bedtime routine prior to bed may also be helpful.	Mrs. Rodriguez sleeps through the night several times a week.
	Help Mrs. Rodriguez with a sponge bath and with oral care; give her a back rub using warm lotion and slow, smooth strokes.	These activities are relaxing.	

continues

Provide a light snack of a warm, noncaffeinated beverage and a plain, easily digested cracker, cookie, or a piece of toast. Be patient and do not rush her.	Hunger or overeating can interfere with sleep.
Question family concerning previous bedtime routines and sleeping habits.	Individuals may have used specific sleep routines throughout their lifetimes, such as sleeping with a night light, having a window open, playing a radio, or wearing socks to bed.
Repeat bedtime routine when Mrs. Rodriguez awakens during night.	Mrs. Rodriguez will think it is time to go to bed.
Encourage a short nap early in the afternoon.	Sleep pattern disturbances may result from overfatigue.
Avoid the use of sleeping medications.	Sleeping medications are seldom effective and may increase confusion, disorientation, and restlessness.

FINANCING ELDER CARE IN THE 21ST CENTURY

Since the 1960s, the U.S. Congress has developed and implemented a series of national entitlement programs to help ensure adequate income, housing, and access to medical care for older Americans. As the number of older clients (those over age 65, particularly those over age 85) continues to rise, caregivers and advocates for elder care should strive to understand the budgetary policies that have influenced and continue to influence the U.S. health care delivery system.

Medicare

Medicare (Title XVIII) is a nationwide health insurance program for Americans who are 65 years of age or older, for persons who are eligible for Social Security disability payments for longer than 2 years, and for certain workers and dependents who need kidney transplants or dialysis. The **Health Care Financing Administration** (HCFA) is the federal agency in charge of administering the Medicare program. The program was enacted as part of the Social Security Act of 1965 and became effective on June 1, 1966. It con-

sists of two separate but coordinated programs: hospital insurance (called part A) and medical insurance (called part B), which covers physician's services, outpatient services, some medical supplies, and some skilled nursing and home health services. Medicare provides basic protection for the cost of health care but does not cover all expenses. Among the expenses *not* covered by Medicare for older Americans are those associated with the following:

- Home health care that does not require skilled personnel (e.g., as of February 1998, expenses for a home health visit [skilled] for the purpose of obtaining a blood sample are not covered).
- Nursing home care (except for skilled care for a limited time)
- Some routine medical checkups and related tests
- Prescription drugs
- Eye and hearing tests and eyeglasses and hearing aids
- Routine dental care and checkups

In the late 1990s, many insurance policies were available to supplement at varying levels the benefits paid by Medicare. This led many older clients to "stack" insurance policies, or to buy numerous overlapping policies for fear of being underinsured. The insurance industry and Congress worked together to outlaw stacking of Medicare supplement policies.

Although there has been some improvement in insurance coverage for preventive screening tests such as mammograms, the lack of reimbursement for prescription drugs continues to significantly burden older Americans, many of whom must choose between costly medications and food.

Medicaid

The Medicaid program was also enacted as part of the Social Security Act of 1966 and is often referred to as Title XIX. This program, which is federally aided and state operated and administered, provides medical benefits to certain indigent, or low-income, Americans. Nursing home bills represent a staggering burden for many older Americans who require nursing care. In 1995, nursing home bills averaged $22,000 per person per year, and projections showed that two-thirds of elders who lived alone would run out of savings after 13 weeks in a nursing home (Gallo, Pulmer, Paveza, & Reichel, 1999). Medicaid takes into account government-determined poverty levels when providing benefits, with coverage being extended to persons who are at certain percentages of the poverty level (e.g., 200% of poverty level, 150% of poverty level, and 100% of poverty level). Long-term care facilities serve both private-pay clients (those whose expenses are paid by themselves, their families, or their long-term care insurance policies) and Title XIX- (Medicaid-) funded clients. Medicaid coverage for long-term care is not available until a person's assets have been depleted to a certain set level. Elder care advocates continue in their efforts to protect the assets of the spouse who is able to stay in the family home after the other spouse must be placed in a nursing home.

To some in the United States, the debate over Social Security, Medicare, and Medicaid financing is viewed as someone else's priority. However, the moral responsibility for providing access to quality services and care for our country's elderly is shared by all Americans. Elder care services should be developed to promote independence yet should provide assistance when needed.

Omnibus Budget Reconciliation Act

The **Omnibus Budget Reconciliation Act** (OBRA), first enacted in 1987 and reenacted in 1990, sought to ensure quality services for older Americans. The act included guidelines for services that were required to be made available to seniors, and promoted the rights of seniors. However, as was the case with all health care costs, elder care costs continued to rise in the United States, and discussions and proposed legislation for financial reforms intensified.

Balanced Budget Act of 1997

Among the most significant influences on the financing of elder care in the past decade is the **Balanced Budget Act** (BBA) of 1997. The BBA replaced cost-based reimbursement for care provided in skilled nursing facilities (SNFs) with a prospective payment system (PPS) based on client assessment within a resource utilization group system (RUGS). Reimbursement for home health services also shifted to a PPS.

The BBA also states that discharge from hospitals to SNFs or home care for 10 common but as yet unpublished diagnosis-related groups (DRGs) is to be considered as a transfer for payment purposes. Medicare's goal was to make a single blended payment that combined the traditional hospital DRG payment and the payment for postacute care services to be shared by the providers.

The intended implications for practice included reduced reimbursement to some SNFs, fewer discharges from hospitals to independent facilities for subacute care or home care, and, thus, encouraged the creation of integrated delivery systems and managed care. In reality, however, it has become more difficult to find placement in SNFs for clients with complex needs, because the new reimbursement system simply does not fund all their health care needs.

These reimbursement and regulatory changes surely represent only the beginning of such efforts to balance resources and need as the U.S. population continues to age. Certainly, significant work lies ahead for advocates of quality elder care in the United States and the world. Nurses will play a vital role in the ensuing debates, for they will see firsthand the positive and negative outcomes of their clients.

CASE STUDY

Mr. Jack Baroni, a 72-year-old male, was admitted to the skilled care facility for rehabilitation following an open reduction, internal fixation of the right hip. Mr. Baroni had fallen while going up the stairs of his home, suffering an intertrochanteric, comminuted fracture of the right femur. He has no recollection of what caused him to fall. He is married and, until his surgery, was working part time as a school-crossing guard. While in the hospital, Mr. Baroni exhibited mental status changes including disorientation and confusion. His wife reports that he never had this problem prior to the surgery. He is continent of bowel and bladder. Mr. Baroni was in relatively good health until the fall. He and his wife agree that he should return home after rehabilitation is complete.

The following questions will guide your development of a nursing care plan for the case study.

1. Identify specific admission assessments that would be required for Mr. Baroni because of his age and condition.
2. Identify complications for which Mr. Baroni is at risk.
3. List interventions to prevent each complication.
4. Cite possible reasons for Mr. Baroni's fall.
5. Describe methods for assessing Mr. Baroni's mental status.
6. Describe possible reasons for his altered mental status.
7. Write three individualized nursing diagnoses and goals for Mr. Baroni.
8. List nursing actions related to altered mental status.
9. List four successful outcomes for Mr. Baroni.
10. Develop a teaching plan for Mr. Baroni.
11. List the community resources Mr. Baroni may need after discharge.

SUMMARY

- The elderly population is rapidly growing.
- Although many stereotypes and myths are associated with aging, elders are in fact very diverse in their characteristics.
- Health maintenance is as important for older adults as it is for younger persons. A healthy lifestyle can enhance the quality of life.
- Many changes are associated with aging. The disorders commonly seen among elders are often the results of pathology and are thus not considered a normal part of aging. However, the risk of acquiring these disorders increases with age.
- Nurses knowledgeable about aging can plan interventions that will prevent complications for which elders are at risk.
- Nurses have a responsibility to advocate for their older clients. Nurses should be active legislatively and should work collaboratively to develop elder-care services that are affordable, provide equal access for all older Americans, and promote optimal wellness and independence.

Review Questions

1. Which of the following is a true statement?

   a. All people eventually become senile if they live long enough.
   b. People lose interest in sex as they age.
   c. Most elders are financially impoverished.
   d. Incontinence is not an expected or normal change of aging.

2. The programmed aging theory states that:

   a. stress causes structural and chemical changes in the body, which, in turn, cause aging.
   b. a genetic clock determines the speed at which people age.
   c. changes in collagen are the cause of aging.
   d. the decreasing ability to produce T-cell differentiation causes aging.

3. The elderly individual can reduce the potential for acquiring RTIs by:

   a. obtaining an influenza vaccine each year.
   b. staying inside throughout the winter months.

c. avoiding exercise.

d. limiting fluid intake.

4. Research indicates that:

a. weight-bearing exercise is not recommended for elders.

b. high-intensity resistance training can improve muscle strength in elders.

c. muscle deterioration in elders is to be expected.

d. walking is the only healthy exercise for elders.

5. Integumentary changes associated with aging include:

a. increased glandular secretions.

b. increased capillary blood flow.

c. increased melanin production.

d. increased vascular fragility.

Critical Thinking Questions

1. What services are essential in a quality elder-care program?

2. How can you advocate as a nurse for your older clients?

3. If you were going to author an Older American client's bill of rights, what things would you include?

4. What myths or stereotypes have you observed that affect the elderly?

WEB FLASH!

- Search federal sites for some of the legislation and policies that are discussed in this chapter and affect elder care (e.g., OBRA and BBA).
- What clinical guidelines are available on the Internet from the government or other sources for the care of elderly clients (e.g., for urinary incontinence or pain treatment)?

REHABILITATION, HOME HEALTH, LONG-TERM CARE, AND HOSPICE

MAKING THE CONNECTION

Refer to the following chapters to increase your understanding of rehabilitation, home health, long-term care, and hospice:

- **Chapter 6, Legal Responsibilities**
- **Chapter 7, Ethical Responsibilities**
- **Chapter 12, Cultural Diversity and Nursing**
- **Chapter 17, Loss, Grief, and Death**

- **Chapter 25, Assessment**
- **Chapter 26, Pain Management**
- **Chapter 28, Nursing Care of the Older Client**

LEARNING OBJECTIVES

Upon completion of this chapter, you should be able to:
- *Define key terms.*
- *List three reasons why there has been a significant change in the growth of nonacute care services.*
- *Discuss the legal/ethical implications of:*
  1. *Limiting aggressive health care services (such as rehabilitation or intensive care) for the elderly as a cost saving measure for the preservation of Medicare funds.*
  2. *Determining nurses' responsibility for accepting decisions made by individuals with questionable mental competency.*
- *Describe the differences between Medicaid and Medicare.*
- *Distinguish among licensure, certification, and accreditation.*
- *Describe the role of the LP/VN as a member of the interdisciplinary health care team in various health care settings.*
- *Discuss the types of clients that would benefit from participation in a rehabilitation program.*
- *Identify the responsibilities of the LP/VN in rehabilitation nursing, nursing in long-term care, in-home care, and hospice.*
- *List the various types of long-term care services.*

KEY TERMS

accreditation	Medicaid
adult day care	Medicare
assisted living	Medigap insurance
certification	rehabilitation
hospice	respite care
licensure	subacute care
long-term care facility	synergy

INTRODUCTION

There has been a strong emergence in the past decade of nonacute health care services. The growth of these services is a reflection of several changes occurring in the United States:

- The Tax Equity and Fiscal Responsibility Act of 1983 initiated the Medicare Prospective Payment system and the diagnosis-related group (DRG) system. This has resulted in the discharge of clients from acute-care hospitals much earlier. Clients, particularly elderly individuals, often require continuing care.
- Lives are being saved that would have been lost a few years ago. Ongoing health care services are often necessary for these individuals.

- The number of Americans over the age of 65 tripled in the 20th century. The risk of acquiring a chronic disease increases as individuals age, requiring health care throughout life.
- The cost of acute care has reached critical proportions. Case management is an attempt to contain costs by assisting people in defining their service needs, locating and arranging services, and coordinating the services of multiple providers. The cost of health care can be managed by controlling client access to services (General Accounting Office, 1994).

These changes have resulted in a vast increase in rehabilitation, home health, long-term care, and hospice services. There is an intermingling of services and settings under each of these categories of care. Rehabilitative services for example, may be provided in an acute-care setting, in a rehabilitation hospital, in a long-term care facility, or in the client's home. Home care may provide the same services that would be available in a subacute care nursing facility. Long-term care refers to both home and community-based services. Hospice care may be provided in the home or institution. While many of the clients requiring these services are elderly, there are an increasing number of services specializing in pediatric care.

LEGAL AND ETHICAL RESPONSIBILITIES

The legal basis for the provision of care in long-term care facilities is found in the Omnibus Budget Reconciliation Act (OBRA) of 1987. This act was legislated after a lengthy study of the care delivery in long-term facilities throughout the country. The major components of the act concern the issues of nursing assistant training, the regulation of the use of physical and chemical restraints, the Minimum Data Set (MDS) as an assessment tool, and the legal foundation for residents' rights. Many of the regulations found in OBRA also apply to home health nursing agencies.

The rights of the health care consumer are regulated for both long-term care and home health care. Before receiving services from either, the consumer must be given a copy of these rights and indicate an understanding of their content (Tables 29–1 and 29–2). In addition to OBRA, there are many other regulatory acts

---

Table 29–1 RESIDENT'S RIGHTS

This is an abbreviated version of the Resident's Rights as set forth in the Omnibus Budget Reconciliation Act. This document must be given to all residents and/or their families prior to admission to any long-term care facility.

1. **The resident has the right to free choice, including the right to:**
   - choose an attending physician
   - full advance information about changes in care or treatment
   - participate in the assessment and care planning process
   - self-administration of medications
   - consent to participate in experimental research
2. **The resident has the right to freedom from abuse and restraints, including freedom from:**
   - physical, sexual, mental abuse
   - corporal punishment and involuntary seclusion
   - physical and chemical restraints
3. **The resident has the right to privacy including privacy for:**
   - treatment and nursing care
   - receiving/sending mail
   - telephone calls
   - visitors
4. **The resident has the right to confidentiality of personal and clinical records.**
5. **The resident has the right to accommodation of needs including:**
   - choices about life
   - receiving assistance in maintaining independence
6. **The resident has the right to voice grievances.**
7. **The resident has the right to organize and participate in family and resident groups.**
8. **The resident has the right to participate in social, religious, and community activities including the right to:**
   - vote
   - keep religious items in the room
   - attend religious services
9. **The resident has the right to examine survey results and correction plans.**
10. **The resident has the right to manage personal funds.**
11. **The resident has the right to information about eligibility for Medicare/Medicaid funds.**
12. **The resident has the right to file complaints about abuse, neglect, or misappropriation of property.**
13. **The resident has the right to information about advocacy groups.**
14. **The resident has the right to immediate and unlimited access to family or relatives.**
15. **The resident has the right to share a room with the spouse if they are both residents in the same facility.**
16. **The resident has the right to perform or not perform work for the facility if it is medically appropriate for the resident to work.**
17. **The resident has the right to remain in the facility except in certain circumstances.**
18. **The resident has the right to personal possessions.**
19. **The resident has the right to notification of change in condition.**

(As determined by Omnibus Budget Reconciliation Act [OBRA] of 1987)

Table 29–2 CLIENT'S RIGHTS IN HOME CARE

Clients receiving home health care services or their families possess basic rights and responsibilities. These include:

The right to:

1. be treated with dignity, consideration, and respect.
2. have their property treated with respect.
3. receive a timely response from the agency to requests for service.
4. be fully informed on admission of the care and treatment that will be provided, how much it will cost, and how payment will be handled.
5. know in advance if they will be responsible for any payment.
6. be informed in advance of any changes in care.
7. receive care from professionally trained personnel, to know their names and responsibilities.
8. participate in planning care.
9. refuse treatment and to be told the consequences of this action.
10. expect confidentiality of all information.
11. be informed of anticipated termination of service.
12. be referred elsewhere if denied services solely based on ability to pay.
13. know how to make a complaint or recommend a change in agency policies and services.

The responsibility to:

1. remain under a doctor's care while receiving services.
2. provide the agency with a complete health history.
3. provide the agency all requested insurance and financial information.
4. sign the required consents and releases for insurance billing.
5. participate in care by asking questions, expressing concerns, stating whether information is not understood.
6. provide a safe home environment in which care is given.
7. cooperate with the doctor, the staff, and other caregivers.
8. accept responsibility for any refusal of treatment.
9. abide by agency policies that restrict duties the staff may perform.
10. advise agency administration of any dissatisfaction or problems with care.

that affect the delivery of care in the settings described in this chapter. These include the Self-Determination Act of 1990, which is a federal regulation, and legislation related to the reporting of client abuse (state regulations).

There is a fine line between what is a legal issue and what is an ethical issue. It is beyond the scope of this chapter to provide answers to the questions arising from such problems. However, these situations are examples of common legal and ethical issues.

1. An 80-year-old client in the third stage of Alzheimer's disease falls and fractures his hip. Should this client be transferred to a rehabilitation hospital for intensive rehabilitation? If not, what are the alternatives?

2. The staff of a long-term care facility suspects that a client was abused by her son before admission to the facility. The son wishes to take the mother home, and the mother is in agreement with this plan. The discharge planner learns that the local social services agency had investigated the client's living situation for abuse prior to the mother's admission. The case worker also suspects abuse but could find nothing objective upon which to build a case. Do the nursing staff and social workers of the facility have a legal or ethical obligation to attempt intervention? If so, what actions should be taken?

3. J.B. is a young adult (23 years old) receiving rehabilitation after suffering a traumatic brain injury

due to a motorcycle accident. He wishes to make decisions concerning his care and treatment. His mental competency is questionable. However, this has not been legally established, and his parents make decisions often in opposition to J.B.'s preferences. What are the legal and ethical responsibilities of the nurse in accepting the decisions of relatives versus client?

4. Mr. A. and Mrs. C. are both residents of a long-term care facility. Mr. A. is married and Mrs. C. is a widow. The two have developed an intimate relationship that appears to be mutually satisfying to them both. Both residents are mentally competent and consenting adults. Mrs. A. is troubled by this and expects the staff to intervene. Does the staff have the right to intervene? If so, does this conflict with the residents' rights?

SOURCES OF REIMBURSEMENT

Medicare and Medicaid have long been traditional sources of reimbursement for care. All health care providers must be certified by both Medicare and Medicaid to receive payment for services rendered. While virtually all hospitals are certified by both Medicare and Medicaid, many long-term care providers, including home health care and skilled care facilities, are not. Clients, families, and hospital discharge planners need to be aware of this when planning continuing care.

Medicare

In 1965, **Medicare** (Title XVIII) was signed into law as an amendment to the Social Security Act and is the source of payment for acute care services for 95% of persons over 65 years old and for permanently disabled individuals who receive Social Security disability benefits (Waid, 1998). Medicare is administered by the federal government through the Health Care Finance Administration (HCFA). Medicare Part A covers inpatient hospital care, home health care, and hospice care. Payment may be made for care in a skilled nursing facility. However, there are many restrictions, and criteria for coverage frequently change. Medicare Part B covers partial costs for physician services, outpatient hospital and rehabilitation care, and certain services and supplies not covered by Part A.

Medicare pays for limited skilled care and rehabilitation services in certified long-term care facilities if the client and the services provided meet specific criteria. Certified home health care agencies may be reimbursed for intermittent visits if the client requires skilled health care by a registered nurse. In 1998, Medicare spent $216.6 billion for the care of its 38.8 million enrollees (HCFA, 2000a).

Medicaid

Medicaid (Title XIX) pays for health services for the aged poor, the disabled, and low-income families with dependent children (Abrams, Beers, & Berkow, 2000). The program is financed by federal and state funds and is administered at the state level. Thus, services provided vary from state to state. Medicaid is currently the primary health financing program for low-income families and disabled individuals. It is a means-tested program, providing funds only when all other financial resources have been exhausted (Waid, 1998). Services covered include inpatient and outpatient hospital care, diagnostic services, physician services, skilled nursing care, and home health services. Medicaid spent $170.6 billion in 1998 (HCFA, 2000a). Medicaid is the principal source of financial assistance for long-term care. Medicaid pays for skilled home health care in all states, and 29 states also cover the optional benefit of personal care in the home. In 1997, home health care and personal care services cost Medicaid $157.1 billion (HCFA, 2000b).

Private Insurance

Sixty-six percent of beneficiaries of Medicare purchase **Medigap insurance** to pay for costs not covered by Medicare. These policies are purchased from private insurance companies. Medigap insurance has been restricted by Congress to a basic plan with nine possible expansions (Abrams et al., 2000). Only 5% of all nursing home care costs are covered by private insurance (HCFA, 2000b). About 30% of costs are paid by the clients and their families, about 9% by Medicare, and 43.5% by Medicaid (HCFA, 2000b). Long-term care insurance is a relatively new concept and the benefits vary greatly depending on the insurance company.

LICENSURE, CERTIFICATION, AND ACCREDITATION

There are a number of processes that have been designed to assure the health care consumer that the facility, agency, or service meets minimal standards of care. **Licensure** is a mandatory system of granting licenses according to specified standards and is regulated by each state. **Certification** is a voluntary process that establishes and evaluates compliance with rules and regulations but is required for any provider who seeks reimbursement from government funds. Because government funding is regulated by the federal government, certification rules are generated by the federal government. **Accreditation** is an additional confirmation of quality and generally indicates that the provider has gone above the minimum standards in the delivery of care and service.

Licensure

All health care facilities must be licensed. Each state has a designated agency (often the Department of Public Health) that is responsible for licensing health care facilities. A team of surveyors visits each facility annually to determine whether the facility is in compliance with the rules and regulations of the state. Noncompliance in any area results in severe sanctions and financial penalties to the institution. The facility is given a limited amount of time to correct any deficiencies. In cases where residents' lives or well-being are threatened, the facility may lose its license to operate.

Certification

Certification is required for any facility that chooses to be reimbursed by government funds, Medicare, and Medicaid. There are regulations that must be met for certification to be granted. HCFA contracts with the state agencies to perform this function. In some states the long-term care survey for licensure and certification is done concurrently. Because there are two regulatory agencies (state and federal), the states have adopted the federal regulations and in some cases have exceeded federal regulations. Certification may not be granted if the facility is not in compliance with regulations. This means the facility will not receive any reimbursement from Medicare or Medicaid funds.

Accreditation

Seeking accreditation is voluntary (not required by law). Accrediting organizations issue standards whereas state/federal licensure and certification agencies issue rules and regulations. The Joint Commission on Accreditation of Healthcare Organizations (JCAHO) has long been accrediting hospitals and skilled nursing facilities. The Commission on Accreditation of Rehabilitation Facilities (CARF) has been accrediting comprehensive inpatient rehabilitation programs since 1966. Facilities like a subacute care unit specializing in rehabilitation may seek accreditation from both commissions.

REHABILITATION

Rehabilitation is a process designed to help individuals reach their optimal level of physical, mental, and psychosocial functioning. This goal is accomplished by preventing complications, modifying the effects of the disability, and increasing independence. By so doing, the individual's self-esteem is maximized, thus increasing quality of life. Rehabilitation is concerned with increasing the client's ability to complete the basic activities of daily living (ADLs) and the instrumental activities of daily living (IADLs). ADLs include grooming and hygiene, eating, dressing, toileting, and mobility. The IADLs include higher-level tasks such as household and money management, using the telephone, and driving a car. For persons who have limited potential for regaining total independence, the goal is to teach the client to manage his or her own care.

The Interdisciplinary Health Care Team

The interdisciplinary health care team (IHCT) is an essential component to any rehabilitation process. The client and family are the focus of the team and are encouraged to participate in the planning of care. The degree to which the family participates is determined by the client. The professional members of the team are selected based on the needs of the client. Physical and occupational therapists, a speech/language pathologist, recreational therapists, rehabilitation nurses, the physician, social workers, dietitians, and mental health professionals are usually required to provide services (Figure 29-1).

Each discipline completes an assessment and pools this information at the care planning conference so that a consensus among members (including the client and family) can be reached. The team process avoids both duplication of services and fragmented care. A holistic approach is utilized so that the client's physical, mental, and psychosocial needs will be identified.

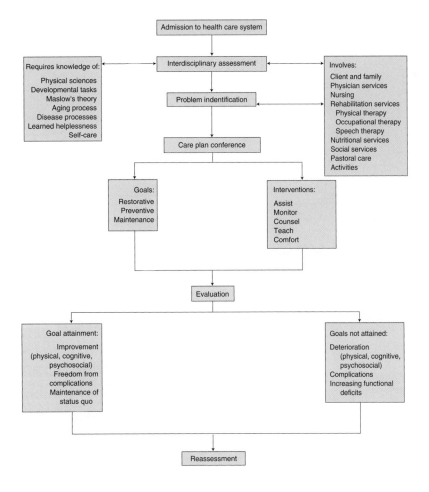

Figure 29-1 The Interdisciplinary Health Care Team Process

Role of the LP/VN

Rehabilitation nursing is a specialty practice and requires specialized knowledge, skills, and attitudes. A sound knowledge base in the anatomy and physiology of the neurological, musculoskeletal, gastrointestinal, and urological systems is a prerequisite. The nurse must have excellent clinical skills in the areas of therapeutic positioning, range of joint motion exercises, transfers, ambulation, and activities of daily living. The nurse is responsible for planning measures to prevent complications such as impaired skin integrity and contractures and to implement interventions for dysphagia, incontinence, and other identified problems.

The nurse is a member of the interdisciplinary team and as such may function as caregiver, counselor, coordinator of care, and client advocate. The nurse needs an understanding of the roles and responsibilities of each discipline and how the nurse interrelates with each discipline. There is a steady demand for rehabilitation nurses in all settings.

Functional Assessment and Evaluation for Rehabilitation

Clients who need rehabilitation are screened before admission to a program. Assessments are completed by health care professionals whose services may be required by the client (Figure 29-2). The purpose of screening is to select the best setting for services. Criteria for admission to a program usually require that the client be:

- Medically stable
- Able to learn
- Able to sit supported for at least 1 hour a day and to actively participate in the program

Interdisciplinary programs may stipulate that the client has disabilities in 2 or more areas of function:

- Mobility
- Performance of ADL
- Bowel and bladder control
- Cognition
- Emotional function
- Pain management
- Swallowing
- Communication

There are a number of standardized assessment instruments that are designed to evaluate motor function, cognition, speech and language, mobility, and the client's performance of activities of daily living. There are additional tools that identify the client's risk for pressure ulcer formation, and potential for bowel and bladder management for incontinence. Refer to the AHCPR publication *Post-Stroke Rehabilitation, Clinical Guideline Number 16*, for a complete description of assessment instruments (Gresham et al., 1995).

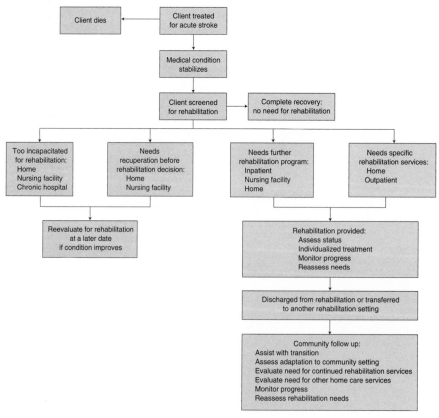

Figure 29-2 Assessing Potential—Stroke Rehabilitation

Rehabilitation Settings

Rehabilitation can be conducted in a variety of settings. Rehabilitation begins during the acute stage of illness when the client's medical condition stabilizes. Continuing rehabilitative services are often needed after discharge from acute care, necessitating transfer to a hospital inpatient program, a skilled nursing facility, an outpatient rehabilitation program, or a home rehabilitation program. Decisions about entry into a rehabilitation program should reflect a consensus among the client, family or significant others, physician, and the rehabilitation program.

Hospital Inpatient Program

Hospitals may have a separate rehabilitation unit, or services may be available in a freestanding hospital specializing in the delivery of rehabilitation services. In either case, the hospitals are staffed by a full range of rehabilitation professionals. Registered nurses and a physician skilled in rehabilitation (physiatrist) are available 24 hours a day. Hospital programs are generally more intense and comprehensive than programs in other settings, requiring greater physical and mental effort from the client.

Skilled Nursing Facility

Skilled nursing facilities often offer rehabilitation services. The facility may be hospital based or community based. The programs are similar to those offered in hospital settings with a full range of services and health care professionals. Physician coverage varies, but professional nursing care is rendered 24 hours a day. The program is usually less intense than a hospital program; this may be a benefit to elderly clients with limited energy resources. Families should research the services available because they differ greatly from one facility to the next.

Outpatient Rehabilitation

Outpatient services are offered by hospital-based rehabilitation programs. The intensity may range from occasional visits to 3 or 4 visits per week. Day hospital programs are another form of outpatient services but require the client to spend several hours a day for 3 to 5 days a week at the hospital. Availability of transportation is a prerequisite for all outpatient programs.

Home Rehabilitation

Some home health agencies provide a full scope of services, including nursing, all therapies, and social services. Service is usually provided on an intermittent basis for medically stable clients. The accessibility of services varies greatly depending on the availability of therapists in the area.

HOME HEALTH CARE

Home care encompasses a number of services delivered to persons in their homes and is the fastest growing segment of health care delivery. The total number of home health care agencies increased by 26% between 1989 and 1994 (Millea, 1995). Clients are receiving intravenous therapy, ventilator care, parenteral nutrition, and chemotherapy at home. Many agencies have nurse specialists on staff for complicated cases involving care required for wounds, intravenous therapy, diabetes, and cardiac or respiratory problems.

Medicare certified agencies (7,747 in 1999) provide intermittent care to persons meeting the criteria for care (NAHC, 2000). A registered nurse may call on the client a specified number of times each week to assess the client's condition, supervise the work of LP/VNs and unlicensed workers, and deliver skilled nursing care. Nursing assistants are assigned to give personal care; check vital signs; and do positioning, transfers, and passive range-of-motion exercises. In addition to nursing staff, the agency may provide therapists and social workers to serve their clients, also on an intermittent basis. These services are time-limited by Medicare and are not reimbursable if the client is not deemed to require skilled care.

The home health agency may provide or arrange with other vendors for services needed by the client. This may include Meals-on-Wheels, homemaker services for light housekeeping tasks, companion services, transportation for outpatient care, intravenous therapy, pain management, and parenteral nutrition. The home health nurse needs to be aware of the availability of respite care because family members may need a break from the rigors of caregiving and may need encouragement from the nurse to do so.

Role of the LP/VN

Although the role of the LP/VN in home care is expanding, current (1994) statistics indicate that LP/VNs make up the smallest number of home health care professionals. There were 254,643 registered nurses, 34,757 LP/VNs, 171,346 home health care assistants, and 48,460 physical therapists working in home care (Millea, 1995). The responsibilities of the LP/VN vary among agencies. All nurses working in home care must have excellent assessment skills and a keen ability to identify actual and potential problems. Working with the family may be a greater challenge than meeting the needs of the client. Teaching the client and family is a major responsibility for the home health nurse. The educated client can assume more control. The client with a chronic health problem will have ongoing needs after the home health care is discontinued. Clients and their family caregivers must know the following:

PROFESSIONAL TIP

Sharps Injuries in the Home
- Significantly more home health workers receive needle injuries than hospital workers do (Jagger & Perry, 2000).
- OSHA cannot regulate private homes.
- Home health employers are responsible for meeting OSHA requirements that are not site specific, including sharps with built-in injury protection.

The disease process
- Complications that may occur
- How to prevent the complications
- Signs and symptoms of the complications
- How to reduce risk factors such as dietary adaptations and exercise programs

Medications
- Actions of medications
- Special administration guidelines such as timing related to meals
- Side effects

Special skills
- Drawing up and administering insulin or other injectables
- Using a blood glucose monitor
- Changing dressings
- Monitoring vital signs
- Using special client care equipment, adaptive devices, and assistive devices

Documentation and communication
- How to keep records for nurse or physician visit; for example, blood glucose, blood pressure, and weight
- Communication with health care providers
- How and when to contact the home health nurse
- How and when to contact the physician
- How and when to contact emergency services

LONG-TERM CARE

Long-term care refers to a spectrum of services provided to individuals who have an ongoing need for health care. Long-term care has traditionally meant a community-based nursing home licensed for skilled or intermediate care. While there is a great demand for this type of care, there is also a market for other levels of health care. It is estimated that by the year 2030, more than 8 million seniors will be residing in nursing homes (American Health Care Association [AHCA], 1998). Currently 1.5 million persons live in 17,000 nursing homes. Of the residents, 90% are over age 65, but 24% are over age 85 (AHCA, 1998).

The increasing population of elderly persons has re-

sulted in tremendous changes in health care delivery. Housing options are often a component of the package of services available. The least restrictive level of care that is appropriate for the client's needs will generally be the most cost effective. The Joint Commission on Accreditation of Healthcare Organizations (JCAHO) has established standards for pain assessment and treatment in long-term care facilities (JCAHO, 2000).

Long-Term Care Facilities

A **long-term care facility** may be licensed for either intermediate care or skilled nursing care. Long-term care facilities provide services to individuals who are not acutely ill, have continuing health care needs, and cannot function independently at home. Intermediate care facilities (ICF) are not certified for reimbursement from Medicare but may be certified for Medicaid funding. Skilled nursing facilities (SNF) are eligible for certification by both Medicare and Medicaid, but not all facilities choose to become certified. These facilities were formerly called nursing homes, rest homes, or convalescent centers. The term *extended care facility* (ECF) refers to any facility that renders care for a long period of time. It has no concrete definition and could refer to either an intermediate or skilled nursing facility. Facilities in every state that receive any government funds from any source are required by law to be in compliance with the OBRA regulations. It is estimated that 2 out of 5 persons in the United States will need long-term care sometime in their lives (AHCA, 1998).

Facilities of today bear little resemblance to those of the 1970s and 1980s. A restorative philosophy of care provides direction for the interdisciplinary team. Emphasis is placed on assisting the client (usually called resident) to attain and maintain the highest level of physical, mental, and psychosocial function. A holistic approach is utilized and families are important members of the care team.

A large number of facilities have special units devoted to the care of residents with specific problems. These units may care for persons with Alzheimer's disease, diabetes, respiratory disorders, wounds, and so on.

Subacute Care

Subacute care is a concept designed to provide services for clients who are out of the acute stage of their illnesses but who still require skilled nursing, monitoring, and ongoing treatments. The clients are not critically ill but do have complex medical needs. Subacute care is intended to fill the gap between the acute care hospital and the traditional long-term care facility (AHCA, 2000).

Subacute care facilities are usually housed in a section of a freestanding long-term care facility. The nurses may have a critical care background or are given additional training to equip them with the skills needed to provide care. Services may include intensive rehabilitation therapies, wound and pain management, care for clients with acquired immunodeficiency syndrome (AIDS), oncology care, postsurgical services, intravenous therapy, nutritional support, peritoneal dialysis, ventilator care, and cardiac monitoring. Many subacute care units specialize in 1 or 2 of these areas. Clients stay from 20 to 30 days. Efficient discharge planning and client teaching are essential components to the plan of care.

Continuing Care Retirement Communities

Continuing Care Retirement Communities (CCRC) are designed to provide continuing levels of care as the individual's health care needs change. These levels include:

- Independent living in apartments located on the campus—housekeeping services and meals are provided
- **Assisted living**—a combination of housing and services for persons who need help with the activities of daily living
- Health care—either short-term for persons recovering from a temporary disorder or permanent for long-term illnesses such as Alzheimer's disease. The health care facility of the CCRC may be licensed as either skilled or intermediate

CCRCs usually charge a fee upon entry to the system and a monthly fee thereafter. The client must give proof of adequate financial resources in order to be accepted into the system. In exchange, individuals have the security of knowing that they will receive care for the remainder of their lives. Most CCRCs stipulate that persons must enter the system when they are able to live independently in the apartments. The health care facility of the CCRC may be certified for Medicaid if clients exhaust their financial resources. The health care facility may be certified for Medicare for clients who are qualified to receive such services. Neither Medicare nor Medicaid will pay for the independent living or assisted living sections of a CCRC.

Assisted Living

Assisted living combines housing and services for persons who require assistance with activities of daily living. Nursing care is not provided. These are persons who cannot live alone but who do not need 24-hour care. It is a less restrictive environment than a long-term care facility and maintains the individual's independence and freedom of choice. This level of care may be offered in a freestanding facility or as a section of a long-term care facility or CCRC as previously described. A monthly fee is charged and covers rent, utilities, housekeeping services, meals, transportation, health promotion, exercise programs, and assistance with ADL (Assisted Living Federation of America [ALFA], 1999).

There are an estimated 30,000 assisted living residences in the United States with more than 1 million residents (ALFA, 1999). The typical resident is a female (single or widowed) 83 years old or older (ALFA, 1999). Assisted living residences are licensed by the state. Costs range from $1,000 to $3,000 per month and are mainly paid from personal funds (AHCA, 1998).

Adult Day Care

Adult day care centers may be located in a separate unit of a long-term care facility, in a private home, or be freestanding. They provide a variety of services in a protective setting for adults who are unable to stay alone but who do not need 24-hour care. The centers are generally open from 7:00 A.M. to 6:00 P.M. 5 days a week and serve 2 or 3 meals a day. A daily or hourly fee is charged with an additional charge for meals. Services may be limited to socialization or may be comprehensive offering modest rehabilitation services and nursing care. Adult day care is often utilized by working persons who have a spouse or parent living with them who cannot be left alone. Fifty percent of clients in day care have some degree of cognitive impairment (NADSA, 2000).

Respite Care

Respite care may be offered by adult day care centers, long-term care facilities, or in private homes. It is intended to provide a break to caregivers and may be utilized a few hours a week, for an occasional weekend, or for longer vacations. Planned activities, meals, and supervision are included in respite care services.

Foster Care

Some states are investigating the use of foster homes for individuals who cannot live independently but who do not require the services of a health care facility. A person with Alzheimer's disease who is mobile but who is unable to stay alone because of cognitive impairment would be a candidate for foster care. The legal structure is similar to the foster home concept for children.

Role of the LP/VN

There are probably more career opportunities available for the LP/VN in long-term care facilities than in the other types of health care described in this chapter. In a small facility the LP/VN might act as supervisor during the night or evening shifts. In larger facilities the LP/VN might be in charge of one unit with a registered nurse as a house supervisor. The nurse needs sharp assessment skills and a sound ability to make nursing judgments based on assessment findings. The LP/VN may also be expected to supervise and coordinate the work of nursing assistants. The nurse may wish to seek additional course work to acquire supervisory skills. LP/VNs may take the Certification Examination for Practical and Vocational Nurses in Long-Term Care (CEPN-LTC™) given by the National Council of State Boards of Nursing (NCSBN). Those who pass the examination are certified in long-term care and may use the initials "CLTC" to signify their certification.

HOSPICE

Hospice is humane, compassionate care provided to clients who can no longer benefit from curative treatment and have 6 months or less to live. The special care is designed to provide sensitivity and support, allowing clients to carry on an alert, pain-free life with other symptoms managed so the last days are spent with dignity and quality of life at home or in a homelike setting. This is sometimes referred to as palliative care.

The first hospice in the United States began in 1974. Today, there are more than 3,000 programs that are estimated to serve 450,000 terminally ill clients and their families each year (National Hospice Organization [NHO], 1999).

The primary physician must refer the client to hospice. Care and support are provided to both client and family by a team consisting of the physician, nurses, counselors, therapists, social worker, aides, and volunteers. The team regards dying as a normal process and does nothing to hasten or postpone death. Relief of pain and other distressing symptoms is provided. The client is supported to live as actively as possible until death. The family is supported to help them cope during the client's illness and in their bereavement after the client's death. Health care workers may also need support as the task of caring for the dying is often quite stressful.

PROFESSIONAL TIP

Hospice Settings

Hospice care may be implemented in a variety of settings: the client's home, a special area of hospitals or nursing homes, or freestanding inpatient facilities. Most clients receive care at home. In 1995, 77% of hospice clients died in their home, 19% died in an institutional facility, and 4% died in other settings (NHO, 1999).

Benefits for hospice are included in most private health care insurance, health maintenance organizations (HMOs), and managed care; Medicare; and in 43 states plus the District of Columbia by Medicaid. For hospice care in 1995, Medicare paid for 65.3% of the clients; private insurance, 12%; Medicaid, 7.8%; indigent (nonreimbursed) care, 4.2%; and other, 10.7% (NHO, 1999). As of 1999, 44 states had licensure laws for hospice programs. Some programs are certified voluntarily by Medicare and accredited by the JCAHO or Community Health Accreditation Program (CHAP) (NHO, 1999).

SAMPLE NURSING CARE PLAN

THE CLIENT REQUIRING REHABILITATIVE CARE

Mr. Jason, 65 years old, was admitted to a skilled nursing facility following hospitalization for a right cerebral hemisphere stroke. He is unable to purposefully change position without assistance. His gag reflex is weakened, swallowing is delayed, and there is coughing after swallowing. Mr. Jason has smoked for 50 years and is still doing so. Rehabilitation was initiated in the hospital. A feeding tube was put in place with the goal to assist Mr. Jason to regain his swallowing ability so the tube can be removed. Mr. Jason frequently expresses his discouragement with his dependency on the staff. He is married and lives in the community with his wife. Mr. Jason had been retired for 1 year before the stroke. Mrs. Jason works full time. Two adult children live in other states. Mrs. Jason hopes that her husband will regain adequate mobility skills so that she can eventually take him home.

Nursing Diagnosis 1 *Impaired Physical Mobility related to left hemiplegia and sensory/perceptual impairments as evidenced by inability to purposefully change position of body without assistance*

PLANNING/GOALS	NURSING INTERVENTIONS	RATIONALE	EVALUATION
Mr. Jason will maintain current level of range of motion in all joints.	Change position at least every 2 hours; place affected extremities out of synergy.	Prevent contracture formation and pressure ulcers. Hemiplegic limbs are flaccid immediately after stroke and then become spastic. **Synergy** patterns (abnor-	Range of joint motion is preserved. Complications related to immobility are prevented. Progress in mobilization is

continues

mal patterns of movement that result from an overactive stretch reflex due to CNS damage) may develop in response to spasticity, causing contractures. Positioning out of synergy avoids contracture formation.

achieved; movement in bed, transfers with 1 to 2 assists, transfer independently, and ambulation are noted.

Mr. Jason will remain free of contractures.	Do passive range-of-motion exercises twice a day on affected extremities. Assist with active range-of-motion exercises on unaffected extremities. Teach to do self-range-of-motion exercises when condition permits.	Range-of-motion exercises maintain joint mobility and prevent contracture formation. Active and self range-of-motion exercises will also increase strength and endurance.	
Mr. Jason will begin program of progressive mobilization.	Teach Mr. Jason to move in bed: – Client begins in supine position with the knees bent and feet flat in bed. – Instruct client to raise the hips by pressing his heels down. – Stabilize the affected limb by exerting pressure downward through the thigh just above the knee while assisting the client to lift the pelvis clear of the bed (Galarneau, 1993). Consult with physical therapist about program for progressive mobilization.	Increases the client's bed mobility. The recovery of a client with a stroke is dependent on the cooperative efforts of several interdisciplinary team members. The physical therapist is an expert in mobility.	

Nursing Diagnosis 2 *Impaired Swallowing related to neuromuscular impairment as evidenced by weakened gag reflex, delayed swallowing, and coughing after swallowing*

PLANNING/GOALS	NURSING INTERVENTIONS	RATIONALE	EVALUATION
Mr. Jason will swallow without aspirating.	Consult with speech/language pathologist in regard to	A video-recorded fluoroscopy is used to make a definitive diag-	There are no signs of aspiration.

continues

video-recorded fluoroscopy for swallowing evaluation.

nosis of impaired swallowing. The results of the evaluation provide a basis for interventions suggested by the speech/language pathologist.

Serve semisolid foods of medium consistency. Use a commercial thickener for liquids. Avoid milk, citrus juices, and water.

These foods require less manipulation in the mouth and allow the client to concentrate on swallowing rather than chewing. Liquids are more manageable when thickened. Water provides minimal sensory stimulation, making it difficult for the client to manage water. Milk and citrus juices stimulate production of saliva.

Allow rest period before eating. Position client at 60°–90° angle before, during, and for 1 hour after eating.

Fatigue increases risk of aspiration.

Maintain head in midline with neck slightly flexed.

This position facilitates the passage of food through the pharynx.

Face the client, avoid haste.

Facing the client allows feeder to evaluate the eating process. If the feeder appears hurried, the client may try to eat faster.

Minimize distractions, keep conversation minimal.

The client's attention must focus only on eating.

Allow Mr. Jason to see and smell food. Give verbal descriptions. Use regular metal teaspoon, give one-half teaspoon at a time.

Sensory cues promote awareness of eating.

Place food on unaffected side of mouth. Teach to hold food in mouth, think about swallowing, and then swallow twice.

Buccal pocketing of food in the cheek on the affected side is common after a stroke.

continues

Nursing Diagnosis 3 *Situational Low Self-Esteem related to changes in functional abilities as evidenced by verbal expression of discouragement*

PLANNING/GOALS	NURSING INTERVENTIONS	RATIONALE	EVALUATION
Mr. Jason will verbalize acceptance of self, situation, and lifestyle changes.	Assess for signs of severe or prolonged grieving.	The client needs to grieve the loss of his former self. Prolonged grieving may indicate need for counseling.	Mr. Jason is progressing through all rehabilitation therapies and presents no signs of prolonged grieving.
	Assess client's interactions with significant others.	Other people may be reinforcing the concepts of helplessness and invalidism.	
	Listen in nonjudgmental fashion to comments about situation.	Each person responds differently to a crisis. Being nonjudgmental builds trust and encourages verbalization of thoughts.	

CASE STUDY

Mrs. Emma James, 72 years old, was admitted to Community Hospital for a left below knee amputation. Mrs. James has been an insulin dependent diabetic for 35 years. The amputation follows a long and unsuccessful period of treatment for venous stasis ulcers. Mrs. James was transferred from the hospital to a rehabilitation hospital on her fourth postoperative day. After 2 weeks at the rehabilitation hospital, she was transferred to a skilled care facility near her home for additional rehabilitation and regulation of the diabetes. She is now ready to be discharged to her home. Mrs. James has a prosthesis and is able to ambulate with a walker. She can perform her ADL with minimal assistance. She was on a sliding scale and blood glucose monitoring 4 times a day while in the long-term care facility. Her physician has now placed her on insulin twice a day with daily blood glucose checks. Her vision is somewhat impaired due to the diabetes. Mrs. James lives alone in a one-story home in a safe residential area. The discharge planner at the skilled care facility has arranged continuing care for Mrs. James through a local home health agency.

The following questions will guide your development of a nursing care plan for the case study.

1. Identify the assessment factors that are most important in planning Mrs. James's care.
2. List the nursing diagnoses that would be applicable to Mrs. James's assessment.
3. Describe the complications for which Mrs. James is at risk.
4. Describe nursing interventions for preventing the complications.
5. What specific actions would you take to prevent a recurrence of venous stasis ulcers?
6. What additional community services does Mrs. James need?
7. What nursing services (frequency of nurse visits, services from a nursing assistant, other home health services) would you plan to meet her needs? Which services would each person provide?
8. Describe the outcomes you would expect for Mrs. James.

SUMMARY

- There has been a significant increase in the growth of nonacute care settings.
- Medicaid (state and federal funds) and Medicare (federal funds) are major sources of health care payment, especially for the elderly and permanently disabled. The availability of these resources in the future is in jeopardy. Alternative funding sources are being explored by state and federal governments.
- Rehabilitation can be provided in a variety of settings.
- There is a need for the services and skills of the LP/VN in all of these health care services. Experience and additional education may be required for employment in special care settings.

Review Questions

1. One reason for the growth in nonacute care health services is:

   a. the diminishing supply of physicians.
   b. an increase in the number of hospitals in the country.
   c. the cost of acute care.
   d. the increase in Medicare reimbursement.

2. Medicare is a reimbursement system for health care providers that:

   a. is based upon the client's personal financial resources.
   b. is available to persons 65 years of age and over or who have been disabled for 2 or more years.
   c. pays the full cost of all medical care.
   d. is managed by each state.

3. Subacute care is most often provided:

   a. in a step-down unit of the hospital.
   b. in a special care unit of a skilled care facility.
   c. for clients who are terminally ill.
   d. for clients who require life support.

4. Which of the following clients would be most likely to benefit from rehabilitation services?

   a. Mr. J, 64 years old, had a stroke, is responsive and stable.
   b. Mrs. B, 89 years old, has Alzheimer's disease in the fourth stage.
   c. Miss Z, 26 years old, is recovering from pneumonia.
   d. Mr. K, 56 years old, has terminal cancer of the lung.

5. Which of the following is a legal requirement for health care facilities that is controlled by each state?

   a. accreditation
   b. certification
   c. licensure
   d. provision of free care

6. As a member of the interdisciplinary health care team, the LP/VN must be able to:

   a. participate in the planning of client care.
   b. plan the appropriate diet for clients.
   c. teach the new amputee how to walk with a prosthesis.
   d. provide alternative methods of communication for the client with recent stroke.

7. In the home health care setting, it is essential that the LP/VN possess skills in:

   a. advanced intravenous therapy.
   b. respiratory therapy treatments.
   c. physical assessment.
   d. planning and providing speech therapy.

8. In a long-term care facility, the LP/VN may serve as the:

   a. charge nurse of a unit.
   b. physical therapist.
   c. clinical nurse specialist.
   d. social worker.

Critical Thinking Question

1. What are the pros and cons related to working for a home health agency, a hospice, or a long-term care facility?

 WEB FLASH!

Search the Internet for the various types of health care discussed in this chapter. What information is available? Is it focused for consumer or provider?

12
Leadership/
Work Transition

Chapter 30
Leadership/Work Transition

LEADERSHIP/ WORK TRANSITION

MAKING THE CONNECTION

Refer to the following chapters to increase your understanding of leadership/work transition:

- **Chapter 5, The Health Care Delivery System**
- **Chapter 6, Legal Responsibilities**
- **Chapter 8, Communication**
- **Chapter 10, Documentation**

LEARNING OBJECTIVES

Upon completion of this chapter, you should be able to:
- *Define key terms.*
- *Outline the skills needed for effective management.*
- *Summarize the five rights of delegation.*
- *Explain factors that must be assessed in establishing priorities of care.*
- *Compare and contrast the roles of the registered nurse, licensed practical/vocational nurse, and unlicensed assistive personnel.*
- *Describe the content and format of résumés.*
- *Outline actions to take prior to a job interview.*

KEY TERMS

accountability	laissez-faire
assignment	leadership
autocratic	management
competency	policy
delegation	procedure
democratic	résumé
job description	

INTRODUCTION

By now you may have mastered the nursing process and demonstrated competency in many of the technical skills you will be required to perform on a daily basis. There are still other skills you will need in order to become competent in practice, however. These are the leadership skills that will allow you to manage yourself and others, delegate and prioritize tasks, and resolve conflicts and problems that may arise in the workplace. As a new graduate, you will not be expected to have yet mastered these skills; rather, they will develop as you progress in your career.

This chapter introduces these leadership skills as well as provides insight into the working environment. It explores the general organizational structure of the health care setting, defines nurses' roles within the health care system, and explores career options. The chapter walks you through the period from graduation to your first day on the job. Included are discussions of the examination process for licensure, preparations for a job search and interview, and continuing education.

LEADERSHIP

Leadership is the ability to direct or motivate others to achieve goals. Many personal qualities are associated with leaders, such as self-direction, flexibility, and assertiveness. Leaders are considered critical thinkers, responsible decision makers, and role models. Often, leaders are considered to possess a vision that directs a group and elicits the group's best efforts (Figure 30-1). Nursing leaders critically examine the way nursing care is delivered and use their power to effect change.

Leadership Styles

Several leadership styles are recognized. The style varies with the personality of the leader. Most often, a leader exhibits some characteristics of each style of leadership, though one style will typically be more dominant. Not all leadership styles are effective in all situations. Three recognized styles of leadership are autocratic, democratic, and laissez-faire.

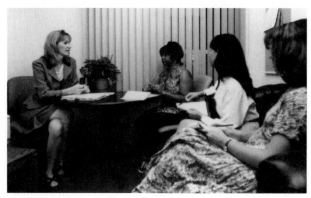

Figure 30-1 Leaders are often effective in unifying and directing groups.

Autocratic

Autocratic leadership is task-oriented and is based on the premise that the leader knows best. This leader is often viewed as controlling and inhibiting of the creativity and autonomy of workers. The leader problem solves and makes decisions without consulting the parties involved. All information is directed downward from leader to workers. The leader exercises responsibility for ensuring the work is done by issuing commands or orders to direct the work force. This leadership form is especially effective in crisis situations or situations requiring a quick response, or when leading a group with limited knowledge. When workers have a certain degree of knowledge, and teamwork is important, this style of leadership is not effective.

Democratic

The underlying belief of the **democratic** style of leadership is that every member of the team should have input (Figure 30-2). Although democratic leadership can be time-consuming, the benefit is seen in increased cooperation and teamwork. Individual workers are encouraged to participate in decision making and to express their viewpoints. The leader acts more as a resource person and facilitator. This approach is less ef-

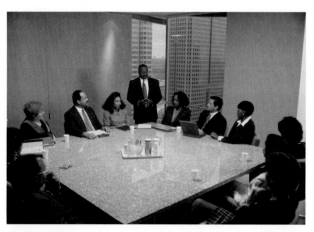

Figure 30-2 A democratic leader asks for input from the team during a brainstorming session. *(Courtesy of Photodisc)*

fective when there is conflict within the group or when time is short.

Laissez-Faire

The **laissez-faire** leadership style is a passive, nondirect approach that gives leadership responsibilities to the group rather than to one person. This style promotes optimal autonomy and creativity in group members. Task achievement is more difficult under this leadership form, so it is not a style of leadership used frequently in health care. The leader is almost unidentifiable, relying on the group's strengths and initiative to accomplish tasks.

Leadership Skills

Many theories of leadership cite several skills needed for effective leadership. These skills include communication, problem solving, self-evaluation, and management.

Communication

Strong communication skills foster trusting relationships with peers, subordinates, superiors, and clients, thus facilitating the leader's ability to motivate others. Additionally, leaders must be able to convey ideas and information clearly, concisely, and persuasively for the leader to effectively implement changes in the delivery of nursing care.

Problem Solving

Problem solving skills incorporate the ability to analyze all aspects of a problem, explore options, find solutions, and implement changes. Problem solving is a careful, deliberate process. Leaders seek information, consult experts, and use available resources to address problematic situations and enhance care.

Self-Evaluation

The self-evaluation skills necessary for effective leadership involve an honest assessment of personal strengths and weaknesses. Following such an assessment, efforts are made to enhance personal growth and development. An unwillingness to critically examine oneself hampers the leader's ability to critically examine, problem solve, and effect change in the workplace.

Management

Management skills involve the accomplishment of tasks either by doing them oneself or directing others to do them. Licensed practical/vocational nurses (LP/VNs) are in positions that require them to manage people and resources used to deliver quality client care.

MANAGEMENT

Management and leadership are closely related concepts. **Management** is the accomplishment of tasks through the effective use of people and resources. Management involves the practical, "nuts and bolts" of getting the job done with the available resources.

Every nurse is a manager. Managing the needs of a group of clients or managing the activities of a group of nursing assistants requires the same skills. Practice and education can help develop the management skills and, potentially, the leadership skills of every nurse.

As managers, LP/VNs are expected to plan, organize, supervise, and monitor the care that is provided to a group of clients. The actual care may be accomplished by the nurse or by others, typically certified nurse assistants (CNAs) or some other type of unlicensed assistive personnel (UAP). Each aspect of management encompasses several components.

- *Planning:* identifying tasks to be accomplished, determining available resources, assessing skill level of workers, identifying problems, and setting priorities
- *Organizing:* making client assignments, ensuring availability of resources, sharing pertinent information, and determining time tables (e.g., of breaks, lunch, completion of certain tasks)
- *Supervising:* directing care provided by others, investigating problems, communicating information, reallocating people and resources as needed, and educating staff as needed
- *Monitoring:* determining whether tasks have been accomplished, assessing need for further action, and ensuring that appropriate documentation is completed

TASK ASSIGNMENT

An array of activities is involved in caring for clients, and all personnel have specific tasks they can facilitate. The ability of a specific staff member to perform a specific task is based on level of education and experience. However, overlap exists, and determining who can legally do what is often confusing.

Tasks of the LP/VN

Registered nurses (RNs) and LP/VNs are individually licensed. Although some overlap exists in the scopes of practice of the LP/VN and the RN, there are also some significant differences. Licensed practical/vocational nurses are dependent practitioners, meaning that an RN, doctor, dentist, or some other health care provider must supervise them. Most often the supervisor is an RN.

In addition to a scope of practice, LP/VNs and RNs have given scopes of competence. Within the scope of practice, there are tasks and responsibilities the individual may or may not be competent to implement. For example, it is within the scope of practice for the LP/VN to perform phlebotomy, but this task does not fall within the scope of competence of every LP/VN.

The scope of competence expands as new skills are acquired, but all skills must fall within the scope of practice.

Licensed practical/vocational nurses are qualified to care for clients with common illnesses and to provide basic and preventive nursing procedures. Licensed practical/vocational nurses can participate in data collection, planning, implementation, and evaluation of nursing care in all settings. In most states, some specific activities are considered beyond the scope of practice of the LP/VN. These activities, with some variances by state, include the following:

- Client assessments (can collect data but not perform physical assessments)
- Independent development of the nursing care plan
- Triage, case management, or mental health counseling
- Intravenous chemotherapy
- Administration of blood and blood products
- Administration of initial doses of any intravenous medication
- Any procedures involving central lines

Tasks of the UAP

Nursing UAP do not have a scope of practice. A task that falls within the protected scope of practice of any licensed profession (including registered nursing and licensed practical/vocational nursing) *cannot* be performed by a UAP. These personnel can perform only those health-related activities for which they have been determined competent to perform. These activities include the following:

- Activities of daily living (feeding, grooming, toileting, ambulating, dressing)
- Vital signs (Figure 30-3)
- Venipuncture
- Glucometer use
- Mouth care and oral suctioning
- Care of hair, skin, and nails

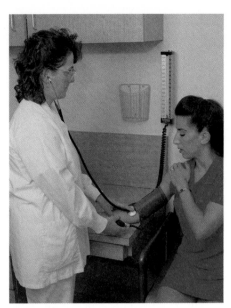

Figure 30-3 Unlicensed assistive personnel (UAP) can assist in many tasks, including measuring vital signs.

- Electrocardiogram measurements
- Applying clean dressings without assessment
- Non-nursing functions (clerical work, transport, cleaning)

DUTY DELEGATION

Delegation is the process of transferring to a competent individual the authority to perform a select task in a select situation. State provisions for the delegation of nursing tasks vary. Some states allow for the delegation of nursing tasks by an RN to both LP/VNs and UAP. In some states, LP/VNs may delegate certain nursing tasks to other LP/VNs or to UAP. Other states restrict delegation to licensed personnel only.

The licensed nurse retains accountability for the delegation. **Accountability** is defined as responsibility for actions and inactions performed by oneself or others. **Assignment**, another term frequently used to describe the transfer of activities from one person to another, involves the downward or lateral transfer of both responsibility and accountability for an activity.

At least one state differentiates between delegating nursing tasks to licensed nurses and assigning tasks to UAP. In New York, a nurse is not legally responsible for the process or outcome of care delegated to another licensed nurse. The nurse does remain responsible for tasks assigned to UAP, however. As an LP/VN, you are responsible for the decisions you make to delegate or assign tasks. Your knowledge of the client, activity, and worker will help you make sound decisions.

In most settings, RNs decide which nursing activities can be delegated or assigned to other licensed nurses (RNs or LP/VNs) and to UAP. Registered nurses and LP/VNs must consider five factors when making the decision to delegate or assign duties:

- *The potential for harm.* Certain nursing activities carry a risk for harming the client. Generally, the more invasive a procedure, the greater the potential for harm. Additionally, some activities carry a greater risk for certain kinds of clients (e.g., cutting the toenails of a diabetic). The greater the potential for harm, the greater the need for a licensed nurse to perform the activity.
- *The complexity of the task.* The cognitive skills and psychomotor skills needed for different nursing tasks vary considerably. As the skills increase in complexity, the level of education and competence becomes more critical. Some activities require a level of nursing assessment and judgment that can be provided only by a licensed professional.
- *The required problem solving and innovation.* As care is delivered, problems may develop. A successful outcome for the client may depend on a complex analysis of the problem and an individualized problem-solving approach. Alternatively, a simple activity may require special adaptation because of the client's condition. As problem solving increases in complexity and the need for innovation grows, so does the likelihood that a licensed nurse should provide the care.
- *The unpredictability of the outcome.* A client's response to an activity may be very predictable. If the client is unstable or the activity is new for the client, however, client response may be unpredictable and unknown. As unpredictability increases, so does the need for a licensed nurse.
- *The required coordination and consistency of the client's care.* Effective planning, coordination, and evaluation of client care requires the nurse to have direct client contact. The more stable the client and the more common the medical diagnosis, the more the care that can generally be delegated to support personnel. The need for a licensed nurse increases as the required coordination needed to delivery quality care increases.

The five rights of delegation provide further direction in making appropriate decisions about delegation. They are as follows:

- *Right Task:* The nurse must determine whether the task should be delegated for a specific client.
- *Right Circumstance:* Factors to consider include the client setting, availability of resources, client's condition, and other considerations.
- *Right Person:* The nurse must ask the question, "Is the right person delegating the right task to the right person to be performed on the right client?"
- *Right Direction/Communication:* A clear, concise description of the task should be conveyed, including all expectations for accomplishing the task.
- *Right Supervision:* Appropriate monitoring, implementation, evaluation, and feedback must be provided.

Registered nurses are frequently responsible for delegating care and assigning clients to the other nursing staff. In some settings, however, LP/VNs make these decisions. Licensed practical/vocational nurses should use the same guidelines to make decisions regarding delegating an activity to another LP/VN or assigning the task to UAP.

CARE PRIORITIZATION

Establishing priorities requires an understanding of the importance of different problems to the nurse, the client, the family, and other health care providers. For example, a client may be impatient to bathe because family is scheduled to visit. The nurse, however, does not want to remove the client's dressing for a bath until the physician has been able to examine the wound. Providing quality care while balancing such competing demands and ensuring completion of all tasks can be challenging.

Information obtained during the change-of-shift report is needed to appropriately establish priorities. This information can be useful in creating a worksheet identifying a list of tasks and target times for accomplishing these tasks. The time allotted for activities varies based on the condition of the client, the availability of support personnel, the availability of supplies, and a number of other factors. The effective use of time is important whether caring for one client, caring for a group of clients, or supervising the activities of others providing care.

While it is useful to get an overview of the day's activities, the clinical setting can change quickly and frequently. This is especially true in acute care settings. The nurse must be flexible and continually evaluate and reorder the priorities of care.

Given the same assignment, nurses will not necessarily establish the priorities of care in exactly the same way. If working closely with an RN, you should determine the priorities as she views them. When supervising UAP, you must be clear about your priorities and expectations. Among the factors that can be examined when establishing priorities are the following:

- *Safety:* You should ascertain whether a safety situation must be addressed immediately. A client experiencing a cardiac arrest, a fall, an insulin reaction, and other situations presenting an imminent threat must be tended to first.
- *Timing:* Medications, tests, and vital signs are frequently ordered at specific times. Often, there is very little flexibility in shifting the times. In hospitals, medications, for example, must be given within a specified time frame, usually ½ hour before or after the established time.
- *Interdependence of events:* You must ascertain whether some activity must occur before another

activity can take place. For example, a fasting blood sugar must be completed before the client receives either insulin or food; blood is drawn a specified time after the medication is given to ascertain the peak level of gentamyacin.
- *Client requests:* Quality care depends on meeting client needs. Some events—showers, bed changings, enema administration, and so on—can be scheduled after consulting with the client regarding personal preferences.
- *Availability of help:* If two people are needed to turn a client, ambulate a client, or provide other care, coordination of the health care team is essential for effective utilization of time. Ascertain which activities require assistance, then consult with coworkers about their availability.
- *Client's status:* Clients vary in the extent to which they can participate in their care. This factor influences the order of executing tasks and the length of time a task takes. A semi-independent client can be performing a task (e.g., bathing) with minimal assistance while the nurse attends to some other need.
- *Availability of resources:* If six clients are supposed to get out of bed and sit in chairs, and only two chairs are available, the clients clearly cannot get out of bed at the same time. Geri-chairs, wheelchairs, and other equipment are sometimes limited. Additionally, tasks may need to be delayed because supplies must be obtained from central supply.

Effectively organizing and establishing priorities with regard to care takes practice. Obtaining answers to certain questions when looking back at the day's events can help you hone this skill: Did you lack information that would have helped you prioritize more effectively? Did you fail to or inaccurately consider the client's status, the availability of help, or other factors? Did you establish priorities and set a schedule without getting client input? Did you fail to coordinate with coworkers? You must learn from experience. Both client and nurse feel the positive benefits of a day that flowed smoothly.

WORKPLACE TRANSITION

A successful employment experience depends on more than nursing knowledge and technical competence. Success requires competence in the particular job position. Success also depends on the nurse's integration into the health care team and the nurse's understanding of the overall health care organization.

The Nursing Team

Within the nursing staff are different team members. Nursing staff includes nursing UAP, CNAs, LP/VNs, RNs, and nurse practitioners (NPs). The roles, levels of education, skills, levels of independence, and lengths

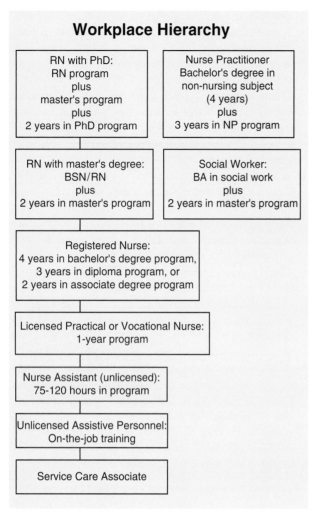

Workplace Hierarchy

RN with PhD:	Nurse Practitioner
RN program plus master's program plus 2 years in PhD program	Bachelor's degree in non-nursing subject (4 years) plus 3 years in NP program

RN with master's degree:	Social Worker:
BSN/RN plus 2 years in master's program	BA in social work plus 2 years in master's program

Registered Nurse:
4 years in bachelor's degree program,
3 years in diploma program, or
2 years in associate degree program

Licensed Practical or Vocational Nurse:
1-year program

Nurse Assistant (unlicensed):
75-120 hours in program

Unlicensed Assistive Personnel:
On-the-job training

Service Care Associate

Figure 30-4 Workplace Hierarchy

of education vary considerably (Figure 30-4). Familiarizing yourself with the roles of other nursing staff will help ensure that your practice conforms to the scope of practice as outlined by law.

PROFESSIONAL TIP

Hierarchy

As defined in the Nursing Practice Acts, or in the state nursing board's rules and regulations, an LP/VN works under the direction of an RN, physician, or dentist. These are the professionals who will directly supervise your work. In some states, the language of the law indicates that "other health care providers" can supervise you. The question is, Who are the other health care providers? In your state, must you follow orders written by a physician's assistant? A nurse practitioner? A physical therapist? The answers vary by state. It is critical that you know who can direct your nursing activities.

Nursing UAP can have a number of different titles including UAP, patient care technician, clinical technician, and nursing assistant. These persons provide hands-on care to clients in addition to performing other duties. None of these personnel has a license to practice. Rather, training is provided by the employer and may last from 2 to 10 weeks. The tasks they are expected to perform are designated by the employer and typically include things such as phlebotomy, electrocardiogram measurement, intake and output reading, bed making, and assisting clients with activities of daily living.

A CNA is also unlicensed. In contrast to other UAP, however, the curriculum and length of training to become a CNA are prescribed. As part of health care reforms in the long-term care setting, the primary employment setting of CNAs, a set curriculum of 100 hours duration must be completed to be certified.

Licensed practical/vocational nurses work very closely with registered nurses. The LP/VN attends a 1-year program and must pass the National Council Licensure Examination for Practical Nurses (NCLEX-PN). The RN is educated in a 3-year hospital-diploma program, a 2-year college associate-degree program, or a 4-year college baccalaureate program and must pass the National Council Licensure Examination for Registered Nurses (NCLEX-RN).

An NP is an RN who has obtained additional education (usually a master's degree) and is certified by the state. The role of the NP typically includes diagnosis and treatment of commonly occurring medical conditions. Outpatient clinics frequently employ NPs. Increasingly, they are also found working in hospitals, long-term care facilities, and rehabilitation centers.

Job Expectations and Responsibilities

Employees are hired to work at a specific site, for example, the fifth floor of the hospital or the internal medicine clinic at the outpatient health facility. The employer's expectations are summarized in job descriptions and in the policy and procedure manual. Although reading these papers is often viewed as bor-

PROFESSIONAL TIP

Unlicensed Personnel

Much controversy surrounds the role of UAP. Concerns have been raised that unlicensed personnel are functioning as de facto licensed nurses in violation of Nursing Practice Acts. Further, serious questions exist about the cost savings and quality of care in light of increased reliance on UAP and a corresponding reduction in licensed nurses. Understanding the role and limitations of UAP is critical.

ing and a waste of time, successful employment depends on understanding job expectations and the employer's policies.

Job Descriptions

A **job description** is a written outline of job responsibilities. Job responsibilities vary from employer to employer. For example, in long-term care facilities, LP/VNs are not routinely expected to bathe clients, as this task is performed by CNAs. In a hospital setting, however, job responsibilities of an LP/VN may include bathing clients. All the job expectations should fall within the scope of practice of the LP/VN.

In addition to summarizing job responsibilities, a job description frequently outlines requirements for the position (e.g., LP/VN, experience preferred), supervisor's title, supervisory responsibilities, and frequency and/or method of evaluation. A job description may also include a list of **competencies**, the specific skills or tasks (e.g., blood glucose monitoring) needed for a particular position. Employers are expected to assess competencies at the time of employment and periodically thereafter, usually annually.

A clear understanding of one's own job description is critical to the safe, effective practice of nursing in the specific employment setting. Failure to meet the job responsibilities as outlined in the job description can result in termination of employment. Familiarity with the job descriptions of supervisors and of persons who you may supervise is also very helpful in ensuring that you have a clear understanding of your role and those things you can expect of others.

Policies and Procedures

The employer's policies and procedures manual is also a very important reference document.

An employer's **policies** are written descriptions of the employer's expectations for handling various situations. Policies often are applicable to everyone working in the facility, rather than being nursing specific. Policies addressing confidentiality, dissemination of client information, handling of suspected cases of abuse, management of client valuables, and so on are common. A review of the policies and procedures manual is often required at the start of employment. A periodic self-initiated review of the manual is useful in ensuring that work performance meets the employer's expectations.

Procedures are step-by-step instructions describing the processes for performing various nursing tasks. Although these nursing procedures will likely be familiar to you, it is important that you perform tasks as directed by your employer. There are usually several correct, safe methods for performing a procedure; the way you were taught in school may vary from your employer's procedure. This may require altering the way you perform certain procedures.

Organizational Chart

An organizational chart is a visual representation of the relationship of one department to another within the facility and/or the relationship of the facility to other facilities in a health care network. Frequently included in the organizational chart are the names and/or titles of department leaders and the lines of authority. This information provides an understanding of the way your department fits into the larger organization.

All employees within a health care facility are part of a large organization. Every organization has a unique organizational culture of commonly held values, beliefs, and expectations directing the work force in the provision of services. For example, the organizational culture of a for-profit freestanding kidney dialysis center will be different from that of a free health clinic. Insights into the organizational culture of any health care facility can be garnered from the organization statement summarizing the facility's mission, vision, values, and goals. Although such statements often seem theoretical and far removed from job responsibilities, they do guide the organization in its provision of services.

FROM STUDENT TO EMPLOYEE

You have completed the licensed practical/vocational nursing educational program (Figure 30-5). Through formal education and clinical supervision, you have studied and learned the skills necessary to become competent in providing client care. Now you are ready to graduate and begin your career as a nurse.

Your first task as a graduate practical nurse is to take and pass the NCLEX-PN examination and obtain your nursing license. After you have obtained your license, you can begin the search for a job. The effort required in the period of time between the job search

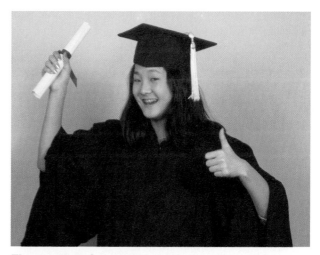

Figure 30-5 Congratulations! You have successfully completed your program. *(Photo courtesy of Tom Stock)*

and employment can be considered a job in and of itself. There are many tasks to complete and skills to master to land your first job as an LP/VN.

STATE BOARD EXAMINATION AND LICENSURE

In some states, you can begin work as a graduate LP/VN. A graduate LP/VN has completed the educational requirements and either is waiting to take the NCLEX-PN or to receive test results and a license. Check with your state board of nursing to learn both the requirements for a temporary license to practice nursing as a graduate LP/VN and any restrictions put on your practice while working under this status. For most students, however, the time after graduation is used to prepare for the state board exams.

The NCLEX-PN

The examination that all practical nurses must pass in order to be licensed is the NCLEX-PN. The NCLEX tests the skills and knowledge required for entry-level practice. The state boards use the results of this examination to determine whether a license will be issued to the graduate. Figure 30-6 lists the steps each graduate must follow in order to take the examination. The NCLEX tests knowledge of client needs such as physiologic and psychological needs, safety, and health promotion, as well as the nursing process, including data collection, planning, and implementation. The test is administered via a computer using a method called computerized adaptive testing (CAT), wherein the computer selects the test questions as you take the examination. You must answer all of the questions as they are presented to you, and you may not skip questions. All of the questions are multiple choice in format. All LP/VN candidates answer a minimum of 85 questions and a maximum of 205 questions during the maximum 5-hour testing period (National Council of State Boards of Nursing, 1997). The results are mailed to the candidate by the state board 1 month or less after the examination. Candidates may retake the examination,

PROFESSIONAL TIP

Temporary Permits

Although it is possible to work during the interim period between NCLEX-PN testing and licensure, most employers will postpone hiring until after you have received your permanent nursing license. Therefore, do not be discouraged if you are unable to obtain employment as a graduate LP/VN during this period.

however, the National Council requires a wait of at least 91 days between testings. Your state board may have other policies related to retaking the exam.

Your License

After you have successfully passed the NCLEX, you will be issued your nursing license from your state board. It is your responsibility to maintain your license according to your state's standards and inform your state board of any changes in name, address, and employment. Once licensed, you are ready to practice.

EMPLOYMENT OPPORTUNITIES

A wide variety of employment opportunities exist for the LP/VN. These range from employment in the traditional settings of hospital and nursing home to less traditional settings such as correctional facilities and hospice care. In 1996, 32% of LP/VNs worked in hospitals, 27% worked in nursing homes, and 13% worked in doctor's offices and clinics (Bureau of Labor

1. Apply to the board of nursing for a license, following instructions from that board.

2. Candidate gets an *NCLEX® Examination Candidate Bulletin* from the board of nursing.

3. Candidate submits a registration form to The Chauncey Group (the National Council's contracted testing service) or registers by phone. The Chauncey Group will acknowledge the candidate's registration my mail.

Note: Candidates seeking licensure from Illinois and Massachusetts do not register directly with The Chauncey Group. Follow registration instructions provided by those boards of nursing.

4. The board of nursing will communicate the candidate's eligibility to test to The Chauncey Group.

5. The Chauncey Group will send the candidate an Authorization To Test (ATT) with a booklet called *Scheduling and Taking your NCLEX® Examination* and a list of test centers.

6. The candidate will call a Sylvan test center and schedule an appointment to test.

7. On the appointed day, the candidate will take the test at a Sylvan Technology Center.

8. Sylvan transmits the test results to The Chauncey Group. After verifying the accuracy of the results, The Chauncey Group transmits them to the designated board of nursing.

9. The board of nursing sends results to the candidate.

Figure 30-6 NCLEX Examination Testing Process (*Reprinted courtesy of the National Council of State Boards of Nursing, Inc.*)

Statistics, 1998). Although the majority of LP/VNs are still employed in traditional settings, increasing opportunities are arising in the nontraditional settings because of changes in health care delivery. An overview of the various employment settings for the LP/VN follows. As a graduate, it is your task to determine the setting that constitutes the best fit for you.

Hospitals

Although the majority of LP/VNs are still working in the hospital setting, it is projected that the number of jobs for LP/VNs in hospitals will decline through the year 2006 (Bureau of Labor Statistics, 1998). Therefore, LP/VNs seeking to enter this setting will meet more competition than in the past. Employment opportunities outside of the client care unit, such as in hospital-based clinics, outpatient care units, and hospital-based long-term care units, are where most LP/VNs will typically find work in the hospital setting.

Long-Term Care Facilities/ Rehabilitation Centers

Employment for LP/VNs in long-term care and rehabilitation settings is projected to grow faster than average through the year 2006 (Bureau of Labor Statistics, 1998). Long-term care will offer the greatest number of new jobs for LP/VNs, due to the growing elderly population. Nurses in this setting will also provide care to clients who have been released by the hospital but who are not yet well enough to go home and who need additional rehabilitative services (Figure 30-7).

Community Health Agencies

In the community health setting, care is provided to clients through established health care programs. These programs are generally funded by local, state, or federal government or by voluntary agencies. Nurses in this setting will generally work in a community clinic or will travel to clients' homes to provide care and education.

Private Duty

Private duty nurses are self-employed, meaning the nurse is hired and paid directly by the client. The nurse works under the direction of a physician but must rely on knowledge and judgment to provide care. Private duty nurses are responsible for handling all matters of licensing and finances on their own.

Home Care Agencies

In the home care setting, care is provided to clients in their own homes. The nurse is generally employed by an agency but will work in the home of an assigned client. This area of nursing is rapidly expanding, due to both a consumer demand for home care and the lowered costs of caring for an individual in the home (Figure 30-8).

Hospice

Hospice nursing care consists of providing comfort to dying clients and their families. The role of the nurse is to alleviate pain and other symptoms but not to provide curative care. The clients in the hospice setting are terminally ill and typically have fewer than 6 months to live. Hospice services are most often rendered in the home, but services can also be offered in other settings.

Occupational Health

Occupational health nursing serves to provide safe working environments in industrial workplaces. Occupational health nurses work within industries and corporations and collaborate with corporate administration to provide health education and promotion to employees in the workplace.

Correctional Facilities

Correctional nursing is the branch of nursing that provides care within prisons, youth detention centers,

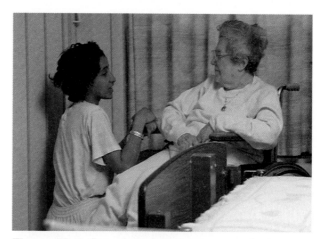

Figure 30-7 Care of elders in long-term care facilities is a growing career opportunity for the LP/VN.

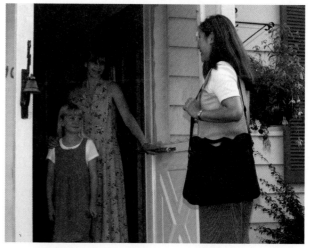

Figure 30-8 Nurses working in home health care agencies must be able to travel to the client's home to provide care.

and probation divisions. Care provided ranges from ambulatory care to emergent care to comprehensive health care.

School

School nursing focuses on providing care to the school-age child. The school nurse serves to promote wellness and identify or prevent problems. Both public and private schools offer opportunities for school nursing.

Parish

Parish nurses provide health care education and support to a congregation. The care is designed to meet the common needs and beliefs of a specified group of people.

Insurance Companies

Nurses working in the insurance setting are often responsible for coding treatments, providing physical examinations for insurance policies, and reviewing medical records.

PREPARING FOR THE JOB HUNT

Job hunting for many people is synonymous with scanning the Sunday want ads. This is not necessarily a bad place to identify potential employers; after all, given that the employer is advertising, they probably are hiring. The problem with relying solely on this approach is that it limits you to the jobs that are available rather than the job you want. Many job openings do not get advertised in the newspaper. Job vacancies exist well before they get advertised. Remember, using this method, you are in competition with all the other job seekers who are relying on want ads to identify employment options.

Other options exist for identifying potential employers. The telephone directory is a great place to identify health care facilities in your area. You are likely to find far more health care facilities in your local area than you ever imagined. All these facilities represent potential employers. Job counselors disagree on the usefulness of telephoning the employers to determine whether job vacancies exist: Some claim that a telephone call is a quick method of determining vacancies, whereas others believe a face-to-face visit to the facility yields better results.

A job club, perhaps formed with your nursing school classmates, is often an effective method of sharing information about employers, vacancies, job requirements, and the like. Additionally, a job club can be a morale booster, if landing that job is somewhat elusive. Your colleagues in the club may also offer in-

sights into those areas of nursing to which they believe you are most suited.

After you have identified potential employers, be persistent in your job hunt. Most importantly, go after that job that looks interesting to you regardless of whether they have a known vacancy. But don't stop there. Apply at many different organizations. Apply not just at different facilities, but at many facilities. Concentrate on small employers. Every health care job seeker has heard about the local large medical center. However, right around the corner from your home may be the less well-known school for developmentally disadvantaged children and waiting there may be your ideal job!

Potential employers can be identified in several other ways. Nursing journals typically advertise positions. Sometimes, your instructors know of positions. The state or local employment office may offer assistance. Professional job placement services are also available. Increasingly, the Internet advertises job openings along with job-hunting information and tips. A little initiative in accessing such resources can prove an immeasurable help in finding the job you want, rather than just any job.

You graduated, passed the NCLEX, and were issued a license to practice; now it is time to begin seeking employment. The job search requires up-front preparation on your part to organize and pinpoint the areas where you would like to concentrate your efforts. After graduation, you must take the following steps to secure a job:

1. Identify your objective.
2. Prepare a résumé.
3. Prepare a cover letter.
4. Prepare a list of references.
5. Prepare a telephone call script.
6. Complete a job application.
7. Prepare for the interview.
8. Prepare a thank you note.

Completing these steps will obtain you the face-to-face meeting (the interview) that will ultimately result in an offer of employment.

Identify Your Objective

A common mistake among job hunters is identifying potential employers as a first step. Most employment counselors advise beginning the job search with *you*. Identify your job target or objective first. If you cannot envision yourself as a medication nurse in a long-term care facility (a very common position for LP/VNs), there is very little reason to apply for such employment in that setting.

Identifying your objective accomplishes two important things. First, once you know your objective, you will know where to focus your efforts in identifying potential employers. Second, you will have a reference on a résumé or during a job interview. You will be prepared to tell prospective employers precisely the ways that you can be of benefit to them.

If you are having difficulty pinpointing your objective, think back to other jobs or volunteer projects in which you have been involved. What skills did you use? What did you like about the job or project? Make a list of your strongest four to six skills: These are the skills you want to use in your new job and that will be valuable in identifying your objective. Ascertain which jobs call for those skills. The skills needed for a particular job can be identified in a number of ways, including the following:

- Talking to people in nursing positions and asking them what they like and do not like about their jobs. During clinical in nursing school, you may have already talked to nurses and have more information than you realize.
- Reading the job descriptions in the classified ads.
- Calling places that employ LP/VNs and asking them to send you a job description.

Once you have matched your skills to the skills required in a particular job, you have effectively identified your job objective.

Prepare a Résumé

The **résumé** is a job-hunting tool that summarizes your employment qualifications. The content of the résumé should be factual, accurate, and honest. The focus should be on verifiable skills or accomplishments that suggest to the employer those things you can do for them should they hire you. The résumé may be targeted toward a specific job, a specific career field (e.g., licensed practical/vocational nursing), or a specific person. Some employers want a résumé, others rely on job applications, and still others ask for both a résumé and a job application.

Regardless of the format selected, the résumé will include the following information:

- Name, address, phone number, and e-mail address, if you have one
- Objective
- Educational experience including names of schools, dates of attendance, and course of study
- Employment history including employers' names and addresses, dates of employment, and descriptions of work experience.

In the course of developing your résumé, make a list of all your past jobs and then decide which jobs you want to include on the résumé. If you have very little work experience, list all jobs on the résumé. Definitely include jobs that show experience related to your job objective. Include unpaid or volunteer work, if it highlights skills and experience needed for the job you are seeking.

Having significant gaps in your employment history may give the impression that you are an unstable worker. Employment gaps can be explained in a number of ways. If the gap resulted because you were in school, include that information. If you did significant volunteer work during that period, describe those activities. Being a full-time parent or a full-time caregiver to a family member is a respectable activity that sufficiently explains gaps in paid employment.

Similarly, make a list of your training and education. You certainly want to include training and education you have completed. If you have an academic degree, include the college, your major, the degree granted, and the date the degree was awarded.

If you have completed only a portion of training, list the courses that are directly related to your objective. The same applies to college courses you may have taken. It is usually not necessary to mention a high school diploma, unless the position you seek calls for one or you have no other higher education.

The next step in creating a résumé is to select a format. The three most common résumé formats are chronological, functional, and combination. Each format contains the same basic information about you, but organized in different ways. Your background and job objective will determine the format you use.

The chronological format highlights your jobs (Figure 30-9). It arranges your work experience in order

Anita Jones, LPN
1234 Pleasant Street
Chicago, Illinois 60000
Telephone: (123) 456-7890

OBJECTIVE:	Position as an LPN in long-term care setting
LICENSE NUMBER:	State of Illinois # _____
PROFESSIONAL EXPERIENCE:	
1992–present	**General Hospital and Medical Center** **Chicago, Illinois**
	Position: LPN, medication nurse Provide direct care as a team member on a 36 bed unit. Distribute and maintain medications. Work in cooperation with nonlicensed team members. Manage nursing outcomes using assistive personnel. Received three letters of commendation for patient care delivery.
1987–1992	**City Teaching Medical Center** Chicago, Illinois
	Position: LPN, general medical unit Provided direct patient care on a 25-bed medical unit. Gained experience caring for geriatric patients. Helped develop unit procedures for shift rotation. Participated in an average of 12 hours of continuing-education contact hours per year.
EDUCATION:	**Chicago State University, Chicago, Illinois** Completed 24 credit hours of course work in BSN prerequisites, focus on physiology and psychology
	Highland Community College, Freeport, Illinois Licensed Practical Nurse, 1987 Class representative to faculty council
RELATED EXPERIENCE:	Lectured 25 preschool students on keeping healthy, repeated program four times
AFFILIATIONS:	Member, NFLPN
REFERENCES:	Available upon request

Figure 30-9 Sample Chronological Résumé

by dates of the jobs you have had. The most recent job is usually listed first. The functional format is organized around your work experience and the skills involved. For example, you may have experience in providing respite care for your aunt, who has sole responsibility for her invalid mother. Additionally, you may have done volunteer work providing respite care for a local hospice, or you may have provided frequent care to your nephew with Down syndrome. These activities could all be listed under one heading that captures the skill of respite care. The résumé style that combines both the chronological and functional format is referred to as the combination format.

Numerous references are available to help you write a résumé. Tips on effective action words, examples of complete résumés, layout options, and other advice on résumé writing can help you create a high-quality résumé. Ask a friend, a teacher, a coworker, a classmate, or someone else to give you feedback on your résumé. Even after you have revised your résumé 10 times, you will be amazed at the degree to which you can still refine it.

The appearance of your résumé is as important as the content. After all, your résumé may provide the employer with their first impression of you. The résumé should be concise enough to fit on one page and must be typed in a neat, readable typeface (e.g., Times Roman). Your final résumé must be absolutely free of typographical or grammatical errors, erasures, grease smudges and fingerprints. Good-quality résumé paper should be used: In health care, white paper is preferred, although ivory can also be used. Avoid using pastel papers and fancy script typefaces. Additionally, avoid logos of any kind. You want to convey competence through a résumé that is professional looking and easy to read.

Prepare a Cover Letter

You should prepare a cover letter to attach to your résumé when applying for a specific position. The letter should be one page in length, refer to the position you are applying for, explain the way you found out about the position, and briefly describe one of your skills that is pertinent to the position. You should also establish a time frame for contacting the prospective employer to follow up on your résumé. Be sure that you do follow up with a call to track the progress of your application. The letter should follow the standard format of a business letter, contain no grammatical or spelling errors, and be on the same quality paper as your résumé. Always use the full name and title of the person to whom you are sending the letter and résumé. You should not use a stock cover letter for all of the positions for which you are applying. The cover letter should always be individualized to the position and the company to which you are applying. Figure 30-10 shows a sample cover letter.

1234 Pleasant Street
Chicago, IL 60000
September 12, 2001

Thomas DiNapoli
Human Resources Manager
St. Anne's Medical Center
P.O. Box 3476
Pittsburgh, PA 15230

Dear Mr. DiNapoli:

I am applying for the position of full-time medication nurse that you advertised in the September 11 *Pittsburgh Press and Post Gazette*. My resume is enclosed.

In the last year I worked with my health care team to establish new procedures and protocols for medication rounds. The procedures have been successfully implemented and I can bring these innovative ideas to your facility.

I would be happy to come in for an interview. I can be reached at (123) 456-7890 and will call you on September 19 to answer any questions you may have.

Sincerely,

Anita Jones, LPN

Enclosure

Figure 30-10 Sample Cover Letter

Prepare a List of References

References are people, such as colleagues, instructors, or employers, who can verify and support your professional and educational background claims.

Through the use of references, prospective employers attempt to verify information you have provided on a job application or your résumé. Employers also use references to gather more information about you. Do not provide references unless the prospective employer requests them. If you must supply references, be sure they are typed and include all pertinent information (name, title, employer, address, and telephone number).

Given the likelihood that a potential employer will ask for references, it is a good idea to always be prepared to provide them. Contact the people you intend to list as references and ask whether they are willing to be references for you. Remember, however, that the willingness of a person to serve as a reference does not guarantee that the information provided will be positive; therefore, ask any prospective references how they may respond to questions that you anticipate from a prospective employer. For example, if the employer asks your nursing school instructor something about your record of tardiness, will the instructor focus on the three times you were late for clinical, or will the instructor comment favorably that you are prompt and efficient in completing your responsibilities?

Choose references who are prepared to comment on the skills you possess and need for the job in question. Provide all references with information about the position for which you applied and the job expectations. This information allows your references to tailor their comments to the demands of the prospective job.

Prepare a Telephone Call Script

A telephone call script outlines the information you want to learn and/or share with prospective employers. Preplanning the telephone call helps you organize the call, ensures that crucial information is learned or given, and generally helps you sound efficient and competent. Consider having several scripts. One script may address a request for information such as job descriptions and vacancies; another may be an introduction about you and an inquiry about the application process; and yet another may focus on the status of your application after you have had an interview. The key is to prepare for any contact with a potential employer, whether it be by phone or in person.

Complete a Job Application

Many employers will simply ask you to complete a job application. The job application should be completed totally and neatly. Most employers balk at job applications that say "see attached résumé" rather than provide the information as requested. Preparation is key. Come with the information you may need to complete an application. Such information typically includes a list of past employers, including addresses, telephone numbers, supervisors' names, and dates of employment. Information about schools you have attended is also generally asked for on a job application. If you are nervous about completing an application "cold," ask the employer to send you a form. Practice completing it at home, so that you are certain you have all the information requested; then the practice application in the trash, and visit the employer to complete the form in person. Figure 30-11 shows a sample job application.

Prepare for the Interview

The interview is a crucial part of the job-search process. An interview is best thought of as an opportunity for you and the interviewer to exchange information. Your task is to convey pertinent information about your skills, abilities, education, and experience. The interviewer's task is to relay information about the particular job and the employer and to evaluate your qualifications. If both parties have fulfilled their responsibilities, appropriate decisions follow. The interviewer decides whether you are the most desirable candidate for the job—and you decide whether you want the job.

Preparation is the key to a successful interview. Well before the actual interview, the stage for a meeting is set. You have determined your objective, identified a potential employer, and filled out a job application or provided a resumé. The prospective employer has screened your information and selected you for an interview. But you still have work to do before the actual interview.

Research the Employer

Part of preparing for an interview involves researching the employer. You want to learn everything you can about the employer. Showing such initiative gives the interviewer the impression that you have a sincere interest in employment with the organization. Information you learn may also help you develop questions to ask the employer or anticipate questions that the employer may ask you.

Application for Employment
(pre-employment questionnaire) (an equal opportunity employer)

Personal Information Date September 20, 2001

Name Anita Jones Social security number 351-44-5751

Present address 1234 Pleasant Street Chicago IL 60000

Permanent address same

Phone No. (123) 456-7890 Are you 18 years or older? yes no

Are you either a U.S. citizen or an alien authorized to work in the United States? yes no

Employment Desired

Position medication nurse Date you can start October 15 Salary desired open

Are you employed now? Yes If so may we inquire of your present employer? Yes

Ever applied to this company before? No where? when?

Referred by Ken Jenkins

Education	Name and location of school attended	No. of years	Did you graduate?	Subjects studied
Grammar school	*Cambden Elementary School District #95*	*8*	*yes*	*general curriculum*
High school	*Cambden High School*	*4*	*yes*	*vocational curriculum, nursing*
College	*Highland Community College*	*1*	*yes*	*LPN*
Trade, business or correspondence school				

Former Employers (list below the last three employers, starting with the last one)

Date, month and year	Name and address of employer	Salary	Position	Reason for leaving
from June 1992 to present	*General Hospital and Medical Center*	*$6.85/hr.*	*medication nurse*	*currently employed*
from June 1987 to May 1992	*City Teaching Medical Center*	*$4.30/hr.*	*nurse*	*part-time only*

Which of these jobs did you like best? *City Teaching Medical Center*
What did you like most about this job? *geriatrics*

References: give the names of the three persons not related to you, whom you have known at least one year

Name			
Denise Thompson			1.5
Phylis Hunter			2.0
Frank Hopkins	Highland Community College - Freeport, IL	nursing instructor	1.0

Figure 30-11 Sample Job Application

Anticipate Questions

Try to anticipate questions the employer may ask you. For example, if after investigating an outpatient clinic, you learn that electrocardiogram and phlebotomy are performed on site, you can be fairly certain that the employer will ask whether you have performed these skills. Typical questions asked by an employer focus on strengths and weaknesses, interest in the position, past experience, future plans, and potential contributions to the open position.

As a general rule, law forbids the employer to ask personal questions. For instance, questions about child care arrangements, plans to have a family, height, weight, and religion are not allowed. With severe limitations, the employer can ask about age (e.g., "Are you over 18 or under 70?") and disabilities or illnesses (e.g., "Is there anything that would interfere with your performance of the job?").

Be Prepared

Anticipate questions and plan your responses. Examine your résumé again. Reflect on your goals. Assess your skills and knowledge. Decide the information you want to convey to the interviewer. Develop complete but concise answers to anticipated questions. Employers have a limited amount of time for interviews and want you to get to the point as quickly as possible.

Bring your résumé and references, even if you have provided these to the potential employer at a prior time. You want to be certain the interviewer has information about you at hand as you talk.

Be prompt for the interview. An overly early arrival will tend to increase your nervousness; and a late arrival is simply unacceptable. Plan your route to the facility ahead of time. Anticipate traffic delays or parking problems. Allow time to compose yourself before the interview.

During the actual interview you want to make a positive impression. Your physical appearance is probably the first thing the interviewer will notice. Dress conservatively, neatly, and clean. You want to project confidence and competence. Excessive jewelry or make-up, trendy body piercing or hairstyle, casual attire, and overdressing tend to detract from the image you want to present.

Attempt to strike a balance between a friendly but not too familiar, professional but not too aloof demeanor. Greet the interviewer by shaking hands, and wait for the interviewer to offer you a seat. Do not smoke or chew gum. Answer questions directly and honestly, but do not ramble on or offer extraneous information (Figure 30-12).

A common tendency is to view the interview as a one-sided interaction—as the employer's opportunity to scrutinize prospective employees. The interviewer's task is to confirm the information you have provided on your job application or resumé. In addition to gathering more detailed information about you, the interviewer is interested in the way you handle yourself and whether you are a good match for the job and the employer. After a screening and selection process, the employer offers employment to the most desirable candidate. But remember, securing employment is a two-sided process: You also are interviewing the interviewer to gather information about the employer, to ascertain whether the job opportunity is the right fit for you.

Any offer of employment you receive can be accepted or rejected. You should already have obtained information about the employer that was enticing enough to cause you to apply for employment. The interview is, however, your opportunity to gather more information about the employer. This information serves as the basis for determining whether you really want the job. Go to the interview with a written list of questions you have for the employer.

Your questions can address a number of topics including orientation, organization of the nursing staff, working conditions, and educational opportunities. For example, How long is the orientation? How often is overtime or floating required? On which unit will I be assigned to work? What are the five most common diagnoses on that unit? What is the ratio of RNs to LP/VNs to UAP? What is the schedule of a normal work week? The list of potential questions is endless.

The advice is often given not to ask about salary and benefits during the first interview. At some point, however, this information becomes crucial to your decision making. If the interviewer does not volunteer information about salary and benefits, at the very least wait until the end of the interview to discuss these matters. Employers want to know you are interested in the work, not just the pay. Thus, you may want to

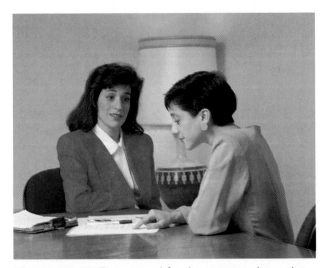

Figure 30-12 Be prepared for the interview; know those things you want to learn and those things you want to share with the interviewer.

consider waiting to learn about salary and benefits until a job offer has been made.

At the end of the interview, you may be offered employment. If you are confident that you want the position, accept the offer. If you have any hesitation, however, inform the employer that you will respond in a day or two. Do not turn the offer down at the interview. Go home, review the information you have available, discuss the offer with relevant people, and then notify the employer. Whether you decide to accept or decline the offer of employment, you should respond to the employer's offer. Even in declining an employment offer, you want to leave a positive impression. You never know when you may encounter that recruiter in the future.

At the end of the interview, shake hands with the interviewer and offer thanks for the interviewer's time and consideration. If you believe you want the job, say so. Statements such as "After our discussion, I am very interested in working here" or "I really want to work with your client population and want the job" indicate your strong interest to the prospective employer.

Prepare a Thank You Note

The thank you note is critical to a successful job search. Always follow up an interview with a thank you note. Some employment counselors suggest you send a thank you note to everyone involved in the interview process. These people may include the person who suggested the employer, the receptionist and, certainly, the person who conducted the interview.

A thank you note can be handwritten or typed. The key is to send it the same day as the interview. The thank you note should be personal: say something about the way the person treated you, the highlights of the interview, or something you forgot to mention during the interview. If the interview confirmed your interest in employment, say so. Even if you decide that the employment setting is not for you, write a thank you anyway. Your career interests may change at some point. Further, employers talk to each other; therefore, you want to leave a good impression any place you seek employment. Figure 30-13 shows a sample thank you note.

A FINAL WORD ABOUT EMPLOYMENT

As a new graduate, financial pressures or a seemingly limited pool of available jobs may influence your job search. You also may be considerably swayed by the advice that you should "get a year of experience in general medical–surgical nursing" before moving on to the job you really want. Financial pressures and the job market may indeed pose some limitations. Further, a year of medical–surgical experience is helpful. But resist taking a job for just these reasons.

1234 Pleasant Street
Chicago, IL 60000
September 26, 2001

Thomas DiNapoli
Human Resources Manager
St. Anne's Medical Center
P.O. Box 3476
Pittsburgh, PA 15230

Dear Mr. DiNapoli:

Thank you for taking the time to speak with me yesterday about the position of medication nurse at St. Anne's Medical Center. I was very impressed with your company, and the job sounds wonderful. I'm more than ever convinced that my experience can benefit your company.

I appreciated the opportunity to meet you and learn about St. Anne's.

Sincerely,

Anita Jones, LPN

Figure 30-13 Sample Thank You Note

As an occupation, licensed practical/vocational nursing offers much variety with regard to employment setting, client age, type of work, number of hours available to work, availability of days and shifts, amount of supervision, and a host of other factors. Such variety will become evident as you investigate available employment options.

A poor fit between the job and your interests, needs, or abilities is a setup for failure. As a newly employed LP/VN, you want to establish an employment record of success and increasing growth in your skills and knowledge. You want to build on your newfound confidence and competence. A thorough and honest evaluation of your strengths and weaknesses, a clearly identified objective, and a careful review of employment options will help ensure satisfying and rewarding employment.

SUMMARY

- Leadership styles are typically classified as autocratic, democratic, or laissez-faire.
- Skills necessary for effective leadership include communication, problem solving, self-evaluation, and management.
- Being a good manager means knowing how and when to assign tasks, delegate duties, prioritize care, and resolve conflict.
- In most instances, the RN will be in charge of delegating tasks to the LP/VN. The decision to delegate a task should be based on the potential for harm, the complexity of the task, the problem solving re-

quired, the unpredictability of the outcome, and the required coordination of care.

- The five rights of delegation include the right task, the right circumstance, the right person, the right direction, and the right supervision.
- Factors to assess when establishing priorities of care include safety, timing of tests and other tasks, interdependency of events, client requests, availability of help, client status, and availability of resources.
- The steps involved in securing a job include identifying your objective, preparing a résumé, preparing a cover letter, preparing a list of references, preparing a telephone call script, completing a job application, preparing for the interview, and preparing a thank you note.

Review Questions

1. The following information should be included on a résumé:

   a. name, address, telephone number, job objective.

   b. information about prior employment, name, family information.

   c. job objective, references, prior education and experiences.

   d. name, address, job objective, availability for interview.

2. Pauline, an LP/VN, is the evening-shift charge nurse on 3B, a 40-bed unit in a long-term care facility. Christine is a CNA from another floor sent to work on 3B for the evening. She asks Pauline when she and the other three CNAs should take their lunch break. Pauline tells her to "work it out between themselves." Pauline is using a style of leadership called:

   a. participatory leadership.

   b. democratic leadership.

   c. autocratic leadership.

   d. laissez-faire leadership.

3. The five rights of delegation include the right

   a. task, time, circumstance, and supervision.

   b. supervision, task, person, and direction.

   c. person, task, time, and direction.

   d. time, task, person, and supervision.

Critical Thinking Questions

1. After a lengthy job search, Alicia secures employment at a long-term care facility. The facility residents are all retired nuns. Alicia enjoys geriatrics, management seemed fair and reasonable, the environment is clean and attractive, and financial benefits are competitive. However, Alicia finds the nuns to be demanding and unappreciative. Additionally, the religious underpinnings of the facility influence her work more than she anticipated. After 2 months, she now dreads going to work. What should she do?

2. Nancy works in a long-term care facility as the evening-shift charge nurse on 4 West. As part of her duties, she makes the client assignments to the CNAs. She also monitors their work and intervenes where necessary to ensure that clients receive safe and appropriate care. Lately, Nancy observes that Martha, a CNA, is not completing all her assigned responsibilities. How should Nancy address this problem?

 WEB FLASH!

- Search the web under broad categories such as *leadership, management, delegation,* and *employment.* What kind of sites do you locate?
- How is your search enhanced when you add qualifiers to narrow the search, such as *nursing, LPN, LVN,* or *UAP?*

Atlas of Nursing Procedures

B1 Handwashing

B2 Use of Personal Protective Equipment (PPE)

B3 Measuring Body Temperature

B4 Assessing Pulse Rate

B5 Assessing Respirations

B6 Assessing Blood Pressure

B7 Weighing Client, Mobile and Immobile

B8 Practicing Proper Body Mechanics

B9 Performing Passive Range-of-Motion Exercises

B10 Assisting a Client with Ambulation

B11 Positioning a Client in Bed

B12 Moving a Client in Bed

B13 Transferring a Client from Bed to Wheelchair

B14 Transferring a Client from Bed to Stretcher with Minimum Assistance/Maximum Assistance

B15 Logrolling a Client with a Turn Sheet

B16 Bedmaking: Unoccupied Bed

B17 Bedmaking: Occupied Bed

B18 Adult Bath

B19 Perineal Care

B20 Catheter Care

B21 Oral Hygiene

B22 Eye Care: Artificial Eye and Contact Lens Removal

B23 Giving a Back Rub

B24 Shaving a Client

B25 Applying Antiembolism Stockings

B26 Positioning and Removing a Bedpan

B27 Applying a Condom Catheter

B28 Administering an Enema (Large; Small/Mini)

B29 Measuring Intake and Output

B30 Urine Collection—Closed Drainage System

B31 Urine Collection—Clean Catch, Female/Male

B32 Collecting Nose, Throat, and Sputum Specimens

B33 Gathering a Stool Specimen

B34 Applying Abdominal, T-, Breast, and Scultetus Binders

B35 Application of Restraints

B36 Clearing an Obstructed Airway

B37 Performing Cardiopulmonary Resuscitation

B38 Admitting a Client

B39 Transferring a Client

B40 Discharging a Client

BASIC PROCEDURES

Procedure B1 Handwashing

Equipment

- Soap
- Sink
- Paper or cloth towels
- Running water

Action	Rationale
1. Remove jewelry. Wristwatch may be pushed up above the wrist (midforearm). Push sleeves of uniform or shirt up above the wrist at midforearm level.	1. Provides access to skin surfaces for cleaning. Facilitates cleaning of fingers, hands, and forearms.
2. Assess hands for hangnails, cuts or breaks in the skin, and areas that are heavily soiled (follow agency policy regarding nail polish and artificial nails)	2. Intact skin acts as a barrier to microorganisms. Breaks in skin integrity facilitate development of infection and should receive extra attention during cleaning.
3. Turn on the water. Adjust the flow and temperature. Temperature of the water should be warm.	3. Running water removes microorganisms. Warm water removes less of the natural skin oils.
4. Wet hands and lower forearms thoroughly by holding under running water. Keep hands and forearms in the down position with elbows straight. Avoid splashing water and touching the sides of the sink.	4. Water should flow from the least contaminated to the most contaminated areas of the skin. Hands are considered more contaminated than arms. Splashing of water facilitates transfer of microorganisms. Touching of any surface during cleaning contaminates the skin.
5. Apply about 5 mL (1 teaspoon) of liquid soap. Lather thoroughly.	5. Lather facilitates removal of microorganisms. Liquid soap harbors less bacteria than bar soap.
6. Thoroughly rub hands together for about 10 to 15 seconds. Interlace fingers and thumbs and move back and forth to wash between digits (Figure B1-1). Rub palms and back of hands with circular motion. Special attention should be provided to areas such as the knuckles and fingernails, which are known to harbor organisms (Figure B1-2).	6. Friction mechanically removes microorganisms from the skin surface. Friction loosens dirt from soiled areas.

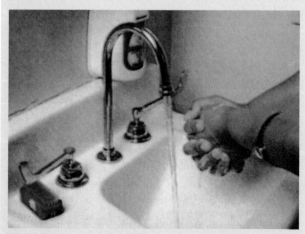

Figure B1-1 Interlace fingers to wash between the digits.

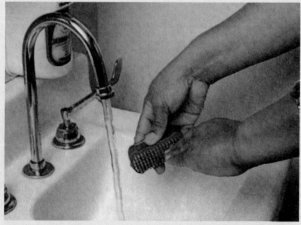

Figure B1-2 Provide special attention to washing knuckles and fingernails (brush may or may not be available).

continued

Action	Rationale
7. Rinse with hands in the down position, elbows straight. Rinse in the direction of forearm to wrist to fingers.	7. Flow of water rinses away dirt and microorganisms.
8. Blot hands and forearms to dry thoroughly. Dry in the direction of fingers to wrist and forearms. Discard the paper towels in the proper receptacle.	8. Blotting reduces chapping of skin. Drying from cleanest (hand) to least clean area (forearms) prevents transfer of microorganisms to cleanest area.
9. Turn off the water faucet with a clean, dry paper towel (Figure B1-3).	9. Prevents contamination of clean hands by a less clean faucet.

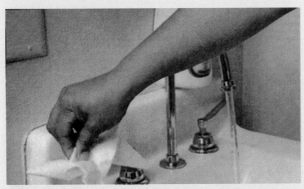

Figure B1-3 Turn off faucet with a clean, dry paper towel.

Procedure B2   Use of Personal Protective Equipment (PPE)

Equipment

- Gloves
- Mask and goggles or face shield
- Gown

Action	Rationale

• *Wash your hands before applying any personal protective equipment (PPE)* •

Applying Gloves (*Note:* If wearing full PPE, gloves are put on last.)

1. Wash hands.	1. Reduces spread of microorganisms.
2. Remove clean gloves from box.	2. Gloves are for one-time use.
3. Put hands into gloves, adjusting fingers for proper fit.	3. Proper fit is important for client care.

Applying Mask

4. Adjust mask over nose and mouth.	4. Ensures proper fit.
5. Tie top strings behind head first, then bottom strings. Or slip elastic over back of head.	5. Keeps mask from falling off.
6. Bend metal nosepiece over bridge of nose.	6. Provides better fit.
7. Replace mask if it becomes significantly damp with exhaled moisture.	7. Moisture can reduce the efficacy of some masks.

continued

Action	Rationale

Applying Protective Eyewear (*Note:* If mask is needed due to potential for splashing, goggles are also needed.)

8. Apply mask first, then apply the goggles or face shield. If eyeglasses are worn, eye protection is still required over eyeglasses to protect sides of eyes.

8. Protects eyes from splashing of body fluids.

Applying Gown (*Note:* If applying complete set of PPE, mask is applied before gown. Gloves are applied after gown.)

9. Hold the clean gown by the neck in front of you, letting it unfold. Do not let it touch the floor.

9. Reduces risk of contamination.

10. Place your arms in the sleeves and slide the gown up to your shoulders (Figure B2-1).

10. Reduces handling of front of gown.

11. Slip your hands inside the neck and grasp the ties. Tie them at the neck (Figure B2-2).

11. Secures gown.

12. Cover your uniform at the back with the gown and tie the ties at the waist. The gown must completely cover your clothing (Figure B2-3).

12. Reduces risk of contamination of nurse.

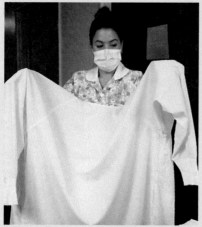

Figure B2-1 Place your arms in the sleeves and slide the gown up to your shoulders.

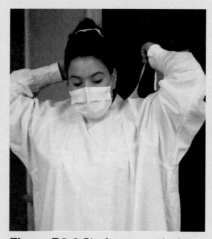

Figure B2-2 Slip fingers inside the neckband and tie gown.

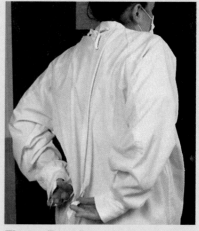

Figure B2-3 Reach behind, overlap the edges of the gown so the uniform is completely covered, and tie the waist ties.

Removing Protective Clothing

Remove PPE in the following order:

- Untie waist tie of the gown.
- Remove gloves.
- Wash your hands.
- Untie the neck tie of the gown and remove the gown.
- Wash your hands.
- Remove protective eyewear (if worn).
- Remove mask.
- Wash your hands.

See detailed procedure, which follows.

continued

Action	Rationale

Removing Gloves (Loosen waist tie on gown before removing gloves.)

13. Grasp the outside of the glove of the non-dominant hand (Figure B2-4).

14. Pull the glove down, turning glove inside out with fingers inside while pulling it off the hand (Figure B2-5).

15. Place this glove in the palm of the gloved hand.

16. Using ungloved hand, reach under remaining glove, and pull glove off from underneath, turning glove inside out, and capturing other glove within (Figure B2-6).

17. Discard gloves according to agency policy.

18. Wash hands.

13. Reduces risk of contaminating hands.

14. Reduces risk of contaminating hands.

15. Reduces risk of contaminating hands.

16. Reduces risk of contaminating hands.

17. Reduces transmission of microorganisms.

18. Reduces risk of transmitting microorganisms.

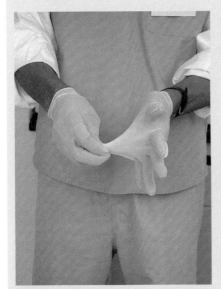

Figure B2-4 With fingers of one hand, grasp glove of other hand.

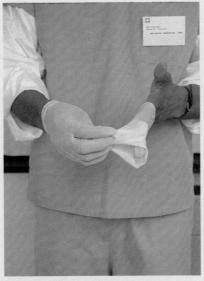

Figure B2-5 Pull the glove down over the hand and the fingers and remove it. The glove is inside out with the contaminated side inside.

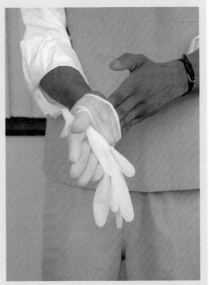

Figure B2-6 Hold the glove just removed in the gloved hand. Insert fingers of the ungloved hand inside the cuff of the other glove.

Removing Gown (*Note:* Waist tie should be loosened before gloves are removed.)

19. Untie neck ties of gown. Loosen gown at shoulders by touching only the inside of the gown (Figure B2-7).

20. Grasp the neck ties and pull the gown down and off, turning inside out.

21. Roll the gown away from your body (Figure B2-8). Discard according to agency policy. Wash your hands.

19. Reduces risk of contaminating clothing.

20. Reduces risk of contaminating clothing.

21. Reduces transmission of microorganisms.

continued

Action	**Rationale**

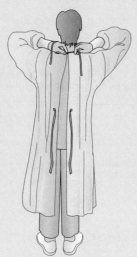

Figure B2-7 Untie neck ties of gown.

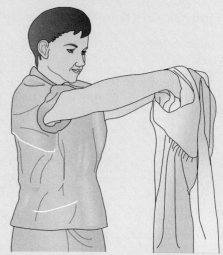

Figure B2-8 Pull the gown down off the arms, being careful that the hands do not touch the outside of the gown. Hold the gown away from your uniform and roll it up with the contaminated side inside. If gown is disposable, place it in the receptacle for contaminated trash. If gown is not disposable, place it in laundry hamper for contaminated linens.

Removing Protective Eyewear

22. Lift protective goggles or face shield away from face. Follow agency policy regarding disposal.

22. In some cases, clean goggles are re-used.

Removing Mask

23. Untie the upper tie first, then the lower tie, or pull the elastic from around the back of the head. Remove the mask by touching only the ties. (*Note:* Never wear a mask around the neck with the lower ties tied around the neck and the upper ties hanging down.

23. Reduces risk of contaminating clothing.

Procedure B3 — Measuring Body Temperature

Equipment

- Thermometer; glass (client's bedside); electronic and disposable protective sheath; disposable (chemical); tympanic
- Lubricant (rectal, glass thermometer)
- Two pairs of nonsterile gloves
- Tissues

Action	**Rationale**

- *Wash your hands* • *Check the client's identification band* •
- *Explain the procedure to the client prior to beginning* •

1. Review medical record for baseline data and factors that influence vital signs.

1. Establishes parameters for client's normal measurements, provides direction in device selection, and determines site to use for measurement. Vital signs are measured in the order of T-P-R and BP, usually without interruptions,

continued

Action	Rationale
	so as to provide the nurse with an objective clinical database to direct decision making.
2. Explain to the client that vital signs will be assessed. Encourage client to remain still and refrain from drinking, eating, or smoking.	2. Encourages participation, allays anxiety, and ensures accurate measurements. Cold or hot liquids or food and smoking alter circulation and body temperature.
3. Assess client's toileting needs and proceed as appropriate.	3. Prevents interruptions during measurements, communicates caring, and promotes client comfort.
4. Gather equipment indicated.	4. Facilitates organized assessment and measurement.
5. Provide for privacy.	5. Decreases embarrassment.
6. Wash hands and don gloves.	6. Hands are washed before and after every contact with a client. Gloves are worn to avoid contact with all bodily secretions and to reduce transmission of microorganisms.
7. Position the client in a sitting or lying position with the head of the bed elevated 45° to 60° for measurement of all vital signs except those designated otherwise.	7. Promotes comfort and site access for all measurements. Activity and movement can elevate heart and respiratory rates.
8. *Oral Temperature: Glass Thermometer*	
a. Select correct color tip of thermometer from client's bedside container.	a. Identifies correct device; a blue color tip usually denotes an oral thermometer.
b. Remove thermometer from storage container and cleanse under cool water.	b. Cleansing removes disinfectant that can cause irritation to oral mucosa. Cool water prevents expansion of the mercury.
c. Wipe thermometer dry with a tissue from bulb's end toward fingertips.	c. Wipe from area of least contamination to most contaminated area.
d. Read thermometer by locating mercury level. It should read 35.5°C (96°F).	d. Thermometer must be below normal body temperature to ensure an accurate reading.
e. If thermometer is not below a normal body temperature reading, grasp thermometer with thumb and forefinger and shake vigorously by snapping the wrist in a downward motion to move mercury to a level below normal.	e. Shaking briskly lowers level of mercury in the column. Because glass thermometers break easily, make sure that nothing in the environment comes in contact with the thermometer when shaking it.
f. Place thermometer in client's mouth under the tongue and along the gumline to the posterior sublingual pocket. Instruct client to hold lips closed.	f. Ensures contact with large blood vessels under the tongue. Prevents environmental air from coming in contact with the bulb.
g. Leave in place as specified by agency policy, usually 3–5 minutes.	g. Thermometer must stay in place long enough to ensure an accurate reading.
h. Remove thermometer and wipe with a tissue away from fingers toward the bulb's end.	h. Mucus on thermometer may interfere with disinfectant solution's effectiveness. Wipe from area of least contamination to most contaminated area.

continued

Action	Rationale
i. Read at eye level and rotate slowly until mercury level is visualized.	**i.** Ensures an accurate reading.
j. Shake thermometer down, and cleanse glass thermometer with soapy water, rinse under cold water, and return to storage container.	**j.** Mechanical cleansing removes secretions that promote growth of microorganisms. Hot water may cause coagulation of secretions and cause expansion of mercury in thermometer.
k. Inform client of temperature reading.	**k.** Promotes client's participation in care.
l. Remove and dispose of gloves in receptacle. Wash hands.	**l.** Reduces transmission of microorganisms.
m. Record reading and indicate site as "OT."	**m.** Accurate documentation by site allows for comparison of data.

9. *Oral Temperature: Electronic Thermometer*

Action	Rationale
a. Place disposable protective sheath over probe.	**a.** Prevents transmission of microorganisms.
b. Grasp top of the probe's stem. Avoid placing pressure on the ejection button.	**b.** Pressure on the ejection button releases the sheath from the probe.
c. Place tip of thermometer under the client's tongue and along the gumline to the posterior sublingual pocket lateral to center of lower jaw (Figure B3-1).	**c.** Sublingual pocket contains superficial blood vessels.

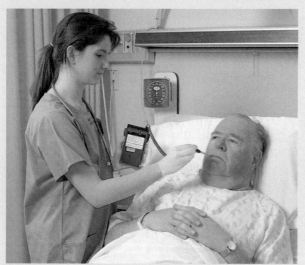

Figure B3-1 Place the tip of thermometer under client's tongue in posterior sublingual pocket lateral to center of lower jaw.

Action	Rationale
d. Instruct client to keep the mouth closed around thermometer.	**d.** Maintains thermometer in proper place and decreases amount of time for an accurate reading.
e. Thermometer will signal (beep) when a constant temperature registers.	**e.** Signal indicates temperature reading.
f. Read measurement on digital display of electronic thermometer. Push ejection button to discard disposable sheath into receptacle and return probe to storage well.	**f.** Reduces transmission of microorganisms. Ensures that the electronic system is ready for next use.

continued

Action	Rationale
g. Inform client of temperature reading.	**g.** Promotes client's participation in care.
h. Remove gloves and wash hands.	**h.** Reduces transmission of microorganisms.
i. Record reading and indicate site "OT."	**i.** Accurate documentation by site allows for comparison of data.
j. Return electronic thermometer unit to charging base plugged into electrical outlet.	**j.** Ensures thermometer is ready for next use.

10. *Rectal Temperature*

Action	Rationale
a. Place client in the Sims' position with upper knee flexed. Adjust sheet to expose only anal area.	**a.** Proper positioning ensures visualization of anus. Flexing knee relaxes muscles for ease of insertion.
b. Place tissues in easy reach. Don gloves.	**b.** Tissue is needed to wipe anus after device is removed.
c. Prepare the thermometer (refer to steps 8b, c, d, and e).	**c.** Same as for steps 8b, c, d, and e.
d. Lubricate tip of rectal thermometer or probe (a rectal thermometer usually has a red cap).	**d.** Promotes ease of insertion of thermometer or probe.
e. With dominant hand, grasp thermometer. With nondominant hand, separate buttocks to expose anus.	**e.** Aids in visualization of anus.
f. Instruct client to take a deep breath. Insert thermometer or probe gently into anus: infant, 1.2 cm (0.5 in.); adult, 3.5 cm (1.5 in.) (Figure B3-2). If resistance is felt, do not force insertion.	**f.** Relaxes anal sphincter. Gentle insertion decreases discomfort to client and prevents trauma to mucous membranes.

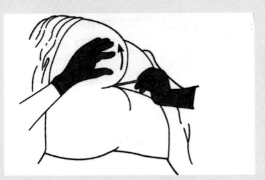

Figure B3-2 Insert probe or rectal thermometer into anus.

Action	Rationale
g. Length of time (refer to step 8g) or signal heard.	**g.** Same as for step 8g.
h. Wipe secretions off glass thermometer with a tissue. Dispose of tissue in a receptacle.	**h.** Removes secretions and fecal material for visualization of mercury level. Prevents transmission of microorganisms.
i. Read measurement and inform client of temperature reading.	**i.** Encourages client participation.
j. While holding glass thermometer in one hand, use other hand to wipe anal area with tissue to remove lubricant or feces and dispose of soiled tissue. Cover client.	**j.** Prevents contamination of clean objects with soiled thermometer, decreases skin irritation, and promotes client comfort. Prevents embarrassment.

continued

Action	Rationale
k. Cleanse thermometer (refer to step 8j).	**k.** Same as for step 8j.
l. Remove and dispose of gloves in receptacle.	**l.** Decreases transmission of microorganisms.
m. Record reading and indicate site as "RT."	**m.** Accurate documentation by site allows for comparison of data.

11. *Axillary Temperature*

a. Remove client's arm and shoulder from one sleeve of gown. Avoid exposing chest.	**a.** Exposes axillary area.
b. Make sure axillary skin is dry; if necessary, pat dry.	**b.** Removes moisture and prevents a false low reading.
c. Prepare thermometer (refer to steps 8b, c, d, and e).	**c.** Same as for steps 8b, c, d, and e.
d. Place thermometer or probe into center of axilla (Figure B3-3A). Fold client's upper arm straight down and place arm across client's chest (Figure B3-3B)	**d.** Puts device in contact with axillary blood supply. Maintains the device in proper position.

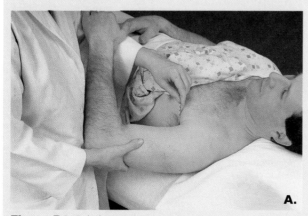 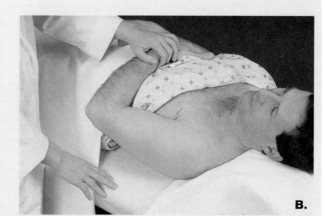

A. B.

Figure B3-3 A. Insert thermometer into center of axilla. B. Place client's arm across chest.

e. Leave glass thermometer in place as specified by agency policy (usually 6–8 minutes). Leave an electronic thermometer in place until signal is heard.	**e.** Device must stay in place long enough to ensure an accurate reading. Signal indicates temperature reading.
f. Remove and read thermometer.	**f.** Allows temperature measurement.
g. Inform client of temperature reading.	**g.** Encourages client participation.
h. Cleanse glass thermometer (refer to steps 8h and 8j) and return to storage container.	**h.** Prevents transmission of microorganisms and breakage of glass thermometer.
i. Assist client with replacing gown.	**i.** Promotes comfort.
j. Record reading and indicate site as "AT."	**j.** Promotes accurate documentation for data comparison.

12. *Disposable (Chemical Strip) Thermometer*

a. Apply tape to appropriate skin area, usually forehead.	**a.** Tape must be in direct contact with the client's skin.

continued

Action	Rationale
b. Observe tape for color changes.	**b.** Color reflects temperature reading (refer to the manufacturer's instructions).
c. Record reading and indicate method.	**c.** Promotes accurate documentation for data comparison.
13. *Tympanic Temperature: Infrared Thermometer*	
a. Position client in Sims' position.	**a.** Promotes access to ear.
b. Remove probe from container and attach probe cover to tympanic thermometer unit.	**b.** Prevents contamination.
c. Turn client's head to one side. For an adult, pull pinna upward and back; for a child, pull down and back. Gently insert probe with firm pressure into ear canal.	**c.** Provides access to ear canal. Gentle insertion prevents trauma to external canal. Firm pressure is needed to ensure probe contact against tympanic membrane.
d. Remove probe after the reading is displayed on digital unit (usually 2 seconds).	**d.** Reading is displayed within seconds.
e. Remove probe cover and replace in storage container.	**e.** Prevents damage to the reusable probe.
f. Return tympanic thermometer to storage unit.	**f.** Recharges batteries of unit.
g. Record reading and indicate site as "ET."	**g.** Promotes accurate documentation for data comparison.

Procedure B4 — Assessing Pulse Rate

Equipment

- Watch with a second hand
- Alcohol swab
- Stethoscope

Action	Rationale
• *Wash your hands* • *Check the client's identification band* • • *Explain the procedure to the client prior to beginning* •	
1. *Radial Pulse*	
a. Inform client of the site(s) at which you will measure pulse.	**a.** Encourages participation and allays anxiety.
b. Flex client's elbow and place lower part of arm across chest.	**b.** Maintains wrist in full extension and exposes artery for palpation. Placing client's hand over chest will facilitate later respiratory assessment without undue attention to your action. (It is difficult for any person to maintain a normal breathing pattern when someone is observing and measuring.)
c. Place your index and middle finger on inner aspect of client's wrist over the radial artery and apply light but firm pressure until pulse is palpated (Figure B4-1).	**c.** Fingertips are sensitive, facilitating palpation of pulse. The nurse may feel own pulse if palpating with thumb. Applying light pressure prevents occlusion of blood flow and pulsation.

continued

Action	Rationale

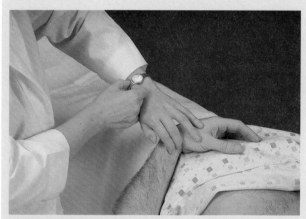

Figure B4-1 Place index and middle finger on inner aspect of client's wrist over the radial artery.

d. Identify pulse rhythm.

e. Determine pulse volume.

f. Count pulse rate by using second hand on a watch:

- For a regular rhythm, count number of beats for 30 seconds and multiply by 2.

- For an irregular rhythm, count number of beats for a full minute, noting number of irregular beats.

2. *Apical Pulse*

a. Raise client's gown to expose sternum and left side of chest.

b. Cleanse earpiece and diaphragm of stethoscope with an alcohol swab.

c. Put stethoscope around your neck.

d. Apex of heart:

- With client lying on left side (optional), locate suprasternal notch.

- Palpate second intercostal space to left of sternum.

- Place index finger in intercostal space, counting downward until fifth intercostal space is located.

- Move index finger along the fifth inter-costal space, left of the midclavicular line to palpate the point of maximal impulse (PMI) (Figure B4-2).

d. Palpate pulse until rhythm is determined. Describe as regular or irregular.

e. Quality of pulse strength is an indication of stroke volume. Describe as normal, weak, strong, or bounding.

f. An irregular rhythm requires a full minute of assessment to count an accurate rate.

a. Allows access to client's chest for proper placement of stethoscope.

b. Decreases transmission of microorganisms from one practitioner to another (earpiece) and from one client to another (diaphragm).

c. Holds stethoscope during palpation.

d. Identification of landmarks facilitates correct placement of the stethoscope at the fifth intercostal space in order to hear point of maximal impulse.

continued

Action	**Rationale**
• Keep index finger of nondominant hand on the PMI.	
e. Inform client that you are going to listen to his heart. Instruct client to remain silent.	e. Elicits client support. Stethoscope amplifies noise.
f. With dominant hand, put earpiece of the stethoscope in your ears and grasp diaphragm of the stethoscope in palm of your hand for 5 to 10 seconds.	f. Dominant hand facilitates psychomotor dexterity for placement of earpiece with one hand. Heat warms metal or plastic diaphragm and prevents startling client.
g. Place diaphragm of stethoscope over the PMI and auscultate for sounds S_1 and S_2 to hear lub-dub sound (Figure B4-3).	g. Movement of blood through the heart valves creates S_1 and S_2 sounds. Listen for a regular rhythm (heartbeats are evenly spaced) before counting.

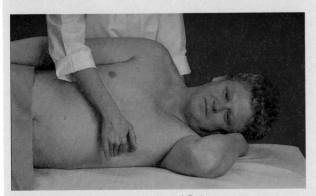

Figure B4-2 Palpating the Apical Pulse

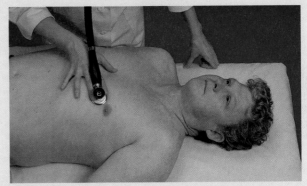

Figure B4-3 Place diaphragm of stethoscope over the PMI to ausculate for sounds. (Supine is alternative position.)

h. Note regularity of rhythm.	h. Establishment of a rhythm pattern determines length of time to count the heartbeats to ensure accurate measurement.
i. Start to count while looking at second hand of watch. Count lub-dub sound as one beat:	i. Ensures sufficient time to count irregular beats.
• For a regular rhythm, count rate for 30 seconds and multiply by 2.	
• For an irregular rhythm, count rate for a full minute, noting number of irregular beats.	
3. *Pedal (dorsalis pedis) Pulse*	
a. Explain to the client that you need to check the circulation in the feet.	a. Encourages client participation and allays anxiety.
b. Position leg flat on the bed with foot in neutral position, or place foot flat on bed.	b. Provides access to artery.
c. Palpate the upper surface (dorsum) of the foot on an imaginary line drawn from the middle of the ankle to a space between the first and second toes.	c. Identifies the location of the artery.
d. Identify pulse rhythm.	d. Palpate pulse until rhythm is determined. Describe as regular or irregular.

continued

Action	Rationale
e. Determine pulse volume.	**e.** Quality of pulse is an indication of peripheral perfusion. Describe as normal, weak, strong, or bounding.
f. Share your findings with client.	**f.** Supports client participation in care.
g. Record by site the rate, rhythm, and, if applicable, number of irregular beats.	**g.** Recording rate and characteristics at bedside ensures accurate documentation.
h. Transfer information to client's record.	**h.** Facilitates communication among members of the health care team.

Procedure B5 — Assessing Respirations

Equipment

- Watch with a second hand

Action	Rationale

• Wash your hands • Check the client's identification band prior to beginning •

Action	Rationale
1. Before replacing client's gown from auscultating heart sounds, assess respirations.	1. Facilitates observation of chest wall and abdominal movements.
2. Place your hand over client's wrist and observe one complete respiratory cycle.	2. Hand rises and falls with inspiration and expiration.
3. Start to count with first inspiration while looking at second hand sweep of watch.	3. Respiratory rate is one complete cycle (inspiration and expiration).
• Infants and children: count a full minute.	• Infants and children usually have an irregular rate.
• Adults: count for 30 seconds and multiply by 2. If an irregular rate or rhythm is present, count for a full minute.	• Respiratory rate reflects number of breaths per minute.
4. Observe depth of respirations by degree of chest wall movement and rhythm of cycle (regular or interrupted).	4. Reveals volume of air movement into and out of the lungs. Describe as shallow, normal, or deep.
5. Replace client's gown.	5. Prevents embarrassment and chilling.
6. Record rate and character of respirations at bedside.	6. Ensures accurate documentation.

Procedure B6 — Assessing Blood Pressure

Equipment

- Alcohol swabs
- Stethoscope
- Sphygmomanometer with proper size cuff

continued

Action	Rationale

• Wash your hands • Check the client's identification band •
• Explain the procedure to the client prior to beginning •

1. Determine which extremity is most appropriate for reading. *Do not* take a pressure reading on an injured or painful extremity or one in which an intravenous line is running. Do not take blood pressure on the operative side of a woman after a mastectomy, or in the arm in which a dialysis shunt is present.	1. Cuff inflation can temporarily interrupt blood flow and compromise circulation in an extremity already impaired or a vein receiving intravenous fluids. Avoids vascular compromise.
2. Select a cuff size that completely encircles upper arm.	2. Provides equalization of pressure on the artery to ensure accurate measurement.
3. Move clothing away from upper aspect of arm.	3. Ensures accurate measurement.
4. Position arm at heart level, extend elbow with palm turned upward.	4. Blood pressure increases when arm is below level of heart and decreases when arm is above level of heart.
5. Make sure bladder cuff is fully deflated and pump valve moves freely.	5. Equipment must function properly to obtain an accurate reading.
6. Locate brachial artery in the antecubital space.	6. Designates placement of stethoscope.
7. Apply cuff snugly and smoothly over upper arm, 2.5 cm (1 in.) above antecubital space with center of bladder over brachial artery (Figure B6-1).	7. Ensures even pressure distribution over brachial artery. Prevents tubing from being constricted and allows visualization of aneroid manometer dial.
8. Connect bladder tubing to manometer tubing. If using a portable mercury-filled manometer, position vertically at eye level.	8. Maintains closed system; supports accurate reading of mercury level in manometer.
9. Palpate brachial artery (Figure B6-2). Turn valve clockwise to close and compress bulb to inflate cuff to 30 mm Hg above point where palpated pulse disappears, then slowly release valve (deflating cuff), noting reading when pulse is felt again.	9. Inflates the cuff's bladder with pressure and temporarily impairs flow of blood through artery. Provides an estimate of maximum pressure required to measure systolic pressure.

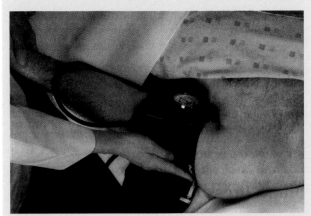

Figure B6-1 Wrap the blood pressure cuff on arm 1 inch above client's brachial pulsation, with bladder centered over brachial artery.

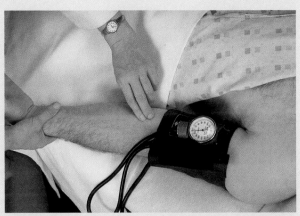

Figure B6-2 Palpate the brachial artery with fingertips below the pressure cuff.

continued

Action	Rationale
10. Insert earpiece of stethoscope into ears with a forward tilt, ensuring diaphragm hangs freely.	**10.** Enhances sound transmission from bell or diaphragm to ears.
11. Relocate brachial pulse with your nondominant hand and place bell or diaphragm directly over pulse. Bell or diaphragm should be in direct contact with skin and should not touch cuff (Figure B6-3).	**11.** Sound heard best directly over artery; decreases muffled sounds that cause inaccurate reading. Bell is more sensitive to low-frequency sound that occurs with pressure release.

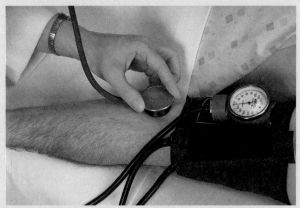

Figure B6-3 Bell Placed over Brachial Artery below Blood Pressure Cuff

Action	Rationale
12. With dominant hand, turn valve clockwise to close. Compress pump to inflate cuff until manometer registers 30 mm Hg above diminished pulse point identified in step 9.	**12.** Prevents air leak during inflation. Ensures the cuff is inflated to a pressure greater than the client's systolic pressure.
13. Slowly turn valve counterclockwise so that mercury falls at a rate of 2–3 mm Hg per second. Listen for five phases of Korotkoff's sounds while noting manometer reading:	**13.** Maintains constant release of pressure to ensure hearing first systolic sound. Identify manometer readings for each of the five phases.
• A faint, clear tapping sound appears and increases in intensity (phase I).	• Identify two consecutive tapping sounds to confirm systolic reading (phase I is systolic).
• Swishing sound (phase II).	
• Intense sound (phase III).	
• Abrupt, distinctive muffled sounds (phase IV).	
• Sound disappears (phase V).	• Phase V is the best index of diastolic blood pressure.
14. Deflate cuff rapidly and completely.	**14.** Prevents arterial occlusion and client discomfort from numbness or tingling.
15. Remove cuff or wait 2 minutes before taking a second reading.	**15.** Releases trapped blood in the vessels.
16. Inform client of reading.	**16.** Promotes client participation in care.
17. Record reading.	**17.** Ensures accuracy.
18. Lower bed, raise side rails, place call light within easy reach.	**18.** Promotes client safety.
19. Put all equipment in proper place.	**19.** Fosters maintenance of equipment.

continued

Action	Rationale
20. Wash hands.	20. Prevents transmission of microorganisms.
21. Document measurements in client's medical record on appropriate form, usually vital signs flow sheet.	21. Vital sign measurements are usually charted on the graphic section of the vital signs form.
22. Compare data with client's baseline and normal range for age group.	22. Provides for comparative data analysis.
23. If any measurements are abnormal, measure again and report abnormal findings to instructor or charge nurse.	23. Reporting abnormal measurements alerts staff to possible problems requiring intervention.

Procedure B7 — Weighing Client, Mobile and Immobile

Equipment

- Scale: standing electronic or balance scale (Figure B7-1); or sling scale (Figure B7-2)
- Plastic cover for sling scale
- Recommended disinfectant
- 1–3 other staff members to assist when using sling scale
- Gloves (when applicable)

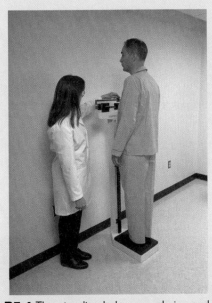

Figure B7-1 The standing balance scale is used to weigh ambulatory clients.

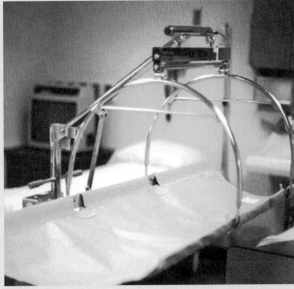

Figure B7-2 The sling scale is used to weigh clients in bed.

Action	Rationale

• Wash your hands • Check the client's identification band •
• Explain the procedure to the client prior to beginning •

Standing Scale

1. Place scale near client.	1. Reduces risk of fall or injury.
2. Turn on scale (if required) and calibrate to zero.	2. Ensures accurate reading.

continued

Action	Rationale
3. Ask client to step up on the scale and stand straight and still. *Electronic scale:* Read weight after digital numbers have stopped fluctuating. *Balance scale:* Slide the scale's weight indicators on the blance beam until the balance rests in the middle. Add the two numbers to read the client's weight.	3. Provides accurate measurement of weight and height. Reading is not accurate when the numbers are still fluctuating. Weights on scale must be balanced to obtain accurate reading.
4. Ask client to step down and assist client back to the bed or chair, if necessary.	4. Reduces risk of injury if client needs assistance.
5. Wipe scale with appropriate disinfectant.	5. Reduces risk of spread of infection.
6. Wash hands.	6. Reduces transmission of microorganisms.

Sling Scale

Action	Rationale
7. Wash hands and put on gloves.	7. Reduces risk of nosocomial infection.
8. Introduce yourself to client and explain what you would like him to do.	8. Builds rapport; involves client in his care.
9. Place plastic covering on sling if available (can usually be ordered in bulk from the manufacturer).	9. Reduces risk of spreading infection between clients.
10. Remove pillows. Turn client to one side and place half of sling on bed next to client with remaining half rolled up against client's back (Figure B7-3).	10. Most accurate weight will be obtained by leaving no other bedding between client and sling.
11. Turn client to other side, and unroll rest of sling so it lies flat beneath client.	11. Turning in this manner maximizes client comfort.
12. Roll the scale over the bed so that the legs of the scale are underneath the bed (Figure B7-4). Open and lock the legs of the scale.	12. Ensures equipment is being used safely to reduce risk of injury.
13. Turn on scale and calibrate to zero.	13. Ensures accurate reading.

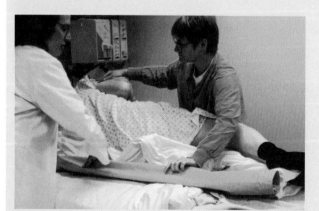

Figure B7-3 Turn client on one side and place sling on the bed.

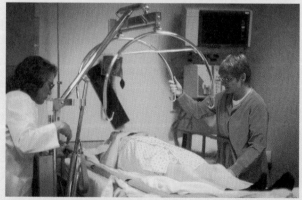

Figure B7-4 After unrolling the rest of the sling under the client, move the scale into position over the bed.

continued

Action	Rationale
14. Lower arms of the scale and slip hooks through holes in sling (Figure B7-5).	14. Attaches sling to scale to obtain weight.
15. Pump scale until sling is completely off the bed (Figure B7-6).	15. Ensures accurate weight.

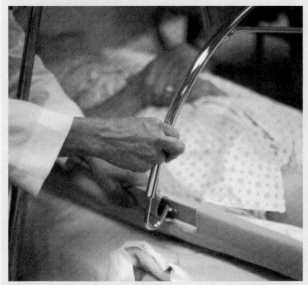

Figure B7-5 Attach the hooks through the holes in the sling.

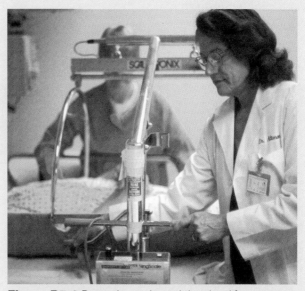

Figure B7-6 Pump the scale until the sling lifts completely off the bed.

Action	Rationale
16. Remind client to remain still. Read weight after digital numbers have stopped fluctuating (Figure B7-7).	16. Reading is not accurate when the numbers are still fluctuating.
17. Lower client back to bed and remove arms of scale from sling (Figure B7-8).	17. Prepare for removal of sling.
18. Unlock legs, return to their original position, and remove scale from bed.	18. Remove equipment to allow staff to remove sling from beneath client.

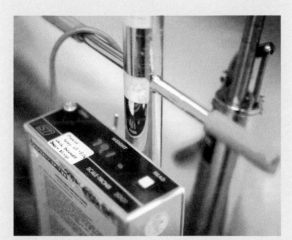

Figure B7-7 Read the weight after the numbers have stopped fluctuating.

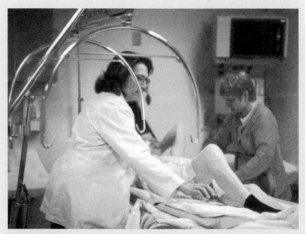

Figure B7-8 Lower the client back to the bed and prepare to remove the sling.

continued

Action	Rationale
19. Turn client from side to side to remove sling from underneath client.	**19.** Remove sling.
20. Realign client with pillows and covers.	**20.** Ensures comfort and privacy.
21. Remove plastic covering from sling and discard per hospital policy.	**21.** Reduces risk of spread of infection.
22. Remove gloves and wash hands.	**22.** Reduces transmission of microorganisms.

Procedure B8 — Practicing Proper Body Mechanics

Equipment

- None required

Action	Rationale
1. Get a firm footing by keeping your feet apart.	**1.** Develops and maintains a stable base.
2. Bend at the knees; avoid bending at the waist. Hold the load close to your body (Figure B8-1).	**2.** Provides greater leverage for lifting.
3. Lift with the leg muscles.	**3.** Uses the strongest muscles, thereby reducing risk of injury.
4. Tighten abdominal muscles to lift.	**4.** Provides greater support to the back.
5. Turn by pivoting your feet, not your trunk, while lifting (Figure B8-2).	**5.** Maintains proper body alignment.
6. If the load is heavy, get help or use a mechanical lift.	**6.** Avoids strain and possible injury.
7. Push, do not pull.	**7.** Prevents back injury.
8. Use wheeled objects (e.g., a wheelchair).	**8.** Eases mobility.
9. Perform health-promoting activities.	**9.** Exercising, maintaining normal weight for height, pacing activities, and relaxing promote good body conditioning.

continued

Action	Rationale
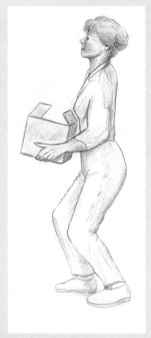	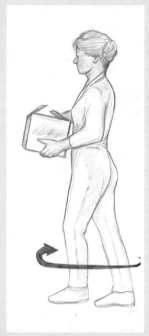
Figure B8-1 Bend knees to lift.	**Figure B8-2** Pivot with feet.

Procedure B9   Performing Passive Range-of-Motion Exercises

Equipment

- Bed with side rails

Action	Rationale
• Wash your hands • Check the client's identification band prior to beginning •	
1. Explain to the client the purposes of range-of-motion (ROM) exercises.	1. Reduces client anxiety and increases cooperation.
2. Elevate the bed.	2. Decrease nurse's muscle strain and promotes proper body mechanics.
3. Assist client to supine position in a warm, comfortable environment.	3. Promotes client's comfort level.
4. Start at head of client and perform ROM exercises down each side of the body.	4. Provides a systematic method to ensure that all body parts are exercised.
5. Repeat each of the following range-of-motion exercises five times in a slow, firm manner. (Cradle client's head with palms of hand; hold the extremities by the long bone areas.)	5. Provides support to each body part, thus reducing strain on muscles and joints.
Head: Rotation—Turn the head from side to side. Flexion and extension—Tilt the head toward the chest and then tilt slightly upward (Figure B9-1). Lateral flexion—Tilt the head on each side so as to almost touch the ear to the shoulder.	

continued

Action	**Rationale**
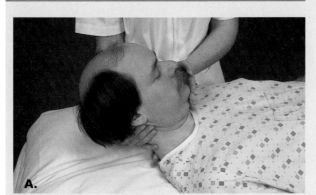	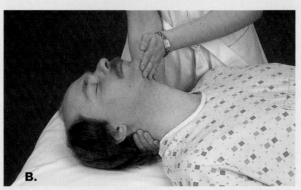

Figure B9-1 Passive ROM Exercises of Head. A. Flexion of neck; B. Extension of neck

Neck: Rotation—Place the client in a sitting position and rotate the neck in a semicircle while supporting the head.

Trunk: Flexion and extension—Bend the trunk forward, straighten the trunk, then extend slightly backward. Rotation—Turn the shoulders forward and return to normal position. Lateral flexion—Tip trunk to left side, straighten trunk, tip to right side.

Have the client resume a supine position.

Arm: Flexion and extension—Extend the arm in a straight position upward toward the head, then downward along the side. Adduction and abduction—Extend the arm in a straight position toward the midline (adduction) and away from the midline (abduction).

Shoulder: Internal and external rotation—Bend the elbow at a 90° angle with the upper arm parallel to the shoulder; rotate the shoulder by moving the lower arm upward and downward.

Elbow: Flexion and extension—Supporting the arm, flex and extend the elbow (Figure B9-2). Pronation and supination—Flex elbow, move the hand in palm-up and palm-down position.

Wrist: Flexion and extension—Supporting the wrist, flex and extend the wrist. Adduction and

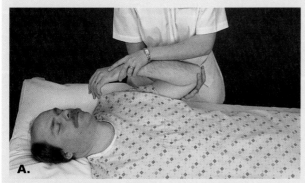	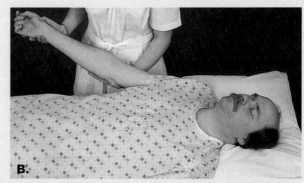

Figure B9-2 Passive ROM Exercises of Elbow. A. Flexion of elbow; B. Extension of elbow

continued

Action	Rationale
abduction—Supporting the lower arm, turn wrist right to left, left to right, then rotate the wrist in a circular motion.	
Hand: Flexion and extension—Supporting the wrist, flex and extend the fingers. Adduction and abduction—Supporting the wrist, spread fingers apart and then bring them close together. Opposition—Supporting the wrist, touch each finger with the tip of the thumb.	
Thumb: Rotation—Supporting the wrist, rotate the thumb in a circular manner.	
Hip and Leg: Flexion and extension—Supporting the lower leg, flex the leg toward the chest and then extend the leg (Figure B9-3). Internal and external rotation—Supporting the lower leg, angle the foot inward and outward.	
Knee: Flexion and extension—Supporting the lower leg, flex and extend the knee.	
Ankle: Flexion and extension—Supporting the lower leg, flex and extend the ankle.	
Foot: Adduction and abduction—Supporting the ankle, spread the toes apart and then bring them close together. Flexion and extension—Supporting the ankle, extend the toes upward and then flex the toes downward.	

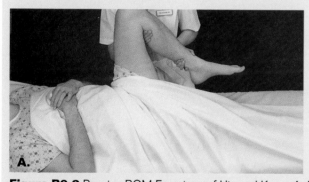 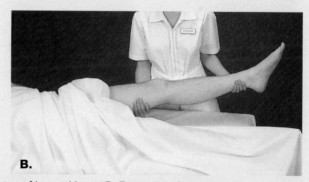

Figure B9-3 Passive ROM Exercises of Hip and Knee. A. Flexion of hip and knee; B. Extension of hip and knee

Procedure B10   Assisting a Client with Ambulation

Equipment

- None required

Action	Rationale
• *Wash your hands* • *Check the client's identification band* • *Explain the procedure to the client prior to beginning* •	
1. Inform client of the purposes and distance of the walking exercise.	1. Reduces client anxiety and increases cooperation.

continued

Action	**Rationale**
2. Elevate the head of the bed and wait several minutes.	2. Prevents orthostatic hypotension.
3. Lower the bed height.	3. Reduces distance client has to step down, thus decreasing risk of injury.
4. With one arm under the client's back and one arm under the client's upper legs, move the client into the dangling position (Figure B10-1).	4. Provides client support and reduces risk of fall.

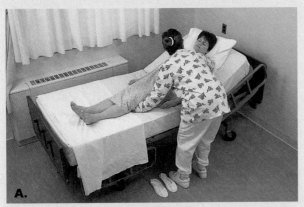 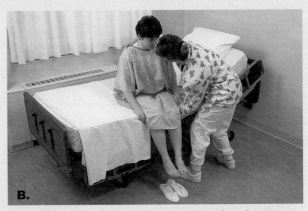

Figure B10-1 Assist the client from a supine to a seated position. A. Place one arm under the client's back and one arm under the client's legs. B. Help the client move into the dangling position.

5. Encourage client to dangle at side of bed for several minutes.	5. Prevents orthostatic hypotension. Allows for assessing tolerance for the sitting position.
6. Stand in front of client with your knees touching client's knees.	6. Prevents client from sliding forward if dizziness or faintness occurs.
7. Place arms under client's axillae (Figure B10-2).	7. Supports client's trunk.

Figure B10-2 Assist client to a standing position by supporting the client's trunk with your arms under the client's axillae.

8. Assist client to a standing position, allowing client time to balance.	8. Reduces risk of fall.
9. Help client ambulate desired distance or distance of tolerance by placing your hand under the client's forearm and ambulating close to the client (Figure B10-3).	9. Provides assistance in achieving ambulatory goals.

continued

Action	Rationale

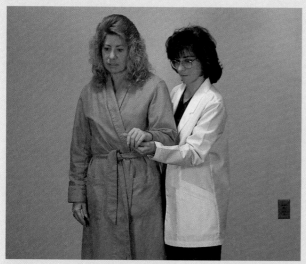

Figure B10-3 Assisting a Client with Ambulation

Action	Rationale
10. At the end of ambulation, assist the client back to bed or to chair beside bed.	10. Allows client to rest.
11. Document client's progress with ambulation.	11. Facilitates communication with members of the health care team.

Procedure B11 — Positioning a Client in Bed

Equipment

- Hospital bed with side rails
- Pillows or foam wedges
- Foot board
- Turn sheet or draw sheet
- Hand cones
- High-top tennis shoes

Action	Rationale
• *Wash your hands* • *Check the client's identification band prior to beginning* •	
1. Inform client of reason for the move and how to assist (if able).	1. Reduces anxiety; helps increase comprehension and cooperation; promotes client autonomy.
2. Elevate bed to highest position.	2. Avoids strain on nurse's back muscles; promotes proper body mechanics.
3. Using two nurses, place turn (or draw) sheet under client's back and head.	3. Decreases shearing, which can precede formation of pressure ulcers.

Fowler's Position

Action	Rationale
4. Place bed in a 15° to 30° angle for low-Fowler's position, 45° to 60° angle for Fowler's position, or 70° to 90° angle for high-Fowler's position.	4. The height of the head of the bed is determined by physician's order, client preference, client tolerance, or client's activity (e.g., eating).
5. If desired, place pillows at small of back, under ankles, under the arms, and under head of client.	5. Promotes client comfort. Pillows under ankles elevate heels to help prevent pressure ulcer formation. Pillows under the arms can assist with lung expansion.

continued

Action	Rationale
6. Slightly elevate the gatch of the lower portion of the bed.	6. Assists in maintaining correct client positioning.
7. Assess client for comfort.	7. Comfort is subjective.
8. Lower height of bed and elevate side rails.	8. Promotes client safety.

Supine Position

Action	Rationale
9. Follow steps 1–3.	
10. Place bed in a flat position.	
11. Place pillows at small of back, under head, and under ankles.	11. Adds to client comfort; relieves pressure on heels.
12. Assess client's comfort level.	12. Comfort is subjective.
13. Lower height of bed and elevate side rails.	13. Promotes client safety.

Side-Lying Position

Action	Rationale
14. Follow steps 1–3.	
15. Place client on side by logrolling (Procedure B15).	15. Places client on side for the proper positioning; reduces flexion of neck and spine.
16. Place a small pillow under client's head. Place pillow or foam wedges behind client's back. Place a pillow between client's legs. Put a pillow tucked by the client's abdomen.	16. Pillows at back and abdomen help maintain side-lying position. Small pillow under head is for comfort. Pillow between legs is for back alignment, comfort, and pressure relief. Pillow at abdomen supports upper arm, thus protecting the upper arm–shoulder joint positioning.
17. Run your hand under the client's dependent shoulder and move the shoulder slightly forward.	17. Removes pressure on upper arm-shoulder joint, promoting comfort.
18. Assess the client for comfort.	18. Comfort is subjective.
19. Lower the bed and elevate the side rails.	19. Promotes client safety.

Prone Position

Action	Rationale
20. Follow steps 1–3.	
21. Assist the client to lie on abdomen.	21. Prepares client to assume prone position.
22. Place a small pillow under client's head; head should be turned to side. The client's arms can be extended near side or flexed toward head. Place a small pillow under chest for female client and for client with a barrel chest.	22. Pillows at head and chest are for comfort. The arms are positioned according to client preference and flexibility. Pillow under chest protects breasts and promotes comfort.
23. Place a small pillow under ankles or have toes placed in space between foot of bed and the mattress.	23. Relieves pressure on toes.
24. Assess client for comfort.	24. Comfort is subjective.
25. Lower the bed and elevate the side rails.	25. Promotes client safety.

General Guidelines for Client Positioning

Action	Rationale
26. Use a hand cone for positioning the hand if needed. Place the cone in hand, with the wider portion near the little finger and the narrow portion nearer the index finger.	26. Helps prevent hand flexion contractures.

continued

Action	Rationale
27. Assess the client's skin frequently (at least every 2 hours) for pressure marks.	**27.** Immobile clients are prone to tissue ischemia with subsequent development of pressure ulcers.
28. Turn client frequently; every 2 hours or less.	**28.** Promotes blood circulation and prevents skin breakdown.
29. Use a footboard or high-top tennis shoes for clients in Fowler's and supine position if indicated.	**29.** Assists in prevention of foot drop.
30. Prepare a turn schedule for each client and place on chart at head of client's bed.	**30.** Stresses to all nursing personnel the importance of turning client frequently.
31. For all clients, be sure call bell is within reach.	**31.** Promotes safety; allows communication.

Procedure B12 Moving a Client in Bed

Equipment

- Hospital bed with side rails
- Turn sheet or draw sheet

Action	Rationale
• *Wash your hands* • *Check the client's identification band prior to beginning* •	
1. Inform client of reason for the move and how to assist (if able).	**1.** Reduces anxiety; helps increase comprehension and cooperation; promotes client autonomy.
2. Elevate bed to high position. Lower head of bed.	**2.** Lessens strain on nurse's back muscles; promotes proper body mechanics.
3. With two nurses, place turn/draw sheet under client's back and head (if not already present).	**3.** Reduces shearing force which can precipitate pressure sores.
4. Nurses stand on each side of client. Position client with knees flexed to push with feet if able to assist with move (Figure B12-1).	**4.** Client assistance lessens strain on nurse's back muscles; promotes client autonomy.
5. Have client use a bed trapeze, if available.	**5.** Lessens shearing force; decreases strain on both client and nurses.

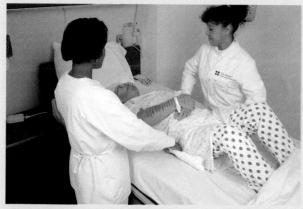

Figure B12-1 Moving Client in Bed: Client Positioned with Knees Flexed

continued

Action	Rationale
6. The lead nurse will give the signal to move. The nurses will lift up on the turn/draw sheet. The move is coordinated to transfer the client up toward the head of the bed.	6. Lessens strain on client and nurses. Reduces shearing force.
7. Position in bed can be maintained using bed gatch, if tolerated by client.	7. Elevated bed gatch maintains position by preventing client from sliding downward.
8. Elevate head of bed, if tolerated by client.	8. Promotes comfort; facilitates eating and drinking; facilitates communication.
9. Assess client for comfort.	9. Comfort is subjective.
10. Lower bed and elevate side rails.	10. Promotes client safety.

Procedure B13 — Transferring a Client from Bed to Wheelchair

Equipment

- Bed
- Wheelchair

Action	Rationale
• Wash your hands • Check the client's identification band prior to beginning •	
1. Inform client about desired purpose and destination.	1. Reduces client anxiety and increases cooperation.
2. Assess client for ability to assist with the transfer and for presence of cognitive or sensory deficits.	2. Promotes safety.
3. Lower the height of the bed.	3. Reduces distance client has to step down, thus decreasing risk of injury.
4. Allow client to dangle for a few minutes.	4. Allows time to assess client's response to sitting; reduces possibility of orthostatic hypotension.
5. Bring wheelchair close to the side of the bed, toward the foot of the bed.	5. Minimizes transfer distance.
6. Lock wheelchair brakes and elevate the foot pedals.	6. Provides stability.
7. Assist client to side of bed until feet touch the floor.	7. Provides guidance and helps client maintain balance.
8. Assist the client to a standing position and provide support.	8. Helps client stand safely and gives time to assess status.
9. Pivot client so client's back is toward the wheelchair (Figure B13-1).	9. Moves client into proper position to be seated.
10. Place client's hands on the arm supports of the wheelchair.	10. Allows client to gain balance and judge distance to seat.
11. Bend at the knees, easing the client into a sitting position (Figure B13-2).	11. Increases stability and minimizes strain on back.

continued

Action	Rationale
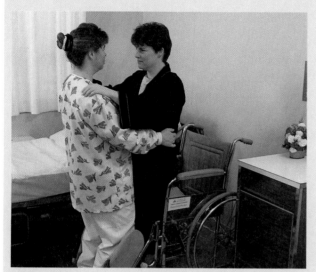	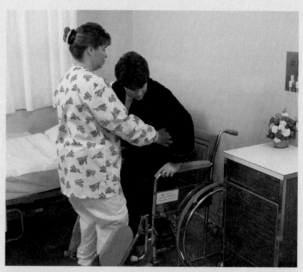
Figure B13-1 Pivot client so back is toward wheelchair.	**Figure B13-2** Ease client into wheelchair.
12. Assist client to maintain proper posture.	12. Broadest, and therefore safest, base of support is with client seated as far back on the seat as possible.
13. Secure the safety belt, place client's feet on feet pedals, and release brakes.	13. Ensures client safety; prepares client for movement.

Procedure B14

Transferring a Client from Bed to Stretcher with Minimum Assistance/Maximum Assistance

Equipment

- Bed
- Pillows
- Stretcher
- Lift Sheet

Action	Rationale
• *Wash your hands* • *Check the client's identification band* •	
1. Inform client about desired purpose and destination.	1. Reduces client anxiety and increases cooperation.
2. Raise the height of bed and lock brakes.	2. Reduces distance nurse must bend, thus preventing back strain; prevents bed from moving.
Minimum Assistance	
3. Instruct client to move to side of bed close to stretcher. Lower side rails of bed and stretcher.	3. Decreases risk of client falling.
4. Stand at outer side of stretcher and push it toward bed. Lock stretcher brakes.	4. Diminishes the gap between bed and stretcher; secures the stretcher position.
5. Instruct client to move onto stretcher with assistance as needed.	5. Promotes client independence.
6. Cover client with sheet or bath blanket. Release brakes of stretcher.	6. Promotes comfort; protects privacy.

continued

Action	**Rationale**
7. Elevate side rails on stretcher and secure safety belts about client.	7. Prevents falls.
8. Stand at head of stretcher to guide it when pushing.	8. Pushing, not pulling, ensures proper body mechanics.

Maximum Assistance

Action	**Rationale**
9. Assess amount of assistance required for transfer. Usually two to four staff members are required for the maximum assisted transfer.	9. Promotes client independence; assures that enough staff are present before beginning transfer.
10. Lock wheels of bed and stretcher (Figure B14-1).	10. Prevents falls.

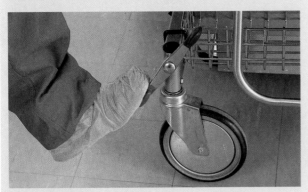

Figure B14-1 Lock wheels on the stretcher.

Action	**Rationale**
11. Have one nurse stand close to client's head.	11. Supports client's head during the move.
12. Logroll the client (see Procedure B15) and place a lift sheet under the client's back, trunk, and upper legs. The lift sheet can extend under the head if client lacks head control abilities.	12. Prevents flexion and rotation of client's hips and spine; maintains correct body alignment.
13. If urinary drainage bag is present, empty it and move it to side of bed closest to stretcher.	13. Prevents risk of urinary infection.
14. Empty all drainage bags (e.g., T-tube, Hemovac, Jackson-Pratt). Secure drainage system to client's gown prior to transfer.	14. Decreases possibility of spills; prevents dislodging of tubes.
15. Move client to edge of bed near stretcher.	15. Prevents dragging, which causes shearing force.
16. Nurse on nonstretcher side of the bed rolls the lift sheet toward the client's side (Figure B14-2).	16. Provides the nurse with stronger gripping surface; provides maximum control of client movement; promotes good body mechanics for nurse.
17. Place pillow overlapping the bed and stretcher.	17. Protects head from injury.
18. One nurse acts as team leader. Client is moved on count of three from team leader. One nurse is on each side of client, one nurse controls client's head. Client is lifted with lift sheet and moved from bed to stretcher by team (Figure B14-3). If client is heavy or difficult to move, it may require several small moves to get client from bed fully onto stretcher.	18. Promotes proper body mechanics and client safety.
19. Secure safety belts and elevate side rails of stretcher.	19. Prevents falls.

continued

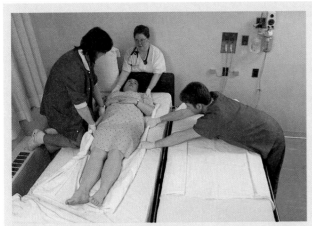

Figure B14-2 Transferring Client with Maximum Assistance; Grasping Lift Sheet

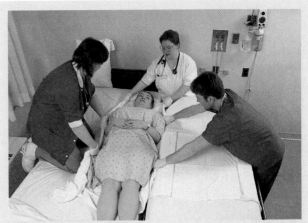

Figure B14-3 Transferring Client with Maximum Assistance; Moving Client from Bed to the Stretcher

Action	Rationale
20. If IV is present, move it from bed IV pole to stretcher IV pole after client transfer.	20. Prevents tubing from being pulled and IV from being dislodged.
21. Document where the client is going on the stretcher and client's response to move.	21. Provides record of client's whereabouts in building.

Procedure B15 — Logrolling a Client with a Turn Sheet

Equipment

- Hospital bed with side rails
- Pillows
- Turn sheet or draw sheet
- Gloves (if chance of exposure to body fluids)

Action	Rationale

• *Wash your hands* • *Check the client's identification band prior to beginning* • *Wear gloves if indicated* •

Action	Rationale
1. Inform client of reason for the move and how to assist (if able).	1. Reduces anxiety; helps increase comprehension and cooperation; promotes client autonomy.
2. Elevate hospital bed to high position.	2. Avoids strain on nurse's back muscles; promotes proper body mechanics.
3. Using one or more staff members; place a turn/draw sheet under the client's back, buttocks, and head (if not already present).	3. Reduces shearing force, which can precipitate pressure ulcer formation.
4. The lead person tells the client and other personnel the direction of the move.	4. Cooperation and coordination place less strain on client and personnel.
5. One person stands on each side of the bed. The lead nurse gives the signal for the move. The staff member on the side of the bed in the direction of the move holds the turn/draw sheet to guide the move. The second staff member applies gentle pressure on client's back toward the direction of the move, assisting client to roll (Figure B15-1).	5. Two persons give more support to client than one person could and are better able to maintain proper alignment of client's spine and neck.

continued

Action	Rationale

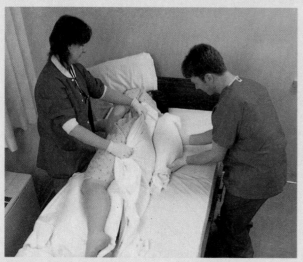

Figure B15-1 Logrolling: Two-Person Move

Action	Rationale
6. Tuck pillows at client's back and abdomen.	6. Maintains side-lying position.
7. Assess the client for comfort and proper alignment.	7. Comfort is subjective.
8. Elevate side rails and lower the bed height.	8. Promotes client safety.
9. This procedure can be reversed to reposition clients on their backs or opposite side.	9. Repositioning can prevent development of pressure sores.

Procedure B16   Bedmaking: Unoccupied Bed

Equipment

- Bottom sheet (fitted, if available)
- Draw sheet (regular top sheet may be used)
- Mattress pad (if available)
- Linen bag hamper outside the room

- Top sheet
- Pillowcase (each pillow on the bed)
- Antiseptic solution, washcloth, and towel
- Nonsterile gloves

Action	Rationale

Unoccupied Bed

Action	Rationale
1. Wash hands.	1. Reduces transmission of microorganisms.
2. Place hamper by client's door if linen bags are not available. Explain procedure to client. Assess condition of blanket and/or bedspread.	2. Provides for proper disposal of soiled linens. Encourages client cooperation. Allows for organization of supplies.
3. Gather linen and gloves. Place linen on a clean, dry surface in reverse order of usage at the client's bedside (pillowcases, top sheet, draw sheet, bottom sheet).	3. Provides easy access to items.
4. Inquire about the client's toileting needs and attend as necessary.	4. Provides for client comfort and prevents interruptions during bedmaking.

continued

Action	Rationale
5. Assist client to a safe, comfortable chair.	5. Increases client's comfort and decreases risk for falls.
6. Don gloves.	6. Decreases risk of infection from soiled, contaminated linens.
7. Position bed: flat, side rails down, adjust height to waist level.	7. Promotes good body mechanics and decreases back strain.
8. Remove and fold blanket and/or bedspread. If clean and reusable, place on clean work area.	8. Keeps reusable bed linens clean.
9. Remove soiled pillowcases by grasping the closed end with one hand and slipping the pillow out with the other. Place soiled cases on top of soiled sheet and put pillows on clean work area.	9. Allows easy removal of the pillowcases without contamination of uniform by soiled linens and keep pillows clean.
10. Remove soiled linens: Start on the side of the bed closest to you; free the bottom sheet by lifting the mattress and rolling soiled linens to the middle of the bed. Go to the other side of the bed, repeat action.	10. Prevents tearing and fanning of linens. Linens are folded from cleanest area to most soiled to prevent contamination.
11. Fold soiled linens: head of bed to middle, foot of bed to middle. Place in linen bag or hamper, keeping soiled linens away from uniform.	11. Fanning linens increases number of microorganisms in air. Folding linens decreases the risk of transmission of infection to others.
12. Check mattress and pad, if used. If the pad is soiled, replace. If the mattress is soiled, clean with an antiseptic solution and dry thoroughly.	12. Reduces transmission of microorganisms.
13. Remove gloves, wash hands.	13. Reduces transmission of microorganisms to clean linens.
14. Open clean bottom sheet lengthwise onto the bed with the seamed side of the sheet toward the mattress. Unfold half of the sheet's width to center crease and smooth the sheet flat (refer to action 15 for placing sheet onto mattress).	14. Facilitates making bed in an organized, time-saving manner by not having to go from one side of the bed to the other.
15. Proceed with placing bottom sheet onto the mattress:	15. Correctly positions bottom sheet.
a. Fitted sheet	
• Position yourself diagonally toward the head of the bed.	• Prevents back strain. Placement of seamed side toward mattress prevents irritation to the client's skin. Proper placement of linens ensures adequate sheeting for all sides of the bed.
• Start at the head with seamed side of the fitted sheet toward the mattress.	
• Lift the mattress corner with your hand closest to the bed; with your other hand, pull and tuck the fitted sheet over the mattress corner; secure at the head and sides.	
• Repeat action at foot of bed.	
b. Flat regular sheet	
• Lay the bottom edge of the sheet on the top of the mattress even with the foot of the bed.	• Ensures proper placement of the sheet so that it can be tightly secured at the top and on both sides of the bed.

continued

Action	**Rationale**

- Allow the sheet to hang 10 inches (25 cm) over the mattress on the side and at the top of the bed.

- Position yourself diagonally toward the head of the bed. Lift the top of the mattress corner with the hand closest to the bed and smoothly tuck the sheet under the mattress (Figure B16-1). | • Prevents straining of back muscles; decreases the chance that the sheet will pull out from under the mattress.

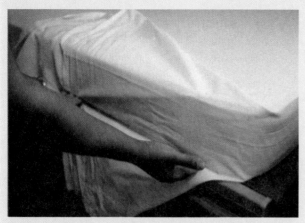

Figure B16-1 Tuck the sheet under the mattress corner.

16. Miter the corner at the head of the bed.

   a. Face the side of bed and lift and lay the top edge of the sheet onto the bed to form a triangular fold (Figure B16-2A).

   b. Tuck lower edge of sheet (hanging free at side of mattress) under mattress.

   c. Grasp the triangular fold, bring it down over the side of the mattress and tuck the sheet smoothly under the mattress (Figure B16-2B). Straighten the free hanging sheet on mattress side.

16. Secures sheet tightly to the mattress; with the triangular fold providing a smooth tuck to keep the linen in place.

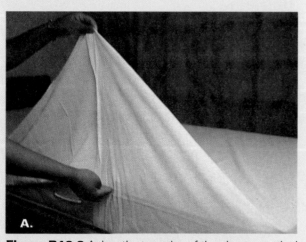
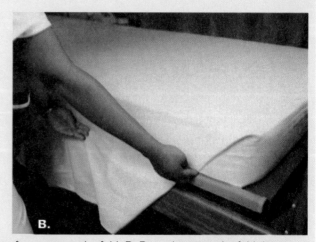

Figure B16-2 A. Lay the top edge of the sheet onto the bed to form a triangular fold. B. Bring the triangular fold down over the side of the mattress and tuck the sheet under the mattress.

continued

Action	Rationale
17. Place draw sheet onto top of bottom sheet and unfold to middle crease. Both sheets should hang 10 inches (25 cm) over the side of the mattress.	**17.** Provides a sheet to lift and move the client in bed without having to use the bottom sheet and remake the bed. Helps to keep bottom sheet clean.
18. Face the side of the bed, palms of hands down. Tuck both the bottom and draw sheets under the mattress. Ensure that the bottom sheet is tucked smoothly under the mattress all the way to the foot of the bed.	**18.** Keeps sheets taut, in place, and wrinkle-free, decreasing the risk of skin irritation.
19. Go to the other side of the bed, unfold the bottom sheet, repeating steps 14 to 16.	**19.** Unfolding decreases air current, which can spread microorganisms.
20. Unfold the draw sheet and grasp the free hanging sides of both the bottom and draw sheets. Pull toward you, keeping your back straight, and with a firm grasp (sheets taut) tuck both sheets under the mattress. Use your arms and open palms to extend the linen under the mattress.	**20.** Uses your body's weight in pulling the sheet taut and prevents strain on your back muscles.
21. Place the top sheet on top of bed and unfold lengthwise, placing the center crease (width) of the sheet in the middle of the bed. Place the top edge of the sheet (seam up) even with the top of the mattress at the head of the bed. Pull the remaining length toward the bottom of the bed.	**21.** Making one side of the bed at a time saves time and movement. Seam will be folded down to prevent contact with the client's skin, which can result in irritation.
22. Unfold and apply the blanket or spread; repeat step 21.	**22.** Provides warmth.
23. Miter the bottom corners as described in action 16.	**23.** Secures linen at the foot of the bed.
24. Face the head of the bed and fold the top sheet and blanket over 6 inches (15 cm). Fan-fold the sheet and blanket (from the head to the middle of the bed).	**24.** Allows the client to get under the covers easily.
25. Apply clean pillowcase on each pillow. With one hand, grasp the closed end of the pillowcase. Gather case and turn it inside out over hand. With same hand, grasp the middle of one end of the pillow. With the other hand, pull the case over the length of the pillow. The corners of the pillow should fit snugly into the corners of the case.	**25.** Keeps clean pillowcase away from your uniform.
26. Return the bed to the lowest position and elevate the head of the bed 30 to 45 degrees. Put side rails up on side, farthest from client.	**26.** Allows the client easy access to the bed. Provides for client safety.
27. Inquire about toileting needs of the client; assist as necessary.	**27.** Saves client energy and provides time to care for the client's needs.
28. Assist the client back into the bed and pull up the side rails; place call light in reach; take vital signs.	**28.** Promotes client safety and a means to call for assistance. Sitting up in a chair and movement may cause changes in the client's vital signs.
29. Document your actions and the client's response during the procedure and to being up in a chair.	**29.** Documents completion of procedure and assessment findings of client's tolerance.

continued

Action	Rationale
Surgical Bed	
30. Follow steps 1–22 Bedmaking: Unoccupied Bed	30. Same as for steps 1–22.
31. Face the head of the bed and fold the top sheet and blanket over 6 inches (15 cm). Face the foot of the bed and fold the top sheet and blanket up so the fold is even with the bottom of the mattress. Standing on the side of the bed where the client will be transferred from the stretcher, face the bed and bring the bottom corner and top corner to the center of the bed, forming a triangle. Fan-fold the top sheet and the blanket to the side of the bed opposite where the stretcher will be placed.	31. Allows easy transfer of client from stretcher into bed without linens getting in the way.
32. Apply clean pillowcase as in step 25, but do not put pillow on the bed.	32. Keeps bed free of obstacles for easy transfer of client; pillow may be contraindicated for client.
33. Maintain bed in high position with head flat.	33. Places bed in proper position to move client from stretcher to bed.
34. Move furniture out of the way to clear a path from doorway to bed.	34. Allows stretcher to be easily brought to bedside.
35. Have the following items available: tissues, emesis basin, blood pressure cuff and stethoscope, IV pole, I&O sheet, and any other equipment specific to client's needs.	35. Ensures supplies and equipment are easily accessible.
36. When client returns, assist with transfer from stretcher to bed (Procedure B14). Pull top sheet and blanket over client. Tuck in top sheet and blanket, leaving room for client's feet.	36. Provides warmth, secures linens, and allows space for feet.
37. Adjust head of bed according to client preference or postoperative orders. When immediate postoperative care is completed, raise side rails, place bed in low position, and put call bell within client's reach.	37. Provides for client safety.
38. Wash hands.	38. Prevents transmission of microorganisms.
39. Document your actions and the client's response.	39. Facilitates communication among members of the health care team.

Procedure B17 Bedmaking: Occupied Bed

Equipment

- Linen hamper
- Pillowcase
- Bath blanket
- Top sheet, draw sheet, bottom sheet
- Blanket
- Gloves if risk of exposure to body fluids

Action	Rationale
• *Wash your hands*	
1. Apply gloves if indicated.	1. Promotes asepsis.
2. Explain procedure to client.	2. Promotes client cooperation.

continued

Action	Rationale
3. Remove top sheet and blanket. Loosen bottom sheet at foot and sides of bed. Lower side rail on side of nurse. Client should be covered with a bath blanket.	3. Facilitates easy removal of linen. Lowering only side rail close to nurse reduces client's risk of falls. Bath blanket prevents exposure and chills.
4. Position client on side, facing away from you. Reposition pillow under head.	4. Provides space to place clean linen.
5. Fan-fold or roll bottom linens close to client toward the center of the bed (Figure B17-1).	5. Maintains soiled linen together. Promotes comfort when client later rolls to other side.
6. Place clean bottom linens with the center fold nearest the client. Fan-fold or roll clean bottom linens nearest client and tuck under soiled linen (Figure B17-2). Maintain an adequate amount of sheet at head for tucking. Sheet should be even with the bottom edge of mattress.	6. Provides for maximum fit of sheets and decreases chance of wrinkles.

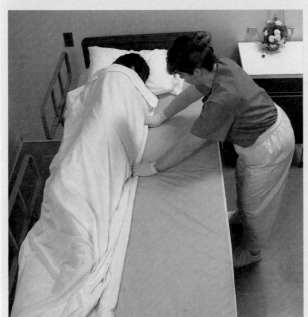

Figure B17-1 Fan-fold or roll the bottom linens close to the client toward the center of the bed.

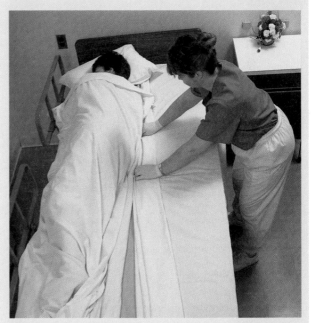

Figure B17-2 Fan-fold the clean bottom linens nearest the client and tuck under the soiled linens.

Action	Rationale
7. Miter bottom sheet at head of bed. To miter, lift mattress and tuck sheet over the edge of the mattress, lift edge of sheet that is hanging to form a triangle and lay upper part of sheet back onto bed; tuck the lower hanging section under the mattress. Tuck the sides of the sheet under the mattress.	7. Holds linens firmly in place.
8. Fold draw sheet in half. Identify the center of the draw sheet and place close to the client. Fan-fold or roll draw sheet closest to client and tuck under soiled linen; refer to Figure B17-3. Smooth linen. Tuck draw sheet under mattress, working from the center to the edges. Draw sheet should be positioned under the lower back and buttocks.	8. Draw sheet facilitates moving and lifting clients while in bed.
9. Log roll client over onto side facing you. Raise side rail.	9. Positions client off soiled linen. Protects client from falling.

continued

Action	Rationale
10. Move to other side of bed. Remove soiled linens by rolling into a bundle and place in linen hamper without touching uniform.	10. Prevents cross-contamination.
11. Unfold/unroll bottom sheet, then draw sheet. Look for objects left in the bed. Grasp each sheet with knuckles up and over the sheet and pull tightly while leaning back with your body weight (Figure B17-4). Client may be positioned supine or side-lying.	11. Tight sheets keep linens wrinkle-free and decrease risk of skin irritation. Leaning back uses body weight for good body mechanics.

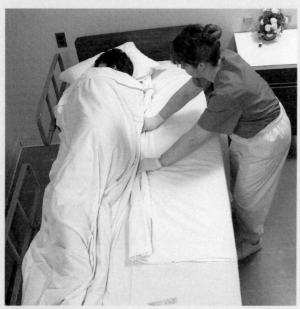

Figure B17-3 Fan-fold the draw sheet close to the client and tucking under the soiled linen.

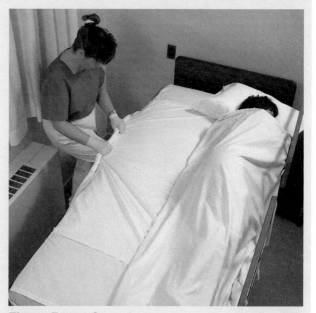

Figure B17-4 Grasp the bottom and draw sheets and pull tightly.

Action	Rationale
12. Place top sheet over client with center of sheet in middle of bed. Unfold top sheet over client. Remove bath blanket left on client to prevent exposure during bedmaking. Place top blanket over client, as you did with the top sheet.	12. Provides client with top sheet and blanket to prevent chilling.
13. Raise foot of mattress and tuck the corner of the top sheet and blanket under. Miter the corner. Repeat with other side of mattress.	13. Secures top sheet and blanket in place.
14. Grasp top sheet and blanket over client's toes and pull upward, then make a small fan-fold in the sheet.	14. Permits client to move feet under the sheets. Provides room under the tight top sheet and blanket.
15. Remove soiled pillowcase. Grasp center of clean pillowcase and invert pillowcase over hand/arm. Maintain grasp of pillowcase while grasping center of pillow. Use other hand to pull pillowcase down over pillow. Place pillow under client's head. While changing pillowcase, client can be instructed to rest head on bed, or place a blanket under client's head.	15. Provides clean pillowcase without shaking pillow or pillowcases. Promotes comfort.
16. Document procedure used to change linen and client's condition during the procedure.	16. Provides documentation of nursing care and assessment of client's status.

Procedure B18   Adult Bath

Equipment

- Bath towels
- Bath blanket
- Soap
- Lotion
- Powder
- Clean linen

- Washcloths
- Washbasin
- Soap dish
- Deodorant
- Clean gown
- Disposable gloves

Action	Rationale

• Wash your hands • Check the client's identification band prior to beginning •

1. Assess client's preferences about bathing.	1. Provides client opportunity to participate in care.
2. Explain procedure to client.	2. Enhances cooperation.
3. Prepare environment. Close doors and windows, adjust temperature, provide time for elimination needs, and provide privacy.	3. Protects from chills during bath and increases sense of privacy.
4. Wash hands. Apply gloves. Gloves should be changed when emptying water basin.	4. Reduces potential for transmission of pathogens.
5. Lower side rail on the side close to you. Position client in a comfortable position close to the side near you.	5. Prevents unnecessary reaching. Facilitates use of good body mechanics.
6. If bath blankets are available, place bath blanket over top sheet. Remove top sheet from under bath blanket (Figure B18-1). Remove client's gown. Bath blanket should be folded to expose only the area being cleaned at that time. (Top sheet may be used instead of bath blanket.)	6. Prevents exposure of client. Promotes privacy; protects from chills.

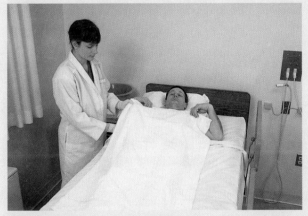

Figure B18-1 Place a bath blanket over the top sheet and remove the sheet from under the blanket.

7. Fill washbasin two-thirds full. Permit client to test temperature of water with his or her hand. Water should be changed when a soapy film develops or water becomes soiled.	7. Prevents accidental burns or chills.

continued

Action	Rationale
8. Make a bath mitten with the washcloth. To make a mitten: grasp the edge of the washcloth with the thumb; fold a third over the palm of the hand; wrap remainder of cloth around hand and across palm, grasping the second edge under the thumb; fold the extended end of the washcloth onto the palm and tuck under the palmar surface of the cloth.	8. Prevents ends of washcloth from dragging across skin. Promotes friction during bath.
9. Wash the face. Ask the client about preference for using soap on the face. Use a separate corner of the washcloth for each eye, wiping from inner to outer canthus (Figure B18-2). Wash neck and ears. Rinse and pat dry. Male clients may want to shave at this time. Provide assistance with shaving as needed.	9. Some clients may not use soap on their face. Using separate corners of washcloth reduces risk of transmitting microorganisms. Patting dry reduces skin irritation and drying.
10. Wash arms, forearms, and hands. Wash forearms and arms using long, firm strokes in the direction of distal to proximal (wrist to upper arm; Figure 18-3). Arm may need to be supported while being washed. Wash axilla. Rinse and pat dry. Apply deodorant or powder if desired. Immerse client's hand into basin of water. Allow hand to soak about 3 to 5 minutes. Wash hands, interdigit area, fingers, and fingernails. Rinse and pat dry.	10. Long strokes promote circulation. Soaking hands softens nails and loosens soil from skin and nails. Strokes directed distal to proximal promote venous return. Powder removes excess moisture.

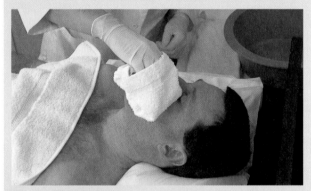

Figure B18-2 Clean the eye with the corner of the washcloth, wiping from the inner to the outer canthus.

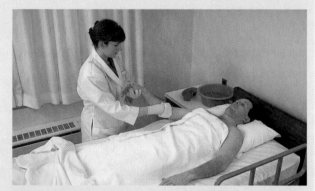

Figure B18-3 Wash forearms and arms in the direction of the wrist to upper arm.

Action	Rationale
11. Wash chest and abdomen. Fold bath blanket down to umbilicus. Wash chest using long, firm strokes. Wash skinfold under the female client's breast by lifting each breast. Rinse and pat dry. Fold bath blanket down to suprapubic area. Use another towel to cover chest area. Wash abdomen using long, firm strokes. Rinse and pat dry. Replace bath blanket over chest and abdomen. Cover chest or abdomen area in between washing, rinsing, and drying to prevent chilling.	11. Promotes privacy and prevents chills. Long strokes promote circulation. Perspiration and soil collect within skin folds.
12. Wash legs and feet. Expose leg farthest from you by folding bath blanket to midline. Bend the leg at the knee. Grasp the heel, elevate the leg from the bed and cover bed with bath towel. Place	12. Supports joint to prevent strain and fatigue. Soaking foot loosens dirt, softens nails, and promotes comfort.

continued

Action	Rationale
washbasin on towel. Place client's foot into washbasin. Allow foot to soak while washing the leg with long, firm strokes in the direction of distal to proximal (ankle to thigh; Figure B18-4). Rinse and pat dry. Clean soles, interdigits, and toes. Rinse and pat dry. Perform same procedure with the other leg and foot.	

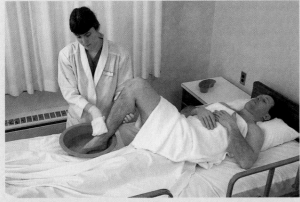

Figure B18-4 Wash the leg and foot in the direction of ankle to thigh.

Action	Rationale
13. Wash back. Assist client into prone or side-lying position facing away from you. Wash the back and buttocks using long, firm strokes. Rinse and pat dry. Give back rub and apply lotion.	13. Exposes back and buttocks for washing. Back rub promotes relaxation and circulation.
14. Perineal care: Assist client to supine position. Perform perineal care (see Procedure B19).	14. Removes genital secretions and oil.
15. Apply lotion and powder as desired. Apply clean gown.	15. Lotion lubricates skin. Powder absorbs excess perspiration.
16. Document skin assessment, type of bath given, and client outcomes and responses.	16. Provides evidence of nursing care.

Procedure B19 — Perineal Care

Equipment

- Bath basin
- Soap
- Two or three washcloths
- Dry bath towel
- Bath blanket
- Waterproof pads
- Toilet tissue
- Lotion or ointment
- Disposable gloves

Action	Rationale
• *Check the client's identification band prior to beginning* •	
1. Explain procedure and purpose to client. Obtain permission. Close door and pull curtain around bed.	1. Promotes cooperation. Provides privacy.
2. Wash hands and apply gloves.	2. Reduces transmission of pathogens.

continued

Action	Rationale
3. Place waterproof pad under client's buttocks. Client may be placed on a bedpan for perineal care. Females usually assume the dorsal recumbent position. Males may assume the dorsal recumbent or supine position with knees and hips flexed.	3. Waterproof pad prevents wetting of linen. Dorsal recumbent position provides maximal visualization of genital area.
4. Expose perineal area. Fold client's gown up above the genital area. Place a bath blanket over the client using a "diamond" draping technique. Corners of bath blanket should point toward the head, sides of body, and between the client's legs. Fold top linen down to the end of the bed. Tuck side corners of bath blanket around client's legs. Lift corner between client's legs to expose perineal area (Figure B19-1).	4. Draping promotes a sense of privacy and decreases exposure.

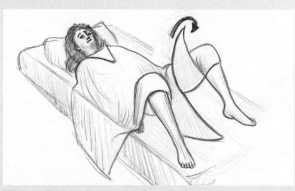

Figure B19-1 Drape the client for perineal care.

Action	Rationale
5. Moisten and lather washcloths. Female: Clean perineal area in the downward direction (from pubic area to rectum). Clean and dry upper thighs. Use separate quarters of the washcloth for each cleaning stroke. Discard soiled washcloths as necessary. Clean the labia majora. Separate the labia majora to clean between the labia majora and labia minora. With the labia separated, clean the clitoris, urethral meatus, and vaginal orifice (Figure B19-2). Rinse the area well with warm water. Pat perineal area dry. Apply lotion to upper thighs. Male: Gently raise penis. May place a bath blanket under the penis. If the client develops an erection, delay perineal care. Gently grasp the shaft of the penis. If the client is uncircumcised, retract the foreskin. Use a circular motion to clean the meatus of the penis and glans in an outward direction (Figure B19-3). Replace the foreskin after cleansing the glans. Clean the shaft of the penis. Rinse penis. Pat glans and shaft of penis dry. Clean and dry scrotum. Scrotum may need to be lifted during cleaning. Discard soiled washcloths as necessary.	5. Cleaning in the direction of the pubic area to rectum reduces risk of transmitting fecal material to the urinary tract. Using clean area of washcloth for each stroke reduces risk of transmitting organisms. Cleaning between the labia removes accumulated smegma. Gentle handling reduces chance of an erection. Smegma accumulates around the foreskin. Replacing of foreskin prevents phimosis. Cleaning moves from area of least to most soiled.

continued

Action	**Rationale**

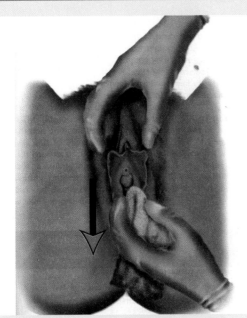

Figure B19-2 Clean the female perineal area.

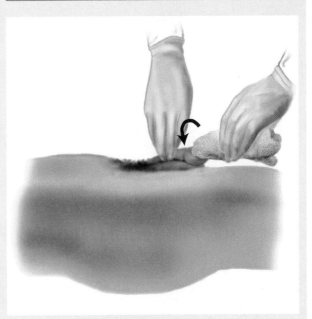

Figure B19-3 Clean the male perineal area.

6. Perform anal care. First remove any fecal material with toilet tissue. Clean perineal area by wiping from genitals to anus with one stroke. Discard soiled washcloths as necessary. Clean anus in circular motion. Rinse anal area. Pat dry.

6. Cleaning fecal material with toilet tissue removes the bulk of soil prior to washing. Cleaning from genitals to anus reduces chances of transmitting fecal microorganisms to urinary tract. Patting dry reduces skin irritation.

7. Remove gloves. Wash hands. Remove bath blanket. Place gown down over genitals. Place top linen on client.

7. Reduces transmission of microorganisms. Covering genitals maintains client's privacy.

8. Document procedure performed, client's response, and assessment findings.

8. Provides evidence of nursing care.

Procedure B20   Catheter Care

Equipment

- Clean gloves
- Waterproof pad to protect linens
- Wash cloths, soap, and water

Action	**Rationale**

• Wash your hands • Check the client's identification band •
• Explain the procedure to the client before beginning •

1. Provide privacy.

1. Protects client dignity.

2. Put on clean gloves.

2. Reduces transmission of microorganisms.

3. Place client in supine position and expose perineal area and catheter.

3. Allows for visualization of field. If unable to visualize the perineal area with the client supine, try placing the client in a side-lying position.

4. Place waterproof pad on bed.

4. Protects linens.

continued

Action	**Rationale**
5. Cleanse periurethral area with soap and water (Figure B20-1). Cleanse meatus in circular motion from the most inner surface to the outside.	5. Soap has antibacterial qualities adequate to clean the area and will usually not irritate the skin or mucous membranes. Moving from the cleanest area out decreases risk of recontamination.

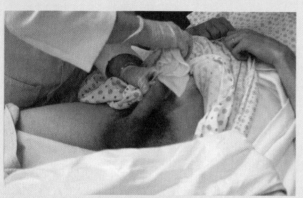

Figure B20-1 Using a washcloth, cleanse the penis and perineal area with soap and warm water.

Action	**Rationale**
6. With clean washcloth, cleanse catheter from meatus to end of catheter, taking care not to pull on catheter.	6. Decreases risk of contamination.
7. Be sure to repeat catheter care anytime the periurethral area becomes soiled with stool or other drainage.	7. Reduces risk of infection.
8. Place linen in proper receptacle for laundry or disposal.	8. Reduces transmission of infection to other clients.
9. Remove gloves and wash hands.	9. Reduces transmission of microorganisms.
10. Document care given.	10. Communicates to other caregivers what care was given.

Procedure B21   Oral Hygiene

Equipment

Brushing and Flossing
- Toothbrush
- Toothpaste
- Emesis basin
- Towel
- Cup of water
- Nonsterile gloves
- Dental floss
- Dental-floss holder
- Mirror
- Lip moisturizer

Denture Care
- Denture brush
- Denture cleaner
- Emesis basin
- Towel
- Cup of water
- Nonsterile gloves
- Tissue
- Denture cup

Special Care Items for Clients with Impaired Physical Mobility or Who Are Unconscious (comatose)
- Soft toothbrush or toothette
- Tongue blade

continued

Equipment *continued*

- 3 × 3 gauze sponges
- Cotton-tip applicators
- Prescribed solution and/or milk of magnesia

- Plastic Asepto syringe
- Suction machine and catheter

Action	Rationale

• Check the client's identification band • Explain the procedure to the client prior to beginning •

Self-Care Client

Flossing and Brushing

Action	Rationale
1. Assemble articles for flossing and brushing.	1. Promotes efficiency.
2. Provide privacy.	2. Relaxes the client.
3. Place client in a high-Fowler's position.	3. Decreases risk of aspiration.
4. Wash hands and don gloves.	4. Reduces microorganism transfer and exposure to body fluids.
5. Arrange articles within client's reach.	5. Facilitates self-care.
6. Assist client with flossing and brushing as necessary. Position mirror and emesis basin near client for use during activity.	6. Flossing and brushing decrease microorganism growth in mouth. Use of mirror permits cleaning back and sides of teeth.
7. Assist client with rinsing mouth.	7. Removes toothpaste and oral secretions.
8. Reposition client, raise side rails, and place call button within reach.	8. Promotes comfort, safety, and communication.
9. Rinse, dry, and return articles to proper place.	9. Promotes a clean environment.
10. Remove gloves, wash hands, and document care.	10. Prevents the transmission of microorganisms and documents nursing care.

Denture Care

Action	Rationale
11. Assemble articles for denture cleaning.	11. Promotes efficiency.
12. Provide privacy.	12. Relaxes the client.
13. Assist client to a high-Fowler's position.	13. Facilitates removal of dentures.
14. Wash hands and don gloves.	14. Reduces microorganism transfer and exposure to body fluids.
15. Assist client with denture removal:	15. Breaks seal created with dentures without causing pressure and injury to oral membranes.
a. Top denture:	
• With tissue, grasp the denture with thumb and forefinger and pull downward.	• Prevents breaking of dentures.
• Place in denture cup.	
b. Bottom denture:	
• Place thumbs on the gums and release the denture. Grasp denture with thumb and forefingers and pull upward.	
• Place in denture cup.	

continued

Action	**Rationale**
16. Apply toothpaste to brush and brush dentures either with cool water in the emesis basin or under running water in the sink.	16. Facilitates removal of microorganisms.
17. Rinse thoroughly.	17. Removes toothpaste.
18. Assist client with rinsing mouth and replacing dentures.	18. Freshens mouth and facilitates intake of solid food.
19. Reposition client, with side rails up and call button within reach.	19. Promotes comfort, safety, and communication.
20. Rinse, dry, and return articles to proper place.	20. Maintains a clean environment.
21. Remove gloves, wash hands, and document care.	21. Prevents the transmission of microorganisms and documents nursing care.

Full-Care Client

Brushing and Flossing

Action	**Rationale**
22. Assemble articles for flossing and brushing.	22. Promotes efficiency.
23. Provide privacy.	23. Relaxes client.
24. Wash hands and don gloves.	24. Reduces microorganism transfer and exposure to body fluids.
25. Position client as condition allows: high-Fowler's, semi-Fowler's, or lateral position with head turned toward side.	25. Decreases risk of aspiration.
26. Place towel across client's chest or under face and mouth if head is turned to one side.	26. Catches secretions.
27. Moisten toothbrush, apply small amount of toothpaste, and brush teeth and gums.	27. Moistens mouth and facilitates plaque removal.
28. Grasp the dental floss in both hands or use a floss holder and floss between all teeth, holding floss against tooth while moving floss up and down sides of teeth (Figure B21-1).	28. Removes plaque and prevents gum disease.
29. Assist the client in rinsing mouth.	29. Removes toothpaste and oral secretions.
30. Reapply toothpaste and brush the teeth and gums using friction in a vertical or circular motion. On inner and outer surfaces of teeth, hold brush at 45 degree angle against teeth and brush from sulcus to crowns of teeth. On biting surfaces, move brush back and forth in short strokes. All surfaces of teeth should be brushed from every angle (Figure B21-2).	30. Permits cleaning of back and sides of teeth and decreases microorganism growth in mouth.
31. Assist the client in rinsing and drying mouth.	31. Removes toothpaste and oral secretions.
32. Apply lip moisturizer, if appropriate.	32. Maintains skin integrity of lips.
33. Reposition client, raise side rails, and place call button within reach.	33. Promotes comfort, safety, and communication.
34. Rinse, dry, and return articles to proper place.	34. Provides an orderly environment.
35. Remove gloves, wash hands, and document care.	35. Prevents transmission of microorganisms and documents nursing care.

continued

Action	**Rationale**

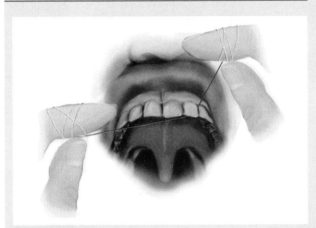

Figure B21-1 Floss teeth.

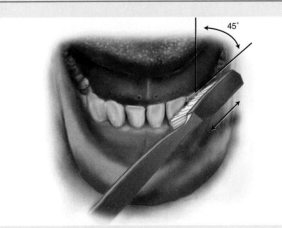

Figure B21-2 Brush teeth.

Clients at Risk for or with an Alteration of the Oral Cavity

Follow actions 22 through 24.

36. Bleeding:	**36.**
a. Assess oral cavity with a padded tongue blade and flashlight for signs of bleeding.	a. Determines if bleeding is present, amount, and specific areas.
b. Proceed with the actions for oral care for a full-care client, except:	
• Do not floss.	
• Use a soft toothbrush, toothette, or a tongue blade padded with 3 × 3 gauze sponges to gently swab teeth and gums.	• Decreases risk of bleeding.
• Dispose of padded tongue blade into a biohazard bag according to agency policy.	• Provides proper disposal of contaminated waste.
• Rinse with tepid water.	• Cleanses mouth.
37. Infection:	**37.**
a. Assess oral cavity with a tongue blade and flashlight for signs of infection.	a. Determines appearance, integrity, and general condition of oral cavity.
b. Culture lesions as ordered.	b. Identifies growth of specific microorganisms.
c. Proceed with the actions for oral care for a full-care client except:	
• Do not floss.	• Prevents irritation, pain, and bleeding.
• Use prescribed antiseptic solution.	• Antiseptic solutions decrease growth of microorganisms.
• Use a tongue blade padded with 3 × 3 gauze sponges to gently swab the teeth and gums.	
• Dispose of padded tongue blade into a biohazard bag according to institutional policy.	• Provides proper disposal of contaminated materials.
• Rinse mouth with tepid water.	• Cleanses mouth.

continued

Action	**Rationale**
38. Ulcerations:	**38.** Same as for action 37.
a. Assess oral cavity with a tongue blade and flashlight for signs of ulcerations.	
b. Culture lesions as ordered.	
c. Proceed with actions for oral care for a full-care client except:	
• Do not floss.	
• Use prescribed antiseptic solution.	
• Use a tongue blade padded with 3×3 gauze sponges to gently swab the teeth and gums.	
• Dispose of padded tongue blade into a biohazard bag according to institutional policy.	
• Rinse mouth with tepid water.	
• Apply solution or paste as prescribed with cotton-tip applicators.	• Provides a coating that promotes healing of the tissue.

Unconscious (Comatose) Client

Action	**Rationale**
39. Follow steps 22 to 24 for full-care client.	**39.** Same as for steps 22 to 24 for full-care client.
40. Explain the procedure to the client.	**40.** Demonstrates respect for the client.
41. Place the client in a lateral position, head turned toward the side.	**41.** Prevents aspiration.
42. Use a floss holder and floss between all teeth.	**42.** Removes plaque and prevents gum disease. Keeps nurse's fingers out of client's mouth.
43. Moisten toothbrush, apply small amount of toothpaste, and brush the teeth and gums as described in step 30.	**43.** Same as for step 30.
44. After flossing and brushing, rinse mouth with an Asepto syringe and perform oral suction (see Procedure 122 for a description of oropharyngeal/nasopharyngeal suctioning).	**44.** Promotes cleansing and removal of secretions and prevents aspiration.
45. Dry the client's mouth.	**45.** Prevents skin irritation.
46. Apply lip moisturizer.	**46.** Maintains skin integrity of lips.
47. Leave the client in a lateral position with head turned toward side for 30 to 60 minutes after oral hygiene care. Remove the towel from under the client's mouth and face.	**47.** Prevents pooling of secretions and aspiration.
48. Dispose of any contaminated items in a biohazard bag. Clean, dry, and return all articles to the appropriate place.	**48.** Provides proper disposal of contaminated materials.
49. Remove gloves, wash hands, and document care.	**49.** Prevents the transmission of microorganisms and documents nursing care.
50. Document type of oral care given and client's response.	**50.** Provides record of care given.

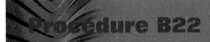

Procedure B22   Eye Care: Artificial Eye and Contact Lens Removal

Equipment

Artificial Eye
- Storage container
- Mild soap
- 3 × 3 gauze sponges
- Cotton balls
- Towel
- Emesis basins
- Eye irrigation syringe (optional)
- Running water
- Nonsterile gloves
- Biohazard bag
- Saline solution

Contact Lenses
- Lens container
- Soaking solution (type used by client)
- Towel
- Suction cup (optional)
- Scotch tape (optional)
- Nonsterile gloves

Action	Rationale
• Wash your hands • Check the client's identification band • *• Explain the procedure to the client prior to beginning •*	

Artificial Eye Removal

1. Inquire about client's care regimen and gather equipment accordingly.	1. Promotes continuity of care.
2. Provide privacy.	2. Relaxes the client.
3. Wash hands; don gloves.	3. Prevents transmission of microorganisms.
4. Place client in a semi-Fowler's position.	4. Facilitates procedure and client participation.
5. Place the cotton balls in emesis basin and half fill with warm tap water.	5. Dry cotton balls could cause irritation.
6. Place 3 × 3 gauze sponges in bottom of second emesis basin, and half-fill with mild soap and tepid water.	6. Gauze serves as padding to prevent breakage of the prosthesis.
7. Grasp and squeeze excess water from a cotton ball. Cleanse the eyelid with the moistened cotton ball, starting at the inner canthus and moving outward toward the outer canthus. After each use, dispose of cotton ball in biohazard bag. Repeat procedure until eyelid is clean (without dried secretions).	7. Eliminating the excess water prevents water from running down the client's face. Cleansing the eyelid prevents contamination of the lacrimal system (inner canthus area). Disposal of cotton balls prevents transmission of micro-organisms to other health care workers.
8. Remove the artificial eye:	8. Promotes removal of artificial eye. Cupping prevents dropping and possible breaking of the eye. Applying pressure will help the prosthesis to slip out.
a. Using dominant hand, raise the client's upper eyelid with index finger and depress the lower eyelid with thumb (Figure B22-1).	
b. Cup nondominant hand under the client's lower eyelid.	
c. Apply slight pressure with index finger between the brow and the artificial eye and remove it.	

continued

Action	**Rationale**

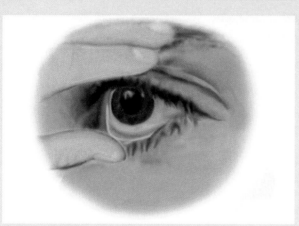

Figure B22-1 Removal of an Artificial Eye

9. Place the artificial eye in the emesis basin that has soap and water.

9. Prevents secretions from adhering to the prosthesis.

10. Grasp a moistened cotton ball and cleanse around the edge of the eye socket. Dispose of the soiled cotton ball into biohazard bag. Keep the prosthesis in the soap-and-water solution.

10. Cleanses the eye socket. Disposal of cotton ball prevents transmission of microorganisms to other health care workers. Keeping eye in solution during cleaning decreases risk of damage.

11. Inspect the eye socket for any signs of irritation, drainage, or crusting.

11. Indicates an infection.

Note: If the client's usual care regimen or physician order requires irrigation of the socket, proceed with step 12; otherwise, go to step 13.

12. Eye socket irrigation:

12.

   a. Lower the head of the bed and place the client in a supine position. Place protector pad on bed; turn head toward socket side and slightly extend neck.

   a. Cleanses the eye socket and removes secretions. Positioning of client facilitates ease in performing the procedure and client comfort.

   b. Fill the irrigation syringe with the prescribed amount and type of irrigating solution (warm tap water or normal saline).

   b. Assures compliance with client's regimen or prescribed orders.

   c. With nondominant hand, separate the eyelids with your forefinger and thumb, resting fingers on the brow and cheekbone.

   c. Keeps the eyelid open and the socket visible.

   d. Hold the irrigating syringe in dominant hand several inches above the inner canthus; with thumb, gently apply pressure on the plunger, directing the flow of solution from the inner canthus along the conjunctival sac.

   d. Prevents injury to the client.

   e. Irrigate until the prescribed amount of solution has been used.

   e. Follows prescription.

   f. Wipe the eyelids with a moistened cotton ball after irrigating. Dispose of soiled cotton ball in biohazard bag.

   f. Promotes cleanliness.

continued

Action	Rationale

g. Pat the skin dry with the towel.

g. Removes moisture.

h. Return the client to a semi-Fowler's position.

h. Promotes comfort.

i. Remove gloves, wash hands, and don clean gloves.

i. Prevents transmission of microorganisms to prosthesis.

13. Rub the artificial eye between index finger and thumb in the basin of warm soapy water.

13. Creates cleaning with friction and prevents breakage of the prosthesis.

14. Rinse the prosthesis under running water or place in the clean basin of tepid water. Do not dry the prosthesis.

Note: Either reinsert the prosthesis (step 15) or store in a container (step 16).

14. Removes soap and secretions. Keeping the artificial eye wet prevents irritation from lint or other particles that might adhere to it and facilitates reinsertion.

15. Reinsert the prosthesis:

15. Facilitates reinsertion of the prosthesis without discomfort to the client.

a. With the thumb of the nondominant hand, raise and hold the upper eyelid open.

a. Opens eye.

b. With the dominant hand, grasp the artificial eye so that the indented part is facing toward the client's nose and slide it under the upper eyelid as far as possible.

b. Assures proper fit.

c. Depress the lower lid.

c. Allows the prosthesis to slide into place.

d. Pull the lower lid forward to cover the edge of the prosthesis.

d. Secures the prosthesis.

16. Place the cleaned artificial eye in a labeled container with saline or tap water solution.

16. Protects the prosthesis from scratches and keeps it clean.

17. Grasp a moistened cotton ball and squeeze out excessive moisture. Wipe the eyelid from the inner to the outer canthus. Dispose of the soiled cotton ball in a biohazard bag.

17. Squeezing the cotton ball removes moisture. Cleansing the eyelid prevents contamination of lacrimal system. Disposal of cotton ball prevents the transmission of microorganisms to other health care workers.

18. Clean, dry, and replace equipment.

18. Promotes a clean environment.

19. Reposition the client, raise side rails, and place call light in reach.

19. Promotes client's comfort, safety, and communication.

20. Dispose of biohazard bag according to agency policy.

20. Prevents the transmission of microorganisms to other health care workers.

21. Remove gloves and wash hands.

21. Same as for step 20.

22. Document procedure, client's response and participation, and client teaching and level of understanding.

22. Demonstrates that the procedure was done and the level of client participation and learning.

Contact Lens Removal

23. Assemble equipment for lens removal.

23. Promotes efficiency.

24. Assess level of assistance needed, provide privacy, and explain the procedure to the client.

24. Level of assistance determines level of intervention. Privacy reduces anxiety. Explanation of procedure promotes cooperation.

25. Wash hands and don gloves.

25. Reduces transfer of microorganisms.

continued

Action	Rationale
26. Assist the client to a semi-Fowler's position.	**26.** Facilitates removal of lens.
27. Drape a clean towel over the client's chest.	**27.** Provides a clean surface and facilitates the location of a lens if it falls during removal.
28. Prepare the lens storage case with the prescribed solution. If storage case is not available, put each lens in a separate sterile specimen cup with saline. Label right and left.	**28.** Hard lenses can be stored dry or in a special soaking solution. Soft lenses are stored in sterile normal saline *without* a preservative.
29. Instruct the client to look straight ahead. Assess the location of the lens. If it is not on the cornea, either you or the client should gently move the lens toward the cornea with pad of index finger.	**29.** Client's position promotes easy removal of lens. Positioning lens on the cornea aids removal. Use of the finger pad of the index finger prevents damage to cornea and lens.
30. Remove the lens. **a.** Hard lens: • Cup nondominant hand under the eye. • Gently place index finger on the outside corner of the eye and pull toward the temple and ask client to blink (Figure B22-2). **b.** Soft lens: • With nondominant hand, separate the eyelid with your thumb and middle finger. • With the index finger of the dominant hand gently placed on the lower edge of the lens, slide the lens downward onto the sclera and gently squeeze the lens. • Release the top eyelid (continue holding the lower lid down) and remove the lens with your index finger and thumb (Figure B22-3).	**30.** Cupping the hand under eye helps to catch the lens and prevent breakage. Pulling corner of the eye tightens eyelid against eyeball. Pressure on upper edge of lens causes lens to tip forward. • Separating the eyelid exposes the lower edge of lens. • Positions lens for easy grasping with the pad of the index finger, which prevents injury to the cornea and lens. Squeezing the lens allows air to enter and release the suction.

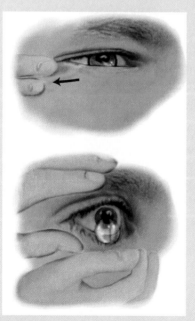

Figure B22-2 Removal of a Hard Contact Lens

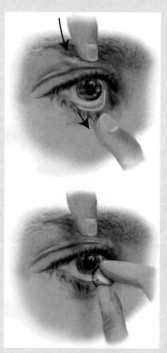

Figure B22-3 Removal of a Soft Contact Lens

continued

Action	Rationale
Note: If step 30 is unsuccessful, secure a suction cup to remove the contact lens. If you are unable to remove the lens, notify the physician.	Suction cup is used to remove a lens from an unconscious or dependent client.
31. Store the lens in the correct compartment of the case ("right" or "left"). Label with the client's name.	31. Storage prevents damage to the lenses and ensures that each lens will be reinserted into the correct eye.
32. Remove the other lens by repeating steps 30 and 31.	32. Same as for steps 30 and 31.
33. Assess eyes for irritation or redness.	33. Signs of corneal irritation.
34. Store the lens case in a safe place.	34. Prevents damage or loss.
35. Dispose of soiled articles; clean and return reusable articles to proper location.	35. Reduces transmission of infection.
36. Reposition the client, raise side rails, and place call light in reach. *Be aware that client may have trouble seeing if eyeglasses are not available.*	36. Promotes client comfort, safety, and communication.
37. Remove gloves and wash hands.	37. Prevents transmission of infection.
38. Document procedure, client's response and assessment findings, and the storage place of the lenses.	38. Documents the removal of lenses, condition of the cornea, and where the lenses are stored.

Procedure B23 — Giving a Back Rub

Equipment

- Quiet environment, free of interruptions, with a comfortable room temperature
- Bath blanket
- Lotion, baby powder, or massage oil
- Comfortable bed or massage table that allows a client to lie in a side-lying or prone position
- Bath towel to absorb excess moisture, oils
- Gloves if necessary

Action	Rationale
• *Check the client's identification band* • *Explain the procedure to the client prior to beginning* •	
1. Wash your hands and don gloves if necessary.	1. Reduces the transmission of microorganisms.
2. Help client to a prone or side-lying position (Figure B23-1).	2. Exposes back and shoulder area.

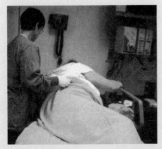

Figure B23-1 Position client in a prone or side-lying position.

continued

Action	**Rationale**
3. Drape the bath blanket, and undo the client's gown exposing the back, shoulder, and sacral area, keeping the remainder of the body covered (Figure B23-2).	3. Prevents chilling and excess exposure.
4. Pour a small amount of lotion in your hand and warm between your palms for a few moments. The lotion bottle can also be submerged in a bowl of warm water for a few minutes to warm the lotion. Baby powder may be substituted for oils or lotions (Figure B23-3).	4. Prevents cold lotion being applied to the body. Some clients may be sensitive to oils or lotions.

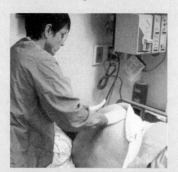

Figure B23-2 Expose the back, shoulder, and sacral area.

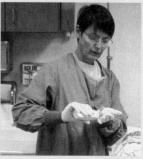

Figure B23-3 Pour lotion on your hand and warm between your palms.

Action	**Rationale**
5. Begin in the sacral area with smooth, circular strokes, moving upward toward the shoulders. Gradually lengthen the strokes (effleurage) to the upper back, scapulae, and upper arms. Apply firm, continuous pressure without breaking contact with the client (Figure B23-4).	5. Applying firm, continuous pressure increases circulation and relaxation.
6. Assess client's back, as you are massaging, for areas of redness and signs of decreased circulation.	6. Monitors for signs of early skin breakdown.
7. Provide a firm, kneading massage (petrissage) to areas of increased tension, if desired, in areas such as the shoulders and gluteal muscles.	7. Firm, kneading strokes can decrease muscle tension, reducing pain and increasing relaxation.
8. Complete the massage with long, very light brush strokes, using the tips of the fingers.	8. A very relaxing stroke; signals end of the massage.

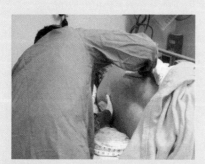

Figure B23-4 Apply firm continuous pressure without breaking contact between your hands and the client's skin.

continued

Action	Rationale
9. Gently pat or wipe excess lubricant off of the client and cover the client.	9. Prevents soiling of the bed with excess lotions and keeps the client warm.
10. Wash hands.	10. Reduces the transmission of microorganisms.
11. Document back rub, client's response to back rub, and any unusual findings.	11. Provides record of care and client's response.

Procedure B24   Shaving a Client

Equipment

- Disposable razor
- Warm water
- Washbasin
- Mirror
- Gloves

- Shaving cream or soap
- Washcloth and bath towel
- After-shave lotion (if the client has no skin irritation and prefers lotion)
- Sharp scissors and comb (if mustache care required)

Action	Rationale
• *Check client's identification band* • *Explain the procedure to the client prior to beginning* •	
1. Wash hands and apply gloves	1. Reduces the transmission of microorganisms.
2. Assist the client to a comfortable position. If the client can shave himself, set up the equipment and supplies, including warm water, and watch the client for safety. Adjust lighting as needed. Follow agency policy.	2. Facilitates comfort and ease of shaving. Encourages autonomy. Facilitates proper body mechanics and prevents injury to client.
3. Place a towel over the client's chest and shoulder.	3. Protects the client and gown from soil.
4. Fill a washbasin with water at approximately 44°C (110°F). Have client check temperature for comfort.	4. Warm water helps to soften the skin and beard; relaxes client.
5. Place the washcloth in the basin and wring out thoroughly. Apply the cloth over the client's entire face.	5. Same rationale as for step 4.
6. Apply shaving cream.	6. Helps soften the whiskers.
7. Take the razor in the dominant hand and hold it at a 45° angle to the client's skin. Start shaving across one side of the client's face. Use the non-dominant hand to gently pull the skin taut while shaving. Use short, firm strokes in the direction of hair growth. Use short, downward strokes over the upper lip area (Figure B24-1).	7. Prevents razor cuts and discomfort during shaving.
8. Rinse the razor in water as cream accumulates.	8. Keeps the cutting edge of the razor clean.
9. Check the face to see if all facial hair is removed.	9. Ensures a neat appearance.
10. After all facial hair is removed, rinse the client's face thoroughly with a moistened washcloth.	10. Promotes comfort and cleanliness.

continued

Action	Rationale

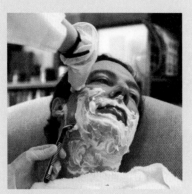

Figure B24-1 Shave with short, firm strokes in the direction the hair grows.

Action	Rationale
11. Pat client's face dry and apply after-shave lotion if desired.	**11.** Promotes skin integrity; stimulates and lubricates the skin.
12. Assist the client to a comfortable position and allow him to inspect the results of your shave with a mirror.	**12.** Facilitates comfort and a sense of control.
13. Dispose of equipment in proper receptacle.	**13.** Equipment should not be shared between clients in accordance with Standard Precautions since disruption of skin and bleeding may occur. The client may, however, keep his own razor. Clean and store it at the bedside.
14. Wash hands.	**14.** Reduces the transmission of microorganisms.
15. Document shaving client, any problems encountered, and client's response.	**15.** Provides record of client's care.

Procedure B25   Applying Antiembolism Stockings

Equipment

- Antiembolism stockings and package directions
- Tape measure
- Powder or cornstarch (if client is not allergic)

Action	Rationale
• *Wash your hands* • *Check the client's identification band* • *Explain procedure to client prior to beginning* •	
1. Review the orders, including the reason for the stockings and the type of stockings ordered (e.g., knee or thigh high).	**1.** Ensures accuracy; facilitates compliance.
2. With the client in a supine position in bed, measure the client's leg for the correct size: • Thigh-high stockings: from Achilles tendon to the gluteal fold, circumference of the midthigh.	**2.** Supine position encourages venous return and decreases swelling, thereby allowing accurate measurement for size of stockings.

continued

Action	Rationale
• Below the knee stockings: from the Achilles tendon to the popliteal fold, circumference of the midcalf.	
3. Compare the obtained measurements with the package insert to ascertain proper size.	3. Correct size is essential for stockings to apply the appropriate pressure for adequate venous return without compromise to circulation.
4. Evenly apply talc or cornstarch to the client's legs and feet if client is not allergic.	4. Allows for smoother appliance of stockings. Powders also absorb moisture.
5. Apply stockings. The best time to apply stockings is early in the morning, before the client gets out of bed, or immediately after surgery. Keep client in supine position until stockings are applied.	5. Feet are less swollen in the morning because the feet have been in a nondependent position during the night.
6. Open the package and turn stockings inside out. Place hands deep enough inside the stockings to grasp the stocking toe.	6. Because stockings contain strong elastic, application can be difficult if not initiated from the bottom up and if stockings are not turned inside out. Wrinkles in stockings can also occur if a systematic approach is not used for application.
7. Hold onto the client's toes with the same hand, invert the stocking with the other hand and pull it over the hand that is holding the client's toes. Remove the hand from the inside of the stocking.	7. See Rationale 6.
8. Hold each side of the stocking and pull the inverted stocking over the client's toes.	8. See Rationale 6.
9. Continuing to hold each side of the stocking, firmly pull the stocking from the client's toes to the heel in one motion. Pull the stockings up by using the thumbs to guide the stockings upward over the ankles and up the client's legs (Figures B25-1 and B25-2).	9. See Rationale 6.
10. Repeat with the other leg.	10. See Rationale 6.

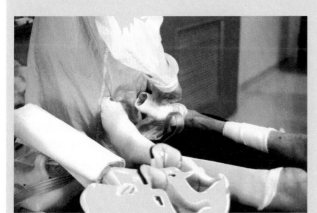

Figure B25-1 Place the stocking over the client's toes and foot.

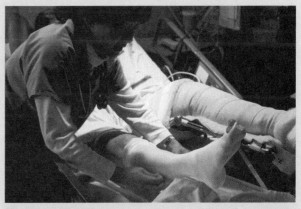

Figure B25-2 Pull the stocking smoothly and evenly up the client's leg.

continued

Action	Rationale
11. Remove any wrinkles in the stockings and smooth over (Figure B25-3).	**11.** Wrinkles can create skin breakdown and constrict the circulation.

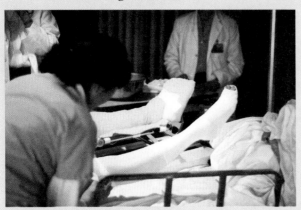

Figure B25-3 Smooth out any wrinkles and make sure the toes are comfortable.

Action	Rationale
12. Wash hands.	**12.** Reduces transmission of microorganisms.
13. Document application of antiembolism stockings.	**13.** Provides record of client care.

Procedure B26   Positioning and Removing a Bedpan

Equipment

- Bedpan (regular or fracture)
- Disposable gloves
- Bedpan cover
- Toilet paper
- Washcloth and towel, soap

Action	Rationale
Positioning a Bedpan	
1. Close curtain or door.	**1.** Provides for privacy.
2. Wash hands, apply gloves.	**2.** Prevents transmission of microorganisms.
3. Lower head of bed so client is in supine position.	**3.** The supine position will increase ability of client to move to side-lying position.
4. Warm bedpan under warm water if needed, powder if necessary.	**4.** For comfort, prevents bedpan from sticking to the skin.
5. If client is able to lift buttocks, place bedpan under buttocks, with lower end near the lower back region (Figure B26-1).	**5.** Ensures proper placement of the bedpan.
6. If client is unable to lift buttocks, assist client to side-lying position using side rail.	**6.** Provides for best position for proper placement of bedpan.
7. While holding the bedpan against the client's buttocks with one hand, help the client to roll onto her back (Figure B26-2).	**7.** Prevents dislocation or misalignment of bedpan. Ensures proper placement of the body before client rolls on top of bedpan.
8. Check placement of bedpan by looking between client's legs.	**8.** May prevent spillage due to misalignment of bedpan.

continued

Action	Rationale

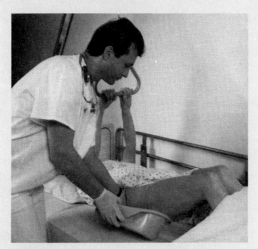

Figure B26-1 Slip the bedpan under the client's buttocks while client lifts herself with the trapeze.

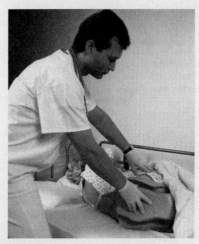

Figure B26-2 Place the bedpan against the client's buttocks and assist client to roll back.

9. If indicated, elevate head of bed to 45° angle.

9. Check physician order; bed remains flat if client has a spinal cord injury or spinal surgery. Elevating the head of bed creates a more normal elimination position.

10. Place call light within reach of client; place side rails in upright position and allow for privacy.

10. Privacy allows for a more comfortable elimination environment; elevated side rails provide for safety.

Removing a Bedpan

11. Wash hands, don gloves.

11. Prevents transmission of microorganisms.

12. Lower head of bed to supine position.

12. Increases client's ability to move to side-lying position.

13. While holding bedpan flat on bed with one hand, roll client to side. Or, if client is strong enough, have her lift buttocks.

13. Prevents possible spillage of bedpan contents.

14. Assist with cleaning or wiping if needed; always wipe from front to back.

14. Client may not be able to clean herself; wiping from front to back decreases chances of cross-contamination from anus to urethra.

15. Empty bedpan, clean it, and store it in proper place; if bedpan is to be emptied outside client's room, cover it during transport.

15. Promotes privacy and decreases the chance of spilling contents.

16. Remove gloves and wash hands.

16. Prevents transmission of microorganisms.

17. Allow client to wash hands.

17. Provides for physical hygiene and comfort.

18. Place call light within reach; recheck that side rails are in the upright position.

18. Ensures client safety and comfort.

19. If client is on I&O, record amount of urine voided.

19. Maintains accurate I&O record.

Procedure B27

Applying a Condom Catheter

Equipment

- Condom catheter
- Collection bag
- Supplies for cleansing skin

- Connecting tubing
- Disposable gloves

Action	Rationale
• *Check the client's identification band* • *Explain the procedure to the client prior to beginning* •	

Action

1. Wash hands and apply gloves.

2. Select an appropriate condom catheter.

3. Cleanse the penile shaft.

4. Inspect the penile shaft for excessive hair.

5. Inspect the penis for altered skin integrity.

6. Stretch the shaft of the penis and unroll the condom to the base of the penis (Figure B27-1). Follow product directions for the application of the sealant (Figure B27-2). A securing strap may or may not be required, depending on the device.

Rationale

1. Reduces risk of contamination.

2. The condom catheter must be sized correctly (refer to manufacturer's recommendations) and have a distal tip that resists twisting and occlusion, and an adhesive that prevents leakage. Latex condom catheters are avoided in men who are allergic to latex and in boys with myelodysplasia.

3. Reduces surface dirt and pathogens.

4. Excessive penile hair is clipped to provide a watertight seal when the condom is applied.

5. Small lesions may be protected by the use of a skin sealant; significant erosions or rashes require consultation with the enterostomal nurse specialist or a dermatologist before proceeding.

6. The condom is applied over the entire penile shaft to maximize a watertight seal; the adhesive may be built into the wall of the condom, or a dual-sided sealant strip may be used to prevent leakage.

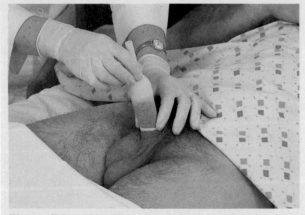

Figure B27-1 Unroll condom catheter to the base of the penis.

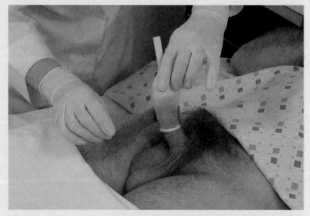

Figure B27-2 Secure the condom catheter with a strap (optional).

7. Attach the condom to the drainage apparatus; either a leg bag or bedside drainage bag.

8. Remove gloves and wash hands.

7. Ensures adequate urine containment.

8. Reduces the risks of contamination.

continued

Action	Rationale
9. Remove and reapply the condom catheter every 24 to 48 hours, or whenever leakage occurs.	**9.** Regular reapplication allows routine inspection of the penile skin and avoids bacterial overgrowth and altered skin integrity under the condom.
10. Document application of condom catheter, any problems encountered, and client's response.	**10.** Provides record of client care and client status.

Procedure B28 [Part 1]   Administering an Enema—Large/Small (Mini)

Equipment

- Enema bag (disposable comes with rectal tip catheter; reusable may need to have rectal tip catheter checked for damage and rectal tip may need to be replaced)
- Towel and washcloth

- Solution per physician's order
- Water-soluble lubricant
- Clean gloves
- Bedpan, commode, or toilet

Action	Rationale
• *Wash your hands* • *Check the client's identification band* • • *Explain the procedure to the client prior to beginning* •	
1. Introduce yourself and explain procedure; close door or curtain.	**1.** Client may be more relaxed if prepared for procedure, told what to expect, and provided with privacy.
2. Prepare the solution; assure temperature is between 99° and 102°F by using a thermometer or placing a few drops on your wrist.	**2.** Avoids harming the intestinal mucosa.
3. Wash hands and don gloves.	**3.** Protects from contamination.
4. Assist client to left side-lying position, with right knee bent.	**4.** Lying flat on left side allows fluid to flow through to colon with contour of bowel.
5. Place bedpan, commode, robe and slippers within easy reach.	**5.** Urgent evacuation of bowels or inability to retain fluid may occur.
6. Hang or hold bag of enema solution 12 to 18 inches above anus.	**6.** This height allows for steady flow of fluid into the client by gravity; a bag placed at a height greater than 18 inches allows for too rapid an infusion rate and could result in cramping or discomfort for the client.
7. Lubricate 4 to 5 inches of catheter tip.	**7.** Eases catheter tip insertion.
8. Separate buttocks, insert catheter tip into anal opening, slowly advance catheter approximately 4 inches.	**8.** Further catheter advancement could cause damage to bowel.
9. Slowly infuse solution via gravity flow; bag height may be increased but should not exceed 18 inches above anal opening (Figure B28-1).	**9.** Rapid infusion caused by bag height over 18 inches may cause cramping and discomfort. Bowel perforation is also a risk.
10. If client complains of increased pain or cramping, or if fluid is not being retained, stop procedure, wait a few minutes, then restart.	**10.** Discomfort may cause poor retention of fluid.

continued

Action	Rationale

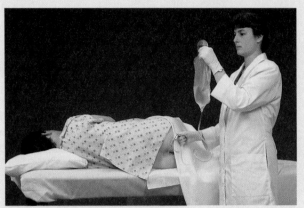

Figure B28-1 Raise the height of the enema container to allow infusion of the solution.

Action	Rationale
11. Clamp tubing when fluid finishes infusing; remove catheter tip.	11. Stops flow of fluid.
12. Assist client to bedpan, commode, or toilet; refer to Procedure B26 for positioning and removing bedpan.	12. If bedpan is used, place client in sitting position. Clients should be instructed to retain fluid for as long as possible.
13. Discard equipment in proper place. If equipment is reusable, properly clean and store it.	13. Prevents spread of microorganisms.
14. Remove gloves and wash hands.	14. Reduces spread of microorganisms.
15. Instruct client to call for assistance when finished eliminating, or if untoward feeling occurs, such as lightheadedness or dizziness.	15. Provides assistance and avoids potential harm to client.
16. Assist client with washing if needed.	16. Promotes client comfort.
17. Document solution given, client's reaction to procedure, and results obtained.	17. Provides information about procedure, client's reaction, and results obtained.

Procedure B28 (Part 2) Administering an Enema (Small/Mini)

Equipment

- Enema—small and mini-enemas come premixed
- Disposable gloves
- Washcloth and towel
- Lubricant
- Bedpan, commode, toilet

Action	Rationale

• Wash your hands • Check the client's identification band •
• Explain the procedure to the client prior to beginning •

Action	Rationale
1. Introduce yourself, explain procedure, close door or curtain.	1. Client may be more relaxed with privacy and knowing what to expect.
2. Place commode next to bed; have robe and slippers available.	2. If client is able to use commode, easy access is necessary due to urgency after enema administration.

continued

Action	Rationale
3. Have bedpan easily available.	3. Bedpan is ready if client is unable to retain fluid.
4. Wash hands and don gloves.	4. Prevents cross-contamination of bacteria.
5. Lower head of bed to flat position.	5. Easier for client to roll to left side.
6. Assist client to roll to left side-lying position with right knee slightly bent.	6. Lying on left side helps solution flow with the contour of the bowel.
7. Remove catheter tip guard; gently squeeze bottle until fluid drips (for mini-enemas, tip needs to be punctured with needle or pin).	7. Most prepared enemas have perforated tips; a gentle squeeze will ensure this.
8. Lubricate catheter tip.	8. Most premixed solutions are prelubricated; however, additional lubrication may be needed.
9. Separate buttocks and insert enema tip into anal opening; gently squeeze contents into rectum.	9. Gentle insertion and infusion lessens risk of undue discomfort and damage to colon.
10. Remove tip and assist to bedpan, commode, or toilet. Ask client to retain fluid for as long as possible, at least 30 minutes.	10. Assistance ensures safe transfer for client. Better results occur when enema is retained for a longer period of time.
11. Dispose of contaminated material in proper receptacles.	11. Prevents contamination.
12. Remove gloves and wash hands.	12. Reduces risk of contamination.
13. Assist client with cleaning if needed.	13. Illness or fatigue may cause some clients to require assistance for cleaning.
14. Document solution given, client's reaction to procedure, and results obtained.	14. Provides information about procedure, client's reaction, and results obtained.

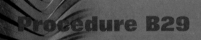

Procedure B29   Measuring Intake and Output

Equipment

- I&O form at bedside
- Glass or cup
- Graduated container for output

- I&O graphic record in chart
- Bedpan, urinal, or bedside commode
- Nonsterile gloves

Action	Rationale
• Check client's identification band prior to beginning •	
1. Wash hands.	1. Reduces potential for transmission of pathogens.
2. Explain purpose of keeping I&O record to client. Explain that:	2. Elicits client support.
• All fluids taken orally must be recorded.	
• Form for recording must be used.	
• Client must void into bedpan, urinal, or "hat" in toilet for collecting urine; not into toilet.	
• Toilet tissue should be disposed of in plastic-lined container, not in bedpan.	

continued

Action	Rationale

Intake

3. Measure all oral fluids in accord with agency policy: e.g., cup = 150 mL, glass = 240 mL.

   3. Provides for consistency of measurement.

4. Record time and amount of all fluid intake in the designated space on bedside form (oral, tube feedings, IV fluids).

   4. Documents fluids.

5. Transfer 8-hour total fluid intake from bedside I&O record to graphic sheet or 24-hour I&O record on client's chart, according to agency policy.

   5. Provides for data analysis of client's fluid status.

6. Record all forms of intake, except blood and blood products, in the appropriate column of the 24-hour record.

   6. Documents intake by type and amount.

7. Complete 24-hour intake record by adding the three 8-hour totals.

   7. Provides consistent data for analysis of client's fluid status over a 24-hour period.

Output

8. Don nonsterile gloves.

   8. Reduces potential for transmission of pathogens.

9. Empty urinal, bedpan, commode "hat," or Foley drainage bag into graduated container and measure. Dispose of urine in toilet or hopper room, according to agency policy.

   9. Provides accurate measurement of urine.

10. Remove gloves and wash hands.

   10. Prevents cross-contamination.

11. Record time and amount of output (urine, drainage from nasogastric tube, drainage tube) on bedside I&O record.

   11. Documents output.

12. Transfer 8-hour output totals to graphic sheet or 24-hour I&O record on the client's chart, according to agency policy.

   12. Provides for data analysis of client's fluid status.

13. Complete 24-hour output record by totaling the three 8-hour totals.

   13. Provides consistent data for analysis of client's fluid status over a 24-hour period.

Procedure B30 — Urine Collection—Closed Drainage System

Equipment

- Rubber band or catheter clamp
- Tape and sign
- Examination gloves
- Sterile specimen container and label
- Sterile packages of 70% isopropanol (anti-infective) or povidone-iodine (antiseptic)
- Sterile 10-mL syringe with 23- or 25-gauge needle

Action	Rationale

• Wash your hands • Check the client's identification band •
• Explain the procedure to the client prior to beginning •

1. Gather equipment.

   1. Promotes efficiency.

2. Manipulate the drainage tubing so that the urine in the tubing goes into the bag.

   2. Facilitates urine to flow into the drainage bag; provides a fresh urine sample.

continued

Action	Rationale
3. Clamp the drainage tubing below the aspiration port; leave clamped 30 to 60 minutes.	**3.** Traps fresh urine in the tubing above the level of the aspiration port.
4. Tape a sign over the client's bed indicating that the Foley catheter's drainage tubing is temporarily clamped for a specimen.	**4.** Communicates to other personnel that the drainage tube is clamped.
5. Wash hands, don gloves.	**5.** Decreases transmission of microorganisms.
6. Provide for privacy.	**6.** Decreases embarrassment.
7. Cleanse the aspiration port with an anti-infective or antiseptic solution; let dry.	**7.** Inhibits growth and reproduction of micro-organisms; povidone-iodine must dry to be effective antiseptic.
8. Remove all air from the needle and syringe.	**8.** Allow for withdrawal of the correct amount of urine.
9. Insert needle into aspiration port at a 45° angle, aspirate 10 mL from port, remove needle.	**9.** Prevents accidental puncture of the catheter wall on distant side of port; provides sufficient urine for analysis.
10. Transfer urine into sterile labeled container, secure lid on container, and place container in a biohazard bag.	**10.** Prevents contamination of sterile specimen, ensures client accuracy, prevents spillage.
11. Place needle and syringe unit into sharps container; *never recap a contaminated needle.*	**11.** Prevents accidental needle sticks.
12. Remove the notice from above the bed after removing clamp from tubing.	**12.** Clamp is no longer in place.
13. Remove and dispose of gloves, wash hands.	**13.** Decreases transmission of microorganisms.
14. Transport specimen to laboratory.	**14.** Prevents growth of bacteria or changes in the urine's analysis.
15. Document collection of urine specimen.	**15.** Provides information on collection of urine specimen.

Procedure B31 — Urine Collection—Clean Catch, Female/Male

Equipment

- Examination gloves
- Sterile collection container and lid, label
- Sterile midstream kit
- 3 antiseptic towelettes or 3 cotton balls saturated with an antiseptic solution

Action	Rationale
• Wash your hands • Check the client's identification band • *• Explain the procedure to the client prior to beginning •*	
1. Gather equipment.	**1.** Promotes efficiency.
2. Don gloves, or ask the client to wash his or her hands.	**2.** Decreases transmission of microorganisms.
3. Provide for privacy.	**3.** Decreases embarrassment.

continued

Action	**Rationale**
4. *Instruct the female client to:*	**4.**
• Sit with legs separated on the toilet.	• Comfortable position, provides access to cleansing the labia.
• Open the sterile container, placing the lid up on a firm surface in easy reach.	• Prevents the inside of the container's lid from touching a soiled surface; prevents contamination of the specimen.
• Use the thumb and forefinger to separate the labia.	• Provides access for cleansing the labia.
• With the labia separated, using a downward stroke, cleanse one side of the labia with the towelette, discard the towelette, repeat procedure on the other side with the second towelette, repeat the procedure down the center with the third towelette, make sure the labia stay separated throughout the procedure (Figure B31-1).	• Prevents contamination of clean area.

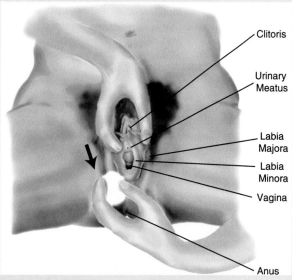

Clitoris
Urinary Meatus
Labia Majora
Labia Minora
Vagina
Anus

Figure B31-1 Client Cleansing Labia

• Begin to urinate into the toilet, place the collection cup under the stream of urine after a good flow of urine has been started. Fill the container half-way with urine.	• Initial flow of urine *is not* collected, can contain bacteria.
Instruct the male client to:	
• Stand in front of the toilet.	• Ensures position of comfort.
• Open the sterile container, placing the lid up on a firm surface in easy reach.	• Prevents the inside of the container's lid from touching a soiled surface; prevents contamination of the specimen.
• Retract foreskin, if necessary.	• Provides access for cleaning penis tip.
• Use a towelette to wipe the tip of the penis in a circular fashion. Repeat with the other two towelettes.	• Prevents contamination of clean area.

continued

Action	Rationale
• Begin to urinate into the toilet. Place the collection cup in the stream of urine, filling the cup approximately half-full.	• Initial flow of urine is not collected, because it can contain bacteria.

For female and male clients

5. Place sterile lid back onto the container, close tightly, label, place in a biohazard bag, and transport to laboratory.	5. Prevents contamination of sterile specimen, prevents spillage, ensures accuracy of client.
6. Remove and dispose of gloves; wash hands.	6. Decreases transmission of microorganisms.
7. Document clean catch urine specimen collected.	7. Informs that clean catch urine specimen has been collected.

Procedure B32   Collecting Nose, Throat, and Sputum Specimens

Equipment

- Two sterile swabs in sterile culture tubes
- Penlight
- Clean, disposable gloves
- Emesis basin or clean container
- Tongue blades
- Facial tissues
- Nasal speculum (optional)
- Sterile specimen cup or sputum specimen container

Action	Rationale
• *Check the client's identification band* • *Explain the procedure to the client prior to beginning* •	
1. Wash hands and put on clean gloves.	1. Reduces transmission of microorganisms.
2. Ask client to sit erect in bed or on chair facing nurse.	2. Provides easy access to nose or throat.
3. Prepare sterile swab for use by loosening top from container.	3. Prevents contamination of swab.

Collecting Throat Culture

4. Ask client to tilt head backward, open mouth, and say "ah."	4. Promotes visualization of pharynx, relaxes throat muscles, minimizes gag reflex.
5. Depress anterior one third of tongue with tongue blade for better visualization (Figure B32-1).	5. Promotes visualization of pharynx, but may induce gag reflex.
6. Insert swab without touching cheek, lips, teeth, or tongue.	6. Prevents contamination of the specimen with oral flora.

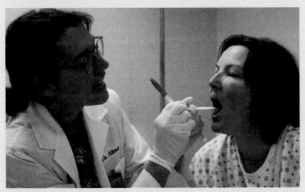

Figure B32-1 Depress the tongue with tongue blade.

continued

Action	Rationale
7. Swab tonsillar area from side to side in a quick, gentle motion (Figure B32-2).	7. Ensures collection of microorganisms.

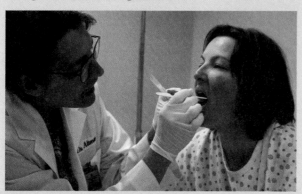

Figure B32-2 Swab the sample area using a quick gentle motion.

Action	Rationale
8. Withdraw swab without touching adjacent structures and place swab in culture tube. Crush ampule at bottom of tube and push swab into liquid medium.	8. Prevents contamination from outside microorganisms and erroneous culture results. Retains microorganisms in the culture tube and ensures the life of bacteria for testing.
9. Secure top to culture tube and label with client's name, according to agency policy.	9. Prevents identification mistakes, promotes accurate diagnosis for client.
10. Discard tongue depressor, place culture tube in biohazard bag, remove gloves and discard. Wash hands.	10. Reduces transmission of microorganisms.
11. Send specimen to laboratory.	11. Provides most accurate results.
12. Document specimen collection.	12. Provides record of physician's order being performed.

Collecting Nose Culture

Action	Rationale
13. Instruct client to blow nose; check nostrils for patency with penlight.	13. Clears nasal passages of mucus containing resident bacteria.
14. Ask client to occlude one nostril and exhale, then occlude the other and exhale.	14. Determines the optimal nasal passage from which to obtain the specimen.
15. Ask client to tilt head back.	15. Promotes visualization of the sinuses.
16. Insert swab into nostril until it reaches the inflamed mucosa and rotate the swab.	16. Ensures the swab will be covered with the appropriate exudate.
17. Withdraw the swab without touching adjacent structures and place swab in culture tube. Crush ampule at bottom of tube and push swab into liquid medium.	17. Prevents contamination from normal nasal flora and erroneous culture results.
18. Secure top to culture tube and label with client's name.	18. Prevents identification mistakes, promotes accurate diagnosis for client.
19. Remove gloves and discard. Wash hands.	19. Reduces transmission of microorganisms.
20. Send specimen to laboratory.	20. Provides most accurate results.
21. Document specimen collection.	21. Provides record of physician's order being performed.

continued

Action	Rationale

Collecting a Sputum Culture

22. Explain to the client that the specimen must be sputum coughed up from the lungs. Saliva is not diagnostic.

22. Promotes client cooperation.

23. Have a sterile specimen cup ready for the sample and some tissues at hand.

23. The specimen must be collected in a sterile cup to prevent contamination.

24. Have the client take several deep breaths and then cough deeply.

24. This helps to loosen secretions so the client will be able to provide a specimen.

25. Have client expectorate the sputum into the sterile cup without touching the inside of the cup.

25. Prevents contamination of the specimen.

26. Place the lid on the specimen container without touching the inside of the lid or the container.

26. Prevents contamination of the specimen.

27. Provide the client with tissues and make him comfortable.

27. Promotes client comfort.

28. Wash hands.

28. Reduces transmission of microorganisms.

29. Label specimen with client's name.

29. Promotes correct diagnosis for client.

30. Send specimen to laboratory.

30. Provides most accurate results.

31. Document sputum collection.

31. Provides record of physician's order being performed.

Procedure B33 — Gathering a Stool Specimen

Equipment

- Clean or sterile bedpan, commode or "hat" for toilet
- Specimen card for occult blood testing, or sterile specimen cup, culture swab, or other special collection device according to test being done and agency policy, and proper identification for specimen

- Gloves
- Two tongue blades
- Paper towel

Action	Rationale

• Wash your hands • Check the client's identification band •

1. Explain that a stool specimen is needed, why it is needed, and how the client can assist.

1. Informs the client and promotes cooperation.

2. Depending on agency policy, assist client as needed to bedside commode or toilet. Have client void before moving bowels. Then, prepare for specimen collection. If client is not ambulatory, use a bedpan.

2. Allows client privacy and the ability to move his bowels in a more normal physiological position.

3. Instruct the client not to contaminate the specimen with urine, vaginal discharge, or toilet paper, if possible.

3. Minimizes risk of skewed laboratory results.

4. Ask the client to notify you as soon as the specimen is available.

4. Reduces the risk of contamination of specimen, allows the nurse to collect a fresh specimen, and reduces embarrassment to client.

continued

Action	Rationale
5. Assist the client with hygiene, help the client back to bed (as required) and ensure his or her comfort before turning attention to specimen.	5. Promotes client cleanliness and dignity.
6. Don gloves, wear gown if client is on isolation or at risk for infectious stool such as vancomycin-resistant enterococcus (VRE).	6. Reduces the risk of transmission of micro-organisms.
7. Assess the stool for color, consistency, and odor, and presence or absence of visible blood or mucus.	7. Facilitates comprehensive client assessment.
8. Using one or two tongue blades (depending on how much specimen is needed and for which test), transfer a representative sample of stool to the specimen card or container, taking care not to contaminate the outside of the container (or the inside of a sterile specimen cup). If using a culture swab, swab in a representative area of stool, particularly if any purulent material is visible. Check with laboratory regarding the volume of stool needed for a particular test.	8. Provides a high-quality sample for optimal results.
9. Close the card, place the lid on the container, or place the swab in the culture tube (according to agency policy) as soon as specimen is collected.	9. Reduces the risk of spread of microorganisms and reduces odor.
10. Place the specimen container in biohazard bag for transport to lab after proper labeling is done according to agency policy. Be careful not to contaminate outside of bag. Provide requisition for test according to agency policy.	10. Properly identifies specimen to client; makes transport of specimen to lab more aesthetic for personnel. Provides client privacy. Reduces spread of microorganisms.
11. Dispose of rest of stool according to agency policy.	11. Reduces spread of microorganisms.
12. Remove gloves and wash hands thoroughly.	12. Reduces spread of microorganisms.
13. Send specimen to laboratory immediately.	13. Maximizes quality of specimen for testing.
14. Document assessment of stool and time of specimen collection and that specimen was sent to laboratory.	14. Facilitates communication among members of the health care team.

Procedure B34 — Applying Abdominal, T-, Breast, and Scultetus Binders

Equipment

- Correct binder for intended purpose
- Safety pins or fasteners

Action	Rationale

• Wash your hands • Check the client's identification band •
• Explain the procedure to the client prior to beginning •

Abdominal Binders

Action	Rationale
1. Choose binder. If a stretch net binder is being used, select the correct circumference, and cut length to fit.	1. The correct size will make the binder most effective.

continued

Action	Rationale
2. Help the client into the proper position to place the binder.	2. Applying binders can be awkward if the client is not positioned correctly.

- For abdominal binders, the client should lie supine, and lift the hips, or position the client on one side, and roll the client onto the binder (Figure B34-1). For stretch net binders, slide the net over the head and neck, or slide the net up from the feet, depending on which is easier for the client.

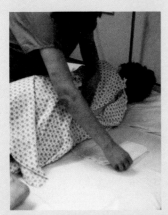

Figure B34-1 Place the binder under the client.

Action	Rationale
3. Wrap the abdominal binder snugly around client's abdomen, starting from the lower abdomen and working upward (Figures B34-2 and B34-3).	3. Correct application allows the client to get the most benefit from the binder.

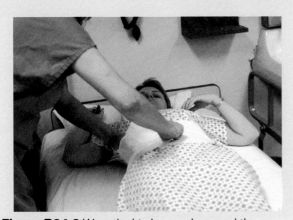

Figure B34-2 Wrap the binder snugly around the abdomen.

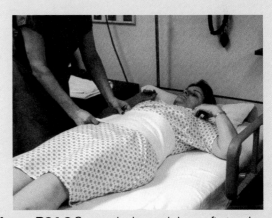

Figure B34-3 Secure the lower abdomen first and work upward.

- Stretch net binders should be adjusted to cover the dressings they will be holding in place.

Action	Rationale
4. Secure binders with fasteners. If the binder does not have Velcro fasteners, secure with safety pins. Stretch net binders cling and stretch over the body part and do not need additional fastening. Check for snug fit.	4. Fasteners will keep binder in place. Be sure that all fasteners are closed securely to prevent possible client injury.

continued

Action	**Rationale**

5. Adjust if necessary. Be sure that binders are not restricting breathing or circulation (Figure B34-4). Be sure that sterile dressings are in place between the binder and any wound (Figure B34-5).

5. Binders that are too tight may make breathing difficult, and may contribute to skin irritation or breakdown. Binders are generally not sterile, so sterile dressings must be in place over the wound.

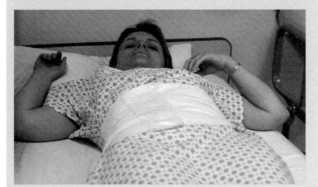

Figure B34-4 Assess the client to be sure the binder does not restrict breathing or circulation.

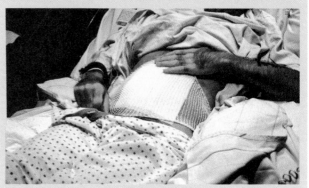

Figure B34-5 If a stretch net binder is used to cover a wound, make sure a sterile dressing is in place between the binder and the wound.

6. Wash hands.

6. Reduces transmission of microorganisms.

T-binder

7. Select the appropriate size binder; choose a single-tail for a female, and a double-tail for a male (Figure B34-6). (A double-tailed binder may be used for a female with a very large dressing.)

7. Proper sizing will keep binder and dressing in place.

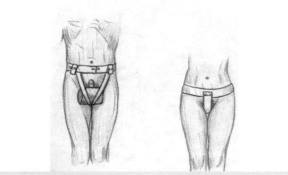

Figure B34-6

8. Place the binder smoothly under the client with the waistband at the waist, and the tail(s) running down the center of the back.

8. Facilitates application.

9. Wrap the waistband around the waist and secure it. Bring the tails up between the legs. For a male, each tail should be placed on either side of the testicles. Secure the tails to the waistband.

9. Secures dressings and promotes client comfort.

10. Wash hands.

10. Reduces transmission of microorganisms.

continued

Action	Rationale

Breast Binder

11. Assist the client to a sitting position.

12. Apply binder, adjusting for a snug fit. Place padding under large breasts, if needed.

13. Adjust if necessary. Be sure that breast binder is not restricting breathing or causing skin irritation.

14. Use adjunctive treatments (e.g., ice packs, analgesics) for additional comfort, if needed.

15. Wash hands.

Scultetus Binder

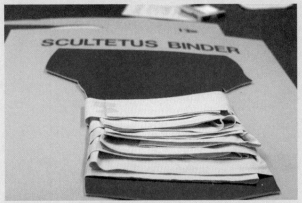

Figure B34-7 Scultetus binder

16. Place the scultetus binder (Figure B34-7) underneath the client, with the upper border no higher than the waist.

17. Bring the tails across the center of the abdomen, one at a time, alternating sides, starting at the bottom. (For a postpartum client, work from the top down.) Each tail should overlap the next lower one by about half the width of tail for maximal support.

18. Secure the last tail with a safety pin or other securing means, depending on the type of scultetus binder used.

19. Wash hands.

20. Document type of binder applied and client's reaction.

---

11. Sitting will allow ease in placement of the binder. If not possible, turn client side-to-side while applying binder.

12. The tightness of the binder will be instrumental in adequate lactation suppression.

13. Breast binders that are too tight may make breathing difficult and/or may contribute to skin irritation or breakdown.

14. If breasts are engorged, adjunctive treatment may be required to increase client's level of comfort.

15. Reduces transmission of microorganisms.

16. If the binder is too high, it will interfere with breathing.

17. Supports the abdomen, and if needed, secures dressings.

18. Keeps the binder in place.

19. Reduces transmission of microorganisms.

20. Informs health care providers of care given.

Procedure B35   Applying Restraints

Equipment

• Restraint

Action	Rationale
• Wash your hands • Check the client's identification band •	
1. Check client's chart for physician's order.	1. Must have physician's order for restraint use. Follow agency policy.
2. Explain rationale for applying restraint. Repeatedly reinforce rationale.	2. Explanations facilitate cooperation.
3. Select the proper type of restraint.	3. Least restrictive restraint that does not interfere with client's health status but provides safety should be selected.
4. Assess skin for irritation.	4. Provides baseline skin assessment.
5. Apply restraint to client assuring some movement of body part. One to two fingers should slide between restraint and client's skin.	5. Maintains adequate circulation and mobility. Prevents skin breakdown.
6. Secure restraint to the bed frame; *do not* tie the straps to the side rail. Use a bow or slip knot that can be readily released in an emergency.	6. Prevents accidental injury to client from moving side rails and decreases client's ability to untie restraints.
7. Assess restraints and skin integrity every 30 minutes. Release restraints at least every 2 hours.	7. Permits muscle exercise. Promotes circulation.
8. Continually assess the need for restraints (at least every 8 hours).	8. Assists in evaluating client's progress and response to restraints.
9. Document application and all assessments according to agency policy.	9. Many regulations govern restraint use.

Procedure B36   Clearing an Obstructed Airway

Equipment

• None required

Action	Rationale
1. Recognize the signs of airway obstruction. In the conscious person, airway obstruction is signaled by the inability to cough, speak, or breathe and often occurs during eating. In the unconscious person, note the absence of respiratory movements and the absence of air movement. A partial obstruction, indicated by high-pitched noises while breathing, a weak ineffective cough, and cyanosis, should be treated as a complete obstruction.	1. Allows you to react quickly and effectively. If the person with a partial airway obstruction has an effective cough, you must observe closely for exacerbation. Prompt intervention is necessary if the person is unable to dislodge the obstruction.

continued

Action	Rationale
2. If the victim is conscious, ask, "Are you choking?" Announce that you can help. Position yourself behind the victim and wrap your arms around the victim's waist.	2. A person who cannot breathe is likely to panic; announcing your intentions will elicit cooperation.
3. Make a fist with one hand. Place the thumb side of the fist against the victim's abdomen just above the umbilicus and well below the xyphoid process. Grasp the fist with the other hand (Figure B36-1).	3. This position allows for rapid compressions of the diaphragm. Avoiding the xyphoid process (lower-most point of the sternum) reduces the risk of internal injury.

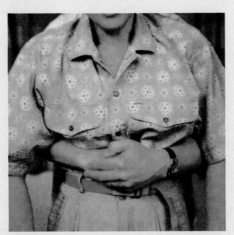

Figure B36-1 Placement of Fist into Abdomen

Action	Rationale
4. Press the fist into the victim's abdomen with quick, upward thrusts. Repeat thrusts until the object is expelled or the victim becomes unconscious.	4. The thrusts should be of sufficient force to produce an artificial cough.
5. If the victim becomes unconscious, lower him to the floor and call for help by activating the Emergency Medical System (EMS) if outside the hospital or the internal emergency call system if inside the hospital.	5. At this point Advanced Life Support equipment and personnel should be mobilized.
6. Place the victim in a supine position. Perform a tongue-jaw lift, followed by a finger-sweep.	6. Potentially opens the airway and removes foreign body.
7. Open airway and try to ventilate; if still obstructed, reposition head and try to ventilate again.	7. Airway must be open for rescue breathing.
8. Kneel astride the victim with your body over the lower trunk or upper legs.	8. This position allows you to apply abdominal thrusts to the unconscious victim.
9. Place the heel of one hand on the victim's abdomen just above the umbilicus but well below the xyphoid process. Place the second hand on top of the first (Figure B36-2).	9. This position allows for rapid compressions of the diaphragm. Avoiding the xyphoid process (lower-most point of the sternum) reduces the risk of internal injury. *Note:* If the rescuer is too short to reach around the victim from behind, this position may also be used for the conscious victim.
10. Press into the abdomen with quick, upward thrusts.	10. The thrusts should be of sufficient force to produce an artificial cough.

continued

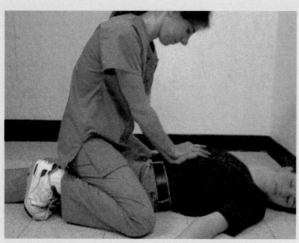

Figure B36-2 Placement of Hands on Abdomen for Unconscious Client

Action	Rationale
11. If the victim is in the late stages of pregnancy or is markedly obese, the hand position may be changed. In this case, place the fist over the midportion of the sternum, avoiding the xyphoid process.	11. A very large abdomen will make effective abdominal thrusts impossible.
12. After five abdominal thrusts in the unconscious victim, open the mouth and sweep with the index finger.	12. Abdominal thrusts may have raised the foreign body up to a level where it can be removed manually.
13. Open the airway using the head tilt–chin lift method (see Procedure B37) and attempt to ventilate. If successful, proceed with cardiopulmonary resuscitation sequence. If unsuccessful, repeat steps 8 through 12 in sequence until successful.	13. Until the obstruction is removed, no other resuscitation efforts will be successful.
14. Document procedure, client's response, and outcome.	14. Communicates care given to health care team.

Procedure B37   Performing Cardiopulmonary Resuscitation

Equipment

- Backboard (optional)
- Personal protective equipment
- Resuscitation mask or face shield

Action	Rationale
1. Determine responsiveness of the victim by tapping or gently shaking and shouting, "Are you OK?"	1. Quickly determines whether an emergency exists. *Note:* If the victim has sustained an injury to the head or neck, to avoid furthering a spinal cord injury, move the victim only if absolutely necessary.
2. If the victim is unresponsive, call out for help and activate the EMS if outside the hospital, or the internal emergency paging system if inside the hospital.	2. Rapid initiation of advanced life support techniques, particularly defibrillation, is associated with increased success of resuscitation.

continued

Action	**Rationale**
3. Position the victim for CPR by placing supine on a firm surface. If in a bed, roll the victim onto his or her side and place firm backboard under the torso, then roll back into a supine position. (Do not waste time searching for backboard if not readily available.)	3. Facilitates airway opening and chest compressions, and the firm surface increases the effectiveness of chest compressions.
4. Open the victim's airway using the head tilt–chin lift method (Figure B37-1) or the jaw thrust. Once the airway is open, place your cheek very close to the victim's mouth; look, listen, and feel for breathing.	4. Removal of the tongue from the posterior oropharynx may restore breathing in the unconscious adult victim. *Note:* If this maneuver restores breathing, place the victim in a side-lying position or continue to hold the airway open and monitor breathing until help arrives.

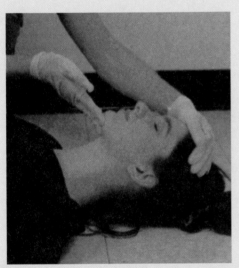

Figure B37-1 Open airway by head tilt–chin lift.

5. If neck injury is present or suspected, open the airway by placing the fingertips of both hands under the angle of the victim's jaw and pulling the jaw forward.	5. Minimizes neck movement but is more difficult to perform.
6. If the victim is not breathing, position your mouth over the victim's mouth, forming an airtight seal. If a resuscitation mask or face shield is available, position it over the victim's mouth according to the product directions.	6. A mask or shield can be used to reduce the exposure of the rescuer to the oral secretions, blood, vomitus of the victim.
7. Give two slow, full breaths. Watch the chest rise as the breath is given, and allow for exhalation after the breath is given.	7. Slow breath delivery improves the distribution of air in the victim's lungs and decreases the risk that air will enter the stomach. Watching the chest rising verifies successful delivery of breaths.
8. Locate the carotid artery in the victim's neck (in the groove between the larynx and the large muscle of the neck). Palpate for at least 5 seconds to determine whether a pulse is present. If a pulse is present, continue to deliver breaths at a rate of 12 per minute, or a breath every 5 seconds.	8. Too-rapid pulse assessment may cause the rescuer to miss a slow or weak pulse. If a pulse is present, chest compression should not be performed.

continued

Action	Rationale
9. If no pulse is present, begin chest compressions: Position yourself over the victim with your shoulders directly over the victim's chest (Figure B37-2). Place the heel of one hand over the lower half of the sternum, avoiding the xyphoid process. Place the second hand directly on top of the first, keeping the fingers up and off of the chest wall. Lock your elbows.	9. Correct hand position maximizes the effectiveness of compressions while minimizing the risk of injuries such as fractured ribs, pneumothorax, and lacerations of internal structures. Correct hand position may be achieved by running the middle finger along the bottom rib toward the sternum until the xyphoid process is felt. Place the opposite hand on the sternum two finger widths above this point.

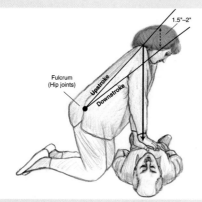

Figure B37-2 Proper Position of Rescuer

Action	Rationale
10. Compress the sternum 1½ to 2 inches, then release fully while maintaining correct hand position. Repeat the compression and release sequence 15 times at a rate equivalent to 80 to 100 compressions per minute.	10. Compression of the sternum forces blood to be ejected from the heart, mimicking normal ventricular systole. Release of the pressure moves blood into the heart, mimicking diastole.
11. After 15 chest compressions, return to the victim's head and open the airway as in step 4. Deliver two slow, full breaths as in steps 6 and 7. Repeat the sequence of 15 compressions to two breaths until help arrives or pulse and breathing are restored.	11. Repeated cycles of breaths and compressions are necessary to deliver oxygenated blood to the vital organs.
12. Reassess for the return of breathing and pulse every few minutes; then resume CPR.	12. In rare instances, breathing and circulation may be restored with CPR. In most circumstances, CPR sustains minimal tissue oxygenation until Advanced Life Support measures are available.

Procedure B38   Admitting a Client

Equipment

- Client education materials
- ID bracelet and bed tag
- Other equipment as dictated by client condition
- Valuables envelope
- Admission kit: wash basin, emesis basin, pitcher, and so on

Action	Rationale
• *Wash your hands* •	
1. Welcome client to unit. Introduce yourself by name and title. Ask client to state his name.	1. Verifies identification.

continued

Action	Rationale
2. Orient client to room and nursing unit. Describe items such as nurse call bell system, location of bathroom, place for clothing, bed controls, television, telephone, visiting hours, meal times, Standard Precautions, and review items in client education materials such as client rights and other written information about the facility.	2. Reduces client anxiety; allows fuller participation in care.
3. Provide privacy for client to change into pajamas or hospital gown, if not already done.	3. Respects client privacy.
4. Show client ID bracelet to double-check proper identification. Attach bracelet to wrist. (This may have been done in Admitting Department.) Review drug allergies and attach allergy bracelet to same wrist, according to agency policy.	4. Confirms client identification; promotes client safety.
5. Document and store client's belongings and valuables according to agency policy.	5. Reduces the risk of loss.
6. Begin nursing assessment, according to agency policy.	6. Starts development of client database.
7. Perform any other actions, as directed by agency policy.	7. Different facilities have different needs, regulations, and guidelines for client admission.

Procedure B39   Transferring a Client

Equipment

- Client medical record (if not electronic)
- Client's medications (if applicable)
- Client's imprinting plate
- Client's belongings
- Old records (if applicable)
- Stretcher or wheelchair

Action	Rationale
• *Wash your hands* • *Check the client's identification band* •	
1. Check to see if order is needed to initiate transfer according to agency policy.	1. Policies differ among facilities.
2. Call nursing unit of new location to see if bed is ready and to give report.	2. Provides continuity of care.
3. Explain the transfer to the client (and family, if appropriate). Answer any questions. Allay anxieties about moving.	3. Keeps client informed and promotes cooperation.
4. Review the valuables and belongings checklist completed on admission. Compare with belongings.	4. Ensures all of client's belongings are transferred with the client. Prevents loss.
5. Gather records and any other equipment that will be transferred with the client, according to agency policy, such as eye drops, other medications, IV pump, respiratory therapy equipment, and so on.	5. Helps make transfer more efficient and reduces multiple trips to new area.

continued

Action	Rationale
6. Transfer client by appropriate vehicle (wheelchair, stretcher). Accompany client to new unit. Transfer care to another staff member in person. Ensure that call bell is within reach or staff member is in room before leaving client.	**6.** Enhances continuity of care. Promotes safety.
7. Document time of transfer and any other information required by agency policy.	**7.** Promotes communication among members of the health care team.
8. Upon return to unit, notify appropriate personnel according to agency policy that client has left the unit. Arrange for personnel to clean the bed and surroundings the client has left.	**8.** Prepares bed for new admission. Reduces transfer of microorganisms.

Procedure B40 Discharging a Client

Equipment

- Any required agency paperwork
- For discharge to home: prescriptions, client instructions

Action	Rationale
• *Wash your hands* • *Check the client's identification band* •	
1. Check for order for discharge.	**1.** Most agency policies require order for discharge.

Discharge to Another Facility

Action	Rationale
2. Complete intra-agency transfer form, according to policy. Be sure to note last time of medication doses. Complete nursing discharge summary. Prepare transfer paperwork, according to policy.	**2.** Facilitates continuity of care. Promotes client safety.
3. Explain discharge to client, and family, if appropriate.	**3.** Includes client in care. Promotes cooperation.
4. Notify receiving agency of impending transfer. Provide report, confirm ability to receive client.	**4.** Facilitates continuity of care. Ensures that new facility will accept client before client leaves current facility.
5. Arrange for transportation to new facility. Call transportation company according to agency policy.	**5.** Reduces waiting time; facilitates continuity of care.
6. Review the valuables and belongings checklist completed on admission. Compare with belongings.	**6.** Ensures all of client's belongings are transferred with the client. Prevents loss.
7. When personnel from transportation company arrive, assist client transfer to stretcher or wheelchair. Provide transportation personnel with required information, such as client's DNR status, for transfer. See that client's belongings accompany client, along with any required paperwork or equipment.	**7.** Provides continuity of care.

continued

Action	**Rationale**
Discharge to Home	
8. Discuss discharge with client, and family, if appropriate. Confirm that discharge teaching has been done. Ask client if there are any questions about self-care at home. If so, follow up with appropriate personnel (typically, RN).	8. Promotes client cooperation. Allays anxiety.
9. LP/VN or RN (according to agency policy) reviews with client: prescriptions to be filled, including telling client when next dose is due based on medications administered in the facility; food and drug interactions and any other essential medication information; care of incision or dressings, if indicated; dietary restrictions or other pertinent information; and when client should make appointment for follow-up with private physician.	9. Promotes continuity of care.
10. Have client/family provide return demonstration of skills required for self-care at home.	10. Demonstrates that learning has occurred.
11. Check that transportation to home is available. Check client room area for any personal belongings.	11. Reduces waiting time.
12. Review valuables and belongings checklist completed on admission. Compare with belongings.	12. Ensures all of client's belongings go home with client. Prevents loss.
13. Complete any paperwork with client, as required by agency policy.	13. Meets regulatory requirements.
14. Escort client to transportation vehicle.	14. Promotes client safety.
For Any Discharge	
15. Document time of discharge and any other information required by agency policy.	15. Promotes communication among members of the health care team.
16. Notify appropriate personnel according to agency policy that client has left the unit. Arrange for personnel to clean the bed and surroundings the client has left.	16. Prepares bed for new admission. Reduces transfer of microorganisms.

Atlas of Nursing Procedures

I1 Surgical Asepsis: Preparing and Maintaining a Sterile Field

I2 Performing Open Gloving and Removal of Soiled Gloves

I3 Performing Urinary Catheterization: Male Client

I4 Performing Urinary Catheterization: Female Client

I5 Irrigating an Open Catheter

I6 Irrigating a Closed Catheter

I7 Changing a Colostomy Pouch

I8 Application of Heat and Cold

I9 Administering an Oral, Sublingual, or Buccal Medication

I10 Withdrawing Medication from an Ampule

I11 Withdrawing Medication from a Vial

I12 Administering an Intradermal Injection

I13 Administering a Subcutaneous Injection

I14 Administering an Intramuscular Injection

I15 Administering an Eye Medication

I16 Instilling an Ear Medication

I17 Applying a Dry Sterile Dressing

I18 Applying a Wet to Dry Dressing

I19 Culturing a Wound

I20 Irrigating a Wound

I21 Administering Oxygen

I22 Performing Nasopharyngeal and Oropharyngeal Suctioning

I23 Performing Tracheostomy Care

I24 Performing Tracheostomy Suctioning

I25 Postoperative Exercise Instruction

I26 Skin Puncture

I27 Assisting a Client with Crutch Walking

I28 Administering Enteral Tube Feedings

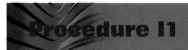

Procedure 11
Surgical Asepsis: Preparing and Maintaining a Sterile Field

Equipment

- Antimicrobial soap for handwashing
- Sterile materials (antiseptic solution, bowl, dressing, instruments)
- Additional sterile supplies (culture swab, gauze, or dressings to complement the type of procedure to be performed)

- Sterile drape (may be contained in dressing tray)
- Sterile solution
- Package of proper-sized sterile gloves
- Container for disposal of waste materials (follow agency policy), colored bag that designates infectious waste products

Action	Rationale

• Wash your hands • Check the client's identification band •
• Explain the procedure to the client prior to beginning •

Action	Rationale

1. Gather equipment for the type of procedure:
 	
  a. Select only clean, dry packages marked sterile, and read listing of contents.
 	
  b. Check the package for integrity and expiration date.
	1. Prevents break in technique during procedure. If the package is moist or outdated, it is considered contaminated and cannot be used.

2. Select a clean area in the client's environment to establish the sterile field.	2. Promotes access to the sterile field during the procedure.
3. Explain procedure to the client; provide specific instructions if client assistance is required during the procedure.	3. Gains client's understanding and cooperation during the procedure.
4. Inquire about and attend to the client's toileting needs.	4. Prevents break in technique during the procedure.
5. Hospital environment: If the procedure is to be performed at the client's bedside, the client should be in a private room or moved to a clean treatment room if available.	5. Minimizes microorganisms in the environment.
6. Home environment: Secure privacy and remove pets from the room.	6. Puts the client at ease and promotes a clean environment.
7. Position client and attend to comfort measures; the client's position should provide the nurse easy access to the area and facilitate good body mechanics during the procedure.	7. Helps the client relax and prevents movement during the procedure; prevents reaching, decreasing the risk of contamination and back strain.
8. Wash hands; refer to Procedure B1.	8. Prevents transmission of infection.
9. Place sterile package (drape or tray) in the center of the clean, dry work area.	9. Prevents reaching over exposed sterile items when wrapper is removed.

Drape

Action	Rationale
10. Open the wrapper, pulling away from the body first.	10. Prevents contamination.
11. Grasp the folded top edge of drape with fingertips of one hand.	11. Edges are considered unsterile.
12. Remove the drape by lifting up and away from all objects while it unfolds; discard the outer wrapper with other hand.	12. If the drape touches an unsterile object, it is contaminated and must be discarded.

continued

Action	**Rationale**
13. With free hand, grasp the other drape corner, keeping it away from all objects.	**13.** Avoids contamination.
14. Lay the drape on the surface, with the drape bottom first touching the surface farthest from you; step back and allow the drape to cover the surface.	**14.** Prevents you from reaching over the sterile field; stepping back decreases risk that drape will touch your uniform.

Tray

15. Remove outer wrapping and place the tray on the work surface so that the top flap of the sterile wrapper opens away from you.	**15.** Prevents reaching over the sterile items.
16. Reach around the tray, not over it. With thumb and index fingertips grasping the wrapper's top flap, gently pull up, then down to open over the surface.	**16.** Only the edges of the field are considered contaminated; pulling up frees the top folded flap.
17. Repeat the same steps to open the side flaps.	**17.** Keeps the arm from reaching over the sterile field.
18. Grasp the corner of the bottom flap with fingertips, step back, and pull flap down (Figure I1-1).	**18.** Creates a sterile work surface.

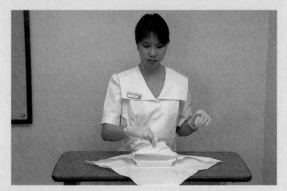

Figure I1-1 Grasp the corner of the bottom flap with fingertips, step back, and pull flap down (gloves not required for this procedure).

Adding Additional Sterile Items to Sterile Field

19. While facing the sterile field, step back, remove the outer wrapper, and grasp the item in your non-dominant hand so that the top flap will open away from you.	**19.** Keeps your dominant hand free; item remains sterile.
20. With your dominant hand, open the flaps as previously described.	**20.** Prevents reaching over the sterile item.
21. With your dominant hand, pull the wrapper back and away from the sterile field (toward your non-dominant arm holding the item) and place the item onto the field.	**21.** Prevents the wrapper from touching the sterile field.
22. When adding additional gauze or dressings to the sterile field, open the package as directed, grasp the top flaps of the wrapper and pull downward as shown in Figure I1-2, then drop the contents onto the center of the field as shown in Figure I1-3.	**22.** Prevents contamination of item and sterile field.

continued

Action	Rationale

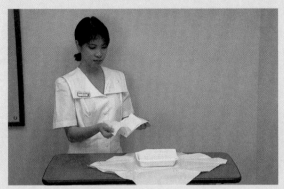

Figure I1-2 Grasp the flaps of the wrapped supply and pull downward.

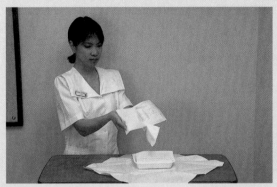

Figure I1-3 Add contents to the sterile field by holding the package 6 inches (15 cm) above the field and allowing the contents to drop onto the field.

Adding Solutions to Sterile Field

23. Read the labels and strengths of all solutions three times prior to pouring.

24. Remove the lid from the bottle of solution and invert the lid onto a clean surface.

25. Hold the bottle, label facing ceiling, 4 to 6 inches (10 to 15 cm) over the container on the sterile field; slowly pour the solution into the container to avoid splashing. Pour from the side of the sterile field. Do not reach over it.

26. Replace the lid on the container, label the container with the date and time, and initial the container.

Using Sterile Gloves

27. Wash hands and perform open gloving (see Procedure I2).

28. Continue with procedure, keeping gloved hands above waist level at all times, touching only items on the sterile field.

29. If using a solution to cleanse a site, use the sterile forceps to prevent contamination of gloves; dispose of forceps after use or process instruments according to agency policy.

30. Postprocedure, dispose of all contaminated items in colored plastic bag.

31. Remove gloves as shown in Procedure I2.

---

23. Ensures proper solution and strength.

24. Inverting the lid prevents contamination of the inner surface.

25. Prevents the label from getting wet. If the solution splashes onto the label, the field is contaminated because moisture conducts microorganisms from the nonsterile surface. Prevents contamination. If the solution splashes out of the container and the drape becomes wet, the field is contaminated.

26. Sterility of the solution will be lost if exposed to air for an extended period of time.

27. Prevents transmission of infection.

28. Decreases chance of contamination.

29. Prevents field contamination.

30. Decreases risk of transmission of infection to all health care workers.

31. Minimizes your risk of contact with infectious wastes on the gloves.

continued

Action	Rationale
32. Reposition the client.	32. Promotes client comfort.
33. Clean the environment; wash hands.	33. Prevents transmission of infection.
34. In the client's medical record, document the procedure, findings (i.e., description of infected area), and the response of the client.	34. Demonstrates compliance with sterile procedure and the effectiveness of therapy.

Procedure 12 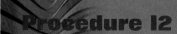 Performing Open Gloving and Removal of Soiled Gloves

Equipment

- Package of proper-sized sterile gloves

Action	Rationale
1. Wash hands (see Procedure B1).	1. Prevents transmission of infection.
2. Read the manufacturer's instructions on the package of sterile gloves; proceed as directed in removing the outer wrapper from the package, placing the inner wrapper onto a clean, dry surface.	2. Manufacturers package gloves differently; the instructions will tell you how to open properly to avoid contamination of the inner wrapper. Any moisture on the surface will contaminate the gloves.
3. Identify right- and left-hand gloves; glove dominant hand first.	3. Dominant hand should facilitate motor dexterity during gloving.
4. Grasp the 2-inch- (5-cm-) wide cuff with the thumb and first two fingers of the nondominant hand, touching only the inside of the cuff.	4. Maintains sterility of the outer surfaces of the sterile glove.
5. Gently pull the glove over the dominant hand, making sure the thumb and fingers fit into the proper spaces of the glove (Figure I2-1).	5. Prevents tearing the glove material; guiding the fingers into proper places facilitates gloving.

Figure I2-1 Pull the glove over the dominant hand.

Action	Rationale
6. With the gloved dominant hand, slip your fingers under the cuff of the other glove, gloved thumb	6. Cuff protects gloved fingers, maintaining sterility.

continued

Action	Rationale

abducted, making sure it does not touch any part of your nondominant ungloved hand.

7. Gently slip the glove onto your nondominant hand, holding the thumb of the fully gloved hand apart from the other fingers and making sure the fingers slip into the proper spaces.

8. With gloved hands, interlock fingers to fit the gloves onto each finger.
When the gloves are soiled, remove by turning inside out as follows:

9. Slip gloved fingers of the dominant hand under the cuff of the opposite hand or grasp the outer part of the glove at the wrist if there is no cuff (Figure I2-2).

7. Contact is made with two sterile gloves; this reduces the risk of contamination from touching the arm.

8. Promotes proper fit over the fingers.

9. Contact is made with two sterile gloves.

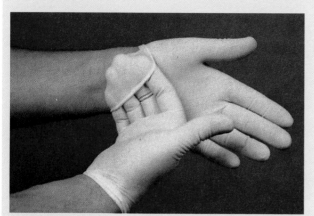

Figure I2-2 Insert gloved fingers under the cuff of the other glove.

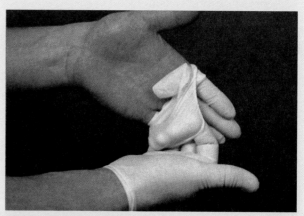

Figure I2-3 Pull the glove down to the fingers and off, turning the glove inside out.

10. Pull the glove down to the fingers and off, turning the glove inside out (Figure I2-3). Hold this glove in gloved hand.

11. Slide two fingers of the bare hand between the wrist and the remaining glove. Slide this glove off, turning it inside out as it is removed, covering first glove removed.

12. Dispose of soiled gloves according to institutional policy and wash hands.

10. Keeps the contaminated surface covered.

11. Keeps the contaminated surface covered.

12. Prevents the transfer of microorganisms.

Procedure I3 — Performing Urinary Catheterization: Male Client

Equipment

- Indwelling catheter with drainage system
- Adequate lighting source
- Blanket or drape
- Warm water
- Forceps

- Sterile catheterization kit
- Disposable gloves
- Soap and washcloth
- Towel
- Tape to secure catheter

continued

Action	**Rationale**

• Wash your hands • Check the client's identification band •
• Explain the procedure to the client prior to beginning •

1. Provide for privacy.	1. Promotes cooperation and client dignity.
2. Set the bed to a comfortable height to work, and raise the side rail on the side opposite you.	2. Promotes proper body mechanics and assures client safety.
3. Assist the client to a supine position with legs slightly spread.	3. Relaxes muscles to facilitate insertion of the catheter.
4. Drape the client's abdomen and thighs, and place the penis over the thighs.	4. Promotes client comfort and warmth.
5. Ensure adequate lighting of the penis.	5. Facilitates proper execution of technique.
6. Wash hands, don disposable gloves, and wash perineal area.	6. Reduces transfer of microorganisms.
7. Remove gloves and wash hands. Choose correct catheter (Figure 13-1).	7. Reduces transfer of microorganisms.
8. Prepare a sterile field, apply sterile gloves, and connect the catheter and drainage system (if necessary).	8. The catheter and drainage system may be pre-connected; otherwise it is connected before catheterization to avoid exposing the client to ascending infection from an open-ended catheter.
9. Gently retract the foreskin (if present) and, using forceps, cleanse the glans penis with a povidone-iodine solution or other antimicrobial cleanser (Figure 13-2).	9. Removes dirt and minimizes the risk of urinary tract infection by removing surface pathogens.

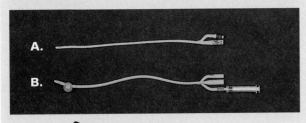
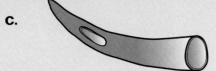

Figure 13-1 Types of Catheters: A. Foley Catheter; B. Three-Way Foley Catheter with Balloon Inflated; C. Coudé Catheter

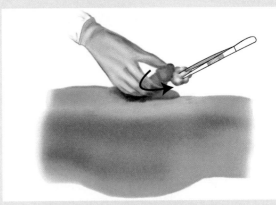

Figure 13-2 Cleanse the glans penis with a cotton ball held with forceps.

10. Inject 10 mL water-soluble lubricant (use a 2% xylocaine lubricant whenever feasible) into the urethra *before* catheter insertion; generously coat the distal portion of the catheter with water-soluble, sterile lubricant.	10. Avoids urethral trauma and discomfort during catheter insertion and facilitates insertion.
11. Hold the penis perpendicular to the body and pull up gently.	11. Facilitates catheter insertion by straightening urethra.
12. Steadily insert the catheter about 8 inches, until urine is noted. Continue inserting until the hub of the catheter (bifurcation between drainage port and retention balloon arm) is met.	12. Ensures adequate catheter insertion before retention balloon is inflated.

continued

Action	Rationale
13. Inflate the retention balloon using manufacturer's recommendations or according to physician orders.	**13.** Ensures retention of the balloon; up to twice the recommended volume of fluid may be inserted safely into the retention balloon if needed.
14. Instruct the client to immediately report discomfort or pressure during balloon inflation; if pain occurs, discontinue the procedure, deflate the balloon, and insert the catheter farther into the bladder.	**14.** Pain or pressure indicates inflation of the balloon in the urethra; further insertion will prevent misplacement and further pain or bleeding.
15. Gently pull the catheter until the retention balloon is snuggled against the bladder neck (resistance will be met) (Figure I3-3).	**15.** Maximizes continuous bladder drainage.

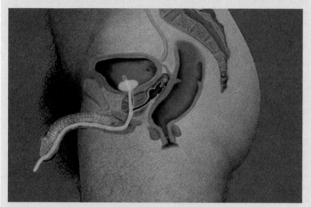

Figure I3-3 Correct Catheter Placement: Male Client

Action	Rationale
16. Secure the catheter to the abdomen or thigh.	**16.** Prevents excessive traction from the balloon rubbing against the bladder neck, inadvertent catheter removal, or urethral erosion.
17. Place the drainage bag below the level of the bladder.	**17.** Maximizes continuous drainage of urine from the bladder (drainage is prevented when the drainage bag is placed above the abdomen).
18. Remove gloves, dispose of equipment, and wash hands.	**18.** Prevents transfer of microorganisms.
19. Help client adjust position.	**19.** Promotes client comfort.
20. Document that catheterization was performed and amount of fluid in retention balloon.	**20.** Informs that catheter is in place; knowing amount of fluid assists when removing catheter.
21. Assess and document the amount, color, odor, and quality of urine.	**21.** Monitors urinary status.

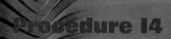

Procedure I4 Performing Urinary Catheterization: Female Client

Equipment

• See Procedure I3

continued

Action	**Rationale**

• Wash your hands • Check the client's identification band •
• Explain the procedure to the client prior to beginning •

1. See Procedure I3, steps 1 and 2.

2. Assist the client to a supine position with legs spread and feet together or to a side-lying position with upper leg flexed.

3. Drape client's abdomen and thighs.

4. Ensure adequate lighting of the perineum.

5. Refer to Procedure I3, steps 6, 7, and 8.

6. Generously coat the distal portion of the catheter with water-soluble, sterile lubricant.

7. Separate the labia and, using forceps, cleanse the periurethral mucosa with a povidone-iodine or other antimicrobial cleanser (Figure I4-1). *Note:* The gloved hand on the labia is no longer sterile.

2. Facilitates visualization of area and promotes client comfort.

3. Promotes client comfort and warmth.

4. Facilitates proper execution of technique.

6. Avoids urethral trauma and discomfort during catheter insertion.

7. Removes dirt and minimizes the risk of urinary tract infection by removing surface pathogens.

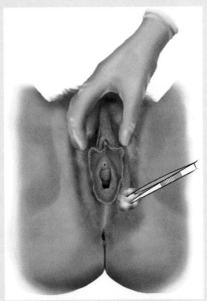

Figure I4-1 Cleanse the periurethral mucosa with a cotton ball held with forceps.

8. With your sterile, gloved hand, gently insert the catheter into meatus until urine is seen in the catheter tubing. Continue inserting for 1 to 3 additional inches.

9. Inflate the retention balloon using manufacturer's recommendations or according to physician orders.

10. Instruct the client to immediately report discomfort or pressure during balloon inflation; if pain occurs, discontinue the procedure, deflate the balloon, and insert the catheter further into the bladder.

8. Ensures adequate catheter insertion before retention balloon is inflated.

9. Ensures retention of the balloon; up to twice the recommended volume of fluid may be inserted safely into the retention balloon if needed.

10. Pain or pressure indicates inflation of the balloon in the urethra; further insertion will prevent misplacement and further pain or bleeding.

continued

Action	Rationale
11. Gently pull the catheter until the retention balloon is snuggled against the bladder neck (resistance will be met) (Figure I4-2).	**11.** Maximizes continuous bladder drainage.

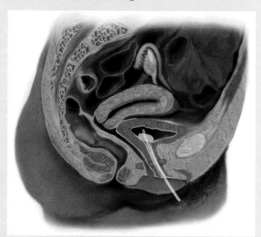

Figure I4-2 Correct Catheter Placement: Female Client

Action	Rationale
12. Secure the catheter to the abdomen or thigh.	**12.** Prevents excessive traction from the balloon rubbing against the bladder neck, inadvertent catheter removal, or urethral erosion.
13. Place the drainage bag below the level of the bladder.	**13.** Maximizes continuous drainage of urine from the bladder (drainage is prevented when the drainage bag is placed above the abdomen).
14. See Procedure I3, steps 18–21.	

Procedure I5 — Irrigating an Open Catheter

Equipment

- Catheter tip irrigation syringe
- Sterile gloves
- Sterile basin
- Sterile solution in amount ordered by physician
- Sterile drape
- 5–10 alcohol wipes

Action	Rationale
• *Wash your hands* • *Check the client's identification band* • • *Explain the procedure to the client prior to beginning* •	
1. Open sterile drape and form a sterile field.	**1.** Promotes sterile environment.
2. Using sterile technique, open and place basin on sterile field.	**2.** Decreases the chances of bacteria being introduced into the bladder.
3. Pour solution into sterile basin. Solution should be no warmer than 99° to 102°F.	**3.** Maintains sterility of the solution.
4. Open syringe, remove tip and fill with solution, then place at opposite end of sterile field away from basin and solution.	**4.** Maintains sterile environment.
5. Open alcohol wipes exposing only half a wipe.	**5.** Facilitates handling of wipe.

continued

Action	Rationale
6. Don sterile gloves.	6. Prevents or inhibits contamination.
7. Clean junction between catheter and drainage tube with alcohol wipes.	7. Prevents contamination when juncture is disconnected.
8. Simultaneously twist and pull catheter and drainage tube apart.	8. Makes disconnection easy.
9. Hold both drainage tube and catheter in nondominant hand; with dominant hand take catheter tip syringe and place into catheter opening. Depending on the amount, syringe may need to be refilled and procedure repeated.	9. Holding both drainage and catheter tubing decreases the chances of falling and cross-contamination.
10. Slowly squeeze solution into the catheter using plunger.	10. Rapid infusion may cause bladder spasms.
11. Clean both tips with alcohol and reconnect.	11. Avoids reintroducing bacteria into catheter system.
12. Drain solution via gravity.	12. Pulling back solution through syringe may cause damage to bladder.
13. Clean work area and dispose of contaminated supplies properly.	13. Maintains safe, clean work environment.
14. Remove gloves and wash hands.	14. Prevents spread of bacteria.
15. Document amount of solution given; amount, color, and clarity of return; and client's response.	15. Provides record of procedure and client's status.

Procedure 16 — Irrigating a Closed Catheter

Equipment

- Three-way indwelling catheter
- Sturdy IV pole
- Gloves
- Irrigation solution
- Large drainage bag
- Wipes

Action	Rationale
• Wash your hands • Check the client's identification band • Explain the procedure to the client prior to beginning •	
1. Obtain irrigation solution from pharmacy as prescribed by the physician.	1. Irrigation solutions are selected for their anti-microbial properties or to remove clots and debris; a hypotonic or hypertonic solution may be absorbed through resected tissue, causing fluid and electrolyte imbalances.
2. Hang solution (1–3 L) from a sturdy IV pole (depending on anticipated rate of irrigation) using one-, two-, or three-port irrigation tubing. Flush tubing to remove air.	2. Relatively rapid irrigation may be used to remove debris or clots from the bladder; slower irrigations are used to treat local infection.
3. Connect the irrigation infusion tubing to the third irrigation port of the three-way catheter; refer to	3. Ensures proper irrigation and simultaneous drainage from the bladder.

continued

Action	Rationale

the product for instructions and identification of the irrigation port (Figure I6-1). Use sterile technique.

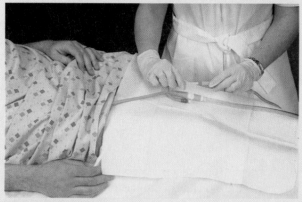

Figure I6-1 Connect the irrigation tubing to the irrigation port of the catheter.

4. Consult the physician concerning the rate of irrigation; *never* slow the irrigation rate because "pink urine" has been observed unless directed by the physician or urologic nurse specialist.

4. Clotting and catheter obstruction following transurethral resection of the prostate or transurethral sphincterotomy frequently occur because the nurse has prematurely slowed the irrigation; a pink solution is expected when an adequate irrigation is being performed; this finding does not mean that all bleeding has stopped.

5. Regularly check the drainage container; empty the bag when filled two-thirds or more.

5. Filling of the drainage bag occurs rapidly and can obstruct the irrigation.

6. Document catheter irrigation; solution and amount used; amount, color, and clarity of return; and client's response.

6. Provides record of procedure and client's status.

Procedure I7　　　Changing a Colostomy Pouch

Equipment

- Appropriate pouch
- Skin barrier (Figure I7-1)
- Pouch clip or rubber band
- Skin paste
- Disposable gloves
- Soap and washcloth
- Warm water

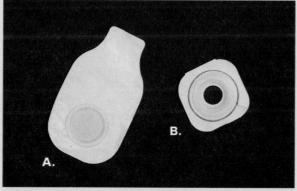

Figure I7-1 Equipment for Application of a Colostomy Pouch: A. Colostomy Pouch; B. Skin Barrier

continued

Action	Rationale

• Wash your hands • Check the client's identification band •
• Explain the procedure to the client prior to beginning •

Action	Rationale
1. Provide for privacy. Include caregivers in instruction if indicated.	1. Promotes cooperation and boosts caregiver confidence in ability to perform procedure.
2. Assist client to a standing (preferable) or sitting position.	2. Facilitates application of pouch by reducing wrinkles.
3. Don gloves.	3. Reduces risk of contamination.
4. Remove the soiled pouch by gently pressing on the skin while pulling the pouch.	4. Avoids trauma to the peristomal skin.
5. Discard the disposable pouch in a plastic bag after removing the clip used to seal the pouch.	5. Minimizes odor associated with the pouch change.
6. Cleanse the skin with soap and warm water. Rinse and dry thoroughly. (Soap may be omitted if the skin is irritated.)	6. Removes fecal material and pathogens and prepares the skin for pouch reapplication.
7. Inspect the peristomal skin for redness, altered skin integrity, or rashes; consult the enterostomal nurse if lesions of the peristomal skin are observed. Tissue or a gauze pad may be placed over stoma to absorb seepage during procedure.	7. Peristomal skin conditions cause morbidity and problems with pouch application unless managed promptly.
8. Remove excessive hair with a safety razor or electric razor as needed.	8. Excessive hair is removed to promote the seal between pouch adhesive and peristomal skin.
9. Inspect the pouch opening and ensure that it fits the stoma; use a pouch pattern to customize the fit if indicated (Figure 17-2).	9. Ensures appropriate-sized pouch and protects the peristomal skin.
10. Apply a skin sealant or skin paste if indicated; apply skin barrier (Figure 17-3).	10. Promotes an effective seal and protects the peristomal skin.
11. Gently apply the pouch and press into place (Figure 17-4). Seal the bottom of the pouch with the clip or a rubber band after air is expelled from the pouch.	11. Prevents leakage of effluent from the pouch.
12. Remove gloves and discard; wash hands.	12. Reduces risk of transfer of microorganisms.
13. Document type and size of pouch; condition of stoma (drainage amount and odor; surrounding skin); and client response.	13. Provides record of client status and condition of stoma.

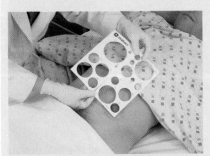

Figure 17-2 Measure the stoma for the colostomy pouch.

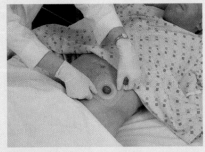

Figure 17-3 Apply the skin barrier to the stoma.

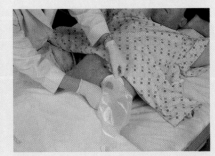

Figure 17-4 Press the pouch into place.

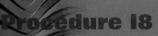

Procedure 18 — Application of Heat and Cold

Equipment

- Heat-producing device with cover
- OR cold-producing device with cover

Action	Rationale
• Wash your hands • Check the client's identification band • *• Explain the procedure to the client prior to beginning •*	
1. Check the order for heat or cold therapy.	1. Ensures correct therapy is used.
2. Prepare the equipment according to manufacturer's instructions before preparing client if it will take time for equipment to become warm or cold.	2. Minimizes exposure time for client.
3. Position the client so that the body part requiring the heat or cold application can be exposed. Expose the body part while covering the rest of the client.	3. Respects client's dignity.
4. Review the circulatory status of the area to be treated and other client factors that can affect tolerance of heat or cold therapy, such as sensory defects. Carefully assess the area to be treated so that changes in appearance can be detected quickly. If open areas of skin exist, check with RN or physician before applying therapy directly to skin. Skin should be clean and dry before applying heat or cold therapy.	4. Promotes client safety by reducing the risk of complications.
5. Apply the heat or cold device on the client after applying cover over the device, according to manufacturer's instructions. (Use waterproof pads to protect linens, if indicated.)	5. Cover protects skin and reduces transfer of microorganisms.
6. Regularly assess the client for any complaints of discomfort, such as pain or burning. The frequency of assessment will depend on the client's underlying condition and experience with heat or cold therapy. If client has any complaints, remove heat or cold therapy immediately and reassess. Be sure the call bell is in reach.	6. Regular assessments will detect problems quickly and prevent injury.
7. Remove the heat or cold after 20 to 30 minutes, or according to physician order or agency policy.	7. Removes heat or cold before rebound phenomenon begins. (With heat application, vasoconstriction occurs to cool the area; with cold application, vasodilation occurs to warm the area.)
8. After removal, record client response to therapy, duration, and type of heat or cold therapy applied.	8. Facilitates communication among members of the health care team.

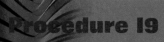

Procedure 19   Administering an Oral, Sublingual, or Buccal Medication

Equipment

- Medication administration record (MAR)
- Medication cart or tray
- Glass of water or juice
- Medication cup
- Medication properly labeled
- Straw (if indicated)

Action	Rationale

Oral Medication

1. Assess the client for potential problems, e.g., absence of a gag reflex.

2. Check the MAR against the physician's written orders.

3. Check for drug allergies.

4. Wash your hands.

5. Prepare the medications for *one client at a time.*

   - Select the correct medication and double check against MAR.

   - Calculate the medication dose, if necessary.

   - Avoid touching the drug while pouring into cup. If unit dose is available leave drug in the wrapper until at the bedside.

   - Prepare liquids by placing the label side of the medicine bottle against the palm of your hand and pouring the liquid at eye level (Figure 19-1).

   - Recheck prepared medications with MAR.

   - Check MAR to make sure all medications to be administered have been prepared.

   - Place medications on the tray or medication cart.

1. Decreases the risk of aspiration.

2. Ensures accuracy in the administration of the medication.

3. Decreases risk of allergic reactions such as hives, urticaria, or anaphylactic shock.

4. Decreases transmission of microorganisms.

5. Ensures that the right client receives the right medications.

   - Increases accuracy.

   - Determines the correct amount of medication to be given.

   - Decreases possibility of contaminating the medication and helps ensure accuracy.

   - Prevents soiling and maintains legibility of the label. Ensures accurate measurement.

   - Ensures right dose, route, and time.

   - Promotes efficiency and decreases risk of error.

   - Prevents spillage.

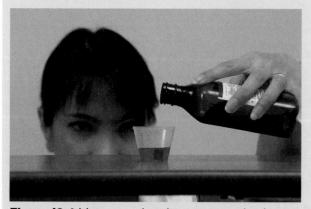

Figure 19-1 Measure oral medications at eye level to ensure accurate measurement.

continued

Action	Rationale
6. Check client's armband before administering the medications.	6. Ensures right client.
7. Identify the drug for the client and its therapeutic purpose.	7. Encourages client cooperation and increases client awareness of what to expect from the medication.
8. Assist client to a sitting position.	8. Prevents aspiration and promotes swallowing of the medication.
9. Offer liquids before and during ingestion of drug.	9. Facilitates downward movement of the medication in digestive system.
10. Remain with the client until all medications have been swallowed.	10. Ensures that all medications have been taken.
11. Wash your hands.	11. Decreases the transmission of microorganisms.

Sublingual Medication

Note: When administering more than one medication, administer the sublingual medication last.

Action	Rationale
12. Follow steps 2–4, 5 (except bullet 4), and 6 and 7.	12. Same as for steps 2–4, 5, and 6 and 7.
13. Don gloves.	13. Protects the nurse from spread of microorganisms.
14. Explain to the client that this medicine is to dissolve under the tongue; it is not to be swallowed. Instruct client to allow tablet to dissolve completely and not to chew the tablet or drink water for an hour.	14. Promotes cooperation; enhances proper drug delivery.
15. Remove tablet from unit dose wrapper (if present), place tablet under client's tongue. (*Note:* If medication is nitroglycerin, have client wet the tablet with saliva before sliding it under the tongue, to speed absorption.)	15. Facilitates drug delivery.
16. Remove gloves and wash hands.	16. Decreases transmission of microorganisms.
17. After administering sublingual medication, check to be sure client did not swallow medication.	17. Swallowing interferes with drug absorption.

Buccal Medication

Note: When administering more than one medication, administer the buccal medication last.

Action	Rationale
18. Follow steps 12 and 13 for sublingual.	18. See Rationales 12 and 13.
19. Explain to client that this medicine is to dissolve between the cheek and gum; it is not to be swallowed. Instruct client to allow tablet to dissolve completely and not to chew or swallow the tablet or drink water while the tablet is in the mouth.	19. Promotes cooperation; enhances proper drug delivery; avoids risk of swallowing tablet.
20. Remove tablet from unit dose wrapper (if present); place tablet between client's cheek and gum.	20. Facilitates drug delivery.
21. Remove gloves and wash hands.	21. Decreases transmission of microorganisms.

continued

Action	Rationale
22. After administering buccal medication, check to be sure client did not swallow medication.	22. Swallowing interferes with drug absorption.
23. Record the administered medications on the MAR.	23. Provides documentation of medication administration.
24. Observe the client for side effects or adverse reactions.	24. Provides identification of potential problems related to the medications administered.

Procedure 110 — Withdrawing Medication from an Ampule

Equipment

- Medication administration record (MAR)
- Sterile syringe and needle
- Extra needle of proper gauge and length in accord with site to be used
- Ampule of prescribed medication
- Sterile gauze or alcohol wipe
- Filter needle (check agency policy)

Action	Rationale
1. Wash your hands.	1. Decreases transmission of microorganisms.
2. Hold the ampule and quickly and lightly tap the top chamber until all fluid flows into the bottom chamber. Alternatively, hold the top chamber between the thumb and fingers, and make a large circle with the outstretched arm.	2. Moves the fluid trapped above the neck of the ampule to the lower chamber of the ampule. Centrifugal force will pull the fluid into the bottom chamber.
3. Place a sterile gauze or alcohol wipe around the neck of the ampule (Figure I10-1).	3. Holds the glass fragments and shields the nurse's fingers from the broken ampule.

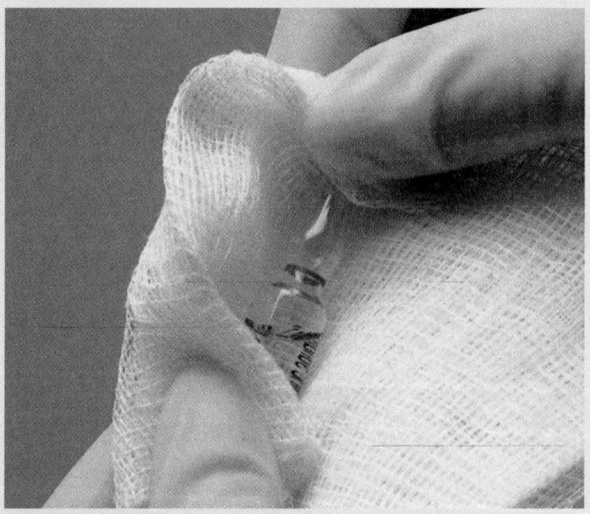

Figure I10-1 Snap open the ampule while holding a wipe or gauze around the neck of the ampule, to protect against glass fragments. (Gloves are optional.)

Action	Rationale
4. Firmly grasp the ampule and quickly snap the top off away from your body. Place the ampule on a flat surface.	4. Directs shattered glass fragments away from the nurse's face and fingers. Prevents spillage of medication.

continued

Action	**Rationale**
5. Withdraw the medication from the ampule, maintaining sterile technique.	**5.** Prevents the transmission of microorganisms.
• Check connection of needle to syringe by turning barrel to right while holding needle guard. *Note:* Some agencies require the use of a filter needle to withdraw medication from an ampule. Follow agency policy.	• Ensures an airtight system.
• Remove needle guard and hold syringe in dominant hand.	• Promotes dexterity.
• With nondominant hand grasp ampule and turn upside down, or hold ampule as shown.	• Provides access to medication.
• Insert the needle into the center of the ampule; do not allow the needle tip or shaft to touch the rim of the ampule.	• Prevents contamination of needle tip or shaft.
• Keep needle tip below level of meniscus (Figure I10-2).	• Prevents air from entering syringe and fluid from leaking out while the ampule is inverted.

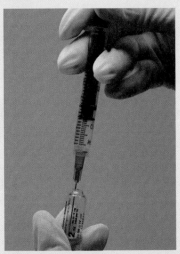

Figure I10-2 Hold the needle point below the level of fluid so the fluid does not leak out. (Gloves are optional.)

• Aspirate the medication by gently pulling on the plunger.	• Allows medication to enter the syringe.
• If air bubbles are aspirated, remove the needle from the ampule. Hold syringe with needle pointing up and tap sides of the syringe. Draw back slightly on plunger, and gently push the plunger upward to eject air. Reinsert the needle in the middle of the ampule and continue to withdraw the medication.	• Prevents loss of medication from the ampule caused from air pressure. Moves air bubbles above the fluid level in the syringe. Pulls medication from needle so only air is ejected from the syringe.
6. Remove excess air from the syringe and check the dosage of medication in the syringe. Recap with one-handed technique.	**6.** Allows for accurate measurement of medication dose; reduces risk of needle stick injury.
7. Change needle and properly discard used needle. Secure needle to syringe by turning the barrel to the right while holding the needle guard.	**7.** Changing needle reduces the risk that the drug will cause irritation to subcutaneous tissue.

Procedure 111   Withdrawing Medication from a Vial

Equipment

- Medication administration record (MAR)
- Sterile syringe and needle
- Alcohol wipe

- Vial of medication
- Sterile needle

Action	Rationale
1. Wash your hands. Gloves are optional.	1. Reduces transmission of microorganisms.

2. Prepare the vial.
 	
  • Mix solution, if needed, by rotating vial between the palms. Do not shake.
 	
  • Open the alcohol wipe.
 	
  • New vial: remove cap from vial of medicine and cleanse the rubber top of the vial.
 	
  • Used vial: cleanse the rubber top of the vial.
	2. Provides access to vial. Removes surface contamination. (*Note:* Manufacturer does not ensure sterility of rubber top.)

3. Prepare syringe:
 	
  • Grasp needle and turn barrel of syringe to the right.
 	
  • Remove the needle cap and pull back on plunger to fill syringe with an amount of air equal to amount of solution to be withdrawn from the vial.
	3. Ensures a closed system.
	
	  • Displaces the solution with air to prevent the formation of a vacuum in the sealed vial.

4. Insert the needle into the center of the upright vial and, while keeping needle above the fluid level, inject air into the vial.	4. Creates positive pressure inside vial to allow accurate withdrawal of medicine. Avoids creating bubbles.
5. Invert vial; keep the vial at eye level and the needle's bevel below the fluid level, and remove the exact amount of medicine while touching only the syringe barrel and plunger tip (Figure I11-1).	5. Prevents contamination of the plunger, barrel, and medicine.

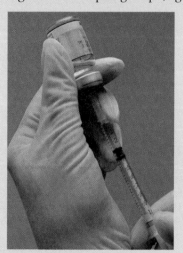

Figure I11-1 Invert the vial and keep the needle below the fluid level.

continued

Action	Rationale
6. Expel air from the syringe while needle remains within the inverted vial after tapping the side of the syringe with your finger.	6. Removes air bubbles created by the dead space in the needle's hub; allows for accurate measurement of the solution.
7. Check the amount of medicine in the syringe.	7. Ensures accurate dose.
8. Turn vial upright and remove the needle.	8. Prevents the leakage of solution from the vial.
9. Replace the needle cap using one-handed technique. Open the sterile package of the new needle. Remove used needle and dispose in the sharps container.	9. Prevents needle stick.
10. Attach the new needle to the syringe by turning the barrel to the right while holding the needle guard.	10. Provides a sharp needle for injection to decrease the client's discomfort.
11. Compare the medication in the syringe with the prescribed dosage in the MAR.	11. Complies with safety standards for ensuring the correct dosage.

Procedure I12 — Administering an Intradermal Injection

Equipment

- Medication administration record (MAR)
- Sterile tuberculin syringe and short bevel, 25 to 27 gauge, ⅜- to ½-inch needle
- Medication
- Alcohol swab and sterile 2 × 2 gauze pad
- Disposable gloves

Action	Rationale
• *Check the client's identification band* • *Explain the procedure to the client prior to beginning* •	
1. Check with the client and the chart for any known allergies.	1. Prevents the occurrence of hypersensitivity reactions such as hives or anaphylactic shock.
2. Check the MAR against the physician's written orders.	2. Ensures accuracy in administration of the correct medication.
3. Wash hands.	3. Reduces transmission of microorganisms.
4. Follow the five rights of drug administration.	4. Promotes client safety.
5. Prepare the medication from an ampule or vial; refer to Procedure I10 or I11 as appropriate. Take the medication to the client's room and place on a clean surface.	
6. Place the client in a comfortable position; provide for privacy.	6. Promotes comfort. Decreases anxiety.
7. Wash hands and don nonsterile gloves.	7. Decreases contact with blood and body fluids.
8. Select and clean the site.	8. Promotes absorption of the drug; reduces trauma to the body's tissue.
• Assess the client's skin for bruises, redness, or broken tissue.	
• Select an appropriate site using appropriate anatomic landmarks.	

continued

Action	**Rationale**
• Cleanse the site with an alcohol wipe using a firm circular motion; cleanse from inside to outside; allow alcohol to dry.	• Aids in the removal of microorganisms on the skin.
9. Prepare the syringe for injection.	9. Ensures correct dosage of medication in the syringe.
• Remove the needle guard.	
• Express any air bubbles from the syringe.	
• Check the amount of solution in the syringe.	
10. Inject the medication.	10. Follows medication prescription.
• Hold the syringe in dominant hand.	
• With nondominant hand, grasp the client's dorsal forearm and gently pull the skin taut on ventral forearm.	• Spreads the skin taut to facilitate needle insertion.
• Insert the needle at a 10° to 15° angle with the bevel facing upward until resistance is felt, and advance the needle approximately 3 mm below the skin surface; the needle's tip should be visible under the skin (Figure I12-1).	• Ensures that medication is injected into the intradermal tissue; initial resistance indicates the needle's tip is going through epidermis.

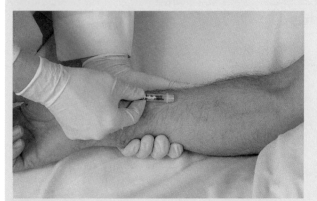

Figure I12-1 Spread the skin taut for an intradermal injection.

• Administer the medication slowly; observe the development of a bleb (small wheal that resembles a mosquito bite).	• Indicates that the medication was injected into the dermis.
• Withdraw the needle.	
• Pat area gently with a dry 2 × 2 sterile gauze pad.	
• Do not massage the area following the removal of the needle.	• Prevents spreading the medication beyond the point of injection.
11. Discard the needle and syringe in a sharps container. *Do not* recap needle.	11. Prevents needle sticks.
12. Remove gloves, dispose in appropriate receptacle, and wash hands.	12. Reduces the spread of microorganisms.
13. Observe for signs of an allergic reaction.	13. Ensures client safety.

continued

Action	Rationale
14. Draw a circle around the perimeter of the bleb with a ball point pen.	**14.** Allows for easy recognition and observation of the injection site.
15. Document medication, route, site, and time of injection on the MAR.	**15.** Provides a written description of the injection site and states the time the medication was administered.

Procedure I13 — Administering a Subcutaneous Injection

Equipment

- Medication administration record (MAR)
- Sterile 3-mL syringe and ⅝-inch needle
- 2 alcohol swabs

- Medication as prescribed
- Disposable gloves

Action	Rationale
• *Check the client's identification band* • *Explain the procedure to the client prior to beginning* •	
1. Check with client and the chart for any known allergies.	**1.** Prevents the occurrence of hypersensitivity reactions such as hives or anaphylactic shock.
2. Check the MAR against the physician's written order.	**2.** Ensures accuracy of administration of the correct medication.
3. Wash your hands.	**3.** Reduces transmission of microorganisms.
4. Follow the five rights of drug administration.	**4.** Promotes client safety.
5. Prepare the medication from an ampule or vial; refer to Procedure I10 or I11 as appropriate. Take medication to the client's room and place on a clean surface.	**5.** Follows medication regimen.
6. Place the client in a comfortable position; provide for privacy.	**6.** Promotes relaxation of the muscles, decreasing discomfort from the injection.
7. Don nonsterile gloves.	**7.** Decreases contact with blood and body fluids.
8. Select and clean the site.	**8.** Promotes absorption of drug when injected into healthy tissue.
• Assess the client's skin for bruises, redness, hard tissue, or broken skin.	
• Cleanse the site with an alcohol swab; cleanse from inside outward.	• Removes the surface microorganisms.
9. Prepare for the injection.	**9.**
• Remove the needle guard and express any air bubbles from the syringe; check the dosage in the syringe.	• Prevents the injection of air into the subcutaneous tissue.
• With dominant hand, hold the syringe like a dart between your thumb and forefingers.	• Decreases risk for accidental contamination of the needle.
• Pinch the subcutaneous tissue between the thumb and forefinger with the nondominant hand. If the client has substantial subcutaneous tissue, spread the tissue taut.	• Ensures insertion of the needle into the subcutaneous tissue.

continued

Action	Rationale
10. Administer the injection.	**10.** Decreases the client's anxiety and the amount of discomfort.
• Insert the needle quickly at a 45° to 90° angle.	
• Release the subcutaneous tissue and grasp the barrel of the syringe with nondominant hand.	
• With dominant hand, aspirate by pulling back on the plunger gently, except when administering a heparin injection.	
• If blood appears, remove needle and discard in a sharps container.	• Indicates needle has entered a blood vessel.
• Inject medication slowly if there is no blood present.	• Prevents the injection of medication into the blood, which causes a faster absorption rate that may be dangerous to the client.
• Remove the needle quickly and lightly massage area with alcohol swab; do not massage the injection site after the administration of heparin.	• Promotes dispersement of medication in the tissues and facilitates absorption.
• Do not recap the needle; discard the needle and syringe in a sharps container.	• Prevents needle sticks.
11. Position client.	**11.** Promotes client comfort.
12. Remove gloves and wash hands.	**12.** Reduces the spread of microorganisms.
13. Record on the MAR the medication, route, site, and time of injection.	**13.** Provides documentation that the medication was administered.
14. Observe the client for any side or adverse effects and assess the effectiveness of the medication at the appropriate time.	**14.** Alerts the nurse to hypersensitivity reactions; the peak plasma level is dependent on the drug's half-life.

Procedure 114 — Administering an Intramuscular Injection

Equipment

- Medication administration record (MAR)
- Sterile 3-ml syringe and long bevel, 20 to 22 gauge, 1- to 2-inch needle (average-sized, adult client receiving a drug in an aqueous solution)
- Medication as prescribed
- Alcohol swab
- 2 × 2 gauze

Action	Rationale
• *Check the client's identification band* • *Explain the procedure to the client prior to beginning* •	
1. Check the MAR against the physician's written orders.	**1.** Ensures accuracy in medication administration.
2. Check with client and the chart for any known allergies.	**2.** Prevents the occurrence of hypersensitivity reactions.
3. Wash hands.	**3.** Reduces the spread of microorganisms.
4. Follow the five rights of drug administration.	**4.** Promotes client safety.

continued

Action	Rationale
5. Prepare the medication from an ampule or vial; refer to Procedure I10 or I11 as appropriate.	**5.** Ensures that all of the medication is expelled from the needle's shaft.
• Add 0.1 to 0.2 mL of air to the syringe.	
• Take medication to the client's room and place on a clean surface.	
6. Place the client in an appropriate position to expose the site.	**6.** Provides access to the site, promotes relaxation of muscles, and decreases the discomfort from the injection.
• Deltoid: sitting position.	
• Ventrogluteal:	
– Side-lying: flex the knee; pivot the leg forward from the hip about 20° so it can rest on the bed.	
– Supine: flex the knee on the injection side.	
– Prone: point toes inward toward each other to internally rotate the femur.	
7. Don nonsterile gloves.	**7.** Decreases contact with blood and body fluids.
8. Select and clean the site.	**8.** Reduces risk of infection.
• Assess the client's skin for redness, scarring, breaks in the skin, and palpate for lumps or nodules.	• Avoids potential problems that may decrease the rate of the drug's absorption.
• Select site using the anatomic landmarks.	• Avoids tissue containing large nerves and blood vessels.
• Cleanse the area with an alcohol swab, cleanse from center outward using friction; wait 30 seconds to allow to dry.	• Removes the surface microorganisms and prevents the introduction of alcohol into subcutaneous tissue to avoid irritation.
9. Prepare for the injection.	**9.** Ensures proper technique.
• Remove the needle cap by pulling it straight off, and expel any air bubbles from the syringe.	• Maintains the sterility of the needle; ensures the correct dosage in the syringe.
• Pull the skin down or to one side (Z-track technique) with nondominant hand.	• Decreases the risk of medication leaking into needle track and the subcutaneous tissue; reduces complications and discomfort.
10. Administer the injection.	**10.** Follows medication prescription.
• Deltoid: quickly insert the needle with a dart-like motion at a 90° angle (Figure I14-1).	
• Ventrogluteal: quickly insert the needle using a dartlike motion and steady pressure at a 90° angle to the iliac crest in the middle of the V (Figure I14-2).	
• Z-track technique: With nondominant hand, pull the skin and subcutaneous tissue about 1 to 1.5 inches (2.5 to 3.5 cm) to one side of the injection site, out of alignment with the underlying muscle (Figure I14-3). (Do not use this technique in the deltoid; the dorsogluteal site in the buttocks is preferred.)	• Allows the medication to be "sealed" in the muscle after injection.

continued

Action	**Rationale**

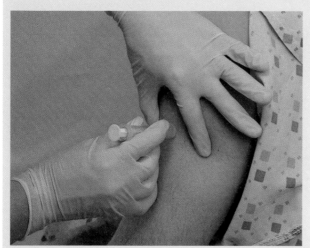

Figure I14-1 Administering Intramuscular Injection into the Deltoid Muscle

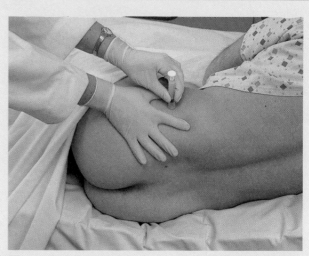

Figure I14-2 Administering Intramuscular Injection into the Ventrogluteal Site

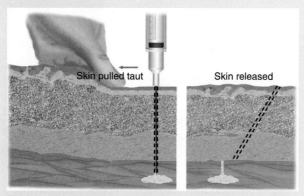

Skin pulled taut   Skin released

Figure I14-3 Administering Intramuscular Injection Using Z-Track Technique.

• While maintaining traction on the skin, insert the needle deeply. Aspirate with the same hand.	• Allows medication to be injected 1 to 1.5 inches to the side of the skin entry site.
• Aspirate by pulling back on the plunger, and observe for blood.	
• If blood appears, remove the needle and discard.	
• If blood does not appear, inject the medication slowly, about 10 sec/mL.	• Promotes comfort and allows time for the tissues to expand and begin absorbing the medication.
• Wait 10 seconds after the medication has been injected, then smoothly withdraw the needle at the same angle of insertion.	• Allows the medication to diffuse through the muscle.
• When finished with Z-track injection, maintain skin traction while removing the needle, then permit skin to return to normal position.	• Releases pressure on tissues and seals medication in muscle.
• Apply gentle pressure at the site with a dry, sterile 2 × 2 gauze; do not massage the injection site. Swab using gentle pressure.	• Decreases tissue irritation.

continued

Action	Rationale
• Discard the needle and syringe in a sharps container; do not recap the needle.	• Prevents needle sticks.
11. Position client for comfort; encourage client receiving ventrogluteal injections to perform leg exercises (flexion and extension).	11. Promotes the absorption of the medication.
12. Remove gloves, wash hands.	12. Prevents transmission of microorganisms.
13. Record on the MAR the medication, dosage, route, site, and time.	13. Provides documentation that the medication was administered.
14. Inspect the injection site within 2 to 4 hours and evaluate the client's response to the medication.	14. Alerts the nurse to hypersensitivity reactions; the peak plasma level is dependent on the drug's half-life.

Procedure 115 — Administering an Eye Medication

Equipment

- Medication administration record (MAR)
- Tissue or cotton ball
- Eye medication
- Nonsterile gloves

Action	Rationale
• *Wash your hands* • *Check the client's identification band* • • *Explain the procedure to the client prior to beginning* •	
1. Check with the client and the chart for any known allergies or medical conditions that would contraindicate use of the drug.	1. Prevents occurrence of adverse reactions.
2. Check the MAR against the physician's written order.	2. Ensures accuracy in administration of the correct medication.
3. Gather the necessary equipment.	3. Promotes efficiency.
4. Follow the five rights of drug administration.	4. Promotes safety.
5. Take the medication to the client's room and place on a clean surface.	5. Decreases risk of contamination of bottle cap.
6. Ask if the client wants to instill own medication.	6. Some clients are used to instilling their own eyedrops.
7. Don nonsterile gloves.	7. Decreases contact with bodily fluids.
8. Place client in a supine position with the head slightly tilted back.	8. Minimizes drainage of medication through the tear duct.

Instilling Eyedrops

Action	Rationale
9. Remove cap from eye bottle and place cap on its side.	9. Prevents contamination of the bottle cap.
10. Squeeze the prescribed amount of medication into the eyedropper. (In some cases, drops will be administered directly from the bottle.)	10. Ensures correct dose.
11. Place a tissue below the lower lid.	11. Absorbs the medication that flows from the eye.

continued

Action	Rationale
12. With dominant hand, hold eyedropper ½ to ¾ inch above the eyeball; rest hand on client's forehead to stabilize.	12. Reduces risk of dropper touching eye structure.
13. Place nondominant hand on cheekbone and expose lower conjunctival sac by pulling on cheek while applying slight pressure to the inner canthus.	13. Stabilizes hand and prevents systemic absorption of eye medication.
14. Instruct the client to look up and drop prescribed number of drops into center of conjunctival sac (Figure I15-1).	14. Reduces stimulation of the blink reflex; prevents injury to the cornea.

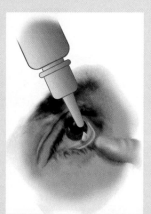

Figure I15-1 To administer an eye medication, gently press the lower lid down and have the client look upward while instilling drops into the lower conjunctival sac.

Action	Rationale
15. Instruct client to gently close and move eyes, but not to squeeze or rub them.	15. Distributes solution over conjunctival surface and anterior eyeball.
16. Recap container.	16. Prevents contamination.
17. Remove gloves, wash hands.	17. Reduces the transmission of microorganisms.
18. Record on the MAR the medication, dosage, route, site (which eye), and time administered.	18. Provides documentation that the medication was given.

Eye Ointment

Action	Rationale
19. Follow steps 1–9.	19. Same as for steps 1–9.
20. Lower lid:	20.
• With nondominant hand, gently separate client's eyelids with thumb and finger, and grasp lower lid near margin immediately below the lashes; exert pressure downward over the bony prominence of the cheek.	• Provides access to the lower lid.
• Instruct the client to look up.	• Reduces stimulation of the blink reflex, and keeps cornea out of way of medication.
• Apply eye ointment along inside edge of the entire lower eyelid, from inner to outer canthus.	• Ensures drug is applied to entire lid.
21. Upper lid:	21.
• Instruct client to look down.	• Keeps cornea out of way of medication.

continued

Action	Rationale

- With nondominant hand, gently grasp client's lashes near center of upper lid with thumb and index finger, and draw lid up and away from eyeball.

- Squeeze ointment along upper lid starting at inner canthus.
  - Ensures medication applied to entire length of lid.

22. Follow steps 15–18.

22. Same as for steps 15–18.

Medication Disk

23. Follow steps 1–8.

23. Same as for steps 1–8.

24. Open sterile package and press dominant, gloved finger against the oval disk so that it lies lengthwise across fingertip. Remove from packet.

24. Promotes sticking of disk to fingertip.

25. Instruct the client to look up.

25. Positions eye to receive disk.

26. With nondominant hand, gently pull the client's lower eyelid down and place the disk horizontally in the conjunctival sac.

26. Allows the disk to automatically adhere to the eye.

- Pull the lower eyelid out, up, and over the disk.

- Instruct the client to blink several times.

- If disk is still visible, repeat previous two steps.

- Once the disk is in place, instruct the client to gently press his or her fingers against closed lid; do not rub eyes or move the disk across the cornea.

- If the disk falls out, wash hands, don gloves, rinse the disk under cool water, and reinsert.

27. If the disk is prescribed for both eyes (OU), repeat steps 24–26.

27. Ensures both eyes are treated at the same time.

28. Follow steps 17–18.

28. Same as for steps 17–18.

Removing an Eye Medication Disk

29. Follow steps 4 and 6–8.

29. Same as for steps 4 and 6–8.

30. Remove the disk.

30.

- With nondominant hand, evert the lower eyelid and identify the disk.
  - Exposes the disk for removal.

- If the disk is located in the upper eye, instruct the client to close the eye, and place your finger on closed eyelid. Apply gentle, long, circular strokes; instruct client to open the eye. Disk should be located in corner of eye. With your fingertip, slide the disk to the lower lid, then proceed.

- With dominant hand, use the forefinger to slide the disk onto the lid and out of the client's eye.

continued

Action	Rationale
31. Remove gloves, wash hands.	31. Reduces transmission of microorganisms.
32. Record on the MAR the removal of the disk.	32. Provides documentation that the disk was removed.

Procedure 116   Instilling an Ear Medication

Equipment

- Medication administration record (MAR)
- Sterile cotton balls, if ordered
- Ear medication
- Tissue

Action	Rationale

• Wash your hands • Check the client's identification band •
• Explain the procedure to the client prior to beginning •

Action	Rationale
1. Check with the client and chart for any known allergies.	1. Prevents the occurrence of hypersensitivity reactions.
2. Check the MAR against the physician's written orders.	2. Ensures accuracy in administration of the correct medication.
3. Follow the five rights of drug administration.	3. Promotes safety.
4. Don nonsterile gloves.	4. Reduces the transfer of microorganisms and decreases contact with bodily fluids.
5. Place the client in a side-lying position with the affected ear facing up.	5. Facilitates the administration of the medication.
6. Straighten the ear canal by pulling the pinna down and back for children or upward and outward for adults.	6. Opens the canal and facilitates introduction of medication.
7. Instill the drops into the ear canal by holding the dropper approximately ½ inch above the ear canal.	7. Prevents injury to the ear canal.
8. Ask the client to maintain the position for 2 to 3 minutes.	8. Allows for distribution of the medication.
9. Place a cotton ball on the outermost part of the canal, if ordered.	9. Prevents the medication from escaping when the client changes to a sitting or standing position.
10. Remove gloves and wash hands.	10. Reduces the transmission of microorganisms.
11. Document the drug, number of drops, time administered, and the ear medicated.	11. Documenting the actions of the nurse will reduce the number of medication errors.

Procedure 117   Applying a Dry Sterile Dressing

Equipment

- Clean disposable gloves
- Moisture-proof bag
- Sterile gloves
- Bath blanket

continued

Equipment *continued*

- Sterile dressing set (if not available, gather the following):
  Sterile drape
  Gauze dressing and ABD pads (surgipads)
  Sterile container for cleansing solution
  Precut gauze if a drain is present
  Cotton-tip swabs
- Cleansing solution (per MD order or agency protocol)
- Adhesive remover
- Tape or Montgomery straps

Action	Rationale
• Check the client's identification band •	
1. Review medical and nursing orders for dressing change procedure and list of needed supplies.	1. A physician's order is needed to use a cleansing solution. Nursing orders will describe individualized client needs such as type and amount of dressing supplies needed.
2. Prepare the client. Assess the client's comfort level and medicate as needed for pain.	2. Dressing changes may cause the client pain.
3. Explain the procedure to the client.	3. Client cooperation is necessary to avoid contamination of the wound. Explanation decreases anxiety and increases cooperation.
4. Position the client. Using a bath blanket, drape the client so that only the wound is exposed.	4. Provides privacy and prevents chilling.
5. Place the moisture-proof bag within easy reach. Make a cuff on the bag by folding the top over.	5. Provides a receptacle for proper disposal of contaminated dressings.
6. Wash hands and don gloves. Remove the soiled dressing.	6. Prevents transmission of microorganisms.
a. If Montgomery straps or a binder was used, untie the tapes. If tape was used, gently remove tape by pulling up small sections at a time while holding down the skin in front of the tape (provides countertraction on the skin). If resistance is met, you may need to use adhesive remover (if skin is torn during tape removal, you have created another wound).	a. Careful removal of adhesive tapes prevents skin breakdown.
b. Carefully remove the outer protective dressing. Then remove the inner layers of gauze. If there is a drain present, use caution so it is not accidentally removed or dislodged.	b. Exposes the wound.
c. Place the soiled dressings in the moisture-proof bag.	c. Provides proper disposal.
d. Remove and dispose of gloves in the moisture-proof bag.	d. Prevents contamination.
7. Assess the wound; note the odor and presence of any drainage	7. The wound needs to be assessed for signs of complications and healing.
8. Open sterile dressing tray or set up sterile supplies on sterile drape. Open cleansing solution (see Procedure I1).	8. Maintains sterile technique.

continued

Action	Rationale
9. Pour solution into sterile basin.	9. Keeps supplies sterile.
10. Wash hands and don sterile gloves.	10. Sterile gloves are needed if the wound is open and if drains are present to prevent introduction of microorganisms.
11. Clean the wound with the cleaning solution. Gauze may be held with the forceps or cotton swabs may be used. Be sure to cleanse from the area least contaminated to the area more contaminated, and use a new swab for each stroke. If a drain is present, cleanse this area last.	11. Always clean from the center of the wound to the outer area or top of incision to bottom to avoid contamination of the wound by pathogens present on surrounding skin surfaces.
12. If a drain is present, apply precut dressing around the drain. Apply a thick second layer of gauze over the drain.	12. Absorbs exudate and isolates drainage from the wound.
13. Apply sterile dressing over wound. Cover with the ABD or surgipad.	13. Provides protection of the wound.
14. Secure the dressing with either tape or the ties from the Montgomery straps (Figure I17-1). Tapes should be placed at the edges of the dressing so that the edges cannot be lifted to expose the wound. Paper tape should be used on clients with thin fragile skin and clients who have sensitive skin.	14. Montgomery straps are used when a wound needs frequent dressing changes to prevent skin breakdown.

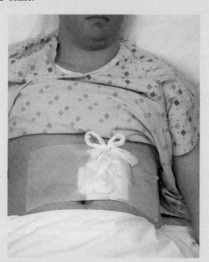

Figure I17-1 Montgomery Straps

Action	Rationale
15. Remove gloves, dispose, and wash hands.	15. Prevents transfer of pathogens.
16. Reassess client following dressing change to determine status and comfort level.	16. Determines effect of dressing change; alerts to any client needs.
17. Document all assessment findings and actions taken.	17. Records information for evaluation of progress of wound healing.

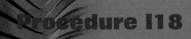

Procedure 118 — Applying a Wet to Dry Dressing

Equipment

- Gather the equipment outlined in Procedure I17, plus:
- Sterile solution
- Fine mesh gauze
- Sterile forceps or sterile cotton swabs

Action	Rationale

• Wash your hands • Check the client's identification band •

Action	Rationale
1. Review medical and nursing orders for dressing change procedure and list of needed supplies.	1. A physician's order is needed to use a cleansing solution. Nursing orders will describe individualized client needs such as type and amount of dressing supplies needed.
2. Prepare the client. Assess the client's comfort level and medicate as needed for pain.	2. Dressing changes may cause the client pain.
3. Explain the procedure to the client.	3. Client cooperation is necessary to avoid contamination of the wound. Explanation increases cooperation by decreasing anxiety.
4. Position the client. Using a bath blanket, drape the client so that only the wound is exposed.	4. Provides privacy and prevents chilling.
5. Place the moisture-proof bag within easy reach. Make a cuff on the bag by folding the top over.	5. Provides a receptacle for proper disposal of contaminated dressings.
6. Remove the soiled dressing and assess the wound as outlined in Procedure I17, steps 6 and 7.	6. Same as for Procedure I17, steps 6 and 7.
7. Open sterile dressing tray. Using aseptic technique, place fine mesh gauze in sterile container. Pour enough cleansing solution into the container to soak gauze. Don sterile gloves.	7. Sterile technique is used to prevent introduction of pathogens into the wound.
8. Clean the wound as described in Procedure I17, step 11.	8. Same as for Procedure I17, step 11.
9. Take one piece of fine mesh gauze and gently squeeze out the solution until the gauze is only slightly moist.	9. If the gauze is too moist, the wound bed can get too soupy, increasing the chance of bacterial growth.
10. Open the gauze and *gently* pack the gauze into the wound, using either forceps or the top of a cotton swab stick. Continue until all surfaces of the wound are in contact with gauze. *Do not* pack the wound too tightly and *do not* overlap wound edges with wet packing.	10. If the wound is packed too tightly, capillaries can be compressed. If the wet packing overlaps the wound edges, it can cause softening and breakdown of tissue.
11. Apply a layer of dry gauze over the wet gauze. Then cover with the ABD or surgipads.	11. Protects wound.
12. Secure the dressing with either tape or Montgomery straps and conclude the procedure (see Procedure I17, steps 14–17).	12. Same as for Procedure I17, steps 14–17.

Procedure 119   Culturing a Wound

Equipment

- Disposable gloves
- Normal saline and irrigation tray
- Moisture-proof container or bag

- Sterile gloves and dressing supplies
- Culture tube and swab
- Sterile gauze

Action	Rationale

• Wash your hands • Check the client's identification band •
• Explain the procedure to the client prior to beginning •

Action	Rationale
1. Don disposable gloves and remove old dressing. Place old dressing in moisture-proof container, and remove and discard gloves. Wash hands again.	1. Prevents transmission of organisms.
2. Open the dressing supplies using sterile technique and don sterile gloves.	2. Maintains sterile environment.
3. Assess the wound's appearance; note quality, quantity, color, and odor of discharge.	3. Provides assessment of the amount and character of the wound's drainage prior to irrigation. Reddened areas and heavy drainage suggest infection.
4. Irrigate the wound with normal saline prior to culturing the wound if agency policy directs; do not irrigate with antiseptic.	4. Irrigation decreases the risk of culturing normal flora and other exudates such as protein; irrigating with an antiseptic prior to culturing may destroy the bacteria.
5. Using a sterile gauze pad, absorb the excess saline then discard the pad.	5. Removal of excess irrigant prevents maceration of tissue due to excess moisture.
6. Remove the culture swab from the culture tube and gently rotate the swab over the granulation tissue. Wipe only once with one swab. Avoid eschar and wound edges.	6. Decreases the chance of collecting superficial skin microorganisms.
7. Replace the swab into the culture tube, being careful not to touch the swab to the outside of the tube. Crush the ampule of medium in the bottom of the tube if present; recap the tube.	7. Avoids contamination with microorganisms. Releases the medium to surround the swab.
8. Wash hands and don sterile gloves. Dress the wound with sterile dressing (see Procedure 117).	8. Prevents contamination of the wound.
9. Label the specimen and arrange to transport the specimen to the laboratory.	9. Ensures proper handling of specimen.
10. Remove gloves and wash hands.	10. Prevents transmission of microorganisms.
11. Document all assessment findings and actions taken.	11. Records information for evaluation and promotes continuity of care.

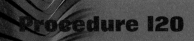

Procedure 120   Irrigating a Wound

Equipment

- Sterile gloves
- Sterile irrigation kit (basin, piston irrigation or bulb syringe, solution container)
- Sterile dressing material to redress the wound after the irrigation procedure

- Disposable gloves
- Irrigation solution (per physician's order)
- Waterproof pad
- Moisture-proof container or bag
- Personal protective equipment (gown, gloves, goggles, mask (or face shield)

Action	Rationale

• Wash your hands • Check the client's identification band •
• Explain the procedure to the client prior to beginning •

Action	Rationale
1. Confirm the physician's order for wound irrigation, note the type and strength of the ordered irrigation solution.	1. Wound irrigation is a dependent nursing action.
2. Assess the client's pain level and medicate with analgesic 30 minutes before procedure if the medication is to be given po or IM.	2. Allows time for medication to be absorbed to increase the analgesic effect.
3. Place a waterproof pad on the bed. Assist the client onto the pad, then assist the client into a position that will allow the irrigant to flow through the wound and into the basin by gravity.	3. Positioning of the client and placement of a waterproof pad will decrease contamination of bed linen.
4. Don the disposable gloves; remove and discard the old dressing in moisture-proof container.	4. Prevents transmission of organisms.
5. Assess the wound's appearance and note quality, quantity, color, and odor of drainage.	5. Provides assessment of the status of the wound.
6. Remove and discard the disposable gloves, and wash hands.	6. Prevents transmission of organisms.
7. Don personal protective equipment except gloves.	7. Protects nurse from pathogens.
8. Prepare the sterile irrigation tray and dressing supplies. Pour the room-temperature irrigation solution into the solution container.	8. Aseptic technique is used to prevent introduction of microorganisms into the wound. Room-temperature solution reduces client discomfort.
9. Don sterile gloves.	9. Promotes sterile environment.
10. Position the sterile basin against the lower edge of the wound to "catch" the irrigant.	10. Decreases possibility of wound contamination.
11. Fill the piston or bulb syringe with irrigant and gently flush the wound. Refill the syringe and continue to flush the wound until the solution returns clear and no exudate is noted.	11. Gently irrigating the wound decreases trauma to granulation tissue.
12. Dry the edges of the wound by patting gently with gauze.	12. Drying the edges of the wound prevents maceration of tissues due to excess moisture.
13. Assess the wound's appearance and drainage.	13. Provides indication of change in wound status.
14. Apply a sterile dressing (see Procedure 117). Remove sterile gloves and wash hands.	14. Application of a sterile dressing protects the wound from microorganisms and trauma.
15. Document all assessment findings and actions taken.	15. Records information for evaluation.

Procedure 121   Administering Oxygen

Equipment

- Oxygen source (wall outlet or tank)
- Humidifier bottle, if used
- Nasal cannula and tubing

- Oxygen regulator or flowmeter
- Nipple adapter for flowmeter, if humidification is not used

Action	Rationale
• Check the client's identification band. •	

Action	Rationale
1. Verify written order for oxygen therapy including method of delivery and flow rate.	1. Oxygen is a drug and its use must be ordered by a physician. Oxygen delivered by nasal cannula is prescribed in flow rates expressed as liters per minute (L/min).
2. Wash hands.	2. Prevents transmission of pathogens.
3. Explain procedure to client. Instruct the client and any other persons in the room to refrain from smoking or lighting matches while oxygen is in use. Check that all electrical equipment in use in the room has been inspected for electrical safety. Post appropriate signs in the room and on the door.	3. Explanation reduces anxiety. Oxygen, while not itself flammable, makes fires burn more readily than they otherwise would, so strict fire safety must be observed. Faulty electrical equipment may produce sparks that could ignite materials nearby.
4. If using a wall outlet as oxygen source, plug flowmeter into outlet by pushing until it snaps into place. If a lock-release button is present, depress it as you insert the flowmeter. • If a tank is used as the oxygen source, the flowmeter should already be attached.	4. Wall outlets are sealed by heavy steel valves that prevent the escape of oxygen from the system. If you hear hissing from the valve, the flowmeter is not fully engaged. • Special tools are used to attach valves to oxygen tanks.
5. If humidification is used, remove the cover from the humidifier bottle to expose the adapter that connects the bottle to the flowmeter. Attach the bottle to the flowmeter by screwing the plastic nut on the adapter to the threaded outlet of the flowmeter.	5. If long-term oxygen therapy is anticipated, flow is 6 L/min or higher, or drying of the respiratory mucosa and/or thick secretions are present, humidification of oxygen is indicated. Short-term and/or low-flow oxygen use, such as during a medical procedure, may not require humidification.
6. If no humidification is used, attach the nipple adapter to the flowmeter by screwing it onto the threaded outlet of the flowmeter.	6. This adapter allows the oxygen tubing to be connected directly to the flowmeter.
7. Attach oxygen tubing to the port on the humidifier bottle or the pointed end of the nipple adapter. Turn on oxygen flow by turning the thumbscrew (wall outlet) or knob (tank).	7. Establishes proper functioning of equipment. If humidifier bottler is used, bubbling of oxygen through the bottle will be noted. In addition, verify flow by feeling for the flow of air from the cannula's nasal prongs.
8. Adjust flow rate to the prescribed amount.	8. As for any drug, correct dosing of oxygen is essential. Both insufficient and excessive amounts can be harmful to the client.
9. Gently position nasal prongs into client's nares, with curves of prongs pointing toward the floor of the nostrils (Figure 121-1).	9. Directs the flow of oxygen into the nasal cavity, where it will mix with inspired room air.

continued

Action	Rationale
10. Loop the cannula tubing over the client's ears; adjust the fit of the tubing by sliding the adjuster upward to hold the cannula in place (Figure I21-2).	10. The fit of the cannula should be secure but not tight. A too-tight fit is uncomfortable, and may cause skin breakdown (especially above the ears).

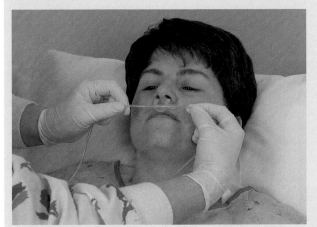

Figure I21-1 Insert cannula prong into nostrils (gloves are optional).

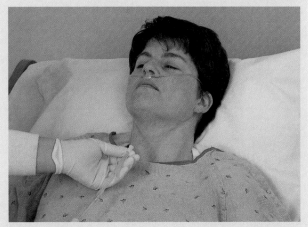

Figure I21-2 Adjust tubing.

Action	Rationale
11. Document the time oxygen is started, the liter flow, and the client's response.	11. Records information for evaluation and promotes continuity of care.
12. Assess the client's nares, face, and ears every 4 hours for signs of skin irritation or breakdown and document your findings. At the same time, inspect the nasal prongs for the presence of nasal secretions or crusts. If needed, wipe the prongs clean with a gauze pad or tissue.	12. Pressure from the tubing or cannula may cause skin breakdown. Accumulated secretions can impair the flow of oxygen.

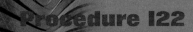

Procedure I22   Performing Nasopharyngeal and Oropharyngeal Suctioning

Equipment

- Suction source (wall suction regulator with collection bottle or portable suction machine)
- Sterile suction kit (contains suction catheter, sterile gloves, sterile solution container; may contain a small container of sterile normal saline)
- Sterile water-soluble lubricant
- Extension tubing connected to suction device
- Small bottle of sterile water or normal saline if not included in kit
- Personal protective equipment: gown, mask and goggles or face shield

Action	Rationale
• *Check the client's identification band* • *Explain the procedure to the client prior to beginning* •	
1. Assess the client's need for suctioning: inability to effectively clear the airway by coughing and expectorating; coarse bubbling or gurgling noises with respiration. Institutional policy will dictate which personnel are authorized to perform this procedure.	1. Suctioning is an uncomfortable and traumatic procedure and should be used only when needed.
2. Choose the most appropriate route (nasopharyngeal or oropharyngeal) for your client.	2. The oropharyngeal approach is easier but requires that the client cooperate; it may also

continued

Action	**Rationale**
If nasopharyngeal approach is considered, inspect the nares with a penlight to determine patency. Alternatively, you may assess patency by occluding each nare in turn with finger pressure while asking the client to breathe through the remaining nare.	produce gagging more readily. The nasopharyngeal route is more effective for reaching the posterior oropharynx but is contraindicated in clients with a deviated nasal septum, nasal polyps, or any tendency toward excessive bleeding (low platelet count, use of anticoagulants, recent history of epistaxis or nasal trauma).
3. Advise the client that suctioning may cause coughing or gagging but emphasize the importance of clearing the airway.	3. Promotes cooperation and reduces anxiety.
4. Wash your hands.	4. Reduces the transmission of pathogens.
5. Position the client in a high Fowler's or semi-Fowler's position.	5. Maximizes lung expansion and effective coughing.
6. If the client is unconscious or otherwise unable to protect his or her airway, place in a side-lying position.	6. Protects the client from aspiration in the event of vomiting.
7. Connect extension tubing to suction device if not already in place, and adjust suction control to between 110 and 120 mm Hg.	7. Excessive negative pressure can cause tissue trauma, whereas insufficient pressure will be ineffective.
8. Put on gown and mask and goggles or face shield.	8. Protects the nurse from splattering of body fluids.
9. Using sterile technique, open the suction kit. Consider the inside wrapper of the kit to be sterile, and spread the wrapper out carefully to create a small sterile field.	9. Produces an area in which to place sterile items without contaminating them.
10. Open a packet of sterile water-soluble lubricant and squeeze out the contents of the packet onto the sterile field.	10. Lubricant will be used to further lubricate the catheter tip if the nasopharyngeal route is used.
11. If sterile solution (water or saline) is not included in the kit, pour about 100 mL of solution into the sterile container provided in the kit.	11. This solution will be used to lubricate the catheter and to rinse the inside of the catheter to clear secretions.
12. If gloves are wrapped, carefully lift the wrapped gloves from the kit without touching the inside of the kit or the gloves themselves. Lay the wrapped gloves down next to the suction kit, and open the wrapper. Put on the gloves using sterile gloving technique (see Procedure I1).	12. The gloves should be kept sterile for handling the sterile suction catheter to avoid introducing pathogens into the client's airway.
13. If a cup of sterile solution is included in the suction kit, open it.	13. This solution will be used to lubricate the catheter and to rinse the inside of the catheter to clear secretions.
14. Designate one hand as *sterile* (able to touch only sterile items) and the other as *clean* (able to touch only unsterile items).	14. Usually, the dominant hand is the sterile hand, while the nondominant hand is clean. This prevents contamination of sterile supplies while allowing you to handle unsterile items.
15. *Using your sterile hand,* pick up the suction catheter. Grasp the plastic connector end between your thumb and forefinger and coil the tip around your remaining fingers.	15. Prevents accidental contamination of the catheter tip.

continued

Action	Rationale
16. Pick up the extension tubing *with your clean hand*. Connect the suction catheter to the extension tubing, taking care not to contaminate the catheter (Figure I22-1).	**16.** The extension tubing is not sterile.

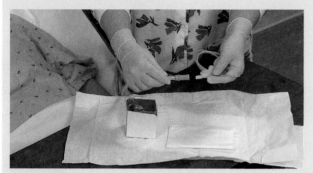

Figure I22-1 Attach catheter to tubing.

Action	Rationale
17. Position your clean hand with the thumb over the catheter's suction port.	**17.** Suction is activated by occluding this port with the thumb. Releasing the port deactivates the suction.
18. Dip the catheter tip into the sterile solution, and activate the suction. Observe as the solution is drawn into the catheter.	**18.** Tests the suction device as well as lubricates the interior of the catheter to enhance clearance of secretions.
19. For oropharyngeal suctioning, ask the client to open his or her mouth. Without activating the suction, gently insert the catheter and advance it until you reach the pool of secretions or until the client coughs. Do not poke catheter in oropharynx.	**19.** To minimize trauma, do not apply suction while the catheter is being advanced.
20. For nasopharyngeal suctioning, estimate the distance from the tip of the client's nose to the earlobe and grasp the catheter between your thumb and forefinger at a point equal to this distance from the catheter's tip.	**20.** Ensures placement of the catheter tip in the oropharynx and not in the trachea.
21. Dip the tip of the suction catheter into the water-soluble lubricant to coat catheter tip liberally.	**21.** Promotes the client's comfort and minimizes trauma to nasal mucosa.
22. Insert the catheter tip into the nare with the suction control port uncovered. Advance the catheter gently with a slight downward slant. Slight rotation of the catheter may be used to ease insertion (Figure I22-2). Advance the catheter to the point marked by your thumb and forefinger.	**22.** Guides the catheter toward the posterior oropharynx along the floor of the nasal cavity.
23. If resistance is met, *do not force the catheter*. Withdraw it and attempt insertion via the opposite nare.	**23.** Forceful insertion may cause tissue damage and bleeding.
24. Apply suction by occluding the suction control port with your thumb; at the same time, slowly rotate the catheter by rolling it between your thumb and fingers while slowly withdrawing it. Apply suction for no longer than 15 seconds at a time.	**24.** Prolonged suction applied to a single area of tissue can cause tissue damage.

continued

Action	Rationale

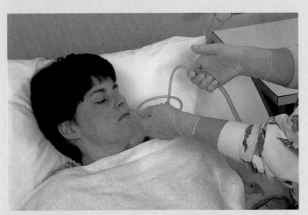

Figure 122-2 Insert catheter into nostril.

25. Repeat step 24 until secretions have been cleared, allowing brief rest periods between suctioning episodes.	25. Promotes complete clearance of the airway.
26. Withdraw the catheter by looping it around your fingers as you pull it out.	26. Allows you to maintain control over the catheter tip as it is withdrawn.
27. Dip the catheter tip into the sterile solution and apply suction.	27. Clears the extension tubing of secretions that would promote bacterial growth and could block tubing.
28. Disconnect the catheter from the extension tubing. Holding the coiled catheter in your gloved hand, remove the glove by pulling it over the catheter. Discard catheter and gloves in an appropriate container.	28. Contains the catheter and secretions in the glove for disposal.
29. Discard remaining supplies in the appropriate container and wash your hands.	29. Prevents the transmission of pathogens.
30. Provide the client with oral hygiene if indicated or desired.	30. Suctioning and coughing may produce an unpleasant taste.
31. Document the procedure, noting the amount, color, and odor of secretions and the client's response to the procedure.	31. Changes in the amount, color, or odor of pulmonary secretions may indicate infection.

Procedure 123   Performing Tracheostomy Care

Equipment

- Tracheostomy care kit (includes two sterile containers, sterile cotton-tip applicators, sterile pipe cleaner, sterile nylon brush, sterile 4 × 4 gauze pads, tweezers, sterile drapes, and tracheostomy ties)
- Two pairs of sterile gloves
- Plastic bag or biohazard container for disposal

- Sterile 0.9% sodium chloride solution
- Hydrogen peroxide solution
- Suction kit and suction equipment (see Procedure 124)
- Sterile precut 4 × 4 drain sponges
- Personal protective devices: gown, mask, and goggles or face shield

continued

Action	Rationale

• Check the client's identification band • Explain the procedure to the client prior to beginning •

Action	Rationale
1. Assist the client to a semi-Fowler's position. Remove pillows from behind the client's head.	1. Semi-Fowler's position allows comfortable access to the tracheostomy site, and removal of pillows reduces neck flexion.
2. Place plastic bag or disposal container within easy reach. Position in an area that does not require crossing over the sterile field or stoma to discard soiled items.	2. Prevents contamination of sterile field or stoma.
3. Place additional items on a clean overbed table or other easily accessible work space.	3. This space will be used to set up a sterile field for the tracheostomy care supplies.
4. Wash your hands.	4. Prevents the transmission of pathogens.
5. Loosen the caps on the bottles of sterile saline and hydrogen peroxide.	5. Permits easy opening of the bottles when ready.
6. Put on goggles, mask (or face shield) and gown.	6. Protects the nurse from splattering of body fluids (sputum).
7. Suction the client's tracheostomy tube (see Procedure I24); then remove the soiled tracheostomy dressing. Note the amount, color, and odor of any drainage around the stoma. Remove the gloves by pulling them over the discarded dressing, and discard the gloves and dressing.	7. Suctioning clears the airway of loose secretions. Inspection of the exudate reveals signs of possible peristomal infection. The old dressing and gloves used for suctioning are discarded to prevent reintroduction of pathogens. Removing the gloves over the old dressing permits containment of infectious exudate (if present).
8. Open the tracheostomy care kit, taking care to avoid touching the inside of the kit.	8. Prevents contamination of sterile items in the kit.
9. Using sterile gloving technique (Procedure I2), put on the gloves supplied in the tracheostomy care kit (if included) or a separate pair of sterile gloves.	9. Maintains sterility of the supplies in the kit.
10. Open the inner wrapper of the tracheostomy care kit to form a sterile field. Separate the two sterile containers and place them on the field. Lay the cotton applicators, pipe cleaners, nylon brush, and sterile 4 × 4 pads on the field. Place the sterile drape on the client's chest, with its upper edge as near to the tracheostomy tube as possible. Fold a tuck of the drape over your fingers as you position the drape.	10. Provides a sterile area in which to work. Prevents contamination of your sterile gloves.
11. Designate one hand as *sterile* (able to touch only sterile items) and the other as *clean* (able to touch only unsterile items).	11. Usually, the dominant hand is the sterile hand, while the nondominant hand is clean. This system prevents contamination of sterile supplies while allowing you to handle unsterile items.
12. *Using your clean hand,* open the bottles of sterile saline and peroxide, laying the caps outside of the sterile field. Pour about 100 mL of saline into one sterile container and about 100 mL of hydrogen peroxide into the other container. Set the bottles down outside of the sterile field. Remove oxygen tubing (if present), if the client can be without humidified oxygen for a short period of time.	12. These solutions will be used to clean the tracheostomy tube's inner cannula. Since the bottles and caps are unsterile, they should not be placed in the sterile field.

continued

Action	Rationale
13. *Using your sterile hand,* pick up a sterile cotton swab and saturate the tip with hydrogen peroxide. Swab the peristomal skin, including the area under the tracheostomy tube's faceplate. If you must touch the tracheostomy tube or the client, do so with your *clean* hand.	**13.** This action removes exudate and other material from the skin to maintain skin integrity.
14. *Using your clean hand,* gently loosen the inner cannula of the tracheostomy tube by twisting the outer ring counterclockwise; then withdraw the inner cannula in a smooth motion. Place the inner cannula into the basin of peroxide. *Note:* some tracheostomy tubes use disposable inner cannulae that would be replaced at this point in the procedure. If replacing a disposable inner cannula, skip to step 18.	**14.** Minimizes trauma to the client's tracheal tissues and reduces reflexive coughing. The hydrogen peroxide serves to dissolve crusted secretions.
15. *Using your sterile hand,* pick up the cannula. Using your clean hand, pick up the nylon brush and scrub to remove any visible crusts or secretions from inside and outside the cannula (Figure I23-1).	**15.** Any secretions retained on the inner cannula may be aspirated into the client's lungs, causing infection and possible airway obstruction. In some cases, the pipe cleaners may be needed to gain access to the inner surface of the cannula.

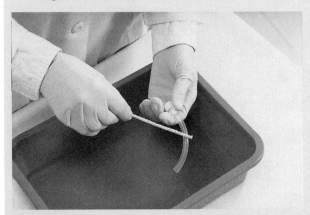

Figure I23-1 Clean lumen and inner cannula.

Action	Rationale
16. Place the cannula into the container of sterile saline. Agitate so that all surfaces are bathed in saline.	**16.** Rinses the peroxide off the cannula before it is returned to the client.
17. Inspect the inner cannula again to be sure it is clean; then remove excess saline from the lumen by tapping the cannula against a sterile surface.	**17.** Fluid trapped in the lumen of the cannula can be aspirated by the client.
18. Gently replace the inner cannula, following the curve of the tube. When fully inserted, lock the inner cannula in place by rotating the external ring clockwise until it clicks into place.	**18.** Minimizes tissue trauma and unintentional displacement.
19. Place a new precut sterile gauze dressing around the stoma, between the faceplate and the skin.	**19.** Protects the skin from irritation and breakdown due to friction with the faceplate and absorbs exudate if present. Using *precut* gauze dressings is important because cutting a regular 4 × 4 gauze will create loose fibers that may be inhaled by the client.

continued

Action	Rationale
20. Inspect the ties or strap securing the faceplate. If damp or soiled, carefully cut them (or loosen the Velcro™ to remove a strap). If cutting ties, be very careful not to cut the pilot balloon to the tracheostomy tube cuff. Remove the ties or strap and inspect the underlying skin for redness or breakdown.	**20.** Ties or straps that are wet contribute to skin breakdown and infection. *Note:* Tracheostomy ties should not be removed or changed for the first 24 hours after tracheostomy tube insertion to prevent dislodgement of the tube and bleeding from the stoma.
21. To replace ties (Figure I23-2), cut a length of twill tape about as long as the circumference of the client's neck. Fold over one end to 1 inch and cut a small (½ inch) slit into the folded end.	**21.** Creates a slit through which the end of the tie can be threaded and secured.

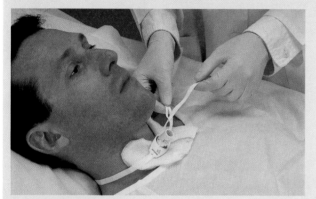

Figure I23-2 Change tracheostomy ties.

Action	Rationale
22. Thread the slit end of the tape through the eye of one side of the tracheostomy faceplate from the underside of the faceplate. Thread the end of the tie through the cut slit and secure it with a knot.	**22.** Creates a secure knot that can be easily cut when the tape needs to be removed and changed.
23. Slip the tape around the client's neck, keeping it smooth and flat against the skin.	**23.** Prevents excessive looseness or bunching of the tape.
24. Bring the loose end of the tape around to the other side of the faceplate. Ask the client to flex his or her neck and slip one of your fingers under the tape as you measure the desired tightness of the tie. (Do not move the head of a client with a neck injury.)	**24.** Flexion of the neck stimulates the increase in neck circumference that occurs with coughing. The tape should be secure but not tight. *Caution: Clients who have had neck surgery or injury should be monitored frequently for tightening of the tape due to neck swelling.*
25. Fold the end of the tape and cut a slit as in step 21, then tie the end as in step 22. Trim off excess tape from the end and knot the cut ends of the tape.	**25.** Prevents fraying of tape ends.
26. To replace a Velcro™ strap: Place new strap behind client's neck and thread ends through faceplate eyelets. Adjust tightness as above and secure Velcro™.	**26.** Velcro™ straps may be more comfortable for some clients and are easier to adjust for proper fit.
27. Reconnect the client to oxygen if necessary and reposition for comfort.	**27.** Restores supplemental oxygen and humidification to the client. *Note:* Some clients may not tolerate removal from supplemental oxygen during the entire tracheostomy care procedure. In this case, an assistant may be needed to intermittently replace and remove oxygen

continued

Action	Rationale
	throughout the procedure. Always work quickly, and continuously assess your client's response to the procedure.
28. Discard soiled items in the appropriate container. Remove and discard soiled gloves. Wash hands.	**28.** Prevents cross-contamination.
29. Document the procedure, noting the appearance of the stomal site and any exudate.	**29.** Increasing exudate or a change in its color or character may indicate infection.

Procedure 124   Performing Tracheostomy Suctioning

Equipment

- Suction source (wall suction regulator with collection bottle or portable suction machine)
- Sterile suction kit (contains suction catheter, sterile gloves, sterile solution container; may contain a small container of sterile normal saline)
- Extension tubing connected to suction device
- Small bottle of sterile water or normal saline if not included in kit
- Personal protective equipment: gown, mask and goggles or face shield

Action	Rationale
• Wash your hands • Check the client's identification band •	
1. Assess the client's need for suctioning: inability to effectively clear the airway by coughing and expectoration or coarse crackles auscultated over the upper airways.	**1.** Suctioning is an uncomfortable and traumatic procedure and should be used only when needed.
2. Explain the procedure to the client. Advise that suctioning may cause coughing; emphasize the importance of clearing the airway.	**2.** Promotes cooperation and reduces anxiety.
3. Position the client in a high Fowler's or semi-Fowler's position.	**3.** Maximizes lung expansion and effective coughing.
4. Connect extension tubing to suction device, if not already in place, and adjust suction control to between 80 and 100 mm Hg.	**4.** Excessive negative pressure can cause tissue trauma, hypoxemia, and atelectasis, whereas insufficient pressure will be ineffective.
5. Put on gown and mask and goggles or face shield.	**5.** Protects nurse from splattering body fluids.
6. Using sterile technique (see Procedure 122), open the suction kit. Consider the inside wrapper of the kit to be sterile, and spread the wrapper out carefully to create a small sterile field.	**6.** Produces an area in which to place sterile items without contaminating them.
7. If sterile solution (water or saline) is not included in the kit, pour about 100 mL of solution into the sterile container provided in the kit.	**7.** This solution will be used to lubricate the catheter and to rinse the inside of the catheter to clear secretions.
8. If gloves are wrapped, carefully lift the wrapped gloves from the kit without touching the inside of the kit or the gloves themselves. Lay the wrapped gloves down next to the suction kit, and open the wrapper. Put on the gloves using sterile gloving technique.	**8.** The gloves should be kept sterile for handling the sterile suction catheter thus avoiding introducing pathogens into the client's airway.

continued

Action	**Rationale**
9. If a cup of sterile solution is included in the suction kit, open it.	9. This solution will be used to lubricate the catheter and to rinse the inside of the catheter to clear secretions.
10. Designate one hand as *sterile* (able to touch only sterile items) and the other as *clean* (able to touch only nonsterile items).	10. Usually the dominant hand is the sterile hand while the nondominant hand is clean. This prevents contamination of sterile supplies while allowing you to handle unsterile items
11. *Using your sterile hand,* pick up the suction catheter. Grasp the plastic connector end between your thumb and forefinger and coil the tip around your remaining fingers.	11. Prevents accidental contamination of the catheter tip.
12. Pick up the extension tubing *with your clean hand.* Connect the suction catheter to the extension tubing, taking care not to contaminate the catheter.	12. The extension tubing is not sterile.
13. Instruct the client to take several slow, deep breaths.	13. Promotes optimal opening of airways and reduces suction-induced hypoxemia. *Note:* Clients should be preoxygenated by taking several deep breaths with supplemental oxygen set at 100% or by delivery of 100% oxygen via manual resuscitation bag. Always return oxygen flow to the prescribed rate after the suctioning procedure is completed.
14. Position your clean hand with the thumb over the catheter's suction port.	14. Suction is activated by occluding this port with the thumb. Releasing the port deactivates the suction.
15. Dip the catheter tip into the sterile solution, and activate the suction. Observe as the solution is drawn into the catheter.	15. Tests the suction device as well as lubricating the interior of the catheter to enhance clearance of secretions.
16. Using your clean hand, remove the oxygen delivery device from the tracheostomy tube and place it on a clean surface.	16. Permits access to the tracheostomy tube. Placing the oxygen device on a clean surface reduces contamination (the sterile glove wrapper may be used for this purpose).
17. Without occluding the suction control port, insert the catheter tip into the tracheostomy tube and advance it until the client coughs or resistance is met (Figure I24-1).	17. To minimize trauma, do not apply suction while the catheter is being advanced.

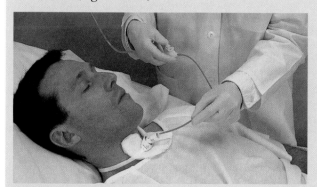

Figure I24-1 Suction tracheostomy.

continued

Action	Rationale
18. Withdraw the catheter slightly.	**18.** Do not want to apply suction when catheter tip is against the carina.
19. Apply suction by occluding the suction control port with your thumb; at the same time, slowly rotate the catheter by rolling it between your thumb and fingers while slowly withdrawing it. Apply suction for no longer than 15 seconds at a time.	**19.** Prolonged suction can cause tissue damage, atelectasis, and hypoxemia.
20. Repeat step 19 until all secretions have been cleared, allowing brief rest periods between suctioning episodes. Encourage client to breathe deeply between suctioning episodes. Provide oxygen between passes of the suction catheter.	**20.** Promotes complete clearance of the airway.
21. Withdraw the catheter and dip it into the cup of sterile saline, applying suction.	**21.** Cleans suction catheter of secretions.
22. Reapply oxygen delivery device.	**22.** Restores supplemental oxygen and humidification.
23. Ask the client to open his or her mouth. Insert the catheter and advance it along the oropharynx until resistance is felt. Apply suction and slowly withdraw the catheter.	**23.** *Note:* At this point the catheter is contaminated. If another suctioning pass into the tracheostomy is needed, a new sterile catheter must be used.
24. Dip the catheter tip into the sterile solution and apply suction.	**24.** Clears the extension tubing of secretions, which would promote bacterial growth.
25. Disconnect the catheter from the extension tubing. Holding the coiled catheter in your gloved hand, remove the glove by pulling it over the catheter. Discard catheter and gloves in an appropriate container.	**25.** Contains the catheter and secretions in the glove for disposal.
26. Discard remaining supplies in the appropriate container.	**26.** Follow institutional policy regarding the disposal of client care supplies.
27. Wash your hands.	**27.** Prevents the transmission of pathogens.
28. Provide the client with oral hygiene if indicated/desired.	**28.** Suctioning and coughing may produce an unpleasant taste.
29. Document the procedure, noting the amount, color, and odor of secretions and the client's response to the procedure.	**29.** Changes in the amount, color, or odor of pulmonary secretions may indicate infection.

Procedure 125   Postoperative Exercise Instruction

Equipment

- Educational materials
- Tissue
- Disposable volume-oriented incentive spirometer or one with disposable mouthpiece
- Pillow
- Nonsterile gloves

continued

Action	Rationale

Action	Rationale
1. Organize equipment.	**1.** Promotes efficiency.
2. Place client in a sitting position.	**2.** Promotes full chest expansion.
3. Demonstrate deep breathing exercise.	**3.** Shows the client how to breathe deeply.
4. Have the client return demonstrate deep breathing:	**4.** Fosters learning.
• Place one hand on abdomen (umbilical area) during inhalation.	• Exerts counterpressure during inhalation.
• Expand the abdomen and rib cage on inspiration.	• Promotes maximum chest expansion.
• Inhale slowly and evenly through your nose until you achieve maximum chest expansion.	• Maintains full expansion of the alveoli.
• Hold breath for 2 to 3 seconds.	• Increases the pressure, preventing immediate collapse of the alveoli.
• Slowly exhale through your mouth until maximum chest contraction has been achieved.	• Promotes maximum chest contraction.
• Repeat the exercise three or four times; allow client to rest.	• Enforces learning.
5. Demonstrate splinting and coughing.	**5.** Shows the client how to raise mucous secretions from the tracheobronchial tree.
6. Don gloves.	**6.** Reduces transmission of microorganisms.
7. Keep the client in a sitting position, head slightly flexed, shoulders relaxed and slightly forward, and feet supported on the floor.	**7.** Promotes full expansion of chest cage and use of accessory muscles to produce a deep, productive cough.
8. Have the client return demonstrate splinting and coughing:	**8.** Fosters learning.
• Have the client slowly raise head and sniff the air.	• Increases the amount of air and helps to aerate the base of the lungs.
• Have the client slowly bend forward and exhale slowly through pursed lips.	• Dries the tracheal mucosa as air flows over it; there is a slight increase in the carbon dioxide level, which stimulates deeper breathing.
• Repeat breathing two or three times.	• Loosens mucous plugs and moves secretions to the main bronchus.
• When the client is ready to cough, have client place a folded pillow against the abdomen (for abdominal incision) and grasp the pillow against the abdomen with clasped hands (Figure I25-1).	• Elevates the diaphragm and expels air in a more forceful cough; supports the abdominal muscles and reduces pain when coughing if the client has an abdominal incision.
• Have client take a deep breath and begin coughing immediately after inspiration is completed by bending forward slightly and producing a series of soft, staccato coughs.	• Removes secretions from the main bronchus.
• Have a tissue ready.	• Provides a tissue for sputum disposal.

continued

Action	**Rationale**

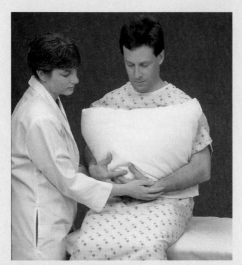

Figure I25-1 Splinting

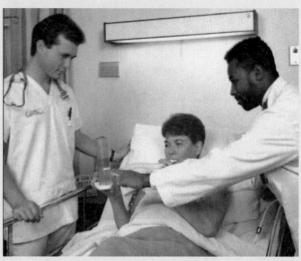

Figure I25-2 Incentive Spirometer

9. Instruct the client on the use of an incentive spirometer (Figure I25-2). Have the client:

- Hold the incentive spirometer upright.

- Take a normal breath and exhale, then seal lips tightly around the mouthpiece; take a slow, deep breath to elevate the balls in the plastic tube, hold the inspiration for at least 3 seconds.

- The client simultaneously receives feedback about the amount of inspired air volume on the calibrated plastic tube.

- Remove the mouthpiece, exhale normally.

- Take several normal breaths.

- Repeat the procedure four to five times.

- Tell client after surgery, incentive spirometer should be used for 10 to 12 breaths every hour, while awake.

- Have the client cough after the incentive effort; repeat Step 8. Have a tissue ready.

- Have client clean mouthpiece under running water and place in clean container (disposable mouthpiece changed every 24 hours).

9. Reinflates the alveoli and removes mucous secretions.

- Promotes proper functioning of the device.

- Allows for greater lung expansion; holding the inspiration increases the pressure, preventing immediate collapse of the alveoli.

- Encourages the client to do respiratory exercises.

- Allows normal expiration.

- Provides client the opportunity to relax.

- Encourages sustained maximal inspiration and loosens secretions.

- Facilitates removal of secretions.

- Prevents transmission of microorganisms.

10. Explain leg and foot exercises (Figure I25-3).

10. Elicits client cooperation.

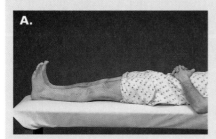 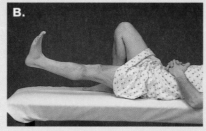 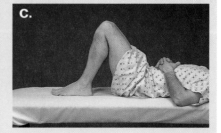

Figure I25-3 Leg Exercises

continued

Action	Rationale
11. Instruct client to return demonstrate in bed:	**11.** Fosters learning of how to improve venous blood return:
• Have the client, with heels on bed, push the toes of both feet toward the foot of the bed (plantar flexion) until the calf muscles tighten, then relax feet. Pull the toes toward the chin (dorsiflexion) until calf muscles tighten, then relax feet (Figure I25-3A).	• Causes contraction and relaxation of the calf muscles.
• With heels on bed, lift and circle each ankle, one at a time, first to the right and then to the left. Repeat three times and relax (Figure I25-3B).	• Causes contraction and relaxation of the quadriceps muscle.
• Flex and extend each knee alternately, sliding foot up along the bed and relax (Figure I25-3C).	• Causes contraction and relaxation of the quadriceps muscles.
12. Instruct clients with orthopedic surgery (e.g., hip surgery) how to use a trapeze bar.	**12.** Facilitates movement in bed without putting pressure on a leg or hip joint.

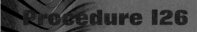

Procedure I26   Skin Puncture

Equipment

- Antiseptic—70% isopropanol or povidone-iodine
- Sterile 2 × 2 gauze
- Sterile lancet
- Hand towel or absorbent pad
- Collection tubes, strip for testing glucose, or other device for testing blood at bedside
- Nonsterile gloves

Action	Rationale
• *Wash your hands* • *Check the client's identification band* • • *Explain the procedure to the client prior to beginning* •	
1. Review client's medical record.	**1.** Verifies physician's order.
2. Prepare supplies:	**2.** Ensures efficiency.
• Open sterile packages.	
• Label specimen collection tubes (if used).	
• Place within easy reach.	
3. Don gloves.	**3.** Decreases the health care provider's exposure to blood-borne organisms.
4. Select site:	**4.** Avoids damage to nerve endings and calloused areas of the skin.
• Lateral aspect of the fingertips in adults/children.	
• Lateral aspect of the heel in infant.	
5. Place the hand or heel in a dependent position; apply warm compresses if fingers or heel are cool to touch.	**5.** Increases the blood supply to the puncture site.
6. Place hand towel or absorbent pad under the extremity.	**6.** Prevents soiling the bed linen.
7. Cleanse puncture site with an antiseptic and allow to dry; use 70% isopropanol if client is allergic to iodine.	**7.** Reduces skin surface bacteria (povidone-iodine must dry to be effective).

continued

Action	**Rationale**
8. With nondominant hand, apply light pressure by gently squeezing the area above/around the puncture site. Do not touch puncture site.	8. Increases blood supply to puncture site; maintains asepsis.
9. With the sterile lancet at a 90° angle to the skin, use a quick stab to puncture the skin (about 2 mm deep) (Figure I26-1).	9. Provides a blood sample with minimal discomfort to the client.

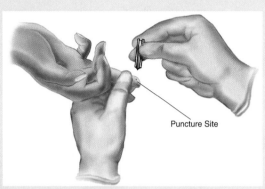

Puncture Site

Figure I26-1 Capillary Puncture of Fingertip

Action	**Rationale**
10. Wipe off the first drop of blood with a sterile 2 × 2 gauze; allow the blood to flow freely.	10. Pressure at the puncture site can cause hemolysis.
11. Collect the blood using tube, strip, or other device. Do not squeeze finger or heel.	11. Pericellular fluid may dilute blood and skew results.
12. Apply pressure to the puncture site with a sterile 2 × 2 gauze.	12. Controls bleeding.
13. Place contaminated articles into a sharps container.	13. Reduces risk for needle stick.
14. Remove gloves; wash hands.	14. Reduces transmission of microorganisms.
15. Position client for comfort with call light in reach.	15. Provides for comfort and communication.
16. Transport specimen to laboratory if indicated, or write results in the medical record.	16. Completes steps to securing specimen.

Procedure I27 Assisting a Client with Crutch Walking

- One pair of crutches
- Gait belt (optional)
- Measuring tape

Action	**Rationale**
1. Review client's medical record.	1. Verifies physician's order.
2. Inform client that you will be assisting with ambulation using crutches.	2. Reduces anxiety; helps increase comprehension and cooperation; promotes client autonomy.
3. Assess client for strength, mobility, range of motion, visual acuity, perceptual difficulties, and balance. *Note:* The nurse and physical therapist often collaborate on this assessment.	3. Helps determine the capabilities of client and amount of assistance required.

continued

Action	**Rationale**
4. Adjust crutches to fit the client. With the client supine, measure from the heel to the axilla. When client is standing, the crutch pad should fit 1.5 to 2 in. below the axilla (Figure I27-1). The hand grip should be adjusted to allow for the client to have elbows bent at 30° flexion.	4. Space between the crutch pad and the axilla prevents pressure on radial nerves. The elbow flexion allows for space between the crutch pad and axilla.

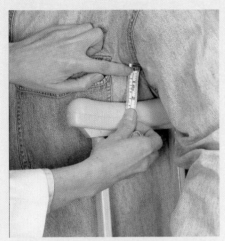

Figure I27-1 Adjusting Crutches to Fit Client

5. Lower the height of the bed.	5. Allows client to sit with feet on floor for stability.
6. Dangle the client at the side of bed for several minutes. Assess for vertigo.	6. Allows for stabilization of blood pressure, thus preventing orthostatic hypotension.
7. Instruct client on method to hold the crutches; that is, with elbows bent 30° and pad 1.5 to 2 in. below the axilla. Instruct client to position crutches lateral to and forward of feet. Demonstrate correct positioning. Tell client to place weight on hands, not axilla.	7. Increase client comprehension and cooperation. Pressure on axilla can cause nerve damage.
8. Apply the gait belt around the client's waist if balance and stability are unreliable.	8. Provides support; promotes client safety.
9. Assist the client to a standing position with crutches. Support as needed.	9. Standing for a few minutes will assist in preventing orthostatic hypotension.
10. Set realistic goals and opportunities for progressive ambulation using crutches.	10. Crutch walking takes up to 10 times the energy required for unassisted ambulation.
11. Consult with a physical therapist for clients learning to walk with crutches.	11. The physical therapist is the expert on the health care team for crutch-walking techniques.

Four-Point Gait

12. Position the crutches 4.5 to 6 in. to the side and in front of each foot. Move the right crutch forward 4 to 6 in. and move the left foot forward, even with the left crutch (Figure I27-2A). Move the left crutch forward 4 to 6 in. and move the right foot forward, even with the right crutch (Figure I27-2B). Repeat the four-point gait.	12. The four-point gait (used for partial or full weight bearing) provides greater stability. Weight bearing is on three points (two crutches and one foot or two feet and one crutch) at all times. The client must be able to bear weight with both legs.

continued

Action	**Rationale**

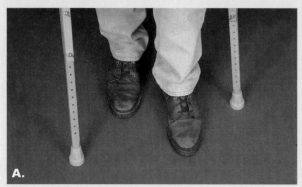
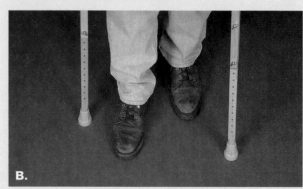

Figure I27-2 Four-Point Gait. A. Moving Right Crutch Forward and Left Foot Forward; B. Moving Left Crutch Forward and Right Foot Forward, Even with Right Crutch

Three-Point Gait

13. Advance both crutches and the weaker leg forward together 4 to 6 in. (Figure I27-3). Move the stronger leg forward, even with the crutches. Repeat the three-point gait.

13. The three-point gait (used for partial or non-weight bearing) provides a strong base of support. This gait can be used if the client has a weak or non-weight-bearing leg.

Two-Point Gait

14. Move the left crutch and right leg forward 4 to 6 in. Move the right crutch and left leg forward 4 to 6 in. Repeat the two-point gait.

14. The two-point gait (used for partial weight bearing) provides a strong base of support. The client must be able to bear weight on both legs. This gait is faster than the four-point gait.

Swing-Through Gait

15. Move both crutches forward together 4 to 6 in. Move both legs forward together in a swinging motion, even with the crutches (Figure I27-4). Repeat the swing-through gait.

15. The swing-through gait (used for people with severe weakness or paralysis of knees or hips) permits a faster pace. This gate requires greater balance and more strength.

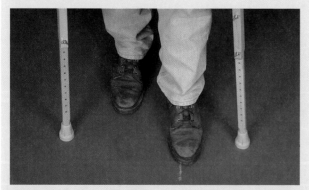

Figure I27-3 Crutch Walking: Three-Point Gait, Advancing Both Crutches and Weaker Leg Forward Together

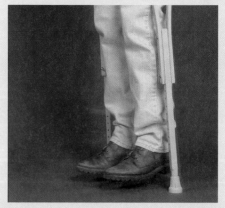

Figure I27-4 Crutch Walking: Swing-Through Gait

Procedure 128   Administering Enteral Tube Feedings

Equipment

- Asepto syringe or 20- to 50-mL syringe
- Clean towel
- Formula
- Water to follow feeding

- Emesis basin
- Disposable gavage bag and tubing
- Infusion pump for feeding tube
- Nonsterile gloves

Action	Rationale

• Wash your hands • Check the client's identification band •
• Explain the procedure to the client prior to beginning •

Action	Rationale
1. Review client's medical record.	1. Verifies physician's prescription for appropriate formula and amount.
2. Gather and assemble equipment. If using a bag, fill with prescribed amount of formula.	2. Promotes efficiency during procedure.
3. Place client on right side in high Fowler's position.	3. Reduces risk of pulmonary aspiration in event client vomits or regurgitates formula.
4. Don nonsterile gloves.	4. Reduces transmission of pathogens from gastric contents.
5. Provide for privacy.	5. Places client at ease.
6. Observe for abdominal distention; auscultate for bowel sounds.	6. Assesses for delayed gastric emptying; indicates presence of peristalsis and ability of GI tract to digest nutrients.
7. Check feeding tube: Insert syringe into adapter port, aspirate stomach contents, and determine amount of gastric residual.	7. Indicates whether gastric emptying is delayed.
• If residual is greater than 50 to 100 mL (or in accordance with agency protocol), hold feeding until residual diminishes.	• Reduces risk of regurgitation and pulmonary aspiration related to gastric distention.
• Instill aspirated contents back into feeding tube.	• Prevents electrolyte imbalance.
8. Administer tube feeding:	8. Provides nutrients as prescribed.

Intermittent—Bolus

Action	Rationale
• Pinch the tubing.	• Prevents air from entering tubing.
• Remove plunger from barrel of syringe and attach to adapter.	• Provides system to delivery feeding.
• Fill syringe with formula (Figure 128-1).	• Allows gravity to control flow rate, reducing risk of diarrhea from bolus feeding.

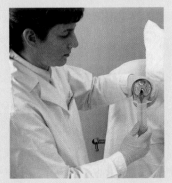

Figure 128-1 Adding Formula to Nasogastric Tube

continued

Action	**Rationale**
• Raise or lower syringe to control rate of feeding.	
• Allow formula to infuse slowly; continue adding formula to syringe until prescribed amount has been administered. Do not allow syringe to empty between fillings.	• Prevents air from entering stomach and reduces risk for gas accumulation.
• Flush tubing with 30 to 50 mL (or prescribed amount) of water.	• Maintains patency of feeding tube.

Intermittent—Gavage Feeding

• Hang bag on IV pole so that it is 18 inches above the client's head.	• Allows gravity to promote infusion of formula.
• Remove air from bag's tubing.	• Prevents air from entering stomach.
• Attach distal end of tubing to feeding tube adapter and adjust drip to infuse over prescribed time.	• Decreases risk of diarrhea.
• When bag empties of formula, add 30 to 60 mL (or prescribed amount) of water; after water is instilled, close clamp.	• Ensures that remaining formula in tubing is administered and maintains patency of tube; prevents air from entering the stomach.
• Wash reusable gavage bag with soap and hot water every 24 hours.	• Decreases risk of multiplication of microorganisms in bag and tubing.

Continuous Gavage

• Check tube placement at least every 4 hours or according to agency policy.	• Ensures that feeding tube remains in stomach.
• Check residual at least every 8 hours or according to agency policy.	• Indicates ability of GI tract to digest and absorb nutrients.
• If residual is greater than 1 to 2 times the hourly rate, hold feeding.	• Reduces risk of regurgitation and pulmonary aspiration related to gastric distention.
• Add prescribed amount of formula to bag for a 3- to 4-hour period; dilute with water if prescribed.	• Provides client with prescribed nutrients and prevents bacterial growth (formula is easily contaminated).
• Hang gavage bag on IV pole.	
• Prime tubing.	• Removes air from tubing.
• Thread tubing through feeding pump and attach distal end of tubing to feeding tube adapter; keep tubing straight between bag and pump.	• Provides for controlled flow rate; prevents loops in tubing.
• Adjust drip rate.	• Infuses formula over prescribed time.
• Monitor infusion rate and signs of respiratory distress or diarrhea.	• Prevents complications associated with continuous gavage.
• Flush tube with water every 4 hours as prescribed or following administration of medications.	• Maintains patency of tube.
• Replace disposable feeding bag at least every 24 hours, in accord with agency's protocol.	• Decreases risks of microorganisms.
• Turn client every 2 hours.	• Promotes digestion and reduces skin breakdown.

continued

Action	Rationale
• Provide oral hygiene every 2 to 4 hours.	• Provides comfort and maintains the integrity of buccal cavity.
9. Administer water as prescribed with and between feedings.	9. Ensures adequate hydration.
10. Clamp proximal end of feeding tube after formula has been administered.	10. Prevents air from entering the tube.
11. Remove gloves and wash hands.	11. Reduces risk of transmission of microorganisms.
12. Record total amount of formula and water administered on I&O form, and client's response to feeding.	12. Documents administration of feeding and achievement of expected outcome; e.g., client tolerates feeding and weight is maintained or increased.

continued

Atlas of Nursing Procedures

A1 Initiating Strict Isolation Precautions

A2 Inserting a Nasogastric or Nasointestinal Tube for Suction and Enteral Feedings

A3 Venipuncture

A4 Preparing an Intravenous Solution

A5 Administering an IV Solution

A6 Administering Medications by IV Piggyback to an Existing IV

A7 Managing IV Therapy and Dressing Change

Procedure A1   Initiating Strict Isolation Precautions

Equipment

- Isolation sign
- Disposable gowns
- Gloves (nonsterile and sterile)
- Tape or bag ties
- Room with sink and running water
- Soap and paper towels
- Water pitcher, cups, and fresh water
- Other supplies relative to client's condition for example, dressings for wound care

- Goggles or face shield
- Disposable cups
- Disposable masks or face shield
- Impermeable bags (linen and trash)
- Disposable vital signs equipment (single-use thermometers, stethoscope, and sphygmomanometer), if available
- Linen
- Specimen containers and labels

Action	Rationale
• *Wash your hands* • *Check the client's identification band* • *Explain the procedure to the client prior to beginning* • *Note: You must don barrier protection before checking the client's ID* •	

1. Review physician orders and agency protocols relative to the type of isolation precautions:
 	
  a. Implement protocol related to the type of disinfectants needed to eliminate specific microorganisms.
 	
  b. Alert housekeeping regarding the room number and type of isolation supplies needed in the room.
 	
  c. Make sure the room has proper ventilation (the door will have to remain closed at all times) and that the bed and other electrical equipment are functioning properly.
	1. Ensures compliance without unnecessary stress being placed on the client and family. Allows housekeeping to have the necessary supplies on their cleaning carts. Provides for client comfort and decreases the spread of microorganisms. Limits the number of personnel coming into the client's room and the client's exposure to microorganisms.

2. Place appropriate isolation supplies outside the client's room and place isolation sign on the door.	2. Ensures staff follows isolation protocol and alerts visitors to check with the nurses' station before entering the room.

3. Gather appropriate supplies to take in the room:
 	
  a. Soap and paper towels
 	
  b. Linen
 	
  c. Impermeable bags
 	
  d. Disposable vital signs equipment, if available
 	
  e. Wound care supplies, if appropriate
	3. Provides for organized care, handwashing, proper isolation, and client care materials. Decreases the spread of microorganisms and the number of times caregivers have to go into and out of the room.

4. Remove jewelry, lab coat, and other items not necessary for providing client care.	4. Decreases the spread of resident and transient microorganisms.
5. Wash hands and don disposable clothing: a. Apply mask by placing the top of the mask over the bridge of your nose (top part of mask has a lightweight metal strip) and pinch the metal strip to fit snugly against your skin.	5. Disposable garments act as a barrier protecting the nurses from contact with pathogens.

continued

Action	**Rationale**

b. Apply cap to cover hair and ears completely, if policy requires cap.

c. Apply gown to cover outer garments completely: Hold gown in front of body and place arms through sleeves (Figure A1-1A). Pull sleeves down to wrist. Tie gown securely at neck and waist (see Figure A1-1B, C).

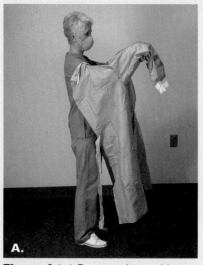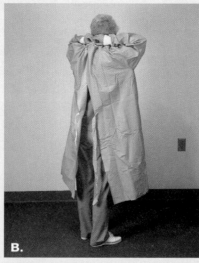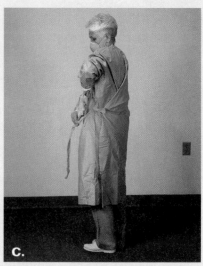

Figure A1-1 Donning disposable gown: A. Hold gown in front of the body and place arms through the sleeves. B. Fasten neck ties. C. Fasten waist ties.

d. Don nonsterile gloves and pull gloves to cover gown's cuff.

e. Don goggles.

6. Enter client's room with all gathered supplies; if client is to receive medications, bring them with you at this time. Arrange and store supplies and equipment.

6. Prevents trips into and out of client room and keeps supplies clean.

7. Assess client and family knowledge relative to client's diagnosed infection and isolation:

7. Client's and family's understanding of isolation procedures will increase their participation in care.

a. Reason isolation initiated

b. Type of isolation

c. Duration of isolation

d. How to apply barrier protection

8. Assess vital signs, administer medications if appropriate, and perform other functions of nursing care to meet the needs of the client. Record assessment data on a piece of paper, avoiding contact with any articles in the client's room.

8. Allows for data collection and the performance of client care measures.

9. Dispose of soiled articles in the impermeable bags, which should be labeled correctly according to contents. If soiled reusable equipment is removed from the room, label bag accordingly.

9. Impermeable bags prevent the leakage of contaminated materials, thereby preventing the spread of infection. Labeling is a warning to other personnel that the contents are infectious.

continued

Action	**Rationale**
10. Double bag soiled linen according to agency policy in an impermeable bag or in plastic linen bag.	10. Double bagging allows the washing of soiled linen without human contact. When linen is double bagged, the first bag is removed prior to washing and the second bag goes into the machine with the dirty linen and dissolves.
11. Replenish supplies before leaving the client's room by having another staff member bring the clean supplies and transfer at the door. Ask client if anything is needed (e.g., juice or personal care items).	11. Decreases the number of times staff members have to go in and out of the room and exposure to microorganisms.
12. Before leaving, let the client know when you will return and make sure call light is accessible.	12. Decreases a feeling of abandonment; provides client with a means of communication.
13. Exiting the isolation room: a. Untie gown at waist. b. Remove one glove by grasping the glove's cuff and pulling down so that the glove turns inside out (glove on glove) and dispose of it. With your ungloved hand, slip your fingers inside the cuff of the other glove, pull it off, inside out, and dispose of it.	13. Gloves are removed inside out to avoid contact with skin. The gown is removed and folded with hands touching only the inside of the garment. Only the ties and the inside of the cap are touched with your hands. All articles are disposed of as soon as they are removed.
c. Grasp and release the ties of the mask, and dispose of it.	c. If a client has a disease spread by airborne pathogens, you may remove the mask last.
d. Release neck ties of the gown and allow the gown to fall forward. Place fingers of dominant hand inside cuff of other hand and pull down over other hand (Figure A1-2A). With gown covered hand, pull gown over the dominant hand (Figure A1-2B). While gown is still on arm, fold outside of gown together, remove, and dispose of it (Figure A1-2C).	

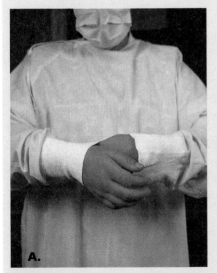 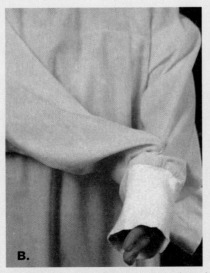 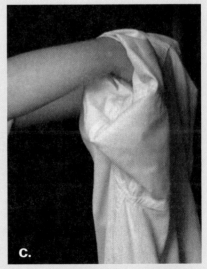

Figure A1-2 Removing disposable gown: A. Place fingers of dominant hand inside the cuff of other hand and pull gown down over other hand. B. With the gown-covered hand, pull gown down over dominant hand. C. As the gown is removed, fold the outside of the gown together and dispose of it.

continued

Action	Rationale
e. Remove cap by slipping your finger under the cap and removing from the front to back and dispose of it.	
14. Wash hands for 10 minutes. Don nonsterile gloves and remove bags from the client's room. Exit room and close door. Dispose of bags according to agency protocol. Remove gloves and wash hands.	**14.** Decreases likelihood of transmission of micro-organisms.

Procedure A2 — Inserting a Nasogastric or Nasointestinal Tube for Suction and Enteral Feedings

Equipment

- Nonsterile gloves
- Cup of ice or water and straw
- Towel and tissues
- Flashlight or penlight
- Hypoallergenic tape, rubber band, safety pin
- 20-mL syringe or asepto syringe
- Disposable irrigation set (optional)
- Wall mount or portable suction equipment as available
- Stethoscope
- Personal protective equipment: gown, gloves, face shield (or goggles and mask)

- Ice chips in an emesis basin
- Water-soluble lubricant
- Tongue blade
- pH chemstrip
- Number 6, 8, 12 French tube for gastric suction (Levine, Salem, or Anderson) or a small-bore feeding tube, 8 or 12 French tube (Keofeed, Dubbhoff, Moss)
- Administration set with pump or controller for feeding tube

Action	Rationale
• *Wash your hands* • *Explain the procedure to the client prior to beginning* • *Check the client's identification band* •	
1. Review client's medical record.	**1.** Confirms physician's prescription for inserting a nasogastric tube; history of nasal or sinus problems.
Nasogastric Tube Insertion	
2. Gather equipment. Place rubber tubes only in basin of ice. Wash hands.	**2.** Promotes efficiency. Stiffens tube for easier insertion. Reduces transfer of microorganisms.
3. Provide for privacy.	**3.** Reduces anxiety.
4. Place client in Fowler's position, at least a 45° angle or higher, with a pillow behind client's shoulders. *Place comatose clients in semi-Fowler's position.*	**4.** Facilitates passage of the tube into the esophagus and swallowing.
5. Place towel over client's chest; put tissues in reach.	**5.** Prevents soiling of gown and bedding; lacrimation can occur during insertion through nasal passages.
6. Examine nostrils and assess as client breathes through each nostril.	**6.** Determines the most patent nostril to facilitate insertion.

continued

Action	Rationale
7. Measure length of tubing needed by using tube as a tape measure (gloves are optional at this step).	**7.** Approximates length of tube needed to reach stomach.

- Measure from end of client's nose to earlobe to xyphoid process of sternum (Figure A2-1).

- If tube is to go below stomach (nasoduodenal or nasojejunal), add an additional 15 to 20 cm.

- Place a small piece of tape on tube to mark length.

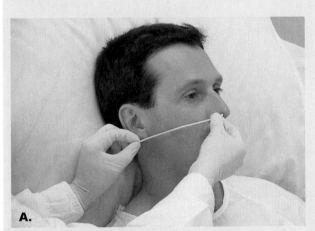

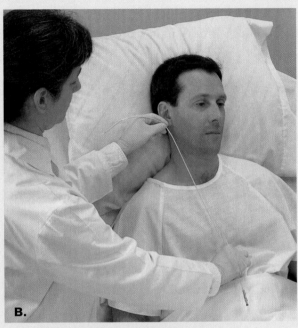

Figure A2-1 A. Measuring From End of Nose to Earlobe; B. Measuring From Earlobe to Xyphoid Process

Action	Rationale
8. Have client blow nose and encourage swallowing of water if level of consciousness and treatment plan permit.	**8.** Clears nasal passage without pushing micro-organisms into inner ear; facilitates passage of tube.
9. Apply personal protective equipment.	**9.** Protects nurse from body fluids.
10. Lubricate first 6 to 8 inches of tube with water-soluble lubricant.	**10.** Facilitates passage into the nares.
11. Insert tube as follows (institutional policy will dictate which personnel are authorized to perform steps 11 to 13):	**11.** Promotes passage of tube with minimal trauma to mucosa.

- Gently pass tube into nostril to back of throat (client may gag); aim tube toward back of throat and down.

- When client feels tube in back of throat, use flashlight or penlight to locate tip of tube.

- Instruct client to flex head toward chest.

- Instruct client to swallow, offer ice chips or water, and advance tube as client swallows.

- If resistance is met, rotate tube slowly with downward advancement toward client's closest ear; do not force tube.

- Ensures tip's placement.

- Opens esophagus and assists in tube insertion after tube has passed through nasopharynx and reduces risk of tube entering trachea.

- Assists in pushing tube past oropharynx.

- Tube may be coiled or kinked or in the oropharynx or trachea.

continued

Action	Rationale
12. Withdraw tube immediately if changes occur in respiratory status.	**12.** Indicates placement of tube in the bronchus or lung.
13. Advance tube, giving client sips of water, until taped mark is reached.	**13.** Assists with tube insertion.
14. Check placement of tube:	**14.** Ensures proper placement in the stomach; pH below 3, tube is in stomach; a pH range of 6 to 7 indicates intestinal sites.

• Attach syringe to free end of tube and aspirate sample of gastric contents and measure with chemstrip pH (Figure A2-2).

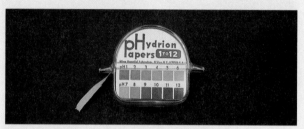

Figure A2-2 For Measuring pH of Aspirate

• Inject 10 mL of air into tube and listen, using a stethoscope, for simultaneous gurgling over epigastrum.

Action	Rationale
15. Leave syringe attached to free end of tube.	**15.** Prevents leakage of gastric contents.
16. If prescribed, obtain x-ray.	**16.** Confirms correct placement; if nasoduodenal or nasojejunal feedings are required, passage through pylorus may require several days.
17. Secure tube with tape as shown in Figure A2-3.	**17.** Prevents tube from becoming dislodged.

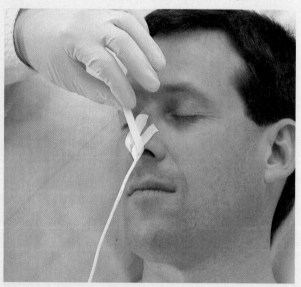

Figure A2-3 Securing Tube to the Client's Nose with Tape

• Split a 4-inch piece of tape to a length of 2 inches and secure tube with tape by placing the intact end of the tape over the bridge of the nose. Wrap split ends around the tube as it exits the nose.

• Prevents trauma to nasal mucosa by reducing pressure on nares.

continued

Action	Rationale
• Place a rubber band, using a slip knot, around the exposed tube (12–18 inches from nose toward chest); after x-ray, pin rubber band to client's gown.	• Allows client movement without causing friction on nares; metal devices are removed for x-rays to prevent artifacts.
18. Instruct client about movements that can dislodge the tube.	18. Reduces anxiety and teaches client how to prevent tugging on tube with head movement.
19. Gastric decompression:	19. Provides for decompression as prescribed by physician; intermittent or continuous suctioning is determined by type of tube inserted.
• Remove syringe from free end of tube and connect tube to suction tubing; set machine on type of suction and pressure as prescribed.	
• Levine tubes are connected to intermittent low pressure.	
• Salem sump or Anderson's tube may be connected to continuous low suction.	
• Observe nature and amount of gastric tube drainage.	• Provides information about patency of tube and gastric contents.
• Assess client for nausea, vomiting, and abdominal distention.	• Indicates effectiveness of intervention.
20. Provide oral hygiene and cleanse nares with a tissue.	20. Promotes comfort.
21. Remove personal protective equipment, dispose of in proper container, and wash hands.	21. Reduces transmission of microorganisms; protects other workers from coming into contact with objects contaminated with body fluids.
22. Position client for comfort, and place call light in easy reach.	22. Promotes comfort and safety.
23. Document:	23. Promotes continuity of care and shows implementation of intervention.
• The reason for the tube insertion.	
• The type of tube inserted.	
• The type (intermittent or continuous) of suctioning and pressure setting.	
• The nature and amount of aspirate and drainage.	
• The client's tolerance of the procedure.	
• The effectiveness of the intervention, such as nausea relieved.	

Insertion of a Small-Bore Feeding Tube

Action	Rationale
24. Follow steps 1 through 8 as stated earlier.	24. See steps 1 through 8.
25. Open adapter cap on tube, snap off end of water vial, and inject water into feeding tube adapter.	25. Activates Keolube lubricant in tube's lumen.
26. Close adapter cap.	26. Ensures a tight fit so water does not leak from adapter site.
27. Check that stylet does not protrude through holes in feeding tube; adjust as necessary.	27. Prevents mucosa trauma.

continued

Action	Rationale
28. Follow steps 9 through 13 as stated earlier.	**28.** See steps 9 through 13.
29. Check placement of tube: • Aspirate gastric contents with Luer-Lok syringe; see Figure A2-4.	**29.** Assures correct placement has been achieved; provides measurement of pH of secretions, as explained in step 14.

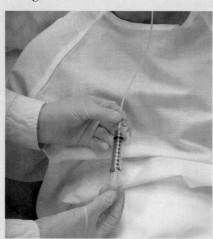

Figure A2-4 Aspirating Gastric Contents with Luer-Lok Syringe with Stylet in Place

Action	Rationale
• Measure pH of aspirate with chemstrip pH.	
30. Leave stylet in place until x-ray confirms placement in case tube needs to be advanced into the duodenum or jejunum.	**30.** Provides a safety measure.
31. Obtain x-ray. Remove stylet from feeding tube after x-ray, and plug open end of tube until feeding.	**31.** Confirms placement of tube prior to instilling formula; prevents gastric juices from seeping out of the tube.
32. Follow steps 20 through 23.	**32.** See steps 20 through 23.
33. Replace small-bore tube every 3 to 4 weeks.	**33.** Prevents obstruction and sepsis of small-bore tubes.

Procedure A3   Venipuncture

Equipment

- Sterile packages of 70% isopropanol (antiseptic) and povidone-iodine (topical antiinfectant)
- Sterile needle and syringe or vacutainer system (20- or 21-gauge needle for cubital vein puncture on an adult)
- Sterile 2 × 2 cotton gauze
- Tourniquet
- Nonsterile gloves
- Bandage or sterile adhesive bandage
- Collecting tubes

continued

Action	Rationale

• Wash your hands • Check the client's identification band •
• Explain the procedure to the client prior to beginning •

1. Place client in a sitting or supine position; lower side rail.

2. Prepare supplies:
   - Open sterile packages.
   - Label specimen tubes with the client's data, according to agency policy.

3. Position arm straight. If possible, place extremity in dependent position.

4. Apply the tourniquet 6 to 10 cm above the elbow. Tourniquet should only obstruct venous blood flow, not arterial. Check for a distal pulse.

5. Select a dilated vein (Figure A3-1). If a vein is not visible, instruct client to open and close a fist; or stroke extremity from proximal to distal, tap lightly over a vein, apply warmth.

1. Promotes client comfort; provides access to the site.

2. Promotes efficiency; ensures accuracy of specimen collection regarding the client's identifying data, date and time of collection.

3. Provides access to vein. Increases venous dilation and visibility.

4. Restricted arterial blood flow prevents venous filling.

5. Assists in veins filling with blood.

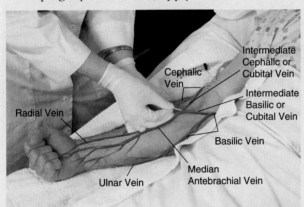

Figure A3-1 Nurse selects site for venipuncture and holds skin taut over site with needle held at 30° angle.

6. Palpate the vein for size and pliancy; be sure it is well seated.

7. Release the tourniquet if it has been on for a lengthy period of time, or if the client is uncomfortable.

8. Cleanse puncture site with isopropanol, let dry and cleanse with povidone-iodine, let dry or wipe with sterile gauze; do not touch site after cleansing. If the client is allergic to iodine, only use isopropanol and cleanse skin for 30 seconds (or according to agency policy).

9. Place equipment in easy reach and position yourself to access the puncture site.

10. Reapply the tourniquet (time should not exceed 3 minutes).

6. Locates a well dilated vein; vein does not roll.

7. Prevents hemoconcentration.

8. Povidone-iodine reduces bacteria on the skin's surface; it must dry to be effective.

9. Promotes efficiency.

10. Restricts blood flow, distends vein.

continued

Action	Rationale
11. Don gloves.	11. Decreases exposure to blood-borne organisms.
12. Perform venipuncture:	12.
• Remove cap from 20- or 21-gauge needle.	• Large-bore needle prevents hemolysis.
• With nondominant hand, stabilize the vein by holding the skin taut over the puncture site (apply downward tension on the forearm with your thumb).	• Prevents the vein from rolling when the needle is pushed against the outer wall of the vein.
• With dominant hand, hold the needle bevel facing upward at an approximately 10° to 30° angle to the arm (refer back to Figure A3-1).	• Provides for a downward movement toward vein.
• Puncture the skin into the straightest part of vein with a steady, moderately fast movement, (When the vein is entered you will feel a slight give and can see blood at the needle's hub.)	• Decreases risk of going through the vein, decreases discomfort.
• Apply moderate negative pressure by puncturing the vacuum tube or by gently retracting the syringe plunger. (When first performing a venipuncture, use a syringe. It takes greater dexterity to puncture the vacuum tube with a two-sided needle; if you apply too much pressure you will go through the vein.)	
13. Remove the tourniquet once blood is flowing into the tube or syringe; collect the specimen(s).	13. Prevents hemolysis.
14. Remove the needle and immediately apply pressure to site for 2 to 3 minutes or 5 to 10 minutes if client is taking anticoagulant medication. Keep the arm straight.	14. Decreases bleeding. Bending the arm can reopen the puncture site.
15. Have the client maintain pressure on the puncture site.	15. Facilitates clotting.
• *Note:* Green stoppers contain sodium heparin (anticoagulant); they must be mixed promptly after collection.	• Prevents coagulation of blood in test tube.
16. Apply a sterile bandage or adhesive bandage to puncture site.	16. Facilitates clotting.
17. If using a needle and syringe, transfer the blood into test tube under moderate pressure.	17. Prevents hemolysis.
18. Dispose the needle or needle-syringe into a sharps container.	18. Prevents needle stick.
19. Remove gloves; wash hands.	19. Decreases transmission of microorganisms.
20. Document venipuncture, amount of blood collected, and client's response.	20. Provides record of venipuncture and client's status.

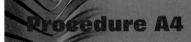

Procedure A4   Preparing an Intravenous Solution

Equipment

- IV solution (bag or bottle)
- Extension set
- IV line filter

- Administration set (vented or nonvented)
- IV pole

Action	Rationale
1. Wash hands before preparing IV equipment.	1. Decreases the transmission of microorganisms.
2. Check the physician's order for the type and amount of solution.	2. Ensures the correct type and amount of fluid.
3. Check IV solution and equipment for expiration dates.	3. Ensures the sterility of the solution and item.
4. Select IV tubing in accord with agency policy.	4. Agency protocols reflect which items of equipment are to be used with specific IV solutions and to complement volume control devices.
5. Prepare IV solution label with client's name, date, time, additives, and your initials (according to agency policy).	5. Provides information to other health care workers relative to when the solution was hung and what additives are infusing in the solution.

Plastic Bag

Action	Rationale
6. Prepare the IV solution bag for administration: • Remove outer wrapper around IV bag of solution. • Inspect bag for tears or leaks by noting any moisture on the protective covering. • Apply gentle pressure and observe for leakage. • Examine solution for discoloration, cloudiness, or particulate matter by holding the bag against a dark and light background; if there is any evidence of contamination, do not use, and return bag to agency's dispensing department.	6. Ensures that solution is free of contamination; contaminated solutions are returned to central supply or pharmacy for manufacturer notification.
7. Remove administration set from the package and close the roller clamp on the IV tubing (Figure A4-1).	7. Prevents solution from escaping into the tubing until the drip chamber on the tubing has been primed.

Figure A4-1 Remove tubing from the package, leaving the protective caps on both ends intact.

continued

Action	**Rationale**
8. Remove the protective cap from the nonvented IV tubing spike and maintain the sterility of the spike.	8. Prepares the sterile spike for insertion into the IV container; IV bags have a vented port.
9. Grasp the port of the IV bag with your nondominant hand. With your dominant hand, remove the plastic tab covering the port (Figure A4-2) and insert the full length of the spike into the bag's port (Figure A4-3).	9. Prevents contamination of both the port and the spike.

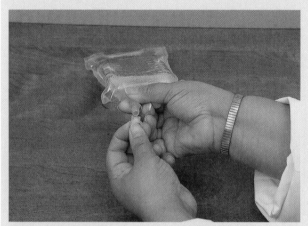

Figure A4-2 Open the IV plastic bag and pull down the plastic tab covering the port with one hand while pinching the port with the other hand.

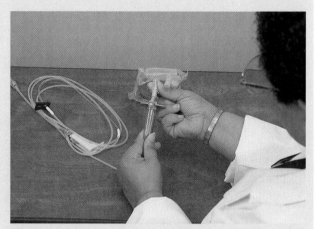

Figure A4-3 Remove the cap from the spike and spike the IV port.

Action	**Rationale**
10. Squeeze and quickly release pressure on the drip chamber of the IV tubing until the chamber is one-third to one-half full. Hang bag on IV pole.	10. Primes the chamber by displacing air with IV solution, allowing half of the chamber to remain free of solution.
11. Connect IV filter to tubing (if required).	11. Reduces the risk for bacteremia and the incidence of infusion phlebitis; tapping the filter as the solution runs through it eliminates any air bubbles trapped in the filter's membrane.
• Remove cap from filter.	
• Fit tubing's male adapter into filter's female connector, and twist to ensure tight connection.	
• Hold filter so connector joint is pointed down.	
• Hold tubing's end tip higher than the tubing's dependent loop to displace the air.	
• Open roller clamp on IV tubing to prime the tubing and filter (Figure A4-4).	
• Tap the filter as the IV solution runs through.	
• Close the roller clamp on the IV tubing.	
12. Replace the cap on the IV tubing's free end.	12. Maintains the sterility of the system.
13. Attach a Dial-a-Flo fluid regulator at the end of the IV tubing if fluids are to be administered with this device. With the cap off the end of the tubing, turn the Dial-a-Flo to the open position, open all the tubing regulator clamps, and clear the tubing of air; close the regulator clamp and replace the cap on the end of the tubing.	13. Controls the rate of infusion.

continued

Action	Rationale

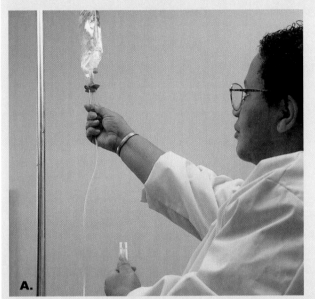

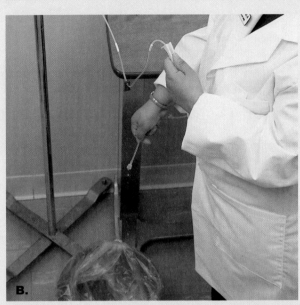

Figure A4-4 A. Prime the IV Tubing. B. Open the roller clamp on the tubing to allow the fluid to enter the tube and expel the air.

14. Tag tubing with date and time and your own initials (according to agency policy).

15. Explain to the client what you are doing before taking the IV equipment into the client's room.

Glass Bottle

16. Follow steps 1–5.
   - Vented tubing is used for glass bottles that are not vented.

17. Prepare the IV solution for administration.
   - Check bottle for cracks or leaks.
   - Remove metal cap, metal disk, and rubber diaphragm from top of glass bottle, or remove protective additive cap if pharmacy has added medications to the IV bottle.
   - Listen for the escape of air when the rubber diaphragm is removed.

18. Close the roller clamp on the IV tubing.

19. Remove the protective cap from the IV tubing spike and maintain the sterility of the spike.

20. Place the glass bottle on a firm surface, and, using firm downward pressure, insert the spike through designated port on the bottle cap.

21. Invert IV bottle (if the bottle is vented, the fluid inside the vent tube will escape), and hang the bottle on an IV pole.

22. Continue steps 10–15.

14. Indicates when tubing replacement is due (no more frequently than every 72 hours, in accord with agency protocol).

15. Elicits client's cooperation.

16. Same as for steps 1–5.

17. Ensures that solution is free of contamination; contaminated solutions are returned to central supply or pharmacy for manufacturer notification. Escape of air indicates the breaking of the vacuum inside the bottle, which will allow the fluid to flow into the tubing.

18. Stops flow of fluid.

19. Prevents contamination.

20. Pressure is required to puncture the rubber stopper in the neck of the IV bottle.

21. Allows gravity to displace the air in the IV tubing when the roller clamp is opened.

22. Same as for steps 10–15.

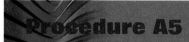

Procedure A5   Administering an IV Solution

Equipment

Adding Solution to a Continuous Infusion Line
• Prepared IV solution and medication

Adding a Solution to an Existing Heparin or PI Lock
• Prepared IV solution system with needleless locking cannula
• Alcohol or iodophor swab

• Needleless injection cap (if one is not in place)
• 2 prefilled syringes of 2 mL each of normal saline
• Nonsterile gloves

Action	Rationale
• Wash your hands • Check the client's identification band • *• Explain the procedure to the client prior to beginning •*	
1. Gather prepared equipment (solution labeled with the client's name, and time-taped for fluids to infuse per hour, according to agency policy.	1. Ensures correct fluids to be administered to the right client at the prescribed infusion rate.
2. Don gloves if you have to perform a venipuncture or connect the tubing to an existing PI. *Gloves are not necessary if you are adding fluids to an existing infusion line.*	2. Decreases risk of transmission of microorganisms.
3. Assess the puncture site.	3. Indicates signs of infiltration or infection.
• Observe for redness and puffiness.	
• Palpate for tenderness.	
4. Check patency of infusion site.	4. Verifies patency of IV system with venous access device in the client's vein.
• Verify that fluid is infusing.	
• If necessary, remove IV container from the pole and lower the container below the level of infusion site.	
• Observe for backflow of blood into the hub of the venous access device.	
• Replace container on IV pole.	

Adding Solution to a Continuous Infusion Line

Action	Rationale
5. Check the date on the tubing tag; if the tubing needs changing, refer to Procedure A4.	5. Indicates when tubing replacement is due.
6. Hang the new bag of fluids on the IV pole and remove the cover from the port.	6. Provides easy access to the fluids.
7. Remove the current infusion bag of fluids from the IV pole.	7. Makes it easier to remove tubing spike.
8. While maintaining aseptic technique, remove the tubing spike from the port of the infusing bag of fluids and reinsert the tubing spike into the port on the new bag of fluids; push the full length of the spike into the port.	8. Maintains the sterility of the IV system.
9. Set the infusion rate.	9. Produces correct drip rate.

continued

Action	Rationale

Manual Rate Regulation

- Open regulator clamp; close slowly while observing the drip chamber until the fluid is dripping at a slow, steady pace.

- Count the number of drops for a full minute; for example, if the drop factor of tubing is 10 drops/mL then the drop rate should be 21 drops/minute to infuse 1000 mL/8 hours (Figure A5-1).

- Determines patency of venous access device.

- Determines number of drops falling per minute.

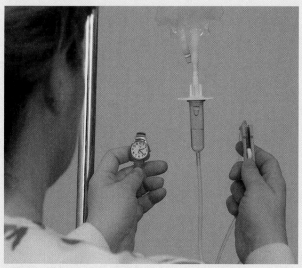

Figure A5-1 Manual Rate Regulation: Counting the Number of Drops for a One-Minute Interval

- Open the regulator clamp slowly to increase the drip flow rate; close the regulator clamp to decrease the drip rate to achieve 21 drops/minute.

- Recount the drop rate after 5 and 15 minutes.

- Proceed to steps 10–17.

- Controls drip rate with regular clamp.

- Detects changes in rate due to expansion and contraction of tubing.

Dial-a-Flo Regulation

- Turn Dial-a-Flo regulator until arrow is aligned with desired volume of fluid to infuse over 1 hour.

- Check drip rate for a full minute.

- Adjust height of IV pole if necessary.

- Recount drip rate after 5 minutes and again after 15 minutes.

- Proceed to steps 10–17.

- Regulates infusion of fluid at the desired rate.

- Verifies calculated drip rate with infusion rate.

- Facilitates flow by gravity.

- Detects changes in rate due to expansion and contraction of tubing.

Infusion Controller or Pump Regulation

- Insert tubing into infusion controller or pump in accord with manufacturer's instruction (Figure A5-2).

- Ensures proper functioning of the device.

continued

Action	**Rationale**

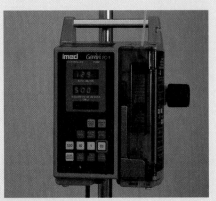

Figure A5-2 IV Tubing Threaded into an Infusion Pump with Controls Set

• Close door to controller or pump and open all tubing clamps and regulators.	• Allows controller or pump to regulate the infusion rate.
• Set machine to regulate the volume to infuse per hour or drops per minute in accord with the type of machine. Also set the total volume to be infused.	• Determines amount of fluid the device will deliver.
• Push the *start* or *on* button.	• Initiates the device's regulation of the fluid flow.
• Proceed to steps 10–17.	

Volume Control Chamber (Buretrol) Regulation

• Close regulators both above and below the chamber.	• Allows for precise release of fluids into the chamber.
• If adding a new Buretrol, open regulator above the chamber and fill the chamber with 10 mL of fluid, close the top regulator, and slowly open the regulator below the chamber to remove air from the tubing. Close the bottom regulator (Figure A5-3).	• Facilitates priming the drip chamber and clearing the tubing below the chamber of air.

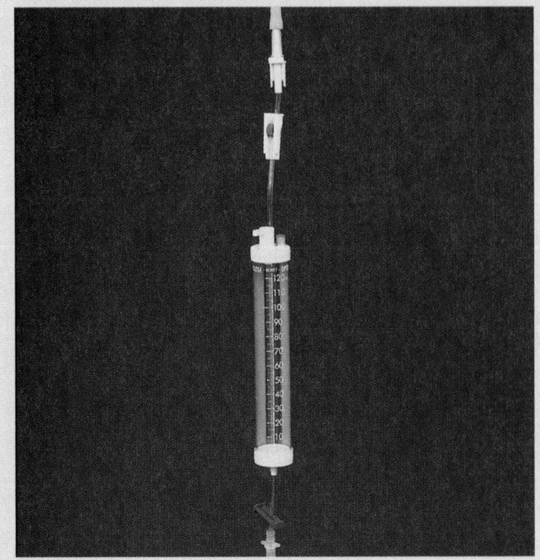

Figure A5-3 Volume Control Chamber

continued

Action	Rationale
• Open the top regulator and fill the chamber with the volume of fluid to infuse in 1 hour or 2 hours if the volume is small.	• Facilitates close monitoring of fluid volume.
• Close top regulator and ensure that air vent is open.	• Allows fluid to escape from the chamber.
• Open bottom regulator and regulate drops to calculated drip rate in accord with the drop factor.	• Determines volume to infuse over an hour.
• Count drip rate for a full minute.	• Verifies rate of infusion.
• Time-tape the chamber if a controller or pump is not used.	• Facilitates easy check of fluid infusion and shows when to add fluid to the chamber.
• Check chamber every 1 to 2 hours depending on the volume placed in the chamber.	• Maintains fluid infusion and prevents air from entering the chamber and tubing if all fluid is infused.
• Proceed with steps 10–17.	
10. On the time tape, write the time the fluids were initiated and your initials.	10. Facilitates easy check of fluid infusion progress as prescribed.
11. Monitor the volume delivered every 1 to 2 hours and compare with the time tape.	11. Ensures the actual volume being delivered.
12. If fluids are not infusing at the prescribed rate as indicated by time tape:	12. Ensures that prescribed amount of fluid is delivered.
• Check setting on controller or pump or Dial-a-Flo and adjust as indicated.	
• Increase height of IV pole.	• Allows gravity to facilitate the drip rate.
• Assess puncture site, reposition the venous access device, lower the IV fluid container below the puncture site and observe for a backflow of blood. Replace container on pole.	• Ensures that venous access device is still in the vein.
13. Instruct client to limit movement of puncture site and to notify a nurse of any problems or discomfort.	13. Facilitates early detection of problems.
14. Apply an armboard as a last resort (Figure A5-4).	14. Immobilizes the extremity receiving the infusion.

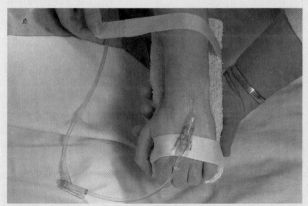

Figure A5-4 Positioning of Client with an IV Armboard

continued

Action	**Rationale**
15. Position the client for comfort and place the call light in easy reach.	**15.** Promotes client comfort and safety.
16. Wash hands and dispose of used supplies.	**16.** Decreases transmission of microorganisms.
17. Document on the client's medical record: • Time of initiation of fluid infusion. • Type and volume of fluid infusing. • Infusion device used, if applicable. • Status of the venous access insertion site. • Problems encountered: for example, if venous access device is repositioned. • Client's tolerance to the fluid infusion. • Client teaching and learning.	**17.** Provides a record of the nursing intervention and the client's response.

Adding a Secondary Line, Additive Bag (IV Piggyback)

Refer to Procedure A6.

Adding a Solution to an Existing Heparin or PI Lock

Action	**Rationale**
18. Follow steps 1–3.	**18.** Same as for steps 1–3.
19. Hang IV solution on IV pole.	**19.** Provides easy access to system.
20. Don nonsterile gloves and cleanse needleless injection port with alcohol or iodophor swab. Allow to dry.	**20.** Reduces risk of transmission of microorganisms.
21. Insert saline syringe into port, slowly aspirate, and observe for blood; flush system and observe for swelling at puncture site.	**21.** Indicates a patent system and, with the presence of blood and lack of swelling, that the needle is probably in the vein.
22. Connect needleless locking cannula into injection port, open tubing clamp, and adjust rate as indicated in step 9.	**22.** Ensures administration of solution at the correct drip rate.
23. Dispose of equipment and gloves in proper receptacle and wash hands.	**23.** Reduces risk of transmission of pathogens.
24. When secondary bag and drip chamber are empty, don gloves, close the clamp, and disconnect the needleless locking cannula from the port's lock.	**24.** Indicates infusion of all of the solution.
25. Flush port with second saline syringe and place sterile needleless injection cap on the port.	**25.** Clears the line and reduces the risk of contaminating the port.
26. Dispose of equipment and gloves in proper receptacle and wash hands.	**26.** Reduces risk of transmission of pathogens.
27. Record fluid administration on MAR and client response in nurses' notes.	**27.** Documents nursing intervention and any client adverse reactions.

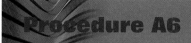

Procedure A6

Administering Medications by IV Piggyback to an Existing IV

Equipment

- Prepared and labeled medication solution bag
- Alcohol swab

- Secondary administration set
- Needle or needleless locking cannula if needleless system used.

Action	Rationale
• *Check the client's identification band* • *Explain the procedure to the client prior to beginning* •	
1. Gather prepared equipment (medication labeled with the client's name, and time tape for fluids to infuse per hour).	1. Ensures correct fluids to be administered to the right client at the infusion rate prescribed by the physician.
2. Wash hands. *Gloves are not necessary if you are adding fluids to an existing infusion line.*	2. Decreases risk of transmission of microorganisms.
3. Assess the puncture site.	3. Indicates signs of infiltration or infection.
• Observe for redness and puffiness.	
• Palpate for tenderness.	
4. Check patency of infusion site.	4. Verifies patency of IV system with venous access device in the client's vein.
• Observe fluid infusing.	
• If necessary, remove IV container from the pole and lower the container below the level of infusion site.	
• Observe for backflow of blood into the hub of the venous access device.	
• Replace container on IV pole.	
5. Secure medication bag and check physician's order and the MAR.	5. Ensures the correct client, medication, dosage, route, and frequency.
6. Check the client's chart for allergies and check the drug compatibility chart.	6. Ensures that the client is not allergic to the drug and that the prescribed drug is compatible with the primary IV solution.
7. Hang the secondary bag on IV pole.	7. Provides easy access for preparation.
8. Add the administration set to the secondary bag and prime the tubing.	8. Removes the air from the tubing.
9. Affix a needleless locking cannula to the end of tubing (Figure A6-1A).	9. Reduces risk of exposure to IV needles.
10. Cleanse needleless Y-site injection port of primary IV tubing closest to infusion site with an alcohol swab, allow to dry.	10. Reduces risk of transmission of microorganisms.
11. Insert needleless locking cannula of secondary bag set into Y-site injection port of primary set (Figure A6-1B).	11. Provides access for infusion and prevents dislodgement of needleless locking cannula.
12. Affix the extension hook to the primary bag on the IV pole so that the primary bag hangs below the level of the secondary bag.	12. Ceases flow of primary solution because of an increased hydrostatic pressure in secondary bag.

continued

Action	Rationale
13. Open clamp of secondary tubing and adjust drip rate to desired infusion rate.	**13.** Allows solution in the secondary bag to infuse at the prescribed drip rate.
• Slowly close the regular clamp while observing the drip chamber until the fluid is dripping at a slow, steady pace (Figure A6-1C).	

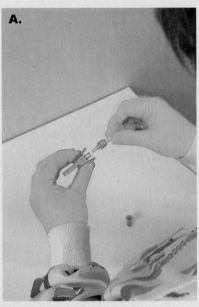
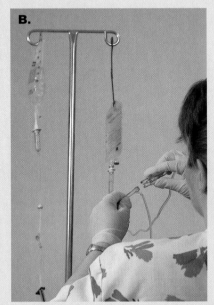
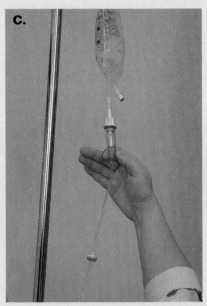

Figure A6-1 Administering Medications by IV Piggyback. A. Connect a needleless locking cannula to a secondary infusion line. B. Connect locking cannula to a Y-site injection port of primary infusion set. C. Monitor the infusion rate. (Gloves are not required for this procedure.)

Action	Rationale
• Count the drops for a full minute, e.g., if the drop factor of tubing is 10 drops/mL then the drop rate should be 10 drops/minute to infuse 50 mL in 50 minutes.	• Determines number of drops falling per minute.
• Recount the drop rate in 5 minutes.	• Detects changes in rate due to expansion and contraction of tubing.
14. Observe client for any signs of adverse reactions to the medication.	**14.** Provides for immediate intervention if client has an adverse reaction.
15. When secondary bag and drip chamber are empty, close the clamp on secondary system, readjust drip rate of primary solution as indicated, and remove the secondary system (or leave in place, according to agency policy).	**15.** Allows the primary solution to infuse at prescribed drip rate.
16. Record medication infusion on the MAR and note any client responses in the nurses' notes.	**16.** Documents the nursing intervention.

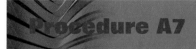

Procedure A7   Managing IV Therapy and Dressing Change

Equipment

Assessing and Changing IV Tubing
- Nonsterile gloves (use for contact with bodily fluids)

- Administration sets (as determined by tubing to be replaced

Troubleshooting an IV System
- Nonsterile gloves
- Sterile needle and 5-cc syringe with 2 mL normal saline or needleless system.

- 70% isopropyl alcohol or povidone-iodine swab (check for client allergy to iodine)

Changing a Gown
- Clean gown

Converting to an Intermittent Infusion Device
- Nonsterile gloves
- Protective pad
- Needleless injection cap

- Sterile needle and 3-cc syringe with 2 mL of normal saline or needleless system

Changing a Peripheral IV Dressing
- Protective pad
- Tape (check for client allergy to tape)
- 70% isopropyl alcohol or povidone-iodine swab (check for client allergy to iodine)
- Antimicrobial ointment

- Sterile IV dressing tray, sterile 2 × 2 gauze dressing, sterile adhesive, or transparent semipermeable membrane dressing and sterile gloves
- Receptacle for contaminated items

Discontinuing an IV Line
- Sterile 2 × 2 gauze
- Tape or Band-Aid

- Nonsterile gloves

Action	Rationale

• Wash your hands • Check the client's identification band •
• Explain the procedure to the client prior to beginning •

1. Gather equipment.	1. Promotes efficiency.
2. Place bed at comfortable working height and lower side rails as necessary.	2. Promotes proper body mechanics and provides access to area.

Managing IV Site

3. Don gloves and assess IV site (according to agency protocol and CDC guidelines) at least every 8 hours for signs and symptoms of complications (phlebitis, infiltration, infection at site, allergic reaction).	3. Decreases risk of contact with bloodborne pathogens; provides early detection of symptoms of complications and appropriate intervention.
4. Assess dressing.	4. Allows for assessment without disrupting in intact IV dressing.
• Determine when dressing was applied by checking date and time written on dressing itself.	
• Observe dressing for moisture.	• Monitors medium for bacterial growth that would render sterile dressing contaminated.
• Observe that dressing is intact.	• Decreases risk of bacterial contamination to venipuncture site from nonadhering dressing.
• Gently palpate over the intact dressing.	• Detects IV site swelling and edema around venipuncture site.

continued

Action	Rationale
• If client complains of tenderness or pain, remove dressing and inspect site.	• Detects early signs of phlebitis.
5. Change dressing immediately if it becomes wet, soiled, or loose.	**5.** Decreases risk of bacterial infection.
6. Observe patency of IV line and needle.	**6.** Ensures proper infusion rate; IV line and needle must be free of kinks, knots, and clots.
• Open roller clamp and observe for rapid flow of fluid into drip chamber; close roller clamp and set drip rate to prescribed flow rate.	• Denotes patency of IV line and prevents fluid overload.
• If fluid does not flow, remove IV container from pole, place below level of infusion site, and observe for blood return.	• Determines patency of needle or cannula and placement of the device in the vein; venous pressure should be greater than IV tubing pressure.
7. Peripheral cannulas are removed and changed to a new site every 48–72 hours.	**7.** Supports CDC recommendations for changing peripheral cannulas to a new site every 48–72 hours to decrease the risk of complications.
8. Change administration sets.	**8.** Promotes compliance with CDC guidelines to prevent infection.
• Use IV sets for blood or blood products only once.	
• Every 24 hours, change tubing for lipids if the solution is infusing continuously; use new tubing with each infusion if solution is infusing intermittently.	
• Every 24 hours, change IV tubing used for hyperalimentation.	
• Routine IV tubing should not be changed more frequently than every 72 hours.	

Troubleshooting an IV system

Action	Rationale
9. Overfilled drip chamber:	**9.** Maintains air in chamber to allow for flow-rate calculation.
• Close drip chamber.	
• Remove container from IV pole and turn it upside down.	
• Squeeze drip chamber until it is one-third to one-half full.	
10. Air in tubing:	**10.** Prevents infusion of air into the bloodstream.
• Observe fluid level in drip chamber.	
• Check tubing connections.	
• Disinfect injection port distal to air.	
• Insert sterile needle and syringe into injection port, and aspirate or use needleless system (if available).	
11. Blood is backing up IV tubing:	**11.** Prevents clot formation at the needle or cannula tip inside the vein.
• Check that IV container is above the level of the infusion site and the heart.	

continued

Action	**Rationale**
• Check security of tubing connections.	
• Check fluid level in tubing chamber and IV container.	
12. IV is positional:	**12.** Maintains bevel of needle or tip of cannula away from the inner lumen of the vein.
• Reposition hand or arm.	
13. Infusion controller or pump alarms:	**13.** Indicates flow problem. Follow agency policy.
• Check device for type of alarm.	
• Follow manufacturer's instructions for each alarm condition.	

Changing a Gown, Continuous IV Infusion in Hand or Arm

Action	**Rationale**
14. Untie back or side of gown.	**14.** Allows gown to slip freely from arms.
15. Remove gown's sleeve from arm and hand without IV.	**15.** Frees the gown for removal from the involved arm.
16. Adjust the tubing to extend over IV hand, then slip the sleeve down arm; avoid tugging on tubing.	**16.** Prevents pressure on the tubing, which could disturb the venipuncture site or dislodge the IV.
17. Place clean gown over client's chest and abdomen.	**17.** Prevents unnecessary exposure and maintains client warmth.
18. Remove IV container from pole and slip sleeve over container, keeping container above client's arm.	**18.** Prevents backflow of blood into tubing.
19. Place your hand up through distal end of clean gown sleeve and grasp container; pull container and tubing out through clean gown sleeve.	**19.** Maintains integrity of the IV system.
20. Hang container on pole and check flow rate.	**20.** Ensures that solution is infusing at prescribed rate.
21. Slip sleeve over client's IV arm and then on other arm; tie gown at back.	**21.** Maintains client's warmth and comfort.

Converting to an Intermittent Infusion Device

Action	**Rationale**
22. Perform steps 1 and 2.	**22.** Same as for steps 1 and 2.
23. Check physician's order.	**23.** Verifies action to establish an intermittent infusion device.
24. Don clean gloves and close roller clamps on tubing.	**24.** Decreases risk of contact with bloodborne pathogens; prevents escape of solution from tubing.
25. Place protective pad under arm or hand with venipuncture site.	**25.** Prevents soiling of bed linen.
26. Open sterile package containing needleless injection cap and place in easy reach near venipuncture site.	**26.** Provides easy access.
27. With your nondominant hand, grasp hub of needle or cannula. With your dominant hand, disconnect IV tubing and attach needleless injection cap to hub.	**27.** Prevents dislodgement of needle or cannula.

continued

Action	**Rationale**
28. While stabilizing hub with nondominant hand, inject needleless injection cap port with 2 mL of normal saline.	**28.** Maintains patency of lock.
29. Discard old tubing and used supplies in receptacle.	**29.** Promotes a clean environment.

Changing a Peripheral IV Dressing

Action	**Rationale**
30. Perform steps 1 and 2.	**30.** Same as for steps 1 and 2.
31. Place protective pad under IV site; don gloves.	**31.** Prevents soiling of bed linens; reduces risk of contact with bloodborne pathogens.
32. Remove transparent or gauze dressing in direction that client's hair grows; keep pressure over IV site and leave in place the tape that secures IV needle or cannula (Figure A7-1).	**32.** Decreases client's discomfort when removing tape; prevents dislodgement of needle or cannula.

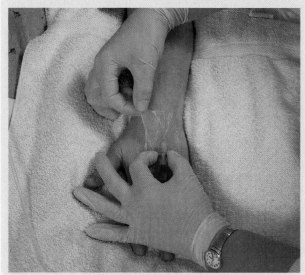

Figure A7-1 Removing Tape from a Peripheral IV. Remove tape with one hand while stabilizing the catheter's hub with the other hand.

Action	**Rationale**
33. Discard dressing and gloves in receptacle; wash hands.	**33.** Reduces risk for transmission of microorganisms.
34. Don gloves; inspect IV site for erythema, edema, infiltration.	**34.** Reduces risk of contact with bloodborne pathogens; denotes complications—for example, phlebitis, infiltration—that would necessitate changing IV site.
35. Cleanse IV site with alcohol or povidone-iodine. Using a circular motion, start at the puncture site and move outward peripherally; allow to dry (1 minute). Apply antimicrobial ointment over IV site, if dictated by agency protocol.	**35.** Reduces skin surface bacteria and prevents cross-contamination from skin bacteria near venipuncture site.
36. Replace tape:	**36.** Allows for stabilization of needle or catheter without tape's covering the insertion site, and eliminates positional flow of IV solution.

continued

Action	Rationale

Butterfly

- Place smallest pieces of tape across wings of butterfly.
- Place another piece of tape across middle to form an H; *or*
- Place piece of tape under wings.
- Cross tape over to form a V.
- Place piece of tape across V.
- Avoid placing tape over insertion site.

Over-the-Needle Catheter (Angiocath)

- With tape edges sticking to your thumb and fingertip, slide small piece of tape under catheter hub with adhesive side up.
- Cross tape over hub to form a U (Figure A7-2).

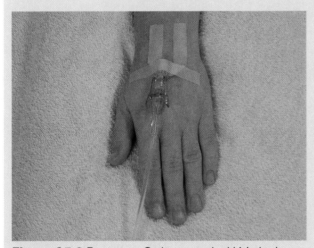

Figure A7-2 Retaping a Catheter via the U Method

- Place another small piece of tape across catheter hub.
- Avoid placing tape over insertion site.

Action	Rationale
37. Apply antimicrobial ointment over IV site if dictated by agency protocol.	37. Prevents transmission of microorganisms.
38. Using aseptic technique, apply transparent or gauze dressing over IV insertion site; avoid wrinkling transparent dressing.	38. Provides protective barrier against bacteria.
39. Place date, time, and your initials directly on dressing.	39. Documents dressing change.
40. Discard soiled items and gloves in receptacle; wash hands.	40. Reduces risk of transmission of microorganisms.
41. Reassess patency of IV system, flow rate, and client's response to dressing change.	41. Validates patency of IV system and infusion of solution at prescribed flow rate.

continued

Action	**Rationale**
42. Record in nurses' notes: time and type of dressing change, nature of venipuncture site, patency, and IV flow rate.	**42.** Documents actions taken and condition of IV site and system.

Discontinuing an IV Line

Action	**Rationale**
43. Perform steps 1 and 2. Don nonsterile gloves.	**43.** Same as for steps 1 and 2.
44. Assess if device is in place before discontinuing.	**44.** Allows for verification of complete removal of device.
45. Close roller clamp on IV tubing. If infusing, note amount of solution left in IV container.	**45.** Prevents spillage of solution when needle or catheter is removed; provides accurate amount of solution infused.
46. Stabilize needle or cannula with nondominant hand and remove tape in direction of hair growth.	**46.** Prevents unnecessary movement that could injure the vein; decreases discomfort when tape is removed.
47. Place sterile 2 × 2 gauze over puncture site and, while applying pressure, quickly and smoothly remove needle or catheter. Avoid pressing down on top of needle point while it is still in the vein.	**47.** Decreases bleeding and prevents injury to the vein.
48. Discard needle or catheter in receptacle.	**48.** Reduces risk of transmission of microorganisms.
49. Apply pressure over puncture site with sterile 2 × 2 gauze until bleeding stops. Apply tape firmly over the gauze; place gloves in receptacle and wash hands.	**49.** Promotes clot formation; keeps puncture site clean.
50. Inspect site for redness, swelling, or hematoma formation. Inspect removed cannula to assure it is intact.	**50.** Determines whether bleeding is occurring in the tissue.
51. Note whether there is any exudate on the catheter tip or at insertion site. Check site again in 15 to 30 minutes.	**51.** May indicate infection. Follow agency policy.
52. Record in nurses' notes time, amount of IV solution left in container when discontinued, and nature of puncture site.	**52.** Documents actions taken; promotes accurate intake recording and documents condition of puncture site.

References/Suggested Readings and Resources

Please note that because Internet resources are of a time-sensitive nature and URL addresses may change or be deleted, resource searches should also be conducted by association and/or topic.

CHAPTER 1
Holistic Care

REFERENCES/SUGGESTED READINGS

American Holistic Nurses' Association. (1994). AHNA Philosophy. *Journal of Holistic Nursing, 12*(3), 350–351.

Cerrato, P. (1998a). Understanding the mind/body link. *RN, 61*(1), 28–31.

Cerrato, P. (1998b). Spirituality and healing. *RN, 61*(2), 49–50.

Dossey, B. (1997). *Core curriculum for holistic nursing.* Gaithersburg, MD: Aspen.

Dossey, B. (1998). Holistic modalities & healing moments. *AJN, 98*(6), 44–47.

Dossey, B. (2000). *Florence Nightingale: Mystic, visionary, healer.* Springhouse, PA: Springhouse.

Dossey, B., & Dossey, L. (1998). Attending to holistic care. *AJN, 98*(8), 35–38.

Dossey, B., Keegan, L., & Guzzetta, C. (1999). *Holistic nursing: A handbook for practice* (3rd ed.). Gaithersburg, MD: Aspen.

Dyer, E. (1998, April 6). Faith & healing. *Corpus Christi Caller-Times.*

Hill, S., & Howlett, H. (1997). *Success in practical nursing: Personal and vocational issues* (3rd ed.). Philadelphia: W. B. Saunders Company.

Hughs, C. (1997). Prayer and healing: A case study. *Journal of Holistic Nursing, 15*(3), 318.

Jerome, A., et al. (1992). Nurse self-awareness in therapeutic relationships. *Pediatric Nursing, 18*(2), 153–156.

Kahn, S., & Saulo, M. (1995). *Healing yourself.* Albany, NY: Delmar.

Kurzen, C. (1997). *Contemporary practical/vocational nursing* (3rd ed.). Philadelphia: Lippincott.

Maslow, A. (1954). *Motivation and personality.* New York: Harper & Row.

National Institutes of Health (NIH). (2000). *Complementary & alternative medicine at the NIH* [On-line]. Available: http://nccam.nih.gov/nccam/ne/newsletter/spring2000.

Rivera-Andino, J., & Lopez, L. (2000). When culture complicates care. *RN, 63*(7), 47–49.

Selye, H. (1956). *The stress of life.* New York: McGraw-Hill.

Taber's cyclopedic medical dictionary. (1997). Philadelphia: F. A. Davis.

Waughfield, C. (1998). *Mental health concepts* (4th ed.). Albany, NY: Delmar.

Webster's new world college dictionary (1997). Springfield, MA: Merriam-Webster.

World Health Organization. (1974). *Chronicle of WHO.* Geneva: Organization Interim Commission.

Wright, K. (1998). Professional, ethical, and legal implications for spiritual care in nursing. *Image: Journal of Nursing Scholarship, 30*(1) 81–83.

RESOURCES

American Holistic Nurses' Association, P.O. Box 2130, Flagstaff, AZ 86003-2130, 800-278-AHNA (1461), http://www.ahna.org; e-mail: AHNA-flag@flaglink.com

National Center for Complementary and Alternative Medicine (NCCAM), Building 31, Room 5B-37, National Institutes of Health, Bethesda, MD 20892, 888-644-6226, http://nccam.nih.gov

Nurse Healers—Professional Associates International, Inc., 3760 South Highland Drive, Suite 429, Salt Lake City, UT 84106, 801-273-3399, http://www.therapeutic-touch.org

VIDEOS

* *Holistic Nursing* (1996), American Holistic Nurses' Association, 800-278-2462
* *At the Heart of Healing: Experiencing Holistic Nursing,* Kineholistic Foundation, 800-255-1914

CHAPTER 2
Critical Thinking

REFERENCES/SUGGESTED READINGS

Baker, C. R. (1996). Reflective learning: A teaching strategy for critical thinking. *Journal of Nursing Education, 35,* 19–22.

Birx, E. (1993). Critical thinking and theory-based practice. *Holistic Nursing Practice, 7* (3).

Brigham, C. (1993). Nursing education and critical thinking: Interplay of content and thinking. *Holistic Nursing Practice, 7* (3).

Brookfield, S. (1993). On impostership, cultural suicide and owners dangers: How nurses learn critical thinking. *Journal of Continuing Education in Nursing, 24* (5), 179–205.

Center for Critical Thinking. (1997). *Critical thinking in living, working & learning (a real time video)* [On-line]. Available: http://www.uncp.edu/home/vanderhoof/criticalthinking.ram

Center for Critical Thinking. (2000, January 25). *A brief history of the idea of critical thinking* [On-line]. Available: http://www.criticalthinking.org/University/univlibrary/cthistory.html

Center for Critical Thinking. (2000, January 25). *Valuable intellectual traits* [On-line]. Available: http://www.criticalthinking.org/University/univlibrary/intraits.html

Chaffee, J. (2000). *Thinking critically* (6th ed.). Boston: Houghton Mifflin College.

Elder, L., & Paul, R. (2000, January 25). *Universal intellectual standards* [On-line]. Available: http://www.criticalthinking.org/University/univlibrary/unistan.html

Ennis, R. H. (1985). A logical basis for measuring critical thinking skills. *Educational Leadership, 43,* 44–48.

Facionè, N. (2000). *Critical thinking assessment in nursing education programs: An aggregate data analysis.* Millbrae, CA: California Academic Press.

Guffey, M. E. (1998). *Five steps to better critical thinking, problem-solving and decision-making skills* [On-line]. Available: http://www.westwords.com/GUFFEY/critical.html

Heaslip, P. (1993, September). Intellectual standards: What are they? *Critical Connections* [Newsletter of the Critical Thinking Interest Group, University College of the Cariboo, Kamloops, B.C.]

Heaslip, P. (1994, November). Defining critical thinking. *Dialogue: A Critical Thinking Newsletter for Nurses, 3.*

Kurfiss, J. (1988). *Critical thinking: Theory, research, practice and possibilities.* Washington, DC: Association for the Study of Higher Education. (ASHE-ERIC Higher Education Report No. 2.)

Miller, M. A., & Malcolm, N. S. (1990). Critical thinking in the nursing curriculum. *Nursing & Health Care, 11,* 66–73.

Norris, S. P., & Ennis, R. H. (1989). *Evaluating critical thinking.* Pacific Grove, CA: Midwest.

Paul, R. (1990). *Critical thinking: What every person needs to survive in a rapidly changing world.* Rohnert Park, CA: Center for Critical Thinking and Moral Critique, Sonoma State University.

Paul, R. (1993). *Critical thinking: How to prepare students for a rapidly changing world.* Santa Rosa, CA: Foundation for Critical Thinking.

Paul, R., & Elder, L. (2000). *Critical thinking: Tools for taking charge of your learning and your life.* Upper Saddle River, NJ: Prentice Hall.

Paul, R., & Elder, L. (2000, January 25). *Helping students assess their thinking* [On-line]. Available: http://www.criticalthinking.org/University/univlibrary/helps.html

Paul, R., & Willsen, J. (1993). *Critical thinking, from an ideal evolves an imperative.* Santa Rosa, CA: Foundation for Critical Thinking.

Saucier, B., Stevens, K., & Williams, G. (2000). Critical thinking outcomes of computer-assisted instruction versus written nursing process. *Nursing and Health Care Perspectives, 21*(5), 240–246.

Scriven, M., & Paul, R. (1996). *Defining critical thinking* [On-line]. (Center for Critical Thinking at Sonoma State University, Rohnert Park, CA). Available: http://www.criticalthinking.org/University/univclass/defining.html

Worrell, P. J. (1990). Metacognition: Implications for instruction in nursing education. *Journal of Nursing Education, 29*(4), 170–175.

RESOURCES

California Academic Press, 217 La Cruz Avenue, Millbrae, CA 94030, 650-697-5628, http://www.calpress.com, email: info@calpress.com

Center for Critical Thinking at Sonoma State University, P. O. Box 220, Dillon Beach, CA 94929, 707-878-9100, http://www.criticalthinking.org

Foundation for Critical Thinking, P.O. Box 220, Dillon Beach, CA 94929, 800-833-3645

International Center for the Assessment of Higher Order Thinking (ICA), 707-878-9100, http://www.criticalthinking.org/icat.html

National Council for Excellence in Critical Thinking, P.O. Box 220, Dillon Beach, CA 94929, 707-878-9100, http://www.criticalthinking.org/ncect.html

CHAPTER 3
Student Nurse Skills for Success

REFERENCES/SUGGESTED READINGS

Brown, J., & Duguid P. (1996, July/August). Universities in the digital age, change. *The Magazine of Higher Learning.*

The Center for New Discoveries in Learning Personal Learning Style Inventory/School Smart Kids. (1998). *Newsletter,* Vol. 1, No. 4 [On-line]. Available: http://www.howtolearn.com/ndil3.html

Chenevert, M. (1995). *Mosby's tour guide to nursing school: A student's road survival kit* (3rd ed.). St. Louis, MO: Mosby.

Chopra, D. (1997, May–June). How can I keep up? *Natural Health,* 208.

Dale, E. (1954). *Audiovisual methods in teaching.* New York: Dryden.

DeLaune S., & Ladner, P. (1998). *Fundamentals of nursing: Standards & practice.* Albany, NY: Delmar.

DeWit, S. (1999). *Saunders student nurse planner.* Philadelphia: W. B. Saunders Company.

Dirkx, J., & Prenger, S. (1997). *A guide for planning and implementing instruction for adults—A theme-based approach.* San Francisco: Jossey-Bass.

Harrington, N., Smith N., & Spratt W. (1996). *LPN to RN transitions.* Philadelphia: Lippincott.

Highfield, M., & Wong, J. (1992, October). How to take multiple-choice tests. *Nursing92, 22*(10) 117–119.

Hoffman, K. (1997). *Effective college planning* (5th ed.). Orchard Park, NY: WNY Collegiate Consortium of Disability Advocates.

Holkeboer, R., and Walker, L. (1999). *Right from the start.* Belmont, CA: Wadsworth.

Korchek, N., & Sides, M. B. (1998). *Successful test-taking; Learning strategies for nurses* (3rd ed.). Philadelphia: Lippincott.

Lagerquist, S., & Billings, D. (1996). *Little, Brown's nursing Q&A critical thinking exercises.* Boston: Little, Brown.

Lesar, T. S. (1998). Errors in the use of medication dosage equations. *Archives of Pediatric Adolescent Medicine, 152*(4), 340–344.

Matthews, K. H. (1997). Learning out of the box: Tuning in to your unique cluster of intelligences, *The Next Step Magazine,* 22–27.

Meltzer, M., & Marcus-Palau, S. (1997). *Learning strategies in nursing: Reading, studying and test taking* (2nd ed.). Philadelphia: W. B. Saunders Company.

Meltzer, M., & Palau, S. M. (1996). *Acquiring critical thinking skills.* Philadelphia: W. B. Saunders Company.

Mind tools: How your learning style affects your use of mnemonics (1998) [On-line]. Available: http://www.mindtools.com/mnem1sty.html

National Center for Learning Disabilities, Inc. (NCLD). (1999, January 24) [On-line]. Information About Learning Disabilities. Available: http://www.ncld.org

Nugent, P. M., & Vitale, B. A. (2000). *Test taking techniques for beginning nursing students* (3rd ed.). Philadelphia: F. A. Davis.

Palau, S. M., & Meltzer, M. (1998). *Learning strategies for allied health students.* Philadelphia: W. B. Saunders Company.

Rubenfeld, M. G., & Scheffer, B. (1998). *Critical thinking in nursing: An interactive approach* (2nd ed.). Philadelphia: Lippincott.

Schank, R. (2000). *Dynamic memory revisited* (2nd ed). Cambridge, UK: Cambridge University Press.

Scott, A., & Fong, E. (1998). *Body structures and functions* (9th ed). Albany, NY: Delmar.

Smith, G. L., Davis, P. E., & Dennerll, J. T. (1999). *Medical terminology: A programmed systems approach* (8th ed.). Albany, NY: Delmar.

Sotiriou, P., & Phillips, A. (1999). *Steps to reading proficiency* (5th ed.). Belmont: Wadsworth.

RESOURCES

The Center for New Discoveries in Learning, P.O. Box 1019, Windsor, CA 95492, 707-837-8180

The Center for New Discoveries in Learning Personal Learning Style Inventory/School Smart Kids Newsletter Vol. 1, No. 4, http://www.howtolearn.com/ndil3.html

Choosing a College for Students with Learning Disabilities, http://www.ldresources.com/education/collegechoice.html

Closing the Gap, A Resource Directory, P.O. Box 68, 526 Main Street, Henderson, MN 56044, 507-248-3294

Directory of Adaptive Technology: Trace Research and Development Center, 5-151 Waisman Center, 1500 Highland Avenue, University of Wisconsin, Madison, WI 53705, 608-262-6966, http://trace.wisc.edu

Identifying Your Best Learning Styles, http://www.marin.cc.ca.us/~don/Study/13styles.html

The Institute for Learning Sciences, Northwestern University, 1890 Maple Avenue, Evanston, IL 60201, 847-491-3500, http://www.ils.nwu.edu

Mind Tools: The Old School House, Yapton, West Sussex, United Kingdom BN18 0DU

Mind Tools: How Your Learning Style Affects Your Use of Mnemonics, http://www.mindtools.com/mnem1sty.html

The National Adult Literacy and Learning Disabilities Center, Academy for Educational Development, 1875 Connecticut Avenue, NW, Washington, DC 20009-1202, 202-884-8185, 800-953-ALLD (953-2553), FAX: 202-884-8429, http://novel.nifl.gov/nalldtop.htm

National Center for Learning Disabilities, Inc., 381 Park Avenue South, Suite 1401, New York, NY 10016, 212-545-7510, 888-575-7373, http://www.ncld.org/

CHAPTER 4
Nursing History, Education, and Organizations

REFERENCES/SUGGESTED READINGS

American Nurses Association. (1990). *Standards for nursing staff development*. Kansas City, MO: Author.

American Nurses Association. (1991). *American Nurses Association bylaws*. Washington, DC: Author.

American Nurses Association. (1998). *Mission statement* [On-line]. Available: http://www.nursingworld.org/about/mission.htm

American Nurses Association. (1999). *About ANA* [On-line]. Available: http://www.ana.org/about/summary/99hodact.htm

Anglin, L. T. (2000). Historical perspectives: Influences of the past. In J. Zerwekh (Ed.), *Nursing today: Transitions and trends* (3rd ed.). Philadelphia: W. B. Saunders Company.

Baker, C. M. (1994). School health: Policy issues. *Nursing & Health Care, 15*(4), 178–184.

Bell, P. (1993). "Making do" with the midwife: Arkansas' Mamie O. Hale in the 1940s. *Nursing History Review,* 155–169.

Bullough, V., & Bullough, B. (1993). Medieval nursing. *Nursing History Review,* 89–104.

Calhoun, J. (1993, March). The Nightingale pledge: A commitment that survives the passage of time. *Nursing & Health Care, 14*(3), 130–136.

Chinn, P. L. (1994). *Developing the discipline: Critical studies in nursing history and professional issues*. Gaithersburg, MD: Aspen.

Cushing, A. (1995, Summer). A historical note on the relationship between nursing and nursing history. *International History Nursing Journal, 1*(1), 57–60.

DeLaune, S., & Ladner, P. (1998). *Fundamentals of nursing: Standards & practice*. Albany, NY: Delmar.

Dossey, B. (1995). Endnote: Florence Nightingale today. *Critical Care Nursing, 15*(4), 98.

Edelman, C. L., & Mandle, C. L. (1998). *Health promotion throughout the lifespan* (4th ed.). St. Louis, MO: Mosby.

Estabrooks, C. A. (1995). Lavinia Lloyd Dock: The Henry Street years. *Nursing History Review, 3,* 143–172.

Guide to Nursing Organizations. (2000). *Nursing2000, 30*(5), 54–56.

Healthy People 2010. (2000). *The prevention agenda* [On-line]. Available: http://www.health.gov/healthypeople/prevagenda/

Johnson, B. S. (1997). *Psychiatric–mental health nursing: Adaptation and growth* (4th ed.). Philadelphia: Lippincott.

Joint Commission on the Accreditation of Healthcare Organizations. (1996). *Accreditation standards and scoring guidelines for hospital-based mental health*. Oak Brook Terrace, IL: Author.

Macrae, J. (1995). Nightingale's spiritual philosophy and its significance for modern nursing. *Image: Journal of Nursing Scholarship, 27*(1), 8–10.

Mason, D. J., & Leavitt, J. K. (1995). The revolution in health care: What's your readiness quotient? *AJN, 95*(6), 50–54.

National Association for Practical Nurse Education and Service, Inc. (1998). *History of NAPNES*. Silver Spring, MD: Author.

National Council of State Boards of Nursing, Inc. (1996). *Creating new national certification examination for LPN/VNs* [On-line]. Available: http://www.ncsbn.org/files/publications/annual reports/ar1996/creatnc.asp

National Council of State Boards of Nursing, Inc. (1998a). *National Council mission and purpose* [On-line]. Available: http://www.ncsbn.org/files/aboutnc.mission.asp

National Council of State Boards of Nursing, Inc. (1998b). *Overview: Programs and services of the National Council* [On-line]. Available: http://www.ncsbn.org/files/aboutnc/overview.asp

National Council of State Boards of Nursing Inc. (1999). *About the National Council* [On-line]. Available: http://www.ncsbn.org/files/aboutnc.asp

National Federation of Licensed Practical Nurses. (2000). *All about NFLPN* [On-line]. Available: http://www.nflpn.org/allaboutnflpn.htm

National League for Nursing. (1995). *Bylaws*. New York: Author.

National League for Nursing. (1998). Research Department, Communication. New York: Author.

National League for Nursing. (2000a). *About NLN* [On-line]. Available: http://www.nln.org/aboutnln/

National League for Nursing. (2000b). *Unofficial, unpublished data from 1998*. Research Department Communication. August 15, 2000.

National League for Nursing History. (1997). Adapted from *The Entry Dilemma* by Shirley H. Fondiller, National League for Nursing. Available: http://www.nln.org/aboutnlninfohistory.htm

Nightingale, F. (1969). *Notes on nursing: What it is and what it is not*. New York: Dover.

Ogren, K. (1994). The risk of not understanding nursing history. *Holistic Nursing Practice, 8*(2), 10.

Secretary's Commission on Nursing. (1988). *Final report*. Washington, DC: Department of Health & Human Services.

Selanders, L. C. (1993). *Florence Nightingale: An environmental adaptation theory*. Newberry Park, CA: Sage.

Silverstein, N. G. (1994). Lillian Wald at Henry Street, 1893–1895. In P. L. Chinn (Ed.), *Developing the discipline: Critical studies in nursing history and professional issues*. Gaithersburg, MD: Aspen.

Strickland, O., & Fishman, D. (1994). *Nursing issues in the 1990s*. Albany, NY: Delmar.

U.S. Department of Health and Human Services. (1996). *The registered nurse population*. Washington, DC: Author.

Wall, B. (1993). Grace under pressure: The nursing sisters of the Holy Cross, 1861–1865. *Nursing History Review,* 71–88.

RESOURCES

American Nurses Association (ANA), 600 Maryland Avenue SW, Suite 100 West, Washington, DC 20024-2571, 202-651-7000, 800-274-4ANA (262), http://www.ana.org

National Association of Practical Nurse Education and Service, Inc. (NAPNES), 1400 Spring Street, Suite 330, Silver Spring, MD 20910, 301-588-2491

National Council of State Boards of Nursing, Inc. (NCSBN), 676 North St. Clair Street, Suite 550, Chicago, IL 60611-2921, 312-787-6555, http://www.ncsbn.org

National Federation of Licensed Practical Nurses, Inc. (NFLPN), 893 U.S. Highway 70 West, Suite 202, Garner, NC 27529, 800-948-2511, http://www.nflpn.org

National League for Nursing (NLN), 61 Broadway, 33rd Floor, New York, NY 10006, 212-363-5555, 800-669-1656, http://www.nln.org

CHAPTER 5
The Health Care Delivery System

REFERENCES/SUGGESTED READINGS

Aiken, L. H. (1995). Transformation of the nursing workforce. *Nursing Outlook, 43*(5), 201–209.

American Nurses Association. (1991). *Nursing's agenda for health care reform.* Kansas City, MO: Author.

American Nurses Association. (1993a, September). *Consumers willing to see a nurse for routine "doctoring" according to Gallup poll* [news release]. Washington, DC: Author.

American Nurses Association. (1993b, September). *States with some form of nurse privileging.* Washington, DC: Author.

American Nurses Association. (1994). *Health care reform and America's nurses: Agenda for change.* Washington, DC: Author.

American Nurses Association. (1995). Managed care: Challenges and opportunities for nursing. *Nursing facts* (Item PR-27). Washington, DC: Author.

Boyd, L., Lowes, R., Guglielmo, W., & Slomski, A. (2000). Advanced practice nursing today. *RN, 63*(9), 57–62.

Centers for Disease Control and Prevention (CDC). (1998). *Combating Complacency—HIV Prevention, Geneva '98. Trends.* Available: http://www.cdcnpin.org

Centers for Disease Control and Prevention (CDC). (2000). *IOM Report—Calling the shots: Immunization finance policies and practice* [On-line]. Available: http://www.cdc.gov/nip/news/IOM-rpt-6-00.htm

Chamberlain, P., Chen, Y., Osuna, E., & Yamamoto, C. (1995). Innovative culture shock prescribed for health care. *Nursing Outlook, 43*(5), 232–234.

Deparle, N. (1998). *The state of the Children's Health Insurance Program.* Health Care Financing Administration. Available: http://www.hcfa.gov/init/testm918.htm

Feldstein, P. J. (1999). *Health care economics* (5th ed.). Albany, NY: Delmar.

Friedman, E. (1997). The uninsured: From dilemma to crisis. In P. Lee & C. Estes (Eds.), *The nation's health* (5th ed.). Boston: Jones & Bartlett.

Grace, H. K. (1997). Can medical costs be contained? In J. C. McCloskey, & H. K. Grace (Eds.), *Current issues in nursing* (5th ed.). St. Louis, MO: Mosby.

Grace, H. K., & Brock, R. M. (1997). Solving the health care dilemma: What will work? In J. C. McCloskey & H. K. Grace (Eds.), *Current issues in nursing* (5th ed.). St. Louis, MO: Mosby.

Haugh, R. (1999). The new consumer. *Hospital Health Network, 73*(12), 30–34, 36.

Health Care Financing Administration (HCFA). (1998). *Medicare and Medicaid expenses, 1997* [On-line]. Available: http://www.hcfa.gov/pubforms/finance/97/ch2n1216.htm

Health Care Financing Administration (HCFA). (2000). The nation's healthcare dollar: 1998 [On-line]. Available: http://www.hcfa.gov/stats/nhe-oact/tables/chart.htm

Health Care News. (2000). Maryland group shows universal coverage can work. *AJN, 100*(8), 20.

Hicks, L. L., & Boles, K. E. (1997). Why health economics? In C. Harrington & C. L. Estes (Eds.), *Health policy and nursing: Crisis and reform in the U.S. health care delivery system* (2nd ed). Boston: Jones & Bartlett.

Hull, K. (1997). Hospital trends. In C. Harrington & C. L. Estes (Eds.), *Health policy and nursing: Crisis and reform in the U.S. health care delivery system* (2nd ed). Boston: Jones & Bartlett.

Kellogg Foundation. (1994, June 24). *How people view their providers. Report of a survey.* Battle Creek, MI: Author.

Lee, P. R., Soffel, D., & Luft, H. (1997). Costs and coverage: Pressures towards health care reform. In P. Lee, C. Estes, & N. Ramsay (Eds.), *The nation's health* (5th ed.). Boston: Jones & Bartlett.

Levit, K. R., Lazenby, H. C., Cowan, C. A., & Letsch, S. W. (1997). National health expenditures. In C. Harrington & C. L. Estes (Eds.), *Health policy and nursing: Crisis and reform in the U.S. health care delivery system* (2nd ed.). Boston: Jones & Bartlett.

Maraldo, P. J. (1997). Nursing's agenda for health care reform. In J. C. McCloskey & H. K. Grace (Eds.), *Current issues in nursing* (5th ed.). St. Louis, MO: Mosby.

McCloskey, J. C., & Grace, H. K. (Eds.). (1997). *Current issues in nursing* (5th ed.). St. Louis, MO: Mosby.

Moyer, M. E. (1997). A revised look at the number of uninsured Americans. In C. Harrington & C. L. Estes (Eds.), *Health policy and nursing: Crisis and reform in the U.S. health care delivery system* (2nd ed.). Boston: Jones & Bartlett.

National Academies. (2000). *Strengthening America's vaccine safety net* [On-line]. Available: http://www.national-academies.org/includes/shots.htm

News. (2000). High public esteem for nurses. *AJN 100*(1), 26.

O'Neil, E. H. (1993). *Health professions education for the future: Schools in service to the nation.* San Francisco: Pew Health Professions Commission.

Parris, N. M., & Hines, J. (1995). Payer and provider relationships: The key to reshaping health care delivery. *Nursing Administration Quarterly, 19*(3), 13–17.

Pearson, L. J. (2000). Annual legislative update: How each state stands on legislative issues affecting advanced nursing practice. *Nurse Practitioner, 25*(1), 16.

Peck, S. P. (1997). Community nursing centers: Implications for health care reform. In J. C. McCloskey & H. K. Grace (Eds.), *Current issues in nursing* (5th ed.). St. Louis, MO: Mosby.

Rowe, J. W. (1996). Health care myths at the end of life. *Bulletin of the American College of Surgeons, 81*(6), 11–18.

Schieber, G. J., Poullier, J. P., & Greenwald, L. M. (1997). U.S. health expenditure performance: An international comparison and data update. In C. Harrington & C. L. Estes (Eds.), *Health policy and nursing: Crisis and reform in the U.S. health care delivery system* (2nd ed.). Boston: Jones & Bartlett.

Society for Ambulatory Care Professionals. (1994). *Glossary of managed care terms: An issue briefing.* Chicago: American Hospital Association.

Stafford, M., & Appleyard, J. (1997). Clinical nurse and nurse practitioners. In J. C. McCloskey & H. K. Grace (Eds.), *Current issues in nursing* (5th ed.). St. Louis, MO: Mosby.

The Robert Wood Johnson Foundation (RWJF). (2000). *Six out of ten parents whose children qualify for low-cost or free health care coverage do not believe their kids are eligible* [On-line]. Available: http://www.coveringkids. org/press_release.html

Tlusty, M. (1994). Higher mortality for women with PCP [brief item]. *Nursing and Health Care, 15*(4), 211.

U.S. Census Bureau. (2000). *Poverty 1999* [On-line]. Available: http://www.census.gov/hhes/poverty/poverty99/tables5. htm

U.S. Department of Health & Human Services. (1993). *Medicare benefits booklet*. Washington, DC: U.S. Government Printing Office.

Vrabec, N. J. (1995). Implications of U.S. health care reform for the rural elderly. *Nursing Outlook, 43*(6), 260–265.

Zerwekh, J., & Claborn, J. C. (1997). *Nursing today: Transitions and trends*. Philadelphia: W. B. Saunders Company.

RESOURCES

American Nurses Association (ANA), 600 Maryland Avenue SW, Suite 100 West, Washington, DC 20024-2571, 800-274-4ANA (262), http://www.ana.com

National Federation of Licensed Practical Nurses, Inc. (NFLPN), 1418 Aversboro Road, Garner, NC 27529, 800-948-2511, http://www.nflpn.org

Society for Ambulatory Care Professionals, One North Franklin, 31st Floor, Chicago, IL 60606, 312-422-3900, http://www.sacp-net.org

CHAPTER 6
Legal Responsibilities

REFERENCES/SUGGESTED READINGS

Badzek, L., & Gross, L. (1999). Confidentiality and privacy: At the forefront for nurses. *AJN, 99*(6), 52–54.

Beare, P., & Myers, J. (1998). *Principles and practices of adult health nursing* (3rd ed.). St. Louis, MO: Mosby.

Becker, B., & Fendler, D. (1994). *Vocational and personal adjustments in practical nursing*. (7th ed.) St. Louis, MO: Mosby.

Bernzweig, E. (1995). *The nurse's liability for malpractice: A programmed course* (6th ed.). St. Louis, MO: Mosby.

Braun, J., & Lipson, S. (1993). *Toward a restraint-free environment*. Baltimore: Health Professions.

Brown, S. (1999). Good Samaritan laws: Protection and limits. *RN, 62*(11), 65.

Calfee, B. (1995). Going before the board: How to prepare yourself. *Nursing95, 25*(3), 56–58.

DeLaune, S., & Ladner, P. (1998), *Fundamentals of nursing: Standards & practice*. Albany, NY: Delmar.

Dempski, K. (2000). Serving as an expert witness. *RN, 63*(2), 65–68.

Dunn, D. (1999). Exploring the gray areas of informed consent. *Nursing99, 29*(7), 41–44.

Eggland, E. (1995). Charting smarter: Using new mechanisms to organize your paperwork. *Nursing95, 25*(9), 35–41.

Flight, M. (1998). *Law, liability, and ethics* (3rd ed.). Albany, NY: Delmar.

Green, A. (1995). Are you at risk for disciplinary action? *AJN, 95*(7), 36–42.

Hill, S., & Howlett, H. (2001). *Success in practical nursing: Personal and vocational issues* (4th ed.). Philadelphia: W. B. Saunders Company.

Hughes, T. (1994). Is your colleague chemically dependent? *AJN, 94*(9), 31–35.

Infante, M. C. (2000). Malpractice may not be your biggest legal risk. *RN, 63*(7), 67–73.

Joint Commission on Accreditation of Healthcare Organizations (JCAHO). (1995). *Accreditation Manual for Hospitals*. Oakbrook Terrace, IL: Author.

Joint Commission on Accreditation of Healthcare Organizations (JCAHO). (2000). *Restraint standards* [On-line]. Available: http://www.jcaho.org/standard/restraint/restraint_stds.html

Keepnews, D. (2000). A systems approach to health care errors. *AJN, 100*(6), 77–78.

LaDuke, S. (2000). The effects of professional discipline on nurses. *AJN, 100*(6), 26–33.

Lee, N. G. (2000). Proving nursing negligence. *AJN, 100*(11), 55–56.

Mayer, T. (1995, April). *Director of nurses' attitudes toward restraint usage in long-term care*. Master's Thesis, Indiana Wesleyan University.

Mitchell, P., & Grippando, G. (1993). *Nursing perspectives and issues* (5th ed.). Albany, NY: Delmar.

Monahan, F.D., Drake, T., & Neighbors, M. (1998). *Nursing care of adults* (2nd ed.). Philadelphia: W. B. Saunders Company.

Moniz, D. M. (1998). Too few staff, too much risk. *RN, 61*(12), 63.

Morris, M. R. (1998). Elder abuse: What the law requires. *RN, 61*(8), 52.

National Council of State Boards of Nursing, Inc. (2000a). What boards of nursing do . . . and what you can do [On-line]. Available: http://www.ncsbn.org/files/consumer/bon.asp

National Council of State Boards of Nursing, Inc. (2000b). Why disciplinary databanks? Why the National Practitioner Data Bank (NPDB)? [On-line]. Available: http://www. ncsbn.org/files/publications/issues/vol171/ddb.171.asp

Professional Update. (2000). JCAHO to amend its new restraint standards. *RN, 63*(7), 14.

Sandler, R. L. (1995). Restraining devices. *AJN, 95*(7), 34–35.

Showers, J. (2000). What you need to know about negligence lawsuits. *Nursing2000, 30*(2). 45–48.

Sullivan, G. H. (2000). Keep your charting on course. *RN, 63*(5), 75–79.

Taylor, C., Lillis, C., & LeMone, P. (1997). *Fundamentals of nursing: The art and science of nursing care* (3rd ed.). Philadelphia: Lippincott.

Ventura, M. (1999a). Staffing issues. *RN, 62*(2), 26–30.

Ventura, M. (1999b). The great multistate licensure debate. *RN, 62*(5), 58–62.

Ventura, M. (1999c). When information must be revealed. *RN, 62*(6), 61.

Walsh, S. M. (1995). Resuscitation decisions: Showing a family the way. *Nursing95, 25*(8), 50–51.

White, L., & Duncan, G. (2001). *Medical surgical nursing: An integrated approach*. Albany, NY: Delmar.

Zerwekh, J., & Claborn, J. C. (1997). *Nursing today: Transitions and trends*. (2nd ed) Philadelphia: W. B. Saunders Company.

RESOURCES

Choice in Dying, Inc., 1035 30th Street NW, Washington, DC 20007, 202-338-9790, 800-989-9455, http://www. choices.org

Health Privacy Project and Consumer Coalition for Health Privacy, 202-687-0880

Living Wills, Films for the Humanities and Sciences, P.O. Box 2053, Princeton, NJ 08543-2053, 800-257-5126

Medcom, Inc., 6060 Phyllis Drive, Cypress, CA 90630, 800-877-1443, http://www.medcomsolutions.com

National EMS Information Exchange, http://naemt.org/ nemsie/immunity.htm

The Verdict Is, Medical Electronic Educational Services, Inc., 930 Pitner Avenue, Evanston, IL 60202, 800-323-9084

CHAPTER 7
Ethical Responsibilities

REFERENCES/SUGGESTED READINGS

American Hospital Association. (1992). *A patient's bill of rights*. Chicago: Author.

Aroskar, M. A. (1994). Politics and ethics in nursing: Implications for education. *Journal of Professional Nursing, 10*(3), 129.

Awong, L., & Miles, A. (1998a). When an adolescent wants to forgo therapy. *AJN, 98*(7), 67–68.

Awong, L., & Miles, A. (1998b). When the physician disregards the patient's expressed wishes. *AJN, 98*(2), 71.

Bandman, E. L., & Bandman, B. (1995). *Nursing ethics through the life span* (3rd ed.). Norwalk, CT: Appleton-Lange.

Beare, G., & Myers, J. (1998). *Adult health nursing* (2nd ed.) St. Louis, MO: Mosby.

Beyea, S., & Nicoll, L. (1999). Using ethical analysis when there is no research. *Aorn Journal, 69*(6), 1261–1263.

Callahan, J. (1994). The ethics of assisted suicide. *Health and Social Work, 19*(4), 237–243.

Curtin, L. (1995). Nurses take a stand on assisted suicide. *Nursing Management, 26*(5), 71–76.

Daly, B. (1999). Ethics: Why a new code? *AJN, 99*(6), 64–66.

Davis, A. J., & Aroskar, M. A. (1997). *Ethical dilemmas and nursing practice* (4th ed.). Norwalk, CT: Appleton-Lange.

DeLaune, S., & Ladner, P. (1998). *Fundamentals of nursing: Standards & practice*. Albany, NY: Delmar.

Edge, R., & Groves, J.R. (1999). *The ethics of health care: A guide for clinical practice* (2nd ed.). Albany, NY: Delmar.

Fowler, M. (1999). Ethics: Relic or resource? The code for nurses. *AJN, 99*(3), 56–58.

Gordon, M., Murphy, C., Candee, D., & Hiltunen, E. (1994). Clinical judgment: An integrated model. *Advances in Nursing Science, 16*(4), 55–70.

Haddad, A. (1995). Ethics in action. *RN, 58*(5), 21–23.

Haddad, A. (1998). Ethics in action. *RN, 61*(3), 21–24.

Haddad, A. (1999a). Ethics in action, *RN, 62*(7), 23–26.

Haddad, A. (1999b). Ethics in action, *RN, 62*(1), 23–26.

International Council of Nurses. (1973). *ICN code for nurses: Ethical concepts applied to nursing*. Geneva, Switzerland: Imprimeries Populaires.

Kennedy-Schwarz, J. (2000). The "ethics" of instinct. *AJN, 100*(4), 71–73.

Kristoff, B., Sellin, S., & Miller, M. (1994). Patients' rights and ethical dilemmas in home care: Incorporation of psychological concepts. *Home Healthcare Nurse, 12*(5), 45–50.

Mitchell, P., & Grippando, G. (1993). *Nursing perspectives and issues*. Albany, NY: Delmar.

National Federation of Practical Nurses, Inc. (NFLPN). (1996). *Nursing practice standards for the licensed practical/vocational nurse*. Garner, NC: Author.

News (2000). Health care fraud in Hawaii. *AJN, 100*(1), 21.

Nguyen, B. (1999). Protecting nurse whistleblowers. *AJN, 99*(12), 71.

Pappas, A. (1997). Ethical issues. In J. Zerwekh & J. Claborn (Eds.), *Nursing today: Transitions and trends*. Philadelphia: W. B. Saunders Company.

Pinch, W. J. (1990). Nursing ethics: Is covering up ever harmless? *Nursing Management, 21*(9), 60–62.

Polston, M. (1999). Whistleblowing: Does the law protect you? *AJN, 99*(1), 26–31.

Raths, L., Harmin, M., & Simon, S. (1978). *Values and teaching* (2nd ed.). Columbus, OH: Merrill.

Rice, V. H., Beck, C., & Stevenson, J. S. (1997). Ethical issues relative to autonomy and personal control in independent and cognitively impaired elders. *Nursing Outlook, 45*(1), 25–34.

Salladay, S. (1998). Ethical problems. *Nursing98, 28*(7), 30.

Schildmeier, D. (1997). Using public opinion to protect nursing practice. *AJN, 97*(3), 56–58.

Sloan, A. (1999). Whistleblowing: There are risks! *RN, 62*(7), 65–68.

Sumodi, V. (1995). Legalization of physician-assisted suicide: Point/counterpoint. *Nursing Forum, 30*(1), 11–17.

Ustal, D. (1993). *Clinical ethics and values: Issues and insights*. East Greenwich, RI: Educational Resources in Health Care.

Wilson, D. M. (1996). Highlighting the role of policy in nursing practice through a comparison of "DNR" policy influences and "No CPR" decision influences. *Nursing Outlook, 44*(6), 272–279.

Wolfe, S. (1999). Ethics on the job: A survey, quality vs. cost. *RN, 62*(1), 28–33.

Zerwekh, J. V. (1997). Do dying patients really need IV fluids? *AJN, 97*(3), 26–30.

Zollo, M. B., & Derse, A. (1997). The abusive patient: Where do you draw the line? *AJN, 97*(2), 31–35.

RESOURCES

American Red Cross, Transplant Services, 2025 E Street NW, Suite 108, Washington, DC 20006, 800-2-TISSUE (84-7783)

The Living Bank International, P.O. Box 6725, Houston, TX 77265, 800-528-2971, http://www.livingbank.org

National Association for Practical Nurse Education and Service, Inc. (NAPNES), 1400 Spring Street, Suite 330, Silver Spring, MD 20901, 301-588-2491

National Federation of Licensed Practical Nurses, Inc. (NFLPN), 1418 Aversboro Road, Garner, NC 27529, 800-948-2511, http://www.nflpn.org

United Network of Organ Sharing (UNOS), 1100 Boulders Parkway, Suite 500, P.O. Box 13770, Richmond, VA 23225-8770, 888-894-6361, 804-330-8541, http://www.unos.org

CHAPTER 8
Communication

REFERENCES/SUGGESTED READINGS

Bailey, D., & Bailey, D. (1997). *Therapeutic approaches to care of the mentally ill* (4th ed.). Philadelphia: F. A. Davis.

Barnsteiner, J. (1996). Newest online journal users: Clinicians. *Reflections, 22*(2), 21.

Barry, P. (1997). *Mental health and mental illness* (6th ed.). Philadelphia: Lippincott.

Brandt, M. (1995, March). Making the CPR vision a reality: Where should you start? *Journal of the American Health Information Management Association, 66*(3), 26–30.

Burtt, K. (1997, November/December). Nurses use telehealth to address rural health care needs, prevent hospitalizations. *The American Nurse, 21*.

DeLaune, S., & Ladner, P. (1998). *Fundamentals of nursing: Standards & practice*. Albany, NY: Delmar.

deWit, S. (1994). *Rambo's nursing skills for clinical practice*. Philadelphia: W. B. Saunders Company.

Estes, M. E. Z. (2002). *Health assessment & physical examination* (2nd ed.). Albany, NY: Delmar.

Frawley, K., & Asmonga, D. (1996). Update on the Medical Records Confidentiality Act. *Journal of the American Health Information Management Association, 67*(1), 12.

Frisch, N., & Frisch, L. (1998). *Psychiatric mental health nursing*. Albany, NY: Delmar.

Gay, K. (1993). *Getting your message across*. New York: Macmillan.

Goldsmith, J. (1996). Computers and nurses changing hospital care. *Reflections, 22*(2), 8–10.

Granade, P. (1997). The brave new world of telemedicine. *RN, 60*(7), 59–62.

Hall, E. (1959). *The silent language*. New York: Doubleday.

Jack, L. (1997). Effective communication. In J. Zerwekh & J. Claborn (Eds.), *Nursing today: Transition and trends* (2nd ed.). Philadelphia: W. B. Saunders Company.

Keller, V., & Baker, L. (2000). Communicate with care. *RN, 63*(1), 32–33.

Kübler-Ross, E. (1969). *On death and dying*. New York: MacMillan.

Kübler-Ross, E. (1975). *Death: The final stage of growth*. Englewood Cliffs, NJ: Prentice Hall.

Kübler-Ross, E. (1978). *To live until we say good-bye*. Englewood Cliffs, NJ: Prentice Hall.

Lorton, L., & Legler, J. (1996). A telemedicine trial. *Journal of the American Health Information Management Association, 67*(1), 40–42.

Lyon, B. (2000). Conquering dysfunctional anxiety: What you say to yourself matters. *Reflections on Nursing Leadership, 26*(4), 33–35.

Medical Records Institute. (1994). Legality of electronic patient record systems. *Toward an electronic patient record, 2*(7).

Meranda, D. (1995). Administrative and security challenges with electronic patient record systems. *Journal of the American Health Information Management Association, 66*(3), 58–60.

Milliken, M. (1998). *Understanding human behavior* (6th ed.). Albany, NY: Delmar.

Ravitch, S. (1996). The Medical Records Confidentiality Act. *For the Record, 8*(9) 8–11.

Rhodes, A. (1995). The need for security with computerized records. *MCN, 20*(6), 299.

Rochman, R. (2000). Are computerized patient records for you? *Nursing2000, 30*(10), 61–62.

Sherman, K. (1994). *Communication and image in nursing*. Albany, NY: Delmar.

Tamparo, C., & Lindh, W. (2000). *Therapeutic communications for health professionals* (2nd ed.). Albany, NY: Delmar.

Telemedicine Research Center. (1997). *What is telemedicine?* Portland, OR: Author.

Waughfield, C. (1998). *Mental health concepts*. Albany, NY: Delmar.

Zolot, J. S. (1999). Computer-based patient records. *AJN, 99*(12), 64–69.

RESOURCES

American Health Information Management Association, 919 North Michigan Avenue, Suite 1400, Chicago, IL 60611-1683, 312-787-2672, http://www.ahima.org

CHAPTER 9
Nursing Process

REFERENCES/SUGGESTED READINGS

Alfaro-LeFevre, R. (1998). *Applying nursing process* (4th ed.). Philadelphia: Lippincott.

Alfaro-LeFevre, R. (1999). *Critical thinking in nursing: A practical approach.* (2nd ed.). Philadelphia: W. B. Saunders Company.

American Nurses Association. (1991). *Standards of nursing practice*. Kansas City, MO: Author.

Bevis, E. O. (1989). *Curriculum building in nursing: A process* (3rd ed., Publication No. 15–2277). New York: National League for Nursing.

Carpenito, L. J. (1999). *Nursing diagnosis: Application to clinical practice* (8th ed.). Philadelphia: Lippincott.

Clark, M. (1998). Implementation of nursing standardized languages NANDA, NIC, and NOC. *On-line Journal of Issues in Nursing* [On-line], 2(2). Available: http://www.nursingworld.org

DeLaune, S., & Ladner, P. (1998). *Fundamentals of nursing: Standards & practice*. Albany, NY: Delmar.

Edelman, C. L., & Mandle, C. L. (1998). *Health promotion throughout the lifespan* (4th ed.). St. Louis, MO: Mosby.

Fry, V. S. (1953). The creative approach to nursing. *AJN, 53*(3), 301–302.

Gebbie, K. M., & Lavin, M. A. (1974). Classifying nursing diagnoses. *AJN, 74*, 250–253.

Gordon, M. (1997). *Manual of nursing diagnoses 1997–1998 edition*. St. Louis, MO: Mosby.

Gordon, M. (1998, September 30). Nursing nomenclature and classification system development. *On-line Journal of Issues in Nursing* [On-line]. Available: http://www.nursingworld.org

Humphrey, C. J. (1998). *Home care nursing* (3rd ed.). Gaithersburg, MD: Aspen.

Iyer, P. W., & Camp, N. H. (1999). *Nursing documentation: A nursing process approach*. St. Louis, MO: Mosby.

Johnson, D. (1959). A philosophy for nursing diagnosis. *Nursing Outlook, 7,* 198–200.

National Federation of Licensed Practical Nurses (NFLPN). (1996). *Nursing practice standards for the licensed practical/vocational nurse*. Garner, NC: Author.

North American Nursing Diagnosis Association (NANDA) (2001). *Nursing diagnoses: Definitions & classifications 2001–2002*. Philadelphia: Author.

Orlando, I. (1961). *The dynamic nurse–patient relationship*. New York: Putnam.

Orem, D. E., Taylor, S. G., & Renpenning, K. (2001). *Nursing: Concepts of practice* (6th ed.). St. Louis, MO: Mosby.

Paul, R. W. (1995). *Critical thinking: How to prepare students for a rapidly changing world*. Santa Rosa, CA: Foundation for Critical Thinking.

Wiedenbach, E. (1963). The helping art of nursing. *AJN, 63*(11), 54–57.

Wilkinson, J. M. (1996). *Nursing process in action: A critical thinking approach*. Redwood City, CA: Addison-Wesley Nursing.

Wilkinson, J. M. (2000). *Nursing diagnosis handbook with NIC interventions and NOC outcomes*. Englewood Cliffs, NJ: Prentice Hall.

Yoder Wise, P. S. (1998). *Leading and managing in nursing* (2nd ed.). St. Louis, MO: Mosby.

Yura, H., & Walsh, M. B. (1967). *The nursing process*. Washington, DC: Catholic University of America Press.

RESOURCES

Center for Nursing Classification, College of Nursing, The University of Iowa, 407 Nursing Building, Iowa City, IA 52242-1121, 319-335-7051, http://www.nursing.uiowa.edu

North American Nursing Diagnosis Association (NANDA), 1211 Locust Street, Philadelphia, PA 19107, 215-545-8105, Fax: 215-545-8107, http://www.nanda.org

Nursing Diagnosis (journal), 1211 Locust Street, Philadelphia, PA 19107, 800-242-6757

CHAPTER 10
Documentation

REFERENCES/SUGGESTED READINGS

Aquilino, M., & Keenan, G. (2000). Having our say: Nursing's standardized nomenclature. *AJN, 100*(7), 33–38.

Burke, L. J., & Murphy, J. (1995). *Charting by exception applications.* Albany, NY: Delmar.

Charting Tips. (1999). Documenting discharges and transfers in long-term care. *Nursing99, 29*(6), 17.

Charting Tips. (1999). Easy as PIE. *Nursing99, 29*(4), 24.

Clark, M. (1998). Implementation of nursing standardized languages NANDA, NIC, and NOC. *On-line Journal of Issues in Nursing, 2*(2) [On-line]. Available: http://www.nursingworld.org

Daly, J., Button, P., Prophet, C., Clarke, M., & Androwich, I. (1997). Nursing interventions classification implementation issues in five test sites. *Computers in Nursing, 15*(1), 23–29.

DeLaune, S., & Ladner, P. (1998). *Fundamentals of nursing: Standards & practice.* Albany, NY: Delmar.

Eggland, E. T., & Heinemann, D. S. (1994). *Nursing documentation: Charting, recording, and reporting.* Philadelphia: Lippincott.

Estes, M. E. Z. (2002). *Health assessment & physical examination* (2nd ed.). Albany, NY: Delmar.

Fiesta, J. (1991). If it wasn't charted, it was done! *Nursing Management, 22*(8), 17.

Grane, N. B. (1995). Documenting a "harmless" medication error. *Nursing95, 25*(4), 80.

Grobe, S. J. (1992). Nursing lexicon and taxonomy: Preliminary categorisation. In K.C. Lun et al. (Eds.), *Med-Info92: Proceedings of the 7th World Congress on Medical Information.* Amsterdam, Netherlands: Elsevier.

Grulke, C. C. (1995). Seven ways to help a student nurse. *AJN, 96* (60), 24L.

Hayes, B., Norris, J., Martin, K. S., & Androwich, I. (1994). Informatics issues for nursing's future. *Advances in Nursing Science, 16*(4), 71–81.

Iowa Interventions Project. (1993). The NIC taxonomy structure. *Image: Journal of Nursing Scholarship, 25*(3), 187–192.

Iyer, P. W., & Camp, N. H. (1999). *Nursing documentation: A nursing process approach* (3rd ed.). St. Louis, MO: Mosby.

Johnson, M. (1998). Overview of the Nursing Outcomes Classification (NOC). *On-line Journal of Nursing Informatics, 2*(2) [On-line]. Available: http://cac.psu.edu/~dxm12/OJNI.htm

Johnson, M., & Maas, M. (1998). Implementing the nursing outcomes classification in a practice setting. *Outcomes Management for Nursing Practice, 2*(3), 99–104.

Johnson, M., Maas, M., & Moorhead, S. (Eds.). (2000). *Nursing outcomes classfication (NOC)* (2nd ed.). St. Louis, MO: Mosby.

Joint Commission on Accreditation of Healthcare Organizations. (1998). *1998 Hospital accreditation standards.* Oakbrook Terrace, IL: Author.

Klenner, S. (2000). Mapping out a clinical pathway. *RN, 63*(6), 33–36.

LaDuke, S. (2000). Spotlight: What you *really* do with this powerful documentation tool. *Nursing2000, 30*(6), 68.

McCloskey, J. C., & Bulechek, G. M. (1994). Standardizing the language for nursing treatments: An overview of the issues. *Nursing Outlook, 42*(2), 56–63.

McCloskey, J. C., & Bulechek, G. M. (1995). Validation and coding of the NIC taxonomy structure. *Image: Journal of Nursing Scholarship, 27*(1), 43–49.

McCloskey, J. C., & Bulechek, G. M. (1998). Nursing interventions classification (NIC): Current status and new directions. *On-line Journal of Nursing Informatics, 2*(2) [On-line]. Available: http://milkman.cac.psu.edu/ndxm12/OJNI.html

McCloskey, J. C., & Bulechek, G. M. (2000). *Nursing interventions classification (NIC)* (3rd ed.). St. Louis, MO: Mosby.

McCloskey, J. C., & Maas, M. (1998). Interdisciplinary team: The nursing perspective is essential. *Nursing Outlook, 46*(4), 157–163.

McConnell, E. (1999). Charting with care. *Nursing99, 29*(10), 68.

National Committee on Vital and Health Statistics (HCVHS) Hearings on Medical Terminology and Code Development. (1999). *Health care terminology: Nursing outcomes classification, The University of Iowa* [On-line]. Available: http://aspe.os.dhhs.gov/NCVHS/990518t4.htm

National Library of Medicine. (2000). *Fact sheet, UMLS* [On-line]. Available: http://www.nlm.nih.gov/pubs/factsheets/umls.html

North American Nursing Diagnosis Association. (2001). *NANDA Nursing diagnoses: Definitions and classification: 2001–2002.* St. Louis, MO: Author.

Oermann, M., & Huber, D. (1999). Patient outcomes: A measure of nursing's value. *AJN, 99*(9), 40–47.

Ozbolt, J. (1998). *From minimum data to maximum impact: Using clinical data to strengthen patient care* [On-line]. Available: http://cti.itc.virginia.edu/~spt2j/707materials/ozbolt98.htm

Ozbolt, J. G., Fruchtnight, J. N., & Hayden, J. R. (1994). Toward data standards for clinical nursing information. *Journal of the American Medical Informatics Association, 1*(2), 175–185.

Rochman, R. (2000). Are computerized patient records for you? *Nursing2000, 30*(10), 61–62.

Simmons, P. B., & Meadors, B. (1995). Eliminating friendly fire: Successful nursing documentation strategies. *Journal of Nursing Staff Development, 11*(2), 79–82.

Smith, L. (2000). How to use focus charting. *Nursing2000, 30*(5), 76.

Springhouse. (1999). *Mastering documentation* (2nd ed.). Springhouse, PA: Author.

Sullivan, G. (2000). Keep your charting on course. *RN, 63*(5), 75–79.

Thompson, C. (1995, May). Writing better narrative notes. *Nursing95, 25*(5), 87.

Tucker, J. L. (1995). Interdisciplinary record improves documentation. *Patient Education Management, 2*(3), 45–47.

Werley, H. H., & Lang, N. M. (1988). The consensually derived nursing minimum data set: Elements and definitions. In H. H. Werley & N. M. Lang (Eds.), *Identification of the nursing minimum data set* (pp. 402–411). New York: Springer.

Wilkinson, J. M. (2000). *Nursing diagnosis handbook with NIC interventions and NOC outcomes.* Englewood Cliffs, NJ: Prentice Hall.

RESOURCES

American Nursing Informatics Association (ANIA), PMB105, 10808 Foothill Boulevard, Suite 160, Rancho Cucamonga, CA 91730, http://www.ania.org

Center for Nursing Classification, NB 407, The University of Iowa, College of Nursing, Iowa City, IA 52252-1121, http://www.nursing.uiowa.edu

North American Nursing Diagnosis Association (NANDA), 1211 Locust Street, Philadelphia, PA 19107, 800-647-9002, http://www.nanda.org

CHAPTER 11
Client Teaching

REFERENCES/SUGGESTED READINGS

American Hospital Association. (1992). *A patient's bill of rights.* Chicago: Author.

Bandura, A. (1977). *Social learning theory.* Englewood Cliffs, NJ: Prentice Hall.

Barnes, L. (1997). Developing educational materials for patients. *MCN—The American Journal of Maternal/Child Nursing, 22*(1), 55.

Beare, P. G., & Myers, J. L. (1998). *Principles and practice of adult health nursing* (3rd ed.). St. Louis, MO: Mosby.

Biddinger, L. A. (1993). Bruner's theory of instruction and preprocedural anxiety in the pediatric population. *Issues in Comprehensive Pediatric Nursing, 16,* 147–154.

Bloom, B. S. (1977). *Taxonomy of educational objectives: The classification of educational goals, handbook I: Cognitive domain.* New York: Longman.

Bruccoliere, T. (2000). How to make patient teaching stick. *RN, 63*(2), 34–38.

Cirone, N. (1997). Patient education handbook. *Nursing97, 27*(8), 44–45.

Cordell, B., & Smith-Blair, N. (1994). Streamlined charting for patient education. *Nursing94, 24*(1), 57–59.

Doak, C. C., Doak, L. G., & Root, J. H. (1996). *Teaching patients with low literacy skills* (2nd ed.). Philadelphia: Lippincott.

Duffy, B. (1997). Using creative teaching process with adult patients. *Home Healthcare Nurse, 15*(2), 102–108.

Edelman, C. L., & Mandle, C. L. (1998). *Health promotion throughout the lifespan* (4th ed.). St. Louis, MO: Mosby.

Freda, M. (1997). Don't give it away. *MCN—The American Journal of Maternal/Child Nursing, 22*(6), 330.

Joint Commission for Accreditation of Healthcare Organizations. (1998). *Accreditation manual.* Chicago: Author.

Jubeck, M. E. (1994). Teaching the elderly: A commonsense approach. *Nursing94, 24*(5), 70–71.

Katz, J. R. (1997). Back to basics: Providing effective patient teaching. *AJN, 97*(5), 33–36.

Knowles, M. S., Holton, E. F., & Swanson, R. A. (1998). *The adult learner* (5th ed.). Houston: Gulf.

Messner, R. L. (1997). Patient teaching tips from the horse's mouth. *RN, 60*(8), 29–31.

Meyers, D. (1997). *Client teaching guides for home health care* (2nd ed.). New York: Aspen.

Muma, R. D., Lyon, B. A., & Newman, T. A. (Eds.). (1996). *Patient education: A practical approach.* New York: McGraw-Hill.

Nightingale, C. (1992). Pointing to the way ahead: Health education for people with learning disabilities. *Professional Nurse, 7*(9), 612–613, 615.

Poroch, D. (1995). The effect of preparatory patient education on the anxiety and satisfaction of cancer patients receiving radiation therapy. *Cancer Nursing, 18*(3), 206–214

Redman, B. K. (1997). *The practice of patient education* (8th ed.). St. Louis, MO: Mosby.

Seley, J. J. (1994). 10 strategies for successful patient teaching. *AJN, 94*(11), 63–65.

Sodeman, W. A. (1999). *Instructions for geriatric patients* (2nd ed.). Philadelphia: W. B. Saunders Company.

Weissman, M., & Jasovsky, D. (1998). Discharge teaching for today's times. *RN, 61*(6), 38–40.

CHAPTER 12
Cultural Diversity and Nursing

REFERENCES/SUGGESTED READINGS

Agre, P., & Spincola, L. (1996). Helping staff meet the needs of a culturally diverse patient population. *Nursing Forum, 23*(2), 347.

Andrews, M., & Boyle, J. S. (1998). *Transcultural concepts in nursing care* (3rd ed.). Philadelphia: Lippincott.

Andrews, M. M. (1997). Cultural diversity and community health nursing. In J. M. Swanson & M. Nies (Eds.), *Community health nursing: Promoting the health of aggregates* (2nd ed., pp. 433–458). Philadelphia: W. B. Saunders Company.

Andrews, M. M., & Bolin, L. (1997). The African American community. In J. M. Swanson & M. Nies (Eds.), *Community health nursing: Promoting the health of aggregates* (2nd ed., pp. 433–458). Philadelphia: W. B. Saunders Company.

Andrews, M. M., & Hanson, P. (1998). Religion, culture, and nursing. In M. M. Andrews & J. Boyle (Eds.), *Transcultural concepts in nursing care* (3rd ed.). Philadelphia: Lippincott.

Boyle, J. (1998). Culture and community. In M. M. Andrews & J. Boyle (Eds.), *Transcultural concepts in nursing care* (3rd ed.). Philadelphia: Lippincott.

Brewer, J. A., & Bonalumi, N. M. (1996). Cultural diversity in the emergency department: Health care beliefs and practices among the Pennsylvania Amish. *Journal of Emergency Nursing, 21*(6), 494–497.

Carpenito, L. J. (1999). *Nursing diagnosis: Application to clinical practice* (8th ed.). Philadelphia: Lippincott.

Clark, M. (1999). *Nursing in the community* (3rd ed.). Stamford, CT: Appleton & Lange.

Davidhizar, R., Dowd, S., & Giger, J. (1998). Educating the culturally diverse health care student. *Nurse Educator, 23*(2), 38–42.

Degazon, C. (2000). Cultural diversity and community health nursing practice. In M. Stanhope & J. Lancaster (Eds.), *Community & public health nursing* (5th ed.). St. Louis, MO: Mosby.

DeLaune, S., & Ladner, P. (1998). *Fundamentals of nursing: Standards & practice.* Albany, NY: Delmar.

Doherty, W. (1992). Private lives, public values. *Psychology Today, 25*(3), 32–27.

Doswell, W., & Erlen, J. (1998). Multicultural issues and ethical concerns in the delivery of nursing care interventions. *Nursing Clinics of North America, 33*(2), 353–361.

Edelman, C., & Mandle, C. (1998). *Health promotion throughout the lifespan* (4th ed.). St. Louis, MO: Mosby.

Edmission, K. W. (1997). Psychosocial dimensions of medical–surgical nursing. In J. M. Black & E. Matassarin-Jacobs (Eds.), *Medical surgical nursing: Clinical management for continuity of care.* Philadelphia: W. B. Saunders Company.

Estin, P. (1999). Spotting depression in Asian patients. *RN, 62*(4), 39–40.

Fawcett, C. (1993). *Family psychiatric nursing.* St. Louis, MO: Mosby.

Galanti, G. (1997). *Caring for patients from different cultures: Case studies from American hospitals* (2nd ed.). Philadephia: University of Pennsylvania Press.

Giger, J., & Davidhizar, R. (1999). *Transcultural nursing: Assessment and intervention* (3rd ed.). St. Louis, MO: C. V. Mosby.

Gonzalez, R. (1999). ANA advocates more diversity in nursing. *AJN, 99*(11), 24.

Grensing-Pophal, L. (1997). Dealing with diversity in the workplace. *Nursing97, 27*(9), 78.

Grossman, D. (1996). Cultural dimensions in home health nursing. *AJN, 96*(7), 33–36.

Grossman, D., & Taylor, R. (1995). Cultural diversity on the unit. *AJN, 95*(2).

Hoeman, S. (1996). Intraethnic diversity. *Home-Healthcare Nurse, 14*(7), 568.

Kelz, R. (1997). *Delmar's English–Spanish pocket dictionary for health professionals*. Albany, NY: Delmar.

Kelz, R. (1999). *Conversational Spanish for health professionals* (3rd ed.). Albany, NY: Delmar.

Kirkpatrick, M., Brown, S., & Atkins, T. (1998). Using the internet to integrate cultural diversity and global awareness. *Nurse Educator, 23*(2), 15–17.

Lee, E. (Ed.). (1997). *Working with Asian Americans: A guide for clinicians*. San Francisco: Richman Area Multi-Services.

Leininger, M. (1996). *Transcultural nursing: Concepts, theories, research, and practices*. Columbus, OH: Greyden.

Lock, D. (1992). *Increasing multicultural understanding: A comprehensive model*. Newbury Park, CA: Sage.

Louie, K. B. (1999). Health promotion interventions for Asian American Pacific Islanders. In L. Zhan (Ed.), *Asian voices* (pp 3–13). Boston: Jones & Bartlett.

Luckmann, J. (1999). *Transcultural communication in nursing*. Albany, NY: Delmar.

Malone, B. (1998). Diversity, divisiveness and divinity. *American Nurse, 30*(1), 5.

Meleis, A. I. (1997). Immigrant transitions and health care: An action plan [News]. *Nursing Outlook, 45*(1), 42.

Morley, P., & Wallis, R. (Eds.). (1978). *Culture and curing: Anthropological perspectives on traditional medical beliefs and practices*. Pittsburgh, PA: University of Pittsburgh Press.

NewsWatch (2000). Delay in seeking MI treatment is tied to social factors. *RN, 63*(10), 20.

Purnell, L., & Paulanka, B. (1997). *Transcultural health care: A culturally competent approach*. Philadelphia: F. A. Davis.

Rivera-Andino, J., & Lopez, L. (2000). When culture complicates care. *RN, 63*(7), 47–49.

Robinson, A. (1994). Spirituality and risk: Toward an understanding. *Holistic Nursing Practice, 8*(2), 1–7.

Shelley, J. (2000). *Spiritual care: A guide for caregivers*. Downers Grove, IL: Inter Varsity.

Sherman, K. (1994). *Communication and image in nursing*. Albany, NY: Delmar.

Singelenberg, R. (1990). The blood transfusion taboo of Jehovah's Witnesses: Origins, development and function of a controversial doctrine. *Social Science Medicine, 31*(4), 515–523.

Smith, L. (1998). Concept analysis: Cultural competence. *Journal of Cultural Diversity, 5*(1), 4–10.

Spector, R. E. (1999). *Cultural diversity in health and illness* (6th ed.). New York: Prentice-Hall.

Spradley, B. W., & Allender, J. A. (1996). *Community health nursing* (4th ed.). Philadelphia: Lippincott.

Stanhope, M., & Knollmueller, R. (1999). *Handbook of community-based and home health nursing practice* (3rd ed.). St. Louis, MO: Mosby.

Stanhope, M., & Lancaster, J. (2000). *Community & public health nursing* (5th ed.). St. Louis, MO: Mosby.

Sue, D. W., & Sue, D. (1999). *Counseling the culturally different: Theory and practice* (3rd ed.). New York: Wiley.

Talabere, L. (1996). Meeting the challenge of culture care in nursing: Diversity, sensitivity, competence, and congruence. *Journal of Cultural Diversity, 3*(2), 53–61.

U.S. Department of Commerce, Bureau of the Census. (1999). *Statistical abstract of the United States: 1999* (112th ed.). Washington, DC: U.S. Government Printing Office.

RESOURCES

Cultural Diversity in Health Care (video), American Journal of Nursing, 345 Hudson Street, New York, NY 10014

CHAPTER 13
Complementary/Alternative Therapies

REFERENCES/SUGGESTED READINGS

Achterberg, J., Dossey, B., & Kolkmeier, L. (1994). *Rituals of healing: Using imagery for health and wellness*. New York: Bantam.

American Association for Therapeutic Humor (AATH). (2000). *Purpose* [On-line]. Available: http://aath.org/home_1.html

Association of Psychophysiology and Biofeedback (AAPB). (1998). *What is biofeedback?* [On-line]. Available: http://www.aapb.org

Astin, J. A. (1998). Why patients use alternative medicine: Results of a national study. *Journal of the American Medical Association, 279*(19), 1,248.

Avis, A. (1999). Aromatherapy in practice. *Nursing Standard, 13*(24), 14–15.

Benson, H. (1975). *The relaxation response*. New York: Morrow.

Borysenko, J., & Borysenko, M. (1994). *The power of the mind to heal*. Carson, CA: Hay House.

Brett, H. (1999). Aromatherapy in the care of older people. *Nursing Times, 95*(33), 56–57.

Brooke, P. (1998). Legal risks of alternative therapies. *RN, 61*(5), 53–58.

Brown, H., Cassileth, B. R., Lewis, J. P., & Renner, J. H. (1994, June 15). Alternative medicine—Or quackery? *Patient Care*, 80–98.

Budesheim, S., Neuberger, G., Kasal, S., Vogel-Smith, K., Hassanein, R., & DeViney, S. (1994). Determinants of exercise and aerobic fitness in outpatients with arthritis. *Nursing Research, 43*, 11–17.

Byers, D. C. (1987). *Better health with foot reflexology*. St. Petersburg, FL: Ingham.

Byrd, C., & Sherrill, J. (1995). The therapeutic effects of intercessory prayer. *Journal of Christian Nursing, 12*(1), 21–23.

Cerrato, P. (1998). Aromatherapy: Is it for real? *RN, 61*(6), 51–52.

Cerrato, P. (1999a). Using designer margarines to control lipid levels. *RN, 62*(10), 67–68.

Cerrato, P. (1999b). Omega-3 fatty acids: Nothing fishy here! *RN, 62*(8), 59–60.

Cerrato, P. (1999c). A radical approach to heart disease. *RN, 62*(4), 65–66.

Cerrato, P. (1999d). Tai chi: A martial art turns therapeutic. *RN, 62*(2), 59–60.

Cerrato, P. (2000). Diet and herbs for BPH? *RN, 63*(2), 63–64.

Cerrato, P. & Rowell, N. (1999). SAMe: A dietary remedy for mind and body? *RN, 62*(12), 61–64.

Chiropractic Arts Center. (1998). *Common questions about chiropractic care* [On-line]. Available: http://www.chiroarts.com/page7.html

Chopra, D. (1998). *Ageless body, timeless mind*. New York: Harmony.

Cousins, N. (1979). *Anatomy of an illness*. New York: Norton.

Cowens, D. (1996). *A gift for healing: How you can use therapeutic touch*. New York: Crown.

DeLaune, S., & Ladner, P. (1998). *Fundamentals of nursing: Standards & practice*. Albany, NY: Delmar.

Dossey, B. M. (1999). The psychophysiology of bodymind healing. In B. M. Dossey, L. Keegan, C. E. Guzzetta, &

L. G. Kolkmeier (Eds.), *Holistic nursing: A handbook for practice* (3rd ed.). Gaithersburg, MD: Aspen.

Dossey, B. M., (1995). Imagery: Awakening the inner healer. In B. M. Dossey, L. Keegan, C. E. Guzzetta, & L. G. Kolkmeier (Eds.), *Holistic nursing: A handbook for practice* (2nd ed.). Gaithersburg, MD: Aspen.

Dossey, B. M. (Ed.). (1997). *Core curriculum for holistic nursing.* Gaithersburg, MD: Aspen.

Dossey, L. (1997). *Healing words: The power of prayer and the practice of medicine.* San Francisco: Harper.

Dossey, L. (1999). *Prayer, healing, and medicine: An evening with Larry Dossey.* Arvada, CO: Lutheran Medical Center Community Foundation, Arvada Center.

Eisenberg, D. (1993). Medicine in a mind/body culture. In B. Moyers (Ed.), *Healing and the mind.* New York: Doubleday.

Evans, B. (1999). Complementary therapies & HIV infection. *AJN, 99*(2), 42–45.

Feuerstein, G. (1998). *Yoga and yoga therapy* [On-line]. Available: http://members.aol.com/yogareserch/yogatherapy.htm

Fonnesbeck, B. (1998). Are you kidding? *Nursing98, 28*(3), 64.

Frisch, N. (1997). Changing of the guard. *Beginnings, 17*(1), 1, 11.

Frisch, N., & Frisch, L. (1998). *Psychiatric mental health nursing.* Albany, NY: Delmar.

Gagne, D., & Toye, R. C. (1994). Decreasing anxiety in psychiatric patients with therapeutic touch. *Archives of Psychiatric Nursing, 8*(3), 184–189.

Gates, R. (1997). Legal issues in alternative medicine. *Alternative Therapies in Clinical Practice, 4*(4), 143.

Guinness, A. (1993). *Family guide to natural medicine: How to stay healthy the natural way.* Pleasantville, NY: Reader's Digest.

Hodge, P., & Ullrich, S. (1999). Does your assessment include alternative therapies? *RN, 62*(6). 47–49.

Hover-Kramer, D. (1996). *Healing touch: A resource for health care professionals.* Albany, NY: Delmar.

Hutchison, C. (1999). Healing touch: An energetic approach. *AJN, 99*(4), 43–48.

Japsen, B. (1995, August 21). Cost-conscious providers take to holistic medicine. *Modern Healthcare,* 138–142.

Kahn, S. (1995). *The nurse's meditative journal: Nurse as healer series.* Albany, NY: Delmar.

Kahn, S., & Saulo, M. (1995). *Healing yourself: A nurse's guide to self-care and renewal.* Albany, NY: Delmar.

Keegan, L. (1994). *The nurse as healer.* Albany, NY: Delmar.

Keegan, L. (1995a). Nutrition, exercise, and movement. In B. M. Dossey, L. Keegan, C. E. Guzzetta, & L. G. Kolkmeier (Eds.), *Holistic nursing: A handbook for practice* (2nd ed., pp. 257–285). Gaithersburg, MD: Aspen.

Keegan, L. (1998). Alternative & complementary therapies. *Nursing98, 28*(4), 50–53.

Keegan, L. (1999). Touch: Connecting with the healing power. In B. M. Dossey, L. Keegan, C. E. Guzzetta, & L. G. Kolkmeier (Eds.), *Holistic nursing: A handbook for practice* (3rd ed.). Gaithersburg, MD: Aspen.

Keegan, L. (2001). *Healing with complementary and alternative therapies.* Albany, NY: Delmar.

Keville, K., & Green, M. (1995). *Aromatherapy: A complete guide to healing art.* Freedom, CA: Crossing.

King, M. O., Pettigrew, A. C., & Reed, F. C. (1999). Complementary, alternative, integrative: Have nurses kept pace with their clients? *Medsurg Nursing, 8*(4), 249–56.

Kolkmeier, L. G. (1999). Relaxation: Opening the door to change. In B. M. Dossey, L. Keegan, C. E. Guzzetta, & L. G. Kolkmeier (Eds.), *Holistic nursing: A handbook for practice* (3rd ed.). Gaithersburg, MD: Aspen.

Krieger, D. (1993). *Accepting your power to heal: The personal practice of therapeutic touch.* Santa Fe, NM: Bear.

Lanfranco, J. (1997). *Acupressure and shiatsu information* [On-line]. Available: http://www.geocities.com/HotSprings/4416/acusci.html

Mackey, R. B. (1995). Discover the healing power of therapeutic touch. *AJN, 95*(4), 27–33.

Marwick, C. (1995). Should physicians prescribe prayer for health? Spiritual aspects of well-being considered. *Journal of the American Medical Association, 273*(20), 1561–1562.

Mason, J. (1999). Massage: The nursing touch. In Healing touch: An energetic approach by C. P. Hutchison. *AJN, 99*(4), 44.

Maxwell, J. (1997). The gentle power of acupressure. *RN, 60*(4), 53–56.

McGhee, P. (1998). Rx: Laughter. *RN, 69*(7), 50–53.

McGhee, P. (1999). *Health, healing, and the amuse system.* (3rd ed.). Dubuque, IA: Kendall/Hunt.

Meehan, T. C. (1993). Therapeutic touch and postoperative pain: A Rogerian research study. *Nursing Science Quarterly, 6*(2), 69–78.

Mentgen, J. (1996). The clinical practice of healing touch. In D. Hover-Kramer (Ed.), *Healing touch: A resource for health care professionals* (pp. 155–165). Albany, NY: Delmar.

Miller, J., & Connor, K. (2000). Going to the dogs . . . for help. *Nursing2000, 30*(11), 65–67.

Mills, E. M. (1994). The effect of low-intensity aerobic exercise on muscle strength, flexibility, and balance among sedentary elderly persons. *Nursing Research, 43,* 206–211.

Mornhinweg, G. C., & Voignier, R. R. (1995). Holistic nursing interventions. *Orthopaedic Nursing, 14*(4), 20–24.

Moyers, B. (1995). *Healing and the mind.* New York: Doubleday.

National Center for Complementary & Alternative Medicine (NCCAM). (2000). *Untitled Document* [On-line]. Available: http://nccam.nih.gov/nccam/an/general/index.html

National Institutes of Health (NIH). (1997). *Acupuncture: NIH consensus statement* [On-line]. Available: http://odp.od.nih.gov/consensus/cons/107.107_intro.htm

National Institutes of Health (NIH). (1998). *About the Office of Alternative Medicine* [On-line] Available: http://altmed.od.nih.gov/oam/about/general.shtml#budget

National Institutes of Health (NIH). (2000). *About the Center for Complementary & Alternative Medicine* (NCCAM). [On-line]. Available: http://altmed.od.nih.gov/nccam/about/general.shtml

Nightingale, F. (1969). *Nursing: What it is and what it is not.* New York: Dover.

Olsen, M., & Sneed, N. (1995). Anxiety and therapeutic touch. *Issues in Mental Health Nursing, 16*(2), 97–108.

O'Neil, C., Avila, J., & Fetrow, C. W. (1999). Herbal medicines: Getting beyond the hype. *Nursing99, 29*(4), 58–61.

Pert, C. (1986). The wisdom of the receptors: Neuropeptides, the emotions, and bodymind. *Advances, 3,* 8–16.

Quinn, J. (1993). Psychoimmunologic effects of therapeutic touch on practitioners and recently bereaved recipients: A pilot study. *Advances in Nursing Science, 15*(4), 13–26.

Renner, J. H., Dillard, J. N., & Edelberg, D. (1999). Should the FDA regulate alternative medicines? *Hospital Health Network, 73*(10), 24.

Rossi, E. L. (1993). *The psychobiology of mind body healing: New concepts of therapeutic hypnosis* (Rev. ed.). New York: Norton.

Schroeder-Shecker, T. (1994). Music for the dying. *Journal of Holistic Nursing, 12*(1), 83–99.

Simons, S. (1997). *Vegetables and fruits: Natural "Phyters" against disease.* Paper presented at the Texas Agricultural Extension service conference.

Snyder, J. R. (1999). Therapeutic touch in hospice care. In Healing touch: An energetic approach by C. P. Hutchison. *AJN, 99*(4), 46.

Spencer, J. W., & Jacobs, J. J. (Eds.) (1999). *Complementary/ alternative medicine: An evidence-based approach.* St. Louis, MO: Mosby.

Stedman, M. (1999). Alternatives: You'd better shop around. *Health, 13*(1), 60–66.

Stevenson, C. (1994). The psychophysiological effects of aromatherapy massage following cardiac surgery. *Complementary Therapies in Medicine, 2*(1), 27.

Sutherland, J. A. (2000). Getting to the point. *AJN, 100*(9), 40–43.

Trevelyan, J. (1993). Aromatherapy. *Nursing Times, 89*(25), 38–40.

Vacca, V. (1998). Back to high touch. *RN, 69*(7), 88.

Walton, J. (1996). Spiritual relationships: A concept analysis. *Journal of Holistic Nursing, 14*(3), 237–250.

Weil, A. (1996). *Spontaneous healing: How to discover and enhance your body's natural ability to maintain and heal itself.* New York: Knopf.

Weil, A. (1998). *Natural health, natural medicine: A comprehensive manual for wellness and self-care* (Rev. ed.). New York: Houghton Mifflin.

Weiss, R. R., & James, W. D. (1997). Allergic contact dermatitis from aromatherapy. *American Journal of Contact Dermatology, 8*(4), 250.

Wetzel, W. (1993). Healing touch as nursing intervention. *Journal of Holistic Nursing, 11*(3), 277–285.

Wilkinson, S. (1995). Aromatherapy and massage in palliative care. *International Journal of Palliative Nursing, 1*(1), 21.

Wilson, D. F. (1995). Therapeutic touch: Foundations and current knowledge. *Alternative Health Practitioner, 1*(1), 55–63.

Worden, J. (1999). *Overview of reflexology* [On-line]. Available: http://www.aol.com/reflexology

Yoga Research and Education Center. (2000). *Frequently asked questions* [On-line]. Available: http://www.yrec.org/faq.html

Zahourek, R. P., & Larkin, D. (1995). Hypnosis and therapeutic suggestion for managing pain and stress. *Alternative Health Practitioner, 1*(19), 43–55.

Zisselman, M. H., Rovner, B. W., Shmuely, Y., & Ferrie, P. (1996). A pet therapy intervention with geriatric psychiatry inpatients. *American Journal of Occupational Therapy, 50*(1), 47–51.

RESOURCES

Acupressure Institute, 1533 Shattuck Avenue, Berkeley, CA 94709, 800-442-2232

The American Association for Therapeutic Humor, 4534 West Butler Drive, Glendale, AZ 85302, 623-934-6068, http://aath.org

American Holistic Nurses' Association, P.O. Box 2130, Flagstaff, AZ 86003-2130, 800-278-2462, http://www.ahna.org

American Massage Therapy Association (AMTA), 820 Davis Street, Suite 100, Evanston, IL 60201, 847-864-0123, http://www.amtamassage.org

American Reflexology Certification Board, P. O. Box 62067, Littleton, CO 80162, 303-933-6921

Association for Applied Psychophysiology and Biofeedback, 10200 West 44th Avenue, Suite 304, Wheat Ridge, CO 80033-2840, 800-477-8892, 303-422-8436, http://www.aapb.org

Colorado Center for Healing Touch, 198 Union Boulevard, Suite 204, Lakewood, CO 80220, 303-989-0581, http://www.healingtouch.net

Holistic Alliance of Professional Practitioners Entrepreneurs Networkers, Inc. (HAPPEN), 1889 West Rose, Stockton, CA 95203, 888-8HAPPEN (42-7736), http://www.happen.org

The Laughter Remedy, 45 North Fullerton, Suite 402, Montclair, NJ 07042, 973-783-8383

Office of Alternative Medicine, OAM Clearinghouse, P.O. Box 8218, Silver Spring, MD 20907-8218, 888-644-6226, http://altmed.od.nih.gov/nccam

Tai Chi Association, 4651 Roswell Road, Atlanta, GA 30342, 404-289-5652, http://tai-chi-association.com

Yoga Research and Education Center, P.O. Box 1386, Lower Lake, CA 95457, 707-928-9898, http://www.yrec.org

CHAPTER 14
The Life Cycle

REFERENCES/SUGGESTED READINGS

American Academy of Child & Adolescent Psychiatry (AACAP). (1998a). *Teenagers with eating disorders* [On-line]. Available: http://www.aacap.org/publications/factsfam/eating.htm

American Academy of Child & Adolescent Psychiatry (AACAP). (1998b). *Teen suicide* [On-line]. Available: http://www.aacap.org/publications/factsfam/suicide.htm

American Academy of Pediatrics. (1998). Guidance for effective discipline. *Pediatrics, 101*(4), 723.

American Academy of Pediatrics (AAP). (2000a). Puberty information for boys and girls [On-line]. Available: http://www.aap.org/family/puberty.htm

American Academy of Pediatrics. (2000b). *2000 red book: Report of the Committee on Infectious Diseases* (23rd ed.). Elk Grove, IL: Author.

American Cancer Society (ACS). (2000). *Cancer facts & figures 2000.* Atlanta, GA: Author.

American Nurses Association. (1990). *Nursing's agenda for health care reform.* Washington, DC: Author.

Beare, P. G., & Myers, J. L. (1998). *Adult health nursing* (3rd ed.). St. Louis, MO: Mosby.

Centers for Disease Control and Prevention. (1999a). *AIDS falls from top fifteen causes of death; teen births, homicides decline; but no change in infant mortality* [On-line]. Available: http://www.cdc.gov/nchs/releases/99news/99news/aidsfall.htm

Centers for Disease Control and Prevention. (1999b). *Teen pregnancy* [On-line]. Available: http://www.cdc.gov/nccdphp/teen.htm

Copenhaver, M. M. (1995). Better late than never: Of reminiscence and resolution. *Journal of Psychosocial Nursing, 33*(7), 18–22.

Davidson, D. A. (1995). Physical abuse of preschoolers: Identification and intervention. *American Journal of Occupational Therapy, 49*(3), 235–243.

de Anda, D., & Smith, M. A. (1993). Differences among adolescent, young adult, and adult callers of suicide help lines. *Social Work, 38*(4), 421–428.

DeLaune, S., & Ladner, P. (1998). *Fundamentals of nursing: Standards & practice,* Albany, NY: Delmar.

Dombeck, M. B. (1995). Dream telling: A means of spiritual awareness. *Holistic Nursing Practice, 9*(2), 37–47.

Edelman, C. L., & Mandle, C. L. (1998). *Health promotion throughout the lifespan* (4th ed.). St. Louis, MO: Mosby.

Eliopoulos, C. (1997). *Gerontological nursing* (4th ed.). Philadelphia: Lippincott.

Erikson, E. (1968). *Childhood and society.* New York: Norton.

Estes, M. E. Z. (2002). *Health assessment & physical examination* (2nd ed.). Albany, NY: Delmar.

Firth, P. A., & Watanabe, S. J. (1996). *Women's health: Instant nursing assessment.* Albany, NY: Delmar.

Foley, D. (1995). *Women's encyclopedia of health & emotional healing.* Emmaus, PA: Rodale.

Forshner, L., & Garza, A. (1999). Childhood vaccines: An update. *RN, 62*(4), 32–36.

Fowler, J. W. (1995). *Stages of faith: The psychology of human development and the quest for meaning.* New York: Harper & Row.

Freud, S. (1961). *Civilization and its discontents.* New York: Norton.

Fuller, J., & Schaller-Ayers, J. (2000). *Health assessment: A nursing approach* (3rd ed.). Philadelphia: Lippincott.

Gilligan, C. (1993). *In a different voice: Psychologic theory and women's development.* Cambridge, MA: Harvard University Press.

Gilligan, C., & Attanucci, D. (1988). Two moral orientations: Gender differences and similarities. *Merrill-Palmer Quarterly, 34*(3), 332–333.

Guyton, A. C., & Hall, J. (1996). *Textbook of medical physiology* (9th ed.). Philadelphia: W. B. Saunders Company.

Hale, P. J. (2000). HIV, hepatitis, and sexually transmitted diseases. In M. Stanhope & J. Lancaster (Eds.), *Community & public health nursing* (5th ed.). St. Louis, MO: Mosby.

Harkness, G. A., & Dincher, J. R. (1999). *Medical–surgical nursing: Total patient care* (10th ed.). St. Louis, MO: Mosby.

Havighurst, R. J. (1972). *Developmental tasks and education.* New York: Longman.

Heriot, C. S. (1999). Developmental tasks and development in the later years of life. In M. Stanley & P. Beare (Eds.), *Gerontological nursing: A health promotion/protection approach* (2nd ed.). Philadelphia: F. A. Davis.

Ineicher, B. (1995). Breastfeeding 2. Strategies to promote breastfeeding in inner cities. *Health Visit, 68*(2), 61–62.

Johnson, B. S. (1995). *Child, adolescent, and family psychiatric nursing.* Philadelphia: Lippincott.

Johnson, B. S. (1997). *Psychiatric–mental health nursing: Adaptation and growth* (4th ed.). Philadelphia: Lippincott.

Kohlberg, L. (1977). *Recent research in moral development.* New York: Holt, Rinehart, & Winston.

Levin, J. D. (1995). *Introduction to alcoholism counseling: A bio-psycho-social approach* (2nd ed.). Washington, DC: Taylor & Francis.

Levinson, D. (1978). *The seasons of a man's life.* New York: Knopf.

Mayo Clinic. (1998a). *Children's snacks: Don't ban them, plan them* [On-line]. Available: http://www.mayohealth.org/mayo/9806/htm/snacks.htm

Mayo Clinic. (1998b). *Vegetarianism: Is it OK for children?* [On-line]. Available: http://www.mayohealth.org/mayo/9807/htm/vegie.htm

Murray, R. B., & Zentner, J. P. (1997). *Health assessment & promotion strategies through the life span* (6th ed.). East Norwalk, CT: Appleton & Lange.

Nugent, E. (1995). Try to remember: Reminiscence as a nursing intervention. *Journal of Psychosocial Nursing, 33*(11), 7–11.

Orpinas, P. K. (1995). The co-morbidity of violence-related behaviors with health-risk behaviors in a population of high school students. *Journal of Adolescent Health, 16*(3), 216–225.

Piaget, J. (1963). *The origins of intelligence in children.* New York: Norton.

Piaget, J., & Inhelder, B. (1969). *The psychology of the child.* New York: Basic.

Randolph, N. (1998). *American nursing review of psychiatric and mental health nursing certification.* Springhouse, PA: Springhouse.

Roye, C. F. (1995). Breaking through to the adolescent patient. *AJN, 95*(12), 19–23.

Sapp, M., & Bliesmer, M. (1999). A health promotion/protection approach to meeting elders' healthcare needs through public policy and standards of care. In M. Stanley & P. Beare (Eds.), *Gerontological nursing: A health promotion/prevention approach.* Philadelphia: F. A. Davis.

Smith, A. (1986). *The body.* New York: Viking Penguin.

Sullivan, H. S. (1953). *Interpersonal theory of psychiatry.* New York: Norton.

U.S. Department of Health & Human Services, Public Health Service. (1990). *Healthy people 2000: National health promotion and disease prevention objectives* (DHHS Publication No. PHS 91-5012). Washington, DC: Author.

Wong, D. L., Hockenberry-Eaton, M., Wilson, D., Winkelstein, M. L., Ahmann, E., & DiVito-Thomas, P. (1999). *Whaley & Wong's nursing care of infants and children* (6th ed.). St. Louis, MO: Mosby.

RESOURCES

American Academy of Pediatrics, 141 Northwest Point Boulevard, Elk Grove Village, IL 60007-1098, 847-434-4000, http://www.aap.org

American Association of Retired Persons, 601 E Street NW, Washington, DC 20049, 800-424-3410, http://www.aarp.com

American Foundation for Suicide Prevention, 120 Wall Street, 22nd floor, New York, NY 10005, 888-333-2377, http://www.afsp.org

American Society on Aging, 833 Market Street, Suite 511, San Francisco, CA 94103, 415-974-9600

Centers for Disease Control and Prevention (CDC), 1600 Clifton Road NE, Atlanta, GA 30333, 404-639-3311, 800-311-3435, http://www.cdc.gov

Gerontological Society of America, 1030 15th Street NW, Suite 25, Washington, DC 20005, 202-842-1275, http://www.geron.org

National Institute of Child Health & Human Development NICHD Clearinghouse, P. O. Box 3006, Rockville, MD 20847, 800-370-2943, http://www.nichd.nih.gov/

Zero to Three: National Center for Infants, Toddlers and Families, 734 15th Street NW Suite 1000, Washington, DC 20005, 202-638-1144, http://www.zerotothree.org

CHAPTER 15
Wellness Concepts

REFERENCES/SUGGESTED READINGS

Baughcum, A. (1998). Mom's beliefs may cause child obesity. *Archives of Pediatric and Adolescent Medicine, 152,* 1010–1014.

Browder, S. (1998). *Attention, women over 50* [On-line]. Available: http://www.seniornews.com/new-choices/article593.html

Brown, E. (1995, August). An inexpensive and painless alternative to colonoscopy? (coprocytobiology). *Medical Update, 19,* 1.

Carey, B. (1996, July/August). The slumber solution. *Health,* 70–75.

Centers for Disease Control and Prevention (CDC). (2000). *Mammography on the rise for women age 50 and over* [On-line]. Available: http://www.od.nih.gov/ormh/press_rel/cdc_report.html

Cerrato, P. (1999). A radical approach to heart disease. *RN, 62*(4), 65–66.

Chase, M. (1996, February 5). Simple handwashing gets new scrutiny for disease control. *The Wall Street Journal,* B1(E&W).

Dixon, B. (1995). *Good health for African Americans.* New York: Random House.

Don't overdo it: Alcohol paradox. (1996, February 5). *Industry Week, 245*(1), 19.

Eastman, P. (1996, January 17). Task force issues new screening guidelines. *Journal of the National Cancer Institute, 88*(3), 74.

Edlin, G., Golanty, E., & McCormack-Brown, K. (1997). *Essentials for health and wellness.* Boston: Jones & Bartlett.

Floyd, P., Mimms, S., & Yelding-Howard, C. (1995). *Personal health: A multicultural approach.* Englewood, CO: Morton.

Hafen, B., & Hoeger, W. (1997). *Wellness: Guidelines for a healthy lifestyle* (2nd ed.). Englewood, CO: Morton.

Health-club hygiene. (1995, November). *Industry Week, 244,* 31.

Hoeger, W., & Hoeger, S. (1995). *Lifetime physical fitness and wellness* (4th ed.). Englewood, CO: Morton.

Hoffman, E. (1996). *Our health, our lives.* New York: Pocket.

Inlander, C., & Moran, C. (1996). *77 Ways to beat colds and flu.* New York: Walker.

Lee, I., & Paffenbarger, R. (1998). Exercise can cut stroke risk 50%. *Stroke, 29,* 2049–2054.

Lyon, B. (2000). Conquering stress. *Reflections on Nursing LEADERSHIP, 26*(1), 22–23, 43.

Malaty, H. (1998). Twin study: *H pylori* tied to hygiene. *American Journal of Epidemiology, 148,* 793–797.

Matthews, K. (1998). Suppressed anger hard on women's hearts. *Psychosomatic Medicine, 60,* 633–638.

National Center for Health Statistics. (1997). *Monthly vital statistics report, 45*(11S2), 23, 40–43 [On-line]. Available: http://www.youfirst.com/risks.htm

Oman, D., & Reed, D. (1998). Religious elderly tend to live longer. *American Journal of Public Health, 88,* 1469–1475.

Osteoporosis, a silent disease, finds a louder voice. (1995, November–December). *Menopause News, 5,* 1.

Payne, W., & Hahn, D. (1998). *Understanding your health* (5th ed.). St. Louis, MO: Mosby.

Poliafico, F. (1999). Abstinence is not the only answer. *RN, 62*(1). 58–60.

Quench strokes with every sip. (1995, October) *Prevention, 47,* 66.

Reed, D. (1998). Four factors predict "Healthy Aging." *American Journal of Public Health, 88,* 1463–1469.

Reichler, G., & Burke, N. (1999). *Active wellness: A personalized 10 step program for a healthy body, mind & spirit.* Time Life Custom Publishing.

Reichman, L., & Mangura, B. (1996, February). State-of-the-art tuberculosis prevention. *Chest, 109,* 301.

Robertson, J. (1996). *Peak-performance living.* New York: HarperCollins.

Seiger, L., Vanderpool, K., & Barnes, D. (1995). *Fitness and wellness strategies.* Dubuque, IA: Brown.

Simon, H. (1992). *Staying well.* Boston: Houghton Mifflin.

Smith, C., & Maurer, F. (1999). *Community health nursing: Theory and practice.* (2nd ed.) Philadelphia: W. B. Saunders Company.

Social stigma of colon and rectal problems thwarts life-saving cancer screenings. (1995, October). *Executive Health's Good Health Report, 32,* 1.

U.S. Department of Agriculture, U.S. Department of Health & Human Services. (2000). *Home and Garden Bulletin No. 232* (5th ed.).

U.S. Department of Health & Human Services. (1990). *Healthy People 2000: National health promotion and disease prevention objectives.* (DHHS Publication No. [PHS] 91-50212). Washington, DC.

U.S. Department of Health & Human Services (USDHHS), Public Health Service. (1998). *Healthy people 2000: National health promotion and disease prevention objectives and first draft healthy people 2010: National health promotion and disease prevention objectives* [On-line]. Available: http://web.health.gov/healthypeople

U.S. Department of Health & Human Services (USDHHS) Public Health Service (2000a). *Healthy people 2010: National Health promotion and disease prevention objectives* [On-line]. Available: http://web.health.gov/healthypeople

U.S. Department of Health & Human Services (USDHHS), Public Health Service (PHS). (2000b). *1998–1999 Progress Review* [On-line]. Available: http://odphp.osophs.dhhs.gov/pubs/hp2000

Wash your hands (to help prevent colds). (1996, January). *Consumer Reports on Health, 2*(1).

Weil, A. (1998). *Natural health, natural medicine* (2nd ed.). Boston: Houghton Mifflin.

RESOURCES

Aerobics and Fitness Association of America, 15250 Ventura Boulevard, Suite 200, Sherman Oaks, CA 91403-3297, 800-446-2322, http://www.aerobics.com/

American Dietetic Association, 216 West Jackson Boulevard, Suite 800, Chicago, IL 60606-6995, 800-366-1655, http://www.eatright.org

American Health Care Association, 1201 L Street, NW, Washington, DC 20005, 202-342-4444, http://www.ahca.org

American Holistic Nurses' Association, P.O. Box 2130, Flagstaff, AZ 86003-2130, 800-278-2462, http://www.ahna.org

Center for Science in the Public Interest, 1875 Connecticut Avenue, NW, Suite 300, Washington, DC 20009-5728, 202-332-9110, http://www.cspinet.org

Centers for Disease Control and Prevention, *Morbidity and Mortality Weekly Report,* http://http://www.cdc.gov/cdc.html

Centers for Disease Control and Prevention, 1600 Clifton Road, NE, Atlanta, GA 30333, 404-639-3311, http://www.cdc.gov

Consumer Product Safety Commission, Washington, DC 20207, 800-638-2772, 800-638-8270 TDD, 800-492-8104 TTD in MD only

Dental Disease Prevention, Centers for Disease Control and Prevention (CDC), 1600 Clifton Road, NE, Atlanta, GA 30333

Environmental Protection Agency (EPA), Public Information Center, 401 M Street, SW, Washington, DC 20466, 800-424-9065, 202-260-2090, http://www.epa.gov

Food and Drug Administration, Office of Consumer Affairs, 5600 Fishers Lane, Rockville, MD 20857, 888-463-6332, http://www.fda.gov

Food and Nutrition Information Center, National Agricultural Library Building, Room 304, 10301 Baltimore Avenue, Beltsville, MD 20705-2351, 301-504-5719, http://www.nal.usda.gov/fnic/

Healthy People 2010, Office of Disease Prevention and Health Promotion, 738-6 Humphrey Building, 200 Independence Avenue SW, Washington, DC 20201, 202-205-8583

Medic Alert Foundation International, P.O. Box 819008, Turlock, CA 95381-1009, 800-344-3226, 209-668-3333, http://www.medicalert.org

National Cholesterol Education Program Information Center, 4733 Bethesda Avenue, Room 530, Bethesda, MD 20814, 301-951-3260

National Council Against Health Fraud, Resource Center, 300 East Pink Hill Road, Independence, MO 64057, 816-228-4595, http://www.ncahf.org

National Health Information Center, P.O. Box 1133, Washington, DC 20013-1133, 800-336-4797, http://nhic-nt.health.org

National Highway Traffic Safety Administration, NES-11 HL, U.S. Department of Transportation, 400 7th Street, SW, Washington, DC 20590, 202-366-9294, Auto Hotline: 800-424-9393, http://www.nhtsa.dot.gov

National Institute for Occupational Safety and Health, Clearinghouse for Occupational Safety and Health Information, Technical Information Branch, 4676 Columbia Parkway, Cincinnati, OH 45226, 800-356-4674

The National Institute on Aging, P.O. Box 8057, Gaithersburg, MD 20898-8057, 800-222-2225, http://www.nih.gov/nia

National Institutes of Health, 9000 Rockville Pike, Bethesda, MD 20892, 301-496-1776, http://www.nih.gov

National League for Nursing, 61 Broadway, New York, NY 10006, 212-363-5555, 800-669-9656, Fax: 212-812-0393, http://www.nln.org

National Safety Council, 1121 Spring Lake Drive, Itasca, IL 60143-3201, 630-285-1121, http://www.national-safety-council.ie

National Wellness Association/National Wellness Institute, 1300 College Court, P.O. Box 827, Stevens Point, WI 54481-0827, 715-342-2961, http://www.wellnesswi.org

National Women's Health Network, 514 Tenth Street, NW, Washington, DC 20004, 202-347-1140

U.S. Department of Agriculture, 14th & Independence Avenue, SW, Washington, DC 20250, 800-535-4555, 202-720-2791, http://www.usda.gov

U.S. Department of Health and Human Services, Office of Disease Prevention and Health Promotion, 638-East Humphrey Building, 200 Independence Avenue, SW, Washington, DC 20201, 202-690-6343, http://www.hhs.gov

World Health Organization, 525 23rd Street, NW, Washington, DC 20037, 202-974-3000, Headquarters Avenue Appia 20, 1211 Geneva 27, Switzerland, http://www.who.int

CHAPTER 16
Stress, Adaptation, and Anxiety

REFERENCES/SUGGESTED READINGS

Aguilera, D. C. (1998). *Crisis intervention: Theory and methodology* (8th ed.). St. Louis, MO: Mosby.

Alfaro-LeFevre, R. (2000). *Critical thinking in nursing: A practical approach* (2nd ed.). Philadelphia: W. B. Saunders Company.

Badger, J. M. (1994). Calming the anxious patient. *AJN, 94*(5), 46–50.

Badger, J. M. (1995). Tips for managing stress on the job. *AJN, 95*(9), 31–33.

Beck, A. (1976). *Cognitive therapy and emotional disorders.* New York: International Universities Press.

Cullen, A. (1995). Burnout: Why do we blame the nurse? *AJN, 95*(11), 23–27.

DeLaune, S. C. (1993). Learned optimism. *Aspen's Advisor for the Nurse Executive, 8*(11), 8.

DeLaune, S. C. (1996). Applying the nursing process for clients with anxiety, somatoform, and dissociative disorders. In H. S. Wilson & C. R Kneisl (Eds.), *Psychiatric nursing* (5th ed., p. 368). Menlo Park, CA: Addison-Wesley.

DeLaune, S., & Ladner, P. (1998). *Fundamentals of Nursing: Standards & practice.* Albany, NY: Delmar.

Fennell, M. E. (1999). Parents in the OR? You Bet! *RN, 62*(12), 38–40.

Freud, S. (1959). Inhibitions, symptoms and anxiety. In J. Strachey (Trans.), *The standard edition of the complete psychological works of Sigmund Freud* (Vol. 20). London: Hogarth.

Frisch, N., & Frisch, L. (1998). *Psychiatric mental health nursing.* Albany, NY: Delmar.

Gillies, D. A. (1994). *Nursing management: A systems approach* (3rd ed.). Philadelphia: W. B. Saunders Company.

Heinrich, K., & Killeen, M. E. (1993). The gentle art of nurturing yourself. *AJN, 93*(10), 41–44.

Holmes, T. H., & Rahe, R. (1967). The social readjustment rating scale. *Journal of Psychosomatic Research, 2,* 213–218.

Kahn, S., & Saulo, M. (1994). *Healing yourself: A nurse's guide to self-care and renewal.* Albany, NY: Delmar.

Keegan, L. (1999). Nutrition, exercise, and movement. In B. M. Dossey, L. Keegan, & C. E. Guzzetta (Eds.), *Holistic nursing: A handbook for practice* (3rd ed.). Gaithersburg, MD: Aspen.

Kneisl, C. R., & Riley, E. (1996). Crisis intervention. In H. S. Wilson & C. R. Kneisl (Eds.), *Psychiatric nursing* (5th ed., pp. 711–731). Menlo Park, CA: Addison-Wesley.

Kobasa, S. C. (1979). Stressful life events, personality and health. An inquiry into hardiness. *Journal of Personality and Social Psychology, 37*(1), 1–11.

Kobasa, S. C., Maddi, S. R., & Kahn, S. (1982). Hardiness and health: A prospective study. *Journal of Personality and Social Psychology, 45*(4), 839–850.

Lauver, D. (1995). Optimism and coping with breast cancer symptoms. *Nursing Research, 44*(4), 202–207.

Lyon, B. L. (2000). Situational anger and self-empowerment. *Reflections on Nursing LEADERSHIP, 26*(3), 36–37.

Mandle, C. L., & Gruber-Wood, R. (1998). Health promotion and the individual. In C. L. Edelman & C. L. Mandle (Eds.), *Health promotion throughout the life-span* (4th ed.). St. Louis, MO: Mosby.

Mayo Clinic. (1999). Stress patrol: Stop tension in its tracks [On-line]. Available: http://www.mayohealth.org/mayo/9912/htm/stress_patrol.htm

Mayo Clinic. (2000a). Dealing with co-worker conflict [On-line]. Available: http://www.mayohealth.org/mayo/9704/htm/stre_1sb.htm

Mayo Clinic. (2000b). Workplace stress: Can you control it? [On-line]. Available: http://www.mayohealth.org/mayo/9704/htm/stress.htm

Meyers, T. A., Eichhorn, D. J., Guzzetta, C. E., Clark, A. P., Klein, J. D., Taliaferro, E., & Calvin, A. (2000). Family presence during invasive procedures and resuscitation. *AJN, 100*(2), 32–40.

North American Nursing Diagnosis Association. (2001). *Nursing diagnoses: Definitions & classification.* 2001–2002. Philadelphia: Author.

Peplau, H. (1952). *Interpersonal relations in nursing.* New York: Putnam.

Selye, H. (1974). *Stress without distress.* New York: New American Library.

Selye, H. (1976). *Stress in health and disease* (Rev. ed.). Boston: Butterworths.

Stubblefield, C. (1995). Optimism: A determinant of health behavior. *Nursing Forum, 30*(1), 19–24.

Sullivan, H. S. (1953). *The interpersonal theory of psychiatry by H. S. Sullivan.* New York: Norton.

Talbott, S. W. (1993). Political analysis: Structure and process. In D. J. Mason, S. W. Talbott, & J. K. Leavitt (Eds.), *Policy and politics for nurses* (2nd ed., pp. 129–148). Philadelphia: W. B. Saunders Company.

Waughfield, C. (1998). *Mental health concepts* (4th ed.). Albany, NY: Delmar.

Wilson, H. S., & Kneisel, C. R. (1996). *Psychiatric Nursing* (5th ed.). Menlo Park, CA: Addison-Wesley.

Woodhouse, D. K. (1993). The aspects of humor in dealing with stress. *Nursing Administration Quarterly, 18*(1), 80–89.

RESOURCES

American Holistic Nurses' Association, P.O. Box 2130, Flagstaff, AZ 86003-2130, 800-278-AHNA (1461), 520-526-2196, http://www.ahna.org

American Institute of Stress, 124 Park Avenue, Yonkers, NY 10703, 914-963-1200, http://www.stress.org

International Stress Management Association, USA Branch, 638 St. Lawrence Avenue, Reno, NV 89509, http://www.stress-management-isma.org/ISMA-USA.html

Stress Reduction Clinic, University of Massachusetts Medical Center, 55 Lake Avenue North, Worcester, MA 01655, 508-856-2656

CHAPTER 17
Loss, Grief, and Death

REFERENCES/SUGGESTED READINGS

American Nurses Association (ANA). (1992). Promotion of comfort and relief of pain in dying patients. In *Compendium of position statements on the nurse's role in end-of-life decisions*. Washington, DC: Author.

Andreas, L. (1998). Controlling pain: Keeping a dying patient comfortable. *Nursing98, 28*(1), 70.

Backer, B. A., Hannon, N. R., & Russell, N. A. (1994). *Death and dying: Understanding and care* (2nd ed.). Albany, NY: Delmar.

Barbus, A. J. (1975). The dying person's bill of rights. *AJN, 75*(1), 99.

Beckel, J. (1996). Resolving ethical dilemmas in long-term care. *Journal of Gerontological Nursing, 22*(1), 20–26.

Boon, T. (1998). Don't forget the hospice option. *RN, 61*(2), 30–33.

Boss, P. (1999). *Ambiguous loss: Learning to live with unresolved grief*. Cambridge, MA: Harvard University Press.

Bowlby, J. (1982). *Attachment and loss: Vol. 2. Separation anxiety and anger*. New York: Basic.

Bral, E. (1998). Caring for adults with chronic cancer pain. *AJN, 98*(4), 27–32.

Carpenito, L. J. (1997). *Handbook of nursing diagnosis* (7th ed.). Philadelphia: Lippincott.

Cerrudo, J. (1998). Letting go of Abuelo. *AJN, 98*(8), 53.

Corless, I., Germino, B., & Pittman, M. (Eds.). (1995). *A challenge for living: Death, dying, and bereavement*. Boston: Jones & Bartlett.

Corr, C., Nabe, C., & Corr, D. (2000). *Death and dying, life and living* (3rd ed.). Belmont, CA: Wadsworth.

Czerwiec, M. (1996). When a loved one is dying: Families talk about nursing care. *AJN, 96*(5), 32–36.

Doka, K., Rushton, C. H., & Thorstenson, T. A. (1994). HealthCare Ethics Forum '94: Caregiver distress: If it is so ethical, why does it feel so bad? *American Association Critical-Care Nurses Clinical Issues, 5*(3), 346–352.

Durham, E., & Weiss, L. (1997). How patients die. *AJN, 97*(12), 41–46.

Edelman, C. L., & Mandle, C. L. (1998). *Health promotion throughout the lifespan* (4th ed.). St. Louis, MO: Mosby.

Engle, G. L. (1961). Is grief a disease? *Psychosomatic Medicine, 23,* 18–22.

Engle, G. L. (1964). Grief and grieving. *AJN, 64*(9), 93–98.

Estes, M. E. Z. (2002). *Health assessment & physical examination* (2nd ed.). Albany, NY: Delmar.

Fauri, D. P., & Grimes, D. R. (1994). Bereavement services for families and peers of deceased residents of psychiatric institutions. *Social Work, 39*(2), 185–190.

Ferrell, B. (1998a). End-of-life care. *Nursing98, 28*(9), 58.

Ferrell, B. (1998b). How can we improve care at the end of life? *Nursing Management, 29*(9), 41–43.

Ferrell, B., Virani, R., Grant, M., Coyne, P., & Uman, G. (2000). End-of-life care: Nurses speak out. *Nursing2000, 30*(7), 54–57.

Forbes, V. (1998). The dying game. *AJN, 98*(9), 50.

Furman, J. (2000). Taking a holistic approach to the dying time. *Nursing 2000, 30*(6), 46–49.

Furman, J., & McNabb, D. (1997). *The dying time: Practical wisdom for the dying and their caregivers*. New York: Bell Tower.

Haynor, P. (1998) Meeting the challenge of advance directives, *AJN, 98*(3), 27–32.

Hellwig, K. (2000). A family lesson in dying. *RN, 63*(12), 32–33.

Hooks, F. J., & Daly, B. J. (2000). Hastening death: Is a natural death always best? *AJN, 100*(5), 56–63.

Hvizdos, D. (2000). The tie that binds: Hanging on by a shoelace. *AJN, 100*(7), 25.

Jaffe, C., & Ehrlich, C. (1997). *All kinds of love: Experiencing hospice*. Amityville, NY: Baywood.

Kübler-Ross, E. (1969). *On death and dying*. New York: Macmillan.

Kübler-Ross, E. (1974). *Questions and answers on death and dying*. New York: Macmillan.

Kübler-Ross, E. (1995). *Death is of vital importance: On life, death, and life after death*. Barrytown, NY: Station Hill.

Kübler-Ross, E. (1997). *Meaning of our suffering*. Barrytown, NY: Barrytown, Ltd.

Lindemann, E. (1944). Symptomatology and management of acute grief. *American Journal of Psychiatry, 101,* 141–148.

Lynn, J., Schuster, J. L., & Kabcenell, A. (2000). *Improving care for the end of life: A sourcebook for health care managers and clinicians*. New York: Oxford University Press.

McCaffery, M., & Pasero, C. (1999). *Pain: Clinical manual for nursing practice* (2nd ed.). St. Louis, MO: Mosby.

McClain, M. E., & Shafer, S. M. (1996). Supporting families after sudden infant death. *Journal of Psychosocial Nursing and Mental Health Services, 34*(4), 30–34.

McGowan, D. (1998). The right to say goodbye. *RN, 61*(5), 84.

North American Nursing Diagnosis Association. (2001). *Nursing diagnoses: Definitions and classification 2001–2002*. Philadelphia: Author.

Pritchett, K., & Lucas, P. (1997a). Death and dying. In B. S. Johnson (Ed.), *Psychiatric–mental health nursing: Adaptation and growth* (4th ed., pp. 206–207). Philadelphia: Lippincott.

Pritchett, K., & Lucas, P. (1997b). Grief and loss. In B. S. Johnson (Ed.), *Psychiatric–mental health nursing: Adaptation and growth* (4th ed., pp. 199–218). Philadelphia: Lippincott.

Puopolo, A. (1999). Gaining confidence to talk about end-of-life care. *Nursing99, 29*(7), 49–51.

Reese, C. D. (1996). Please cry with me: Six ways to grieve. *Nursing96, 26*(8), 56.

Rhymes, J. (1993). Hospice care in the nursing home. *Nursing Home Medicine, 1*(6), 14–16, 22–24.

Roach, S. S., & Nieto, B. C. (1997). *Healing and the grief process*. Albany, NY: Delmar.

Rodebaugh, L., Schwindt, R., & Valentine, F. (1999). How to handle grief with wisdom, *Nursing99, 29*(10), 52–53.

Smith-Stoner, M., & Frost, A. (1998). Coping with grief and loss: Bringing your shadow self into the light. *Nursing98, 28*(2), 49–50.

Smith-Stoner, M., & Frost, A. (1999). How to build your "hope skills." *Nursing99, 29*(9), 49–51

Taylor, M. (1995). Benefits of dehydration in terminally ill clients. *Geriatric Nursing, 16*(6), 271–272.

Taylor, P., & Ferszt, G. (1994). Letting go of a loved one. *Nursing94, 24*(1), 55–56.

Ufema, J. (1995a). How to help dying clients feel "safe." *Nursing95, 25*(9), 59.

Ufema, J. (1995b). Insights on death and dying. *Nursing95, 25*(11,12), 19, 22–23.

Ufema, J. (1999). Reflections on death and dying. *Nursing99, 29*(6), 56–59.

Ufema, J. (2000a). Death & dying: Bedside vigils. *Nursing2000, 30*(7), 26.

Ufema, J. (2000b). Death & dying: Seeking closure. *Nursing2000, 30*(8), 28.

Ufema, J. (2000c). Death & dying: Setting goals, withholding nutrition, will to die. *Nursing2000, 30*(9), 66–67.

Vanderbeek, J. (2000). Till death do us part: A firsthand account of family presence. *AJN, 100*(2), 44.

Wong, M. M. (1996). *The 1996 national directory of bereavement support groups and services.* Forest Hills, NY: ADM.

Worden, J. W. (1991). *Grief counseling and grief therapy: A handbook for the mental health practitioner* (2nd ed.). New York: Springer.

RESOURCES

Americans for Better Care of the Dying, 4125 Albemarle Street NW, Suite 210, Washington, DC 20016, 202-895-9485, http://www.abcd-caring.org

American Nurses Association Center for Ethics and Human Rights, 600 Maryland Avenue, Suite 100 West, Washington, DC 20024, 800-274-4262, http://www.nursingworld.org/readroom/position

Association for Death Education & Counseling, 342 North Main Street, Hartford, CT 06117, 860-586-7503, http://www.adec.org

Choice in Dying, 475 Riverside Drive, Room 1852, New York, NY 10115, 800-989-9455, http://www.choices.org

Hospice Foundation of America, 2001 S. Street NW #300, Washington, DC 20009, 800-854-3402, http://www.hospice foundation.org

Last Acts, 325 West Huron, Suite 300, Chicago, IL 60610, 312-642-8652, http://www.lastacts.org

The National Hospice and Palliative Care Organization, 1700 Diagonal Road, Suite 300, Alexandria, VA 22314, 703-837-1500, http://www.nhpco.org

CHAPTER 18
Basic Nutrition

REFERENCES/SUGGESTED READINGS

American Heart Association. (1999). *Non-AHA-Approved Diets.* [On-line]. Available: http://www.deliciousdecisions.org/ff/tsd_nondiets_fad.html

Barrett, S. (1998). *Dietary reference intakes (DRIs): New guidelines for calcium and related nutrients* [On-line]. Available: http//www.quackwatch.com/03healthpromotion/dr01.html

Centers for Disease Control and Prevention. (1997). Update: Prevalence of overweight among children, adolescents, and adults—United States, 1988–1994. *MMWR, 46*(9), 199.

Cerrato, P. (1999). When food is the culprit. *RN, 62*(6), 52–56.

Cobb, M. (1997). Improving your patient's nutritional status. *Nursing97, 27*(6), 32hhr,32hh6.

Costello, M. (1996). Home health nutrition. *MedSurg Nursing, 5*(4), 229–238.

Craig, W. (1997). Phytochemicals: Guardians of our health. *Journal of the American Dietetic Association, 97*(10 Suppl. 2), S199–S204.

DeLaune, S., & Ladner, P. (1998). *Fundamentals of nursing: Standards & practice.* Albany, NY: Delmar.

Dudek, S. (1997). *Nutrition handbook for nursing practice* (3rd ed.). Philadelphia: Lippincott.

Dudek, S. G. (2000). Malnutrition in hospitals: Who's assessing what patients eat? *AJN, 100*(4), 36–42.

Estes, M. E. Z. (2002). *Health assessment & physical examination* (2nd ed.). Albany, NY: Delmar.

Frankel, E., Waterhouse, A., & Teissedra, P. (1995). Principal phenolic phytochemicals in selected California wine and their antioxidant activity in inhibiting oxidation of human low-density lipoproteins. *Journal of Agricultural & Food Chemistry, 43*, 890–894.

Gravely, M. (1993, Spring/Summer). Answering your questions on nutrition and nutrition labeling. *Food News for Consumers.* USDA, Food Safety and Inspection Service.

Institute of Medicine. (1997). *Dietary reference intakes for calcium, phosphorus, magnesium, vitamin D, and fluoride* [On-line]. Available: http//www2.nas.edu/whatsnew/276a.html

Institute of Medicine. (1998). *Dietary reference intakes: Thiamin, riboflavin, niacin, vitamin B$_6$, folate, vitamin B$_{12}$ pantothenic acid, biotin, and choline* [On-line]. Available: http//www2.nas.edu/whatsnew/287e.html

Kohn-Keeth, C. (2000). How to keep feeding tubes flowing freely. *Nursing2000, 30*(3), 58–59.

Kurtzwell, P. (1998). Staking a claim to good health [On-line]. Available: http://www.fda.gov/fdca/features/1998/698_labl.html

Lee, R., & Nieman, D. (1997). *Nutritional assessment* (2nd ed.). Columbus, OH: WCB/McGraw-Hill.

Loan, T., Magnuson, B., & Williams, S. (1998). Debunking six myths about enteral feeding. *Nursing98, 28*(8), 43–48.

McConnell, E. (1998). Administering parenteral nutrition. *Nursing98, 28*(7), 18.

National Academy of Sciences. (1989). *Recommended dietary allowances: 10th edition.* Washington, DC: National Academy.

Position of the American Dietetic Association: Phytochemicals and functional foods. (1995). *Journal of the American Dietetic Association, 95*, 493–498.

Sharpe, P., McGrath, L., McClean, E., Young, I., & Archbold, G. (1995). Effect of red wine consumption on lipoprotein (a) and other risk factors for atherosclerosis. *QJM, 88*, 101–108.

Simons, S. (1997). *Vegetables and fruits: Natural "phyters" against disease.* Texas Agriculture Extension Service.

Stanfield, P. (1997). *Nutrition and diet therapy* (3rd ed.). Boston: Jones & Bartlett.

Steinmetz, K., & Potter, J. (1996). Vegetables, fruit, and cancer prevention: A review. *Journal of the American Dietetic Association, 96*, 1027–1036.

Townsend, C. & Roth, R. (2000). *Nutrition & diet therapy.* (7th ed.). Albany, NY: Delmar.

U.S. Food & Drug Administration (FDA). (1999). The food label [On-line]. Available: http://www.fda.gov/opacom/backgrounders/foolaabel/newlabel.html

USDA. (2000). *Nutrition and your health: Dietary guidelines for Americans* (5th ed., Home and Garden Bulletin, No. 232). Washington, DC: United States Department of Agriculture and United States Department of Health and Human Services.

USDA. (1996). *The food guide pyramid* (Home and Garden Bulletin, No. 252). Washington, DC: United States Department of Agriculture, Center for Nutrition Policy and Promotion.

Washington, H. (1998). The vitamin revolution. *Health, 12*(6), 104–110.

Wilkes, G. (2000). Nutrition: The forgotten ingredient in cancer care. *AJN, 100*(4), 46–51.

Williams, S. (2001). *Basic nutrition and diet therapy* (11th ed.). St. Louis, MO: Mosby.

RESOURCES

American Dietetic Association, 216 West Jackson Blvd., Chicago, IL 60606-6995, 312-899-0040, 800-877-1600, Fax: 312-899-1979, http://www.eatright.org, e-mail: webmaster@eatright.org

Food and Nutrition Board, Institute of Medicine, 2101 Constitution Avenue, NW, Washington, DC 20418, 202-334-2169

Food and Nutrition Information Center, USDA/National Agricultural Library, 10301 Baltimore Boulevard, Room 304, Beltsville, MD 20705-2351, 301-504-5755, http://www.nal.usda.gov/fnic/

Food Safety Education and Communication Office, 1400 Independence Avenue, SW, Room 1180, Washington, DC 20250, Food Safety Hotline: 800-332-4010

CHAPTER 19
Rest and Sleep

REFERENCES/SUGGESTED READINGS

American Psychiatric Association (APA). (2000). *DSM-IV.* Washington, DC: Author.

American Academy of Sleep Medicine (NASM). (2000). *Insomnia* [On-line]. Available: http://www.aasmnet.org

Brown, W. (1997). *What sleep disturbances do preschool children experience?* (From "Best Practices" series) [On-line]. Available: http://www.psychlink.com/resourc/consultn/article 28.html

Carter, A. (1997). *Restless legs syndrome (RLS)* [On-line], Clinical Reference Systems. Available: http://www.realage.com/Library/M_behavior.htm

Coleman, R. M. (1986). *Wide awake at 3:00 AM: By choice or by chance?* New York: Freeman.

Cooper, P. (1998). *Insomnia* [On-line], Clinical Reference Systems. Available: http://www.realage.com/Library/M_behavior.htm

Coren, S. (1997). *Sleep thieves: An eye-opening exploration into the science and mysteries of sleep.* New York: Free.

DeRoin, D. (1997). *Snoring* [On-line]. Clinical Reference Systems. Available: http://www.realage.com/Library/M_behavior.htm

Hogstel, M. O. (1994). *Nursing care of the older adult* (3rd ed.). Albany, NY: Delmar.

McCaffery, M., & Pasero. (1999). *Pain: Clinical manual for nursing practice* (2nd ed.). St. Louis, MO: Mosby.

McNeil, R. Padrick, K., & Wellman, J. (1986). "I didn't sleep a wink." *AJN, 86*(1), 26–27.

Merritt, S. L. (2000). Putting sleep disorders to rest. *RN, 63*(7), 26–30.

Morgan, D. (1996). *Sleep secrets for shift workers & people with off-beat schedules.* Duluth, MN: Whole Person Associates.

National Sleep Foundation (NSF). (1998). *Why Target Sleep?* [On-line]. Available: http://www.sleepfoundation.org

National Sleep Foundation (NSF). (2000a). *ABCs of ZZZs* [On-line]. Available: http://www.sleepfoundation.org/publications/ZZZs.html

National Sleep Foundation (NSF). (2000b). *Facts about PLMS* [On-line]. Available: http://www.sleepfoundation.org/publications/fact_plms.html

National Sleep Foundation (NSF). (2000c). *Facts about restless legs* [On-line]. Available: http://www.sleepfoundation.org/publications/fact_rls.html

National Sleep Foundation (NSF). (2000d). *The nature of sleep* [On-line]. Available: http://www.sleepfoundation.org/publications/nos.html

National Sleep Foundation (NSF). (2000e). *Sleep & aging* [On-line]. Available: http://www.sleepfoundation.org/publications/sleepage.html

National Sleep Foundation (NSF). (2000f). *Sleep apnea* [On-line]. Available: http://www.sleepfoundation.org/publications/sleepap.html

National Sleep Foundation (NSF). (2000g). *Sleep strategies for shift workers* [On-line]. Available: http://www.sleepfoundation.org/publications/1999shiftworker.html

National Sleep Foundation (NSF). (2000h). *Sleep and the traveler* [On-line]. Available: http://www.sleepfoundation.org/publications/travel.html

Nordenberg, T. (1998). *Tossing and turning no more: How to get a good night's sleep* [On-line]. Available: http://www.fda.gov/fdac/features/1998/498_sleep.html

North American Nursing Diagnosis Association. (2001). *Nursing diagnoses: Definitions and classification, 2001–2002.* Philadelphia: Author.

Pillow Firmness Key to Sleeping Well. (1998). [On-line]. Available: http://www.thirdage.com

Simpson, C. (1996). *Coping with sleep disorders.* New York: Rosen.

Sorrell, J. (1999). Taking steps to calm restless legs syndrome. *Nursing99, 29*(9), 60–61.

Summerfield, C. (1998). *Napping: Men have the edge* [On-line]. Available: http://www.thirdage.com/health

RESOURCES

American Sleep Apnea Association, 2025 Pennsylvania Avenue, NW, Washington, DC 20006, 202-293-3650, http://www.nicom.com/~asaa/

American Academy of Sleep Medicine, 1610 14th Street NW, Suite 300, Rochester, MN 55901, http://www.asda.org

National Sleep Foundation, 1522 K Street, NW, Suite 510, Washington, DC 20005, 202-347-3471, http://www.sleepfoundation.org, E-mail: natsleep@erols.com

CHAPTER 20
Safety/Hygiene

REFERENCES/SUGGESTED READINGS

Bouman, C. C. (1998). Functions of the immune system. In J. Myers & P. Beare, *Adult Health Nursing* (3rd ed.). St. Louis, MO: Mosby.

Carpenito, L. (1999). *Handbook of nursing diagnosis* (8th ed). Philadelphia: Lippincott.

Carroll, P. (1998). Preventing nosocomial pneumonia. *RN, 61*(6), 44–47.

Centers for Disease Control and Prevention (CDC). (2000). Falls: An increasing danger to the elderly. *Morbidity and Mortality Weekly Report (MMWR) 49*(RR-02), 1–12.

Easterling, M. (1990). Which of your clients is heading for a fall? *RN, 53*(1), 56–58.

Eriksson, J. H. (1995). *Oncologic nursing* (2nd ed.). Springhouse, PA: Springhouse.

Food and Drug Administration. (1996). *FDA safety alert: Entrapment hazards with hospital bed side rails* [On-line]. Available: http://http://www.fda.gov/cdrh/bedrails.html

Guyton, A. C., & Hall, J. (1996). *Textbook of medical physiology* (9th ed.). Philadelphia: W. B. Saunders Company.

Joint Commission on Accreditation of Healthcare Organizations. (2000). *2000 hospital accreditation standards* (HAS). Oakbrook Terrace, IL: Author.

McCloskey, J. C., & Bulecheck, B. M. (2000). *Nursing interventions classification* (NIC) (3rd ed.). St. Louis, MO: Mosby.

National Institute for Occupational Safety & Health (NIOSH). (2000). *About NIOSH research and services* [On-line]. Available: http://www.cdc.gov/niosh/about.html

North American Nursing Diagnosis Association. (2001). *Nursing diagnoses: Definitions and classification 2001–2002*. Philadelphia: Author.

Richman, D. (1998). To restrain or not to restrain? *RN, 61*(7), 55–60.

Salladay, S. (1998). Severing the ties that bind. *Nursing98, 28*(5), 30.

Shaffer, S. (1997). Protective mechanisms. In S. Otto (Ed.), *Oncology nursing* (3rd ed.). St. Louis, MO: Mosby.

Stanhope, M., & Knollnueller, R. (2000). *Handbook of community-based and home health nursing practice: Tools for assessment, intervention, and education* (3rd ed.). St. Louis, MO: Mosby.

Stillwell, E. (1991). Nurses' education related to the use of restraints. *Journal of Gerontological Nursing, 17*(2), 23–25.

Sullivan-Marx, E. M. (1994). Delirium and physical restraint in the hospitalized elderly. *Image: The Journal of Nursing Scholarship, 26*, 295–300.

U.S. Department of Labor. (1999). *Workplace fire safety* [On-line]. Available: http://www.cdc.gov/niosh/nasd/docs2/oa14000.html

Walker, B. (1998). *Injury prevention for the elderly: Preventing falls*. Gaithersberg, MD: Aspen.

Walker, B. (1998). Preventing falls. *RN, 61*(5), 40–42.

Whedon, M., & Shedol, P. (1989). Prediction and prevention of patient falls. *Image: The Journal of Nursing Scholarship, 21*(2), 108–114.

RESOURCES

Consumer Product Safety Commission, Washington, DC 20207, 800-638-2772

Environmental Protection Agency, Public Information Center, 401 M Street SW, Washington, DC 20460, 202-260-2090, http://www.epa.gov

Food and Drug Administration, Office of Consumer Affairs, 5600 Fishers Lane, Rockville, MD 20857, 888-463-6332, http://www.fda.gov

Joint Commission on Accreditation of Healthcare Organizations (JCAHO), One Renaissance Boulevard, Oakbrook Terrace, IL 60181, 630-792-5000, http://www.jcaho.org

National Institute for Occupational Safety and Health, Clearinghouse for Occupational Safety and Health Information, Technical Information Branch, 4676 Columbia Parkway, Cincinnati, OH 45226, 800-356-4674

CHAPTER 21
Infection Control/Asepsis

REFERENCES/SUGGESTED READINGS

Association for Professionals in Infection Control and Epidemiology, Inc. (APIC). (1999). *Infection control tips on handwashing* [On-line]. Available: http://www.apic.org/html/cons/washtips/html

Association for Professionals in Infection Control and Epidemiology (APIC). (1999). *Infection control—A few ounces of prevention* [On-line]. Available: http://www.apic.org/html/cons/icdesc.html

Beaumont, E. (1997). Technology scoreboard: Focus on infection control. *AJN, 97*(12), 51–54.

Benenson, A. S. (Ed.). (1995). *Control of communicable diseases in man* (16th ed.). Washington, DC: American Public Health Association.

Benner, J. (1998). Combating infection: Help from the web. *Nursing98, 28*(11), 71–72.

Berlinguer, G. (1992). The interchange of disease and health between the old and new worlds. *American Journal of Public Health, 82*(10), 1407–1414.

Black, J. M., & Matassarin-Jacobs, E. (1997). *Medical–surgical nursing: Clinical management for continuity of care* (5th ed.). Philadelphia: W. B. Saunders Company.

Bouman, C. C. (1998). Functions of the immune system. In J. Myers & P. Beare, *Adult health nursing* (3rd ed.). St. Louis, MO: Mosby.

Centers for Disease Control and Prevention (CDC). (1991). *Recommendations for preventing transmission of human immunodeficiency virus, hepatitis B virus to patients during exposure—prone invasive procedures*. Washington, DC: U.S. Government Printing Office.

Centers for Disease Control and Prevention. (1992). *Principles of epidemiology: Agent, host, environment* (2nd ed.). Atlanta, GA: Public Health Practice Program Office.

Centers for Disease Control and Prevention. (2000). Hospital-acquired infections hit fewer ICU patients. *Morbidity and Mortality Weekly Report, 49*(8), 149.

Combating Infection. (1997). Tackling disease transmission. *Nursing97, 27*(7), 65.

Compliance Control Center. (1998). *Hand-transmitted infection* [On-line]. Available: http:\\users.aol.com/comcontrol/cc12htm

DeLaune, S., & Ladner, P. (1998). *Fundamentals of nursing: Standards & practice*. Albany, NY: Delmar.

Department of Labor. (1991). Bloodborne pathogens rules and regulations. *Federal Register, 58*, 64175–64182.

Ellner, P. D., & Neu, H. C. (1992). *Understanding infectious disease*. St. Louis, MO: Mosby.

Finkelstein, L., & Mendelson, M., with Bailey, E. (1998). Exposure to bloodborne pathogens. *AJN, 98*(3), 67–68.

Guyton, A. C., & Hall, J. (1995). *Textbook of medical physiology* (9th ed.). Philadelphia: W. B. Saunders Company.

Hartstein, A. (1995). Control of methicillin-resistant *Staphylococcus aureus* in a hospital and an intensive care unit. *Infection Control and Hospital Epidemiology, 16*(7), 405–411.

Hegner, B., & Caldwell, E. (1999). *Nursing assistant: A nursing process approach* (8th ed.). Albany, NY: Delmar.

Hospital Infection Control Practices Advisory Committee (HICPAC). (1995). Recommendations for preventing the spread of vancomycin resistance. *Infection Control and Hospital Epidemiology, 16*(2), 105–113.

Ikeda, R., et al. (1995). Nosocomial tuberculosis: An outbreak of a strain resistant to seven drugs. *Infection Control and Hospital Epidemiology, 16*(3), 152–159.

Infection Control Update 1997. (1997). How to prevent IV catheter contamination. *Nursing97, 27*(6), 60.

Infectious Disease. (2000). Blood contamination in 50% of reusable tourniquets. *AJN, 100*(4), 17.

Inman, W. B. (2000). Combating infection: Pathogens invade 21st century. *Nursing2000, 30*(8), 22–24.

National Center for Infectious Disease (NCID). (1997). *Sterilization or disinfection of medical devices: General principles* [On-line]. Available: http://www.cdc.gov/ncidod/diseases/hip/sterilgp.htm

Nicolle, L. E., & Garibaldi, R. A. (1995). Infection control in long-term-care facilities. *Infection Control and Hospital Epidemiology, 16,* 348–353.

North American Nursing Diagnosis Association (NANDA). (2001). *Nursing diagnoses: Definitions & classification 2001–2002.* Philadelphia: Author.

OSHA Regulations (1996). *Bloodborne pathogens 1910.1.3. (d)(4)(111)(A)(1)* [On-line]. Available: http://http://www.osha.gov/oshstd_data/1910_1030html

Porche, D. J. (1991). Universal precautions. In R. L. Nichols, N. E. Hyslop, & J. G. Bartlett (Eds.), *Decision making in surgical sepsis.* Philadelphia: Decker.

Porche, D. J. (1998). Nursing management of adults with immune disorders. In J. Myers & P. Beare (Eds.), *Adult health nursing* (3rd ed.). St. Louis, MO: Mosby.

Pugliese, G. (1994). EPA begins testing hospital disinfectants as sterilant testing program nears completion. *Infection Control and Hospital Epidemiology, 16*(4), 248–250.

Pugliese, G. (1995). Nursing home fined $75,000 for isolating patient for 9 months. *Infection Control and Hospital Epidemiology, 16*(7), 418.

Satterfield, N. (1995). CDC publishes draft guidelines for isolation. Association for Professionals in Infection Control and Epidemiology, Inc. *Newsletter, 6*(1), 1–2.

Voss, A., & Widner, A.F. (1997). No time for handwashing!? Handwashing versus alcoholic rub: Can we afford 100% compliance? *Infection Control and Hospital Epidemiology, 18*(3), 205–208.

Weltman, A. C., Short, L. J., & Mendelson, M. H. (1995). Disposal-related sharps injuries at a New York City teaching hospital. *Infection Control and Hospital Epidemiology, 16*(5), 268–274.

RESOURCES

Association for Professionals in Infection Control and Epidemiology, Inc. (APIC), 1275 K Street, NW, Suite 1000, Washington, DC 20005-4006, 202-789-1890, http://www.apic.org

Environmental Protection Agency (EPA), Disinfectant Hotline, 401 M Street, SW, Washington, DC 20460-0003, 800-447-6349, Antimicrobial Program Branch, 703-305-7443

Hospital Infection Program (HIP), Office of the Director, HIP Mailstop A07, National Center for Infectious Diseases, Centers for Disease Control and Prevention, 1600 Clifton Rd., Atlanta, GA 30333, http://www.cdc.gov/ncidod/hip/

National Foundation for Infectious Diseases, 4733 Bethesda Ave., Suite 750, Bethesda, MD 20814, 301-656-0003, http://www.nfid.org

Society for Healthcare Epidemiology of America, 19 Mantua Road, Mt. Royal, NJ 08061, 609-423-0087

CHAPTER 22
Standard Precautions and Isolation

REFERENCES/SUGGESTED READINGS

Borton, D. (1996). Gloves on or off. *Nursing96, 26*(9), 46.

Borton, D. (1997). Isolation precautions: Clearing up the confusion. *Nursing97, 27*(1), 49.

Centers for Disease Control and Prevention (CDC). (1975). *Isolation techniques for use in hospitals* (2nd ed.), (HHS [CDC] Publication No. 80-8314). Washington, DC: U.S. Government Printing Office.

Centers for Disease Control and Prevention (CDC). (1985). Recommendations for preventing transmission of infection with human T-lymphotropic virus type III/lymphadenopathy-associated virus in the workplace. *Morbidity and Mortality Weekly Report (MMWR), 34,* 681–686, 691–695.

Centers for Disease Control and Prevention (CDC). (1987). Recommendations for prevention of HIV transmission in health-care settings. *MMWR, 36*(2S), 1S–18S.

Centers for Disease Control and Prevention (CDC). (1988). Update: Universal precautions for prevention of transmission of human immunodeficiency virus, hepatitis B virus, and other blood borne pathogens in health-care settings. *MMWR, 37,* 377–382, 387–388.

Centers for Disease Control and Prevention (CDC). (1996). Guideline for isolation precautions in hospitals. In *Guidelines for the prevention and control of nosocomial infections.* Atlanta, GA: Author.

Centers for Disease Control and Prevention (CDC)/ Hospital Infection Control Practices Advisory Committee (HICPAC). (1997a). *Part I: Evolution of isolation practices* [On-line]. Available: http://www.cdc.gov/ncidod/hip/isolat/isopart1.htm

Centers for Disease Control and Prevention (CDC)/ Hospital Infection Control Practices Advisory Committee (HICPAC). (1997b). *Part II. Recommendations for isolation precautions in hospitals* [On-line]. Available: http://www.cdc.gov/ncidod/hip/isolat/isopart2.htm

Centers for Disease Control and Prevention (CDC)/ Hospital Infection Control Practices Advisory Committee (HICPAC). (1997c). *Table I. Synopsis of types of precautions and patients requiring precautions* [On-line]. Available: http://www.cdc.gov/ncidod/hip/isolat/isotab_1.htm

Centers for Disease Control and Prevention (CDC)/ Hospital Infection Control Practices Advisory Committee (HICPAC). (1997d). *Table II. Clinical syndromes warranting additional emperic precautions to prevent transmission of epidemiologically important pathogens pending confirmation of diagnosis* [On-line]. Available: http://www.cdc.gov/ncidod/hip/isolat/isotab_2.htm

Centers for Disease Control and Prevention (CDC)/ Hospital Infection Control Practices Advisory Committee (HICPAC). (1997e). *Appendix A: Type and duration of precautions needed for selected infections and conditions* [On-line]. Available: http://www.cdc.gov/ncidod/hip/isolat/isoapp_a.htm

Department of Labor. (1991). Bloodborne pathogens rules and regulations. *Federal Register, 58,* 64175–64182.

Gage, N. D., Landon, J. F., & Sider, M. T. (1959). *Communicable disease.* Philadelphia, PA: F. A. Davis.

Garner, J. S. (1984). Comments on CDC guideline for isolation precautions in hospitals, 1984. *American Journal of Infection Control, 12,* 163.

Garner, J. S., & Simmons, B. P. (1983). *CDC Guideline for Isolation Precautions in Hospitals* (HHS [CDC] Publication No. 83-8314). Atlanta, GA: U.S. Department of Health and Human Services, Public Health Service, Centers for Disease Control. *Infection Control* (1983) 4:245–325; and *American Journal of Infection Control* (1984) 12:103–163.

Haley, R. W., Garner, J. S. & Simmons, B. P. (1985). A new approach to the isolation of patients with infectious diseases: Alternative systems. *Journal of Hospital Infection, 6,* 128–138.

Haley, R. W., & Shachtman, R. H. (1980). The emergence of infection surveillance and control programs in U.S. hospitals: An assessment, 1976. *American Journal of Epidemiology, 111,* 574–591.

Hospital Infection Control Practices Advisory Committee (HICPAC). (1995). Recommendations for preventing the spread of Vancomycin resistance. *Infection Control and Hospital Epidemiology, 16*(2), 105–113.

Lynch, P., Jackson, M. M., Cummings, J., & Stamm, W. E. (1987). Rethinking the role of isolation practices in the prevention of nosocomial infections. *Annals of Internal Medicine, 107,* 243–246.

Lynch, T. (1949). *Communicable disease nursing.* St. Louis, MO: Mosby.

National Communicable Disease Center. (1970). *Isolation techniques for use in hospitals* (1st ed., PHS Publication No. 2054). Washington, DC: U.S. Government Printing Office.

North American Nursing Diagnosis Association. (2001). *Nursing diagnoses: Definitions & classification 2001–2002.* Philadelphia: Author.

Occupational Safety and Health Administration (OSHA). (1991). Occupational exposure to bloodborne pathogens: Final rule, 29CRF 1919;1030. *Federal Register, 56,* 64175.

Porche, D. J. (1991). Universal precautions. In R. L. Nichols, N. E. Hyslop & J. G. Bartlett (Eds.), *Decision making in surgical sepsis.* Philadelphia: Decker.

Porche, D. J. (1998). Nursing management of adults with immune disorders. In P. Beare & J. Myers (Eds.), *Adult health nursing* (3rd ed.). St. Louis, MO: Mosby.

Satterfield, N. (1995). CDC publishes draft guidelines for isolation. *Association for Professionals in Infection Control and Epidemiology, Inc. Newsletter, 6*(1), 1–2.

Schaffner, W. (1980). Infection control: Old myths and new realities. *Infection Control, 1,* 330–334.

RESOURCES

Centers for Disease Control and Prevention, 1600 Clifton Road, Atlanta, GA 30333, 404-639-3311, http://www.cdc.gov

CHAPTER 23
Fluid, Electrolyte, and Acid–Base Balance
REFERENCES/SUGGESTED READINGS

Bulechek, G., & McCloskey, J. (1999). *Nursing interventions: Effective nursing treatments* (3rd ed). Philadelphia: W. B. Saunders Company.

Castiglione, V. (2000). Hyperkalemia. *AJN, 100*(1), 55–56.

Clayton, K. (1997). Cancer-related hypercalcemia: How to spot it how to manage it. *AJN, 97*(5), 42–48.

Cohen, B., & Wood, D. (2000). *Memmler's the human body in health & disease* (9th ed.). Philadelphia: Lippincott.

Cook, L. (1999). The value of lab values. *AJN, 99*(5), 66–75.

DeLaune, S., & Ladner, P. (1998). *Fundamentals of nursing: Standards & practice.* Albany, NY: Delmar.

Estes, M. E. Z. (2002). *Health assessment & physical examination* (2nd ed.). Albany, NY: Delmar.

Hartshorn, J., Lamborn, M., & Noll, M. (1997). *Introduction to critical care nursing* (2nd ed.). Philadelphia: W. B. Saunders Company.

Hogstel, M. (1994). *Nursing care of the older adult* (3rd ed.). Albany, NY: Delmar.

Incredibly Easy! Understanding hypokalemia. *Nursing2000, 30*(11), 74–76.

I.V. therapy: Update97. (1997). *Nursing97, 27*(11), 60–61.

Josephson, D. L. (1999). *Intravenous infusion therapy for nurses: Principles and practice.* Albany, NY: Delmar.

Kee, J. L. (1998). *Laboratory and diagnostic tests with nursing implications.* Englewood Clifs, NJ: Prentice Hall.

Kee, J., & Paulanka, B. (1999). *Fluids and electrolytes with clinical applications* (6th ed.). Albany, NY: Delmar.

Mader, S. (1997). *Understanding human anatomy & physiology* (3rd ed.). Dubuque, IA: Brown.

Marieb, E. (1997). *Essentials of human anatomy & physiology* (5th ed.). Redwood City, CA: Cummings.

Martini, F., & Welch, K. (1997). *Fundamentals of anatomy and physiology* (4th ed.). Englewood Cliffs, NJ: Prentice-Hall.

Masoorli, S. (1995). Know the pitfalls of I.V. therapy. *NSO Risk Advisor, 20*(2), 1,4.

McConnell, E. (1999). Performing pulse oximetry. *Nursing99, 29*(11), 17.

McFarland, M., & Grant, M. (1994). *Nursing implications of laboratory tests* (3rd ed.). Albany, NY: Delmar.

Memmler, R., Cohen, B., & Wood, D. (1996). *The human body in health and disease* (8th ed.). Philadelphia: J. B. Lippincott.

Noe, D., & Rock, R. (1994). *Laboratory medicine.* Baltimore: Williams & Wilkins.

North American Nursing Diagnosis Association (NANDA). (2001). *Nursing diagnoses: Definitions & classification 2001–2002.* Philadelphia: Author.

Scanlon, V., & Sanders, T. (1999). *Essentials of anatomy and physiology* (3rd ed.). Philadelphia: F. A. Davis.

Schmidt, T. C., & Williams-Evans, S. A. (2000). How to recognize hypokalemia. *Nursing2000, 30*(2), 22.

Sensi-Scott, A., & Fong, E. (1998). *Body structures and functions* (9th ed.). Albany, NY: Delmar.

Tasota, F., & Wesmiller, S. (1998). Balancing act: Keeping blood pH in equilibrium. *Nursing98, 28*(12), 34–40.

Thibodeau, G. (1999). *Structure & function of the body* (10th ed.). St. Louis, MO: Mosby.

White, J., & Barnes, R. (1983). *Hands on biology, manual* (2nd ed.). Corpus Christi, TX: L P Enterprises.

White, V. (1997). Hyperkalemia. *AJN, 97*(6), 35.

Wong, F. (1999). A new approach to ABG interpretation. *AJN, 99*(8), 34–36.

RESOURCES

Intravenous Nurses Society, Fresh Pond Square, 10 Fawcett Street, Cambridge, MA 02138, 617-441-3008, http://www.ins1.org

CHAPTER 24
Medication Administration
REFERENCES/SUGGESTED READINGS

American Hospital Formulary Service. (1996). *AHFS drug information 96.* Bethesda, MD: American Society of Hospital Pharmacists.

American Nurses Association. (1997, March/April). *American Nurse, 29*(2), 11.

Behrman, R. E., Kliegman, R., & Arvin, A. M. (Eds.). (1996). *Nelson textbook of pediatrics* (15th ed.). Philadelphia: W. B. Saunders Company.

Beyea, S. C., & Nicoll, L. H. (1996). Back to basics: Administering IM injections the right way. *AJN, 96*(1), 34–35.

Bulechek, G.M., & McCloskey, J.C. (2000). *Nursing interventions: Essential nursing treatments* (3rd ed.). Philadelphia: W. B. Saunders Company.

Charting Tips. (2000). Documenting IV therapy, part I. *Nursing2000, 30*(2), 73.

Charting Tips. (2000). Documenting IV therapy, part II. *Nursing2000, 30*(3), 83.

Daniels, J., & Smith, L. (1999). *Clinical calculations* (4th ed.). Albany, NY: Delmar.

Drug information for the health care professional (17th ed.). (1997). Rockville, MD: USP Convention.

Ellenberger, A. (1999). Starting an IV line. *Nursing99, 29*(3), 56–59.

Fitzpatrick, L., & Fitzpatrick, T. (1997). Blood transfusion: Keeping your patient safe. *Nursing97, 27*(8), 34–41

Goldy, D. (1998). Circulatory overload secondary to blood transfusion. *AJN, 98*(7), 33.

Hadaway, L. C. (1999a). Choosing the right vascular access device, part I. *Nursing99, 29*(2), 18.

Hadaway, L. C. (1999b). Choosing the right vascular access device, part II. *Nursing99, 29*(7), 28–29.

Hadaway, L. C. (1999c). IV infiltration: Not just a peripheral problem. *Nursing99, 29*(9), 41–47.

Hartshorn, J., Lamborn, M., & Noll, M. (1997). *Introduction to critical care nursing* (2nd ed.). Philadelphia: W. B. Saunders Company.

I.V. therapy: Update97. (1997). *Nursing97, 27*(11), 60–61.

Josephson, D. L. (1999). *Intravenous infusion therapy for nurses: Principles and practice.* Albany, NY: Delmar.

Kee, J., & Paulanka, B. (1999). *Fluids and electrolytes with clinical applications* (6th ed.). Albany, NY: Delmar.

Larouere, E. (1999). Deaccessing an implanted port. *Nursing99, 29*(6), 60–61.

Lehne, R. (1998). *Pharmacology for nursing care* (3rd ed.). Philadelphia: W. B. Saunders Company.

Macklin, D. (2000). Removing a PICC. *AJN, 100*(1), 52–54.

Matheny, N., Wehrle, M. A., Wiersema, L., & Clark, J. (1998). Testing feeding tube placement: Ascultation vs. pH method. *AJN, 98*(5), 37–42.

McConnell, E. (1998). Giving medications through an enteral feeding tube. *Nursing98, 28*(3), 6.

McConnell, E. (1999). Administering a Z-track IM injection. *Nursing99, 29*(1), 26.

North American Nursing Diagnosis Association. (2001). *Nursing diagnoses: Definitions and classification 2001–2002.* Philadelphia: NANDA.

Obenour, P. (1998). Administering an S.C. medication continuously. *Nursing98, 28*(6), 20.

Pickar, G. (1996). *Dosage calculation* (5th ed.). Albany, NY: Delmar.

Remington: The science and practice of pharmacology (19th ed.). (1995). Easton, PA: Mack.

Rice, J. (1998). *Medications & mathematics for the nurse* (8th ed.). Albany, NY: Delmar.

Saxton, D., & O'Neill, N. (1998). *Math and meds for nurses.* Albany, NY: Delmar.

Shannon, M., Wilson, B., & Stang, C. (1999). *Appleton & Lange's 1999 drug guide.* Norwalk, CT: Appleton & Lange.

Spratto, G., & Woods, A. (2002). *PDR nurse's handbook 2002.* Albany, NY: Delmar.

Springhouse Corporation. (2000). *Nursing2000 drug handbook.* Springhouse, PA: Author.

Wilson, B., & Shannon, M. (1997). *Dosage calculations: A simplified approach* (3rd ed.). Norwalk, CT: Appleton & Lange.

Wise, M. (1997). Understanding needle-free access devices. *Nursing97, 27*(7), 32.

RESOURCES

Intravenous Nurses Society, Fresh Pond Square, 10 Fawcett Street, Cambridge, MA 02138, 616-441-3008, http://www.ins1.org

U.S. Pharmacopeia, 12601 Twinbrook Parkway, Rockville, MD 20852, 800-822-8772, http://www.usp.gov

CHAPTER 25
Assessment

REFERENCES/SUGGESTED READINGS

American Heart Association (AHA). (1987). *Recommendations for human blood pressure determination.* (AHA Publication No. 701005). Dallas, TX: Author.

Andresen, G. (1998). Assessing the older patient. *RN, 61*(3), 46–55.

Bickley, L. S. (1999). *A guide to physical examination and history taking* (7th ed.). Phildelphia: Lippincott.

Bosley, C. L. (1995). Assessing cardiac output: Don't stop at the heart. *Nursing95, 25*(9), 43–45.

Crow, S. (1997). Your guide to gloves. *Nursing97, 27*(3), 26–28.

DeLaune, S., & Ladner, P. (1998). *Fundamentals of nursing: Standards & practice.* Albany, NY: Delmar.

Estes, M. E. Z. (2002). *Health assessment & physical examination* (2nd ed.). Albany, NY: Delmar.

Firth, P., & Watanabe, S. (1996). *Women's health.* Albany, NY: Delmar.

Fuller, J., & Schaller-Ayers, J. (1999). *Health assessment: A nursing approach.* Philadelphia: Lippincott.

Gallauresi, B. A. (1998). Pulse oximeters. *Nursing98, 28*(9), 31.

Hanson, C. (1996). *Delmar's instant nursing assessment: Gerontologic.* Albany, NY: Delmar.

Heery, K. (2000). Straight talk about the patient interview. *Nursing 2000, 30*(6), 66–67.

Hodge, P., & Ullrich, S. (1999). Does your assessment include alternative therapies? *RN, 62*(6), 47–49.

Joint Commission on Accreditation of Healthcare Organizations (JCAHO). (2000a). *Comprehensive accreditation manual for hospitals (CAMH) revised pain management standards* [On-line]. Available: http://www.jcaho.org/standard/pm_hap.html

Joint Commission on Accreditation of Healthcare Organizations (JCAHO). (2000b). *Pain assessment and management standards* [On-line]. Available: http://www.jcaho.org/standard/pm_coll.html

Karch, A. M., & Karch, F. E. (2000). When a blood pressure isn't routine. *AJN, 100*(3), 23.

Kirton, C. A. (1997). Assessing bowel sounds. *Nursing97, 27*(3), 64.

Klingman, L. (1999). Assessing the female reproductive system. *AJN, 99*(8), 37–43.

Klingman, L. (1999). Assessing the male genitalia. *AJN, 99*(7), 47–50.

Lazar, J. S., & O'Conner, B. B. (1997). Talking with patients about their use of alternative therapies. *Complementary and Alternative Therapies in Primary Care, 24*(4), 699.

Murray, R. B., & Zentner, J. P. (1997). *Health assessment and promotion through the lifespan* (6th ed.). Norwalk: Appleton & Lange.

O'Hanlon-Nichols, T. (1997). Basic assessment series: The adult cardiovascular system. *AJN, 97*(12), 34–40.

O'Hanlon-Nichols, T. (1998). Basic assessment series: Musculoskeletal system. *AJN, 98*(6), 48–52.

O'Hanlon-Nichols, T. (1998). Basic assessment series: Gastrointestinal system. *AJN, 98*(4), 48–53.

O'Hanlon-Nichols, T. (1998). Basic assessment series: The adult pulmonary system. *AJN, 98*(2), 39–45.

O'Hanlon-Nichols, T. (1999). Neurologic assessment. *AJN, 99*(6), 44–50.

Owen, A. (1998). Respiratory assessment revisited. *Nursing98, 28*(4), 48–49.

Rice, K. L. (1998). Sounding out blood flow with a Doppler device. *Nursing98, 28*(9), 56–57.

Rice, K. L. (1999). Measuring thigh BP. *Nursing99, 29*(8), 58–59.

Taylor, C., Lillis, C., & LeMone, P. (1997). *Fundamentals of nursing: The art and science of nursing care* (3rd ed.). Philadelphia: Lippincott.

Warner, P., Rowe, T., & Whipple, B. (1999). Shedding light on the sexual history. *AJN, 99*(6), 34–40.

Weber, J. (1997). *Health assessment in nursing.* Philadelphia: Lippincott.

CHAPTER 26
Pain Management

REFERENCES/SUGGESTED READINGS

Acello, B. (2000a). Meeting JCAHO standards for pain control. *Nursing2000, 30*(3), 52–54.

Acello, B. (2000b). Facing fears about opioid addiction. *Nursing2000, 30*(5), 72.

Adler, P., Good, M., Roberts, B., & Snyder, S. (2000). The effects of tai chi on older adults with chronic arthritis pain. *Journal of Nursing Scholarship, 32*(4), 377.

Agency for Health Care Policy and Research. (1992). *Clinical practice guideline: Acute pain management: Operative or medical procedures and Trauma.* (AHCPR Publication No. 92–0032). Rockville, MD: U.S. Department of Health and Human Services.

Agency for Health Care Policy and Research. (1994). *Clinical practice guideline: Management of cancer pain.* (AHCPR Publication No. 94–0592). Rockville, MD: U.S. Department of Health and Human Services.

American Pain Society. (1999). *Principles of analgesic use in the treatment of acute pain and cancer pain* (4th ed.). Glenview, IL: Author.

Beecher, H. K. (1956). Relationship of significance of wound to pain experienced. *JAMA, 161,* 1609–1613.

Berkowitz, C. (1997). Epidural pain control—Your job, too. *RN, 60*(8), 22–27.

Bonica, J. J. (Ed.). (1990). *The management of pain* (2d ed.). Philadelphia: Lea & Febiger.

Brand, P., & Yancey, P. (1993). *Pain: The gift nobody wants.* New York: HarperCollins.

Brown, J., Horn, J., Calbert, J., & Nolan-Goslin, K. (1999). A question of pain. *Nursing99, 29*(10), 48–51.

Chapman, G. F. (1999). Documenting a pain assessment. *Nursing99, 29*(11), 25.

Cleeland, C. S., Gonin, R., Hatfield, A. K., Edmonson, J. H., Blum, R. H., Stewart, J. A., & Pandya, K. J. (1994). Pain and its treatment in outpatients with metastatic cancer. *New England Journal of Medicine, 330,* 592–596.

Collins, P. M., Auclair, M., Butler, E., Hush, M., Bernstein, B. J., Aguirre, F., & Huston, M. (2000). Educating staff about pain management *AJN, 100*(1), 59.

Compton, P. (1999). Managing a drug abuser's pain. *Nursing99, 29*(5), 26–28.

Cousins, N. (1991). *Anatomy of an illness as perceived by the patient.* Toronto: Bantam.

Derby, S. A. (1999). Opioid conversion guidelines for managing adult cancer pain. *AJN, 99*(10), 62–65.

Donovan, M., Dillon, P., & McGuire, L. (1987). Incidence and characteristics of pain in a sample of medical-surgical inpatients. *Pain, 30,* 69–78.

Faries, J. (1997a). Taking another route to pain relief. *Nursing97, 27*(6), 28.

Faries, J. (1997b). Assessing pediatric pain. *Nursing97, 27*(8), 18.

Faries, J. (1998a). Easing your patient's postoperative pain. *Nursing98, 28*(6), 58–60.

Faries, J. (1998b). Making a smooth switch from IV analgesia. *Nursing98, 28*(7), 26.

Feinberg, S. D. (2000). Complex regional pain syndrome. *AJN, 100*(12), 23–24.

Gordon, D., & Ward, S. (1995). Correcting patient misconceptions about pain. *AJN, 95*(7), 43–45.

Haddad, A. (2000). Ethics in action: Treating pain in substance abusers. *RN, 63*(1), 21–24.

Joint Commission on Accreditation of Healthcare Organizations (JCAHO). (1999). Joint Commission focuses on pain management [On-line]. Available: http://www.jcaho.org/news/nb207.html

Joint Commission on Accreditation of Healthcare Organizations (JCAHO). (2000a). Comprehensive accreditation manual for hospitals (CAMH) revised pain management standards [On-line]. Available: http://www.jcaho.org/standard/pm_hap.html

Joint Commission on Accreditation of Healthcare Organizations (JCAHO). (2000b). Pain assessment and management standards [On-line]. Available: http://www.jcaho.org/standard/pm_coll.html

Juarez, G. (1995). When culture clashes with pain control. *Nursing95, 25*(5), 90.

Kedziera, P. (1998). The two faces of pain. *RN, 61*(2), 45–46.

Liebeskind J., & Melzack, R. (1987). The International Pain Foundation: Meeting a need for education in pain management. *Pain, 30,* 1–2.

Loeb, J. L. (1999). Pain management in long-term care. *AJN, 99*(2), 48–52.

Markey, B. T., & Graham, M. (1997). Management of chronic pain with epidural steriods. *AORN Journal, 65*(4), 791.

Mattson, J. E. (2000). The language of pain. *Reflections on Nursing LEADERSHIP, 26*(4), 10–14.

McCaffery, M. (1979). *Nursing management of the patient with pain* (2nd ed.). Philadelphia: Lippincott.

McCaffery, M. (1999a). Pain control. *AJN, 99*(8), 18.

McCaffery, M. (1999b). Understanding your patient's pain tolerance. *Nursing99, 29*(12), 17.

McCaffery, M., & Beebe, A. (1999). *Pain: Clinical manual for nursing practice* (2nd ed.). St. Louis, MO: Mosby.

McCaffery, M. & Ferrell, B. R. (1999). Opioids and pain management. *Nursing99, 29*(3), 48–52.

McCaffery, M., & Pasero, C. (1999). *Pain: Clinical manual* (2nd ed.). St. Louis, MO: Mosby.

McDevitt, M. J. (1995). A(TENS)tion! *Nursing95, 25*(12), 46–47.

McGuire, D. B., Yarbro, C. H., & Ferrell, B. R. (1995). *Cancer pain management* (2d ed.). Boston: Jones & Bartlett.

Melzack, R., & Wall, P. D. (1965). Pain mechanisms: A new theory. *Science, 150,* 971–979.

Merskey, J., & Bogduk, N. (Eds.). (1994). *Classification of chronic pain* (2nd ed., pp. 209–214). Task Force on Taxonomy. Seattle, WA: IASP.

Morrison, C. (2000). Fear of addiction: Balancing the facts and concerns about opioid use. *AJN 100*(7), 81.

North American Nursing Diagnosis Association. (2001). *Nursing diagnoses: Definitions & classification, 2001–2002.* Philadelphia: Author.

Pasero, C. (1999). Using superficial cooling for pain relief. *AJN, 99*(3), 48–52.

Pasero, C. (2000a). Oral patient-controlled analgesia. *AJN, 100*(3), 24.

Pasero, C. (2000b). Continuous local anesthetics. *AJN, 100*(8), 22–23.

Pasero, C., & McCaffery, M. (2000a). Reversing respiratory depression with naloxone. *AJN, 100*(2), 26.

Pasero, C., & McCaffery, M. (2000b). When patients can't report pain. *AJN, 100*(9), 22–23.

Portenoy, R. K., Payne, R, et al. (1999). Oral transmucosal fentanyl citrate (OTFC) for the treatment of breakthrough pain in cancer patients: A controlled dose titration study. *Pain, 79,* 303.

Poulain, P., Langlade, A., & Goldberg, J. (1997). Cancer pain management in the home. *Pain Clinical Updates, 5*(1). Internet access: http://www.halcyon.com/iasp/PCU97a.html.

Schecter, N. L., Berde, C. B., & Yaster, M. (Eds.). (1993). *Pain in infants, children, and adolescents.* Baltimore, MD: Williams & Wilkins.

Scholz, M. (2000). Managing constipation that's opioid-induced. *RN, 63*(6), 103.

Spratto, G., & Woods, A. (2000). *PDR® Nurse's Drug Handbook™*. Albany, NY: Delmar.

Stevens, B. (1994). Nursing management of pain in children. In C. L. Betz, M. M. Hunsberger, & S. Wright (Eds.), *Family-centered nursing care of children* (2nd ed.). Philadelphia: W. B. Saunders Company.

Strevy, S. (1998). Myths and facts about pain. *RN, 61*(2), 42–45.

Thomas, M., & Lundeberg, T. (1996). Does acupuncture work? *Pain Clinical Updates, 4*(3). Internet access http://www.halcyon.com/iasp/PCU96c.html.

Travell, J. G., & Simons, D. G. (1983, 1998). *Travell & Simon's myofascial pain and dysfunction: The trigger point manual* (2nd ed.), (Vols. 1 & 2). Baltimore: Lippincott.

Vasudevan, S. V. (1993). *Pain: A four letter word you can live with*. Milwaukee, WI: Montgomery Media.

Wong, D. L., Hockenberry-Eaton, M., Wilson, D., & Winkelstein, M. L. (1999). *Whaley & Wong's nursing care of infants and children* (6th ed.). St. Louis, MO: Mosby.

World Health Organization. (1986). *Cancer pain relief*. Geneva, Switzerland: Author.

World Health Organization. (1990). Cancer pain relief and palliative care. *Report of a WHO expert committee [World Health Organization Technical Report Series, 804]*. Geneva, Switzerland: Author.

RESOURCES

Agency for Health Care Policy and Research (AHCPR), Office of Health Care Information, Executive Office Center, Suite 501, 2101 East Jefferson St., Rockville, MD 20852, http://www.ahcpr.gov

AHCPR Clearinghouse, P.O. Box 8547, Silver Spring, MD 20907-8547, 800-358-9295, http://www.ahcpr.gov

- Clinical Practice Guideline for managing acute pain. Available in three formats: (1) The clinical practice guideline (Publication No. 92-0032); (2) Quick reference guides (Adults—No. 92-0019 and Pediatric—No. 92-0020); and (3) Pain Control after Surgery: A Patient's Guide (No. 92-0021)
- Clinical Practice Guideline for managing cancer pain. Available in three formats: (1) The clinical practice guideline (Publication No. 94-0592); (2) Quick reference guides (Adults—No. 94-0593 and Pediatric—No. 92-0594); and (3) Patient's Guide (No. 94-0595)

American Chronic Pain Association, P.O. Box 850, Rocklin, CA 95677-0850, 916-632-0922, http://www.theacpa.org/

American Pain Society (APS), 4700 W. Lake Avenue, Glenview, IL 60025, 847-375-4715, http://www.ampainsoc.org

American Society of Pain Management Nurses, 7794 Grow Drive, Pensacola, FL 32514, 850-473-0233

International Association for the Study of Pain (IASP), 909 Forty-third Street NE, Suite 306, Seattle, WA 98105-6020, 206-547-6409, http://www.halcyon.com/iasp

Joint Commission on Accreditation of Healthcare Organizations (JCAHO), One Renaissance Boulevard, Oakbrook Terrace, IL 60181-4294, 630-792-5000, http://www.jcaho.org

National Chronic Pain Outreach Association, P.O. Box 274, Millboro, VA 24460-0274, 540-862-9437

National Committee on Treatment of Intractable Pain, P.O. Box 9553, Friendship Station, Washington, DC 20016-1553, 202-944-8140

National Headache Foundation, 428 W. St. James Place, 2nd Floor, Chicago, IL 60614-2750, 888-843-5552, http://www.headaches.org

National Hospice and Palliative Care Organization, 1700 Diagonal Road, Suite 300, Alexandria, VA 22304, 703-837-1500, http://www.nhpco.org

Nursing Research and Education/City of Hope Pain Resource Center, 1500 East Duarte Road, Duarte, CA 91010, 626-359-8111 ext. 3829, http://mayday.coh.org

Journals

Chronic Pain Letter, Box 1303, Old Chelsea Station, New York, NY 10011

The Clinical Journal of Pain, Lippincott Williams & Wilkins, 2275 Washington Square, Philadelphia, PA 19106, 800-638-3030

The Journal of Pain and Symptom Management, Elsevier Publishing Co., Inc., Journal Fulfillment Department, P.O. Box 882, Madison Square Station, New York, NY 10160-0200

Pain, International Association for the Study of Pain, 909 Forty-third Street NE, Suite 306, Seattle, WA 98105-6020, 206-547-6409

CHAPTER 27
Diagnostic Tests

REFERENCES/SUGGESTED READINGS

Ahmed, D. S. (2000). Hidden factors in occult blood testing. *AJN, 100*(12), 25.

Beattie, S. (1999). Cut the risks for cardiac cath patients. *RN, 62*(1), 50–54.

Cook, L. (1999). The value of lab values: Incorporate lab results into the nursing diagnosis. *AJN, 99*(5), 66–75

Dammel, T. (1997). Fecal occult-blood testing: Looking for hidden danger. *Nursing97, 27*(7), 44–45.

DeLaune, S., & Ladner, P. (1998). *Fundamentals of nursing: Standards & practice*. Albany, NY: Delmar.

Ernst, D. (1999). Collecting blood culture specimens. *Nursing99, 29*(7), 56–58.

Gallauresi, B. (1998). Pulse oximeters. *Nursing98, 28*(9), 31.

Gibbar-Clements, T., Shirrell, D., & Free, C. (1997). PT and APTT: Seeing beyond the numbers. *Nursing97, 27*(7), 49–51.

Guyton, A. C., & Hall, J., (2000). *Textbook of medical physiology* (10th ed.). Philadelphia: W. B. Saunders Company.

Hill, J., & Newton, J. (1998). Contrast echo: Your role at the bedside. *RN, 61*(10), 32–35.

Hospital Nursing Section. (1995). Interpreting ECF waveform components. *Nursing95, 25*(6), 32C-32F.

Kee, J. L. (1998). *Laboratory and diagnostic tests with nursing implications* (5th ed.). Upper Saddle River, NJ: Prentice Hall.

Laxson, C., & Titler, M. (1994). Drawing coagulation studies from arterial lines: An integrated literature review. *American Journal of Critical Care, 3*(1), 16–23.

McFarland, M., & Grant, M. (1994). *Nursing implications of laboratory tests* (3rd ed.). Albany, NY: Delmar.

Montes, P. (1997). Managing outpatient cardiac catheterization. *AJN, 97*(8), 34–37.

Ryan, D. (2000). Is it an MI?: A lab primer. *RN, 63*(2), 26–30.

Shortall, S. P., & Perkins, L. A. (1999). Interpreting the ins and outs of pulmonary function tests. *Nursing99, 29*(12), 41–46.

Siconolfi, L. (1995). Clarifying the complexity of liver function test. *Nursing95, 25*(5), 39–44.

Somerson, S., Husted, C., & Sicilia, M. (1995). Insights into conscious sedation. *AJN, 95*(6), 26–33.

Wolfe, S. (1997). The great mammogram debate. *RN, 60*(8), 41–44.

Wong, F. W. H. (1999). A new approach to ABG interpretation. *AJN, 99*(8), 34–36.

RESOURCES

National Library of Medicine, http://www.nlm.nih.gov (then click on "Search MEDLINE")

National Network of Libraries of Medicine (NN/LM) Regional Medical Libraries, 800-338-7657

CHAPTER 28
Nursing Care of the Older Client

REFERENCES/SUGGESTED READINGS

Administration on Aging (AoA). (2000). The Administration on Aging and the Older American's Act. [On-line]. Available: http://www.aoa.dhhs.gov/aoa/pages/aoafact.html

American Association of Retired Persons (AARP). (1998). *A profile of older Americans.* Washington, DC: Department of Health and Human Services.

Andersen, C. (1999). *Antecedents, correlates, and impact of violent behaviors in the elderly VA client.* Unpublished thesis, University of Iowa, Iowa City, IA.

Bahr, Sr. R. T. (1994). An overview of gerontological nursing. In M. Hogstel (Ed.), *Nursing care of the older adult* (3rd ed., pp. 2–25). Albany, NY: Delmar.

Burggraf, V., & Barry, R. (2001). What the future holds for gerontology. *Nursing2001, 31*(1), 52.

Fetters, C. (1994). *Standard of care on wandering.* Knoxville, IA: Department of Veterans Affairs Medical Center, Division of Nursing.

Gallo, J., Fulmer, T., Paveza, G., & Reichel, W. (1999). *Handbook of geriatric assessment* (3rd ed.). Gaithersburg, MD: Aspen.

Hoban, S. (2000). Elder abuse and neglect. *AJN, 100*(11), 49–50.

Hogstel, M. (Ed.). (1994). *Nursing care of the older adult* (3rd ed.). Albany, NY: Delmar.

Maas, M., Buckwalter, K., & Hardy, M. (1991). *Nursing diagnosis and new interventions for the elderly.* Redwood City, CA: Addison-Wesley.

McCloskey, J., & Bulechek, G. (1999). *Nursing interventions classifications (NIC)* (3rd ed.). St. Louis, MO: Mosby.

Morris, M. R. (1998). Elder abuse: What the law requires. *RN, 61*(8), 52–53.

National Council on Aging (NCOA). (2000). Facts about older Americans. [On-line]. Available: http://www.ncoa.org/news/mra_2000/factsheet.html

Needham, J. F. (1995). *Gerontological nursing.* Albany, NY: Delmar.

Peskin, B. (1999). *Beyond the zone.* Houston, TX: Noble.

Social Security Administration (SSA). (2000). The president signs the "Senior Citizens' Freedom to Work Act of 2000." [On-line]. Available: http://www.ssa.gov/legislation/legis_bulletin_040700.html

Stiegel, L. A. (1995). *Recommended guidelines for state courts handling cases involving elder abuse.* Washington, DC: American Bar Association.

Wilkinson, J. (1999). *A family caregiver's guide to planning and decision making for the elderly.* Minneapolis, MN: Fairview.

Wolfe, S. (1998). Look for signs of abuse. *RN, 61*(8), 48–51.

Yen, P. K. (1995). Maximizing calcium intake. *Geriatric Nursing, 16*(2), 92–93.

RESOURCES

The Administration on Aging (AoA), Elder Abuse and Prevention and Treatment, 330 Independence Avenue, SW, Washington, DC 20201, 202-619-7501, http://www.aoa.ggov/abuse/default.htm

The Administration on Aging (AoA), U.S. Department of Health and Human Services, 330 Independence Avenue SW, Washington, DC 20201, 202-619-0724, http://www.aoa.dhhs.gov

American Association of Geriatric Psychiatry, 7910 Woodmont Avenue, Suite 1050, Bethesda, MD 20814-3004, 301-654-7850, http://www.aagpgpa.org

American Association of Retired Persons (AARP), 601 East Street NW, Washington, DC 20049, 800-424-3410, http://www.aarp.org

American Nurses Association (ANA), Council on Gerontological Nursing Practice, 600 Maryland Avenue SW, Suite 100W, Washington, DC 20024, 800-274-4262, http://www.nursingworld.org

Department of Health and Human Services, Public Health Service, Agency for Healthcare Research and Quality, Executive Office Center, 200 Independence Avenue, SW, Washington, DC 20201, 202-619-0257, 877-696-6775, http://www.dhhs.gov, http://www.ahcpr.gov

National Center on Elder Abuse, 1225 I Street, NW, Suite 725, Washington, DC 20005, 202-898-2586, http://www.elderabusecenter.org

National Council on Aging, Inc. (NCOA), 409 3rd Street, SW, Washington, DC 20024, 800-424-9046, http://www.ncoa.org

CHAPTER 29
Rehabilitation, Home Health, Long-Term Care, and Hospice

REFERENCES/SUGGESTED READINGS

Abrams, W. B., Beers, M. H., & Berkow, R. (Eds.). (2000). *The Merck manual of geriatrics* (3rd ed.). Whitehouse Station, NJ: Merck Research Laboratories.

American Association of Retired Persons (AARP). (1998). *A profile of older Americans.* Washington, DC: U.S. Department of Health and Human Services.

American Health Care Association (AHCA). (1998). The looming crisis [On-line]. Available: http://www.ahca.org

American Health Care Association (AHCA). (2000). Nursing facility subacute care: The quality and cost-effective alternative to hospital care [On-line]. Available: http://www.ahca.org/who/pubsubac.htm

Assisted Living Federation of America (ALFA). (1999). What is assisted living [On-line]. Available: http://www.alfa.org

Barker, E. (1999). Life care planning. *RN, 62*(3), 58–61.

Benefield, L. (1996). Making the transition to home care nursing. *AJN, 96*(10), 47–49.

Boon, T. (1998). Don't forget the hospice option. *RN, 61*(2), 30–33.

Bral, E. (1998). Caring for adults with chronic cancer pain. *AJN, 98*(4), 26–32.

Diaz, D. (1995). Geriatric UPDATE 95. *Nursing95, 25*(3), 62–64.

General Accounting Office (1994). *Long-term care reform.* (GAO)/HEHS–94–227). Washington DC: U.S. General Accounting Office.

Gresham, G. E., Duncan, P. W., Stason, W. B., et al. (1995, May). *Post stroke rehabilitation.* Clinical Practice Guideline, No. 16, Rockville, MD: U.S. Department of Health and Human Services. Public Health Service Agency for Health Care Policy and Research. AHCPR Publication No. 95–0062.

Grove, N. (1997). Helping families select a nursing home. *RN, 60*(3), 37–40.

Health Care Financing Administration (HCFA). (2000a). Highlights: National Health Care Expenditures, 1998 [On-line]. Available: http://www.hcfa.gov/stats/nke-oact/hilites.htm

Health Care Financing Administration (HCFA). (2000b). National Health Expenditures Projection [On-line]. Available: http://www.hcfa.gov/stats/NHE-Proj/proj1998/tables

Hospice Education Institute (1999). Definition of palliative care [On-line]. Available: http://www.hospiceworld.org

Jagger, J., & Perry, J. (2000). Preventing sharps injuries in the home. *Nursing2000, 30*(12), 73.

Joint Commission on Accreditation of Healthcare Organizations (JCAHO). (2000). Pain Assessment and Management Standards [On-line]. Available: http://www.jcaho.org/standard/pm_coll.html

Kazanowski, M. (1997). A commitment to palliative care: Could it impact assisted suicide? *Journal of Gerontologic Nursing, 23*(3), 36–42.

Kennison, M. (1999). A case study in care. *RN, 62*(1), 46–48.

Lattanzi-Licht, M. E. (1998). *The hospice choice: In pursuit of a peaceful death.* New York: Simon and Schuster/Fireside.

Loeb, J., & Pasero, C. (2000). JCAHO standards in long-term care. *AJN, 100*(5), 22–23.

Millea, K. (1995). Home health care UPDATE 95. *Nursing95, 25*(7), 57–59.

National Adult Day Services Association (NADSA). (2000). Adult day services fact sheet. [On-line]. Available: http://www.ncoa.org/nadsa/ADS_factsheet.htm

National Association for Home Care (NAHC). (1999). Hospice [On-line]. Available: http://www.nahc.org/HAA

National Association for Home Care (NAHC). (2000). Basic statistics about home care. [On-line]. Available: http://www.nahc.org/consumer/hcstats.html

National Hospice Organization (NHO). (1999). The basics of hospice [On-line]. Available: http://www.nho.org

National Institute on Aging (NIA). (1996). Planning for long-term care [On-line]. Available: http://www.nih.gov/nia/health/pubpub/longterm.htm

Puopolo, A. (1999). Gaining confidence to talk about end-of-life care. *Nursing99, 29*(7), 49–51.

Skokal, W. (2000). IV push at home? *RN, 63*(10), 26–29.

Ufema, J. (1999). Reflections on death and dying. *Nursing99, 29*(6), 56–59.

Waid, M. O. (1998). Brief summaries of Medicare and Medicaid [On-line]. Available: http://www.hcfa.gov/medicare/ormedmed.htm

RESOURCES

American Association of Homes and Services for the Aging (AAHSA), Suite 500, 901 E Street NW, Washington, DC 20004-2011, 202-783-2242, http://www.aahsa.org

American Association of Retired Persons (AARP), 601 E Street NW, Washington, DC 20049, 202-434-6190, 800-424-3410, http://www.aarp.org

American Health Care Association (AHCA), 1201 L Street NW, Washington, DC 20005, 202-842-4444, http://www.ahca.org

American Hospital Association (AHA), Chicago Headquarters (CH), One North Franklin, Chicago, IL 60606, 312-422-3000, http://www.aha.org

American Hospital Association (AHA), Washington Office (WO), 325 Seventh Street NW, Washington, DC 20004, 202-638-1100, 800-424-4301, http://www.aha.org

Assisted Living Federation of America, Suite 400, 10300 Eaton Place, Fairfax, VA 22030, 703-691-8100, http://www.alfa.org

Association of Rehabilitation Nurses (ARN), 4700 W. Lake Avenue, Glenview, IL 60025-1485, 800-229-7530, 847-375-4710, http://www.rehabnurse.org

Department of Health and Human Services (DHHS), 200 Independence Avenue, SW, Washington, DC 20201, 202-619-0257, 877-696-6775, http://www.hhs.gov/

Foundation for Hospice & Home Care, 519 C Street NE, Washington, DC 20002, 302-547-6586

Health Care Financing Administration (HCFA), 7500 Security Boulevard, Baltimore, MD 21244, 800-638-6833, http://www.hcfa.gov

Home Healthcare Nurses Association, 7794 Grow Drive, Pensacola, FL 32514, 850-474-1066, 800-558-4462, http://www.hhna.org

Hospice Association of America (HAA), 228 Seventh Street SE, Washington, DC 20003, 202-546-4759, http://www.nahc.org/HAA

Hospice Education Institute, 190 Westbrook Road, Essex, CT 06426-1510, 860-767-1620, 800-331-1620, http://www.hospiceworld.org

Hospice Foundation of America (HFA), 2001 S Street NW #300, Washington, DC 20009, 800-854-3402, http://www.hospicefoundation.org

National Adult Day Services Association (NADSA), 409 Third Street, SW, Washington, DC 20024, 202-479, 6682, http://www.ncoa.org/nadsa

National Association for Home Care (NAHC), 228 Seventh Street SE, Washington, DC 20003, 202-547-7424, http://www.nahc.org

National Citizens' Coalition for Nursing Home Reform, Suite 202, 1424 16th Street NW, Washington, DC 20036-2211, 202-332-2275, http://www.nccnhr.org

National Hospice and Palliative Care Organization (NHPCO), 1700 Diagonal Road, Suite 300, Alexandria, VA 22314, 703-243-5900, http://www.nhpco.org

National Rehabilitation Association, 633 S. Washington Street, Alexandria, VA 22314, 703-836-0850, http://www.nationalrehab.org

National Rehabilitation Information Center (NARIC), 1010 Wayne Avenue, Suite 800, Silver Spring, MD 20910-5633, 301-562-2400, 800-346-2742, http://www.naric.com

Nursing Home Information Service, National Council of Senior Citizens, 8403 Colesville Road, Suite 1200, Silver Spring, MD 20910, 310-578-8800, 888-3-SENIOR, http://www.ncscinc.org

CHAPTER 30
Leadership/Work Transition

REFERENCES/SUGGESTED READINGS

Bernzweig, E. P., & Bernzwell, C. P. (1996). *The nurse's liability for malpractice: A programmed course* (6th ed.). St. Louis, MO: Mosby.

Bolles, R. N. (1997). *What color is your parachute? A practical manual for job-hunters & career-changers.* Berkeley, CA: Ten Speed.

Brent, N. J. (1997). *Nurses and the law: A guide to principles and application.* Philadelphia: W. B. Saunders Company.

Bureau of Labor Statistics. (1998). 1998–99 *Occupational outlook handbook.* Chicago, IL: Author.

Catalano, J. T. (1996). *Contemporary professional nursing.* Philadelphia: F. A. Davis.

Catalano, J. T. (1999). *Nursing now!: Today's issues, tomorrow's trends* (2nd ed.). Philadelphia: F. A. Davis.

Guido, G. W. (2000). *Legal and ethical issues in nursing* (3rd ed.). Englewood Cliffs, NJ: Prentice Hall.

Haft, T. (1997). *Job notes: Resumes*. New York: Princeton Review.

Hansten, R. I., & Washburn, M. J. (1998). *Clinical delegation skills. A handbook for professional practice*. Gaithersburg, MD: Aspen.

Joint Commission on Accreditation of Healthcare Organizations. (1998). *Addressing staffing needs for patient care: Solutions for hospital leaders*. Oakbrook Terrace, IL: Author.

Marino, K. (1997). *Just resumes: 200 powerful and proven successful resumes to get that job* (2nd ed.). New York: Wiley.

Marquis, B. L., & Huston, C. J. (1999). *Leadership roles and management functions in nursing theory and application* (3rd ed.). Philadelphia: Lippincott.

Mattera, M. D. (Ed.). (1997). Ace the all-important job interview. *Nursing opportunities 1997*. Montvale, NJ: Medical Economics.

National Council of State Boards of Nursing. (1996). *Delegation: Concepts and decision-making process*. Chicago, IL: Author.

National Council of State Boards of Nursing, Inc. (1997). *NCLEX candidate examination bulletin*. Chicago, IL: Author.

National Council of State Boards of Nursing (NCSBN) (1997). *The five rights of delegation* [On-line]. Available: http://www.ncsbn.org/files/uap/fiverights.pdf

National Council of State Boards of Nursing, Inc. (1999). *1998 profiles of member boards*. Chicago, IL: Author.

New York State Nurses Association. (1998a). LPNs and the practice of nursing. *Report the official newsletter of the New York State Nurses Association, 29*(9), 3.

New York State Nurses Association. (1998b). Responsibility for delegated and assigned care. *Report the official newsletter of the New York State Nurses Association, 29*(5), 3.

Office of the Professions. (1995). *Nursing handbook*. Albany, NY: New York State Education Department.

Parker, Y. (1996). *Damn good resume guide: A crash course in resume writing* (3rd ed.). Berkeley, CA: Ten Speed.

Parkman, C. A. (1996). Delegation: Are you doing it right? *AJN, 96*(9), 43–47.

Trandel-Korenchuk, D. M. (1997). *Nurses and the law* (5th ed.). Gaithersburg, MD: Aspen.

Wilkinson, A. P. (1998). Nursing malpractice. *Nursing98, 28*(6), 34–38.

RESOURCES

National Council of State Boards of Nursing (NCSBN), 676 North Saint Clair Street, Suite 550, Chicago, IL 60611-2921, 312-787-6555, http://www.ncsbn.org

Appendix A: NANDA Nursing Diagnoses 2001–2002

Activity Intolerance
Risk for Activity Intolerance
Impaired Adjustment
Ineffective Airway Clearance
Latex Allergy Response
Risk for Latex Allergy Response
Anxiety
Death Anxiety
Risk for Aspiration
Risk for Impaired Parent/Infant/Child Attachment
Autonomic Dysreflexia
Disturbed Body Image
Risk for Imbalanced Body Temperature
Bowel Incontinence
Effective Breastfeeding
Ineffective Breastfeeding
Interrupted Breastfeeding
Ineffective Breathing Pattern
Decreased Cardiac Output
Caregiver Role Strain
Risk for Caregiver Role Strain
Impaired Verbal Communication
Decisional Conflict (Specify)
Parenteral Role Conflict
Acute Confusion
Chronic Confusion
Constipation
Perceived Constipation
Risk for Constipation
Ineffective Coping
Ineffective Community Coping
Readiness for Enhanced Community Coping
Defensive Coping
Compromised Family Coping
Disabled Family Coping
Readiness for Enhanced Family Coping
Ineffective Denial
Impaired Dentition
Risk for Delayed Development
Diarrhea
Risk for Disuse Syndrome
Deficient Diversional Activities
Disturbed Energy Field
Impaired Environmental Interpretation Syndrome

Adult Failure to Thrive
Risk for Falls
Dysfunctional Family Processes: Alcoholism
Interrupted Family Processes
Fatigue
Fear
Deficient Fluid Volume
Excess Fluid Volume
Risk for Deficient Fluid Volume
Risk for Imbalanced Fluid Volume
Impaired Gas Exchange
Anticipatory Grieving
Dysfunctional Grieving
Delayed Growth and Development
Risk for Disproportionate Growth
Ineffective Health Maintenance
Health-Seeking Behaviors (Specify)
Impaired Home Maintenance
Hopelessness
Hyperthermia
Hypothermia
Disturbed Personal Identity
Functional Urinary Incontinence
Reflex Urinary Incontinence
Stress Urinary Incontinence
Total Urinary Incontinence
Urge Urinary Incontinence
Risk for Urge Urinary Incontinence
Disorganized Infant Behavior
Risk for Disorganized Infant Behavior
Readiness for Enhanced Organized Infant Behavior
Ineffective Infant Feeding Pattern
Risk for Infection
Risk for Injury
Risk for Perioperative-Positioning Injury
Decreased Intracranial Adaptive Capacity
Deficient Knowledge
Risk for Loneliness
Impaired Memory
Impaired Bed Mobility
Impaired Physical Mobility
Impaired Wheelchair Mobility
Nausea
Unilateral Neglect

Noncompliance

Imbalanced Nutrition: Less than Body Requirements

Imbalanced Nutrition: More than Body Requirements

Risk for Imbalanced Nutrition: More than Body Requirements

Impaired Oral Mucous Membrane

Acute Pain

Chronic Pain

Impaired Parenting

Risk for Impaired Parenting

Risk for Peripheral Neurovascular Dysfunction

Risk for Poisoning

Post-Trauma Syndrome

Risk for Post-Trauma Syndrome

Powerlessness

Risk for Powerlessness

Ineffective Protection

Rape-Trauma Syndrome

Rape-Trauma Syndrome: Compound Reaction

Rape-Trauma Syndrome: Silent Reaction

Relocation Stress Syndrome

Risk for Relocation Stress Syndrome

Ineffective Role Performance

Bathing/Hygiene Self-Care Deficit

Dressing/Grooming Self-Care Deficit

Feeding Self-Care Deficit

Toileting Self-Care Deficit

Chronic Low Self-Esteem

Situational Low Self-Esteem

Risk for Situational Low Self-Esteem

Self-Mutilation

Risk for Self-Mutilation

Disturbed Sensory Perception (Specify: Visual, Auditory, Kinesthetic, Gustatory, Tactile, Olfactory)

Sexual Dysfunction

Ineffective Sexuality Patterns

Impaired Skin Integrity

Risk for Impaired Skin Integrity

Sleep Deprivation

Disturbed Sleep Pattern

Impaired Social Interaction

Social Isolation

Chronic Sorrow

Spiritual Distress

Risk for Spiritual Distress

Readiness for Enhanced Spiritual Well-Being

Risk for Suffocation

Risk for Suicide

Delayed Surgical Recovery

Impaired Swallowing

Effective Therapeutic Regimen Management

Ineffective Therapeutic Regimen Management

Ineffective Community Therapeutic Regimen Management

Ineffective Family Therapeutic Regimen Management

Ineffective Thermoregulation

Disturbed Thought Processes

Impaired Tissue Integrity

Ineffective Tissue Perfusion (Specify Type: Renal, Cerebral, Cardiopulmonary, Gastrointestinal, Peripheral)

Impaired Transfer Ability

Risk for Trauma

Impaired Urinary Elimination

Urinary Retention

Impaired Spontaneous Ventilation

Dysfunctional Ventilatory Weaning Response

Risk for Other-Directed Violence

Risk for Self-Directed Violence

Impaired Walking

Wandering

Appendix B: Recommended Childhood Immunization Schedule United States, January–December 2001

From Morbidity and Mortality Weekly Report, *50* 8–9, (2001, January 12).

Age

Vaccine	Birth	1 mo	2 mos	4 mos	6 mos	12 mos	15 mos	18 mos	24 mos	4–6 yrs	11–12 yrs	14–18 yrs
Hepatitis B[†]	Hep B #1	Hep B #2			Hep B #3						Hep B	
Diphtheria and tetanus toxoids and pertussis[§]			DTaP	DTaP	DTaP		DTaP			DTaP	Td	
H. influenzae type b[¶]			Hib	Hib	Hib	Hib						
Inactivated Polio[**]			IPV	IPV	IPV	IPV				IPV		
Pneumococcal conjugate[††]			PCV	PCV	PCV	PCV						
Measles-mumps-rubella[§§]						MMR				MMR	MMR	
Varicella[¶¶]						Var					Var	
Hepatitis A[***]									Hep A in selected areas			

☐ Range of recommended ages for vaccination.

⬭ Vaccines to be given if previously recommended doses were missed or were given earlier than the recommended minimum age.

▨ Recommended in selected states and/or regions.

Childhood Immunization Schedule — Continued

* This schedule indicates the recommended ages for routine administration of currently licensed childhood vaccines as of November 1, 2000, for children through age 18 years. Additional vaccines may be licensed and recommended during the year. Licensed combination vaccines may be used whenever any components of the combination are indicated and the vaccine's other components are not contraindicated. Providers should consult the manufacturer's package inserts for detailed recommendations.

† **Infants born to hepatitis B surface antigen (HBsAg)-negative mothers** should receive the first dose of hepatitis B vaccine (Hep B) by age 2 months. The second dose should be administered at least 1 month after the first dose. The third dose should be administered at least 4 months after the first dose and at least 2 months after the second dose, but not before age 6 months. **Infants born to HBsAg-positive mothers** should receive Hep B and 0.5 mL hepatitis B immune globulin (HBIG) within 12 hours of birth at separate sites. The second dose is recommended at age 1–2 months and the third dose at age 6 months. **Infants born to mothers whose HBsAg status is unknown** should receive Hep B within 12 hours of birth. Maternal blood should be drawn at delivery to determine the mother's HBsAg status; if the HBsAg test is positive, the infant should receive HBIG as soon as possible (no later than age 1 week). **All children and adolescents (through age 18 years)** who have not been immunized against hepatitis B should begin the series during any visit. Providers should make special efforts to immunize children who were born in or whose parents were born in areas of the world where hepatitis B virus infection is moderately or highly endemic.

§ The fourth dose of diphtheria and tetanus toxoids and acellular pertussis vaccine (DTaP) may be administered as early as age 12 months, provided 6 months have elapsed since the third dose and the child is unlikely to return at age 15–18 months. Tetanus and diphtheria toxoids (Td) is recommended at age 11–12 years if at least 5 years have elapsed since the last dose of diphtheria and tetanus toxoids and pertussis vaccine (DTP), DTaP, or diphtheria and tetanus toxoids (DT). Subsequent routine Td boosters are recommended every 10 years.

¶ Three *Haemophilus influenzae* type b (Hib) conjugate vaccines are licensed for infant use. If Hib conjugate vaccine (PRP-OMP) (PedvaxHIB or ComVax [Merck]) is administered at ages 2 and 4 months, a dose at age 6 months is not required. Because clinical studies in infants have demonstrated that using some combination products may induce a lower immune response to the Hib vaccine component, DTaP/Hib combination products should not be used for primary immunization in infants at ages 2, 4 or 6 months unless approved by the Food and Drug Administration for these ages.

** An all-inactivated poliovirus vaccine (IPV) schedule is recommended for routine childhood polio vaccination in the United States. All children should receive four doses of IPV at age 2 months, age 4 months, between ages 6 and 18 months, and between ages 4 and 6 years. Oral poliovirus vaccine should be used only in selected circumstances (1).

†† The heptavalent pneumococcal conjugate vaccine (PCV) is recommended for all children age 2–23 months. It is also recommended for certain children age 24–59 months (2).

§§ The second dose of measles, mumps, and rubella vaccine (MMR) is recommended routinely at age 4–6 years but may be administered during any visit, provided at least 4 weeks have elapsed since receipt of the first dose and that both doses are administered beginning at or after age 12 months. Those who previously have not received the second dose should complete the schedule no later than the routine visit to a health-care provider at age 11–12 years.

¶¶ Varicella vaccine (Var) is recommended at any visit on or after the first birthday for susceptible children, (i.e., those who lack a reliable history of chickenpox [as judged by a health-care provider] and who have not been immunized]). Susceptible persons aged ≥13 years should receive two doses given at least 4 weeks apart.

*** Hepatitis A vaccine (Hep A) is recommended for use in selected states and/or regions, and for certain high-risk groups. Information is available from local public health authorities (3).

Additional information about the immunization schedule is available on the National Immunization Program World-Wide Web site, http://www.cdc.gov/nip, or by telephone, (800)232-2522 (English) or (800)232-0233 (Spanish).

Appendix C: Abbreviations, Acronyms, and Symbols

ʒ	dram
℥	ounce
ɱ	minum
ā	before
AARP	American Association of Retired Persons
AAT	animal-assisted therapy
AATH	American Association for Therapeutic Humor
ABC	airway, breathing, circulation
ABD	abdomen, abdominal
ABG	arterial blood gases
a.c.	before meals
ACIP	Advisory Committee on Immunization Practices
ACS	American Cancer Society
ACTH	adrenocorticotropic hormone
AD	Alzheimer's disease
AD	right ear
ad lib	freely, as desired
ADA	Americans with Disabilities Act
ADH	antidiuretic hormone
ADL	activities of daily living
ADN	associate degree nurse (nursing)
AEB	as evidenced by
AFP	alpha-fetoprotein
AHA	American Hospital Association
AHCA	American Health Care Association
AHCPR	Agency for Health Care Policy and Research
AHNA	American Holistic Nurses' Association
AHRQ	Agency for Healthcare Research and Quality
AI	adequate intake
AIDS	acquired immunodeficiency syndrome
AIDS	autoimmune deficiency syndrome
AJN	*American Journal of Nursing*
ALFA	Assisted Living Federation of America
ALT	alanine aminotransferase
AMA	against medical advice
AMA	American Medical Association
ANA	American Nurses Association
ANA	antinuclear antibody
AoA	Administration on Aging
AP	anterior/posterior
AP	apical pulse
APIC	Association for Practitioners in Infection Control and Epidemiology
APRN	advance practice registered nurse
APS	Adult Protective Services
APS	American Pain Society
APTT	activated partial thromboplastin time
AROM	active range of motion
AS	left ear
ASA	acetylsalicylic acid
ASO	antireptolysin-O
AST	aspartate aminotransferase
AT	axillary temperature
ATC	around the clock
ATP	adenosine triphosphatase
AU	both ears
B₁ (B_1)	thiamine
B₂ (B_2)	riboflavin

B₆ (B_6)	pyridoxine
B₁₂ (B_{12})	cobolomine
BBA	Balanced Budget Act
BE	base excess
bid	twice a day
BMD	bone mineral density
BMI	body mass index
BMR	basal metabolic rate
BP	blood pressure
BPH	benign prostatic hypertrophy
BPM	beats per minute
BSA	body surface area
BSE	breast self-examination
BSI	body substance isolation
BSN	bachelor of science in nursing
BUN	blood urea nitrogen
c	cup
c̄	with
C	Celsius
Ca	calcium
Ca⁺ (Ca^+)	calcium ion
CaCl₂ ($CaCl_2$)	calcium chloride
CAD	coronary artery disease
CAI	computer-assisted instruction
CAM	complementary/alternative medicine
C & S	culture and sensitivity
cap	capsule
CARF	Commission on Accreditation of Rehabilitation Facilities
CAT	computed axial tomography
CAT	computerized adaptive testing
CBC	complete blood count
CBD	common bile duct
CBE	charting by exception
cc	cubic centimeter
CCRC	continuing care retirement community
CCU	coronary care unit
CDC	Centers for Disease Control and Prevention
CEA	carcinoembryonic antigen
CEPN-LTC™	Certification Examination for Practical and Vocational Nurses in Long-Term Care
CEU	continuing education unit
CHAP	Community Health Accreditation Program
CHD	coronary heart disease
CHF	congestive heart failure
CHIP	Children's Health Insurance Program
CHO	carbohydrate (carbon, hydrogen, oxygen)
CHON	protein (carbon, hydrogen, oxygen, nitrogen)
CK or CPK	creatine kinase or creatine phosphokinase
Cl	chlorine
Cl⁻ (Cl^-)	chloride ion
CLTC	certified in long-term care
cm	centimeter
CN	cranial nerve
CNA	certified nursing assistant
CNM	certified nurse midwife
CNO	community nursing organization
CNS	central nervous system

CNS	clinical nurse specialist
Co	cobalt
CO_2	carbon dioxide
CO_2^-	carbon dioxide ion
COBRA	Comprehensive Omnibus Budget Reconciliation Act
COOH	carboxyl group
COPD	chronic obstructive pulmonary disease
CPAP	continuous positive airway pressure
CPNP	Council of Practical Nursing Programs
CPR	cardiopulmonary resuscitation
CPR	computerized patient record
Cr	chromium
CRNA	Certified Registered Nurse Anesthetist
CRP	C-reactive protein
CSF	cerebrospinal fluid
CSM	circulation, sensation, motion
CT	computed tomography
Cu	copper
CVA	cerebrovascular accident
CVC	central venous catheter
D_5W	dextrose 5% in water
D & C	dilatation and curettage
DAR	document, action, response
dc	discontinue
DDB	Disciplinary Data Bank
DDS	doctor of dental surgery
DEA	Drug Enforcement Agency
DHHS	Department of Health and Human Services
DIC	disseminated intravascular coagulation
DICC	dynamic infusion cavernosometry and cavernosography
dL	deciliter
DMD	doctor of dental medicine
DNA	deoxyribonucleic acid
DNR	do not resuscitate
DO	doctor of osteopathy
DPAHC	durable power of attorney for health care
dr	dram, or ʒ
DRG	diagnosis-related group
DRI	dietary reference intake
DSM-IV	*Diagnostic and Statistical Manual of Mental Disorders,* 4th edition
DST	dexamethasone suppression test
DT	delirium tremens
DTaP	diphtheria, tetanus, acellular pertussis
DTP	diphtheria, tetanus, pertussis
DVT	deep vein thrombosis
EAR	estimated average requirement
ECF	extended care facility
ECF	extracellular fluid
ECG (EKG)	electrocardiogram
ED	emergency department
EDTA	ethylenediaminetetraacetic acid
EEG	electroencephalograph
EGD	esophagogastroduodenoscopy
EKG	electrocardiogram
ELISA	enzyme-linked immunosorbent assay
elix	elixir
EMG	electromyogram
EMLA	eutectic (cream) mixture of local anesthetics
EMS	emergency medical services
EMT	emergency medical technician
EMT-P	emergency medical technician-paramedic
EPA	Environmental Protection Agency
EPO	exclusive provider organization
ER	emergency room
ERCP	endoscopic retrograde cholangiopancreatogram
ERG	electroretinogram
ERT	estrogen replacement therapy
ESR	erythrocyte sedimentation rate
ET	ear (tympanic) temperature
EVAD	explantable venous access device
F	fahrenheit
FAS	fetal alcohol syndrome
FBS	fasting blood sugar
FCA	False Claims Act
FDA	Food and Drug Administration
fe	iron
$FeSO_4$	iron sulfate
fl	fluid
Fl	fluorine
FOBT	fecal occult blood test
FSH	follicle-stimulating hormone
ft	foot or feet
g	gram
GAO	General Accounting Office
GAS	general adaptation syndrome
GCS	Glasgow Coma Scale
g/dL	grams per deciliter
GED	general education development
GER	gastroesophageal reflux
GFR	glomerular filtration rate
GGT (GGTP)	gammaglutamy transpeptidase
GH	growth hormone
GHb	glycosylated hemoglobin
GI	gastrointestinal
gr	grain
gtt	drop
GTT	glucose tolerance test
gtt/min	drops per minute
GU	genitourinary
h	hour(s)
H^+	hydrogen ion
H_2CO_3	carbonic acid
H_2O	water
H&H	hemoglobin and hematocrit
HB5AG	hepatitis B surface antigen
HBV	hepatitis B virus
HCFA	Health Care Financing Administration
hCG	human chorionic gonadotropin
HCl	hydrochloric acid, hydrochloride
HCO_3^-	bicarbonate ion
Hct	hematocrit
HCV	hepatitis C virus
HDL	high density lipoprotein
HDV	hepatitis D virus
Hep B	hepatitis B
Hg	mercury
Hgb	hemoglobin
Hgbs	hemoglobins
HICPAC	Hospital Infection Control Practices Advisory Committee
HIS	hospital information system
HIV	human immunodeficiency virus
HLA	human leukocyte antigen
HMO	health maintenance organization
HPO_4	phosphate
HR	heart rate
HRSA	Health Resources and Services Administration
h.s.	hour of sleep
I	iodine
IADL	instrumental activities of daily living

I&O	intake and output	**MgSO₄**	magnesium sulfate
IASP	International Association for the Study of Pain	**MI**	myocardial infarction
ICF	intermediate care facility	**min**	minute
ICF	intracellular fluid	**mL**	milliliter
ICN	International Council of Nurses	**mm³**	cubic millimeter
ICU	intensive care unit	**mm Hg**	millimeters of mercury
ID	identification	**MMR**	measles, mumps, rubella
ID	intradermal	**Mn**	manganese
IgG	immunoglobulin G	**Mo**	molybdenum
IgM	immunoglobulin M	**MOM**	Milk of Magnesia
IHCT	interdisciplinary health care team	**mOsm/kg**	milliosmoles/kilogram
IM	intramuscular	**MRI**	magnetic resonance imaging
in	inch	**MRSA**	methicillin-resistant *staphylococcus aureus*
INR	International Normalized Ratio	**MS**	morphine sulfate
I&O	intake and output	**MSDS**	material safety data sheet
IOL	intraocular lens	**MUGA**	multi-gated acquisition
IOM	Institute of Medicine	**N₂**	nitrogen
ITT	insulin tolerance test	**Na**	sodium
IV	intravenous	**Na⁺**	sodium ion
IVAD	implantable vascular access device	**Na₂SO₄**	sodium sulfate
IVP	intravenous push, intravenous pyelogram	**NaCl**	sodium chloride
IVPB	intravenous piggyback	**NADSA**	National Adult Day Services Associations
JCAHO	Joint Commission on Accreditation of Healthcare Organizations	**NaH₂PO₄**	sodium dihydrogen phosphate
K	potassium	**Na₂HPO₄**	disodium phosphate
K⁺	potassium ion	**NAHC**	National Association for Home Care
kcal	kilocalorie	**NaHCO₃**	sodium bicarbonate
KCl	potassium chloride	**NaHPO₄**	sodium monohydrogen phosphate
kg	kilogram	**NANDA**	North American Nursing Diagnosis Association
KS	ketosteroids	**NaOH**	sodium hydroxide
KUB	kidneys/ureters/bladder	**NAPNE**	Natonal Association of Practical Nurse Education
KVO	keep vein open	**NAPNES**	National Association for Practical Nurse Education and Services
L	liter	**NCCAM**	National Center for Complementary & Alternative Medicine
LAS	local adaptation syndrome	**NCHS**	National Center for Health Statistics
lb	pound	**NCLEX**	National Council Licensure Examination
LDH	lactic dehydrogenase	**NCLEX-PN**	National Council Licensure Examination—Practical Nurse
LDL	low density lipoprotein	**NCLEX-RN**	National Council Licensure Examination—Registered Nurse
LE	lupus erythematosus	**NCLD**	National Center for Learning Disabilities
LES	lower esophageal sphincter	**NCOA**	National Council on Aging
LFT	liver function test	**NCSBN**	National Council of State Boards of Nursing
LH	luteinizing hormone	**NCVHS**	National Committee on Vital and Health Statistics
LLQ	left lower quadrant	**NF**	*National Formulary*
LMP	last menstrual period	**NFLPN**	National Federation of Licensed Practical Nurses, Inc.
L/min	liters per minute	**NG**	nasogastric
LOC	level of consciousness	**NH₂**	amino group
LP	lumbar puncture	**NHO**	National Hospice Organization
LP/VN	licensed practical/vocational nurse	**NIA**	National Institute on Aging
LPN	licensed practical nurse	**NIC**	Nursing Interventions Classification
LUQ	left upper quadrant	**NIH**	National Institutes of Health
LVN	licensed vocational nurse	**NIS**	nursing information system
m	meter	**NLEA**	Nutrition, Labeling, and Education Act
m²	square meter	**NLN**	National League for Nursing
MAO	monoamine oxidase	**NLNAC**	National League for Nursing Accrediting Commission
MAOI	monoamine oxidase inhibitor	**NMDS**	nursing minimum data set
MAR	medication administration record	**NOC**	Nursing Outcomes Classification
mcg (or μg)	microgram	**NP**	nurse practitioner
MD	doctor of medicine	**NPDB**	National Practitioner Data Bank
MDI	metered-dose inhaler	**NPO**	*nil per os,* Latin for "nothing by mouth"
MDR	multidrug-resistant	**NREM**	non-rapid eye movement
MDR-TB	multidrug-resistant tuberculosis	**NS**	normal saline
MDS	minimum data set		
mEq	milliequivalent		
mEq/L	milliequivalents per liter		
mg	milligram		
Mg	magnesium		
Mg⁺⁺	magnesium ion		
MgCl	magnesium chloride		

NSAID	nonsteroidal anti-inflammatory drug		**PTT**	partial thromboplastin time
NSF	National Sleep Foundation		**PVD**	peripheral vascular disease
O₂	oxygen		**q**	*quaque,* Latin for "every"
OAM	Office of Alternative Medicine		**qd**	every day
O&P	ova and parasite		**qh**	every hour
OBRA	Omnibus Budget Reconciliation Act		**qid**	four times a day
OD	right eye		**qod**	every other day
OH	hydroxyl		**qs**	quantity sufficient
OR	operating room		**q2h**	every 2 hours
ORIF	open reduction/internal fixation		**qt**	quart
OS	left eye		**R (Resp)**	respiration
OSHA	Occupational Safety and Health Administration		**RAIU**	radioactive iodine uptake
OT	occupational therapist		**RAST**	radio allergosorbent test
OT	oral temperature		**RBC**	red blood count, red blood cell
OTC	over-the-counter		**RD**	registered dietician
OU	both eyes		**RDA**	recommended dietary allowance
oz	ounce		**REM**	rapid eye movement
p̄	after		**RF**	rheumatoid factor
P	phosphorus		**RLQ**	right lower quadrant
P	pulse		**RLS**	restless leg syndrome
PA	physician's assistant		**RN**	registered nurse
PA	posterioanterior		**RNA**	ribonucleic acid
PaCO₂	partial pressure of carbon dioxide		**RNFA**	registered nurse first assistant
PaO₂	partial pressure of oxygen		**ROM**	range of motion
Pap	Papanicolaou test		**ROS**	review of systems
p.c.	after meals		**RPh**	registered pharmacist
PCA	patient-controlled analgesia		**RPR**	rapid plasma reagin
PCO₂ (PaCO₂)	partial pressure of carbon dioxide		**RR**	recovery room
PCP	primary care provider		**RSV**	respiratory syncytial virus
PCR	polymerase chain reaction		**R/T**	related to
PDPH	postdural puncture headache		**RT**	rectal temperature
PEG	percutaneous endoscopic gastrostomy		**RT**	respiratory therapist
PERRLA	pupils equal, round, reactive to light and accommodation		**RTI**	respiratory tract infection
PET	positron emission tomography		**RUGS**	resource utilization group system
PFT	pulmonary function test		**RUQ**	right upper quadrant
pH	potential hydrogen		**RWJF**	Robert Wood Johnson Foundation
PICC	peripherally inserted central catheter		**s̄**	without
PIE	problem, implementation, evaluation		**S**	sulfur
PKU	phenylketonuria		**SAMe**	S-adenosylmethionine
PLMS	periodic limb movements in sleep		**SaO₂**	oxygen saturation
PMI	point of maximum intensity		**SBC**	school-based clinic
PMR	progressive muscle relaxation		**SC/SQ**	subcutaneous
PMS	premenstrual syndrome		**SCHIP**	State Children's Health Insurance Program
PNI	psychoneuroimmunology		**Se**	selenium
PNS	peripheral nervous system		**SGOT**	serum glutamate oxaloacetate transaminase
po	*per os,* Latin for "by mouth"		**SGPT**	serum glutamic pyruou transaminase
PO₂ (PaO₂)	partial pressure of oxygen		**SL**	sublingual
PO₄⁻⁻	phosphate ion		**SNF**	skilled nursing facility
POMR	problem-oriented medical record		**SOAP**	subjective data, objective data, assessment, plan
POR	problem-oriented record		**SOAPIE**	subjective data, objective data, assessment, plan, implementation, evaluation
PPBS	post prandial blood sugar			
PPE	personal protective equipment		**SOAPIER**	subjective data, objective data, assessment, plan, implementation, evaluation, revision
PPG	post prandial glucose			
PPO	preferred provider organization		**SPF**	sun protection factor
PPS	prospective payment system		**s̄s̄**	one half
PRA	plama renin activity		**SSA**	Social Security Administration
PRL	prolactin level		**STAT**	*statim,* Latin for "immediately"
PRN	*pro re nata,* Latin for "as required"		**STD**	sexually transmitted disease
PRO	peer review organization		**supp**	suppository
PROM	passive range of motion		**susp**	suspension
PSA	prostate specific antigen		**SW**	social worker
PSDA	Patient Self-Determination Act		**T**	temperature
PSP	phenolsulfonphtalein		**T₃**	triiodothyronine
pt	pint		**T₄**	thyroxine
PT	physical therapist		**tab**	tablet
PT	prothrombin time		**TAC**	tetracaine, adrenaline, cocaine
PTH	parathyroid hormone		**TB**	tuberculosis
PTSD	post-traumatic stress disorder		**Tbsp**	tablespoon

Td	tetanus/diphtheria
TDD	telecommunication device for the deaf
TEFRA	Tax Equity Fiscal Responsibility Act
TENS	transcutaneous electrical nerve stimulation
TF	tube feeding
THA	total hip arthroplasty
TIA	transient ischemic attack
TIBC	total iron binding capacity
t.i.d.	three times a day
TMJ	temporomandibular joint
t.o.	telephone order
TPN	total parenteral nutrition
TPR	temperature, pulse, respirations
Tr or tinct	tincture
TRH	thyrotropin-releasing hormone
TSE	testicular self examination
TSH	thyroid-stimulating hormone
tsp	teaspoon
U	unit
U/L	unit per liter
UA	routine urinalysis
UAP	unlicensed assistive personnel
UIS	Universal Intellectual Standards
UTI	urinary tract infection
UL	upper intake level

UMLS	Universal Medical Language System
U-100	100 units insulin per cc
UPP	urethra pressure profile
URQ	upper right quadrant
USDHHS	United States Department of Health and Human Services
USP	*United States Pharmacopeia*
USPHS	United States Public Health Service
UTI	urinary tract infection
VA	Veterans Administration, Veterans Affairs
VAD	ventricular assist device, vascular access device
VAS	Visual Analog Scale
VDRL	venereal disease research laboratory
VLDL	very low-density lipoprotein
VMA	vanilymandelic acid
VRE	vancomycin-resistant enterococci
VS	vital signs
WASP	white, Anglo-Saxon, Protestant
WBC	white blood cell, white blood count
WHO	World Health Organization
WNL	within normal limits
WPM	words per minute
wt	weight
Zn	Zinc

Appendix D: English/Spanish Words and Phrases

Being able to say a few words or phrases in the client's language is one way to show that you care. It lets the client know that you as a nurse are interested in the individual. There are three rules to keep in mind regarding the pronunciation of Spanish words.

- If a word ends in a vowel, or in *n* or *s,* the accent is on the next to the last syllable.
- If the word ends in a consonant other than *n* or *s,* the accent is on the last syllable.
- If the word does not follow these rules, it has a written accent over the vowel of the accented syllable.

Courtesy phrases, names of body parts, and expressions of time and numbers are included in this section for quick reference. The English version will appear first, followed by the Spanish translation and Spanish pronunciation.

Courtesy Phrases

Please	Por favor	Por fah-**vor**
Thank-you	Grácias	**Grah**-the-as
Good morning	Buénos dias	Boo-**ay**-nos **dee**-as
Good afternoon	Buénas tardes	Boo-**ay**-nas **tar**-days
Good evening	Buénas noches	Boo-**ay**-nas **no**-chays
Yes/No	Si/no	See/no
Good	Bien	Be-en
Bad	Mal	Mahl
How many?	¿Cuántos?	¿Coo-**ahn**-tos?
Where?	¿Dónde?	¿**Don**-day?
When?	¿Cuándo?	¿Coo**ahn**-do?

Body Parts

abdomen	el abdomen	el ab-doh-men
ankle	el tobillo	el to-**beel**-lyo
anus	el ano	el **ah**-no
anvil (incus)	el yunque	el **yoon**-kay
appendix	el apéndice	el ah-**pen**-de-thay
aqueous humor	el humor acuoso	el oo-**mor** ah-coo-**o**-so
bladder	la vejiga	lah vay-**nee**-gah
brain	el cerebro	el thay-**ray**-bro
breast	el pecho	el **pay**-cho
buttock	la nalga	lah **nahl**-gah
calf	la pantorrilla	lah pan-tor-**reel**-lyah
cervix	la cerviz	lah ther-**veth**
cheek	la mejilla	lah may-**heel**-lyah
chin	la barbilla	lah bar-**beel**-lyah
choroid	la coroidea	lah co-ro-e-**day**-ah
ciliary body	el cuerpo ciliar	el coo-**err**-po the-le-**ar**
clitoris	el clítoris	el **clee**-to-ris
coccyx	el coxis	el **coc**-sees
conjunctiva	la conjuntiva	lah con-hoon-**tee**vah
cornea	la córnea	lah **cor**-nay-ah
penis	el pene	el **pay**-nay
prostrate gland	la próstata	lah **pros**-ta-tah
pupil	la pupila	lah poo-**pee**-lah
rectum	el recto	el **rec**-to
retina	la retina	lah ray-**tee**-nah
sclera	la esclerótica	lah es-clay-**ro**-te-cah

scrotum	el escroto	el es-**cro**-to
seminal vesicle	la vesícula seminal	lah vay-**see**-coo-lah say-me-**nahl**
shoulder	el hombro	el **om**-bro
small intestine	el intestino delgado	el in-tes-**tee**-no del-**gah**-do
spinal cord	la médula espinal	lah **may**-doo-lah es-pe-**nahl**
spleen	el bazo	el **bah**-tho
stirrup (stapes)	el estribo	el es-**tree**-bo
stomach	el estómago	el es-**toh**-mah-go
temple	la sien	lah se-**ayn**
testis	el testículo	el tes-**tee**-coo-lo
thigh	el muslo	el **moos**-lo
thorax	el tórax	el **to**-rax
tongue	la lengua	lah **len**-goo-ah
trachea	la tráquea	lah **trah**-kay-ah
upper extremities	las extremidades superiores	las ex-tray-me-**dahd**-es soo-pay-re-**or**-es
ureter	el uréter	el oo-**ray**-ter
uterus	el útero	el **oo**-tay-ro
vagina	el vagina	lah vah-**hee**-nah
vitreous humor	el humor vítreo	el oo-**mor vee**-tray-o
wrist	la muñeca	lah moo-**nyay**-cah

Expressions of Time, Calendar, and Numbers

after meals	después de comer	des-poo-**es** day co-**merr**
at bedtime	al acostarse	al ah-cos-**tar**-say
before meals	antes de comer	**ahn**-tes day co-**merr**
daily	el diario	el de-**ah**-re-o
date	la fecha	lah **fay**-chah
day	el dia	el **dee**-ah
every hour	a cada hora	ah **cah**-dah **o**-rah
hour (time)	la hora	lah **o**-rah
how often	cada cuánto tiempo	**cah**-dah coo-**ahn**-to te-**em**-po
noon	el mediodia	el may-de-o-**dee**-ah
now	ahora	ah-**o**-rah
once	una vez	**oo**-nah veth
today	hoy	**oh**-e
tomorrow	mañana	mah-**nyah**-nah
tonight	esta noche	**es**-tah **no**-chay
week	la semana	lah say-**mah**-nah
year	año	**a**-nyo
Sunday	el domingo	el do-**meen**-go
Monday	el lunes	el **loo**-nes
Tuesday	el martes	el **mar**-tes
Wednesday	el miércoles	el me-**err**-co-les
Thursday	el jueves	el hoo-**ay**ves
Friday	el viernes	el ve-**err**-nes
Saturday	el sábado	el **sah**-bah-do
zero	cero	**thay**-ro
one	uno	**oo**-no
two	dos	dose
three	tres	trays
four	cuatro	coo-**ah**-tro
five	cinco	**theen**-co
six	seis	**say**-ees
seven	siete	se-**ay**-tay
eight	ocho	**o**-cho
nine	nueve	noo-**ay**-vay
ten	diez	de-**eth**

Nursing Care Sentences and Questions

What is your name?
¿Como se llama usted?
¿**Co**-mo say **lyah**-mah oos-**ted?**

I am a student nurse.
Soy estudiente enfermera(o).
Soy es-too-de-**ahn**-tay en-fer-**may**-ra(o).

My name is . . .
Mi nombre es . . .
Mee **nom**-bray es . . .

Do you need a wheelchair?
¿Necesita usted una silla de rueda?
¿Nay-thay-**se**-ta oos-**ted oo**-nah **seel**-lyah day
    roo-**ay**-dah?

How do you feel?
¿Como se siente?
¿**Co**-mo say se-**ayn**-tah?

When is your family coming?
¿Cuándo viene su familia?
¿Coo-**ahn**-do vee-**en**-nah soo fah-**mee**-le-ah?

This is the call light.
Esta es la luz para llamar a la enfermera.
Es-tah es lah looth **pah**-ra lyah-**mar** a lah
    en-fer-**may**-ra.

If you need anything, press the button.
Si usted necesita algo, oprima el botón.
See oos-**ted** nay-thay-**se**-ta **ahl**-go o-pre-**ma** el
    bo-**tone.**

Do not turn without calling the nurse.
No se voltee sin llamar a la enfermera.
No say **vol**-tay seen lyah-**mar** a lah en-fer-**may**-ra.

The side rails on your bed are for your protection.
Los rieles del costado están para su protección.
Los re-**el**-es del cos-**tah**-do es-**tahn pah**-ra soo
    pro-tec-the-**on.**

Please do not try to lower or climb over the side rail.
Por favor no pretenda bajarlos (barjarlas) o treparse
    sobre ellos.
Por fah-**vor** no pray-**ten**-dah ba-**har**-los o
    tray-**par**-say **so**-bray **ayl**-lyos.

The head nurse is . . .
La jefa de enfermeras es . . .
La **hay**-fay day en-fer-**may**-ras es . . .

Do you need more blankets or another pillow?
¿Necesita usted más frazadas u orta almohada?
¿Nay-thay-**si**-ta oos-**ted** mahs frah-**thad**-dahs oo
    o-trah al-mo-**ah**-dah?

You may not smoke in the room.
No se puede fumar en el cuarto.
No say poo-**ay**-day foo-**mar** en el coo-**ar**-to.

Do you want me to turn on (turn off) the lights?
¿Quiere usted que encienda (apague) la luz?
¿Ke-**ay**-ray oos-**ted** day en-the-**en**-dah (a-**pah**-gay)
    lah looth?

Are you thirsty?
¿Tiene usted sed?
¿Tee-**en**-nah oos-**ted** sayd?

Are you allergic to any medication?
¿Es usted alérgico(a) a alguna medicina?
¿Es oos-**ted** ah-**lehr**-hee-co(a) ah ah-**goo**-nah nay-de-
    thee-nah?

You may take a bath.
Usted puede bañarse.
Oos-**ted** poo-**ay**-day bah-**nyar**-say.

Do not lock the door, please.
No cierre usted la puerta con llave, por favor.
No the-**err**-ray oos-**ted** lah poo-**err**-tah con **lyah**-vay
    por fah-**vor.**

Call if you feel faint or in need of help.
Llame si usted se siente débil o si necesita ayuda.
Lyah-mah see oos-**ted** say se-**ayn**-tah **day**-bil o see
    nay-thay-**se**-ta ah-**yoo**-dah.

Call when you have to go to the toilet.
Llame cuando tenga que ir al inodoro.
Lyah-mah coo-**ahn**-do **ten**-gah kay eer al in-o-**do**-ro.

I will give you an enema.
Le pondré una enema.
Lay pon-**dray oo**-nah ay-**nay**-mah.

Turn on your left (right) side.
Voltese a su lado izquierdo (derecho).
Vol-**tay**-say ah soo **lah**-do ith-ke-**er**-do(dah) (day-**ray**-
    cho[cha]).

Here is an appointment card.
Aqui tiene usted una tarjeta con la información
    escrito.
Ah-**kee** tee-**en**-nah oos-**ted oo**-nah tar-**hay**-tah con
    lah in-for-mah-the-**on** es-**cree**-to.

You are going to be discharged (released) today.
A usted le van a dar de alta hoy.
Ah oos-**ted** lay vahn ah dar day **ahl**-tah **oh**-e.

How did this illness begin?
¿Como empezó esta enfermedad?
¿**Co**-mo em-pa-**tho es**-tah en-fer-may-**dahd**?

Is the pain better after the medicine?
¿Siente usted alivio depués de tomar la medicina?
¿Se-**ayn**-tah oos-**ted** al-**lee**-ve-o des-poo-**es** day to-**mar** lah may-de-**thee**-nah?

Where is the pain?
¿Que la duele? (or) Dónde le duele?
¿Kay lah doo-**ay**-le? (or) **Don**-day lay doo-**ay**-le?

Do you have pains in your chest?
¿Tiene usted dolores in el pecho?
¿Tee-**en**-nah oos-**ted** do-**lor**-es en el **pay**-cho?

Are you in pain now?
¿Tiene usted dolores ahora?
¿Tee-**en**-nah oos-**ted** do-**lor**-es ah-**o**-rah?

Is it constant pain or does it come and go?
¿Es un dolor constante o va y vuelve?
¿Es oon do-**lor** cons-**tahn**-tay o vah ee voo-**el**-vah?

Is there anything that makes the pain better?
¿Hay algo que lo alivie?
¿**Ah**-ee **ahl**-go kay lo al-**le**-ve?

Is there anything that makes the pain worse?
¿Hay algo que lo aumente?
¿**Ah**-ee **ahl**-go kay lo ah-oo-**men**-tay?

Where do you feel the pain?
¿Dónde siente usted el dolor?
¿**Don**-day se-**ayn**-tah oos-**ted** el do-**lor**?

Point to where it hurts.
Apunte usted por favor, adonde le duele.
Ah-**poon**-tay oos-**ted** por fah-**vor** ah-**don**-day lay doo-**ay**-le.

Show me where it hurts.
Enséñeme usted donde le duele.
En-**say**-nah-may oos-**ted don**-day lay doo-**ay**-le.

Is the pain sharp or dull?
¿Es agudo o sordo el dolor?
¿Es ah-**goo**-do o **sor**-do el do-**lor**?

Do you know where you are?
¿Sabe usted donde esta?
¿Sah-**bay** oos-**ted don**-day es-**tah**?

You are in the hospital.
Usted está en el hospital.
Oos-**ted** es-**tah** en el os-pee-**tahl**.

You will be okay.
Usted va a estar bien.
Oos-**ted** vah a es-**tar** be-en.

Do you have any drug reactions?
¿Tiene usted alguna sensibilidad a productos químicos?
¿Te-**en**-nah oos-**ted** al-**goo**-nah sen-se-be-le-**dahd** a pro-**dooc**-tos **kee**-me-cos?

Have you seen another doctor or native healer for this problem?
¿Ha visto usted a otro médico o curandero tocante a este problema?
¿Ah **vees**-to oos-**ted** a o-tro **may**-de-co o coo-ran-**day**-ro to-**cahn**-tay a **es**-ah pro-**blay**-mah?

Have you vomited?
¿Ha vomitado usted?
¿Ah vo-me-**tah**-do oos-**ted**?

Do you have any difficulty in breathing?
¿Tiene usted alguna dificultad para respirar?
¿Te-**en**-nah oos-**ted** ah-**goo**-nah de-fe-cool-**tahd pah**-ra res-pe-**rar**?

Do you smoke?
¿Fuma usted?
¿Foo-**mar** oos-**ted**?

How many per day?
¿Cuántos al dia?
¿Coo-**ahn**-tos al **dee**-ah?

For how many years?
¿Por cuántos años?
¿por coo-**ahn**-tos **a**-nyos?

Do you awaken in the night because of shortness of breath?
¿Se despierta usted por la noche por falta de respiración?
¿Say des-pee-**err**-tah oos-**ted** por lah **no**-chay por **fahl**-tah day res-pe-rah-the-**on**?

Is any part of your body swollen?
¿Tiene usted alguna parte del cuerpo hinchada?
¿Te-**en**-nah oos-**ted** ah-**goo**-nah **par**-tay del coo-**err**-po in-**chah**-da?

How much water do you drink daily?
¿Cuántos vasos de agua bebe usted diariamente?
¿Coo-**ahn**-tos **vah**-sos day **ah**-goo-ah **bay**-be oos-**ted** de-ah-re-ah-**men**-tay?

Are you nauseated?
¿Tiene náusea?
¿Te-**en**-nah **nah**-oo-say-ah?

Are you going to vomit?
¿Va a vomitar?
¿Vah a vo-me-**tar**?

When was your last bowel movement?
¿Cuánto tiempo hace que evacúa usted?
¿Coo-**ahn**-to te-**em**-po **ah**-the kay ay-vah-**coo**-ah oos-**ted**?

Do you have diarrhea?
¿Tiene usted diarrea?
¿Te-**en**-nah oos-**ted** der-ar-**ray**-ah?

How much do you urinate?
¿Cuánto orina usted?
¿Coo-**ahn**-to o-**re**-nah oos-**ted**?

Did you urinate?
¿Orinó usted?
¿O-re-**no** oos-**ted**?

What color is your urine?
¿De qué color es la orina?
¿Day kay co-**lor** es lah o-**re**-nah?

Call when you have to go to the toilet.
Llame usted cuando tenga que ir al inodoro.
Lyah-mah oos-**ted** coo-**ahn**-do **ten**-gah kay eer al in-o-**do**-ro.

I need a urine specimen from you.
Necesito una muestra de orina de usted.
Nay-thay-**se**-to **oo**-nah moo-**ays**-trah day o-**re**-nah day oos-**ted**.

We will put a tube in your bladder so that you can urinate.
Le pondremos un tubo en la vejiga para que puede orinar.
Lay pon-**dray**-mos un **too**-be en lah vay-**hee**-gah **pah**-rah kay poo-**ay**-day o-re **nar**.

When was your last menstrual period?
¿Cuándo fue se última menstruación?
¿Coo-**ahn**-do foo-**ay** soo **ool**-te-mah mens-troo-ah-the-**on**?

Are you bleeding heavily?
¿Está sangrando mucho?
¿Es-**tah** san-**grahn**-do **moo**-cho?

Take off your clothes, please
Desvístase usted, por favor.
Des-**ves**-tah-say oos-**ted** por-fah-**vor.**

Just relax.
Relaje usted el cuerpo.
Ray-**lah**-he oos-**ted** el coo-**err**-po.

I am going to listen to your chest.
Voy a escucharle el pecho.
Voye a es-coo-**char**-lay el **pay**-cho.

Let me feel your pulse.
Déjeme tomarle el pulso.
Day-ha-me to-**bar**-lay el **pool**-so.

I am going to take your temperature.
Voy a tomarle la temperatura.
Voye a to-**mar**-lay lah tem-pay-rah-**too**-rah.

Lie down, please.
Acuéstese, por favor.
Ah-coo-**es**-tah-say por fah-**vor.**

Do you understand?
¿Me comprende usted?
¿May com-**pren**-day oos-**ted?**

That's right.
Así. Bien.
Ah-**see.** Be-en.

You are doing very well.
Usted va muy bien.
Oos-**ted** vah **moo**-e **be**-en.

Do not take any medicine from home.
No tome usted ninguna medicina traída de su casa.
No **to**-may oos-**ted** nin-**goon**-ay may-de-**thee**-nah trah-**ee**-dah day soo **cah**-sah.

I am going to give you an injection.
Voy a ponerle ana inyección.
Voye a po-**nerr**-lay **oo**-nah in-yec-the-**on.**

Take a sip of water.
Tome usted un traguito de agua.
To-may oos-**ted** un trah-**gee**-to day **ah**-goo-ah.

Very good. That was fine.
Muy bien. Excelente.
Moo-e **be**-en. Ex-thay-**len**-tay.

Don't be nervous.
No se ponga nervioso(a).
No say **pon**-gah ner-ve-**o**-so(ah).

Do you feel dizzy?
¿Se siente vertigo?
¿Say see-**ayn**-tah **verr**-to-go?

Please lie still.
Quédese inmóvil, por favor.
Kay-day-say in-**mo**-veel por fah-**vor.**

You must drink lots of liquids.
Usted debe tomar muchos líquidos.
Oos-**ted day**-bay to-**mar moo**-chos **lee**-ke-dos.

References

Kelz, R. K. (1982.) *Conversational Spanish for Medical Personnel.* Albany, NY: Delmar.
Velazquez de la Cadena, M., Gray, E., & Iribas, J. (1985). *New Revised Velazquez Spanish and English Dictionary.* Clinton, NJ: New Win Publishing, Inc.

Glossary

Abduction Lateral movement away from the body.

Ability Competence in an activity.

Absorption Passage of a drug from the site of administration into the bloodstream; Process whereby the end products of digestion pass through the epithelial membranes in the small and large intestines and into the blood or lymph system.

Abuse Incident involving some type of violation to the client; Misuse, excessive, or improper use of a substance, the absence of which does not cause withdrawal symptoms.

Accommodation Component of cognitive development that allows for readjustment of the cognitive structure (mindset) in order to take in new information.

Accountability Responsibility of actions and inactions performed by oneself or others.

Accreditation Process by which a voluntary, nongovernmental agency or organization appraises and grants accredited status to institutions and/or programs or services that meet predetermined structure, process, and outcome criteria.

Acculturation Process of learning norms, beliefs, and behavioral expectations of a group.

Acid Any substance that in a solution yields hydrogen ions bearing a positive charge.

Acidosis Condition characterized by an excessive number of hydrogen ions in a solution.

Acquired Immunity Formation of antibodies (memory B cells) to protect against future invasions of an already experienced antigen.

Active Euthanasia Process of taking deliberate action that will hasten a client's death.

Active Listening Process of hearing spoken words and noting nonverbal behaviors.

Activities of Daily Living Basic care activities that include mobility, bathing, hygiene, grooming, dressing, eating, and toileting.

Actual Nursing Diagnosis Nursing diagnosis that indicates that a problem exists; composed of the diagnostic label, related factors, and signs and symptoms.

Acupressure Technique of releasing blocked energy within an individual when specific points (tsubas) along the meridians are pressed or massaged by the practitioner's fingers, thumbs, and heel of the hands.

Acupuncture Technique of application of heat and needles to various points on the body to alter the energy flow.

Acute Pain Discomfort identified by sudden onset and relatively short duration, mild to severe intensity, and a steady decrease in intensity over several days or weeks.

Adaptation Ongoing process whereby individuals use various responses to adjust to stressors and change.

Adaptive Energy Inner forces that an individual uses to adapt to stress (phrase coined by Selye).

Adaptive Measure Measure for coping with stress that requires a minimal amount of energy.

Addiction Overwhelming preoccupation with obtaining and using a drug for its psychic effects; used interchangeably with dependence.

Adjuvant Medication Drug used to enhance the analgesic efficacy of opioids, treat concurrent symptoms that exacerbate pain, and provide independent analgesia for specific types of pain.

Administrative Law Law developed by those persons who are appointed to governmental administrative agencies and who are entrusted with enforcing the statutory laws passed by the legislature.

Adolescence Developmental stage from the ages of 12 years to 20 years that begins with the appearance of the secondary sex characteristics (puberty).

Adult Day Care Provision of a variety of services in a protective setting for adults who are unable to stay alone, but who do not need 24-hour care.

Advance Directive Written instruction for health care that is recognized under state law and is related to the provision of such care when the individual is incapacitated.

Adventitious Breath Sound Abnormal sound, including sibilant wheezes (formerly wheezes), sonorous wheezes (formerly rhonchi), fine and course crackles (formerly rales), and pleural friction rubs.

Affect Outward expression of mood or emotions.

Affective Domain Area of learning that involves attitudes, beliefs, and emotions.

Afferent Nerve (Pain) Pathway Ascending spinal cord pathway that transmits sensory impulses to the brain.

Agent Entity capable of causing disease.

Agglutination Clumping together of red blood cells.

Agglutinin Specific kind of antibody whose interaction with antigens is manifested as agglutination.

Agglutinogen Any antigenic substance that causes agglutination by the production of agglutinin.

Agnostic Individual who believes that the existence of God cannot be proved or disproved.

Airborne Precautions Measures taken in addition to Standard Precautions and for clients known to have or suspected of having illnesses spread by airborne droplet nuclei.

Airborne Transmission Transfer of an agent to a susceptible host through droplet nuclei or dust particles suspended in the air.

Algor Mortis Decrease in body temperature after death, resulting in lack of skin elasticity.

Alkalosis Condition characterized by an excessive loss of hydrogen ions from a solution.

Allergy Altered reaction of the tissues of some individuals to substances that in similar amounts are harmless to other people.

Alopecia Partial or complete baldness or loss of hair.

Alternative Therapy Therapy used instead of conventional or mainstream medical practices.

Anabolism Constructive process of metabolism whereby new molecules are synthesized and new tissues are formed, as in growth and repair.

Analgesia Pain relief without producing anesthesia.

Analgesic Substance that relieves pain.

Analysis Breaking down the whole into parts that can be examined.

Analyte Substance that is measured.

Aneurysm Weakness in the wall of a blood vessel.

Angiocatheter Intracatheter with a metal stylet.

Angiography Visualization of the vascular structures through the use of fluoroscopy with a contrast medium.

Anion Ion bearing a negative charge.

Anorexia Nervosa Psychiatric disorder of self-imposed starvation that results in a 15% or more loss of body weight.

Anthropogenic State reflecting changes in the relationship between humans and their environment.

Anthropometric Measurements Measurements of the size, weight, and proportions of the body.

Antibody Immunoglobulin produced by the body in response to bacteria, viruses, or other antigenic substances.

Anticipatory Grief Occurrence of grief work before an expected loss actually occurs.

Anticipatory Guidance Information, teaching, and guidance given to a client in anticipation of an expected event.

Antigen Any substance identified by the body as nonself.

Antioxidant Substance that prevents or inhibits oxidation, a chemical process wherein a substance is joined to oxygen.

Anxiety Subjective response that occurs when a person experiences a real or perceived threat to well-being; a diverse feeling of dread or apprehension.

Aphasia Inability to communicate; often the result of a brain lesion.

Aromatherapy Therapeutic use of concentrated essences or essential oils that have been extracted from plants and flowers.

Arterial Blood Gases Measurement of levels of oxygen, carbon dioxide, pH, partial pressure of oxygen (PO_2 or PaO_2), partial pressue of carbon dioxide (PCO_2 or $PaCO_2$), saturation of oxygen (SaO_2), and bicarbonate (HCO_3) in arterial blood.

Arteriography Radiographic study of the vascular system following the injection of a radiopaque dye through a catheter.

Ascites Abnormal accumulation of fluid in the peritoneal cavity.

Asepsis Absence of microorganisms.

Aseptic Technique Collection of principles used to control and/or prevent the transfer of pathogenic microorganisms from sources within (endogenous) and outside (exogenous) the client.

Aspiration Procedure performed to withdraw fluid that has abnormally collected or to obtain a specimen; also inhalation of regurgitated gastric contents into the pulmonary system.

Assault Threat to do something that may cause harm or be unpleasant to another person.

Assessment First step in the nursing process; includes systematic collection, verification, organization, interpretation, and documentation of data.

Assessment Model Framework that provides a systematic method for organizing data.

Assignment Downward or lateral transfer of both responsibility and accountability for an activity.

Assimilation Component of cognitive development that involves taking in new experiences or information.

Assisted Living Combination of housing and services for persons who require assistance with activities of daily living.

Assisted Suicide Situation wherein another person provides a client with the means to end his own life.

Assumption Belief or attitude that one takes for granted in a situation that requires action or resolution.

Atheist Individual who does not believe in God or any other deity.

Atherosclerosis Cardiovascular disease of fatty deposits on the inner lining, the tunica intima, of vessel walls.

Atom Smallest unit of an element which still retains the properties of that element and which cannot be altered by any chemical change.

Attitude Manner, feeling, or position toward a person or thing.

Attribute Characteristic that belongs to an individual.

Audible Wheeze Wheeze that can be heard without the aid of a stethoscope.

Auditory Learner Person who learns by processing information through hearing.

Auscultation Physical examination technique that involves listening to sounds in the body that are created by movement of air or fluid.

Autocratic Leadership style that is task oriented and based on the premise that the leader knows best.

Autonomy Self-direction; Ethical principle based on the individual's right to choose and the individual's ability to act on that choice.

Autopsy Examination of a body after death by a pathologist to determine cause of death.

Bacteremia Condition of bacteria in the blood.

Bactericide Bacteria-killing chemicals; found in tears.

Balanced Budget Act Federal law enacted in 1997 that replaced cost-based reimbursement for care in skilled nursing facilities with a prospective payment system based on client assessment within a resource utilization group system.

Barium Chalky-white contrast medium.

Barrier Precautions Use of personal protective equipment, such as masks, gowns, and gloves, to create a barrier between the person and the microorganisms and thus prevent transmission of the microorganism.

Basal Metabolism Energy needed to maintain essential physiological functions such as respiration, circulation, and muscle tone, when a person is at complete rest physically, digestively, and mentally.

Base Substance that when dissociated produces ions that will combine with hydrogen ions.

Baseline Level Lab value that serves as a reference point for future value levels.

Battery Unauthorized or unwanted touching of one person by another.

Beneficence Ethical principle based on the duty to promote good and prevent harm.

Bereavement Period of grief following the death of a loved one.

Bias Mental inclination or leaning.

Bioavailability Readiness to produce a drug effect.

Bioethics Application of general ethical principles to health care.

Biofeedback Measurement of physiological responses that yields information about the relationship between the mind and body and helps clients learn the way to manipulate these responses through mental activity.

Biologic Response Modifier Agent that destroys malignant cells by stimulating the body's immune system.

Biological Agent Living organism that invades a host, causing disease.

Biological Clock Internal mechanism capable of measuring time in a living organism.

Biopsy Excision of a small amount of tissue.

Body Image Individual's perception of physical self, including appearance, function, and ability.

Body Mass Index Measurement used to ascertain whether a person's weight is appropriate for height; calculated by dividing the weight in kilograms by the height in meters squared.

Body Mechanics Use of the body to move or lift objects.

Bodymind Inseparable connection and operation of thoughts, feelings, and physiological functions.

Bonding Rapid process of attachment, parent to infant, that takes place during the sensitive period, the first 30 to 60 minutes after birth.

Borborygmi High-pitched, loud, rushing sounds produced by the movement of gas in the liquid contents of the intestine.

Bradycardia Heart rate less than 60 beats per minute in an adult.

Bradykinesia Slowness of voluntary movement and speech.

Bradypnea Respiratory rate of 10 or fewer breaths per minute.

Breakthrough Pain Sudden, acute, temporary pain that is usually precipitated by a treatment, a procedure, or unusual activity of the client.

Bronchial Sound Loud, tubular, hollow-sounding breath-sound normally heard over the sternum.

Bronchovesicular Sound Breath sound normally heard in the area of the scapula and near the sternum; medium in pitch and intensity, with inspiratory and expiratory phases of equal length.

Bruxism Grinding of teeth during sleep.

Buffer Substance that attempts to maintain pH range, or hydrogen ion concentration, in the presence of added acids or bases.

Bulimia Nervosa Psychiatric disorder characterized by episodic binge-eating followed by purging.

Burnout State of physical and emotional exhaustion that occurs when caregivers deplete their adaptive energy.

Butterfly Needle Wing-tipped needle.

Calorie Amount of heat required to raise the temperature of 1 gram of water 1 degree Celsius.

Capitated Rate Preset fee based on membership rather than services provided; payment system used in managed care.

Carrier Person who harbors an infectious agent but has no symptoms of disease.

Catabolism Destructive process of metabolism whereby tissues or substances are broken into their component parts.

Cataplexy Sudden loss of muscle control.

Categorical Imperative Concept that states that one should act only if the action is based on a principle that is universal.

Catharsis Process of talking out one's feelings; "getting things off the chest" through verbalization.

Cation Ion bearing a positive charge.

Ceiling Effect Medication dosage beyond which no further analgesia occurs.

Centering Process of bringing oneself to an inward focus of serenity; done before beginning an energetic touch therapy treatment.

Central Line Venous catheter inserted into the superior vena cava through the subclavian or internal or external jugular vein.

Certification Voluntary process that establishes and evaluates standards of care; mandatory for any health care services receiving federal funds.

Chain of Infection Phenomenon of the development of an infectious process.

Change Dynamic process whereby an individual's response to a stressor leads to an alteration in behavior.

Change Agent Person who intentionally creates and implements change.

Charting by Exception Documentation method that requires the nurse to document only deviations from preestablished norms.

Chemical Agent Substance that interacts with a host, causing disease.

Chemical Name Precise description of the drug's composition (chemical formula).

Chemical Restraint Medication used to control client behavior.

Cheyne-Stokes Respirations Breathing characterized by periods of apnea alternating with periods of dyspnea.

Cholesterol Sterol produced by the body and used in the synthesis of steroid hormones.

Chronic Acute Pain Discomfort that occurs almost daily over a long period, has the potential for lasting months or years, and has a high probability of ending; also known as progressive pain.

Chronic Nonmalignant Pain Discomfort that occurs almost daily, has been present for a least 6 months, and ranges in intensity from mild to severe; also known as chronic benign pain.

Chronic Pain Discomfort generally identified as long term (lasting 6 months or longer) that is persistent, nearly constant, or recurrent, and that produces significant negative changes in a person's life.

Chronobiology Science of studying biorhythms.

Chyme Acidic, semi-fluid paste found in the gastrointestinal tract.

Circadian Rhythm Biorhythm that cycles on a daily basis.

Civil Law Law that deals with relationships between individuals.

Clean Object Object on which there are microorganisms that are usually not pathogenic.

Cleansing Removal of soil or organic material from instruments and equipment used in providing client care.

Client Advocate Person who speaks up for or acts on behalf of the client.

Client Behavior Accident Mishap resulting from the client's behavior or actions.

Clinical Observing and caring for living clients.

Coarse Crackle Moist, low-pitched crackling and gurgling lung sound of long duration.

Cognitive Domain Area of learning that involves intellectual understanding.

Cognitive Reframing Stress management technique whereby the individual changes a negative perception of a situation or event to a more positive, less threatening perception.

Colic Condition of acute abdominal pain.

Colonization Multiplication of microorganisms on or within a host that does not result in cellular injury.

Communicable Agent Infectious agent transmitted to a client by direct or indirect contact, via vehicle, vector, or airborne route.

Communicable Disease Disease caused by a communicable agent.

Communication The sending and receiving of a message.

Comorbidity Simultaneous existence of more than one disease process within an individual.

Competency Specific skill or task needed for a particular position.

Complementary Therapy Therapy used in conjunction with conventional medical therapies.

Complete Protein Protein containing all nine essential amino acids.

Complicated Grief Grief associated with traumatic death such as death by homicide, violence, or accident; survivors suffer emotions of greater intensity than those associated with normal grief.

Compound Combination of atoms of two or more elements.

Comprehensive Assessment Type of assessment that provides baseline client data, including a complete health history and current needs assessment.

Compromised Host Person whose normal defense mechanisms are impaired and who is therefore susceptible to infection.

Computed Tomography Radiological scanning of the body with x-ray beams and radiation detectors to transmit data to a computer that transcribes the data into quantitative measurement and multidimensional images of the internal structures.

Concept Mental picture of abstract phenomena that serves to organize observations related to those phenomena.

Conditioning Teaching a person a behavior until it becomes an automatic response; method of conserving adaptive energy.

Confidential Private or secret.

Confidentiality Nondisclosure of the identity of or personal information about an individual.

Congruence Agreement between two things.

Conscious Sedation Minimally depressed level of consciousness during which the client retains the ability to maintain a continuously patent airway and to respond appropriately to physical stimulation or verbal commands.

Consciousness State of awareness of self, others, and surrounding environment.

Constitutional Law Law that defines and limits the power of government.

Contact Precautions Measures taken in addition to Standard Precautions for clients known to have or suspected of having illnesses easily spread by direct client contact or by contact with fomites.

Contact Transmission Physical transfer of an agent from an infected person to a host through direct contact with that person, indirect contact with an infected person through a fomite, or close contact with contaminated secretions.

Contract Law Enforcement of agreements among private individuals.

Contrast Medium Radiopaque substance that facilitates roentgen (x-ray) imaging of the body's internal structures.

Convalescent Stage Time period in which acute symptoms of an infection begin to disappear until the client returns to the previous state of health.

Crackle Abnormal breath sound that resembles a popping sound, heard on inhalation and exhalation; not cleared by coughing.

Crenation Condition wherein cells decrease in size, shrivel and wrinkle, and are no longer functional when in a hypertonic solution.

Criminal Law Law concerning acts of offense against the welfare or safety of the public.

Crisis Acute state of disorganization that occurs when the individual's usual coping mechanisms are no longer effective. Stressor that forces an individual to respond and/or adapt in some way.

Crisis Intervention Specific technique used to assist clients in regaining equilibrium.

Critical Pathway Comprehensive, standard plan of care for a specific case situation.

Critical Period Time of the most rapid growth or development in a particular stage of the life cycle during which an individual is most vulnerable to stressors of any type.

Critical Thinking Mode of thinking—about any subject, content, or problem—whereby the thinker improves the quality of his or her thinking by skillfully taking charge of the structures inherent in thinking and imposing intellectual standards (or a level of degree of quality) upon them.

Cultural Assimilation Process whereby individuals from a minority group are absorbed by the dominant culture and take on the characteristics of the dominant culture.

Cultural Diversity Differences among people that result from racial, ethnic, and cultural variables.

Culture Dynamic and integrated structures of knowledge, beliefs, behaviors, ideas, attitudes, values, habits, customs, languages, symbols, rituals, ceremonies, and practices that are unique to a particular group of people. Growing of microorganisms to identify a pathogen.

Curing Ridding one of disease.

Cutaneous Pain Discomfort caused by stimulation of the cutaneous nerve endings in the skin.

Cyanosis Bluish discoloration of the skin and mucous membranes observed in lips, nail beds, and earlobes.

Cytology Study of cells.

Data Clustering Process of putting data together in order to identify areas of the client's problems and strengths.

Death Rattle Breathing sound in the period preceding death caused by a collection of secretions in the larynx.

Decomposition Chemical reaction wherein the bonding between atoms in a molecule is broken and simpler products are formed.

Defamation Use of words to harm or injure the personal or professional reputation of another person.

Defense Mechanism Unconscious operation that protects the mind from anxiety.

Defining Characteristics Collected data; also known as signs and symptoms, subjective and objective data, or clinical manifestations.

Deglutition Swallowing of food.

Dehiscence Complication of wound healing wherein the wound edges separate.

Dehydration Condition wherein more water is lost from the body than is being replaced.

Delegation Process of transferring to a competent individual the authority to perform a selected task.

Delirium Cognitive changes or acute confusion of rapid onset (less than 6 months).

Dementia Organic brain pathology characterized by losses in intellectual functioning and a slow onset (longer than 6 months).

Democratic Leadership style in which all members have input in decision making.

Dental Caries Cavities.

Deontology Ethical theory that considers the intrinsic significance of an act as the criterion for determination of good.

Dependent Nursing Intervention Nursing action that requires an order from a physician or other health care professional.

Depersonalization Treating an individual as an object rather than as a person.

Development Behavioral changes in functional abilities and skills.

Developmental Tasks Certain goals that must be achieved during each developmental stage of the life cycle.

Dialysis Mechanical means of removing nitrogenous waste from the blood by imitating the function of the nephrons; involves filtration and diffusion of wastes, drugs, and excess electrolytes and/or osmosis of water across a semipermeable membrane into a dialysate solution.

Didactic Systematic presentation of information.

Diet Therapy Treating a disease or disorder with a special diet.

Dietary Prescription/Order Order written by the physician for food, including liquids.

Diffusion Process whereby a substance moves from an area of higher concentration to an area of lower concentration.

Dirty Object Object on which there is a high number of microorganisms, some that are potentially pathogenic.

Discharge Planning Planning that involves critical anticipation and planning for the client's needs after discharge.

Discipline Branch of learning, field of study, or occupation requiring specialized knowledge.

Disciplined Trained by instruction and exercise.

Disenfranchised Grief "Grief that is not openly acknowledged, socially sanctioned, or publicly shared" (Doka, Rushton, & Thorstenson, 1994).

Disinfectant Chemical solution used to clean inanimate objects.

Disinfection Elimination of pathogens, with the exception of spores, from inanimate objects.

Distraction Technique of focusing attention on stimuli other than pain.

Distress Subjective experience that occurs when stressors evoke an ineffective response.

Distribution Movement of drugs from the blood into various body fluids and tissues.

Documentation Written evidence of: the interactions between and among health care professionals, clients and their families, and health care organizations; the administration of tests, procedures, treatments, and client education; and the result of or client's response to diagnostic tests and interventions.

Dominant Culture Group whose values prevail within a society.

Down Syndrome Congenital chromosomal abnormality; also called trisomy 21.

Droplet Precautions Measures taken in addition to Standard Precautions for clients known to have or suspected of having serious illnesses spread by large particle droplets.

Drug Allergy Hypersensitivity to a drug.

Drug Incompatibility Undesired chemical or physical reaction between a drug and a solution, between two drugs, or between a drug and the container or tubing.

Drug Interaction Effect one drug can have on another drug.

Drug Tolerance Reaction that occurs when the body becomes accustomed to a specific drug and requires larger doses of the drug to produce the desired therapeutic effects.

Durable Power of Attorney for Health Care Legal document designating who may make health care decisions for a client when that client is no longer capable of decision making.

Dysarthria Difficult and defective speech due to a dysfunction of the muscles used for speech.

Dysfunctional Grief Persistent pattern of intense grief that does not result in reconciliation of feelings.

Dysphasia Impairment of speech resulting from damage to the speech center in the brain.

Dyspnea Difficulty breathing as observed by labored or forced respirations through the use of accessory muscles in the chest and neck.

Edema Detectable accumulation of increased interstitial fluid.

Efferent Nerve (Pain) Pathway Descending spinal cord pathway that transmits sensory impulses from the brain.

Electrocardiogram Graphic recording of the heart's electrical activity.

Electroencephalogram Graphic recording of the brain's electrical activity.

Electrolyte Element or compound that, when dissolved in water or another solvent, dissociates (separates) into ions (electrically charged particles).

Element Basic substance of matter.

Embryonic Stage Developmental stage that occurs during the first 2–8 weeks after fertilization of a human egg.

Empathy Capacity to understand another person's feelings or perception of a situation.

Empowerment Process of enabling others to do for themselves.

Empty Calories Calories that provide few nutrients.

Encephalitis Inflammation of the brain.

Encoding Laying down tracks in areas of the brain to enhance the ability to recall and utilize information.

Endemic Occurring continuously in a particular population and having low mortality.

Endorphins Group of opiate-like substances produced naturally by the brain which raise the pain threshold, produce sedation and euphoria, and promote a sense of well-being.

Endoscopy Visualization of a body organ or cavity through a scope.

Energetic-Touch Therapy Technique of using the hands to direct or redirect the flow of the body's energy fields and thus enhance balance within those fields.

Enriched Descriptor for food in which nutrients that were removed during processing are added back in.

Enteral Instillation Administration of drugs through a gastrointestinal tube.

Enteral Nutrition Feeding method meaning both the ingestion of food orally and the delivery of nutrients through a gastrointestinal tube, but generally meaning the latter.

Epidemic Infecting many people at the same time and in the same geographic area.

Epidural Analgesia Analgesics administered via a catheter that terminates in the epidural space.

Equipment Accident Accident resulting from the malfunction or improper use of medical equipment.

Erythema Redness of the skin that may be caused by inflammation of tissues or by sunburn.

Ethical Dilemma Situation wherein there is a conflict between two or more ethical principles.

Ethical Principle Widely accepted code, generally based on the humane aspects of society, that directs or governs actions.

Ethical Reasoning Process of thinking through what one ought to do in an orderly, systematic manner based on principles.

Ethics Branch of philosophy concerned with determining right from wrong on the basis of a body of knowledge.

Ethnicity Cultural group's perception of itself or a group identity.

Ethnocentrism Assumption of cultural superiority and an inability to accept other cultures' ways of organizing reality.

Etiology Related cause of or contributor to a problem.

Euglycemia Normal blood glucose level.

Eupnea Easy respirations with a rate of breaths per minute that is age-appropriate.

Eustress Stress that results in positive outcomes.

Euthanasia Intentional action or lack of action that causes the merciful death of someone suffering from a terminal illness or incurable condition; derived from the Greek word *euthanatos,* which literally means "good or gentle death."

Evaluation Fifth step in the nursing process; involves determining whether client goals have been met, partially met, or not met.

Evisceration Complication of wound healing characterized by a complete separation of wound edges accompanied by visceral protrusion.

Exclusive Provider Organization Organization wherein care must be delivered by the plan in order for clients to receive reimbursement for health care services.

Excretion Elimination of drugs or waste products from the body.

Exophthalmos Marked protrusion of the eyeballs resulting from increased orbital fluid behind the eyeballs.

Expected Outcome Detailed, specific statement that describes the methods through which a goal will be achieved and that includes aspects such as direct nursing care, client teaching, and continuity of care.

Expressed Contract Conditions and terms of a contract given in writing by the concerned parties.

Extracellular Fluid Fluid outside of the cells; includes interstitial, intravascular, synovial, cerebrospinal, and serous fluids; aqueous and vitreous humor; and endolymph and perilymph.

False Imprisonment Situation wherein a person is made to wrongfully believe that he cannot leave a place.

Fat-Soluble Vitamin Vitamin requiring the presence of fats for its absorption from the gastrointestinal tract into the lymphatic system and for cellular metabolism: vitamins A, D, E, and K.

Fee for Service System in which the health care recipient directly pays the provider for services as they are provided.

Feedback Response from the receiver of a message so that the sender can verify the message.

Felony Crime of a serious nature that is usually punishable by imprisonment in a state penitentiary or by death.

Fetal Alcohol Syndrome Condition wherein fetal development is impaired by maternal consumption of alcohol.

Fetal Stage Intrauterine developmental period from 8 weeks to birth.

Fidelity Ethical concept based on faithfulness and keeping promises.

Fight-or-Flight Response State wherein the body becomes physiologically ready to defend itself by either fighting or running away from the danger.

Filtration Process of fluids and the substances dissolved in them being forced through the cell membrane by hydrostatic pressure.

Flashback Rushing of blood back into intravenous tubing when a negative pressure is created on the tubing. Reliving of an original trauma as if the individual were currently experiencing it.

Flora Microorganisms which occur or have adapted to live in a specific environment, such as intestinal, skin, vaginal, or oral flora.

Flow Rate Volume of fluid to infuse over a set period of time.

Fluoroscopy Immediate, serial images of the body's structure or function.

Focus Charting Documentation method using a column format to chart data, actions, and responses.

Focused Assessment Type of assessment that is limited in scope in order to focus on a particular need or health care problem or on potential health care risks.

Fomite Object contaminated with an infectious agent.

Formal Contract Written contract that cannot be changed legally by an oral agreement.

Formal Teaching Teaching that takes place at a specific time, in a specific place, and on a specific topic.

Fortified Descriptor for food in which nutrients not naturally occurring in the food are added to it.

Fracture Break in the continuity of a bone.

Fraud Wrong that results from a deliberate deception intended to produce unlawful gain.

Free Radical Unstable molecule that alters genetic codes and triggers the development of cancer growth in cells.

Gate Control Pain Theory Theory that proposes that the cognitive, sensory, emotional, and physiologic components of the body can act together to block an individual's perception of pain.

General Adaptation Syndrome Physiologic response that occurs when a person experiences a stressor.

Generic Name Name assigned by the U.S. Adopted Names Council to the manufacturer who first develops a drug.

Genogram A method of visualizing family members, their birth and death dates or ages, and specific health problems.

Genuineness Sincerity.

Germicide Chemical that can be applied to both animate and inanimate objects for the purpose of eliminating pathogens.

Germinal Stage Developmental stage that begins with conception and lasts approximately 10 to 14 days.

Gerontological Nursing Specialty within nursing that addresses and advocates for the special care needs of older adults.

Gerontologist Specialist in gerontology in advanced practice nursing, geriatric psychiatry, medicine, and social services.

Gerontology Study of the effects of normal aging and age-related diseases on human beings.

Gingivitis Inflammation of the gums.

Gluconeogenesis Conversion of amino acids into glucose.

Glycogenesis Conversion of glucose into glycogen.

Glycogenolysis Conversion of glycogen into glucose.

Goal Objective that outlines the desired resolution of the nursing diagnosis over a longer period of time, usually weeks or months.

Good Samaritan Law Law that provides protection to health care providers by assuring them of immunity from civil liability when care is provided at the scene of an emergency and the caregiver does not intentionally or recklessly cause the client injury.

Grief Series of intense physical and psychological responses that occurs following a loss; a normal, natural, necessary, and adaptive response to a loss.

Grief Work Process whereby the bereaved experiences freedom from attachment to the deceased, becomes reoriented to the environment where the deceased is no longer present, and establishes new relationships.

Growth Quantitative (measurable) changes in the physical size of the body and its parts.

Half-life Time it takes the body to eliminate half of the blood concentration level of the original dose of medication.

Halitosis Bad breath.

Handwashing Rubbing together of all surfaces and crevices of the hands using a soap or chemical and water, followed by rinsing in a flowing stream of water.

Haustra Sac-like pouches of the colon.

Healing Process that activates the individual's recovery forces from within.

Healing Touch Energy-based therapeutic modality that alters the energy fields through the use of touch, thereby affecting physical, mental, emotional, and spiritual health.

Health According to the World Health Organization, the state of complete physical, mental, and social well-being, not merely the absence of disease or infirmity.

Health Care Delivery System Mechanism for providing services that meet the health-related needs of individuals.

Health Care Financing Administration Federal agency in charge of administering the Medicare program.

Health Care Surrogate Law Law enacted by some states that provides a legal means for decision making in the absence of advance directives.

Health Continuum Range of an individual's health, from highest health potential to death.

Health History Review of the client's functional health patterns prior to the current contact with a health care agency.

Health Maintenance Organization Prepaid health plan that provides primary health care services for a preset fee and focuses on cost-effective treatment methods.

Hearing Act or power of receiving sounds.

Hematuria Blood in the urine.

Hemolysis Breakdown of red blood cells and the release of hemoglobin.

History Study of the past, including events, situations, and individuals.

Holistic Whole; includes physical, intellectual, sociocultural, psychological, and spiritual aspects as an integrated whole.

Homeostasis Balance or equilibrium among the physiologic, psychological, sociocultural, intellectual, and spiritual needs of the body.

Hospice Humane, compassionate care provided to clients who can no longer benefit from curative treatment, and have 6 months or less to live.

Host Simple or complex organism that can be affected by an agent.

Human Immunodeficiency Virus (HIV) Retrovirus that causes AIDS.

Humoral Immunity Type of immunity dominated by antibodies.

Hydrostatic Pressure Pressure that a fluid exerts against a membrane; also called filtration force.

Hygiene Science of health.

Hypergylcemia Condition wherein the blood glucose level becomes too high as a result of the absence of insulin.

Hypersomnia Alteration in sleep pattern characterized by excessive sleep, especially in the daytime.

Hypertonic Solution Solution that has a higher molecular concentration than the cell; also called a hyperosmolar solution.

Hyperventilation Breathing characterized by deep, rapid respirations.

Hypervolemia Increased circulating fluid volume.

Hypnosis Altered state of consciousness or awareness resembling sleep and during which a person is more receptive to suggestion.

Hypoglycemia Condition wherein the blood glucose level is exceedingly low.

Hypotonic Solution Solution that has a lower molecular concentration than the cell; also called hypo-osmolar solution.

Hypoventilation Breathing characterized by shallow respirations.

Hypovolemia Abnormally low circulatory blood volume.

Hypoxemia Decreased oxygen level in the blood.

Idiosyncratic Reaction Highly unpredictable response that may be manifested by an overresponse, an underresponse, or an atypical response.

Illness Stage Time period when the client is manifesting specific signs and symptoms of an infectious agent.

Imagery Relaxation technique of using the imagination to visualize a pleasant, soothing image.

Immunization Process of creating immunity or resistance to infection in an individual.

Impaired Nurse Nurse who is habitually intemperate or is addicted to the use of alcohol or habit-forming drugs.

Implantable Port Device made of a radiopague silicone catheter and a plastic or stainless steel injection port with a self-sealing silicone-rubber septum.

Implementation Fourth step in the nursing process; involves the execution of the nursing plan of care formulated during the planning phase.

Implied Contract Contract that recognizes a relationship between parties for services.

Incident Report Risk-management tool used to describe and report any unusual event that occurs to a client, visitor, or staff member.

Incomplete Protein Protein with one or more of the essential amino acids missing.

Incubation Period Time interval between the entry of an infectious agent in the host and the onset of symptoms.

Independent Nursing Intervention Nursing action initiated by the nurse that does not require direction or an order from another health care professional.

Infancy Developmental stage from the end of the first month to the end of the first year of life.

Infection Invasion and multiplication of pathogenic microorganisms in body tissue that results in cellular injury.

Infectious Agent Microorganism that causes infection.

Infiltration Seepage of foreign substances into the interstitial tissue, causing swelling and discomfort at the IV site.

Inflammation Nonspecific cellular response to tissue injury.

Informal Teaching Teaching that takes place any time, any place, and whenever a learning need is identified.

Informed Consent Legal form signed by a competent client and witnessed by another person that grants permission to the client's physician to perform the procedure described by the physician and that demonstrates the client's understanding of the benefits, risks, and possible complications of the procedure, as well as alternate treatment options.

Ingestion The taking of food into the digestive tract, generally through the mouth.

Initial Planning Development of a preliminary plan of care by the nurse who performs the admission assessment and gathers the comprehensive admission assessment data.

Insomnia Difficulty in falling asleep initially or in returning to sleep once awakened.

Inspection Physical examination technique that involves thorough visual observation.

Instrument of Healing Means by which healing can be achieved, performed, or enhanced.

Insulin Pancreatic hormone that aids in both the diffusion of glucose into the liver and muscle cells, and the synthesis of glycogen.

Intellectual Wellness Ability to function as an independent person capable of making sound decisions.

Interdependent Nursing Intervention Nursing action that is implemented in a collaborative manner with other health care professionals.

Interstitial Fluid Fluid in tissue spaces around each cell.

Intracath Plastic tube for insertion into a vein.

Intracellular Fluid Fluid within the cells.

Intradermal Injection into the dermis.

Intramuscular Injection into the muscle.

Intrapsychic Theory Developmental approach based on an individual's unconscious processes.

Intrathecal Analgesia Administration of analgesics into the subarachnoid space.

Intravascular Fluid Fluid consisting of the plasma in the blood vessels and the lymph in the lymphatic system.

Intravenous Injection into a vein.

Intravenous Therapy Administration of fluids, electrolytes, nutrients, or medications by the venous route.

Invasive Accessing the body tissues, organs, or cavities through some type of instrumentation procedure.

Ion Atom bearing an electrical charge.

Ischemic Pain Discomfort resulting when the blood supply of an area is restricted or cut off completely.

Isolation Separate from other persons, especially those with infectious diseases.

Isotonic Solution Solution that has the same molecular concentration as does the cell; also called an isosmolar solution.

Isotope Atom of the same element that has a different atomic weight (i.e., different numbers of neutrons in the nucleus).

IV Push (bolus) Method of administering a large dose of medication in a relatively short time, usually 1–30 minutes.

Jet Lag Time required for the biological clock to adjust to a new time.

Job Description Written outline of job responsibilities.

Judgment Ability to evaluate alternatives to arrive at an appropriate course of action.

Justice Ethical principle based on the concept of fairness extended to each individual.

Justify To prove or show to be valid.

Kardex Summary worksheet reference of basic client care information.

Ketosis Condition wherein acids called ketones accumulate in the blood and urine, upsetting the acid–base balance.

Kilocalorie Equivalent to 1,000 calories.

Kinesthetic Learner Person who learns by processing information through touching, feeling, and doing.

Laissez-faire Leadership style that is passive and nondirect.

Law That which is laid down or fixed.

Leadership Ability to direct or motivate others to achieve goals.

Learning Act or process of acquiring knowledge and/or skill in a particular subject; assimilation of information with a resultant change in behavior.

Learning Plateau Peak in the effectiveness of teaching and depth of learning.

Learning Style Individual preference for receiving, processing, and assimilating information about a particular subject.

Leukocytosis Increased number of white blood cells.

Leukopenia Decreased number of white blood cells.

Liability Obligation one has incurred or might incur through any act or failure to act.

Libel Written words that harm or injure the personal or professional reputation of another person.

Licensure Mandatory system of granting licenses according to specified standards.

Life Review Form of reminiscence wherein a client attempts either to come to terms with conflict or to gain meaning from life and die peacefully.

Lipid Organic compound that is insoluble in water but soluble in organic solvents such as ether and alcohol; also known as fats.

Lipoprotein Blood lipid bound to protein.

Listening Interpreting the sounds heard and attaching meaning to them.

Liver Mortis Bluish-purple discoloration of the skin, usually at pressure points, that is a by-product of red blood cell destruction.

Living Will Legal document that allows a person to state preferences about the use of life-sustaining measures should she be unable to make her wishes known.

Local Adaptation Syndrome Physiologic response to a stressor (e.g., trauma, illness) affecting a specific part of the body.

Localized Infection Infection limited to a defined area or single organ.

Logic Formal principles of a branch of knowledge (such as nursing).

Long-Term Care Facility Health care facility that provides services to individuals who are not acutely ill, have continuing health care needs, and cannot function independently at home.

Long-Term Goal Statement written in objective format and demonstrating an expectation to be achieved in resolution of the nursing diagnosis over a long period of time, usually weeks or months.

Loss Any situation, either actual, potential, or perceived, wherein a valued object or person is changed or is no longer accessible to the individual.

Lumbar Puncture Aspiration of cerebrospinal fluid from the subarachnoid space.

Lymphokine Chemical substance released by sensitized lymphocytes (T cells) that assists in antigen destruction.

Magnetic Resonance Imaging Imaging technique that uses radiowaves and a strong magnetic field to make continuous cross-sectional images of the body.

Maladaptive Measure Measure used to avoid conflict or stress.

Malpractice Negligent acts on the part of a professional; relates to the conduct of a person who is acting in a professional capacity.

Managed Care System of providing and monitoring care wherein access, cost, and quality are controlled before or during delivery of services.

Management Accomplishment of tasks through the effective use of people and resources.

Maslow's Hierarchy of Needs Theory of behavioral motivation based on needs; includes physiologic, safety and security, love and belonging, self-esteem, and self-actualization needs.

Mastication Chewing food into fine particles and mixing the food with enzymes in saliva.

Material Principle of Justice Rationale for determining those times when there can be unequal allocation of scarce resources.

Matter Anything that occupies space and possesses mass.

Maturation Process of becoming fully grown and developed; involves physiologic and behavioral aspects.

Maturational Loss Loss that occurs as a result of moving from one developmental stage to another.

Medicaid Government title program (XIX) that pays for health services for the aged, poor, disabled, and low-income families with dependent children.

Medical Asepsis Practices that reduce the number, growth, and spread of microorganisms.

Medical Diagnosis Clinical judgment by the physician that identifies or determines a specific disease, condition, or pathological state.

Medical Model Traditional approach to health care wherein the focus is on treatment and cure of disease.

Medicare Amendment (Title XVIII) to the Social Security Act that helps finace the health care of persons over 65 years old and for permanently disabled younger persons who receive Social Security disability benefits.

Medigap Insurance Insurance plan for persons with Medicare that pays for health care costs not covered by Medicare.

Meditation Quieting of the mind by focusing the attention.

Menarche Onset of the first menstrual period.

Metabolic Rate Rate of energy utilization in the body.

Metabolism Sum total of all the biological and chemical processes in the body.

Metacognition Process of examining the way we think.

Middle Adulthood Developmental stage from the ages of 40 years to 65 years.

Minority Group Group of people that constitute less than a numerical majority of the population and who, because of their cultural, racial, ethnic, religious, or other characteristics, are often labeled and treated differently from others in the society.

Misdemeanor Offense that is less serious than a felony and may be punished by a fine or by sentence to a local prison for less than 1 year.

Mixed Agonist-Antagonist Compound that blocks opioid effects on one receptor type while producing opioid effects on a second receptor type.

Mixture Substances combined in no specific way.

Mnemonic Method to aid in association and recall; a memorable sentence created from the first letters of a list of items to be used to recall the items later.

Mode of Transmission Process that bridges the gap between the portal of exit of the infectious agent from the reservoir or source, and the portal of entry of the susceptible "new" host.

Modulation Central nervous system pathway that selectively inhibits pain transmission by sending signals back down to the dorsal horn of the spinal cord.

Molecule Atoms of the same element that unite with each other.

Monounsaturated Fatty Acid forms a glycerol ester with a double or triple bond; nuts, fowl, and olive oil.

Moral Maturity Ability to decide for oneself what is "right."

Morbidity Illness.

Mortality Death.

Mortuary Funeral home.

Mourning Period of time during which grief is expressed and resolution and integration of the loss occur.

Myofascial Pain Syndrome Group of muscle disorders characterized by pain, muscle spasm, tenderness, stiffness, and limited motion.

Narcolepsy Sleep alteration manifested as sudden uncontrollable urges to fall asleep during the daytime.

Narrative Charting Story format of documentation that describes the client's status, the interventions and treatments, and the client's response to treatments.

Necrosis Tissue death as the result of disease or injury.

Neglect Situation wherein a basic need of the client is not being provided.

Negligence General term referring to careless acts on the part of an individual who is not exercising reasonable or prudent judgement.

Neonatal Period First 28 days of life following birth.

Neuralgia Paroxysmal pain that extends along the course of one or more nerves.

Neuropeptide Amino acid produced in the brain and other sites in the body that acts as a chemical communicator.

Neurotransmitter Chemical substance produced by the body that facilitates nerve-impulse transmission.

Nociceptor Receptive neuron for painful sensations.

Noninvasive Descriptor for procedure wherein the body is *not* entered with any type of instrument.

Nonmaleficence Ethical principle based on the obligation to cause no harm to others.

Nonverbal Communication Sending a message without words; sometimes called body language.

Nosocomial Infection Infection that is acquired in the hospital or other health care facility and was not present or incubating at the time of the client's admission.

Noxious Stimulus Underlying pathology that causes pain.

Nursing An art and a science that assists individuals to learn to care for themselves whenever possible; also involves caring for others when they are unable to meet their own needs.

Nursing Audit Process of collecting and analyzing data to evaluate the effectiveness of nursing interventions.

Nursing Care Plan Written guide that organizes data about a client's care into a formal statement of the strategies that will be implemented to help the client achieve optimal health.

Nursing Diagnosis Second step in the nursing process; a clinical judgement about individual, family, or community (aggregate) responses to actual or potential health problems/life processes.

Nursing Intervention Action performed by a nurse that helps the client achieve the results specified by the goals and expected outcomes.

Nursing Intervention Classification Standardized language for nursing interventions.

Nursing Minimum Data Set Elements contained in clinical records and abstracted for studies on the effectiveness and costs of nursing care.

Nursing Outcomes Classification Standardized language for nursing outcomes.

Nursing Practice Act Statute that is enacted by the legislature of a state and that outlines the scope of nursing practice in that state.

Nursing Process Systematic method of providing care to clients, consisting of five steps: assessment, diagnosis, outcome identification and planning, implementation, and evaluation.

Nutrition All of the processes (ingestion, digestion, absorption, metabolism, and elimination) involved in consuming and utilizing food for energy, maintenance, and growth.

Obesity Weight that is 20% or more above the ideal body weight.

Objective Data Observable and measurable data that are obtained through standard assessment techniques performed during the physical examination and through laboratory and diagnostic tests.

Occult Blood Blood in the stool that can be detected only through a microscope or by chemical means.

Older Adulthood Developmental stage occurring from the age of 65 years until death.

Oliguria Diminished production of urine.

Omnibus Budget Reconciliation Act Federal law first enacted in 1989 to provide for rights and clinical guidelines to ensure quality health services for older Americans.

Oncology Study of tumors.

Ongoing Assessment Type of assessment that includes systematic monitoring and observation related to specific problems.

Ongoing Planning Continuous updating of the client's plan of care.

Onset of Action Time it takes the body to respond to a drug after administration.

Opinion Subjective belief.

Oppression Condition wherein the rules, modes, and ideals of one group are imposed on another group.

Orthophea Difficulty breathing while lying down.

Orthostatic Significant decrease in blood pressure that results when a person moves from a lying or sitting (supine) position to a standing position.

Osmolality Measurement of the total concentration of dissolved particles (solutes) per kilogram of water.

Osmolarity Concentration of solutes per liter of cellular fluid.

Osmosis Movement of a solvent, usually water, through a semipermeable membrane, from a region of higher concentration to a region of lower concentration.

Osmotic Pressure Pressure exerted against the cell membrane by the water inside a cell.

Oxidation Chemical process of combining with oxygen.

Oxidized Joined with oxygen.

Pain Unpleasant sensory and emotional experience associated with actual or potential tissue damage or described in terms of such.

Pain Threshold Level of intensity at which pain becomes appreciable or perceptible.

Pain Tolerance Level of intensity or duration of pain that a person is willing to endure.

Palliative Relief of symptoms, such as pain, without altering the course of disease.

Palliative Care Care that relieves symptoms, such as pain, but does not alter the course of disease.

Palpation Physical examination technique that uses the sense of touch to assess texture, temperature, moisture, organ location and size, vibrations and pulsations, swelling, masses, and tenderness.

Papanicolaou Test Smear method of examining stained exfoliative cells.

Paracentesis Aspiration of fluid from the abdominal cavity.

Parasomnia Condition characterized by profoundly disturbed sleep due to behavioral or physiologic events.

Parenteral Any route other than the oral-gastrointestinal tract.

Parenteral Nutrition Feeding method whereby nutrients bypass the small intestine and enter the blood directly.

Passive Euthanasia Process of cooperating with the client's dying process.

Patency Being freely opened.

Pathogen Microorganism that causes disease.

Pathogenicity Ability of a microorganism to produce disease.

Patient-Controlled Analgesia Device that allows the client to control the delivery of intravenous or subcutaneous pain medication in a safe, effective manner through a programmable pump.

Peak Plasma Level Highest blood concentration of a single dose of a drug until the elimination rate equals the rate of absorption.

Peer Assistance Program Rehabilitation program that provides an impaired nurse with referrals, professional and peer counseling support groups, and assistance and monitoring back into nursing.

Perception Ability to experience, recognize, organize, and interpret sensory stimuli.

Percussion Physical examination technique that uses short, tapping strokes on the surface of the skin to create vibrations of underlying organs.

Perfectionism Overwhelming expectation of being able to get everything done.

Perineal Care Cleansing of the external genitalia and perineum and the surrounding area.

Peristalsis Coordinated, rhythmic, serial contraction of the smooth muscles of the gastrointestinal tract.

Permeability Ability of a membrane to permit substances to pass through it.

Phantom Limb Pain Neuropathic pain that occurs after amputation with pain sensations referred to an area in the missing portion of the limb.

Pharmacokinetics Study of the absorption, distribution, metabolism, and excretion of drugs to determine the relationship between the dose of a drug and the drug's concentration in biological fluids.

Phlebitis Inflammation in the wall of a vein without clot formation.

Phlebotomist Individual who performs venipuncture.

Phlebotomy Removal of blood from a vein.

Phospholipid Lipid composed of glycerol, fatty acids, and phosphorus; the structural component of cells.

Physical Agent Factor in the environment capable of causing disease in a host.

Physical Restraint Equipment that reduces the client's movement.

Physical Wellness Healthy body that functions at an optimal level.

Phytochemical Physiologically active compound present in plants in very small amounts that gives plants flavor, odor, and color.

PIE Charting Documentation method using the problem, intervention, evaluation (PIE) format.

Piggyback Addition of an intravenous solution to infuse concurrently with another infusion.

Planning Third step of the nursing process; includes both the formulation of guidelines that establish the proposed course of nursing action in the resolution of nursing diagnoses and the development of the client's plan of care.

Plateau Level at which a drug's blood concentration is maintained.

Pleural Effusion Collection of fluid within the pleural cavity.

Pleural Friction Rub Abnormal breath sound that is creaky and grating in nature and is heard on inspiration and expiration.

Pneumothorax Condition wherein air or gas accumulates in the pleural space of the lungs, causing the lungs to collapse.

Point-of-Care Charting Documentation system that allows health care providers to gain immediate access to client information at the bedside.

Poison Any substance that when taken into the body interferes with normal physiologic functioning; may be inhaled, injected, ingested, or absorbed by the body.

Policy Written description of employer's expectations for handling various situations.

Polypharmacy Problem of clients taking numerous prescription and over-the-counter medications for the same or various disease processes, with unknown consequences from the resulting combinations of chemical compounds and cumulative side-effects.

Polyunsaturated Fatty Acid Forms a glycerol ester with many carbons unbanded to hydrogen atoms; fish, corn, sunflower seeds, soybeans, cotton seeds, and safflower oil.

Port-a-Cath Port that has been implanted under the skin with a catheter inserted into the superior vena cava or right atrium through the subclavian or internal jugular vein.

Portal of Entry Route by which an infectious agent enters the host.

Portal of Exit Route by which an infectious agent leaves the reservoir.

Post-mortem Care Care given immediately after death before the body is moved to the mortuary.

Postprandial After eating.

Preadolescence Developmental stage from the ages of approximately 10 years to 12 years.

Preferred Provider Organization Type of managed care model wherein member choice is limited to providers within the system.

Prenatal Period Developmental stage beginning with conception and ending with birth.

Presbycusis Sensorineural hearing loss associated with aging.

Preschool Period Developmental stage from the ages of 3 years to 6 years.

Prescriptive Authority Legal recognition of the ability to prescribe medications.

Prevention Hindering, obstructing, or thwarting a disease or illness.

Primary Care Care focused on promoting wellness and preventing illness or disability.

Primary Care Provider Health care provider whom a client sees first for health care, typically a family practitioner (physician/nurse), internist, or pediatrician.

Primary Health Care Client's point of entry into the health care system; includes assessment, diagnosis, treatment, coordination of care, education, prevention services, and surveillance.

Primary Prevention All practices designed to keep health problems from developing.

Primary Source Major provider of information about a client.

Privacy Includes the right to be left alone, to choose care based on personal beliefs, to govern body integrity, and to choose when and how sensitive information is shared (Badzek & Gross, 1999).

Problem-Oriented Medical Record Documentation method focusing on the client's problem and using a structured, logical format to narrative charting, called SOAP (subjective data, objective data, assessment, plan).

Procedure Step-by-step instruction describing the process for performing various nursing tasks.

Process Series of steps or acts that leads to the accomplishment of a goal or purpose.

Procrastination Intentionally putting off or delaying something that should be done.

Prodromal Stage Time interval from the onset of nonspecific symptoms until specific symptoms of the infectious process begin to manifest.

Professional Boundaries Limits of the professional relationship that allow for a safe, therapeutic connection between the professional and the client.

Progressive Muscle Relaxation Stress management strategy in which muscles are alternately tensed and relaxed.

Prospective Payment Predetermined rate paid for each episode of hospitalization based on the client's age and principle diagnosis and the presence or absence of surgery or comorbidity.

Protocol Series of standing orders or procedures that should be followed under certain specific conditions.

Proxemics Study of the space between people and its effect on interpersonal behavior.

Psychological Wellness Enjoyment of creativity, satisfaction of the basic need to love and be loved, understanding of emotions, and ability to maintain control over emotions.

Psychomotor Domain Area of learning that involves performance of motor skills.

Psychoneuroimmunology Study of the complex relationship among the cognitive, affective, and physical aspects of humans.

Puberty Emergence of secondary sex characteristics that signals the beginning of adolescence.

Public Law Law that deals with an individual's relationship to the state.

Purulent Exudate Discharge that occurs with severe inflammation accompanied by infection; also called pus.

Pulse Amplitude Measurement of the strength or force exerted by the ejected blood against the arterial wall with each contraction.

Pulse Deficit Condition in which the apical pulse rate is greater than the radial pulse rate.

Pulse Rate Indirect measurement of cardiac output obtained by counting the number of peripheral pulse waves over a pulse point.

Pulse Rhythm Regularity of the heart beat.

Pyorrhea Periodontal disease.

Race Grouping of people based on biological similarities such as physical characteristics.

Radiography Study of x-rays or gamma ray-exposed film through the action of ionizing radiation.

Rapport Bond or connection between two people that is based on mutual trust.

Readiness for Learning Evidence of willingness to learn.

Reasoning Use of the elements of thought to solve a problem or settle a question.

Recurrent Acute Pain Discomfort marked by repetitive painful episodes that may recur over a prolonged period or throughout a client's lifetime.

Referred Pain Discomfort from the internal organs that is felt in another area of the body.

Reflective Introspective.

Rehabilitation Process designed to assist individuals to reach their optimal level of physical, mental, and psychosocial functioning.

Religious Support System Group of ministers, priests, rabbis, nuns, or lay persons who are able to meet clients' spiritual needs in the health care setting.

Resident Flora Microorganisms that are always present, usually without altering the client's health.

Respite Care Care and service that provides a break to caregivers and is utilized for a few hours a week, for an occasional weekend, or for longer periods of time.

Rest State of relaxation and calmness, both mental and physical.

Restless Leg Syndrome Condition characterized by uncomfortable sensations of tingling or crawling in the muscles, and twitching, burning, prickling, or deep aching in the foot, calf, or upper leg when at rest (lying or sitting).

Restraint Protective device used to limit the physical activity of a client or to immobilize a client or extremity.

Résumé Tool that summarizes employment qualifications.

Resuscitation Support measures implemented to restore consciousness and life.

Reverse Isolation Barrier protection designed to prevent infection in clients who are severely compromised and highly susceptible to infection; also known as protective isolation.

Review of Systems Brief account of any recent signs or symptoms related to any body system.

Rigor Mortis Stiffening of the body that occurs 2 to 4 hours after death as a result of contraction of skeletal and smooth muscles.

Risk for Infection State wherein an individual is at increased risk for being invaded by pathogenic organisms.

Risk Nursing Diagnosis Nursing diagnosis indicating that a problem does not yet exist but that specific risk factors are present; composed of the diagnostic label followed by the phrase "Risk for" and a list of the specific risk factors.

Satiety Feeling of adequate fullness from food.

School-Age Period Developmental stage from the ages of 6 years to 10 years.

Sebum Oily substance secreted by the sebaceous glands of the skin.

Secondary Care Care focused on diagnosis and treatment after the client exhibits symptoms of illness.

Secondary Source Data source other than the client; can include family members, other health care providers, or medical records.

Sedation Reduction of stress, excitement, or irritability via some central nervous system depression.

Self-Awareness Consciously knowing how the self thinks, feels, believes, and behaves at any specific time.

Self-Care Deficit State wherein an individual is not able to perform one or more activities of daily living.

Self-Concept Individual's perception of self; includes self-esteem, body image, and ideal self.

Self-Efficacy Belief in one's ability to succeed in attempts to change behavior.

Semipermeable Membrane Membrane that allows passage of only certain substances.

Sensitivity Susceptibility of a pathogen to an antibiotic.

Sensory Overload State of excessive and sustained multisensory stimulation manifested by behavior change and perceptual distortion.

Shaman Folk healer-priest who uses natural and supernatural forces to help others.

Shamanism Practice of entering altered states of consciousness with the intent of helping others.

Short-Term Goal Objective that outlines the desired resolution of the nursing diagnosis over a short period of time, usually a few hours or days (less than a week).

Shroud Covering for the body after death.

Sibilant Wheeze Abnormal breath sound that is high pitched and musical in nature and is heard on inhalation and exhalation.

Single-Payer System Health care delivery model wherein the government is the only entity to reimburse.

Situational Loss Loss that occurs in response to external events that are usually beyond the individual's control.

Slander Words that are communicated verbally to a third party and that harm or injure the personal or professional reputation of another.

Sleep State of altered consciousness during which an individual experiences fluctuations in level of consciousness; minimal physical activity; and general slowing of the body's physiologic processes.

Sleep Apnea Syndrome wherein breathing periodically ceases during sleep for a period of 30–60 seconds; often associated with heavy snoring.

Sleep Cycle Sequence of sleep that begins with the four stages of no rapid eye movement (NREM) sleep in order, with a return to stage 3 and then stage 2, followed by passage into the first rapid eye movement (REM) stage.

Sleep Deprivation Prolonged inadequate quality and quantity of sleep.

Snellen Chart Chart containing various-sized letters with standardized numbers at the end of each line of letters.

Snoring Noisy breathing during sleep.

SOAP Charting Documentation method using subjective data, objective data, assessment, and plan.

Sociocultural Wellness Ability to appreciate the needs of others and to care about one's environment and the inhabitants of it.

Somatic Pain Nonlocalized discomfort originating in tendons, ligaments, and nerves.

Somnambulism Sleepwalking.

Sonorous Wheeze Abnormal breath sound that is low pitched and snoring in nature and is louder on expiration.

Source-Oriented Charting Narrative recording by each member (source) of the health care team on a separate record.

Specific Order Order written in a client's medical record or nursing care plan by a physician or nurse especially for that individual client; not used for any other client.

Spiritual Wellness Inner strength and peace.

Spiritual Care Recognition of spiritual needs and the assistance given toward meeting spiritual needs.

Spiritual Needs Individual's desire to find meaning and purpose in life, pain, and death.

Spirituality Relationships with one's self, with others, and with a higher power or divine source.

Spore Bacteria in a resistant stage that can withstand unfavorable environments.

Stable Alert with vital signs within the client's normal range.

Staff Development Delivery of instruction to assist the nurse in achieving the goals of the employer.

Standard Level or degree of quality.

Standard Precautions Preventive practices to be used in the care of all clients in hospitals regardless of their diagnosis or presumed infection status.

Standards of Practice Guidelines established to direct nursing care.

Standing Order Standardized intervention written, approved, and signed by a physician that is kept on file within health care agencies to be used in predictable situations or in circumstances requiring immediate attention.

Statutory Law Law enacted by legislative bodies.

Stereotyping Beliefs that all people within the same racial, ethnic, or cultural group act alike and share the same beliefs and attitudes.

Sterile Without microorganisms.

Sterile Conscience Individual's personal sense of honesty and integrity with regard to adherence to the principles of aseptic technique, including prompt admission and correction of any errors and omissions.

Sterile Field Area surrounding the client and the surgical site that is free from all microorganisms; created by draping of the work area and the client with sterile drapes.

Sterilization Total elimination of all microorganisms including spores.

Stock Supply Medications dispensed and labeled in large quantities for storage in the medication room or nursing unit.

Stomatitis Inflammation of the oral mucosa.

Stress Nonspecific response to any demand made on the body (Selye, 1974).

Stress Test Measure of a client's cardiovascular response to exercise.

Stressor Any situation, event, or agent that produces stress.

Stridor High-pitched, harsh sound heard on inspiration when the trachea or larynx is obstructed.

Subacute Care Short-term, aggressive care for clients who are out of the acute stage of illness but who still require skilled nursing, monitoring, and ongoing treatment.

Subcutaneous Injection into the subcutaneous tissue.

Subjective Data Data from the client's point of view, including feelings, perceptions, and concerns.

Surgical Asepsis Practices that eliminate all microorganisms and spores from an object or area.

Susceptible Host Person who lacks resistance to an agent and is thus vulnerable to disease.

Synthesis Chemical reaction when two or more atoms, called reactants, bond and form a more complex molecular product. Putting data together in a new way.

Systemic Infection Infection that affects the entire body with involvement of multiple organs.

Tachycardia Heart rate in excess of 100 beats per minute in an adult.

Tachypnea Respiratory rate greater than 24 beats per minute.

Teaching Active process wherein one individual shares information with another as a means to facilitate learning and thereby promote behavioral changes.

Teaching Strategy Technique to promote learning.

Teaching–Learning Process Planned interaction that promotes a behavioral change that is not a result of maturation or coincidence.

Telemedicine Use of communications technology to transmit health information from one location to another.

Teleology Ethical theory that states that the value of a situation is determined by its consequences.

Teratogenic Substance Substance that can cross the placental barrier and impair normal growth and development.

Tertiary Care Care focused on restoring the client to the state of health that existed before the development of an illness; if unattainable, then care directed to attaining the optimal level of health possible.

Tertiary Prevention Treatment of an illness or disease after symptoms have appeared so as to prevent further progression.

Therapeutic Communication Communication that is purposeful and goal directed, creating a beneficial outcome for the client.

Therapeutic Massage Application of pressure and motion by the hands with the intent of improving the recipient's well-being.

Therapeutic Procedure Accident Accident that occurs during the delivery of medical or nursing interventions.

Therapeutic Touch Technique of assessing alterations in a person's energy fields and using the hands to direct energy to achieve a balanced state.

Thoracentesis Aspiration of fluid from the pleural cavity.

Time Management System to help meet goals through problem solving.

Toddler Period Developmental stage beginning at approximately 12 to 18 months of age, when a child begins to walk, and ending at approximately age 3 years.

Tolerance Decreased sensitivity to subsequent doses of the same substance; an increased dose of the substance is needed to produce the same desired effect.

Tort Civil wrong committed by a person against another person or property.

Tort Law Enforcement of duties and rights among individuals and independent of contractual agreements.

Touch Means of perceiving or experiencing through tactile sensation.

Toxic Effect Reaction that occurs when the body cannot metabolize a drug, causing the drug to accumulate in the blood.

Trade (Brand) Name Name assigned a drug by the pharmaceutical company. Always capitalized.

Transcutaneous Electrical Nerve Stimulation Process of applying a low-voltage electrical current to the skin through cutaneous electrodes.

Transducer Instrument that converts electrical energy to sound waves.

Transduction Noxious stimulus that triggers electrical activity in the endings of afferent nerve fibers (nociceptors).

Transient Flora Microorganisms that attach to the skin for a brief period of time but do not continuously live on the skin.

Transmission Process whereby the pain impulse travels from the receiving nociceptors to the spinal cord.

Transmission-Based Precautions Practices designed for clients documented as, or suspected of, being infected with highly transmissible or epidemiologically important pathogens for which additional precautions beyond Standard Precautions are required to interrupt transmission in hospitals.

Triglyceride Lipid compound consisting of three fatty acids and a glycerol molecule.

Trocar Sharply pointed surgical instrument contained in a cannula.

Turgor Normal resiliency of the skin.

Type and Cross-Match Laboratory test that identifies the client's blood type (e.g., A or B) and determines the compatibility of the blood between potential donor and recipient.

Ultrasound Use of high-frequency sound waves to visualize deep body structures; also called an echogram or sonogram.

Uncomplicated Grief Grief reaction that normally follows a significant loss.

Unilateral Neglect Failure to recognize or care for one side of the body.

Unit Dose Form System of packaging and labeling each dose of medication by the pharmacy, usually for a 24-hour period.

Utility Ethical principle that states that an act must result in the greatest degree of good for the greatest number of people involved in a given situation.

Vaccination Inoculation with a vaccine to produce immunity against specific diseases.

Value System Individual's collection of inner beliefs that guides the way the person acts and helps determine the choices the person makes.

Values Principles that influence the development of beliefs and attitudes.

Values Clarification Process of analyzing one's own values to better understand those things that are truly important.

Variations Goals not met or interventions not performed according to the time frame; also called variances.

Vector-Borne Transmission Transfer of an agent to a susceptible host by animate means such as mosquitoes, fleas, ticks, lice, and other animals.

Vehicle Transmission Transfer of an agent to a susceptible host by contaminated inanimate objects such as food, milk, drugs, and blood.

Venipuncture Puncturing of a vein with a needle to aspirate blood.

Veracity Ethical principle based on truthfulness (neither lying nor deceiving others).

Verbal Communication Using words, either spoken or written, to send a message.

Vesicant Agent that may produce blisters and tissue necrosis.

Villi Finger-like projections that line the small intestine.

Virulence Frequency with which a pathogen causes disease.

Visceral Pain Discomfort felt in the internal organs.

Visual Learner Person who learns by processing information through seeing.

of melanocytes; appears as milk-white patches on the skin.

Vitamin Organic compounds essential to life and health.

Void Process of urine elimination.

Walking Rounds Reporting method used when members of the care team walk to each client's room and discuss care with each other and with the client.

Water Soluble Vitamin Vitamin that must be ingested daily in normal quantities because it is not stored in the body: vitamins C and B-complex.

Wellness State of optimal health wherein an individual moves toward integration of human functioning, maximizes human potential, takes responsibility for health, and has greater self-awareness and self-satisfaction.

Wellness Nursing Diagnosis Nursing diagnosis that indicates the client's expression of a desire to obtain a higher level of wellness in some area of function; composed of the diagnostic label preceded by the phrase "potential for enhanced."

Whistleblowing Calling attention to unethical, illegal, or incompetent actions of others.

Young Adulthood Developmental stage from the ages of 21 years through approximately 40 years.

Index

Note: Page numbers in *italics* indicate figures. Page numbers followed by "t" indicate a table.

A

Abdominal assessment, 542–544, *544*
Abilities, recognizing, 27, 27
Absorption
  drug process, 487
  nutrition process, 344
Abused clients, assessment
    considerations, 534
Acceptance, stage of dying , 328–329,
  328t
Accidents, 401–402
Accommodation, definition, 254
Accountability, 672
Accreditation, nursing, 61
Accreditation, nonacute health care
    services, 656–657
Acculturation, definition, 207
Accuracy vs. inaccuracy, 18
Acid, definition, 462
Acid-base balance, 469–473, 472t
  nursing process, 473–479
Acidic environment, immune system,
  436
Acidosis, 462, 472
Acquired immunity, immune response,
  437
Acquired immunodeficiency syndrome,
  82
Active listening, 130, 131
Active transport, 465
Activities of daily living (ADLs), 628
Actual nursing diagnosis, 151, 152t
Acupressure, 236–237, 567
Acupuncture, 228, 568, 569t
Acute pain, 549–550, 550t
Adaptation, 254, 302–303
Adaptive energy, 300
Adaptive grieving, 326
Adaptive measures, 302–303
Adequacy vs. inadequacy, 19
Adjuvant medications, pain relief,
  560–561, *561*
Adolescents
  client teaching, 192–193
  complementary therapies, 243t
  growth and development, 269t–270t,
    270–273
  home safety, 406
  nutritional needs of, 368
  perception of death, 322t
  preadolescence, 268–270, 269t–270t,
    271
Adult day care, 661
Advance directive, 100, 166, 326, 327
Advanced practice registered nurse
  (APRN), 61, 84

Adventitious breath sounds, 542
Affective domain, 187, 187t
  teaching methods applicable in, 191
Afferent pain pathways, 551
African Americans
  advance directives, 326
  health beliefs of, 209–211, 210t
Age. *See also* Aging, Life cycle
    considerations, specific age groups
  as factor affecting loss, grief, and
    death, 321–323, 322t
  as factor affecting pain experience,
    554
  as factor affecting safety, 401–402
  as factor affecting sleep, 389–390,
    392
Agency for Health Care Policy and
    Research (AHCPR), 83–84
Agent, in chain of infection, *430*, 430,
    433–434, 435
Agglutination, 581
Agglutinins, 581
Agglutinogens, 581
Aging, 626
  health, 628–632
  myths and realities, 625–627
  physiological changes, 632–645
  theories of, 625, 626t
Agnostics, 215
AIDS (acquired immunodeficiency
    syndrome), 82
Airborne precautions, *451*, 452t
Airborne transmission, in chain of
    infection, 431, 431t
Alcohol
  abuse, 9
  use, as health factor, 292
  use, as sleep factor, 389
Algor mortis, 335
Allergies
  food, 375
  health history, 530
Alkalosis, definition, 462, 472, 473
Alternative therapy, definition, 227.
    See also Complementary/alternative
    therapies
Alzheimer's disease (AD), 641–642
American Cancer Society, 71
American Heart Association, 71
American Holistic Nurses' Association,
  (AHNA), 4
American Journal of Nursing (AJN), 57
American Medical Association (AMA),
  71
American Nurses Association (ANA), 56,
  63, 64t, 71

American Red Cross, 52t
Ampules, for injection, 503–504, *504*
Anabolism, metabolic process, 344
Analgesia, definition, 562
Analgesics, 548, 560–564, *561*
Analysis, definition, 149
Analytes, definition, 577
Ancient Greece,
    alternative/complementary
    therapies in, 228
Anger, stage of dying, 328, 328t
Angiocatheter, 508
Angiography, radiological test, 605
Animal-assisted therapy, 241–242
Anion, definition, 461, 581
Anorexia nervosa, definition, 271
Anthropogenic, conditions for infection,
  433
Anthropometric measurements, 376
Antibodies, 437, 581
Anticipatory grief, 321
Antigens, 435, 581
Antioxidants, 238
Anxiety, 303–306
  definition, 44, 303
  nursing process, 308–312
  as sleep factor, 388
  test-taking, 44–45
Aphasia, 139
Apothecary system, of measurement,
  490, 491t, 491–492
Arithmetic, basic skill, 29
Aromatherapy, 239–241, 241t
Arterial blood gases, 471, 579
Arteriography, radiological test, 605
Arthritis, degenerative, 638
Ascites, definition, 614
Asepsis, 440
Aseptic technique, 440–441, 447
Asian Americans
  advance directives, 326
  health beliefs of, 210t, 211
Aspiration, 500, 610
Aspiration/biopsy procedures, 610–615,
  612t–613t, *614*, *615*
Assault and battery, 94t, 94–95
Assessment, 146–149, 527–546
  standard form, *528–529*
Assignment, 672
Assimilation, definition, 254
Assisted living, 661
Assisted suicide, 118
Assistive devices, for walking, 412–414
Associate Degree in Nursing (AND), 61
Assumptions, 20, 158
Atheists, 215

Atherosclerosis, definition, 350
Atom, definition, 458
Attitude, 10, 26–28
Attribute, 26
Auditory learning style, 33, 33t, 34t
Auscultation, assessment technique, 532
Autocratic leadership, 670
Autonomy, 51, 110t, 110–111
Autopsy, 336

B
Baccalaureate degree program, 61
Bachelor of Science in Nursing (BSN), 61
Back rubs, 420
Bacteremia, definition, 599
Bacteria, 428
Bactericides, immune response, 436
Balanced Budget Act (BBA) of 1997, 650
Ballard, Lucinda, 57
Bargaining, stage of dying , 328, 328t
Barium studies, radiological test, 605
Barrier precautions, 449
Barton, Clara, 52t
Basal metabolism, 345
Base, definition, 462
Basic skills. *See* Skills
Bathing needs of client, 418–419, 628
Baths, types of, 419
Beard and mustache care, client hygiene, 422
Beard, Richard Olding, 58
Beck, Aaron, 310–311
Behavioral pain response, 558
Beneficence, 110t, 112
Bereavement, definition, 318
Bias, definition, 158
Bicarbonate buffer system, 463
Bioavailability, definition, 484
Bioethics, 110
Biofeedback, 233, 567, 569t
Biographical data, assessment tool, 498–499
Biological agent, in chain of infection, 430
Biological clock, 387–388
Biological variation, 217, 217t
Biopsy, 611
    aspiration/biopsy procedures, 610–615, 612t–613t, *614*, *615*
Biorhythms, 387
Bladder management techniques, 644t
Blood-borne pathogens, Standard Precautions, 450–451
Blood
    chemistry, laboratory tests, 581
    culture, laboratory test, 599
    enzymes, 581
    lipid level, 581, 596
    glucose, 581
    pressure, vital sign measurement, *535*, 536t, 538, *538*

transfusion, 514–515, 515t
Blue Cross and Blue Shield, 58
Body image, hygiene practices, 402
Body fluids, balance of, 465–468, *466*
Body mass index (BMI), 377, 377t
Body mechanics, 8, 414
Body-movement strategies, 231t, 233–234
Body systems model, 149
Body water and body size, 461
Bodymind, 230
Bolus (IV push), 513–514, *514*
Bonding, neonatal, 258
Bone marrow aspiration/biopsy, 614
Borborygmi, bowel sounds, 543
Bowlby, John, 319
Bradley, Richard, 58
Bradycardia, 536
Bradypnea, 537
Brand name, of drugs, 485
Breakthrough pain, definition, 332
Breast assessment, 542
Breast cancer, controllable factors of, 295
Breastfeeding, 364–365
Breckenridge, Mary, 57, 85
Bronchial sounds, 541
Bronchovesicular sounds, 541–542
Brown, Esther Lucille, 59
Brown report, 59
Buccal medications, 485–487, 486t, 500–501
Buddhism, 217
    death and dying issues, 333t
Buffer systems, 463, 469
Buffers, definition, 462
Bulimia nervosa, 271
Burnout, professional, 312
Butterfly needles, 508

C
Calcium, 469
Calories, 345, 360, 360t
Cambodian, dietary factors, 363
Cancer, controllable factors of, 295, 295t
Cane, assistive walking device, 412–413
Capillary puncture, 580
Capitated rates, 77
Carbohydrates, necessary nutrients, 347–349
Cardiovascular assessment, 541, *541*
Cardiovascular system, and aging, 633–634
Care prioritization, 673
Caring-based theory, 113
Carotid pulse assessment, 537
Carriers, in chain of infection, 431
Case studies
    assessment, 545
    client teaching, 203
    communication, 143
    complementary/alternative therapies, 244

critical thinking, 23
cultural diversity, 223
dying client, 340
ethical issues, 121
fluid, electrolyte, and acid-base balance, 481
genogram, 296
growth and development, 279
HIV-positive client, 383
infection control, 444
legal issues, 106
malpractice vs. negligence, 97
medication administration, 522
nonacute health care services, 665
nursing care of the older client, 651
nutrition, 383
pain management, 571
safety/hygiene, 424
sleep disturbance, 397
standard of care, 97
Standard Precautions, 454
stress and anxiety, 315
Catabolism, metabolic process, 344
Cataplexy, sleep disturbance, 391
Cataracts, controllable factors of, 295
Catharsis, 310
Catheter sepsis, 512
Catholics, 216
    death and dying issues, 333t
    dietary factors, 363
Cation, definition, 461, 581
Ceiling effect, of analgesia, 562
Center for Critical Thinking, 14, 17
Centering, therapeutic intervention, 236, 237t
Centers for Disease Control and Prevention (CDC), 8
Cerebrospinal fluid aspiration, 614–615, *615*
Certification Examination for Practical and Vocational Nurses in Long-Term Care (CEPN-LTC), 67
Certification, nonacute health care services, 656
Chain of infection, 429–435, *430*
Change, as response to stress, 306–308, 308t
Change agent, 308
Channel, communication, 126, 126t
Charting. *See* Documentation, Documentation methods
Charting by exception (CBE), 171
Chemical agent, in chain of infection, 430
Chemical name, of drugs, 485
Chemical restraints, 412
Cheyne-Stokes respirations, 335
Children. *See also* Growth and development
    access to health care, 82
    communication, factors affecting, 138
    client teaching, 192

medication administration, 493–494, 506, 507

nutritional needs of, 239, 366–367, 367t

pain management, 557, 564, 565

play therapy, 242

perception of death, 322t

promoting wellness, 266

Children's Health Insurance Program (CHIP), 78, 79

China, alternative/complementary therapies in, 228

Chinese, dietary factors, 362

Chiropractic therapy, 234

Chloride, definition, 470

Choking prevention, 418

Cholesterol, 349, 350

Christian Scientists, 216

Chronic acute pain, 551

Chronic congestive heart failure, 634

Chronic nonmalignant pain, 551

Chronic obstructive pulmonary disease (COPD), 633

Chronic pain, 549, 550t, 551

Chronobiology, 387

Chyme, digestive product, 344

Civil law, 90–92, 91t

Circadian rhythms, 387

Clarity vs. lack of clarity, 17–18

Clean object, infection control, 441

Clean-voided specimen, urine, 580

Cleansing, infection control, 433

Client behavior accident, 401

Client identification, 408–409

Client placement, Standard Precautions, 451

Client teaching, 185–203. *See also* Learning styles, Teaching-learning process

  ability to learn, 188

  adolescents, 192, 193

  advance directives, 100

  anxiety, methods to reduce, 388

  bottle-feeding, 261

  breastfeeding, 364

  children, 192

  children, promoting wellness in, 266

  cultural considerations, 200

  culturally sensitive teaching guidelines, 220

  dietary considerations for elders, 370

  dietary guidelines, 291

  digoxin toxicity, 634

  food allergies, 375

  guided imagery, 232

  guidelines for effective, 201

  health practices, crucial, 294

  home health care, 194

  informed consent, 99

  jet lag, 388

  literacy assessment, 188

  medical jargon, 195

medication administration, sublingual and buccal, 500

medication administration, tampon use, 519

medication information, written, 500

middle-aged adults, self-care for, 277

nursing bottle syndrome, 365

nutrition, 10

nutrition, blood cholesterol, 350

nutrition, cow's milk for infants, 365

nutrition, fats, 349

nutrition, honey for infants, 365

nutrition, introducing new foods, 365

nutrition, natural or synthetic vitamins, 355

nutrition, toddler, 264

older adults, 193

pain at night, 556

pain management, 562

pain management, hot or cold applications, 567

pain management, timed-release tablets, 565

Pap smear, 600

parents and newborn, 259

postarterial puncture, 579

pregnancy and medications, 257

preventing accidental poisonings, 418

preventing choking, 367

preventing food-borne diseases, 291

preventing infant accidents, 262

progressive muscle relaxation, 231

self-administration, metered-dose inhaler, 518

sleep disturbance, managing, 394, 395

Standard Precautions, 449

teaching a family caregiver, 334

thought stopping/cognitive reframing, 310

wellness, 11

women, suppressed anger in, 284

Client-care equipment, Standard Precautions, 450

Clients' rights, 115–116

  home health care, 655t

Clinical, definition, 61

Closed-drainage system, urine collection, 580

Code for LP/VNs, 115t

Code for Nurses (International Council of Nurses), 116t

Cognitive-behavioral interventions, pain relief, 565–567, 569t

Cognitive dimension, human development, 252, 254, 255t

Cognitive domain, 187, 187t

  teaching methods applicable in, 190

Cognitive reframing technique, 306, 310–311

  pain relief, 566, 569t

Cognitive status, assessment tool, 499

Cold application, pain relief, 567, 569t

Colds and flu, controllable factors of, 295

Colic, 553

Colonization, of microorganisms, 429

Comfort, as sleep factor, 388, 389

Communicable agents, 429

Communicable diseases, 429

Communication, 125–144. *See also* Health care team communication, Nurse-client communication, Therapeutic communication

  channels, 126t

  congruency of messages, 129

  cultural differences, 126, 128, 129, 135, 136, 212

  documentation, 163–167

  health care team, 140–142

  impairments, 138–139

  influences on, 126, 128–129

  leadership skill, 670

  methods, 127–128, 135

  process of, 125–126, *127*

  professional boundaries, 137

  psychosocial aspects of, 134

  self, 142–143

  style, 135

  telemedicine, 142

Community health agency, 677

Community health services, 84–85

Community/home health care

  assessment, 147

  assessment, electronic sphygmomanometers, 538

  blood temperature, for transfusion, 514

  burn prevention, 415

  central line, 580

  client autonomy, 111

  client teaching, 194, 195t

  client's rights, 117

  clients at risk for infection, 442

  culturally sensitive care, 214

  death at home, 335

  disinfection, 434

  documentation, 167

  documentation form, *198*

  documentation using Kardex, 175

  dying client, 335

  effectiveness of care, 158

  equipment to increase client comfort, 332

  fire prevention, 415

  as health care setting, 72t

  home safety for elders, 279

  home safety risk appraisal, 406

  isolation, 453

  meal preparation resources, 374

  measuring I&O, considerations for, 477

  medications, dose conversion, 493

  medications, proper storage and use of, 417

Community/home health care (cont.)
  nasal inhalers, 516
  nursing interventions, taxonomy of, 179
  nutritional status, 635
  reduced cost, 82
  reducing stressors, 305
  standing orders, 157
  sterilization, 434
  telemedicine, 142
  urine collection, 580
Community nursing center, as health care setting, 73t
Community nursing organization (CNO), 85
Comorbidity, definition, 78
Competencies, 675
Complementary/alternative therapies, 227–245, 231t
  historical influences, 228–229
  holism, 230
  life cycle stages, 243t
  mind/body medicine and research, 229–230
  modern trends, 229–230
  nursing process, 230–242
  practical use of, 230, 242–243
  safety and efficacy of, 242–243
Complementary therapy, definition, 227
Completeness vs. incompleteness, 19
Complicated grief, 324
Compound, definition, 460
Comprehensive assessment, 147
Comprehensive Omnibus Budget Reconciliation Act (COBRA), 167
Compromised host, in chain of infection, 430, 432
Computed tomography (CT), 604, 605
Computer activities, teaching method, 191
Concept, definition, 13
Concepts, in reasoning, 20t, 21
Conclusions, in reasoning, 20t, 21–22
Conditioning, coping with stress, 302
Confidentiality, 95, 142
Conscious sedation, 577
Consequences, in reasoning, 20t, 22
Consent. See Informed consent
Consistency vs. inconsistency, 18
Constipation, elderly client, 629, 635–636
Contact precautions, 451, 452t
Contact transmission, in chain of infection, 431, 431t
Continuing Care Retirement Communities (CCRC), 661
Continuing education units (CEUs), 63
Contrast media, 600, 604
Controlled substances, 484t, 497
Convalescent stage, infectious process, 438

Coping measures, 302
Correctional facilities, employment opportunities, 677–678
Coughing, immune response, 436
Council of Practical Nursing Programs (CPNP), 66
Cover letter preparation, 680, 680
Crackles, breath sounds, 542
Crenation, definition, 464
Crisis and stress, 303, 304t
Critical listening, 16–17
Crisis intervention, 311, 312
Critical pathway, 160, 175
Critical period, of development, 250
Critical reading, 15–16, 16t, 46
Critical speaking, 17
Critical thinking, 13–24, 14, 14t
  activities to practice, 15, 22, 43–44
  nursing process, 23, 158, 159t
  skills, 15
  traits that support, 22
Critical thinking questions
  advance directives, 108
  blood transfusion, 523
  client teaching, 203
  communication barriers, 144
  communication, with unconscious adult, 144
  complementary/alternative therapies, 243t
  critical thinking, 24
  cultural beliefs about death, 341
  cultural beliefs, 225
  decision-making process, 48
  diagnostic tests, 621
  documentation (charting), 184
  documentation and legal issues, 184
  dying clients, nursing care for, 341
  elderly clients, 652
  ethical dilemmas, 122, 203
  fluid imbalance, 482
  holistic care, 12
  human development, 280
  hygiene, perineal care, 425
  infection control, 445
  informed consent, 108
  leadership, 684
  living will, 122
  medication administration, 523
  noise as safety factor, 425
  nonacute health care services, 666
  nursing interventions, 161
  nursing process, 159t, 161
  nutrition and obesity, 384
  pain categories, 572
  pain management, 572
  physical assessment, 546
  safety, use of restraints, 425
  self-care, 316
  serum levels, 482
  sleep, 398
  stress and anxiety, 316

  value systems, differing, 280
  vitamin supplements, 384
  work transition, 684
Critical writing, 17
Cross-contamination prevention, 516
Crutches, assistive device, 413
Cryotherapy, pain relief, 567, 569t
Cultural assessment interview guide, 219
Cultural assimilation, 207
Cultural beliefs. See also Cultural considerations, Religion, specific cultural groups
  health care, 208–209
  hygiene, 402
  nutrition, 361–363
  pain experience, 554
Cultural considerations
  adaptive measures, 302
  advance directives, 326
  aging, 626
  assault and battery charges, 94
  assessment, cleanliness, 534
  assessment, genitourinary, 544
  assessment, skin color, 541
  barriers to health care services (client beliefs), 80
  client teaching, overcoming sociocultural barriers, 190
  death, rituals following, 325
  environmental control, 213
  eye contact, 128
  family interaction patterns, 140
  gestures, 135
  growth and development, 251
  hygiene, 403, 422
  individuality, 207
  infant feeding method, 261
  learning and culture, 200
  music and culture, 242
  pain, language barrier, 557
  pain perception, 558
  sharing culture, 206
  sleep, cultural and societal expectations, 389
  smoke-free facilities, 113
  spiritual well-being, 285
  subculture, 209
  wellness, parents' beliefs about feeding children, 291
Cultural diversity, 205–225
  areas of, 207
  coworkers, 218
  definition, 206
  nurse sensitivity to, 208, 214
Culture
  biological variations, 217, 217t
  characteristics of, 208
  components of, 207–208
  definition, 10, 206
  dominant, 207
  social organization, 213–217

Culture and sensitivity (C&S) tests, 599–600
Cutaneous pain, 549
Cutaneous stimulation, pain relief, 567, 569t
Cyanosis, 531
Cytology, 600

D

Daily requirements, nutrition, 346t. *See also* specific nutrients
Data, 147–149, 148, 148t
  forms for recording, 175–178
  nursing diagnosis, 151
  in reasoning, 20t, 21
Data, action, and response (DAR), 171
Death and dying, 326–240. *See also* Family, Loss, Grief
  advance directives, 326, 327
  cultural considerations, 326
  Dying Person's Bill of Rights, *330*
  impending death, 334–335
  legal issues, 327, 336
  nurse's self-care, 336–337
  nursing care after death, 335–336
  nursing care of dying client, 327, 329–334
  stages of, 327–329, 328t
"Death rattle," 335
Decision making, in nursing process, 159
Decomposition, chemical, 460
Defamation, 94t, 95
Defense mechanisms, immune system, 435–438
Defense mechanisms, psychological, 303, 304t
Defining characteristics, definition, 150–151
Deglutition, digestive process, 344
Dehydration, 347, 467, 476
  in children, 347
  in elderly clients, 347, 474, 636
Delegation, 672
Democratic leadership, 670
Demonstration, teaching method, 191
Denial
  defense mechanism, 304t
  stage of dying, 327, 328t
Dental care, elderly clients, 636
Deontology, 113
Dependent nursing interventions, 154
Depersonalization, definition, 306
Depression
  elderly clients, 642
  stage of dying, 328, 328t
Depth vs. superficiality, 19
Dental caries, 295, 421
Dental exam, as health factor, 293
Development, definition, 250. *See also* Growth and development
Developmental tasks, 250, 253t–254t

Developmental stage. *See* Age
Dialysis, definition, 464
Diabetes, insulin levels, 348
Diabetes Mellitus type 2, 637
Diffusion, definition, 463–464, *464*
Diagnosis. *See also* Nursing diagnosis
  critical thinking question, 159t
  medical vs. nursing, 149–50, 150t
Diagnosis-related group (DRG), 71, 78, 79, 167
Diagnostic data. *See also* Diagnostic testing
  as health factor, 293
  fluid, electrolyte, and acid-base balance, 471, 472t, 474–475
  infection indicators, 440
  medication administration, 499
  nutritional assessment, 378
  safety/hygiene assessment, 405
Diagnostic departments, 74
Diagnostic testing. *See also* Laboratory tests
  aspiration/biopsy, 610–615, 612t–613t, *614, 615*
  client care, 574–577, 576t, 578t
  electrodiagnostic studies, 608–610, 609t
  endoscopic procedures, 610, 611t
  magnetic resonance imaging (MRI), 607, 607t
  other tests, 615t–620t
  preparing client, 574, 575t
  radioactive studies, 607, 607t–608t
  radiological studies, 600–606, 600, 601t–604t, *605*
  ultrasonography, 606, 606t
Didactic, 61
Diet
  as health factor, 290, 291, 296–297
  as sleep factor, 389
Diet history, assessment tool, 376
Diet therapy, 378–380
Dietary guidelines, 358–361
  for Americans, 361t
  four food groups (historical), 358
  food guide pyramid, 358–360, *359*
  recommended dietary allowance (RDA), 360–361
Dietary prescription/order, 378–379
Dietary reference intake (DRI), 360
Diets, hospital, 379–380
Digestion, nutrition process, 344
Digestive system, 344–345, *345*
Diploma nursing program, 61
Dirty object, infection control, 441
Disabled clients
  Americans with Disabilities Act (ADA), 91–92
  assessment considerations, 534
Discharge planning, 152
Discharge summary, 178, *178*
Discipline, definition, 13

Disciplined, 13
Discussion, teaching method, 190, 191
Disenfranchised grief, 321
Disinfectants, infection control, 433–434
Disinfection, infection control, 433–434
Displacement, defense mechanism, 304t
Distraction, noninvasive pain relief, 566, 569t
Distress, opposed to eustress, 302
Distribution, drug process, 487
Dix, Dorothea, 52t
Documentation, 163–184. *See also* Documentation forms, Documentation methods, Reporting
  abbreviations, 169
  assessment, 149, 156–157
  client teaching, 195, *196–198*
  correcting an error in, *168*
  description of documents, 165t
  elements of effective, 168–170
  general guidelines, 168t
  home health care, 167
  legal considerations, 98, 99, 166
  medication administration, 494, *495, 496*
  Nursing Interventions Classification (NIC), 179–180
  nursing minimum data set (NMDS), 179
  Nursing Outcomes Classification (NOC), 180
  nursing process, 168
  pain assessment, 559, *559*
  purposes of, 164–167
  reimbursement, 167
  Unified Medical Language System (UMLS), 179
  when to chart, 167
Documentation forms, 175–178
  client teaching, *196–198*
  discharge summary, 178, *178*
  flow sheets, 175–178, *176–177*
  Kardex, 175
  nurses' progress notes, 178
Documentation methods, 170–175
  charting by exception (CBE), 171
  computerized, 173–174
  critical pathway, 175
  focus charting, 171, *174*
  PIE charting, 171, *173*
  point-of-care charting, 175
  problem-oriented charting, 171
  problem-oriented medical record (POMR), 171
  narrative charting, 171
  SOAP charting, 171, *172*
  source-oriented charting, 171
Dominant culture, 207
Do-not-resuscitate (DNR) orders, 100, 327
Dosage. *See* Medication

Dressing, elderly client, 628–629
Droplet precautions, *451*, 452t
Drowning prevention, 418
Drug abuse, 9, 292, 389
    as factor affecting pain experience, 554
Drug allergy, 488
Drug history, assessment tool, 498
Drug tolerance, 488
Drugs. *See also* Drug abuse, Medication action, 485–489
    documentation, 494, *495,* 496
    incompatibilities, 513
    interaction, 488
    legislation, 484–485, 484t
    nomenclature, 485
    safe administration, 494–497
    side effects and adverse reactions, 488
    standards, 484–485
    supply and storage, 497
    types of preparations, 486t
Durable power of attorney for health care (DPAHC), 102, *103*
Duration, of pain, 556
Duty delegation, 672–673
Dye injection studies, radiological test, 605–606
Dying. *See* Death and Dying
Dying Person's Bill of Rights, *330*
Dysarthria, 139
Dysfunctional grief, 320–321, 322t, 325
Dysphasia, 139
Dyspnea, 537
Dyspneic clients, positioning, 537

E
Ear care, client hygiene, 422–423
Ear medications, 516
Eating disorders, 271, 368
Eating, elderly client, 629
Edema, excess fluid symptom, 474, 475, 476t
    immune response, 437
Efferent pain pathways, 551
Elder abuse, 645
Elder care, financing, 649–650
Elderly clients. *See also* Older adulthood
    abuse of, 645
    access to health care, 83
    assessment considerations, 534
    client teaching, 193
    communication, factors affecting, 138
    complementary therapies, 243t
    dietary considerations, 370, 629, 630, 635
    disease prevention, 631
    essential oils, 240
    exercise, 233, 629
    financing care of, 649–650
    health care needs, meeting, 85
    home safety, 279

pain management, 554, 564, 565
physiological changes, 632–645
skin turgor and dehydration, 474
sleep and aging, 392
strengths, 630, 631
Electrocardiogram (ECG or EKG), 608–610, 609t
Electrodiagnostic studies, 608–610, 609t
Electroencephalogram (EEG), 610
Electroencephalography, 610
Electrolytes, 461t, *461,* 468–470, 472, 581
Electronic sphygmomanometers, 538, 539t
Elements, 458, 459t
Elimination, immune response, 436
Embryonic stage, 257
Emotional state, as safety factor, 402
Emotional wellness, 284
Empathy, 131–132
Employee right-to-know laws, 401
Employment opportunities, 676–678
Empowerment, 52
Empty calories, definition, 360
Encoding, 40
Endemic, definition, 448
Endocrine system, aging, 637
Endorphin, definition, 311t, 551
Endoscopy, definition, 610
Endoscopic procedures, 610, 611t
Energetic-touch therapies, 234–237, *235*
Engle, George L, 319, 320t
Enriched, food products, 359
Enteral instillation, of medication, 501–502
Enteral nutrition, 380–381, *381*
Environment, as sleep factor, 388, 389, 394
Environmental barriers, in client teaching, 189, 189t
Environmental control, Standard Precautions, 450
Enzymes, 581
Epidemic, definition, 448
Epidural analgesia, 564–565
Equipment accident, 401
Erikson, Erik, 252
    stages of psychosocial development, 253t
Error, documentation of, *168,* 170
Erythema, immune response, 436, 437t
Ethical responsibilities, 109–122
    bioethics, 110
    client's rights, 115–116
    codes, 115, 115t, 116t
    committees, 120
    death and dying, 327
    decision making, *119,* 119–120
    dilemmas, 116, 118
    nonacute health care services, 654–655, 654t, 655t

principles, 110t, 110–113
    theories, 113–114
Ethics, concept of, 110
Ethnicity, definition, 206
Ethnocentrism, 207
Etiology
    cultural diversity, 208–209
    definition, 150
Euglycemia, definition, 348
European Americans
    advance directives, 326
    health beliefs of, 209, 210t
Europeans, dietary factors, 362
Eustress, 301–302
Euthanasia, 118, 327
Evaluation, 157–158, 158t, 159t
Exams, preparing for, 42–43
Exclusive provider organization (EPO), 77, 77t, 78
Excretion
    digestive process, 345
    drug process, 488
Exercise
    as health factor, 290–291, 292
    complementary/alternative intervention, 233
    elderly clients, 233, 629
    infection control, 435
    pain relief, 568
    physiological benefits of, 311t
    stress management, 310, 311t
Expected outcome, definition, 153, 153t
Extended care facility, as health care setting, 72t
External barriers, client teaching, 189, 189t
Extracellular fluid, definition, 346, 466
Extremity assessment, 544–545
Eye care, client hygiene, 422
Eye contact, 128
Eye exam
    assessment tool, 539, *539*
    as health factor, 293
Eye medications, 516
Eye protection, Standard Precautions, 450

F
Face shield, Standard Precautions, 450
FACES pain rating scale, 557
Fads, influence on nutrition, 363–364
Fairness vs. bias, 19
Faith healing, 238
Falls, 405t, 409–414, 410t
False imprisonment, 94t, 95
Family
    cultural differences, 213
    death and dying issues, 334, 336
    interaction patterns, 140
    nurse-client communication, 138
Far East, alternative/complementary therapies in, 228

Fats, necessary nutrients, 349–350
Fee-for-service, health care delivery, 72, 76
Feedback, communication, 126
Fetal alcohol syndrome (FAS), 257
Fetal stage, 257
Fidelity, 110t, 112–113
Fight-or-flight response, 301
Filtration, 465
Flashback, IV solution, 512
Flexner, Abraham, 58
Flexner report, 58
Flora, infection control, 428, 436
Flow rate, for IV solution, 511
Flow sheets, 175–178, *176–177*
Fluid and electrolyte balance, 465–468
    nursing process, 473–479
Fluid therapy, 478–479
Fluoroscopy, 600
Focus charting, 171, *174*
Focused assessment, 147
Folk medicine, 209, 210t
Fomites, in chain of infection, 431
Food
    allergies, 375–376, 498
    drug interactions, 488
    labeling, 373, *373*
    quality, 373, 374t
    safety, 374, *375*
Food-borne illnesses, 374–375
Food frequency questionnaire, assessment tool, 376
Food guide pyramid, 358–360, *359*
    food plan for children, 367t
Food record, assessment tool, 376
Foot and toenail care, client hygiene, 420, 421
Forced fluids, fluid imbalance, 478
Formal lecture, teaching method, 190
Formal teaching, 186
Fortified, food products, 359
Foster care, 661
Fowler, J. W., 255
    stages of faith, 256t
Fractured hip, elderly client, 638
Free radicals, 238
Functional assessment, for rehabilitation, 658, *658*
Functional Health Patterns, Gordon's, 149
Fungi, definition, 429
Fraud, 95
Freud, Sigmund, 252
    stages of psychosexual development, 252t

G
Games, teaching method, 191
Gases, in human body, 461
Gastrointestinal (GI) system
    aging, 634–636
    assessment of, 542–544
    body fluid balance, 467

Gate control pain theory, 553
Gender roles, and cultural differences, 213–214
General adaptation syndrome, *300*, 300–301
Generic name, of drugs, 485
Genitourinary assessment, 544
Genogram, 294, *294*, 296
Germicide, infection control, 434
Germinal stage, 257
Gerontological nursing, 624–625
Gerontologist, definition, 623
Gerontology, definition, 623
Gingivitis, client oral hygiene, 421
Glaucoma, controllable factors of, 295
Gloves, Standard Precautions, 450
Glycogenesis, definition, 348
Glycogenolysis, definition, 348
Goals, nursing process, 152–153, 153t
Goldmark report, 59
Goldmark, Josephine, 59
Good Samaritan laws, 92
Gordon's Functional Health Patterns, 149
Gown, Standard Precautions, 450
Grief
    definition, 318
    factors affecting, 321–324, 322t, 323t, 324t
    reactions during, 320t
    nursing care of grieving client, 324–326
    theories of, 319
    types of, 320–321
Grief work, 319
Grooming, 6–7, 628
Growth and development, 250–256
    adolescence, 269t–270t, 270–273
    factors influencing, 251
    infancy, 259–262, 260t
    middle adulthood, 275–277, 275t–276t
    neonatal period, 257–259, 258t
    nutritional needs, 364–370
    older adulthood, 277–279, 278t
    preadolescence, 268–270, 269t–270t, 271
    prenatal period, 156–257
    preschool period, 264–266, 265t
    principles of, 250, 250t
    school-age period, 266–267, 267t
    theoretical perspectives, 251–256
    toddler period, 262–264, 263t
    young adulthood, 273–275, 273t–274t
Guided imagery, mind/body technique, 232t, 232
    pain relief, 566, 569t

H
Hair assessment, 539
Hair care, client hygiene, 421–422
Hale, Mamie, 57

Halitosis, client hygiene, 421
Handwashing, infection control, 8, 261, 433, 441, 449
Havighurst, Robert, 252
    developmental stages and tasks, 253t–254t
Head assessment, 539–540
Head-to-toe assessment, 532–545
Healer, qualities of a, 4–5
Healing, 4, 230
Healing prayer, 238
Healing touch, 236
Health, definition, 4, 283–284
Health
    environmental influences, 292
    factors affecting, 289–294
    genetics and human biology, 289, 290t
    nutrition, 371
    personal behavior, 289–292
Health care, 292–294
    access, 79–80
    barriers to services (client beliefs), 80
    costs, 60, 79, 79
    initiatives, 59–60
    quality, 60, 80
    reform, 60, 76
    services, 69–70
Health care delivery system, 63, 69–86. *See also* Health insurance
    challenges within, 80–83
    departments/units, 73–74
    personnel, 73–74
    private and public sectors, 71–72
    services, 73–74
    settings, 72t–73t, 81
    trends affecting, 85t
Health care economics, 76–80. *See also* Health insurance
    ethical issues of, 82, 119
Health Care Financing Administration (HCFA), 78
Health Care Surrogate Law, 327
Health care team, 74–76, 75t, 76t. *See also* Interdisciplinary health care team
Health care team communication, 140–142
Health continuum, 5
Health history, 147
    assessment tool, 528–531
    fluid, electrolyte, and acid-base balance, 473
    safety and hygiene, 403–403
Health insurance, 76–79
    early 20th-century, 58
    Source of the Nation's Health Dollar in 1998, *76*
Health maintenance organizations (HMOs), 77t, 77–78
    definition, 60, 77
Health promotion, 285–286, 287t–288t

Health status, growth/development factor, 251

Healthy living, guidelines for, 294–297, 295t

Healthy People 2000, 63, 64t, 285–286, 287t–288t

Healthy People 2010, 286, 287t–288t

Hearing impaired client, communication with, 139, 645

Hearing, aging, 645

Heart disease, controllable factors of, 294, 295t

Heat and cold application, pain relief, 567, 569t

Height measurement, 539

Hematocrit index, 474

Hematuria, 577

Hemoglobin index, 474

Hemolysis, definition, 464

Henry Street Settlement, 56, *56*, 57, 58

Heparin lock, 509, *514*

Herbal therapy, 239, 240t

Herbs, medicinal value of, 240t

Heredity, growth/development factor, 251

Herpes zoster, elderly client, 639

Hierarchy of needs, *5*, 5–6, 148–149, 152t

Hinduism, 217
    death and dying issues, 333t
    dietary factors, 363

Hippocrates, 52t, 53

Hispanic Americans
    advance directives, 326
    health beliefs of, 210t, 211

History
    definition, 51
    events influencing nursing evolution, 52t–53t
    of nursing process, 146

Holism, 230

Holistic
    definition, 4
    framework for nursing, 256
    nature of human beings, *256*

Holistic care, 3–12, 69, 230

Home care agency, 677

Home health care, 654–656, 654t, 655t, 659–660. *See also* Community/home health care

Home rehabilitation, 659

Homelessness, access to health care, 82–83

Homeostasis, 4, 300, 458

Hormones, effects on tissues, 290t

Hospice care, 334, 654–656, 654t, 655t, 662
    as health care setting, 72t, 662, 677

Hospital inpatient program, 659

Hospital, 72t, 677

Host, in chain of infection, *430*, 432–433

Household system, of measurement, 491–492, *491*, 491t

Human development, dimensions of, 251–256. *See also* Growth and development

Human energy field, *235*

Humor, as complementary therapy, 241
    pain relief, 566

Humoral immunity, immune response, 437

Hydration, body process, 461

Hydrostatic pressure, 465

Hygiene
    assessment, 403–405, 404t, 405t
    elderly clients, 628
    factors influencing practice of, 402–403
    infection control, 434
    key interview questions about, 403
    nursing interventions, 418–423
    self-care deficit, 407, 407t, 409t

Hyperalimentation, 470

Hypercalcemia, 469

Hypercalcemic crisis, 469

Hyperchloremia, 470

Hyperglycemia, 348

Hyperkalemia, 468

Hypermagnesemia, 469

Hypernatremia, 468

Hyperphosphatemia, 470

Hypersomnia, sleep disturbance, 390

Hypertension, 634

Hypertonic solution, 464

Hyperventilation, 537

Hypervolemia, 512

Hypnosis, 233, 568, 569t

Hypocalcemia, 469

Hypochloremia, 470

Hypodermic syringe, 502, *503*

Hypoglycemia, 348

Hypokalemia, 468

Hypomagnesemia, 469, 470

Hyponatremia, 468

Hypophosphatemia, 470

Hypotonic solution, 464

Hypoventilation, 537

Hypoxemia, 472

I

Idiosyncratic reaction, to drugs, 488

Illness prevention, 286–289

Illness stage, infectious process, 438

Imagery, mind/body technique, 232t, 232

Immune system, 435–438

Immunizations
    as health factor, 293
    hepatitis B vaccine, 293
    infection control, 435

Impaired nurse, 105–106

Implantable port, 509, 580

Implementation, 154–157, 159t
    institutional care plan, *155*

Implications, in reasoning, 20t, 22

Incident report, 102, 104–105, 182–183

Incontinence, urinary, 643, 643t, *643*, 644t

Incubation period, infectious process, 438

Independent practice, vs. managed care, 77t

India, alternative/complementary therapies in, 228–229

Indian, dietary factors, 362

Industrial clinic, as health care setting, 73t

Infants
    growth and development, 259–262, 260t
    nutritional needs of, 364–366

Infection control, 427–445
    breaking the chain of infection, 433–435
    cleansing, 433
    disposal of materials, 442
    eye care, 422, 644
    handwashing, first line of defense, 433
    handwashing and infant care, 261
    herpes zoster, 639
    measuring weight, 539
    needle disposal, 442
    nursing process, 439–442
    skin integrity, 639
    Standard Precautions, 449, 532
    TB, 633
    venipuncture, 511

Infection
    causes of, 428–429
    chain of, 429–435, *430*
    definition, 429
    process of, 438

Infectious agents, 429

Infectious diseases, 433

Inferences, in reasoning, 20t, 21

Infiltration, 479, 512

Inflammation, immune response, 436–437, 437t

Inflammatory process, immune response, 436–437, 437t

Informal teaching, 186–187

Information, in reasoning, 20t, 21

Informed consent, 98–100
    client autonomy, 111
    documentation, 166
    form for medical and surgical procedures, *101*

Ingestion, nutrition process, 344

Inhalants, medication, 486t, 487, 516

Initial planning, 152

Injections. *See* Parenteral medications

Insomnia, 390

Inspection, assessment tool, 531

Institute of Research and Service in Nursing Education Report, 59
Instrument of healing, 230
Insulin syringe, 502, *503*
Insulin, 348
Insurance companies, employment opportunities, 678
Insurance plans. *See* Health insurance
Intake and output (I&O), 473, 477–478
Integumentary system, aging, 638–641, *640*, 640t
Intellectual wellness, 10, 284
Intensity, of pain, 556, *556*
Interdependent nursing interventions, 154
Interdisciplinary health care team (IHCT), 657, *657*
Intermittent infusion, 513
Interpersonal skills, client teaching, 194–195
Interpersonal theory, 252, 254t
Interstitial fluid, definition, 346, 466
Interventions. *See* Nursing interventions
Interview, job hunt, 681–683
Intracath, 508
Intracellular fluid (ICF), definition, 346, 466
Intradermal (ID) injection, 487, *502*, 504, *504*
Intramuscular (IM) injection, 487, *502*, *505*, 505–506, *506*
Intrapsychic theory, 252, 252t, 253t–254t
Intrathecal analgesia, 564–656
Intravascular fluid, 466
Intravenous (IV) injection, 506–514
  definition, 487
  equipment, 507, *508*, 509, *509*
  insertion, *502*, 510, *510*
Intravenous (IV) therapy, 478, 506–514, 507t
Intravenous drug therapy, 512–514
Invasion of privacy, 94t, 95–96
Invasive, definition, 574
Ion, definition, 460–461
Ischemic pain, 553
Islam, 216
  death and dying issues, 333t
  dietary factors, 363
Isolation, infection control, *451*, 451–453
Isotonic solution, 464
Isotopes, definition, 459
Italians, dietary factors, 362
IV push (bolus), 513–514, *514*

J
Japanese, dietary factors, 362
Jehovah's Witnesses, 216
  death and dying issues, 333t
Jet lag, 388
Job application, 681
Job description, 675

Job hunting, 678–683
Job interview, 681–683
Job opportunities, 676–678
Joint Commission on Accreditation of Healthcare Organizations (JCAHO), 60, 166–167
  agenda for change, 60
  pain management standards, 554
Judaism, 216
  death and dying issues, 333t
  dietary factors, 363
Judgments, 15
Jugular vein distention, 474
Justice, 110t, 112
Justify, 19

K
Kardex, 175
Ketorolac, contraindications, 563
Ketosis, 348–349
Kohlberg, Lawrence, 254–255
  stages of moral development, 255t
Kidneys
  acid-base balance, 471
  body fluid balance, 467
Kilocalories, 345
Kinesthetic learning style, 33, 33t, 34t
Knowledge base, client teaching, 194
  hygiene practices, 403
Kubler-Ross, Elizabeth, 327–329, 328t

L
Laboratory data. *See* Diagnostic data
Laboratory tests
  blood tests, 581, 582t–583t, 583t–595t, 595
  culture and sensitivity (C&S) tests, 599–600
  specimen collection, 577–581
  stool tests, 599, 599t
  urine tests, 595–599, *595*, 596t–598t
Lactation, nutritional needs during, 370
Lactose intolerance, 349
Laissez-faire leadership, 670
Loatian, dietary factors, 363
Local anesthesia, 565
Localized infection, 438
Location, of pain, 556
Leadership, 669–671
Learning. *See also* Client teaching
  basic assumptions about, 187
  common beliefs about, 189
  definition, 25, 185
  developmental level, 188
Learning disability, 33
Learning domains, 187, 187t
Learning plateau, 188
Learning styles, 32–34, 33t, 34t, 35t, 189
Legal concepts, 90–92
Legal responsibilities, 89–108
  death and dying, 327, 336
  elder abuse, reporting, 645

federal antifraud laws, 96–97
  issues in practice, 93
  medication administration, 498
  nonacute health care services, 654–655, 654t, 655t
  professional liability, 93, 105
  state reporting requirements, 97
  tort law, 93–96, 94t
Liability, 93, 105
Licensed practical nurse (LPN)
  program of study, 60–61
Licensed practical/vocational nurse (LP/VN), 61
  nursing practice standards for, 62t
  roles of, 76t, 658, 659, 661
  tasks of, 671
Licensed vocational nurse (LVN)
  program of study, 60–61
Licensure
  nursing, 676
  nonacute health care services, 656
Life cycle, 249–280
  nutritional needs during, 364–370
  stages of, 256–279
Life cycle considerations
  access to health care (children), 82
  access to health care (elderly clients), 83
  assessment (older clients), 534
  blood transfusion, initial assessment, 515
  body water and body size, 461
  coping ability, 302
  death, talking with children about, 322
  death and dying, 328
  dehydration, 347
  drug action and dosing, 489
  essential oils (elderly clients), 240
  exercise (elderly clients), 233
  health care needs (elderly clients), 83
  learning ability and developmental level, 188
  macrobiotic diets (children and pregnant women), 239
  medication administration, choosing IV equipment, 507
  medication administration, locating vein, 510
  medication administration, primary site for IM injection, 506
  medication administration, selecting needle gauge, 509
  nutrition, 9, 10
  nutrition, children and cholesterol, 350
  nutrition, vitamins, 352
  pain assessment, children, 557
  pain management, effects of meperidine (Demerol), 564
  pain management, injections and children, 565

Life cycle considerations (*cont.*)
    pain management, opioids and the elderly, 565
    pain, elderly clients, 554
    proteins, 350
    REM sleep, 387
    skin turgor, elderly clients, 474
    teaching adolescents, 193
    teaching children, 192
    teaching older adults, 193
    vitamins and minerals, poison risk to children, 417
Life experience, growth/development factor, 251
Life-prolonging procedures declaration, *104*
Life review, 328
Lifestyle
    assessment component, 499
    as safety factor, 402
    as sleep factor, 388–389
Lindemann, Erich, 319
Linen, Standard Precautions, 450
Lipids, definition, 349
Lipoproteins, 581
Listening, basic skill, 30
    active, 130, 131
Literacy, 188
Liver mortis, 335
Living will, 102, *104*
Local adaptation syndrome (LAS), 301
Logic, 15
Logical vs. illogical, 19
Long-term care, 654–656, 654t, 655t, 660–661
Long-term care facility, 660, 677. *See also* Extended care facility
Long-term goal, 153, 153t
Loss, 318
    factors affecting, 321–324, 322t, 323t, 324t
Love and belonging needs, 5,6
Low-back pain, controllable factors of, 295
Lumbar puncture (LP, "spinal tap"), 614
Lungs, body fluid balance, 467
Lymphokines, immune response, 437

M

Macrobiotic diet, 239
Magnesium, 469–470
Magnetic resonance imaging (MRI), 607, 607t
Mahoney, Mary, 57
Maladaptive measures, 303
Malpractice, 94t, 96, 97
Managed care, 63, 77t, 77–78
    organization as health care setting, 73t
    vs. independent practice, 77t
Management, 670–671

Manipulation strategies, complementary/alternative interventions, 233–234
Mask, Standard Precautions, 450
Maslow's hierarchy of needs, *5*, 5–6, 148–149, 152t
Maslow, Abraham, 5
Massage, therapeutic, 235, 420, 567
Mastication, digestive process, 344
Material safety data sheet (MSDS), 401
Mathematics, basic skill, 29
Matter, definition, 458
Maturation, learning principle, 188, 250
Maturational loss, 318
Meals, assisting client with, 380–381
Measurement conversions, dosage systems, 491t, 491–493
Medicaid, 59, 78–79, 650, 655–656
Medical asepsis, infection control, 441
Medical diagnosis, 150
    vs. nursing diagnosis, 149–150, 150t
Medical history, assessment tool, 498–499
Medical record documents, 165t
Medicare, 59, 78, 79, 649–650, 655–656
Medication. *See also* Drugs
    administration preparation and routes, 485–487, 486t
    compliance, 497–498
    dose calculations, 493–494, *494*
    dose equivalents, 491–494, *491*, 491t, *494*
    error, documentation of, 170
    expiration date, 504
    injury risk, 405t
    legal considerations, 498
    management, 485
    nursing process, 498–520
    orders, 489–490
    sleep and safety, 389
    weight and measurement of, 490–491, 490t
Medicinal therapies, 238–239
Medigap insurance, 656
Meditation, 231
Menarche, 268
Mental health, elderly client, 641
Mental status and affect, assessment of, 540
Mentholated rubs, pain relief, 567
Meperidine (Demerol), 564
Messages, communication, 126
    congruency of, 129–130
Mental wellness, 284
Metabolic acidosis, 472
Metabolic alkalosis, 472–473
Metabolic rate, 345, 470
Metabolism
    drug process, 487
    nutritional process, 344–345
Metacognition, 43
Metric system, 490, 490t, 491t

Mexicans, dietary factors, 362
Middle adulthood
    growth and development, 275–277, 275t–276t
    home safety, 406
    nutritional needs, 368–369
    sleep and aging, 392
Middle Easterners, dietary factors, 362
Mind/body techniques, 231t, 231–233
Minerals, necessary nutrients, 355–358, 355t–357t, 358t
Minority group, 207
Mixture, definition, 460
Mobility, 402, 628
Mode of transmission, in chain of infection, *430*, 431, 431t, 435
Modulation, of pain impulse, 554
Molecule, definition, 460
Monounsaturated fatty acids, definition, 350
Moral dimension, human development, 254, 255t
Moral maturity, 254
Morbidity, definition, 55
Mormons, 216
    death and dying issues, 333t
    dietary factors, 363
Mortality, definition, 55
Mortuary, 336
Motivation, learning principle, 187–188
Mourning, definition, 318
Mucous membranes, immune response, 436
Musculoskeletal system
    aging, 637–638
    assessment, 544–545
Music therapy, 242
Mustache and beard care, client hygiene, 422
Myofascial pain syndromes, 551

N

Narcolepsy, sleep disturbance, 390–391
Narcotics, storage, 497
Narrative charting, 171
Nasal medications, 516–517, *517*
National Center for Complementary and Alternative Medicine (NCCAM), 4
    definition of holistic care, 4
National Association of Practical Nurse Education and Service, Inc. (NAPNES), 63, 65t
National Council Licensure Examination (NCLEX), 60–61
    NCLEX-PN, 61, 67, 676, *676*
    NCLEX-RN, 61, 67
National Council of State Boards of Nursing, Inc. (NCSBN), 66t, 66–67
National Federation of Licensed Practical Nurses, Inc. (NFLPN), 61, 63, 65t, 66, 71
    standards of nursing practice, 62t

National Institutes of Health (NIH), 4
National League for Nursing Accrediting Commission (NLNAC), 66
National League of Nursing Education (NLN), 56, 65t–66t, 71
Native Americans
    death and dying issues, 333t
    dietary factors, 361
    health beliefs of, 210t, 211
    religious beliefs of, 216
Neck assessment, 539, 540
Necrosis, 581
Needle-free system, 509, *509*
Needles, 503, *503*, 508, 509
Negligence, 94t, 96, 97
Neonatal period, growth and development, 257–259, 258t
Nerve block, pain relief, 568
Neuralgia, pain type, 551
Neurological system
    aging, 641–642
    assessment, 540
Neuropeptides, 229–230
Neurosurgery, pain relief, 568
Neurotransmitters, 229–230
Nicotine. *See* Smoking
Night terrors, sleep disturbance, 391
Nightingale, Florence, 52t, 54–55, *55*
Nightingale pledge, 112t
Nociceptors, 551
Noise pollution, 418
Nonacute health care services, 653–666
    role of LP/VN, 658, 659, 661
Noninvasive, definition, 574
Nonmaleficience, 110t, 111
Nonopioids, 563
Nonspecific immune defense, 436
Nonverbal communication, 127–128, 135, 139
North American Nursing Diagnosis Association (NANDA), 149, 179
Nose assessment, 540
Nose care, client hygiene, 423
Nosocomial infection, 438–439, 447
Note taking, 41–42
Nothing by mouth (NPO), 379, 478
Noxious stimulus, 549
NREM sleep, 386–387, *387*
Nurse
    as client advocate, 120
    as whistleblower, 120–121
    self-care during grief, 336–337
Nurse-client communication, 137–140
Nurses, positive perception of, 81
Nurses' progress notes, 178
Nursing
    agenda for health care reform, 83, 83t
    definition, 5
    historical overview, 51–60, 52t–53t
    practice standards for LP/VNs, 62t
    professional misconduct in, 97–98
    reforms in, 53t, 54–60

    roles, 75–76, 76t
    student nurse skills for success, 25–48
    women's movement, 56
Nursing audit, 157–158
Nursing bottle syndrome, 365
Nursing care plan, 154, *155–156*
Nursing care plan samples
    client at risk for infection, 443–444
    client at risk for injury, 423–424
    client experiencing anxiety, 314–315
    client requiring rehabilitative care, 662–665
    client with altered nutrition, 382–383
    client with Alzheimer's disease (AD), 646–649
    client with chronic pain, 569–570
    client with deep vein thrombosis, 520–522
    client with excess fluid volume, 479
    client with trouble sleeping, 395–396
    family with ineffective coping, 221–223
    terminally ill client, 337–340
Nursing diagnosis, 149–152
    North American Nursing Diagnosis Association (NANDA), 149
    vs. medical diagnosis, 149–150, 150t
Nursing education, 57–63, 62t
Nursing interventions, 153–157
    taxonomy of, 179
    vs. nursing activities, 179
Nursing Interventions Classification (NIC), 179–180
Nursing minimum data set (NMDS), 179
Nursing organizations, 63–67
Nursing Outcomes Classification (NOC), 180
Nursing practice acts (state), 166
Nursing process, 145. *See also* specific topics
    assessment, 146–149
    diagnosis, 149–152
    documentation, 168
    evaluation, *157*, 157–158, 158t
    implementation, 154–157
    interventions, 153–154
    planning and outcome identification, 152–154
    steps, 146, *146*
Nursing team, 673–674, *674*
Nursing units, 73
Nutrients, 345–358
Nutrition, 343–384. *See also* Dietary guidelines, Weight management
    definition, 344
    factors influencing, 361–364
    health, 371
    in adolescence, 368
    in childhood, 366–367, 367t
    in infancy, 364–366, 364, 365
    in middle adulthood, 368–369

    in older adulthood, 369, 370, 630
    in young adulthood, 368–369
    infection control, 435
    nurse's role in meeting client's needs, 344
    nursing process, 376–381, 377t, *378*
    physical indicators of nutritional status, 377t
    physiology of, 344–345, *345*
    sleep promotion, 394
    wellness, 9, 10
Nutritional support, 380–381, *381*
Nutritional therapies, 238–239
Nutting, Adelaide, 57, 58, 59

O

Obesity, 372
Objective data, 148, 148t
Occupation, as safety factor, 402
Occupational health nursing, 677
Occupational health, Standard Precautions, 450–451
Occult blood, 599
Older adulthood. *See also* Age, Aging, Elderly clients
    growth and development, 277–279, 278t
    home safety, 406
    nutritional needs, 369, 370, 635
Olguria, definition, 604
Omnibus Budget Reconciliation Act (OBRA), 650, 654
Ongoing assessment, 147
Ongoing planning, 152
Onset of action, of drugs, 485
Onset, of pain, 556
Opinion, 15
Opioids, 563–564, 565
Oppression, 207
Oral assessment, 540
Oral care, for client hygiene, 420–421, 478
Oral medications, 485–487, 486t, 500–501
Orders, telephone, 181–182, *182*
Organ donation, 336
    religious beliefs, 333t
Organization, learning principle, 188
Organizational chart, 675
Orthodox religion, 216
    death and dying issues, 333t
    dietary factors, 363
Orthostatic hypotension, 538
Osmolality, 474–475
Osmolarity, 475
Osmosis, definition, 464, *464, 465*
Osmotic pressure, 464
Osteoporosis, 294–295, 637–638
Oucher pediatric pain intensity scale, *557*
Outcome identification. *See* Planning and outcome identification

Outpatient health care setting, 72t
Outpatient rehabilitation, 659
Over-the-counter (OTC) drugs, 498
Oxidation, metabolic process, 344, 470
Oxygen use, fire prevention, 416

P

Pain
  acute vs. chronic, 550t
  categories of, 549–551
  common myths, 549, 549t
  definition, 548
  factors affecting experience of, 554
  "fifth" vital sign, 538–539
  physiology of, 551–554, *552*
  purpose of, 551
Pain assessment tools, *555, 556, 557*
Pain intensity scales, *556, 557*
Pain management
  JCAHO standards, 554
  nursing process, 554–569
  pharmacological interventions,
    560–565, *561*
  noninvasive interventions, 565–568,
    569t
  sleep disturbance, 394–395
Pain threshold, definition, 555
Pain tolerance, definition, 555
Palliative care, definition, 330
Palpation, assessment tool, 531
Papanicolaou test (Pap smear), 600
Paracentesis, 614
Parasites, 599
Parasomnia, sleep disturbance, 391
Parenteral medications, 485, 487,
    502–514
  intradermal, *502, 504, 504*
  intramuscular, *502, 505,* 505–506,
    506
  intravenous, *502,* 506–514, 507t, *510*
  subcutaneous, *502, 504,* 504–505
Parenteral fluids, 506–507, 507t
Parenteral nutrition, 381
Parish, employment opportunities, 678
Participation, learning principle, 188
Passive transport, 463–465
Patency, medication administration, 501
Pathogenicity, 428
Pathogens, 428–429
Patient Admission Data Base, *528–529*
Patient-controlled analgesia (PCA), 564
Patient's Bill of Rights, 116, 117t–118t
Peak plasma level, of drugs, 485
Peer assistance programs, 106
Peer review organization (PRO), 167
Perception, of pain, 553, 558
Perceptual alterations, as safety factor,
    402
Percussion, assessment technique, 532,
    532t
Perfectionism, 28, 28t, 36
Peripheral vascular disease, 634

Perineal care, client hygiene, 420
Periodic limb movements in sleep
    (PLMS), 392
Periodontal disease, controllable factors
    of, 295
Peripheral intravenous (PI) lock, 509
Peristalsis, digestive process, 344
Permeability, definition, 463
Personal care, as health factor, 291
Personal preferences, hygiene practices,
    402–403
Pet therapy, 241–242
pH, definition, 462
Phantom limb pain, 551
Pharmacokinetics, 487–488
Pharmacological interventions, sleep
    promotion, 394–395
Pharmacology, 485–487
Phlebitis, 508, 512
Phlebotomist, definition, 578
Phosopholipids, definition, 349
Phosphate, definition, 470
Phosphate buffer system, 463
Physical agent, in chain of infection,
    430
Physical exam
  assessment tool, 531–532, *533*
  fluid, electrolyte, and acid-base
    balance, 473
  as health factor, 293
  infection control, 439–440
  medication administration, 499
  safety and hygiene, 404
Physical restraints, 412, *413*
Physical wellness, 6, 285
  as sleep factor, 390
Physiological barriers, client teaching,
    189t, 190
Physiological dimension, human
    development, 251
Physiological needs, 5
  of dying client, 330–332
Physiological pain response, 558
Phytochemicals, 238
Piaget, Jean, 252, 254
  phases of cognitive development, 255t
PIE charting, 171, *173*
Piggybacked, 511, 513, *513*
Planning and outcome identification,
    152–154
Plants, medicinal use of, 239
Plateau, drug administration, 485
Play therapy, 242
Pleural friction rub, breath sound, 542
Pneumothorax, definition, 614
Point-of-care charting, 175
Point of view, in reasoning, 20t, 21
Policies, employer's, 675
Political correctness, 136
Polypharmacy, definition, 632
Polyunsaturated fatty acids, definition,
    350

Port-a-cath, 580
Portal of exit, in chain of infection, *430,*
    432, 434–435
Post-mortem care, 335–336
Posture, 8
Potassium, 468
Potassium chloride, and safety, 468
Poverty, and access to health care,
    82–83
Practical nurse, historical definition, 57
Practical nurse's pledge, 112t
Prayer, healing, 238
Preadolescence, 268–270, 269t–270t,
    271
Precision vs. imprecision, 18
Preferred provider organization (PPO),
    77, 77t, 78
Prefilled single-dose syringe, 502
Pregnancy, 256–257, 370
Prenatal period, growth and
    development, 256–257
Preschoolers
  growth and development, 264–266,
    265t
Prescription drugs, 498. *See also* Drugs,
    Medication
Prescriptive authority, 81
Pressure ulcers, 639, *640,* 640t
Prevention, *See* Illness prevention
Primary care, 70, 70t
Primary care provider, 60, 77
Primary health care, 60, 78
Primary nutritional disease, 371
Primary prevention, 289
Primary source, of data, 147
Private duty nurse, 677
Private sector, in health care delivery,
    72
PRN (as needed) orders, 490
Problem definition, in reasoning, 20
Problem-oriented charting, 171
Problem-oriented medical record, 171
Problem solving. *See also* Critical
    thinking, Reasoning
  leadership skill, 670
  nursing process, 158–159, 159t
Procedures, employer's, 675
Procrastination, 36
Prodomal stage, infectious process, 438
Professional boundaries, 137
Professional liability, 105
Professional misconduct, 97–98
Professional tips
  "anxiety buster," 45
  "strict" I&O, 477
  30-second vacation, 45
  abbreviations (in documentation),
    169
  accidents in health care setting, 401
  adolescents, working with, 271
  adopted clients, 147
  advance directives, 100

aging, predictors for healthy, 285
assessment, abdomen, 542
assessment, abnormal breath odors, 540
assessment, blood pressure contraindications, 538
assessment, carotid pulse, 537
assessment, positioning dyspneic clients, 537
attending lectures, 42
autonomy, 111
biorhythms, 387
calcium and vitamin D, 469
client teaching, evaluation of effectiveness, 202
client teaching, guidelines for effective, 201
client teaching, medical jargon, 195
client teaching, overcoming barriers, 190
client teaching, physiological comfort and learning, 190
communication barriers, 134
communication, assertive, 135
communication, importance of immediate, 166
communication, objectivity, 140
communication, when clients block, 134
complementary/alternative therapy, contraindications for touch, 235
complementary/alternative therapy, preparation for chiropractic, 234
complementary/alternative therapy, use of humor, 241
complementary/alternative therapy, use of medicinal plants, 239
complementary/alternative therapy, use of, 230
consent from sedated clients, 166
consent in emergencies, 99
consent in special situations, 100
creatinine excretion, 378
critical thinking, 22
cultural diversity, families, 213
cultural diversity, non-native speakers, 212
cultural sensitivity, 208
culturally appropriate care, 220
culturally diverse coworkers, 218
defense mechanisms, 303
dehydration, signs and symptoms of, 347
diagnostic testing, cultures, 599
diagnostic testing, arterial blood gases, 579
diagnostic testing, blood lipid level, 596
diagnostic testing, capillary puncture, 580
diagnostic testing, computed tomography, 604

diagnostic testing, contrast media, 600
diagnostic testing, CSF pressure, 615
diagnostic testing, documentation of specimen-collection difficulties, 577
diagnostic testing, drugs, 595
documenting an incident report, 182
dying client, adjuvant therapy for, 332
dying client, assessment of, 329
dying client, planning care for, 329
elderly client, bowel patterns, 629
elderly client, COPD, 633
elderly client, identifying strengths, 631
elderly client, neurological system, 641
elderly client, reporting abuse of, 645
elderly client, tuberculosis, 632, 633
electrolyte shift, 472
ethical care, 120
evaluation, variables to consider in, 395
feeding client, 380
feeding visually impaired client, 380
fluid replacement, 478
food-drug interactions, 369
Good Samaritan laws, 92
grief, identifying dysfunctional, 321
grief, nurse's self-care during, 337
grieving, adaptive, 326
hygiene, bathing, 419
hygiene, eye care for the comatose client, 422
hygiene, foot and toenail care, 421
hygiene, oral care for the unconscious client, 421
hygiene, perineal care, 420
hygiene, tub or shower bath, 419
hyperalimentation, 470
hypercalcemic crisis, 469
hyperphosphatemia, 470
hypokalemia, 468
infection control, bedridden client, 435
infection control, drug-resistant organisms, 439
infection control, nosocomial infections, 438
infection control, questions related to, 440
infectious diseases, 433
insulin levels, diabetic clients, 348
lactose intolerance, 349
learning disabilities, 33
learning evaluation, 202
learning needs assessment, 200
learning, 26
learning, common beliefs about, 189
loss of gastric juices, 476
LP/VN services, 671

mammograms, 293
medication administration, catheter sepsis, 512
medication administration, enteral tube instillation, 501
medication administration, enteral tube management, 502
medication administration, expiration date, 504
medication administration, inserting CVC, 510
medication administration, nose drops, 517
medication administration, reasonable answer, 493
medication administration, rectal suppositories, 518, 519
medication administration, setting volume, 511
medication administration, special considerations, 486
medication administration, systemic effects of eye drops, 516
medication administration, transfusion reaction, 515
medication administration, vaginal suppositories, 520
medications, expired, 530
memory and activity, 41
metabolic alkalosis, 473
mnemonics, 41
mouthwashes, 478
noise control in hospitals, 394
nursing diagnosis, benefits of, 151
nursing diagnosis, data, 151
nursing practice act/title act, 92
nursing process, 147
nutrition, daily allowance of protein, 352
nutrition, determining alterations in, 635
nutrition, enriched or fortified foods, 355
nutrition, labeling of vitamins, minerals, and herbs, 358
nutrition, nurse's role in, 344
nutrition, preventing eating disorders, 368
nutrition, snacks, 367
nutrition, vegetarians and protein, 352
nutritional history, 376
nutritional needs of infants, 364
opening a food tray, 379
pain management, cognitive-behavior interventions, 566
pain management, using distraction, 566
pain medication, Ketorolac, 563
pain medication, nonopioid, 563
pain medication, opioids and constipation, 564

Professional tips (*cont.*)
  pain, effect on sleep, 558
  pain, location of, 556
  pain, sensation of, 553
  post-mortem care, 336
  professional hierarchy, 674
  professional memberships, 67
  psychological interventions for clients
    in isolation, 453
  pulse oximeter reading, 471
  restraints, key elements of
    documentation, 412
  safety and hygiene, key interview
    questions about, 403
  safety, oxygen use, 416
  safety, workplace, 401
  self-nurturing, 11
  serum calcium, 469
  sharps injuries, in home, 660
  shift report, 180
  sleep apnea, 391
  sleep deprivation, 386
  sleep history, 393
  sleep in the United States, 388
  sleep, providing environmental
    comfort, 389
  sleep-impaired client, communicating
    with, 393
  speaking, 32
  Standard Precautions, exposure
    incident, 449
  stress reduction, promoting client
    control, 306
  stress, anticipatory, 301
  stress, managing professional, 313
  temperature conversion, 536
  temperature of fluids, 478
  temporary permits, 676
  therapeutic communication, 133
  time orientation, 135
  time wasters, 36
  toddlers, health care for, 262
  unlicensed personnel, 674
  urine osmolality, 475
  vaccine, hepatitis B, 293
  values clarification, 115
  wellness, moderate exercise reduces
    stroke risk, 292
Progress notes, 178
Progressive muscle relaxation, 566
Projection, defense mechanism, 304t
Prospective payment, 78
Prospective payment system (PPS),
  167
Protestants, 215–216
  death and dying issues, 333t
Protein, necessary nutrient, 350–352
Protein buffers, 463
Protocol, 156
  diagnostic testing, 575t, 576t, 578t
Protozoa, definition, 429
Proxemics, 136

Psychological barriers, client teaching,
  189t, 190
Psychological wellness, 10
Psychomotor domain, 187, 187t
  teaching methods applicable in, 191
Psychoneuroimmunology (PNI), 229
Psychosocial dimension, human
  development, 251
Psychosocial needs, 332, 630
Psychotherapy, 568, 569t
Puberty, 268
Public health, 84
Public law, 90, 90t
Public sector, in health care delivery,
  71, *71*
Public/private sector, in health care
  delivery, 71, 84
Puerto Ricans, dietary factors, 362
Pulse
  amplitude, 536
  deficit, 436–537
  points, *536, 537t*
  rate, 536
  rhythm, 536
  vital sign measurement, *535,*
    536–537, 536t, 537t
Pulse oximeter reading, 471
Purpose, in reasoning, 20
Purulent exudate (pus), immune
  response, 437
Pyorrhea, client oral hygiene, 422

Q

Quality, of pain, 556
Question-and-answer session, teaching
  method, 190

R

Race, definition, 206
Radiation, for pain relief, 568
Radioactive studies, 607, 607t–608t
Radiography, 600, *605*
Radiological studies, 600–606, 600,
  601t–604t, *605*
Random collection, urine, 580
Rapport, 130
Rationalization, defense mechanism,
  304t
Reaction formation, defense
  mechanism, 304t
Readiness, learning principle, 188, 192
Reading, basic skill, 29
Reasoning, 14, 19–22, 20t
Receiver, communication, 126
Recommended dietary allowance
  (RDA), 360–361
Rectal medications, 485, 486t, 518–519,
  519
Recurrent acute pain, 550
References, for job hunt, 680–681
Referred pain, 549, *550*
Reflective, 13

Reflexology, 237, *238*
Refusal of treatment, 119
Registered nurse (RN)
  program of study, 60–61
  roles of, 76t
  vs. trained nurse, 56
Regression, defense mechanism, 304t
Rehabilitation center, 677
Rehabilitative care, 70, 654–659, 654t,
  655t, *657, 658*
Reinforcement, learning principle, 188
Relaxation techniques, 231–232, 310,
  394
  pain relief, 566, 569t
Relevance, learning principle, 187
Relevance vs. irrelevance, 18
Religion, 214–217 *See also* Cultural
  beliefs, specific cultural groups,
  specific religious groups
  communication, 138
  influence on nursing, 54
  influence on nutrition, 363
  loss, grief, and death, 323, 325, 333t
  organ donation, 333t
  spiritual needs and care, 215
Religious support system, 215
REM movement disorder, sleep
  disturbance, 391
REM sleep, 368–387, *387*
Repetition, learning principle, 188–189
Reporting, 180–183, *182*
Reproductive system, aging, 636–637
Reservoir, in chain of infection, *430,*
  430–431, 433–435
Resident (normal) flora, 428
Resident's Rights (OBRA), 654t
Respirations, vital sign measurement,
  535,, 536t, 537–538
Respiratory system
  acid-base balance, 470–471, 472
  acidosis, 472
  aging, 632–633
  alkalosis, 472
  assessment, 541–542, *543*
  medications, 485, 486t, 486, 487,
    517–518
  tract infections, 632–633
Respite care, 661
Rest
  definition, 385
  factors affecting, 388–390
  nursing process, 392–393
  physiology of, 386–387
  wellness, 9
Restless leg syndrome, 392
Restraints, for client safety, 411–412,
  413
Restricted fluids, fluid imbalance, 478
Résumé preparation, 679–680, *679*
Resuscitation, definition, 327
Return demonstration, teaching
  method, 191

Reverse isolation, 453
Review of systems (ROS), 530–531
Richards, Linda, 52, 57
Rickettsia, 429
Rigor mortis, 335
Risk assessment, safety and hygiene, 404–405, 404t, 405t, 406
Risk for infection, nursing diagnosis, 440, 442
Risk for injury, planning for client at, 409t
Risk nursing diagnosis, 151, 152t
Robb, Isabel Hampton, 56
Role play, teaching method, 190–191
Rural primary care hospital (RPCH), as health care setting, 73t

S
Safety, 399–425
    aromatherapy, 241
    as health factor, 292
    aspirin, 417
    assessment for allergies, 530
    bathroom hazards, 414
    blood transfusion incompatibilities, 515
    body mechanics, 414
    car seats, 259
    cleaning carts, 417
    client care, 400, 401
    contrast media, 604
    cross-contamination prevention, 516
    diagnostic testing, 574
    drug amount calculations, 492
    drug form substitution, 485
    drug safety considerations, 496
    enteral tube placement, 501
    factors affecting, 401–402
    fire prevention, 414–415, 416t
    fluid measurements, 473
    home safety for elders, 279
    home, work, and travel, 296
    hospital equipment, 416
    immunizations, 113
    incubation period, 438
    ischemic pain, 553
    latex allergies, 450
    magnesium level, 470
    marking IV bag, 509
    massage precautions, 235
    medications and sleep, 389
    medications, 417
    medications, guidelines for safe administration, 496
    metric system, 490
    noise pollution, 418
    nursing process, 403–423
    oxygen and smoking, 633
    palpation, 531
    panic, client experiencing, 309
    poisoning, 417, 418
    potassium chloride, 468
    pregnancy, tobacco and alcohol use during, 257
    prepping skin for venipuncture, 511
    radiation exposure, 417
    radioactive iodine and urine collection, 577
    removing glasses before charting, 477
    restraints, 411–412, *413*
    shaving, 422
    stool collection, 581
    suicide prevention, 273
    TENS contraindications, 568
    toys for toddlers, 264
    tub bath, 419
    urine collection and Standard Precautions, 580
    workplace, 401
    x-rays, 600
Safety and hygiene, nursing process, 403–405, 404t, 405t
Safety and security needs, 5,6
Safety awareness, 409
Salt, definition, 462
Scalp assessment, 539
Scarcity of resources, 119
Scheduled orders, medication, 489–490
Schools, employment opportunities, 678
School-age children, growth and development, 266–267, 267t
School-based clinic (SBC), 72t
Schools, as health care setting, 72t
Sebum, immune response, 436
Secondary care, 70, 70t
Secondary nutritional disease, 371
Secondary prevention, 289
Secondary source, of data, 147
Self-actualization needs, 5,6
Self-awareness, definition, 6
    client teaching, 194–195
Self-care, theory of, 149
Self-concept, 6–7, 251
    self-fulfilling cycle, *251*
Self-efficacy, definition, 187
Self-esteem needs, 5,6
Self-evaluation, leadership skill, 670
Self-image, creating positive, 26–27
Self-regulatory techniques, 231t, 231–233
Self-talk, 310
Selye, Hans, 299–301
Semipermeable membrane, 463
Sender, communication, 126
Sensory alterations
    aging, 644–645
    safety factor, 402
Sensory overload, 418
Sensory status, assessment tool, 499
Serum
    albumin, 475
    calcium, 469
    electrolytes, 581
    osmolality, 475
Seventh Day Adventists, dietary factors, 363
Sexual relationship, as health factor, 291
Sexually transmitted diseases, controllable factors of, 295
Shamanism, 229
Shaving, client hygiene, 422
Shiatsu, 236–237
Shift report, 180
Short-term goal, 153, 153t
Shroud, 336
Sibilant wheezes, 542
Sickle-cell anemia, controllable factors of, 295
Side rails, 411, *411*
Significance vs. triviality, 19
Single-dose orders, medication, 489
Single-payer system, 76
Single point of entry, 77–78
Situational loss, 318
Situational theory, 113
Skilled nursing facility, 659
Skills
    developing basic, 28–32
    student nurse, 25–48
Skin, body fluid balance, 467, 474
Skin assessment, 540, 541
Skin cancer, elderly client, 641
Skin integrity
    elderly client, 639, *640*, 640t
    risk appraisal, 404t
Skin turgor, 474
Skinfold measurement, assessment tool, 377, *378*
Sleep
    definition, 385
    disturbances, 390–392, 394
    factors affecting, 388–390, 392
    medications, safety issues, 389
    nursing process, 392–395
    physiology of, 386–387
Sleep apnea, 391, 392
Sleep cycle, 387, *387*
Sleep deprivation, 386, 391
Sleep history, 393
Sleep patterns, alterations in, 390–392
Sleeptalking, 391
Sleepwalking, 391
Smoking, 8–9, 113
    as health factor, 291–292
    as sleep factor, 389
Sneezing, immune response, 436
Snoring, 391
SOAP charting, 171, *172*
Social organization, 213–217
Social practices, hygiene, 402
Social wellness, 285
Sociocultural barriers, client teaching, 189, 189t
Sociocultural wellness, 10

Socioeconomic status
  hygiene, 403
  nutrition, 363
Sodium, 468
Solutions, medications, 486t
Somatic pain, 549
Somnambulism, sleep disturbance, 391
Sonorous wheeze, 542
Source-oriented charting, 171
Southern U.S., dietary factors, 362
Space, in communication, 136
Speaking, basic skill, 31–32
Specialized client care units, 73
Specific immune defense, 437–438
Specific order, 155
Specificity vs. vagueness, 18
Specimen collection, 577–581
Speech impaired client, communication
    with, 139
Spinal tap, 614
Spiritual dimension, human
    development, 255–256, 256t
Spiritual needs, of dying client, 333,
    333t
Spiritual therapies, 237–238. See also
    Shamanism
Spiritual wellness, 285
Spores, definition, 428
Sputum culture, laboratory test, 600
Stable, client status, 577
Staff development, 61
Standard Precautions (CDC/HICPAC),
    449–451, 452t
  definition, 449
  handwashing, 8, 449
  historical perspective, 447–449
Standards, intellectual, 14. See also
    Universal intellectual standards
    (UIS)
Standards of care, 83–84
Standards of practice, 92–93
Standing order, 155–156, 157
Stat orders, medication, 489
State board examination and licensure,
    676
State nursing practice acts, 166
Stereotyping, 207
Sterile attire, donning, 441–442
Sterile field and equipment, 441
Sterile specimen, urine, 580
Sterile technique, infection control, 441
Sterilization, 434
Stock supplied, drugs, 497
Stomatitis, client oral hygiene, 421
Stool
  collection, 581
  culture, laboratory test, 600
  tests, 599, 599t
Stress, 297, 299–303
  anticipatory, 301
  as effect of illness, 305–306
  change, as response to, 306–308

definition, 299
  disorders related to, 306t
  general adaptation syndrome (GAS),
    300, 300–301
  local adaptation syndrome (LAS), 301
  managing professional, 312–313, 313t
  manifestations of, 301t
  nursing process, 308–312
Stress level, as health factor, 291, 297
Stress management techniques,
    310–311, 311t, 312
  for nurses, 312–313, 313t
Stress test, 610
Stressor, definition, 299
Strider, breath sound, 542
Study planning, 39–41
Study strategies, 38–43
Study techniques, learning styles, 35t
Subacute care, 660–661
Subcutaneous (SC or SQ) injection, 487,
    504, 504–505
Subjective data, 147, 148t
Sublimation, defense mechanism, 304t
Sublingual medications, 485–487, 486t,
    500–501
Suffocation prevention, 418
Suicide, loss and grief, 324
Sullivan, Henry Stack, 252
  interpersonal model of personality
    development, 254t
Summary report, 180
Sunburn, controllable factors of, 295
Superstitions, influence on nutrition,
    364
Supervised practice, teaching method,
    191
Support services, 74
Suppression, defense mechanism, 304t
Surgical asepsis, infection control, 441
Surgical attire, donning, 441–442
Surgical handwashing, infection control,
    441
Surgical unit, 74
Susceptible host, in chain of infection,
    430, 432
Synthesis, definition, 149, 460
Syringes, 502–504, 503, 505
Systemic infection, 438
Tachycardia, 536
Tachypnea, 537

T
Tai chi, 234
Task assignment, client care, 671–672
Teaching, 185. See also Client teaching
Teaching-learning process, 185–191.
    See also Client teaching
  nursing process, 195–202, 199
Tearing, immune response, 436
Telemedicine, 142
Teleology, 113
Telephone call script, job hunt, 681

Telephone reports and orders, 181–182,
    182
Temperature, vital sign measurement,
    534, 535, 536
Teratogenic substance, 257
Terminally ill clients, complementary
    therapies, 243t. See also Death and
    dying
Tertiary care, 70, 70t
Tertiary prevention, 289
Tests. See Diagnostic data
Test-taking skills, 44–45
  improving, 45–48
Thai, dietary factors, 363
Thalassemia, controllable factors of, 295
Thallium test, 610
Thank you note, job hunt, 683, 683
Theory of self-care, 149
Therapeutic communication, 130–134
Therapeutic massage, 235
Therapeutic procedure accident, 401
Therapeutic touch, 236, 237t
Therapy departments, 74
Third-party payment, definition, 58
Thirst, body fluid balance, 468
Thompson, Thomas, 58
Thoracentesis, 614, 614
Thoracic assessment, 541–542
Thought stopping. See Cognitive
    reframing
Three-part statement, 150–151, 151t
Throat (swab) culture, 599–600
Time management, 34–38
Time orientation, 135
Timed collection, urine, 580
Tobacco use. See Smoking
Toddlers
  growth and development, 262–264,
    263t
Toileting, elderly client, 629
Tolerance, to pain medication, 562
Topical medications, 485, 486t, 487,
    515–516
Tort law, 91, 91t, 94t
Touch, 234, 235
Toxic effect, of drugs, 488
Trade name, of drugs, 485
Trained nurse, 56
Transcutaneous Electrical Nerve
    Stimulation (TENS), 567–568, 569t
Transdermal analgesia, 565
Transducer, 606
Transduction, of pain impulse, 553
Transient flora, 428
Transient ischemic attack, elderly client,
    642
Transmission-Based Precautions, 451,
    451
Transmission, of pain impulse, 553–554
Trigylcerides, definition, 349
Trocar, surgical instrument, 614
Tube feeding, 478

Tuberculin syringe, 502, *503*
Tuberculosis, 295, 632, 633
Turgor, skin, 474
24-hour recall, assessment tool, 376
Two-part statement, 150, 151t
Type and crossmatch, blood test, 581

U
Ultrasonography, 606, 606t
Ultrasound, definition, 606
Uncomplicated grief, 320
Unified Medical Language System
    (UMLS), 179
Unit dose form, of drugs, 497
United States Department of Health and
    Human Services (HHS), 71
United States Public Health Service
    (USPHS), 71
Universal intellectual standards (UIS),
    15, 15t, 17–19, 22
Unlicensed assistive personnel (UAP),
    671–672, *674*, 674
Urinary system
    aging, 642–644, 643t, *643*, 644t
    tract infections, 295, 600, 643–644
Urine
    collection, 580–581
    culture, 600
    osmolality, 475
    pH, 475, 595
    tests, 595–599, *595*, 596t–598t
Urobilinogen, 599

V
Vaccination, immune response, 437–438
Vaginal medications, 519, *519,* 520

Values and ethics, 114–115
Values clarification, 114, 115
Variations, in documentation, 175
Vascular access device, (VAD), 509
Vectorborne transmission, in chain of
    infection, 431t, 432
Vehicle transmission, in chain of
    infection, 431, 431t
Venipuncture, 577, 578–579
Veracity, 110t, 112
Verbal communication, 127
Vesicant, 512
Vesicular sounds, 542
Veterans Administration (VA), 71
Vials, for injection, 503–504, *504*
Vietnamese, dietary factors, 363
Villi, digestive system, 344
Virulence, 428
Viruses, 428–429
Visceral pain, 549
Vision, aging, 644
Visiting nurses associations, 58–59
Visual learning style, 33, 33t, 34t
Visually impaired client
    communication with, 138–139
    feeding, 380
Vital signs, measurement of, 534–538,
    535, 536t, *536*, 537t
Vitamin D and calcium, 469
Vitamins, necessary nutrients, 352–355,
    352t, 353t–354t
Vocational wellness, 284

W
Wald, Lillian, 56, 58, 85
Walker, assistive walking device, 413

Walking rounds, 181
Water
    amount in body, 461
    homeostasis, 461
    necessary nutrient, 346–347, *346*
Weight management, 371–373
Weight measurement, 539
Wellness, definition, 5, 284
    areas of, 284–285
    guidelines for healthy living,
        294–297, 295t
Wellness nursing diagnosis, 151, 152t
Wheelchair, assistive walking device, 413
Whistleblowing, 120–21
WHO analgesic ladder, *561*
Women's movement, 56
Wong/Baker FACES pain rating scale,
    557
Worden, J. William, 319
Workplace hierarchy, 674, *674*
Workplace transition, 673–675
World Health Organization (WHO), 4
    definition of health, 4, 283–284
Writing, basic skill, 30, 31t

Y
Yin and yang, 211
Yoga, 233–234
Young adulthood
    growth and development, 273–275,
        273t–274t
    nutritional needs, 368–369

Z
Zimmerman, Anne, 60
Z-track injection, 505–506, *506*